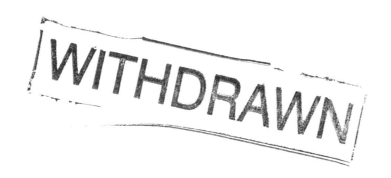

SIDE EFFECTS OF DRUGS ANNUAL

VOLUME 38

SIDE EFFECTS OF DRUGS ANNUAL

VOLUME 38

A worldwide yearly survey of new data
in adverse drug reactions

Editor

SIDHARTHA D. RAY, PHD., FACN
Manchester University College of Pharmacy, Natural and Health Sciences, USA

ELSEVIER AMSTERDAM • BOSTON • HEIDELBERG • LONDON • NEW YORK • OXFORD
PARIS • SAN DIEGO • SAN FRANCISCO • SINGAPORE • SYDNEY • TOKYO

Elsevier
Radarweg 29, PO Box 211, 1000 AE Amsterdam, Netherlands
The Boulevard, Langford Lane, Kidlington, Oxford OX5 1GB, United Kingdom
50 Hampshire Street, 5th Floor, Cambridge, MA 02139, United States

First edition 2016

Notices

Knowledge and best practice in this field are constantly changing. As new research and experience broaden our understanding, changes in research methods, professional practices, or medical treatment may become necessary.

Practitioners and researchers must always rely on their own experience and knowledge in evaluating and using any information, methods, compounds, or experiments described herein. In using such information or methods they should be mindful of their own safety and the safety of others, including parties for whom they have a professional responsibility.

To the fullest extent of the law, neither the Publisher nor the authors, contributors, or editors, assume any liability for any injury and/or damage to persons or property as a matter of products liability, negligence or otherwise, or from any use or operation of any methods, products, instructions, or ideas contained in the material herein.

ISBN: 978-0-444-63718-5
ISSN: 0378-6080

For information on all Elsevier publications
visit our website at https://www.elsevier.com/

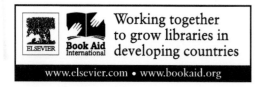

Working together
to grow libraries in
developing countries

www.elsevier.com • www.bookaid.org

Publisher: Zoe Kruze
Acquisition Editor: Zoe Kruze
Editorial Project Manager: Shellie Bryant
Production Project Manager: Surya Narayanan Jayachandran
Cover Designer: Victoria Pearson Esser

Typeset by SPi Global, India

Contributors

Alexander Accinelli School of Pharmacy and Health Professions, University of Maryland at Eastern Shore, Princess Anne, MD, USA

Asima N. Ali Campbell University CPHS, Buies Creek; Wake Forest Baptist Health—Internal Medicine OPD Clinic, Winston-Salem, NC, USA

Laura J. Baumgartner Department of Clinical Sciences, Touro University California College of Pharmacy, Vallejo, CA, USA

Robert D. Beckett Manchester University College of Pharmacy, Natural, and Health Sciences, Fort Wayne, IN, USA

Renee A. Bellanger Department of Pharmacy Practice, University of the Incarnate Word, Feik School of Pharmacy, San Antonio, TX, USA

Nicholas T. Bello Department of Animal Sciences, School of Environmental and Biological Sciences, Rutgers, The State University of New Jersey, New Brunswick, NJ, USA

Skye Bickett Medical Librarian. Assistant Director of Library Services, PCOM, Suwanee, GA, USA

Adrienne T. Black 3E Company, Warrenton, VA, USA

Alison Brophy Ernest Mario School of Pharmacy, Rutgers, The State University of New Jersey, Piscataway; Saint Barnabas Medical Center, Livingston, NJ, USA

Maria Cardinale Ernest Mario School of Pharmacy, Rutgers, The State University of New Jersey, Piscataway; Saint Peter's University Hospital, New Brunswick, NJ, USA

Saira B. Chaudhry Ernest Mario School of Pharmacy, Rutgers-The State University of New Jersey, Piscataway, NJ, USA

James Chue Clinical Trials and Research Program, Edmonton, AB, Canada

Pierre Chue University of Alberta, Edmonton, AB, Canada

Karyn I. Cotta Department of Pharmaceutical Sciences, South University School of Pharmacy, Savannah, GA, USA

Bryony Coupe Asthma & Allergy Group, Swansea University Medical School, Institute of Life Science 1, Swansea University, Swansea, United Kingdom

Kendra M. Damer Butler University College of Pharmacy and Health Sciences, Indianapolis, IN, USA

Gwyneth A. Davies Asthma & Allergy Group, Swansea University Medical School, Institute of Life Science 1, Swansea University, Swansea, United Kingdom

Teresa DeLellis Department of Pharmacy Practice, College of Pharmacy, Natural and Health Sciences, Manchester University, Fort Wayne, IN, USA

Rahul Deshmukh Department of Pharmaceutical Sciences, College of Pharmacy, Rosalind Franklin University of Medicine and Science, North Chicago, Il, USA

Sujana Dontukurthy New York Methodist Hospital, Brooklyn, NY, USA

Kirk Evoy College of Pharmacy, The University of Texas at Austin, Austin; School of Medicine, University of Texas Health Science Center San Antonio, Pharmacotherapy Education and Research Center, San Antonio, TX, USA

Jingyang Fan Department of Pharmacy Practice, SIUE School of Pharmacy, Edwardsville, IL, USA

Elizabeth Flockton Royal Liverpool Hospital, Liverpool, United Kingdom

Cynthia E. Franklin Department of Pharmaceutical Sciences, University of the Incarnate Word, Feik School of Pharmacy, San Antonio, TX, USA

Lynn Frendak Department of Pharmacy, Johns Hopkins Bayview Medical Center, Baltimore, MD, USA

Jason C. Gallagher Temple University, Philadelphia, PA, USA

Nidhi Gandhi Department of Pharmacy Practice, PCOM School of Pharmacy, Suwanee, GA, USA

Tatsuya Gomi Department of Radiology, Ohashi Medical Center, Toho University, Tokyo, Japan

Joshua P. Gray Department of Science, United States Coast Guard Academy, New London, CT, USA

Andrew L. Griffiths Asthma & Allergy Group, Swansea University Medical School, Institute of Life Science 1, Swansea University, Swansea, United Kingdom

Kristopher G. Hall Department of Pharmaceutical Sciences, Manchester University College of Pharmacy, Natural and Health Sciences, Fort Wayne, IN, USA

Makoto Hasegawa Department of Radiology, Ohashi Medical Center, Toho University, Tokyo, Japan

Christopher S. Holaway Department of Pharmacy Practice, PCOM School of Pharmacy, Suwanee, GA, USA

Sandra L. Hrometz Department of Pharmaceutical Sciences, Manchester University College of Pharmacy, Natural and Health Sciences, Fort Wayne, IN, USA

I-Kuan Hsu Department of Clinical Sciences, Touro University California College of Pharmacy, Vallejo, CA, USA

Eric J. Ip Department of Clinical Sciences, Touro University California College of Pharmacy, Vallejo, CA, USA

Jason Isch PGY2 Ambulatory Care, Saint Joseph Health System, Mishawaka, IN, USA

Abhishek Jha Royal Liverpool Hospital, Liverpool, United Kingdom

Carrie M. Jung Butler University College of Pharmacy and Health Sciences; Eskenazi Health, Indianapolis, IN, USA

Allison Kalstein New York Methodist Hospital, Brooklyn, NY, USA

Spinel Karas Department of Pharmacy Practice, School of Pharmacy and Pharmaceutical Sciences, State University of New York at Buffalo, Buffalo, NY, USA

Sipan Keshishyan Department of Pharmacy Practice, Manchester University College of Pharmacy, Natural and Health Sciences, Fort Wayne, IN, USA

Madan K. Kharel School of Pharmacy and Health Professions, University of Maryland at Eastern Shore, Princess Anne, MD, USA

Nicole Kiehle Department of Pharmacy, Johns Hopkins Bayview Medical Center, Baltimore, MD, USA

Vladlena Kovalevskaya Department of Pharmaceutical Sciences, Manchester University College of Pharmacy, Natural and Health Sciences, Fort Wayne, IN, USA

Justin G. Kullgren Department of Pharmacy, The Ohio State University Wexner Medical Center, Columbus, OH, USA

Dirk W. Lachenmeier Chemisches und Veterinäruntersuchungsamt (CVUA) Karlsruhe, Karlsruhe, Germany

Bonnie Lau Department of Clinical Sciences, Touro University California College of Pharmacy, Vallejo; Department of Emergency Medicine, Kaiser Permanente Santa Clara Medical Center, Santa Clara; Department of Emergency Medicine, Stanford University School of Medicine, Palo Alto, CA, USA

Tina C. Lee University of the Incarnate Word Feik School of Pharmacy, San Antonio, TX, USA

Linda Lim College of Pharmacy, The University of Texas at Austin, Austin; School of Medicine, University of Texas Health Science Center San Antonio, Pharmacotherapy Education and Research Center, San Antonio, TX, USA

Tristan Lindfelt Department of Clinical Sciences, Touro University California College of Pharmacy, Vallejo, CA, USA

Mei T. Liu Jersey City Medical Center, Jersey City, NJ, USA

Megan E. Maroney Rutgers University Ernest Mario School of Pharmacy, Piscataway, NJ, USA

Ashley Martinelli Department of Pharmacy, Johns Hopkins Bayview Medical Center, Baltimore, MD, USA

Mark Martinez Department of Pharmacy Practice, PCOM School of Pharmacy, Suwanee, GA, USA

Dianne May University of Georgia College of Pharmacy on Augusta University Campus, Augusta, GA, USA

Cassandra Maynard Department of Pharmacy Practice, SIUE School of Pharmacy, Edwardsville, IL, USA

Renee McCafferty Department of Pharmacy Practice, Manchester University College of Pharmacy, Natural and Health Sciences, Fort Wayne, IN, USA

Dayna S. McManus Department of Pharmacy Services, Yale-New Haven Hospital, Yale University, New Haven, CT, USA

Calvin J. Meaney Department of Pharmacy Practice, School of Pharmacy and Pharmaceutical Sciences, State University of New York at Buffalo, Buffalo, NY, USA

Philip B. Mitchell School of Psychiatry, University of New South Wales; Black Dog Institute, Sydney, NSW, Australia

Vicky V. Mody Department of Pharmaceutical Sciences, PCOM School of Pharmacy, Suwanee, GA, USA

Kaitlin Montagano Department of Pharmaceutical Sciences, Manchester University College of Pharmacy, Natural and Health Sciences, Fort Wayne, IN, USA

Toshio Nakaki Department of Pharmacology, Teikyo University School of Medicine, Tokyo, Japan

Anjan Nan Department of Pharmaceutical Sciences, University of Maryland Eastern Shore School of Pharmacy, Princess Anne, MD, USA

Diane Nguyen Department of Pediatrics, Baylor College of Medicine, Houston, TX, USA

John D. Noti Allergy and Clinical Immunology Branch, Health Effects Laboratory Division, National Institute for Occupational Safety and Health, Centers for Disease Control and Prevention, Morgantown, WV, USA

Igho J. Onakpoya Nuffield Department of Primary Care Health Sciences, Oxford, United Kingdom

Michael G. O'Neil Department of Pharmacy Practice, Drug Diversion, Pain Management and Substance Abuse Specialist, South College School of Pharmacy, Knoxville, TN, USA

Yekaterina Opsha Ernest Mario School of Pharmacy, Rutgers, The State University of New Jersey, Piscataway; Saint Barnabas Medical Center, Livingston, NJ, USA

Sreekumar Othumpangat Allergy and Clinical Immunology Branch, Health Effects Laboratory Division, National Institute for Occupational Safety and Health, Centers for Disease Control and Prevention, Morgantown, WV, USA

Harish Parihar Department of Pharmacy Practice, PCOM School of Pharmacy, Suwanee, GA, USA

Deepa Patel Department of Pharmacy Practice, PCOM School of Pharmacy, Suwanee, GA, USA

Punam B. Patel Department of Clinical Sciences, Touro University California College of Pharmacy, Vallejo, CA, USA

Michelle M. Peahota Infectious Diseases, Thomas Jefferson University Hospital, Philadelphia, PA, USA

Alan Polnariev College of Pharmacy, University of Florida, Gainesville, FL, USA

Hanna Raber College of Pharmacy, The University of Utah, Salt Lake City, UT, USA

Sushma Ramsinghani Department of Pharmaceutical Sciences, University of the Incarnate Word, Feik School of Pharmacy, San Antonio, TX, USA

Sidhartha D. Ray Department of Pharmaceutical Sciences, Manchester University College of Pharmacy, Natural and Health Sciences, Fort Wayne, IN, USA

David Reeves Department of Pharmacy Practice, College of Pharmacy and Health Sciences, Butler University; Department of Pharmacy, St. Vincent Indianapolis Hospital, Indianapolis, IN, USA

Lucia Rivera Lara Departments of Neurology, Anesthesiology, and Critical Care Medicine, Johns Hopkins Medicine, Baltimore, MD, USA

Nicholas Robinson Manchester University College of Pharmacy, Natural, and Health Sciences, Fort Wayne, IN, USA

Lauren K. Roller Department of Clinical Sciences, Touro University California College of Pharmacy, Vallejo, CA, USA

Lucia Rose Infectious Diseases, Cooper University Hospital, Camden, NJ, USA

Audrey Rosene Manchester University College of Pharmacy, Natural, and Health Sciences, Fort Wayne, IN, USA

Christina Seeger University of the Incarnate Word, Feik School of Pharmacy, San Antonio, TX, USA

Mona U. Shah Department of Pharmacy, Falls Church, VA, USA

Ajay N. Singh Department of Pharmaceutical Sciences, South University School of Pharmacy, Savannah, GA, USA

Michel R. Smith School of Pharmacy and Health Professions, University of Maryland at Eastern Shore, Princess Anne, MD, USA

Thomas Smith Manchester University College of Pharmacy, Fort Wayne, IN, USA

Jonathan Smithson School of Psychiatry, University of New South Wales; Black Dog Institute, Sydney, NSW, Australia

Brian Spoelhof Department of Pharmacy, Johns Hopkins Bayview Medical Center, Baltimore, MD, USA

Lisa V. Stottlemyer Wilmington VA Medical Center, Wilmington, DE; Pennsylvania College of Optometry, Elkins Park, PA, USA

Kalee Swanson Department of Pharmaceutical Sciences, Manchester University College of Pharmacy, Natural and Health Sciences, Fort Wayne, IN, USA

Fred R. Tejada School of Pharmacy and Health Professions, University of Maryland at Eastern Shore, Princess Anne, MD, USA

Kelan L. Thomas Touro University California College of Pharmacy, Vallejo, CA, USA

Sonia Thomas Department of Pharmacy Practice, PCOM School of Pharmacy, Suwanee, GA, USA

Sara N. Trovinger Department of Pharmacy Practice, Manchester University College of Pharmacy, Natural and Health Sciences, Fort Wayne, IN, USA

Kirby Welston AU Medical Center/University of Georgia College of Pharmacy, Augusta, GA, USA

Andrea L. Wilhite Manchester University College of Pharmacy, Natural, and Health Sciences, Fort Wayne, IN, USA

Zhiqian Wu Department of Pharmaceutical Sciences, PCOM School of Pharmacy, Suwanee, GA, USA

Joel Yarmush New York Methodist Hospital, Brooklyn, NY, USA

Matthew R. Zahner Drug Safety and Research Development, Pfizer, Groton, CT, USA

Contents

Preface

Side Effects of Drugs: Annual (SEDA) is a yearly publication focused on existing, new and evolving side effects of drugs encountered by a broad range of healthcare professionals including physicians, pharmacists, nurse practitioners, and advisors of poison control centers. This 37th edition of SEDA includes analyses of the side effects of drugs using both clinical trials and case-based principles which include encounters identified during bedside clinical practice over the 18 months since the previous edition. SEDA seeks to summarize the entire body of relevant medical literature into a single volume with dual goals of being comprehensive and of identifying emerging trends and themes in medicine as related to side effects and adverse drug effects (ADEs).

With a broad range of topics authored by practicing clinicians and scientists, SEDA is a comprehensive and reliable reference to be used in clinical practice. The majority of the chapters include relevant case studies that are not only peer-reviewed but also have a forward-looking, learning-based focus suitable for practitioners as well as students in training. The nationally known contributors believe this educational resource can be used to stimulate an active learning environment in a variety of settings. Each chapter in this volume has been reviewed by the editor, experienced clinical educators, actively practicing clinicians and scientists to ensure the accuracy and timeliness of the information. The overall objective is to provide a framework for further understanding the intellectual approaches in analyzing the implications of the case studies and their appropriateness when dispensing medications, as well as interpreting adverse drug reactions (ADRs), toxicity and outcomes resulting from medication errors.

This issue of SEDA is the first to include perspectives from pharmacogenomics/pharmacogenetics and personalized medicine. Due to the advances in science, the genetic profiles of patients must be considered in the etiology of side effects, especially for medications provided to very large populations. This marks the first phase of genome-based personalized medicine, in which side effects of common medications are linked to polymorphisms in one or more genes. A focus on personalized medicine should lead to major advances for patient care

and awareness among clinicians to deliver the most effective medication for the patient. This modality should considerably improve 'appropriate medication use' and enable the clinicians to pre-determine "good versus the bad responders", and help reduce ADRs. Overall, clinicians will have a better control on 'predictability and preventability' of ADEs induced by certain medications. Over time, it is anticipated that pharmacogenetics and personalized medicine will become an integral part of the practice sciences. SEDA will continue to highlight the genetic basis of side effects in future editions.

The collective wisdom, expertise and experience of the editor, authors and reviewers were vital in the creation of a volume of this breadth. Reviewing the appropriateness, timeliness and organization of this edition consumed an enormous amount of energy by the authors, reviewers and the editor, which we hope will facilitate the flow of information inter-professionally among health practitioners, professionals in training, and students, and will ultimately improve patient care. Scanning for accuracy, rebuilding and reorganizing information between each edition is not an easy task; therefore, the editor had the difficult task of accepting or rejecting information. The editor will consider this undertaking worthwhile if this publication helps to provide better patient care; fulfills the needs of the healthcare professionals in sorting out side effects of medications, medication errors or adverse drug reactions; and stimulates interest among those working and studying medicine, pharmacy, nursing, physical therapy, chiropractic, and those working in the basic therapeutic arms of pharmacology, toxicology, medicinal chemistry and pathophysiology.

Editor of this volume gratefully acknowledge the leadership provided by the former editor Prof. J.K. Aronson, all the contributors and reviewers, and will continue to maintain the legacy of this publication by building on their hard work. The editor would also like to extend special thanks for the excellent support and assistance provided by Ms. Zoe Kruze (Publisher, serials and series) and Ms. Shellie Bryant (Editorial Project Manager) during the compilation of this work.

Sidhartha D. Ray
Editor

Special Reviews in SEDA 38

Table of Essays, Annuals 1–37

SEDA	Author	Country	Title
1	M.N.G Dukes	The Netherlands	The moments of truth
2	K.H. Kimbel	Germany	Drug monitoring: why care?
3	L. Lasagna	USA	Wanted and unwanted drug effects: The need for perspective
4	M.N.G. Dukes	The Netherlands	The van der Kroef syndrome
5	J.P. Griffin, P.F. D'Arcy	UK	Adverse reactions to drugs—the information lag
6	I. Bayer	Hungary	Science vs practice and/or practice vs science
7	E. Napke	Canada	Adverse reactions: some pitfalls and postulates
8	M.N.G. Dukes	Denmark	The seven pillars of foolishness
9	W.H.W. Inman	UK	Let's get our act together
10	S. Van Hauen	Denmark	Integrated medicine, safer medicine and "AIDS"
11	M.N.G. Dukes	Denmark	Hark, hark, the fictitious dogs do bark
12	M.C. Cone	Switzerland	Both sides of the fence
13	C. Medawar	UK	On our side of the fence
14	M.N.G. Dukes, E. Helsing	Denmark	The great cholesterol carousel
15	P. Tyrer	UK	The nocebo effect—poorly known but getting stronger
16	M.N.G. Dukes	Denmark	Good enough for Iganga?
17	M.N.G. Dukes	Denmark	The mists of tomorrow
18	R.D. Mann	UK	Databases, privacy, and confidentiality—the effect of proposed legislation on pharmacoepidemiology and drug safety monitoring
19	A. Herxheimer	UK	Side effects: Freedom of information and the communication of doubt
20	E. Ernst	UK	Complementary/alternative medicine: What should we do about it?
21	H. Jick	USA	Thirty years of the Boston Collaborative Drug Surveillance Program in relation to principles and methods of drug safety research
22	J.K. Aronson, R.E. Ferner	UK	Errors in prescribing, preparing, and giving medicines: Definition, classification, and prevention
23	K.Y. Hartigan-Go, J.Q. Wong	Philippines	Inclusion of therapeutic failures as adverse drug reactions
24	IPalmlund	UK	Secrecy hiding harm: case histories from the past that inform the future
25	L. Marks	UK	The pill: untangling the adverse effects of a drug
26	D.J. Finney	UK	From thalidomide to pharmacovigilance: a Personal account
26	L.L.Iversen	UK	How safe is cannabis?
27	J.K. Aronson	UK	Louis Lewin—Meyler's predecessor
27	H. Jick	USA	The General Practice Research Database
28	J.K. Aronson	UK	Classifying adverse drug reactions in the twenty-first century
29	M. Hauben, A. Bate	USA/Sweden	Data mining in drug safety
30	J.K. Aronson	UK	Drug withdrawals because of adverse effects
31	J. Harrison, P. Mozzicato	USA	MedDRA®: The Tale of a Terminology
32	K. Chan	Australia	Regulating complementary and alternative medicines

Abbreviations

The following abbreviations are used throughout the SEDA series.

2,4-DMA	2,4-Dimethoxyamfetamine
3,4-DMA	3,4-Dimethoxyamfetamine
3TC	Lamivudine (dideoxythiacytidine)
ADHD	Attention deficit hyperactivity disorder
ADP	Adenosine diphosphate
ANA	Antinuclear antibody
ANCA	Antineutrophil cytoplasmic antibody
aP	Acellular pertussis
APACHE	Acute physiology and chronic health evaluation (score)
aPTT	Activated partial thromboplastin time
ASA	American Society of Anesthesiologists
ASCA	*Anti-Saccharomyces cerevisiae* antibody
AUC	The area under the concentration versus time curve from zero to infinity
$AUC_{0\to x}$	The area under the concentration versus time curve from zero to time x
$AUC_{0\to t}$	The area under the concentration versus time curve from zero to the time of the last sample
AUC_τ	The area under the concentration versus time curve during a dosage interval
AVA	Anthrax vaccine adsorbed
AZT	Zidovudine (azidothymidine)
BCG	Bacillus Calmette Guérin
bd	Twice a day (bis in die)
BIS	Bispectral index
BMI	Body mass index
CAPD	Continuous ambulatory peritoneal dialysis
CD [4, 8, etc]	Cluster of differentiation (describing various glycoproteins that are expressed on the surfaces of T cells, B cells and other cells, with varying functions)
CI	Confidence interval
C_{max}	Maximum (peak) concentration after a dose
$C_{ss.max}$	Maximum (peak) concentration after a dose at steady state
$C_{ss.min}$	Minimum (trough) concentration after a dose at steady state
COX-1 and COX-2	Cyclo-oxygenase enzyme isoforms 1 and 2
CT	Computed tomography
CYP (e.g. CYP2D6, CYP3A4)	Cytochrome P450 isoenzymes
D4T	Stavudine (didehydrodideoxythmidine)
DDC	Zalcitabine (dideoxycytidine)
DDI	Didanosine (dideoxyinosine)
DMA	Dimethoxyamfetamine; *see also* 2,4-DMA, 3,4-DMA
DMMDA	2,5-Dimethoxy-3,4-methylenedioxyamfetamine
DMMDA-2	2,3-Dimethoxy-4,5-methylenedioxyamfetamine
DTaP	Diphtheria + tetanus toxoids + acellular pertussis
DTaP-Hib-IPV-HB	Diphtheria + tetanus toxoids + acellular pertussis + IPV + Hib + hepatitis B (hexavalent vaccine)
DT-IPV	Diphtheria + tetanus toxoids + inactivated polio vaccine
DTP	Diphtheria + tetanus toxoids + pertussis vaccine
DTwP	Diphtheria + tetanus toxoids + whole cell pertussis
eGFR	Estimated glomerular filtration rate
ESR	Erythrocyte sedimentation rate
FDA	(US) Food and Drug Administration
FEV_1	Forced expiratory volume in 1 s
FTC	Emtricitabine
FVC	Forced vital capacity
G6PD	Glucose-6-phosphate dehydrogenase
GSH	Glutathione
GST	Glutathione S-transferase
HAV	Hepatitis A virus
HbA_{1c}	Hemoglobin A_{1c}
HbOC	Conjugated Hib vaccine (Hib capsular antigen polyribosylphosphate covalently linked to the nontoxic diphtheria toxin variant CRM197)
HBV	Hepatitis B virus

HDL, LDL, VLDL	High-density lipoprotein, low-density lipoprotein, and very low density lipoprotein (cholesterol)
Hib	*Haemophilus influenzae* type b
HIV	Human immunodeficiency virus
hplc	High-performance liquid chromatography
HPV	Human papilloma virus
HR	Hazard ratio
HZV	Herpes zoster virus vaccine
ICER	Incremental cost-effectiveness ratio
Ig (IgA, IgE, IgM)	Immunoglobulin (A, E, M)
IGF	Insulin-like growth factor
INN	International Nonproprietary Name (rINN = recommended; pINN = provisional)
INR	International normalized ratio
IPV	Inactivated polio vaccine
IQ [range], IQR	Interquartile [range]
JE	Japanese encephalitis vaccine
LABA	Long-acting beta-adrenoceptor agonist
MAC	Minimum alveolar concentration
MCV4	4-valent (Serogroups A, C, W, Y) meningococcal Conjugate vaccine
MDA	3,4-Methylenedioxyamfetamine
MDI	Metered-dose inhaler
MDMA	3,4-Methylenedioxymetamfetamine
MenB	Monovalent serogroup B meningoccocal vaccine
MenC	Monovalent serogroup C meningoccocal conjugate vaccine
MIC	Minimum inhibitory concentration
MIM	Mendelian Inheritance in Man (see http://www.ncbi.nlm.nih.gov/omim/607686)
MMDA	3-Methoxy-4,5-methylenedioxyamfetamine
MMDA-2	2-Methoxy-4,5-methylendioxyamfetamine
MMDA-3a	2-Methoxy-3,4-methylendioxyamfetamine
MMR	Measles + mumps + rubella
MMRV	Measles + mumps + rubella + varicella
MPSV4	4-Valent (serogroups A, C, W, Y) meningococcal polysaccharide vaccine
MR	Measles + rubella vaccine
MRI	Magnetic resonance imaging
NMS	Neuroleptic malignant syndrome
NNRTI	Non-nucleoside analogue reverse transcriptase inhibitor
NNT, NNT_B, NNT_H	Number needed to treat (for benefit, for harm)
NRTI	Nucleoside analogue reverse transcriptase inhibitor
NSAIDs	Nonsteroidal anti-inflammatory drugs
od	Once a day (omne die)
OMIM	Online Mendelian Inheritance in Man (see http://www.ncbi.nlm.nih.gov/omim/607686)
OPV	Oral polio vaccine
OR	Odds ratio
OROS	Osmotic-release oral system
PCR	Polymerase chain reaction
PMA	Paramethoxyamfetamine
PMMA	Paramethoxymetamfetamine
PPAR	Peroxisome proliferator-activated receptor
ppb	Parts per billion
PPD	Purified protein derivative
ppm	Parts per million
PRP-CRM	*See* HbOC
PRP-D-Hib	Conjugated Hib vaccine(Hib capsular antigen polyribosylphosphate covalently Linked to a mutant polypeptide of diphtheria toxin)
PT	Prothrombin time
PTT	Partial thromboplastin time
QALY	Quality-adjusted life year
qds	Four times a day (quater die summendum)
ROC curve	Receiver-operator characteristic curve
RR	Risk ratio or relative risk
RT-PCR	Reverse transcriptase polymerase chain reaction
SABA	Short-acting beta-adrenoceptor agonist
SMR	Standardized mortality rate
SNP	Single nucleotide polymorphism
SNRI	Serotonin and noradrenaline reuptake inhibitor
SSRI	Selective serotonin reuptake inhibitor

SV40	Simian virus 40
Td	Diphtheria + tetanus toxoids (adult formulation)
Tdap:	Tetanus toxoid + reduced diphtheria toxoid + acellular pertussis
tds	Three times a day (ter die summendum)
TeMA	2,3,4,5-Tetramethoxyamfetamine
TMA	3,4,5-Trimethoxyamfetamine
TMA-2	2,4,5-Trimethoxyamfetamine
t_{max}	The time at which C_{max} is reached
TMC125	Etravirine
TMC 278	Rilpivirine
V_{max}	Maximum velocity (of a reaction)
wP	Whole cell pertussis
VZV	*Varicella zoster* vaccine
YF	Yellow fever
YFV	Yellow fever virus

ADRs, ADEs and SEDs: A Bird's Eye View

Sidhartha D. Ray*,1, Kelan L. Thomas†, David F. Kisor*

*Department of Pharmaceutical Sciences, Manchester University College of Pharmacy, Natural and Health Sciences, Fort Wayne, IN, USA

†Department of Clinical Sciences, Touro University California College of Pharmacy, Vallejo, CA, USA

1Corresponding author: sdray@manchester.edu

INTRODUCTION

Adverse drug events (ADEs), drug-induced toxicity and side effects are a significant concern. ADEs are known to pose significant morbidity, mortality, and cost burden to society; however, there is a lack of strong evidence to determine their precise impact. The landmark Institute of Medicine (IOM) report *To Err is Human* implicated adverse drug events in 7000 annual deaths at an estimated cost of $2 billion [1]. However, the US Department of Health and Human Services estimates 770 000 people are injured or die each year in hospitals from ADEs, which costs up to $5.6 million each year per hospital excluding the other accessory costs (e.g., hospital admissions due to ADEs, malpractice and litigation costs, or the costs of injuries). Nationally, hospitals spend $1.56–5.6 billion each year, to treat patients who suffer ADEs during hospitalization [2]. A second landmark study suggests that approximately 28% of ADEs are preventable, through optimization of medication safety and distribution systems, provision and dissemination of timely patient and medication information, and staffing assignments [3]. Subsequent recent investigations suggest these numbers might be conservative estimates of the morbidity and mortality impact of ADEs [4].

Analysis of ADEs, ADRs, Side Effects and Toxicity

A recent report suggested that ADEs and/or side effects of drugs occur in approximately 30% of hospitalized patients [5]. The American Society of Health-System Pharmacists (ASHP) defines medication misadventures as unexpected, undesirable iatrogenic hazards or events where a medication was implicated [6]. These events can be broadly divided into two categories: (i) medication errors (i.e., preventable events that may cause or contain inappropriate use), (ii) adverse drug events (i.e., any injury, whether minor or significant, caused by a medication or lack thereof). Another significant ADE generating category that can be added to the list is: lack of incorporation of pre-existing condition(s) or pharmacogenetic factors. This work focuses on adverse drug events; however, it should be noted that adverse drug events may or may not occur secondary to a medication error.

The lack of more up to date epidemiological data regarding the impact of ADEs is largely due to challenges with low adverse drug event reporting. ASHP recommends that health systems implement adverse drug reaction (ADR) monitoring programs in order to (i) mitigate ADR risks for specific patients and expedite reporting to clinicians involved in care of patients who do experience ADRs and (ii) gather pharmacovigilance information that can be reported to pharmaceutical companies and regulatory bodies [7]. Factors that may increase the risk for ADEs include polypharmacy, multiple concomitant disease states, pediatric or geriatric status, female sex, genetic variance, and drug factors, such as class and route of administration. The Institute for Safe Medication Practices (ISMP) defines high-alert medications as those with high risk for harmful events, especially when used in error [8]. Examples include antithrombotic agents, cancer chemotherapy, insulin, opioids, and neuromuscular blockers.

Terminology

ADEs may be further classified based on expected severity into adverse drug reactions (ADRs) or adverse effects (also known as side effects). ASHP defines ADRs as an "unexpected, unintended, undesired, or excessive response to a drug" resulting in death, disability, or harm [7]. The World Health Organization (WHO) has traditionally defined an ADR as a "response to a drug which is noxious and unintended, and which occurs at doses normally used"; however, another proposed definition, intended to highlight the seriousness of ADRs, is "an appreciably harmful or unpleasant reaction, resulting from an intervention related to the use of a medicinal product, which predicts hazard from future administration and warrants prevention or specific treatment, or alteration of the dosage regimen, or withdrawal of the product" [9]. Under all definitions, ADRs are distinguished from side effects in that they generally necessitate some type of modification to the patient's therapeutic regimen. Such modifications could include discontinuing treatment, changing medications, significantly altering the dose, elevating or prolonging care received by the patient, or changing diagnosis or prognosis. ADRs include drug allergies, immunologic hypersensitivities, and idiosyncratic reactions. In contrast, side effects, or adverse effects, are defined as "expected, well-known reaction resulting in little or no change in patient management" [7]. Side effects occur at predictable frequency and are often dose-related, whereas ADRs are less foreseeable [9,10].

Two additional types of adverse drug events are drug-induced diseases and toxicity. Drug-induced diseases are defined as an "unintended effect of a drug that results in mortality or morbidity with symptoms sufficient to prompt a patient to seek medical attention, require hospitalization, or both" [11]. In other words, a drug-induced disease has elements of an ADR (i.e., significant severity, elevated levels of patient care) and adverse effects (i.e., predictability, consistent symptoms). Toxicity is a less precisely defined term referring to the ability of a substance "to cause injury to living organisms as a result of physicochemical interaction" [12]. This term is applied to both medication and non-medication types of substances, while "ADRs," "side effects," and "drug-induced diseases" typically only refer to medications. When applied to medication use, toxicity typically refers to use at higher than normal dosing or accumulated supratherapeutic exposure over time, while ADRs, side effects, and drug-induced diseases are associated with normal therapeutic use.

Although the title of this monograph is "Side Effects of Drugs," this work provides emerging information for all adverse drug events including ADRs, side effects, drug-induced diseases, toxicity, and other situations less clearly classifiable into a particular category, such as effects subsequent to drug interactions with other drugs, foods, and cosmetics. Pharmacogenetic considerations have been incorporated in several chapters as appropriate and subject to availability of literature.

Adverse drug reactions are described in SEDA using two complementary systems, EIDOS and DoTS [13–15]. These two systems are illustrated in Figures 1 and 2 and general templates for describing reactions in this way are shown in Figures 3–5. Examples of their use have been discussed elsewhere [16–20]. As the clinicians are becoming more cognizant about different types of ADRs, reports in this arena are growing faster than one can imagine; few recent articles are listed for reference [21].

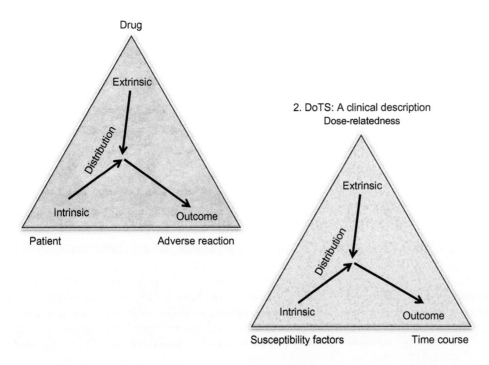

FIGURE 1 Describing adverse drug reactions—two complementary systems. Note that the triad of drug–patient–adverse reaction appears outside the triangle in EIDOS and inside the triangle in DoTS, leading to Figure 2.

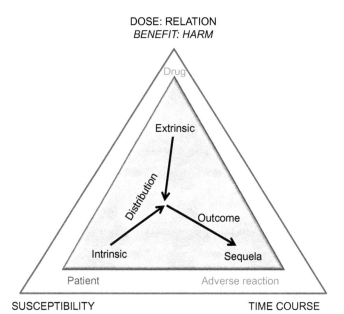

DOSE: RELATION
BENEFIT: HARM

SUSCEPTIBILITY   TIME COURSE

FIGURE 2 How the EIDOS and DoTS systems relate to each other. Here the two triangles in Figure 1 are superimposed, to show the relation between the two systems. An adverse reaction occurs when a drug is given to a patient. Adverse reactions can be classified mechanistically (EIDOS) by noting that when the Extrinsic (drug) species and an Intrinsic (patient) species are co-Distributed, a pharmacological or other effect (the Outcome) results in the adverse reaction (the Sequela). The adverse reaction can be further classified (DoTS) by considering its three main features—its Dose-relatedness, its Time-course, and individual Susceptibility.

EIDOS

The EIDOS mechanistic description of adverse drug reactions [15] has five elements:

- the Extrinsic species that initiates the reaction (Table 1);
- the Intrinsic species that it affects;
- the Distribution of these species in the body;
- the (physiological or pathological) Outcome (Table 2), which is the adverse effect;
- the Sequela, which is the adverse reaction.

Extrinsic species: This can be the parent compound, an excipient, a contaminant or adulterant, a degradation product, or a derivative of any of these (e.g. a metabolite) (for examples see Table 1).

Intrinsic species: This is usually the endogenous molecule with which the extrinsic species interacts; this can be a nucleic acid, an enzyme, a receptor, an ion channel or transporter, or some other protein.

Distribution: A drug will not produce an adverse effect if it is not distributed to the same site as the target species that mediates the adverse effect. Thus, the pharmacokinetics of the extrinsic species can affect the occurrence of adverse reactions.

Outcome: Interactions between extrinsic and intrinsic species in the production of an adverse effect can result in physiological or pathological changes (for examples see Table 2). Physiological changes can involve either increased actions (e.g. clotting due to tranexamic acid) or decreased actions (e.g. bradycardia due to β(beta)-adrenoceptor antagonists). Pathological changes can

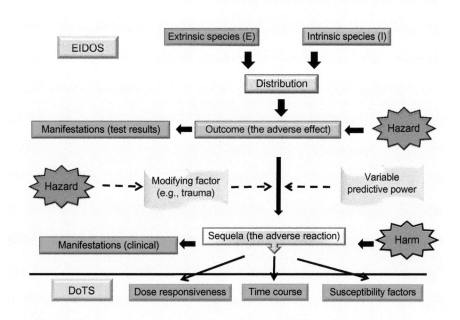

FIGURE 3 A general form of the EIDOS and DoTS template for describing an adverse effect or an adverse reaction.

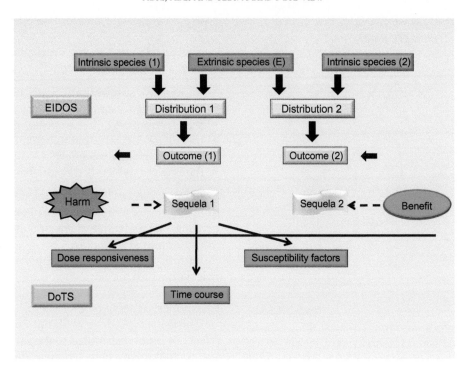

FIGURE 4   A general form of the EIDOS and DoTS template for describing two mechanisms of an adverse reaction or (illustrated here) the balance of benefit to harm, each mediated by a different mechanism.

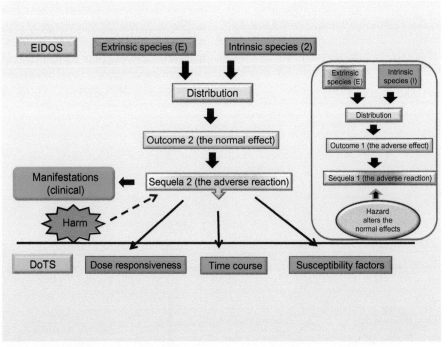

FIGURE 5   A general form of the EIDOS and DoTS template for describing an adverse drug interaction.

involve cellular adaptations (atrophy, hypertrophy, hyperplasia, metaplasia and neoplasia), altered cell function (e.g. mast cell degranulation in IgE-mediated anaphylactic reactions) or cell damage (e.g. cell lysis, necrosis or apoptosis).

Sequela: The sequela of the changes induced by a drug describes the clinically recognizable adverse drug

reaction, of which there may be more than one. Sequelae can be classified using the DoTS system.

DoTS

In the DoTS system (SEDA-28, xxvii–xxxiii; 1,2) adverse drug reactions are described according to the

TABLE 1 The EIDOS Mechanistic Description of Adverse Drug Effects and Reactions

Feature	Varieties	Examples
E. Extrinsic species	1. The parent compound	Insulin
	2. An excipient	Polyoxyl 35 castor oil
	3. A contaminant	1,1-Ethylidenebis[1-tryptophan]
	4. An adulterant	Lead in herbal medicines
	5. A degradation product formed before the drug enters the body	Outdated tetracycline
	6. A derivative of any of these (e.g. a metabolite)	Acrolein (from cyclophosphamide)
I. The intrinsic species and the nature of its interaction with the extrinsic species		
(a) Molecular	1. Nucleic acids	
	(a) DNA	Melphalan
	(b) RNA	Mitoxantrone
	2. Enzymes	
	(a) Reversible effect	Edrophonium
	(b) Irreversible effect	Malathion
	3. Receptors	
	(a) Reversible effect	Prazosin
	(b) Irreversible effect	Phenoxybenzamine
	4. Ion channels/transporters	Calcium channel blockers; digoxin and Na^+–K^+–ATPase
	5. Other proteins	
	(a) Immunological proteins	Penicilloyl residue hapten
	(b) Tissue proteins	N-acetyl-p-benzoquinone-imine (paracetamol [acetaminophen])
(b) Extracellular	1. Water	Dextrose 5%
	2. Hydrogen ions (pH)	Sodium bicarbonate
	3. Other ions	Sodium ticarcillin
(c) Physical or physicochemical	1. Direct tissue damage	Intrathecal vincristine
	2. Altered physicochemical nature of the extrinsic species	Sulindac precipitation
D. Distribution	1. Where in the body the extrinsic and intrinsic species occur (affected by pharmacokinetics)	Antihistamines cause drowsiness only if they affect histamine H_1 receptors in the brain
O. Outcome (physiological or pathological change)	The adverse effect (see Table 2)	
S. Sequela	The adverse reaction (use the Dose, Time, Susceptibility [DoTS] descriptive system)	

Dose at which they usually occur, the Time-course over which they occur, and the Susceptibility factors that make them more likely, as follows:

- *Relation to dose*
  - Toxic reactions (reactions that occur at supratherapeutic doses)
  - Collateral reactions (reactions that occur at standard therapeutic doses)
  - Hypersusceptibility reactions (reactions that occur at subtherapeutic doses in susceptible individuals)
- *Time course*
  - Time-independent reactions (reactions that occur at any time during a course of therapy)

TABLE 2   Examples of Physiological and Pathological Changes in Adverse Drug Effects (Some Categories Can Be Broken Down Further)

Type of change	Examples
1. Physiological changes	
(a) Increased actions	Hypertension (monoamine oxidase inhibitors); clotting (tranexamic acid)
(b) Decreased actions	Bradycardia (beta-adrenoceptor antagonists); QT interval prolongation (antiarrhythmic drugs)
2. Cellular adaptations	
(a) Atrophy	Lipoatrophy (subcutaneous insulin); glucocorticosteroid-induced myopathy
(b) Hypertrophy	Gynecomastia (spironolactone)
(c) Hyperplasia	Pulmonary fibrosis (busulfan); retroperitoneal fibrosis (methysergide)
(d) Metaplasia	Lacrimal canalicular squamous metaplasia (fluorouracil)
(e) Neoplasia	
– Benign	Hepatoma (anabolic steroids)
– Malignant	
– Hormonal	Vaginal adenocarcinoma (diethylstilbestrol)
– Genotoxic	Transitional cell carcinoma of bladder (cyclophosphamide)
– Immune suppression	Lymphoproliferative tumors (ciclosporin)
3. Altered cell function	IgE-mediated mast cell degranulation (class I immunological reactions)
4. Cell damage	
(a) Acute reversible damage	
– Chemical damage	Periodontitis (local application of methylenedioxymetamfetamine [MDMA, 'ecstasy'])
– Immunological reactions	Class III immunological reactions
(b) Irreversible injury	
– Cell lysis	Class II immunological reactions
– Necrosis	Class IV immunological reactions; hepatotoxicity (paracetamol, after apoptosis)
– Apoptosis	Liver damage (troglitazone)
5. Intracellular accumulations	
(a) Calcification	Milk-alkali syndrome
(b) Drug deposition	Crystal-storing histiocytosis (clofazimine) Skin pigmentation (amiodarone)

- *Time-dependent reactions*
  - Immediate or rapid reactions (reactions that occur only when drug administration is too rapid)
  - First-dose reactions (reactions that occur after the first dose of a course of treatment and not necessarily thereafter)
  - Early tolerant and early persistent reactions (reactions that occur early in treatment then either abate with continuing treatment, owing to tolerance, or persist)
  - Intermediate reactions (reactions that occur after some delay but with less risk during longer term therapy, owing to the 'healthy survivor' effect)
  - Late reactions (reactions the risk of which increases with continued or repeated exposure)
  - Withdrawal reactions (reactions that occur when, after prolonged treatment, a drug is withdrawn or its effective dose is reduced)
  - Delayed reactions (reactions that occur at some time after exposure, even if the drug is withdrawn before the reaction appears)

- *Susceptibility factors*
  - Genetic (Ex. Variations in expression of certain drug-metabolizing enzymes)
  - Age (newborn, pediatric, young adult, adult and old age)
  - Sex (gender differences—hormonal variations)
  - Physiological variation (e.g. weight, pregnancy)
  - Exogenous factors (for example the effects of other drugs, devices, surgical procedures, food, phytochemicals & nutraceuticals, alcoholic beverages, smoking)
  - Diseases (ongoing but latent with no clinical signs, pre-existing and obvious)
  - Environmental factors (drinking water containing trace chemicals; breathing polluted air)

WHO Classification

Although not systematically used in Side Effects of Drugs Annual, the WHO classification, used at the Uppsala Monitoring Center, is a useful schematic to consider in assessing ADRs and adverse effects. Possible classifications include:

- Type A (dose-related, "augmented"), more common events that tend to be related to the pharmacology of the drug, have a mechanistic basis, and result in lower mortality;
- Type B (non-dose-related, "bizarre"), less common, unpredictable events that are not related to the pharmacology of the drug;
- Type C (dose-related and time-related, "chronic"), events that are related to cumulative dose received over time;
- Type D (time-related, "delayed"), events that are usually dose-related but do not become apparent until significant time has elapsed since exposure to the drug;
- Type E (withdrawal, "end of use"), events that occur soon after the use of the drug;
- Type F (unexpected lack of efficacy, "failure"), common, dose-related events where the drug effectiveness is lacking, often due to drug interactions;

REFERENCES ON ADVERSE DRUG REACTIONS

[1] Kohn, LT, Corrigan JM, Donaldson MS, editors. *To Err is Human: Building a Safer Health System*. Washington, DC National Academy Press; 1999: 1–8.

[2] US Department of Health & Human Services Report: http://archive.ahrq.gov/research/findings/factsheets/errors-safety/aderia/ade.html.

[3] Leape LL, Bates DW, Cullen DJ, et al. Systems analysis of adverse drug events. JAMA. 1995; 274 (1):35–43.

[4] James JT. A new, evidence-based estimate of patient harms associated with hospital care. J Patient Saf. 2013; 9(3):122–128.

[5] Wang G, Jung K, Winnenburg R, Shah NH. A method for systematic discovery of adverse drug events from clinical notes. J Am Med Inform Assoc. 2015 Jul 31. pii: ocv102. doi: 10.1093/jamia/ocv102.

[6] American Society of Health-Systems Pharmacists. Positions. Medication Misadventures. http://www.ashp.org/DocLibrary/BestPractices/MedMisPositions.aspx.

[7] American Society of Health-Systems Pharmacists. Guidelines. ASHP Guidelines on adverse drug reaction monitoring and reporting. http://www.ashp.org/DocLibrary/BestPractices/MedMisGdlADR.aspx.

[8] Institute for Safe Medication Practices. ISMP list of high-alert medications in acute care settings. http://www.ismp.org/Tools/institutionalhighAlert.asp.

[9] Edwards IR, Aronson JK. Adverse drug reactions: Definitions, diagnosis, and management. Lancet. 2000; 356:1255–59.

[10] Cochrane ZR, Hein D, Gregory PJ. Medication misadventures I: adverse drug reactions. In: Malone PM, Kier KL, Stanovich JE, Malone MJ, editors. Drug Information: A Guide for Pharmacists, 5th edition. New York, NY: McGraw-Hill; 2013.

[11] Tisdale JE, Miller DA, editors. Drug-Induced Diseases: Prevention, Detection, and Management. 2nd edition. Bethesda, MD: American Society of Health-System Pharmacists; 2010.

[12] Wexler P, Abdollahi M, Peyster AD, et al., editors. Encyclopedia of Toxicology. 3rd edition. Burlington, MA: Academic Press, Elsevier; 2014.

[13] Aronson JK, Ferner RE. Joining the DoTS. New approach to classifying adverse drug reactions. BMJ. 2003; 327:1222–1225.

[14] Aronson JK, Ferner RE. Clarification of terminology in drug safety. Drug Saf. 2005; 28(10):851–870.

[15] Ferner RE, Aronson JK. EIDOS: a mechanistic classification of adverse drug effects. Drug Saf. 2010; 33(1):13–23.

[16] Callréus T. Use of the dose, time, susceptibility (DoTS) classification scheme for adverse drug reactions in pharmacovigilance planning. Drug Saf. 2006; 29(7):557–566.

[17] Aronson JK, Price D, Ferner R.E. A strategy for regulatory action when new adverse effects of a licensed product emerge. Drug Saf. 2009; 32(2):91–98.

[18] Calderón-Ospina C, Bustamante-Rojas C. The DoTS classification is a useful way to classify adverse

drug reactions: a preliminary study in hospitalized patients. Int J Pharm Pract. 2010; 18(4):230–235.

[19] Ferner RE, Aronson JK. Preventability of drug-related harms. Part 1: A systematic review. Drug Saf. 2010; 33(11):985–994.

[20] Aronson JK, Ferner RE. Preventability of drug-related harms. Part 2: Proposed criteria, based on frameworks that classify adverse drug reactions. Drug Saf. 2010; 33(11):995–1002.

[21] Saini VK, Sewal RK, Ahmad Y, Medhi B. Prospective Observational Study of Adverse Drug Reactions of Anticancer Drugs Used in Cancer Treatment in a Tertiary Care Hospital. Indian J Pharm Sci., 2015; 77(6):687–93.

[22] White RS; Thomson Reuters Accelus. Pharmaceutical and Medical Devices: FDA Oversight. Issue Brief Health Policy Track Serv. 2015; 28:1–97.

[23] Davies EA, O'Mahony MS. Adverse drug reactions in special populations—the elderly. Br J Clin Pharmacol., 2015; 80(4):796–807.

[24] Mouton JP, Mehta U, Parrish AG, et al. Mortality from adverse drug reactions in adult medical inpatients at four hospitals in South Africa: a cross-sectional survey. Br J Clin Pharmacol., 2015; 80(4):818–26.

[25] Bouvy JC, De Bruin ML, Koopmanschap MA. Epidemiology of adverse drug reactions in Europe: a review of recent observational studies. Drug Saf., 2015; 38(5):437–53.

[26] Bénard-Laribière A, Miremont-Salamé G, Pérault-Pochat MC, et al. Incidence of hospital admissions due to adverse drug reactions in France: the EMIR study. (EMIR Study Group on behalf of the French network of pharmacovigilance centres). Fundam Clin Pharmacol., 2015; 29(1):106–11.

PHARMACOGENOMIC CONSIDERATIONS

Introduction

Advances in genomic medicine have fostered an increased public interest in precision (personalized) medicine, while the field of pharmacogenomics provides an opportunity to identify clinically important genetic variants that alter drug efficacy or ADR risk. However, the cost and turn-around-time of genetic tests have slowed the routine use of pharmacogenetic testing for clinical decision-making. It is anticipated that clinicians' education and attitudes toward pharmacogenetic testing may be vital to the success of health system implementation.

It has been suggested that pharmacogenetic profiles of patients be analyzed when administering and tailoring drug therapy.

The past decade has witnessed an explosion in the development, implementation and availability of genetic testing. Compelling statistics on ADRs remain a primary component for driving such testing. In the United States, ADRs occur in nearly 10% of patients taking prescription medications in the ambulatory setting and cause estimated 100 000 deaths annually in hospitalized patients [1,2]. Although many nongenetic factors, such as age, organ function, concomitant therapy, drug interactions, and pathophysiology of the disease, influence the effects of medications, it has been projected that genetics can account for 20–95% of variability in drug disposition and effects [3]. More than one-fourth of primary care patients take a medication commonly implicated in ADRs and metabolized by enzymes with a known "poor metabolizer" genetic variant [4]. The United States Food and Drug Administration (FDA) has made considerable efforts to inform prescribers about drugs with pharmacogenomic information in their labeling [5]. Information pertaining to pharmacogenomics is indicated on the labels of over 150 drugs, and it has been estimated that 25% of outpatients take at least one drug with pharmacogenomic information in the labeling [5,6].

Definition of Pharmacogenomics

The U.S. Food and Drug Administration defines pharmacogenomics (PGx) as the study of variations of DNA and RNA characteristics as related to drug response, whereas pharmacogenetics (PGt), being a subset of PGx, is defined as the study of variations in DNA sequence as related to drug response [7]. Pharmacogenomics is also referred to as the study of the scientific area of drug–gene(s) interaction. The interaction between a drug and a gene product (e.g., functional protein) affecting an individual's response to the drug represents a clear application of the EIDOS mechanism description; an adverse drug reaction when the drug–gene interaction produces a collateral reaction due to susceptibility factors as described using the DoTS system [8].

The gene products affecting individual drug response include receptors, target enzymes, drug transporters and drug-metabolizing enzymes [9]. Gene variants, a consequence of single nucleotide polymorphisms (SNPs) or insertions or deletions (indels), among other DNA alterations or duplications can result in outcomes with deleterious effects. These effects range from an exaggerated clinical response, e.g. increased bleeding as can be seen with warfarin in an individual with decreased production of the target enzyme vitamin K epoxide reductase subunit 1 (VKORC1; A/A genotype), or in an individual

TABLE X Drug (Extrinsic)–Gene (Intrinsic) Interactions and Example Outcomes with Prescribing Information Recommendations

Drug–gene(s) interaction	Example Gene variant[a] Diplotype Metabolizer phenotype[b]	Effect on drug response	Pharmacokinetic consequences[b]	Prescribing information recommendations
Azathioprine and 6-mercaptopurine–TPMT [14]	TPMT*2, *3A, *3B, *3C or *4 *2/*3A Poor metabolizer (PM)	Increased risk of severe myelosuppression	Increased active metabolite exposure: higher thioguanine nucleotide metabolite concentrations	Testing should be considered if patients develop severe toxicity, since substantial dose reductions may be required
Carbamazepine–HLA-B [12]	HLA-B*15:02 negative/HLA-B*15:02 positive HLA-B*15:02 positive[c]	Increased risk of severe cutaneous reactions like SJS and TEN	None	Testing should be performed in patients of Asian ancestry before initiation
Clopidogrel–CYP2C19 [15,16]	CYP2C19*2 or *3 *2/*2 PM	Increased risk of adverse cardiovascular events like thrombosis	Decreased active metabolite exposure: ~40% lower AUC for active metabolite	Testing can be used as an aid to determine therapeutic strategy
Codeine–CYP2D6 [11,17]	CYP2D6*1xN or *2xN *1/*2xN UM	Increased risk of respiratory depression	Increased active metabolite exposure: ~1.5-fold higher AUC for morphine	Codeine is contraindicated for pain management in pediatric patients undergoing adenotonsillectomy due to case reports of death
Warfarin–CYP2C9 [10,18]	CYP2C9*2 or *3 *3/*3 PM	Increased risk of over-anticoagulation and bleeding	Increased drug exposure: ~3-fold higher AUC for S-warfarin	Decreased daily dosage recommendations based on genotypes with variant

[a] "Star" nomenclature [13].
[b] AUC = area under the plasma drug concentration–time curve.
[c] Carrier status.

who is a CYP2C9 poor metabolizer, being exposed to higher warfarin concentrations to death, e.g. respiratory arrest due to morphine overdose following the administration of codeine in CYP2D6 ultrarapid metabolizers [10,11]. Another example of a drug–gene interaction resulting in a life-threatening adverse effect involves carbamazepine with its increased risk of Stevens–Johnson Syndrome (SJS) and Toxic Epidermal Necrolysis (TEN) for individuals with the human leukocyte antigen (HLA)-B*15:02 allele, which is a genetic variant that encodes a cell surface protein involved in presenting antigens to the immune system [12]. These drug–gene interactions may result in collateral reactions, due to intrinsic susceptibility factors, since the adverse outcomes are seen at standard therapeutic doses.

Perhaps the most studied drug–gene interactions are related to the activity of drug-metabolizing gene elements, such as cytochrome P450 enzymes (CYPs) and thiopurine methyl transferase (TPMT). Variants of these genes may result in altered drug metabolism and changes in pharmacokinetic parameters, which may influence the required maintenance dose of a given drug. Table X presents examples of gene variants and the effects on drug response, including pharmacokinetic consequences and prescribing information recommendations.

The intrinsic genetic susceptibility factors can influence an individual's response to standard doses of a given drug. In Table X examples below, the collateral reactions can potentially result in life-threatening outcomes. As technology allows, preemptive genetic testing of patients may allow for appropriate drug and dose selection to decrease the risk of adverse drug reactions.

Readers are advised to refer to specific literature pertaining to a drug or a class of drugs to gain further insights into this field. Several references are provided [19–36].

REFERENCES ON PHARMACOGENOMIC CONSIDERATIONS

[1] Taché SV, Sönnichsen A, Ashcroft DM. Prevalence of adverse drug events in ambulatory care: a systematic review. Ann Pharmacother. 2011; 45(7–8):977–989.

[2] Lazarou J, Pomeranz B, Corey PN. Incidence of adverse drug reactions in hospitalized patients: a meta-analysis of prospective studies. JAMA. 1998; 279(15):1200–1205.

[3] Evans WE., McLeod HL. Pharmacogenomics: Drug Disposition, Drug Targets, and Side Effects. N Engl J Med 2003; 348:538–549

[4] Grice GR, Seaton TL, Woodland AM, McLeod HL. Defining the opportunity for pharmacogenetic intervention in primary care. Pharmacogenomics. 2006; 7(1):61–65.

[5] U.S. Food and Drug Administration. Table of pharmacogenomic biomarkers in drug labeling. Available from: http://www.fda.gov/drugs/scienceresearch/researchareas/pharmacogenetics/ucm083378.htm.

[6] Frueh FW, Amur S, Mummaneni P, et al. Pharmacogenomic biomarker information in drug labels approved by the United States food and drug administration: prevalence of related drug use. Pharmacotherapy. 2008; 28(8):992–998.

[7] U.S. Food and Drug Administration. Definitions for Genomic Biomarkers, Pharmacogenomics, Pharmacogenetics, Genomic Data and Sample Coding Categories. Available from: http://www.fda.gov/downloads/drugs/guidancecompliance regulatoryinformation/guidances/ucm073162.pdf.

[8] Aronson JK, Ferner RE. Joining the DoTS. New approach to classifying adverse drug reactions. BMJ. 2003; 327:1222–5.

[9] Ma Q, Lu AYH. Pharmacogenetics, pharmacogenomics, and individualized medicine. Pharmacol Rev. 2011; 63(2):437–459.

[10] Johnson JA, Gong L, Whirl-Carrillo M, et al. Clinical Pharmacogenetics Implementation Consortium guidelines for CYP2C9 and VKORC1 genotypes and warfarin dosing. Clin Pharmacol Ther. 2011; 90(4):625–629.

[11] Crews KR, Gaedigk A, Dunnenberger HM, et al. Clinical Pharmacogenetics Implementation Consortium guidelines for cytochrome P450 2D6 genotype and codeine therapy: 2014 update. Clin Pharmacol Ther. 2014; 95(4):376–82.

[12] Leckband SG, Kelsoe JR, Dunnenberger HM, et al. Clinical Pharmacogenetics Implementation Consortium guidelines for HLA-B genotype and carbamazepine dosing. Clin Pharmacol Ther. 2013; 94(3):324–8.

[13] Robarge JD, Li L, Desta Z, Nguyen A, Flockhart DA. The star-allele nomenclature: retooling for translational genomics. Clin Pharmacol Ther. 2007; 82(3):244–8.

[14] Relling MV, Gardner EE, Sandborn WJ, et al. Clinical Pharmacogenetics Implementation Consortium guidelines for thiopurine methyltransferase genotype and thiopurine dosing. Clin Pharmacol Ther. 2011; 89(3):387–91.

[15] Scott SA, Sangkuhl K, Stein CM, et al. Clinical Pharmacogenetics Implementation Consortium guidelines for CYP2C19 genotype and clopidogrel therapy: 2013 update. Clin Pharmacol Ther. 2013; 94(3):317–23.

[16] Erlinge D, James S, Duvvuru S, et al. Clopidogrel metaboliser status based on point-of-care CYP2C19 genetic testing in patients with coronary artery disease. Thromb Haemost. 2014; 111 (5):943–50.

[17] Kirchheiner J, Schmidt H, Tzvetkov M, et al. Pharmacokinetics of codeine and its metabolite morphine in ultra-rapid metabolizers due to CYP2D6 duplication. Pharmacogenomics J. 2007; 7(4):257–65.

[18] Flora DR, Rettie AE, Brundage RC, Tracy TS. CYP2C9 Genotype-Dependent Warfarin Pharmacokinetics: Impact of CYP2C9 Genotype on R- and S-Warfarin and Their Oxidative Metabolites. J Clin Pharmacol. 2016; doi: 10.1002/jcph.813.

[19] Hertz DL, Rae J. Pharmacogenetics of cancer drugs. Annu Rev Med. 2015; 66:65–81.

[20] Dunnenberger HM, Crews KR, Hoffman JM, et al. Preemptive clinical pharmacogenetics implementation: current programs in five US medical centers. Annu Rev Pharmacol Toxicol. 2015; 55:89–106.

[21] Aithal GP. Pharmacogenetic testing in idiosyncratic drug-induced liver injury: current role in clinical practice. Liver Int. 2015; 35(7):1801–8.

[22] Cuzzoni E, De Iudicibus S, Franca R, et al. Glucocorticoid pharmacogenetics in pediatric idiopathic nephrotic syndrome. Pharmacogenomics. 2015; 16(14):1631–48.

[23] Aceti A, Gianserra L, Lambiase L, et al. Pharmacogenetics as a tool to tailor antiretroviral therapy: A review. World J Virol. 2015; 4(3):198–208.

[24] Sahu RK, Singh K, Subodh S. Adverse Drug Reactions to Anti-TB Drugs: Pharmacogenomics Perspective for Identification of Host Genetic Markers. Curr Drug Metab. 2015; 16(7):538–52.

[25] Higgins GA, Allyn-Feuer A, Handelman S, et al. The epigenome, 4D nucleome and next-generation neuropsychiatric pharmacogenomics. Pharmacogenomics. 2015; 16(14):1649–69.

[26] Niemeijer MN, van den Berg ME, Eijgelsheim M, et al. Pharmacogenetics of Drug-Induced QT Interval Prolongation: An Update. Drug Saf. 2015; 38(10):855–67.

[27] Perwitasari DA, Atthobari J, Wilffert B. Pharmacogenetics of isoniazid-induced hepatotoxicity. Drug Metab Rev., 2015; 47(2):222–8.

[28] Roberts RL, Barclay ML. Update on thiopurine pharmacogenetics in inflammatory bowel disease. Pharmacogenomics. 2015; 16(8):891–903.

[29] Seripa D, Panza F, Daragjati J, Paroni G, Pilotto A. Measuring pharmacogenetics in special groups: geriatrics. Expert Opin Drug Metab Toxicol. 2015; 11(7):1073–88.

[30] Chan SL, Jin S, Loh M, et al. Brunham LR. Progress in understanding the genomic basis for adverse drug reactions: a comprehensive review and focus on the role of ethnicity. Pharmacogenomics. 2015;16 (10):1161–78.

[31] Jarjour S, Barrette M, Normand V, et al. Genetic markers associated with cutaneous adverse drug reactions to allopurinol: a systematic review. Pharmacogenomics. 2015; 16(7):755–67.

[32] Błaszczyk B, Lasoń W, Czuczwar SJ. Antiepileptic drugs and adverse skin reactions: An update. Pharmacol Rep. 2015 Jun; 67(3):426–34.

[33] Zhou ZW, Chen XW, Sneed KB, et al. Clinical association between pharmacogenomics and adverse drug reactions. Drugs. 2015; 75(6):589–631.

[34] Sousa-Pinto B, Pinto-Ramos J, Correia C, et al. Pharmacogenetics of abacavir hypersensitivity: A systematic review and meta-analysis of the association with HLA-B*57:01. J Allergy Clin Immunol. 2015; 136(4):1092–4.e3.

[35] Pellegrino P, Falvella FS, Perrone V, et al. The first steps towards the era of personalised vaccinology: predicting adverse reactions. Pharmacogenomics J. 2015; 15(3):284–7.

[36] Goulding R, Dawes D, Price M, et al. Genotype-guided drug prescribing: a systematic review and meta-analysis of randomized control trials. Br J Clin Pharmacol. 2015; 80(4):868–77.

IMMUNOLOGICAL REACTIONS

The immunological reactions are diverse and varied but considered specific. Nearly five decades ago, Karl Landsteiner's ground-breaking work "The Specificity of Serological Reactions" set the standard in experimental immunology. Several new discoveries in immunology in the twentieth century, such as, 'CD' receptors (cluster of differentiation), recognition of 'self' versus 'non-self', a large family of cytokines and antigenic specificity became instrumental in describing immunological reactions. The most widely accepted classification divides immunological reactions (drug allergies or otherwise) into four pathophysiological types, namely, anaphylaxis (immediate type or Type I hypersensitivity), antibody-mediated cytotoxic reactions (cytotoxic type or Type II hypersensitivity), immune complex-mediated reactions (toxic-complex syndrome or Type III hypersensitivity), and cell-mediated immunity (delayed-type hypersensitivity or Type IV hypersensitivity). Although Gell and Coomb's classification was proposed more than 30 years ago, it is still widely used [1–3].

Type I Reactions (IgE-Mediated Anaphylaxis; Immediate Hypersensitivity)

In type I reactions, the drug or its metabolite interacts with IgE molecules bound to specific type of cells (mast cells and basophils). This triggers a process that leads to the release of pharmacological mediators (histamine, 5-hydroxytryptamine, kinins, and arachidonic acid derivatives), which cause the allergic response. Mounting of such a reaction depends exclusively upon exposure to the same assaulting agent (antigen, allergen or metabolite) for the second time and the severity depends on the level of exposure. The clinical effects [2] are due to smooth muscle contraction, vasodilatation, and increased capillary permeability. The symptoms include faintness, light-headedness, pruritus, nausea, vomiting, abdominal pain, and a feeling of impending doom (angor animi). The signs include urticaria, conjunctivitis, rhinitis, laryngeal edema, bronchial asthma and pulmonary edema, angioedema, and anaphylactic shock; takotsubo cardiomyopathy can occur, as can Kounis syndrome (an acute coronary episode associated with an allergic reaction). Not all type I reactions are IgE-dependent; however, under circumstances, adverse reactions that are mediated by direct histamine release have conventionally been called anaphylactoid reactions, but are better classified as non-IgE-mediated anaphylactic reactions. Cytokines, such as, IL-4, IL-5, IL-6 and IL-13, either mediate or influence this class of hypersensitivity reaction. Representative agents that are known to induce such reactions include: Gelatin, Gentamicin, Kanamycin, Neomycin, Penicillins, Polymyxin B, Streptomycin and Thiomersal [1–3].

Type II Reactions (Cytotoxic Reactions)

Type II reactions involve circulating immunoglobulins G or M (or rarely IgA) binding with cell surface antigens (membrane constituent or protein) and interacting with an antigen formed by a hapten (drug or metabolite) and subsequently fixing complement. Complement is then activated leading to cytolysis. Type II reactions often involve antibody-mediated cytotoxicity directed to the membranes of erythrocytes, leukocytes, platelets, and probably hematopoietic precursor cells in the bone marrow. Drugs that are typically involved are methyldopa (hemolytic anemia), aminopyrine (leukopenia), and heparin (thrombocytopenia) with mostly hematological consequences, including thrombocytopenia, neutropenia, and hemolytic anemia [1–3].

Type III Reactions (Immune Complex Reactions)

In type III reactions, formation of an immune complex and its deposition on tissue surface serve as primary initiators. Occasionally, immune complexes bind to endothelial cells and lead to immune complex deposition with subsequent complement activation in the linings of blood vessels. Circumstances that govern immune formation or immune complex disease remain unclear to date, and it usually occurs without symptoms. The clinical symptoms of a type III reaction include serum sickness (e.g., β-lactams), drug-induced lupus erythematosus (eg, quinidine), and vasculitis (e.g., minocycline). Type III reactions can result in acute interstitial nephritis or serum sickness (fever, arthritis, enlarged lymph nodes, urticaria, and maculopapular rashes) [1–3].

Type IV Reactions (Cell-Mediated or Delayed Hypersensitivity Reactions)

Type IV reactions are initiated when hapten–protein antigenic complex-mediated sensitized T lymphocytes meet the assaulting immunogen for the second time; usually this leads to severe inflammation. Type IV reactions are exemplified by contact dermatitis. Pseudoallergic reactions resemble allergic reactions clinically but are not immunologically mediated. Examples include asthma and rashes caused by aspirin and maculopapular erythematous rashes due to ampicillin or amoxicillin in the absence of penicillin hypersensitivity. Few other entities that can initiate this reaction are: sulfonamides, anticonvulsants (phenytoin, carbamazepine, and phenobarbital), NSAIDs (aspirin, naproxen, nabumetone, and ketoprofen), antiretroviral agents and cephalosporins [1–4].

Other Types of Reactions

Several types of adverse drug reactions do not easily fit into Gell and Coomb's classification scheme. These include most cutaneous hypersensitivity reactions (such as toxic epidermal necrolysis), 'immune-allergic' hepatitis and hypersensitivity pneumonitis. Another difficulty is that allergic drug reactions can occur via more than one mechanism; picryl chloride in mice induces both type I and type IV responses. Although other classification schemes have evolved over time, Gell and Coomb's system remains the most widely utilized scheme. Several articles are included in this review to serve as a pointer to this field [4–12].

REFERENCES

[1] Coombs RRA, Gell PGH. Classification of allergic reactions responsible for clinical hypersensitivity and disease. In: Gell PGH, Coombs RRA, Lachmann PJ, editors. Clinical Aspects of Immunology. London: Blackwell Scientific Publications; 1975. pp. 761–81.

[2] Schnyder B, Pichler W. Mechanisms of Drug-Induced Allergy. Mayo Clin Proc. Mar 2009; 84(3): 268–272.

[3] Boyman O, Comte D, Spertini F. Adverse reactions to biologic agents and their medical management. Nat Rev Rheumatol., 2014 Aug 12. doi: 10.1038/nrrheum.2014.123. [Epub ahead of print].

[4] Brown SGA. Clinical features and severity grading of anaphylaxis. J Allergy Clin Immunol 2004; 114(2): 371–6.

[5] Johansson SGO, Hourihane JO, Bousquet J, Bruijnzeel-Koomen C, Dreborg S, Haahtela T, Kowalski ML, Mygind N, Ring J, van Cauwenberge P, van Hage-Hamsten M, Wüthrich B. A revised nomenclature for allergy. An EAACI position statement from the EAACI nomenclature task force. Allergy 2001; 56(9): 813–24.

[6] Uzzaman A, Cho SH. Chapter 28: Classification of hypersensitivity reactions. Allergy Asthma Proc. 2012 May–Jun; 33 Suppl 1:S96–9.

[7] Descotes J, Choquet-Kastylevsky G. Toxicology, 2001; 158(1–2):43–9. Gell and Coombs's classification: is it still valid?

[8] Corominas M, Andrés-López B, Lleonart R. Severe adverse drug reactions induced by hydrochlorothiazide: A persistent old problem. Ann Allergy Asthma Immunol., 2016; 117(3):334–5.

[9] Velicković J, Palibrk I, Miljković B, et al. Self-reported drug allergies in surgical population in Serbia. Acta Clin Croat. 2015; 54(4):492–9.

[10] Yip VL, Alfirevic A, Pirmohamed M. Genetics of immune-mediated adverse drug reactions: a comprehensive and clinical review. Clin Rev Allergy Immunol., 2015; 48(2–3):165–75.

[11] Agúndez JA, Mayorga C, García-Martin E. Drug metabolism and hypersensitivity reactions to drugs. Curr Opin Allergy Clin Immunol. 2015; 15(4):277–84.

[12] Wheatley LM, Plaut M, Schwaninger JM. et al. Report from the National Institute of Allergy and Infectious Diseases workshop on drug allergy. J Allergy Clin Immunol., 2015; 136(2):262–71.e2.

ANALYSIS OF TOXICOLOGICAL REACTIONS

Potentiation Reactions

This type of reaction occurs only when one non-toxic chemical interacts with another non-toxic chemical, or one non-toxic chemical interacts with another toxic chemical at low doses (subtoxic, acutely toxic). An alternate interpretation could be when two drugs are taken together and one of them intensifies the action of the other. In such scenarios, if the final outcome is high toxicity, then the final outcome is called a potentiation (increasing the toxic effect of 'Y' by 'X'). Theoretically, it can be expressed as: $x + y = M$ $(1 + 0 = 4)$.

Examples: (i) When chronic or regular alcohol drinkers consume therapeutic doses of acetaminophen, it can lead to alcohol-potentiated acetaminophen-induced hepatotoxicity (cause: ethanol-induced massive CYP2E1 induction in the liver); (ii) Avoid iron supplements in patients on doxorubicin therapy to prevent possible potentiation of doxorubicin-induced cardiotoxicity (cause: hydroxyl radical formation and redox cycling of doxorubicin); (iii) Phenergan®, an antihistamine, when given with a painkilling narcotic such as Demerol® can intensify its effect; therefore, reducing the dose of the narcotic is advised; (iv) Ethanol potentiation of CCl4-induced hepatotoxicity; (v) Use of phenytoin and calcium-channel blockers combination should be used with caution. Representative references from each category of toxic reactions are provided below:

Synergistic Effect

Synergism is somewhat similar to potentiation. When two drugs are taken together that are similar in action, such as barbiturates and alcohol, which are both depressants, an effect exaggerated out of proportion to that of each drug taken separately at the given dose may occur (mathematically: $1 + 1 = 4$). Normally, taken alone, neither substance would cause serious harm, but if taken together, the combination could cause coma or death. Another established example: when smokers get exposed to asbestos.

Additive Effect

Additive effect is defined as a consequence which follows exposure to two or more physicochemical agents which act jointly but do not interact, or commonly, the total effect is the simple sum of the effects of separate exposure to the agents under the same conditions. This could be represented by $1 + 1 = 2$: (i) one example would be barbiturate and a tranquilizer when given together before surgery to relax the patient; (ii) toxic effect on bone marrow that follows after AZT+Ganciclovir or AZT+Clotrimazole administration.

Antagonistic Effects

Antagonistic effects are when two drugs/chemicals are administered simultaneously or one followed by the other, and the net effect of the final outcome of the reaction is negligible or zero. This could be expressed by $1 + 1 = 0$. An example might be the use of a tranquilizer to stop the action of LSD.

Examples: (i) When ethanol is administered to methanol-poisoned patient; (ii) NSAIDs administered to diuretics (hydrochlorothiazide/Furosemide): Reduce diuretics effectiveness; (iii) Certain β-blockers (INDERAL®) taken to control high blood pressure and heart disease counteract β-adrenergic stimulants, such as Albuterol®.

REFERENCES

[1] Ray SD, Mehendale HM. Potentiation of CCl4 and CHCl3 hepatotoxicity and lethality by various alcohols. Fundam Appl Toxicol. 1990; 15(3):429–40.

[2] Gammella, E., Maccarinelli, F., Buratti, P., et al. The role of iron in anthracycline cardiotoxicity. Front Pharmacol. 2014; 5:25. doi: 10.3389/fphar.2014.00025. eCollection 2014.

[3] NLM's Toxlearn tutorials: http://toxlearn.nlm.nih.gov/Module1.htm.

[4] NLM's Toxtutor (visit interactions): http://sis.nlm.nih.gov/enviro/toxtutor/Tox1/a42.htm.

[5] Smith MA, Reynolds CP, Kang MH, et al. Synergistic activity of PARP inhibition by talazoparib (BMN 673) with temozolomide in pediatric cancer models in the pediatric preclinical testing program. Clin Cancer Res., 2015; 21(4):819–32.

[6] Niu F, Zhao S, Xu CY, et al. Potentiation of the antitumor activity of adriamycin against osteosarcoma by cannabinoid WIN-55,212-2. Oncol Lett. 2015; 10(4):2415–2421.

[7] Calderon-Aparicio A, Strasberg-Rieber M, Rieber M. Disulfiram anti-cancer efficacy without copper overload is enhanced by extracellular H2O2 generation: antagonism by tetrathiomolybdate. Oncotarget. 2015; 6(30):29771–81.

[8] Zajac J, Kostrhunova H, Novohradsky V, et al. Potentiation of mitochondrial dysfunction in tumor cells by conjugates of metabolic modulator dichloroacetate with a Pt(IV) derivative of oxaliplatin. J Inorg Biochem. 2016; 156:89–97.

[9] Nurcahyanti AD, Wink M. Cytotoxic potentiation of vinblastine and paclitaxel by L-canavanine in human cervical cancer and hepatocellular carcinoma cells. Phytomedicine. 2015; 22(14):1232–7.

[10] Lu CF, Yuan XY, Li LZ, et al. Combined exposure to nano-silica and lead-induced potentiation of oxidative stress and DNA damage in human lung epithelial cells. Ecotoxicol Environ Saf. 2015; 122:537–44.

[11] Kuchárová B, Mikeš J, Jendželovský R, et al. Potentiation of hypericin-mediated photodynamic therapy cytotoxicity by MK-886: focus on ABC transporters, GDF-15 and redox status. Photodiagnosis Photodyn Ther. 2015; 12(3):490–503.

[12] Djillani A, Doignon I, Luyten T, et al. Potentiation of the store-operated calcium entry (SOCE) induces phytohemagglutinin-activated Jurkat T cell apoptosis. Cell Calcium. 2015; 58(2):171–85.

GRADES OF ADVERSE DRUG REACTIONS

Drugs and chemicals may exhibit adverse drug reactions (ADR, or adverse drug effect) that may include unwanted (side effects), uncomfortable (system dysfunction), or dangerous effects (toxic). ADRs are a form of manifestation of toxicity, which may occur after over-exposure or high-level exposure or, in some circumstances, after exposure to therapeutic doses but often with an underlying cause (pre-existing condition). In contrast, 'Side effect' is an imprecise term often used to refer to a drug's unintended effects that occur within the therapeutic range [1]. Risk–benefit analysis provides a window into the decision-making process prior to prescribing a medication. Patient characteristics such as age, gender, ethnic background, pre-existing conditions, nutritional status, genetic predisposition or geographic factors, as well as drug factors (e.g., type of drug, administration route, treatment duration, dosage, and bioavailability) may profoundly influence ADR outcomes. Drug-induced adverse events can be categorized as unexpected, serious or life-threatening.

Adverse drug reactions are graded according to intensity, using a scheme that was originally introduced by the US National Cancer Institute to describe the intensity of reactions to drugs used in cancer chemotherapy [2]. This scheme is now widely used to grade the intensity of other types of adverse reactions, although it does not always apply so clearly to them. The scheme assigns grades as follows:

- Grade 1 ≡ mild;
- Grade 2 ≡ moderate;
- Grade 3 ≡ severe;
- Grade 4 ≡ life-threatening or disabling;
- Grade 5 ≡ death.

Then, instead of providing general definitions of the terms "mild", "moderate", "severe", and "life-threatening or disabling", the system describes what they mean operationally in terms of each adverse reaction, in each case the intensity being described in narrative terms. For example, hemolysis is graded as follows:

- Grade 1: Laboratory evidence of hemolysis only (e.g. direct antiglobulin test; presence of schistocytes).
- Grade 2: Evidence of red cell destruction and ≥2 g/dl decrease in hemoglobin, no transfusion.
- Grade 3: Transfusion or medical intervention (for example, steroids) indicated.

- Grade 4: Catastrophic consequences (for example, renal failure, hypotension, bronchospasm, emergency splenectomy).
- Grade 5: Death.

Not all adverse reactions are assigned all grades. For example, serum sickness is classified as being of grade 3 or grade 5 only; i.e. it is always either severe or fatal.

The system is less good at classifying subjective reactions. For example, fatigue is graded as follows:

- Grade 1: Mild fatigue over baseline.
- Grade 2: Moderate or causing difficulty performing some activities of daily living.
- Grade 3: Severe fatigue interfering with activities of daily living.
- Grade 4: Disabling.

Attribution categories can be defined as follows:

(i) Definite: The adverse event is clearly related to the investigational agent(s).
(ii) Probable: The adverse event is likely related to the investigational agent(s).
(iii) Possible: The adverse event may be related to the investigational agent(s).
(iv) Unlikely: The adverse event is doubtfully related to the investigational agent(s).
(v) Unrelated: The adverse event is clearly NOT related to the investigational agent(s).

REFERENCES

[1] Merck Manuals: http://www.merckmanuals.com/professional/clinical_pharmacology/adverse_drug_reactions/adverse_drug_reactions.html.

[2] National Cancer Institute. Common Terminology Criteria for Adverse Events v3.0 (CTCAE). 9 August, 2006. http://ctep.cancer.gov/protocolDevelopment/electronic_applications/docs/ctcaev3.pdf.

FDA PREGNANCY CATEGORIES/ CLASSIFICATION OF TERATOGENICITY

On June 30, 2015 the FDA implemented the "Pregnancy and Lactation Labeling Rule (PLLR)" that will apply to new prescription drugs and biologic products submitted after this date, while labeling approved on or after June 30, 2001 will be phased in gradually.

Prior to the PLLR the FDA had established five categories to indicate the potential of a drug to cause birth defects if used during pregnancy. The categories were determined by the reliability of documentation and the risk to benefit ratio. They did not take into account any risks from pharmaceutical agents or their metabolites in breast milk. The pregnancy categories were:

Category A: Adequate and well-controlled studies have failed to demonstrate a risk to the fetus in the first trimester of pregnancy (and there is no evidence of risk in later trimesters).

Example drugs or substances: levothyroxine, folic acid, magnesium sulfate, liothyronine.

Category B: Animal reproduction studies have failed to demonstrate a risk to the fetus and there are no adequate and well-controlled studies in pregnant women.

Example drugs: metformin, hydrochlorothiazide, cyclobenzaprine, amoxicillin, pantoprazole.

Category C: Animal reproduction studies have shown an adverse effect on the fetus and there are no adequate and well-controlled studies in humans, but potential benefits may warrant use of the drug in pregnant women despite potential risks.

Example drugs: tramadol, gabapentin, amlodipine, trazodone, prednisone.

Category D: There is positive evidence of human fetal risk based on adverse reaction data from investigational or marketing experience or studies in humans, but potential benefits may warrant use of the drug in pregnant women despite potential risks.

Example drugs: lisinopril, alprazolam, losartan, clonazepam, lorazepam.

Category X: Studies in animals or humans have demonstrated fetal abnormalities and/or there is positive evidence of human fetal risk based on adverse reaction data from investigational or marketing experience, and the risks involved in use of the drug in pregnant women clearly outweigh potential benefits.

Example drugs: atorvastatin, simvastatin, warfarin, methotrexate, finasteride.

Category N: FDA has not classified the drug.

Example drugs: aspirin, oxycodone, hydroxyzine, acetaminophen, diazepam.

Examples of drugs approved since June 30th, 2015 showing various new pregnancy and lactation subsections in their labels [3]:

Addyi (flibanserin)—indicated for generalized hypoactive sexual desire disorder (HSDD) in premenopausal women.
Descovy (emtricitabine and tenofovir alafenamide fumarate)—indicated for HIV-1 infection.
Entresto (sacubitril and valsartan)—indicated for heart failure.
Harvoni (ledipasvir and sofosbuvir)—indicated for chronic viral hepatitis C infection (HCV).
Praluent (alirocumab)—indicated for heterozygous familial hypercholesterolemia, or patients with atherosclerotic heart disease who require additional lowering of LDL-cholesterol.

REFERENCES

[1] Doering PL, Boothby LA, Cheok M. Review of pregnancy labeling of prescription drugs: is the current system adequate to inform of risks? Am J Obstet Gynecol 2002; 187(2): 333–9.

[2] Ramoz LL, Patel-Shori NM. Recent changes in pregnancy and lactation labeling: retirement of risk categories. Pharmacotherapy, 2014; 34(4):389–95. doi: 10.1002/phar.

[3] Drugs.com: http://www.drugs.com/pregnancy-categories.html.

Clinicians are suggested to be aware of the information contained in the following literature originating from regulatory agencies:

[4] FDA/CDER SBIA Chronicles. Drugs in Pregnancy and Lactation: Improved Benefit-Risk Information. January 22, 2015. URL: http://www.fda.gov/downloads/Drugs/DevelopmentApprovalProcess/SmallBusinessAssistance/UCM431132.pdf.

[5] FDA Consumer Articles. Pregnant? Breastfeeding? Better Drug Information Is Coming. Updated: December 17, 2014. URL: https://www.drugs.com/fda-consumer/pregnant-breastfeeding-better-drug-information-is-coming-334.html.

[6] FDA News Release. FDA issues final rule on changes to pregnancy and lactation labeling information for prescription drug and biological products. December 3, 2014. URL: http://www.fda.gov/NewsEvents/Newsroom/PressAnnouncements/ucm425317.htm.

[7] Mospan C. New Prescription Labeling Requirements for the Use of Medications in Pregnancy and Lactation. CE for Pharmacists. Alaska Pharmacists Association. April 15, 2016. URL: http://www.alaskapharmacy.org/files/CE_Activities/0416State_CE_Lesson.pdf.

[8] Australian classification: https://www.tga.gov.au/australian-categorisation-system-prescribing-medicines-pregnancy#.U038WfmSx8E.

CONCLUSION

Adverse drug events, including ADRs, side effects, drug-induced diseases, toxicity, pharmacogenetics and immunologic reactions, represent a significant burden to patients, health care systems, and society. It is the goal of *Side Effects of Drugs Annual* to summarize and evaluate important new evidence-based information in order to guide clinicians in the prevention, monitoring, and assessment of adverse drug events in their patients. The work provides not only a summary of this essential new data, but suggestions for how it may be interpreted and implications for practice.

1

Central Nervous System Stimulants and Drugs That Suppress Appetite

Matthew R. Zahner*, Nicholas T. Bello†,1

*Drug Safety and Research Development, Pfizer, Groton, CT, USA
†Department of Animal Sciences, School of Environmental and Biological Sciences, Rutgers, The State
University of New Jersey, New Brunswick, NJ, USA
1Corresponding author: ntbello@aesop.rutgers.edu

The studies and cases described herein supplement Meyler's Side Effects of Drugs: The International Encyclopedia of Adverse Drug Reactions and Interactions. The purpose of this supplement is to provide a concise reference of the newly available literature to support the existing information regarding the known adverse effects of commonly prescribed medications or abused drugs. The information covers peer-reviewed publications from January 2015 to December 2015.

Amphetamine and Amphetamine Derivates [SEDA-34, 1; SEDA-35, 1; SEDA 36, 1; SEDA 37, 1]

Key to abbreviations of amphetamines

MA: methamphetamine
MDA: 3,4-methylenedioxyamphetamine
MDMA: 3,4-methylenedioxymetamphetamine

Studies

Data collected from the U.S. National Poison Center found that there were 23 553 cases of toxicity from lisdexamfetamine (LD), dextroamphetamine/amphetamine extended release (DXR), and dextroamphetamine/amphetamine immediate release (DIR) from 2007 to 2012. The most frequently reported adverse effects were agitation (19.8% for LD, 21.7% for DXR, and 25.1% for DIR), tachycardia (19.2% for LD, 22.8% for DXR, and 23.9%for DIR) and hypertension (7.2% for LD, 9.6% for DXR, and 9.1% for DIR). Less frequent, but more severe adverse effects were seizures (0.44% for LD, 0.29% for DXR, and 0.51% for DIR), conduction disturbances (0.24% for LD, 0.19% for DXR, and 0.31% for DIR), dysrhythmias (0.21% for LD, 0.29% for DXR, and 0.24% for DIR), and hypotension (0.06% for LD, 0.13% for DXR, and 0.26% for DXR) [1M].

Intentional or accidental toxicity from amphetamine, related derivates, and analogues (ARDA) frequently results in agitation and psychosis, as well as hyperadrenergic (e.g., hypertension and tachycardia) states. These conditions are often treated with other medications. In a systematic review inclusive of 81 studies (*n* = 835 subjects), the pharmacological treatment of ADRA toxicity was examined. Antipsychotic medications, such as haloperidol and aripiprazole, had the strongest evidence (i.e., controlled clinical randomized trials) to support their use in the reduction of ARDA-induced agitation and psychosis. Additional evidence (i.e., non-randomized clinical trials and case-controlled studies) was found for the use of benzodiazepines, such as lorazepam. For ARDA-induced hyperadrenergic states, strongest evidence supported the use of β-adrenoceptor antagonists, such as metoprolol and atenolol and the α2-adrenoceptor agonist, clonidine [2M].

Methamphetamine (MA) is a commonly abused drug during pregnancy. In a prospective study of pregnant women measuring birth outcomes, subjects were divided into MA exposed (*n* = 144) and non-MA exposed (*n* = 107). Gestational age was shorter (*p* < 0.05) for MA exposed (38.5 ± 2 weeks) compare with non-MA exposed (39.1 ± 2.1 weeks) pregnancies. The adjusted OR for preterm delivery (<37 weeks) for other drugs besides MA was 2.40 (CI: 1.01–6.00; *p* < 0.05), MA-positive at birth was 3.54 (CI: 1.02–11.66; $p < 0.05$), and delayed prenatal care 1.07 (CI: 1.01–1.15; $p < 0.05$) [3C].

Brain-derived neurotrophic factor (BDNF) has been implicated in substance abuse. The association between three single nucleotide polymorphisms (SNP) of the BDNF gene (rs16917204, rs16917234, and rs2030324) and impulsivity in MA-abusers ($n = 200$) and healthy controls ($n = 219$) was examined. While there were no significant difference in allele frequency and genotype among MA-abusers and controls, there was a negative association ($p < 0.05$) for the C-C-T haplotype (for rs16917204, rs16917234, and rs2030324, respectively) and MA abuse. The OR for C-C-T haplotype in MA abuser was 0.394 (CI: 0.195–0.797). There was a genotype effect for the rs2030324 SNP for motor impulsivity ($p < 0.05$). Those MA abusers with CC genotype had lower motor impulsivity scores than those with TT and CT genotypes [4C].

Cases

- Two cases were reported of maxillary sinus manifestations in MA abusers. A 27-year-old female with a history of MA use had two radicular cysts that compressed the maxillary sinus. The right abscess also compressed the nasal cavity. Following surgery to drain the abscesses and 2 weeks after discharge, the patient made a full recovery. A 21-year-old female that abused MA by inhalation had right facial swelling and tenderness to palpation of the right maxillary canine. Patient was given a short dose of clindamycin, but left against medical advice to inhale MA. The risk of MA-induced oral and sinus infections is believed to result from sympathomimetic action on vasculature and salivary glands to reduce regional blood flow and saliva production [5A].

- Infant death was associated with MA use during pregnancy and delivery. Toxicology reported a concentration of 1.60 mg/l of MA in the blood of the stillborn infant [6A].

- Two cases were reported of complications resulting from penile injection of MA. A 47-year-old male with a history of prior penile complications, HIV, hepatitis C, and diabetes mellitus was presented to emergency room. He arrived with severe penile pain, fevers, and scrotal swelling. Several days prior, he reportedly injected MA into his corpus cavernosum. Surgical drainage of penile abscesses (*Streptococcus viridans* spp.) was performed, and patient was treated with IV vancomycin and ertapenem. Patient was discharged after 2 weeks. A 33-year-old male presented at the emergency room with fever, chills, and sharp penile pain. Onset of symptoms began the same day as MA injections into his penis. Following surgical drainage of penile abscess, the patient initially began IV vancomycin and ertapenem, but developed a sensitive Group A *Streptococcus* spp.

Patient was discharged with amoxicillin/clavulanate for 14 days [7A]. Both cases noted the rarity of the injections site and resulting abscess.

- A 42-year-old man arrived at the emergency with emaciation and dehydration. After 1.5 h, his ECG revealed an elevated S-T segment. Blood markers for myocardial damage were severely elevated, such that CK-MB mass levels were 131.4 ng/ml (normal < 4.94 ng/ml) and troponin T hs was 204.4 ng/l (normal < 14 ng/l). Patient was diagnosed with an acute myocardial infarction and shortly died. Autopsy reported reveals amphetamine concentration of 269.5 ng/ml (toxicity > 500 ng/ml) [8A].

- Drug-induced Parkinsonism developed in a 32-year male recovering MA user. Patient had recurrent psychotic episodes of auditory hallucination with intent for self-harm. He was prescribed IM-injections of haldol decanoate (initially 100 mg followed by 50 mg a week later). Afterwards, he was admitted into a drug rehabilitation program, but left after a few days to restarted MA use for 5 days. He had acute onset of bilateral hand tremors, excess salivation, tongue protrusion, trouble swallowing, and truncal rigidity. Patient was admitted to hospital and prescribed oral diphenhydramine. Parkinsonian symptoms resolved after 1 week [9A].

- Superior mesenteric artery (SMA) syndrome developed in a 30-year-old woman with ADHD. She increased her dosage of dextroamphetamine/amphetamine for an unspecified time and developed acute weight loss, which precipitated SMA syndrome. She was treated for gastric compression with nasogastric tubing feeding and anti-emetic medications until she could tolerate normal feeding. Patient resumed normal weight at 8-month follow-up [10A].

- Lisdexamfetamine use was noted in spontaneous coronary artery dissection (SCAD). A 22-year-old male with ADHD was prescribed lisdexamfetamine for 5 months. He presented in the emergency with severe chest pain and elevation in troponin levels (< 0.05–24 µg/l). Computed coronary angiogram revealed decreased density in the proximal left anterior descending artery. Treatment with aspirin, statin, carvedilol, and lisinopril for 6 months resolved the SCAD pathology [11A].

Ecstasy (3,4-Methylenedioxy-N-Methylamphetamine; MDMA)

Studies

A prospective longitudinal study of infants with ($n = 28$) or without ($n = 68$) MDMA prenatal exposure measured developmental outcomes for the first 2 years of life. MDMA-exposed infants were stratified based on

MDMA use 1 month before and during pregnancy into heavy (averaged 1.3 tablets/three trimesters; $n = 13$) or light (averaged 0.7 tablets/three trimesters; $n = 15$). At 12- and 24-month time intervals, there were more pronounced motor delays in the infants from mothers classified as heavy user than the those infants without MDMA prenatal exposure [12C].

Cases

- Several cases report acute liver failure with MDMA use. The first case was a 24-year-old male presented with jaundice in the eyes, nausea, fatigue, and tiredness. Patient had taken 5 ecstasy tablets in 2 days a week prior to visit. Blood measurements indicated hepatic pathology, and he developed 3–4 hepatic encephalopathy after 10 days. Patient underwent a liver transplant 3 days later. Two weeks post-transplant, the patient died from sepsis. The second case was an 18-year-old male presented with fatigue, tiredness, and jaundice of the eyes. Patient ingested 1 ecstasy tablet 1 week prior to visit. Patient developed 1–2 hepatic encephalopathy after 1 week and underwent a liver transplant without complications. He recovered and was discharged. The third case was a 21-year presented with fatigue, tiredness, and nausea. Patient ingested 1 ecstasy tablet 1 week prior to visit. Blood measurements indicated hepatic pathology without hepatic encephalopathy. Patient was treated with ursodeoxycholic acid and 5% dextrose fluid without complications and was discharged [13A].
- A 20-year-old female was admitted to the hospital unresponsive and hyperpyrexic after ingesting MDMA. Patient had extensive hepatic portal vein pneumatosis with marked loss of hepatic volume. She required multiple organ system supportive care. Patient was discharged after 28 days with normal liver function [14A].
- Oral angioedema developed following MDMA ingestion. A 30-year-old male had progressive dyspnea, dsyphagia, and impaired phonation 1 h after consumption of MDMA. Hydrocortisone and epinephrine administration failed to improve the condition. Treatment with icatibant (30 mg) resolved angioedema within 8 h. Improvement with icatibant, a selective antagonist of bradykinin type 2 receptor, suggested bradykinin-mediated edema caused by MDMA [15A].
- MDMA and amphetamine associated hypoglycemia with hyperinsulinemia. A 29-year-old female with a history of depression and polysubstance abuse was found minimally responsive. Initially her blood glucose was 20 mg/dl, and she had hyperinsulinemia. Following IV dextrose treatment for 3 days, her blood glucose levels stabilized and she fully recovered. Her

urine tested positive for cannabis, amphetamine, and MDMA. No known mechanisms were noted for the drug-induced hypoglycemia [16A].
- Thrombotic thrombocytopenic purpura (TTP) developed in a 36-year-old male chronic MDMA user. Patient complained of fever, difficult speech, cognitive changes, and red rashes on his legs. Blood pressure and heart rate were elevated, but heart was in normal rhythm. Examination of blood revealed he had anemia and thrombocytopenia, increased lactate dehydrogenase, indirect bilirubin, creatinine kinase, transaminases (twofold), and reticulocytes. Patient had intensively used MDMA for 10 years and was diagnosed with MDMA-induced TPP. A plasmapheresis regimen was performed, and he was treated with methylprednisolone and vincristine. Patient had normal blood values at 3-month follow-up [17A].

Methylphenidate [SEDA-34, 5; SEDA-35, 1; SEDA-36, 1; SEDA-37, 1]

Studies

The acute effects of initial dosing of methylphenidate immediate release (MPH-IR) on cardiovascular outcomes were examined in drug-naïve children and adolescents (mean age 12.14 ± 2.6 years old) with ADHD ($n = 54$). Two hours after administration of MPH-IR (5 mg/kg), there was an elevation in systolic blood pressure (+5.2 mm Hg), diastolic blood pressure (+3.9 mm Hg), and heart rate (+7.2 bpm) from pre-drug baseline. There were no abnormalities in ECG measurements were noted, but there was an increase in TpTe/QTc ratio from pre-drug baseline [18c].

A two-phase methylphenidate (Ritalin LA), a spheroidal oral drug absorption system (SODAS) formulation, was assesses in 12-week observational study in children (mean age 10.9 ± 2.5 years old) with ADHD ($n = 262$). The SODAS formulation releases 50% of methylphenidate immediately and 50% after 4 h after oral administration. A total of 63 adverse events (AE) were reported in 13.7% of patients. However, 28 (10.7%) of the total AE were considered drug related with 1 AE (0.4%) considered serious requiring hospitalization due to sleepiness, decreased activity, and anorexia. The System Organ Classes (SOC) affected were metabolism and nutrition (4.2%), psychiatric (3.8%), nervous system disorders (3.8%) and gastrointestinal disorders (3.1%). The most commonly AE reported were anorexia (4.2%), abdominal pain (1.5%), and nausea (1.5%) [19C].

Cases

- A 24-year-old female with a 5-month remission of depression began methylphenidate extended release (MPH-XR; 18 mg/day) treatment of ADHD inattentive subtype. Six days after initiating MPH-XR, the patient experienced suicidal ideation, and MPH-XR was discontinued [20A].

- Recurrent episodes of spontaneous pneumothorax were reported in 19-year-old male with ADHD receiving oral methylphenidate (20 mg/day). The first episode was reported 1 year after initiating methylphenidate. The second episode was reported after 3 years. Methylphenidate was discontinued and no new episodes of pneumothorax were reported [21A]. The mechanisms remain unclear between long-term treatment oral methylphenidate and pneumothorax, but others have noted a higher prevalence of basilar panlobular emphysema in intravenous methylphenidate abusers [22A].
- An 11-year-old male with ADHD and Tourette syndrome had been receiving methylphenidate (titrated to 54 mg/day) for 2 years. After an episode of cardiac arrest, a cardiac MRI revealed a previous infarction on the left ventricle, which resulted in an easily induced ventricular tachycardia. No other agent or heritable factors were suspected in causing the infarction. Methylphenidate was discontinued. He was implanted with cardioverter defibrillator and metoprolol succinate (100 mg) [23A].
- Acute dystonia developed in 15-year-old female with ADHD 9 days after initiation of modified-release methylphenidate (27 mg). Patient developed involuntary extensor muscle contraction of her right hand and wrist (approximately 4 h). She had associated tension and pain. Intramuscular diazepam (5 mg) resolved the dystonia. A few years earlier, she had a similar reaction to immediate-release methylphenidate [24A].
- An adolescent male with ADHD and oppositional behaviors was being treated with risperidone (3 mg/day) and modified-release methylphenidate (54 mg/day). He developed a dystonic reaction following interruption of methylphenidate treatment. The dystonic reactions of licking, tongue movement, and tension with difficult mouth closing were resolved with restarting methylphenidate treatment [25A].
- Intravenous methylphenidate (30 mg) resulted in chest pain and elevation in ST segment on ECG recording in 40-year-old male. Chest pain initiated 15 min after self-injection. Troponin T levels were elevated to 0.352 ng/ml after 12 h (reference range <0.01 ng/ml). Patient was diagnosed with anterolateral ST-elevation myocardial infarction. He received standard cardiac care and was discharge after 4 days [26A].
- A 9-year-old male developed daytime bruxism 2 days after initiating methylphenidate (18 mg/day). Bruxism resolved when methylphenidate was discontinued. Symptoms were re-established with the restart of methylphenidate [27A].
- A 7-year-old male with ADHD had a sudden onset of involuntary movements, recurrent spontaneous limb movements, and ataxic gait. Meningoencephalitis was suspected, but the patient did not have a fever. His blood values and lumbar puncture were also unremarkable. The patient had begun methylphenidate 3 months earlier and 1 month prior recently double his daily dose (10 mg). At 36 h after discontinuation of methylphenidate, the patient had no residual neurological symptoms and was discharged [28A].

METHYLXANTHINES

Caffeine [SEDA-15, 588; SEDA-32, 14; SEDA-33, 11; SEDA-34, 6; SEDA-36, 1; SEDA-37, 1]

Studies

The association between pregnancy loss and caffeine/coffee intake was examined in a meta-analysis of case-controlled and cohort 26 studies. Twenty studies were of caffeine and 8 studies were of coffee. Caffeine consumption was associated with pregnancy loss (OR 1.32; CI 1.24–1.40). When data were stratified based on use, the association was significant in moderate (150–300 mg/day) and heavy users (>301 mg/day), but not light users (<150 mg/day). For coffee consumption, there was also an association with pregnancy loss (OR 1.31; CI 1.15–1.50). The association remained for heavy users (>4 cups/day), but not for moderate (2–3 cups/day) or light (<2 cups/day) coffee drinkers [29M].

Cases

- Caffeine-induced psychotic symptoms were reported in several cases. A 32-year-old male diagnosed with paranoid schizophrenia had been maintained for 3 years with olanzapine (20 mg/day) and haloperidol (10 mg/day). He experienced an increase in psychotic episodes after consuming 3 or 4 cups of coffee daily (207–276 mg/day) for 3 weeks. Psychotic episodes improved after the discontinuation of coffee. A 32-year-old male habitual coffee drinker with no known psychiatric illness experienced manic symptoms, reduced sleep, and increased activity over a 1-week period. These symptoms were preceded by 2 weeks of excessive caffeine consumption (537.5–762.5 mg/day). Manic-symptoms resolved with caffeine discontinuation. One year later, the patient experience similar manic-like episodes after 2 weeks of heavy caffeine consumption [30A]. Recurrent visual hallucinations were reported in 61-year-old male habitually consuming 5–20 packets/day of over-the-counter aspirin (845 mg/packet) and caffeine (65 mg/packet) analgesic [31A]. A 69-year-old female with bipolar disorder not otherwise specified (NOS), mood disorder NOS, alcohol use disorder in remission, and hypothyroidism was being treated with clonazepam (0.25 mg) and zolpidem (5 mg). Excessive caffeine consumption negatively affected her mixed maniac state and caused paranoid episodes [32A].

- A 27-year-old female had an anaphylactic episode after ingesting candy containing 42 mg of caffeine. She was diagnosed with caffeine hypersensitivity after a specific serum IgE test revealed a positive reaction for 5 and 50 mg/ml of caffeine [33A].
- A sudden loss of vision in the right eye was reported in a 26-year-old male after consuming 2 energy drinks (250 ml) on an empty stomach. He was diagnosed with a transient ischemic attack and his vision fully resolved in 4 h [34A].
- A 20-year-old female with ADHD and bipolar disorder attempted suicide with ingestion of undisclosed amount of concentrated caffeine. She was found agitated and vomiting and received medical attention 1–2 h after ingestion. Ventricular defibrillation developed shortly after arrival at the emergency room and return to spontaneous circulation (ROSC) was achieved after defibrillation. She developed 24 episodes pulseless ventricular tachycardia several minutes apart. Each ventricular tachycardia episodes was several minutes apart and required defibrillation for ROSC. After 80 min, the tachydysrhythmia was stabilized. Serum caffeine concentration was 240 µg/ml 4 h after arrival (as a reference, 300 mg of caffeine ingestion peaks serum caffeine at 6–9 µg/ml at 1 h) [35A].

Selective Norepinephrine Reuptake Inhibitors Atomoxetine [SEDA-34, 4; SEDA-36, 1; SEDA-37, 1]

Studies

Allele status of cytochrome P450 2D6 (CYP2D6) produces a variability in atomoxetine metabolism. The frequencies of treatment-emergent adverse effects (TEAE) were assessed in subjects after receiving 12-week open-label treatment of atomoxetine (titrated up to 80 or 100 mg/day by 8 weeks). Adult ADHD subjects were grouped according to genotype into metabolizer groups: ultra-rapid or extensive (UM/EM; $n = 1039$), intermediate (IM; $n = 780$), and poor (PM; $n = 117$). Comparing PM with non-PM (UM/EM and IM), PM had increase in dry mouth (29.1% vs. 15.9%; $p < 0.001$), erectile dysfunction (19.4% vs. 7.2%; $p = 0.002$), and urinary retention (6.0% vs. 0.7%; $p < 0.001$). The frequency of dry mouth

was also higher comparing IM with EM/UM (19.6% vs. 13.1%, $p < 0.001$) [36MC].

The time to onset and resolution of TEAE were examined during a 25-week withdrawal of atomoxetine. In two 12-week phases (pre-randomization), adult ADHD subjects received atomoxetine (titrated up to 80 or 100 mg/day) and then in a double-blind design (post-randomization) continued to receive atomoxetine ($n = 266$) or received placebo ($n = 258$) for 25 weeks. During the pre-randomization period, sexual dysfunction was reported in 12.6% of male subjects with 25.5% of those subjects discontinued the study. The time of onset to sexual dysfunction on average was 12 days, 45.9% of cases resolved within 90 days, and approximately 20% were unresolved. Small increases in diastolic blood pressure (BP) and heart rate were observed after the pre-randomization and diastolic BP returned to baseline 3 weeks after atomoxetine discontinuation. Heart rate was reduced after 3 weeks but continued to drop during the post-randomization period returning to baseline at 17 weeks after initiating placebo treatment [37C].

Cases

- A 12-year male with Tourette syndrome presented with moderately painful penile erection for 10 h. Atomoxetine was the suspected causative agent; patient was switched to clonidine without episode of priapism [38A].
- A 10-year female recently developed depigmentation on the medial aspect of her right eyebrow. She was recently diagnosed with ADHD 6 weeks prior and had begun atomoxetine (increased to 40 mg/day after 1 week). Patient's parents refuse to discontinue atomoxetine and a 3-month follow-up her localized depigmentation was unchanged [39A].

VIGILANCE PROMOTING DRUGS

Modafinil and Armodafinil [SEDA-34, 6; SEDA-36, 1; SEDA-37, 1]

Studies

Armodafinil as an adjunctive therapy was assessed in adult patients with major depressive episodes associated with bipolar I disorder. Patients were randomized to receive armodafinil (150 mg/day; $n = 232$), armodafinil (200 mg/day; $n = 30$) or placebo ($n = 230$) to their maintenance medications for 8 weeks. The most common TEAE for 150 mg/day of armodafinil were headache (16% vs 13% in placebo group), nausea (7% vs. 2% in placebo group), diarrhea (5% vs 6% in placebo group), and insomnia (5% vs 3% in placebo group). Diarrhea and dry mouth were the most common TEAE for the 200 mg/day armodafinil dose. Discontinuation due to adverse effects occurred in 8% (150 mg/day armodafinil), 7% (200 mg/day armodafinil), and 5% (placebo) of subjects [40C].

Armodafinil was assessed in binge eating disorder (BED) subjects in a 10-week randomized placebo-controlled trial. BED subject received with armodafinil (150–250 mg/day; $n=30$) or placebo ($n=30$). Armodafinil was associated with increase in pulse rate at the end of 10 weeks (5.5 bpm compared with −2.6 bpm in placebo group). One armodafinil patient developed a marked elevation in blood pressure (128/64–210/100 mm Hg) in 2 days. Blood pressure normalized after discontinuation of armodafinil. The most common TEAE were feeling jittery, which was reported in 30% of armodafinil-treated subject compared with 0% in the placebo group ($p < 0.001$) [41c].

Cases

- Two cases of fixed drug eruptions were reported with modafanil use. A 23-year-old male had been using modafinil (200 mg/day) for mental alertness developed recurrent mouth erosions. Discontinuation of modafinil and application of triamcinolone acetonide oral paste resolved the mouth erosion. A 19-year-old male had a recurrent red annular painful mark on his right palm. Patient had been taking modafinil (100 mg/day) to maintain alertness for medical school. Rash resolved in 36 h after discontinuation of modafinil and application of mometasone furoate cream [42A].
- A 34-year-old male with recurrent depression and alcohol addiction for 11 years had modafinil (200 mg/day) added to his current treatment regimen. After 6 months, the patient escalated his modafinil dose to 35 tablets per day (3500 mg/day). Modafinil was acquired at other outpatient clinics and purchased online [43A]. Treatment strategies included increasing duloxetine (90 mg/day) and carbamazepine (600 mg/day) to gradual reduce modafinil daily intakes [43A].
- A 23-year-old male was receiving modafinil (200 mg/day) for hypersomnolence and fatigue after methamphetamine withdrawal. After 6 months, the patient was admitted to the hospital for methamphetamine psychosis, and it was discovered he escalated his modafinil dose (400 mg/day). Patient demonstrate dependency by increased his use of modafinil and his reluctance to discontinue the medication [44A].
- A 46-year-old female receiving modafinil (200–300 mg/day) for hypersomnolence for 1 year developed a compulsive gambling problem. Patient was switched from modafinil to methylphenidate and gambling pathology resolved within 1 month [45A].
- A 44-year-old male with schizoaffective disorder in partial remission was receiving risperidone (4 mg/day) and amisulpride (400 mg/day). Patient was

experiencing excessive lethargy and sleepiness that was impairing his shift work. He was prescribed modafinil (200 mg/day). The patient, however, began using modafinil (100 mg) every 3–4 h to overcome somnolence during shift work and escalated his modafinil (1200 mg/day) dose for the past 6 months. He reported a dependence on modafinil. Modafinil was gradually reduced over 1 month to 100 mg every 2–3 days, and he was started on bupropion and clonazepam [46A].

DRUGS THAT SUPPRESS APPETITE [SEDA-34, 8; SEDA-36, 1; SEDA-37, 1]

Lorcaserin [SEDA-37, 1]

Case

A 39-year-old male with history of major depressive disorder, generalized anxiety disorder, diabetes, obesity, hypertension, hyperlipidemia, obstructive sleep apnea, and gastroesophageal reflux disease was enrolled into a psychopharmacology clinic. He was taking metformin (1000 mg/day), insulin (180 units/day, via insulin pump), simvastatin (40 mg/day), benazepril–hydrochlorothiazide (20–25 mg/day), and omeprazole (20 mg/day). He was also taking escitalopram (20 mg/day) and clonazepam (0.5 mg as needed) for 8 months to treat his psychiatric disorders. Upon admission, he was started on lorcaserin (10 mg/twice/day). After 8 days, he began to experience depression, hopelessness, insomnia, and anhedonia. After 2 more weeks, these symptoms worsened and he had suicidal ideation. The subject did not meet the Hunter Criteria for serotonin syndrome [47R] and reported no experiences of clonus, agitation, tremor, or fever. Despite weight loss (3–4 kg), lorcaserin was discontinued. Within 5 days, the subject reported an improvement in mood and suicide ideation [48A].

Phentermine [SEDA-34, 8; SEDA-36, 1; SEDA-37, 1]

Case

A 49-year-old obese (BMI 33 kg/m^2) female with a history of migraine without aura presented with unremittent migraines occurring twice a week and typically lasted 24–36 h. Typical treatment consisted of subcutaneous sumatriptan (6 mg/day) and oral ondansetron (4 mg/day). Sodium valproate (500 mg) was administered twice daily and atenolol (50 mg/day). However, this also failed to relieve the migraines. Topiramate (25 mg) was administered daily and increased by 25 mg every 2 weeks to a maximum of 50 mg twice a day. After 10 days of treatment, the patient experienced increased appetite accompanied by constant intrusive thoughts of food. She gained 7 kg during the first 5 weeks of treatment. Over the next 3 months, her waist circumference increased from 90 to 125 cm. However, because topiramate treatment alleviated the severe migraines, she remained on it despite the weight gain and appetite stimulation. A temporary cessation of topiramate led to a return of the frequency of migraines. Combination of topiramate (25–50 mg twice daily as previously prescribed) and phentermine (30 mg/day, controlled release) was administered after approval for a 1-month off-label drug trial. No appetite stimulation was reported with this combinational therapy [49A].

Phentermine/Topiramate Extended Release (XR) [SEDA-37, 1]

Studies

Gastric emptying, fasting and postprandial gastric volume, satiation via nutrient drink test, satiety via ad libitum feeding, gastrointestinal hormones, and psychological traits were assessed in a prospective study with 328 normal-weight, overweight, or obese adults. Obesity was positively associated with fasting gastric volume, accelerated gastric emptying, and higher postprandial levels of glucagon-like peptide 1. Retrospective analysis of data from 181 adults to determine associations between body mass index and waist circumference was performed using similar approaches. Obesity was associated with higher volume to fullness and satiety with abnormal waist circumference. In a cohort of 24 volunteers, the effect of phentermine/topiramate XR in order to validate associations between quantitative traits and response to weight loss therapy. The combination of phentermine/topiramate XR caused significant weight loss, slowed gastric emptying, decreased calorie intake, and weight loss [50C].

Case

- A 39-year-old normal weight (BMI 23.4 kg/m²) female arrived in the emergency room with acute bilateral vision loss and eye pain. Symptom onset was 2 h prior to visit. One week prior, she began phentermine (3.75 mg)/topiramate (23 mg) in an extended release formulation. Ophthalmological examination revealed she had an acute, nonpupillary block, secondary angle closure glaucoma. She was treated with atropine (1%; twice/day), brimonidine (0.2%)/timolol (0.5%; twice/day) and difluprednate ophthalmic emulsion (0.05% every 2 h). Phentermine/topiramate treatment was also discontinued. At 2-week follow-up, bilateral secondary angle closure was resolved [51A].

Topiramate has been associated with acute bilateral secondary angle-closure glaucoma [52A].

Parasympathomimetics [SEDA-34, 9; SEDA-36, 1; SEDA-37, 1]

In a worldwide pharmacovigilance study to investigate adverse drug reactions caused by cholinesterase inhibitors used for Alzheimer's, donepezil, rivastigmine, and galantamine were extracted from reports between 1998 and 2013. A total of 43753 adverse events were reported. Of these 60.1% were reported from women, and the mean age was 77.4±9.1 years. Rivastigmine and donepezil were each involved in 41.4% of the reports, whereas galantamine was involved in 17.2%. The highest reported adverse events were neuropsychiatric (31.4%), gastrointestinal (15.9), general (11.9%), and cardiovascular (11.7) in nature. The most serious adverse events were neuropsychiatric (34.0%), general (14.0), cardiovascular (12.1%), and gastrointestinal (11.6%) [53MC].

Rivastigmine [SEDA-34, 10; SEDA-36, 1; SEDA-37, 1]

Studies

A 24-week retrospective analysis was conducted to assess the efficacy, safety and tolerability of high dose (13.3 mg/day) vs. low dose (4.6 mg/day) rivastigmine patch in subjects with severe Alzheimer's dementia with or without co-administration of memantine (up to 20 mg/day). TEAE were related to the dose of rivastigmine and unrelated to co-administration of memantine. In this regard, the most common adverse events reported by subjects who received 13.3 mg/day rivastigmine patch and memantine were application site erythema (13.4%), agitation (12.9%), and application site dermatitis (9.2%). In subjects who received 13.3 mg/day rivastigmine patch without memantine, the most common adverse events were urinary tract infection (13.0%), application site erythema (13.0%) and agitation (9.4%). In subjects who received 4.6 mg/day rivastigmine patch and memantine, the most common adverse events were agitation (13.8%), application site erythema (12.9%) and urinary tract infection (8.8%). In those who received 4.6 mg/day rivastigmine patch without memantine, the most common adverse events were agitation (14.8%), urinary tract infection (10.6%) and application site dermatitis (10.6%). In both the 13.3 and 4.6 mg/day rivastigmine groups, the proportion of patients who discontinued due to adverse events was slightly higher in subjects that did not receive memantine compared with those who did receive memantine [54C].

Cases

- An 83-year-old female with heart failure was admitted to the hospital. She had been taking prednisone (5 mg/day) for myalgia and rivastigmine (4.5 mg/day) by transdermal patch for dementia with Lewy bodies. On admission to the hospital, her blood pressure was 118/58 mm Hg, pulse 93 bpm and temperature 36.5 ° C. She was intubated immediately to control severe hypoxia. On her ninth day after admission, she experienced recurrent sinus arrest just after inspiring sputum. The sinus arrest associated with sputum inspiration did not occur after the rivastigmine was removed. Autonomic dysfunction is a common feature of dementia with Lewy bodies. The present patient's sinus arrest may have been caused by sputum inspiration induced by a vagal reflex in the presence of the acetylcholinesterase and butyrylcholinesterase, rivastigmine [55A].

- A nonverbal 81-year-old female with severe dementia, hypertension, cardiac arrhythmia, coronary artery disease, and deep venous thrombosis, presented with involuntary movements. She was on a pacemaker due to sick sinus arrhythmia and was taking amiodarone, metoprolol, and rivaroxaban. Additionally, the subject was on patch rivastigmine 9.5 mg/24 h since August 2009. For 4 months prior, her dose was 4.6 mg/24 h and had the dose increased again to 13.3 mg/24 h. One month later, the subject developed involuntary movements initially of the left lower extremity and then of the right extremity as well. CT scan of the brain showed no lesions indicating that this was not secondary to stroke. EEG was performed to rule out epileptic activity. Levetiracetam (250 mg) and risperidone (1 mg) were subsequently administered but failed to alleviate the involuntary movements. Neither cranial CT nor any biochemical or hematological marker revealed any information towards the cause of the movements. The only change to the patients' medical care over the previous 3 months was the increase in dosage of transdermal rivastigmine from 9.5 mg/24 h to 13.3 mg/24 h. Rivastigmine were subsequently discontinued, and the uncontrolled movements were diminished within 6 days. A one-time challenge with 13.3 mg/24 h led to the reemergence of the uncontrolled movements. The patch was discontinued, and the movements did not return [56A].

Donepezil [SEDA-34, 10; SEDA-36, 1; SEDA-37, 1]

Studies

A retrospective clinical cohort study to analyze the effect of combinational therapy of donepezil plus memantine or galantamine plus memantine in 123 Alzheimer's dementia patients already receiving cholinesterase inhibitors was conducted. Adverse effects were reported in 13 subjects. In the memantine plus donepezil group 7 subjects reported adverse events and 6 dropped out of the study. In the memantine plus galantamine group 6 subjects reported adverse events and all 6 dropped out of the study. The mean age of these 53 subjects was 77.8 ± 7.8 years, and 19 subjects were male and 34 were female [57c].

A 6-month multicenter study was conducted to determine the tolerability of switching from oral donepezil or rivastigmine to transdermal applications. The study consisted of 174 subjects that switched to the transdermal patch. Of those 174 subjects, 99 switched due to loss of efficacy, 57 due to tolerability issues, and 18 attributed to both. Prior to switching, patients were taking oral cholinesterase inhibitors for an average of 25.4 ± 19 months. The mean oral dose of donepezil ($n=100$) was 8.0 ± 2.6 mg/day, and the mean dose of rivastigmine ($n=74$) was 5.5 ± 1.8 mg/day. After switching to the patch rivastigmine, 59 subjects reported the following adverse events: skin reaction ($n=28$), gastrointestinal (13), heart related (5), and unspecified (13). Of the subjects that reported adverse events, 31 of them discontinued the study. The subjects citied skin reaction (16), gastrointestinal (5), heart related (1) and unspecified (9) [58C].

A phase II clinical study to determine the efficacy of donepezil was conducted in 43 elderly subjects with mild Alzheimer's dementia. In those subjects, 4 months of donepezil resulted in improved gait velocity and trail making tests but not stride time variability, all of which are measures of motor activity. There were no major adverse events reported. However, in this study, 6 subjects were withdrawn for medical intolerance. Five of those subjects experienced gastrointestinal symptoms, and one experienced vivid dreams and sleep disturbances [59c].

Cases

- A 72-year-old female was recently diagnosed with probable major neurocognitive disorder due to Alzheimer's disease. She had a 1-month history of cognitive and behavioral disorganization, pressured speech, delusions, insomnia, agitation, and violent behavior. This behavior developed within 1 week of increasing her dosage of donepezil from 5 to 10 mg/day. Donepezil was discontinued. She was treated with risperidone (titrated up to 1.5 mg/day) and tapered off risperidone by 10-week follow-up without maniac episodes [60A].

- An 80-year-old female with Alzheimer's disease developed polymorphic ventricular tachycardia requiring cardiopulmonary resuscitation. Incidence occurred following an increase in donepezil dosage from 5 to 10 mg/day. Donepezil discontinuation normalized cardiac activity [61A].

- An 80-year-old female with Alzheimer's disease experienced drug-induced lupus erythematosus 1 month after starting donepezil (10 mg/day). Patient was switched to memantine (20 mg/day), and the rash and myalgia completly disappeared. Several months later, the patient ran out of memantine and took some donepezil that she still possessed. The symptoms of lupus erythematosus reappeared shortly after restarting donepezil [62A].
- A 76-year-old male with Alzheimer's disease, hypothyroidism, gastric esophageal reflux (GERD), chronic obstructive pulmonary disease, benign prostate hyperplasia, and mild normocytic anemia developed intractable hiccups. Intermittent hiccups began with treatment with donepezil (5 mg/day) at bedtime. The hiccups worsened with an increase in donepezil dosage (15 mg/day). Patient suffered complications related to GERD and thoracic and lumbar compression fracture and was removed from donepezil for 6 days. During this time the hiccups subsided, hiccups resumed following restarting donepezil treatment [63A].
- A 79-year-old female with Alzheimer's disease began treatment with donepezil (5 mg/day). After 2 months, the dosage was increased to 10 mg/day. Two weeks after initiating the donepezil (10 mg/day), the patient complained of increased libido. The increased libido was accompanied by insomnia. Discontinuation of donepezil resolved the increased libido and insomnia in 3 days [64A].

Galantamine [SEDA-36, 1; SEDA-37, 1]

Studies

In a study examining the physiological and neurobehavioral effect of cholinesterase inhibition was reported consisting of 84 healthy men ($n=37$) with a mean age of 25.85 years that ranged from 18 to 38 years and non-pregnant, non-lactating women ($n=47$) with a mean age of 23.67 years that ranged from 18 to 37 years. In the subjects that completed the study, the frequency of symptom reporting was consistently low. However, on the first post-drug symptom checklist (110 min after drug administration), frequency of nausea was higher after galantamine ($n=4$ of 12) compared with that of the placebo group. One female subject withdrew 90 min after galantamine 8 mg administration citing moderate nausea and dizziness [65c].

References

[1] Kaland ME, Klein-Schwartz W. Comparison of lisdexamfetamine and dextroamphetamine exposures reported to U.S. poison centers. Clin Toxicol (Phila). 2015;53(5):477–85 [M].

[2] Richards JR, Albertson TE, Derlet RW, et al. Treatment of toxicity from amphetamines, related derivatives, and analogues: a systematic clinical review. Drug Alcohol Depend. 2015;150:1–13 [M].

[3] Wright TE, Schuetter R, Tellei J, et al. Methamphetamines and pregnancy outcomes. J Addict Med. 2015;9(2):111–7 [C].

[4] Su H, Tao J, Zhang J, et al. The analysis of BDNF gene polymorphism haplotypes and impulsivity in methamphetamine abusers. Compr Psychiatry. 2015;59:62–7 [C].

[5] Faucett EA, Marsh KM, Farshad K, et al. Maxillary sinus manifestations of methamphetamine abuse. Allergy Rhinol (Providence). 2015;6(1):76–9 [A].

[6] Sakai K, Iwadate K, Maebashi K, et al. Infant death associated with maternal methamphetamine use during pregnancy and delivery: a case report. Leg Med (Tokyo). 2015;17(5):409–14 [A].

[7] Gaither TW, Osterberg EC, Awad MA, et al. Surgical intervention for penile methamphetamine injections. Case Rep Urol. 2015;2015:467683 [A].

[8] Smedra A, Szustowski S, Berent J. Amphetamine-related myocardial infarction in a 42-year old man. Arch Med Sadowej Kryminol. 2015;65(3):173–81 [A].

[9] Matthew BJ, Gedzior JS. Drug-induced parkinsonism following chronic methamphetamine use by a patient on haloperidol decanoate. Int J Psychiatry Med. 2015;50(4):405–11 [A].

[10] Fazio RM, Chen O, Eldarawy W. Superior mesenteric artery syndrome associated with rapid weight loss attributed to amphetamine abuse. Case Rep Gastrointest Med. 2015;2015:817249 [A].

[11] Afzal AM, Sarmast SA, Weber NA, et al. Spontaneous coronary artery dissection in a 22-year-old man on lisdexamfetamine. Proc (Bayl Univ Med Cent). 2015;28(3):367–8 [A].

[12] Singer LT, Moore DG, Min MO, et al. Developmental outcomes of 3,4-methylenedioxymethamphetamine (ecstasy)-exposed infants in the UK. Hum Psychopharmacol. 2015;30(4):290–4 [c].

[13] Atayan Y, Cagin YF, Erdogan MA, et al. Ecstasy induced acute hepatic failure. Case reports. Acta Gastroenterol Belg. 2015;78(1):53–5 [A].

[14] Maharaj R, Pingitore A, Menon K, et al. Images of the month: MDMA-induced acute liver failure and transient abdominal pneumatosis. Am J Gastroenterol. 2015;110(7):963 [A].

[15] Escalante FA, Del Bano F, Supervia A. MDMA-induced angioedema treated with icatibant. Clin Toxicol (Phila). 2015;53(10):1148–9 [A].

[16] Carrera P, Iyer VN. Profound hypoglycemia with ecstasy intoxication. Case Rep Emerg Med. 2015;2015:483153 [A].

[17] Kayar Y, Kayar NB, Gangarapu V. Thrombotic thrombocytopenic purpura and focal segmental glomerulosclerosis associated with the use of ecstasy. Indian J Crit Care Med. 2015;19(4):230–2 [A].

[18] Lamberti M, Italiano D, Guerriero L, et al. Evaluation of acute cardiovascular effects of immediate-release methylphenidate in children and adolescents with attention-deficit hyperactivity disorder. Neuropsychiatr Dis Treat. 2015;11:1169–74 [c].

[19] Haertling F, Mueller B, Bilke-Hentsch O. Effectiveness and safety of a long-acting, once-daily, two-phase release formulation of methylphenidate (Ritalin (R) LA) in school children under daily practice conditions. Atten Defic Hyperact Disord. 2015;7(2):157–64 [C].

[20] Macaluso M, Larson CA. The first published case report of an adult woman who developed suicidal ideation as an adverse event related to methylphenidate use. Prim Care Companion CNS Disord. 2015;17(2) 10.4088/PCC.14l01739, [A].

[21] Boonsarngsuk V, Suwatanapongched T. A case of recurrent pneumothorax related to oral methylphenidate. J Thorac Dis. 2015;7(8):E255–7 [A].

[22] Ward S, Heyneman LE, Reittner P, et al. Talcosis associated with IV abuse of oral medications: CT findings. AJR Am J Roentgenol. 2000;174(3):789–93 [A].

[23] Munk K, Gormsen L, Kim WY, et al. Cardiac arrest following a myocardial infarction in a child treated with methylphenidate. Case Rep Pediatr. 2015;2015:905097 [A].

[24] Tekin U, Soyata AZ, Oflaz S. Acute focal dystonic reaction after acute methylphenidate treatment in an adolescent patient. J Clin Psychopharmacol. 2015;35(2):209–11 [A].

[25] Guler G, Yildirim V, Kutuk MO, et al. Dystonia in an adolescent on risperidone following the discontinuation of methylphenidate: a case report. Clin Psychopharmacol Neurosci. 2015;13(1):115–7 [A].

[26] Hay E, Shklovski V, Blaer Y, et al. Intravenous methylphenidate: an unusual way to provoke ST-elevation myocardial infarction. Am J Emerg Med. 2015;33(2):313.e1–3 [A].

[27] Sivri RC, Bilgic A. Methylphenidate-induced awake bruxism: a case report. Clin Neuropharmacol. 2015;38(2):60–1 [A].

[28] Snell LB, Bakshi D. Neurological adverse effects of methylphenidate may be misdiagnosed as meningoencephalitis. BMJ Case Rep. 2015; pii: bcr2014207796, [A].

[29] Li J, Zhao H, Song JM, et al. A meta-analysis of risk of pregnancy loss and caffeine and coffee consumption during pregnancy. Int J Gynaecol Obstet. 2015;130(2):116–22 [M].

[30] Wang HR, Woo YS, Bahk WM. Caffeine-induced psychiatric manifestations: a review. Int Clin Psychopharmacol. 2015;30(4):179–82 [A].

[31] Golden LE, Sassoon P, Caceda R. A case report of late onset psychosis with dementia and aspirin and caffeine addiction. Schizophr Res. 2015;168(1–2):591–2 [A].

[32] Krankl JT, Gitlin M. Caffeine-induced mania in a patient with caffeine use disorder: a case report. Am J Addict. 2015;24(4):289–91 [A].

[33] Sugiyama K, Cho T, Tatewaki M, et al. Anaphylaxis due to caffeine. Asia Pac Allergy. 2015;5(1):55–6 [A].

[34] Dikici S, Saritas A, Kilinc S, et al. Does an energy drink cause a transient ischemic attack? Am J Emerg Med. 2015;33(1):129.e5–6 [A].

[35] Laskowski LK, Henesch JA, Nelson LS, et al. Start me up! Recurrent ventricular tachydysrhythmias following intentional concentrated caffeine ingestion. Clin Toxicol (Phila). 2015;53(8):830–3 [A].

[36] Fijal BA, Guo Y, Li SG, et al. CYP2D6 predicted metabolizer status and safety in adult patients with attention-deficit hyperactivity disorder participating in a large placebo-controlled atomoxetine maintenance of response clinical trial. J Clin Pharmacol. 2015;55(10):1167–74 [MC].

[37] Upadhyaya H, Tanaka Y, Lipsius S, et al. Time-to-onset and -resolution of adverse events before/after atomoxetine discontinuation in adult patients with ADHD. Postgrad Med. 2015;127(7):677–85 [C].

[38] Armstrong WR, Grimsby GM, Jacobs MA. Pediatric priapism secondary to psychotherapeutic medications. Urology. 2015;86(2):376–8 [A].

[39] Bilgic O, Bilgic A. Possible atomoxetine-induced vitiligo: a case report. Atten Defic Hyperact Disord. 2015;7(3):179–81 [A].

[40] Ketter TA, Yang R, Frye MA. Adjunctive armodafinil for major depressive episodes associated with bipolar I disorder. J Affect Disord. 2015;181:87–91 [C].

[41] McElroy SL, Guerdjikova AI, Mori N, et al. Armodafinil in binge eating disorder: a randomized, placebo-controlled trial. Int Clin Psychopharmacol. 2015;30(4):209–15 [c].

[42] Ghoshal L, Sinha M. Fixed drug eruptions with modafinil. Indian J Pharmacol. 2015;47(2):224–6 [A].

[43] Cengiz Mete M, Senormanci O, Saracli O, et al. Compulsive modafinil use in a patient with a history of alcohol use disorder. Gen Hosp Psychiatry. 2015;37(2):e7–8 [A].

[44] Dhillon R, Wu X, Bastiampillai T, et al. Could modafinil be a drug of dependence? Aust N Z J Psychiatry. 2015;49(5):485–6 [A].

[45] George WT, Varghese R, Khawaja S. New onset of compulsive gambling associated with modafinil: a case report. Prim Care Companion CNS Disord. 2015;17(1) [A].

[46] Krishnan R, Chary KV. A rare case modafinil dependence. J Pharmacol Pharmacother. 2015;6(1):49–50 [A].

[47] Dunkley EJ, Isbister GK, Sibbritt D, et al. The Hunter serotonin toxicity criteria: simple and accurate diagnostic decision rules for serotonin toxicity. QJM. 2003;96(9):635–42 [R].

[48] Rakofsky JJ, Tang Y, Dunlop BW. Depression worsening associated with lorcaserin: a case report. J Clin Psychopharmacol. 2015;35(6):747–8 [A].

[49] Johnson JL, Rolan PE. Paradoxical topiramate-induced hyperphagia successfully treated with phentermine in a woman with migraine. J Clin Neurosci. 2015;22(8):1363–4 [A].

[50] Acosta A, Camilleri M, Shin A, et al. Quantitative gastrointestinal and psychological traits associated with obesity and response to weight-loss therapy. Gastroenterology. 2015;148(3):537–546.e4 [C].

[51] Grewal DS, Goldstein DA, Khatana AK, et al. Bilateral angle closure following use of a weight loss combination agent containing topiramate. J Glaucoma. 2015;24(5):e132–6 [A].

[52] Fraunfelder FW, Fraunfelder FT, Keates EU. Topiramate-associated acute, bilateral, secondary angle-closure glaucoma. Ophthalmology. 2004;111(1):109–11 [A].

[53] Kroger E, Mouls M, Wilchesky M, et al. Adverse drug reactions reported with cholinesterase inhibitors: an analysis of 16 years of individual case safety reports from VigiBase. Ann Pharmacother. 2015;49(11):1197–206 [MC].

[54] Grossberg GT, Farlow MR, Meng X, et al. Evaluating high-dose rivastigmine patch in severe Alzheimer's disease: analyses with concomitant memantine usage as a factor. Curr Alzheimer Res. 2015;12(1):53–60 [C].

[55] Muto S, Kawano H, Nakatomi D, et al. Sinus arrest as a result of rivastigmine in an elderly dementia with Lewy bodies patient. Geriatr Gerontol Int. 2015;15(2):229–30 [A].

[56] Diaz MC, Rosales RL. A case report on dyskinesia following rivastigmine patch 13.3 mg/24 hours for Alzheimer's disease: perspective in the movement disorders spectrum following use of cholinesterase inhibitors. Medicine (Baltimore). 2015;94(34): e1364 [A].

[57] Matsuzono K, Hishikawa N, Ohta Y, et al. Combination therapy of cholinesterase inhibitor (donepezil or galantamine) plus memantine in the Okayama Memantine Study. J Alzheimers Dis. 2015;45(3):771–80 [c].

[58] Cagnin A, Cester A, Costa B, et al. Effectiveness of switching to the rivastigmine transdermal patch from oral cholinesterase inhibitors: a naturalistic prospective study in Alzheimer's disease. Neurol Sci. 2015;36(3):457–63 [C].

[59] Montero-Odasso M, Muir-Hunter SW, Oteng-Amoako A, et al. Donepezil improves gait performance in older adults with mild Alzheimer's disease: a phase II clinical trial. J Alzheimers Dis. 2015;43(1):193–9 [c].

[60] Hategan A, Bourgeois JA. Donepezil-associated manic episode with psychotic features: a case report and review of the literature. Gen Hosp Psychiatry. 2015;38:115.e1–4 [A].

[61] Kitt J, Irons R, Al-Obaidi M, et al. A case of donepezil-related torsades de pointes. BMJ Case Rep. 2015; published online 5 October 2015, [A].

[62] Manzo C, Putignano S. Drug-induced lupus erythematosus associated with donepezil: a case report. Age Ageing. 2015;44(6):1062–3 [A].

[63] McGrane IR, Shuman MD, McDonald RW. Donepezil-related intractable hiccups: a case report. Pharmacotherapy. 2015;35(3): e1–5 [A].

[64] Segrec N, Zaman R, Pregelj P. Increased libido associated with donepezil treatment: a case report. Psychogeriatrics. 2015;16(1):70–2 [A].

[65] Morasch KC, Aaron CL, Moon JE, et al. Physiological and neurobehavioral effects of cholinesterase inhibition in healthy adults. Physiol Behav. 2015;138:165–72 [c].

2

Antidepressant Drugs

Jonathan Smithson*,†, *Philip B. Mitchell**,†,1

*School of Psychiatry, University of New South Wales, Sydney, NSW, Australia
†Black Dog Institute, Sydney, NSW, Australia
1Coresponding author: phil.mitchell@unsw.edu.au

GENERAL

Hematological

Selective serotonin reuptake inhibitor (SSRI) antidepressants have been associated with increased risk of bleeding events, including gastrointestinal (GI), intracranial and postpartum hemorrhage. Further major reports have been published recently.

GASTROINTESTINAL BLEEDING

As noted in previous editions (SEDA-36, 11; SEDA-37, 16), there have been consistent reports of an increased risk of upper GI bleeding (UGIB) associated with SSRIs, with the risk increased when co-prescribed with NSAIDs, anticoagulants or antiplatelet agents. Due to a lack of prospective randomized controlled trials and uncertainty as to the nature of the risk, the clinical implications of these observations remain unclear [1E]. However, findings have been reasonably consistent in terms of both the magnitude of the association with SSRIs, and the size of the additional risk from co-prescribed drugs such as NSAIDs and aspirin.

Cheng et al. examined the incidence of UGIB and lower GI bleeding (LGIB) among users of SSRIs and serotonin–noradrenaline reuptake inhibitors (SNRIs) and controls using national health insurance data over a 10-year period [2C]. They identified 9753 subjects who were taking either of these antidepressant classes (8809 SSRIs and 944 SNRIs), comparing them with 39012 controls matched for age, sex, and time of enrolment. Cheng et al. found that SSRI users, but not SNRI users, had significantly higher incidences of both UGIB and LGIB than controls ($P < 0.001$; log-rank test). After adjusting for age, sex, comorbidities and other medications, SSRI use remained associated with an increased

risk of both UGIB (HR 1.97; 95% CI: 1.67–2.31) and LGIB (HR: 2.96, 95% CI: 2.46–3.57).

This association between SSRIs and UGIB was also examined in a meta-analytic review of 22 cohort and case–control studies conducted by Jiang et al. [3M]. A significant but modest association between SSRIs and UGIB was found (OR 1.55; 95% CI [1.35–1.78]; $P < 0.001$). The authors confirmed that concomitant use of NSAIDs or antiplatelet agents further increased the magnitude of the association. They concluded that the risk of UGIB attributable to SSRI was minimal in "low-risk" SSRI users, with a 'number needed to harm' (NNH) of 760. When other risk factors for UGIB were present, they found a greater risk—reporting a NNH of 160 if SSRIs and NSAIDs were used concurrently. The simultaneous use of PPIs negated this increased risk. The investigators concluded that clinicians should consider the potential risks of UGIB against the merits of SSRIs and avoid NSAID use where possible.

INTRACRANIAL HEMORRHAGE

Shin et al., using a retrospective nationwide matched cohort study of 4145226 people, sought to evaluate the risk of intracranial hemorrhage (ICH) among patients treated with antidepressants and non-steroid anti-inflammatory drugs (NSAIDs), compared with the risk among those treated with antidepressants alone [4C]. Using nationwide health insurance data over a 4-year period, the study examined patients without a diagnosis of cerebrovascular disease in the previous year, who had commenced antidepressants for the first time. Comparing the risk of ICH with antidepressants alone or in combination with NSAIDS, to the risk with no antidepressants, the authors found that the combined use of antidepressants and NSAIDs was associated with an increased risk of intracranial hemorrhage within

30 days—a rate significantly greater than that found for antidepressants alone (HR 1.6, 95% CI 1.32–1.85). No differences were found between the antidepressant classes.

POSTPARTUM HEMORRHAGE

A major review and retrospective cohort study have examined the association between antidepressant use in pregnancy and postpartum hemorrhage (PPH). In the context of pro-hemorrhagic effects of SSRIs, concerns persist regarding the use of antidepressants during pregnancy and the risk of PPH. Bruning et al. conducted a systematic review of this association [5R], identifying four studies (previously described in SEDA-36 and -37) for inclusion. Using the Newcastle–Ottawa scale for assessing quality, 3 were considered "good" quality and 1 "satisfactory". Two studies reported an increased incidence of PPH, while the other two found no overall increased risk. They concluded that the evidence for this association remains inconclusive.

Grzeskowiak et al. investigated the association between antidepressant use in late gestation and PPH in a retrospective cohort study of 30 198 deliveries over a 6-year period [6C]. The authors calculated adjusted relative risks (aRRs) for PPH, comparing 588 women with late-gestation exposure to antidepressants, 1292 women with a psychiatric illness but no antidepressant use, and 28 348 unexposed control women. They found that, compared with the controls, women using antidepressants in late gestation had an increased risk of PPH (aRR 1.53; 95% CI 1.25–1.86). No increased risk was found in women with a psychiatric illness without antidepressant use. In sensitivity analyses, late gestation antidepressant exposure was associated with an increased risk of both severe PPH (aRR 1.84; 95% CI 1.39–2.44) and postpartum anemia (aRR 1.80; 95% CI 1.46–2.22).

Reproductive System (Pregnancy, Development and Infancy)

Malm et al. [7C] have examined the relationship between use of SSRIs in pregnancy and subsequent pregnancy complications, taking into account the psychiatric conditions leading to the SSRI usage. The authors examined a national register population-based prospective birth cohort including 845 345 national singleton live births over a 15-year period to 2010. Subjects were categorised into: SSRI exposure ($n = 15 729$); unexposed to SSRIs but with psychiatric diagnoses ($n = 9652$); and without exposure to medication or psychiatric diagnoses ($n = 31 394$). Pregnancy outcomes for SSRI users were compared to those in the unexposed groups, with and without psychiatric diagnoses. 12 817 women were prescribed SSRIs in the first trimester or 30 days prior to gestation, with 9322 (59.3%) receiving two or more

prescriptions. Compared to offspring of un-medicated mothers *with* psychiatric disorders, children of mothers who received SSRIs during pregnancy had a lower risk for late preterm birth (OR 0.84, 95% CI 0.74–0.96), very preterm birth (OR = 0.52, 95% CI 0.37–0.74) and Cesarean section (OR 0.70, 95% CI = 0.66–0.75). However, they found that the offspring of SSRI-treated mothers, when compared with mothers with a psychiatric diagnosis but who were on no medication, had a higher risk for neonatal complications, including low Apgar score (OR 1.68, 95% CI = 1.34–2.12) and a greater likelihood of requiring neonatal care unit monitoring (OR 1.24, 95% CI = 1.14–1.35). When compared against the offspring of unexposed mothers without psychiatric illness, the offspring of SSRI-treated mothers and unexposed mothers with psychiatric disorders both had an increased risk of a number of adverse pregnancy outcomes, including Cesarean section and need for monitoring in a neonatal care unit.

To summarise, Malm et al. found that SSRI use during pregnancy was associated with a lower risk of late preterm/very preterm birth and Cesarean sections when compared with offspring of women who had an untreated psychiatric illness whilst pregnant; however, there was conversely a higher associated risk of neonatal maladaptation. They interpreted their findings as providing evidence for a protective role of SSRIs against some deleterious reproductive outcomes, which they speculated might be mediated by reducing maternal depressive symptoms.

SPONTANEOUS ABORTION/MISCARRIAGE

Johansen et al. examined miscarriage rates in a 13-year national register study using a Scandinavian Patient, Birth, Psychiatric Registers and National Prescription database which included 1 191 164 pregnancies [8C].

They found that pregnancies exposed to SSRIs during or before pregnancy were more likely—compared to those without exposure—to result in first-trimester miscarriage, hazard rate (HR) = 1.08 [95% CI 1.04–1.13] and HR = 1.26 [95% CI 1.16–1.37], respectively. They observed no differences for second-trimester miscarriages. Interestingly, SSRI-exposed pregnancies without maternal depression and/or anxiety were less likely to result in first-trimester miscarriage than unexposed pregnancies with such conditions, HR = 0.85 [95% CI 0.76–0.95]. In pregnancies positive for SSRI exposure, maternal lifestyle and mental health profile were less healthy compared to unexposed pregnancies. The authors concluded that confounding by psychiatric indication and lifestyle in pregnancy may explain the association between SSRI use and miscarriage.

TERATOGENESIS—CARDIAC MALFORMATIONS

Although atrial septal defects, ventriculo-septal defects and right ventricular outflow tract obstruction have been repeatedly reported to be associated with SSRIs in early pregnancy, controversy persists as to the nature of this association. Four large-scale studies have recently confirmed such findings; however, the possibility of confounding by indication and the result of sibling analyses have raised doubts as to causation.

Bérard et al. conducted an updated meta-analysis and systematic review of the literature to November 2015 on the risk of cardiac malformations associated with gestational exposure to paroxetine [9M]. Identifying 23 suitable studies, the investigators found that, compared to non-exposure, first-trimester use of paroxetine was associated with an increased risk of any major congenital malformations (pooled OR 1.23, 95% CI 1.10, 1.38; $n = 15$ studies) and any major cardiac malformations (pooled OR 1.28, 95% CI 1.11, 1.47; $n = 18$ studies). The specific cardiac defects significantly associated with paroxetine were: bulbus cordis anomalies and abnormalities of cardiac septal closure (pooled OR 1.42, 95% CI 1.07, 1.89; $n = 8$ studies), atrial septal defects (pooled OR 2.38, 95% CI 1.14, 4.97; $n = 4$ studies) and right ventricular outflow track defects (pooled OR 2.29, 95% CI 1.06, 4.93; $n = 4$ studies).

In an attempt to clarify if these defects were specific to paroxetine or related to the indication of depression, Bérard et al. examined (in a further study) the association between first-trimester exposure to sertraline and the risk of congenital malformations in a cohort of depressed women [10C]. They studied 18 493 pregnancies where the mother was either depressed or anxious in a 12-year population-based cohort. The mothers were either sertraline-exposed, non-sertraline SSRI-exposed, non-SSRI exposed, or not exposed to any antidepressants. During the first trimester, 366 mothers were exposed to sertraline, 1963 to other SSRIs, and 1296 to non-SSRI antidepressants. The authors found that sertraline was not significantly associated with an overall increased risk of major malformations but was associated with an increased risk of both atrial/ventricular defects (RR, 1.34; 95% CI, 1.02–1.76; 9 exposed cases), and craniosynostosis (premature fusion of one or more cranial sutures) (RR, 2.03; 95% CI, 1.09–3.75; 3 exposed cases). They also found that exposure to other SSRIs during the first trimester was also associated with craniosynostosis (RR, 2.43; 95% CI, 1.44–4.11; 19 exposed cases) and musculoskeletal defects (RR, 1.28; 95% CI, 1.03–1.58; 104 exposed cases), leading them to conclude that (i) sertraline during the first trimester was associated with an increased risk of atrial/ventricular defects and craniosynostosis above and beyond the effects of maternal depression, and (ii) non-sertraline SSRIs were associated with an increased risk of craniosynostosis and musculoskeletal defects.

Reefhuis et al. re-examined previously reported associations between peri-conceptional use of SSRIs and birth defects using an expanded dataset from the National Birth Defects Prevention Study [11MC]. The final dataset comprised 17 952 mothers of infants with birth defects and 9857 mothers of infants without birth defects. Using Bayesian analysis, they were unable to confirm any of the previously reported birth defects associated with sertraline (even though this was the most commonly used SSRI in this sample). However, high posterior odds ratios excluding the null value were observed for five birth defects with paroxetine (anencephaly 3.2, 95% credible interval 1.6–6.2; atrial septal defects 1.8, 1.1–3.0; right ventricular outflow tract obstruction defects 2.4, 1.4–3.9; gastroschisis 2.5, 1.2–4.8; and omphalocele 3.5, 1.3–8.0) and two defects with fluoxetine (right ventricular outflow tract obstruction defects 2.0, 1.4–3.1 and craniosynostosis 1.9, 1.1–3.0).

Furu et al. used a 14-year multi-national population register-based cohort to assess whether use of specific SSRIs or venlafaxine in early pregnancy was associated with an increased risk of birth defects, particularly cardiovascular, whilst accounting for lifestyle or familial confounding [12C]. The full cohort included mothers giving birth to 2.3 million live singletons, including a sibling cohort of 2288 singleton live births. The authors conducted sibling-controlled analyses including sibling pairs discordant for exposure to SSRIs or venlafaxine and birth defects. They found that of 36 772 infants exposed to any SSRI in early pregnancy, 3.7% ($n = 1357$) had a birth defect compared with 3.1% of 2 266 875 unexposed infants, yielding a covariate adjusted odds ratio of 1.13 (95% CI 1.06–1.20). In the sibling-controlled analysis, the adjusted odds ratio was not significant. The odds ratios for any cardiac birth defect with use of any SSRI or venlafaxine was 1.15 (95% CI 1.05–1.26) in the covariate adjusted analysis, but was not significant in the sibling-controlled analysis. In the specific case of atrial and ventricular septal defects, the adjusted odds ratio was 1.17 (1.05–1.31). They found that exposure to any SSRI or venlafaxine increased the prevalence of right ventricular outflow tract obstruction defects, with an adjusted odds ratio of 1.48 (1.15–1.89). However, in the sibling-controlled analysis, the adjusted odds ratio was not significant. It is difficult to interpret the non-significant sibling-controlled findings of this study, as while they may indicate shared (non-antidepressant) environmental factors, the findings may rather reflect low statistical power in light of the relatively small sibling sample size.

Wemakor et al. sought to determine the specificity of association between first-trimester exposure to SSRIs and specific congenital heart defects (CHD) and other congenital anomalies (CA) in a population-based case–control study [13MC]. They used 12 national registries covering a 14-year period; the total sample comprised 2.1 million births which included live births, fetal deaths from 20 weeks gestation, and terminations of pregnancy for fetal anomalies. The investigators found that SSRI exposure in the first trimester was associated with CHD overall (any SSRI OR adjusted for registry 1.41, 95% CI 1.07–1.86; fluoxetine adjOR 1.43 95% CI 0.85–2.40; and paroxetine adjOR 1.53, 95% CI 0.91–2.58) and with severe CHD (adjOR 1.56, 95% CI 1.02–2.39), particularly Tetralogy of Fallot (adjOR 3.16, 95% CI 1.52–6.58) and Ebstein's anomaly (adjOR 8.23, 95% CI 2.92–23.16). They also observed significant associations between SSRI exposure and anorectal atresia/stenosis (adjOR 2.46, 95% CI 1.06–5.68), gastroschisis (adjOR 2.42, 95% CI 1.10–5.29), renal dysplasia (adjOR 3.01, 95% CI 1.61–5.61), and clubfoot (adjOR 2.41, 95% CI 1.59–3.65). While reporting these associations, the authors made the caveat that they could not exclude confounding by indication or associated factors.

PERSISTENT PULMONARY HYPERTENSION OF THE NEWBORN (PPHN)

The association between the use of SSRIs during pregnancy and subsequent risk of persistent pulmonary hypertension of the newborn (PPHN) was first raised over a decade ago but remains controversial. In 2006, the US Food and Drug Administration (FDA) issued a public health advisory [14S], based on a single published study [15C]. Subsequent conflicting findings have led to the FDA qualifying its position, stating that it is premature to reach any conclusion about a possible link between SSRI use in pregnancy and PPHN [16S].

In an effort to clarify this association, Huybrechts et al. conducted a large-scale cohort study nested in the 2000–2010 data from 46 US states and Washington, DC [17C], comprising the largest study to date which has examined for rates of PPHN in newborns exposed to antidepressants. 128 950 women (3.4% of the total cohort) obtained one or more prescriptions for antidepressants in late pregnancy. Of these, 102 179 (2.7%) were prescribed an SSRI and 26 771 (0.7%) a non-SSRI antidepressant. Overall, 7630 infants who were not exposed to antidepressants received a diagnosis of PPHN (20.8; 95% CI, 20.4–21.3 per 10 000 births), compared with 322 infants exposed to SSRIs (31.5; 95% CI, 28.3–35.2 per 10 000 births) and 78 infants exposed to non-SSRIs (29.1; 95% CI, 23.3–36.4 per 10 000 births). For the unadjusted analysis, the odds ratio for risk of PPHN with SSRIs compared to infants not exposed to antidepressants was 1.51 (95% CI, 1.35–1.69); however, after restricting the analysis to women with depression and adjusting for the high-dimensional propensity score, the odds ratio was a non-significant 1.10 (95% CI, 0.94–1.29). For non-SSRI antidepressants, the respective unadjusted and adjusted odds ratios were 1.40 (95% CI, 1.12–1.75) and 1.02 (95% CI, 0.77–1.35), respectively. When the outcome was restricted to 'primary PPHN' (PPHN typically presenting soon after birth with hypoxaemia in a baby with clinically and radiologically normal lungs), the adjusted odds ratio for SSRIs was a significant 1.28 (95% CI, 1.01–1.64), while for non-SSRI antidepressants, this was non-significant 1.14 (95% CI, 0.74–1.74). The investigators considered their findings to be consistent with a possible increase in risk of PPHN in the infants of mothers who used of SSRIs in late pregnancy. However, they noted that the absolute risk was small, being more modest than suggested in previous studies.

Autism

The relationship between autistic spectrum disorder (ASD) and *in utero* exposure to SSRIs continues to be controversial. In SEDA-37, we noted some evidence for an approximate doubling of risk, with the risk being greater with first-trimester exposure and longer exposure *in utero*. The nature of the association remains unclear; some studies suggest that this apparent effect may reflect rather the impact of maternal depression, or other confounding variables.

A large-scale population register study and a further meta-analysis have recently been published. Boukhris et al. examined the risk of ASD, according to trimester of exposure, in the offspring of children whose mothers were prescribed an SSRI during pregnancy, taking into account maternal depression [18C].

They conducted a register-based study of a population-based cohort, which included data on all pregnancies and children in Québec from January 1, 1998 to December 31, 2009. The sample was comprised of 145 456 singleton full-term live births whose mothers were covered by the government health insurance board of Québec during pregnancy and the preceding year. They found that over 904 000 person-years of follow-up, 1054 children (0.7%) received a diagnosis of ASD; with boys outnumbering girls by a ratio of about 4:1. The average age of children at the end of follow-up was 6.24 years (SD 3.19). After adjusting for potential confounders, they found that the use of SSRIs during the second and/or third trimester was significantly associated with an increased risk of ASD ($n=22$ exposed infants; adjusted HR, 2.17; 95% CI, 1.20–3.93). This increased risk persisted after taking into account maternal history of depression (adjusted HR, 1.75; 95% CI, 1.03–2.97).

In a critical analysis of the association between antidepressant use in pregnancy and ASD, Man et al. found an increased risk, albeit with uncertain causality [19M]. The authors included four case–control studies in their meta-analysis, with the adjusted odds ratios from these studies being 1.81 (95% CI [1.47–2.24]).

Bone Density, Fracture Risk and Falls

Both cross-sectional and prospective studies continue to report an association between the use of serotonergic antidepressants and both decreased bone mineral density and increased fracture risk. While animal models suggest a role of serotonin in bone metabolism, the nature of the association in patients remains unclear. Similarly, while recent reviews have noted an association between SSRIs and falls [20S,21S], its nature remains unclear and insufficient to infer causation at this time. Both depression and antidepressant medications appear to independently increase fall risk [22C].

Using data from a claims database over a 12-year period, female patients aged 40–64 years and initially without a diagnosis of a mental illness were compared with a cohort who had been commenced on H2 antagonists or proton-pump inhibitors (PPIs) [23C]. The risk of fractures among new users of SSRIs was compared to those commenced on H2 antagonists or PPIs. Primary analyses allowed for a 6-month lag to account for any delay in the onset of an effect on bone mineral density after initiation of medications. The authors found that fracture rates were higher among the 137 031 women commenced on SSRIs compared with the 236 294 initiated on either H2 antagonists or PPIs. Hazard ratios for SSRIs vs H2 antagonists or PPIs over 1, 2 and 5 years were 1.76 (95% CI 1.33–2.32), 1.73 (95% CI 1.33–2.24) and 1.67 (95% CI 1.30–2.14), respectively. The authors concluded that, in an effect sustained over time, SSRIs appear to increase fracture risk among middle-aged women without baseline psychiatric disorders.

To further examine this association, Wang et al. conducted a population-based nested case–control study examining for the association between serotonergic antidepressants (including SSRIs and SNRIs) and risk of fracture [24C]. This was the first study to investigate this association in a nationwide representative cohort of ethnic Chinese. Using 9 years of data from their National Health Insurance Research Database, the authors defined the study cohort as patients receiving 3 or more prescriptions of antidepressants. They identified 8250 patients with a first admission for fracture matching them with 33 000 controls, matched by age, sex, and date of cohort entry. Current users of serotonergic antidepressants were found to have an increased risk of fracture (adjusted odds ratio (aOR) 1.16 [95% CI 1.07–1.25]), with the risk of fracture comparable between SSRI and SNRI users.

Past studies of adult patients have suggested a negative association between the use of SSRIs and bone mineral density (BMD), increased rate of bone loss and a greater risk of fractures, although the nature of the association remains unclear. Feuer et al. sought to investigate any association between the use of SSRIs and bone mass in adolescents [25C]. They conducted a cross-sectional analysis of 5 years of data from the National Health and Nutrition Examination Study. The sample comprised 4303 participants aged 12–20 years. 62 subjects used SSRIs and were assessed for total femur, femoral neck and lumbar spine bone mineral content (BMC). BMD was assessed via dual-energy X-ray absorptiometry (DXA). In order to account for the potential confounding effect of anorexia nervosa (which may be treated with SSRIs), individuals with a Body Mass Index of less than the 5th percentile were excluded. SSRI use was found to be an independent predictor of bone mass after adjustment for age, sex, height and weight Z score, socioeconomic status, physical activity, serum cotinine (a major metabolite of nicotine and surrogate for smoking status) and ethnicity. Further analysis with multivariable adjustment found that total femur BMC was 8.8% lower in SSRI users than in non-users (mean difference 2.98 g, $SE \pm 0.105$ g, $P = 0.0006$), and total femur BMD was 6.1% lower (mean difference 0.06 g/cm^2, $SE \pm 0.002$ g/cm^2, $P = 0.016$). Femoral neck BMC and BMD and lumbar spine BMC were also negatively associated with SSRI use, with the lumbar spine BMC being 7% lower among SSRI users (mean difference 0.97 g, $SE \pm 0.048$ g, $P = 0.02$) and BMD was 3.2% lower (mean difference 0.03 g/cm^2, $SE \pm 0.015$ g/cm^2, $P = 0.09$) compared to non-users. In a sub-analysis, individuals treated for more than 6 months were found to have similar results. Furthermore, adolescents treated with SSRIs had lower DXA measurements of their total femur and lumbar spine.

In a prospective cohort study of 488 community dwelling patients aged 70–90 years, Kvelde et al. [26C] followed subjects for 1 year to examine fall risk. In univariate analyses, the presence of depressive symptoms (RR = 1.50; 95% CI = 1.06–2.11), antidepressants (RR = 1.56; 95% CI = 1.08–2.27), high physiological fall risk (RR = 1.61; 95% CI = 1.20–2.15) and poor executive functioning (RR = 1.40; 95% CI = 1.05–1.88) wase each identified as significant risk factors for falls. Multivariate analyses demonstrated that depressive symptoms and antidepressant use were independent risks, and furthermore were also independent of high physiological risk and poor executive functioning in predicting falls, the risk of which increased with the number of risk factors present. Participants with any two risk factors had a 55% increase in risk (RR = 1.55; 95% CI = 1.17–2.04), while those with three or four risk factors had a 144% increase (RR = 2.44; 95% CI = 1.75–3.43).

Suicide/Self-Harm

In a large register-based study in general practice, Coupland et al. [27C] examined the association between treatment with particular antidepressants and rates of suicide, attempted suicide or self-harm in subjects with depression. In this cohort study, 238 963 patients between 20 and 64 years of age who received a first diagnosis of depression were followed over time. They were classified according to antidepressant class (tricyclic and related antidepressants; SSRIs; and 'other antidepressants'), dose and duration of use. Within the first 5 years of follow-up, 198 cases of suicide and 5243 cases of attempted suicide or self-harm occurred. Coupland et al. found no difference in the likelihood of suicide between tricyclic and related antidepressants compared with SSRIs; however, the suicide rate was significantly increased during treatment with 'other antidepressants' when compared with the SSRI group (adjusted HR 2.64, 95% CI 1.74–3.99). Interestingly, the hazard ratio for suicide was significantly increased for mirtazapine compared with citalopram (adjusted HR 3.70, 95% CI 2.00–6.84). When considering rates of attempted suicide or self-harm, no significant difference was found between tricyclic antidepressants and SSRIs. However, the rate of attempted suicide or self-harm was again significantly higher for 'other antidepressants' compared to SSRIs (adjusted HR 1.80, 95% CI 1.61–2.00). When compared with citalopram, the adjusted hazard ratios for attempted suicide or self-harm were significantly increased for venlafaxine (1.85, 95% CI 1.61–2.13), trazodone (1.73, 95% CI 1.26–2.37), and mirtazapine (1.70, 95% CI 1.44–2.02) and significantly reduced for amitriptyline (0.71, 95% CI 0.59–0.85). The investigators observed that the absolute risk of attempted suicide or self-harm over a 1-year period ranged from 1.02% for amitriptyline to 2.96% for venlafaxine. Rates of attempted suicide or self-harm were highest in the first 28 days after starting treatment and remained increased for the first 28 days after stopping treatment. Interestingly, adjusted hazard ratios for completed suicide tended to increase with dose for selective serotonin reuptake inhibitors ($P = 0.02$), but not for tricyclic antidepressants ($P = 0.6$) or other antidepressants ($P = 0.9$).

The investigators commented upon the number of suicide events being small, and therefore leading to imprecise estimates. They noted further that as this was an observational study, their findings may reflect indication biases and residual confounding from both differing characteristics of patients prescribed these drugs and the severity of depression. Their observation of greatest risk during both the 28 days after initiation or cessation of treatment led them to emphasize the need for careful monitoring during these periods.

Stroke

Wang et al. conducted a population-based nested case–control study using a national universal health care claims database [28C] to examine for an association between antidepressant exposure and risk of stroke. The study sample was comprised of 19 825 adult patients who survived a first admission for stroke, of whom a further 3536 cases were hospitalized with a recurrence of stroke. The authors found, using a multivariate conditional logistic regression model, that the use of any tricyclic antidepressant (TCA) was associated with a 1.41-fold (95% CI, 1.19–1.67) increased risk of stroke recurrence, whereas SSRIs or other antidepressants showed no such association. Furthermore, ceasing TCAs abruptly within 30 days of the first stroke was associated with a 1.87-fold (95% CI, 1.22–2.86) increased risk of recurrence compared to patients on no antidepressants, with this risk falling with discontinuation after longer periods. The risk of recurrent stroke risk associated with the use of a TCA was not dose- or duration dependent.

SELECTIVE SEROTONIN RE-UPTAKE INHIBITORS (SSRIs) [SED-15, 3109; SEDA-31, 18; SEDA-32, 33; SEDA-33, 26; SEDA-34, 17; SEDA-35, 30; SEDA-36, 14]

Citalopram and Escitalopram

DYSTONIA

Escitalopram has been previously associated with one case report of paroxysmal cervical dystonia [29A] and another of oculogyric dystonia [30A]. A case of escitalopram-induced progressive cervical dystonia has been recently reported [31A].

Mr. R, a 78-year-old man with no prior psychiatric history, was treated for depression with citalopram 10 mg daily after 4 months of treatment for Waldenström macroglobulinemia. After 2 weeks of nausea, elevated anxiety and insomnia, citalopram was discontinued, and escitalopram 5 mg daily commenced with clonazepam 0.25 mg nocte. Due to persistent anxiety after 6–8 weeks, escitalopram was increased to 10 mg daily, and clonazepam to 0.25–0.5 mg nocte as needed. Within days of the increase of escitalopram the patient noticed mild neck stiffness, worsening over 3 weeks. As this was partly attributed to anxiety, escitalopram was increased further to 15 mg daily. Five days later, he presented to the emergency room with worsened neck stiffness, a markedly decreased lateral range of motion, persistent neck flexion with incomplete ability to extend, and severe neck pain. Medical evaluation failed to identify underlying medical, neurologic, or toxic causes of nuchal rigidity. Treatment with diphenhydramine 75 mg intravenously resulted in rapid improvement with reduction in pain and an improvement in range of motion.

SEROTONIN AND NORADRENALINE RE-UPTAKE INHIBITORS (SNRIS)

Venlafaxine and Desvenlafaxine [SED-15, 3614; SEDA-31, 22; SEDA-32, 35; SEDA-33, 32; SEDA-34, 20; SEDA-35, 32; SEDA-36, 19]

Venlafaxine

HYPOGLYCEMIA IN OVERDOSE

Treatment with a variety of antidepressants has been associated with disturbances in glucose metabolism. Some investigators have noted that hypoglycemia is more often associated with antidepressants with a high affinity for the serotonin reuptake transporter such as fluoxetine and sertraline [32A, 33A].

Hypoglycemia has not been previously reported with therapeutic doses of venlafaxine; however, there have been two case reports of severe hypoglycemia in venlafaxine overdose, both of which were attributed to increased insulin levels [34A, 35A]. A third case of hypoglycemia in venlafaxine overdose has been reported where insulin levels were normal [36A].

A depressed 42-year-old woman weighing 70 kg was admitted to the emergency room 4 h after taking of 9.0 g of venlafaxine in a suicide attempt. On presentation, she was somnolent and had mydriasis, tremor and tachycardia. Her initial serum glucose level was 2.6 mmol/L. All other laboratory results, including hepatic and renal tests, were within normal limits. The hypoglycemia was treated with 50 mL of 50% glucose. Gastric lavage was performed and activated charcoal administered. Immediately afterwards, she had a grand mal seizure. A continuous infusion of 10% glucose was started at 250 mL/h. Subsequently intermittent hypoglycemia (0.9–3.2 mmol/L) with neurological signs requiring treatment with 50 mL of 50% glucose or 200 mL sugared tea was recorded seven times during her hospitalization, the last episode occurring 40 h after venlafaxine ingestion whilst still receiving glucose infusion. Plasma insulin and C-peptide level measurement by immune-radiometric assays were within the normal range during the episodes of hypoglycemia. Toxicological analysis of the serum by LC–MS/MS revealed 14.7 mg/L of venlafaxine 14 h after ingestion (therapeutic range 0.07–0.27 mg/L). Afterwards, serum venlafaxine concentration decreased with a prolonged half-life of 15 h. No ethanol or other medications were found.

The authors noted that in this case of venlafaxine overdose, the patient experienced prolonged normo-insulinemic hypoglycemia which was resistant to glucose therapy suggesting that the increased rate of glucose uptake from the blood by the peripheral tissues (increased glucose disposal rate) may have been clinically important. Prolonged hypoglycemia persisted despite a continuous glucose infusion of 6 mg/kg/min, whilst insulin levels remained in the normal range. They noted that hypoglycemia with normal insulin levels and a glucose infusion rate at twice the recognized glucose disposal rate could be explained only by increased glucose uptake, probably due to the venlafaxine overdose. They recommended that in venlafaxine overdose, other causes of hypoglycemia should be excluded and that glucose levels should be monitored continuously as hypoglycemia after venlafaxine overdose may persist for up to 48 hours.

Duloxetine

Although SSRIs are not infrequently associated with the syndrome of inappropriate antidiuretic hormone secretion (SIADH), there have been relatively few reported cases of serotonin–noradrenaline reuptake inhibitors (SNRIs) causing SIADH-induced hyponatremia.

A 76-year-old woman had recently been prescribed duloxetine for fibromyalgia. She presented to hospital with abdominal pain and constipation and was found to have adynamic ileus. Her sodium was 124 mmol/L and declined to 118 mmol/L; she was euvolemic. Evaluation for other causes of hyponatraemia yielded negative results. Three days after the cessation of duloxetine her sodium increased to 130 mmol/L [37R].

OTHER ANTIDEPRESSANTS

Vortioxetine

Vortioxetine is a new antidepressant which was approved by the US FDA for the treatment of major depressive disorder in September 2013. It is a serotonin reuptake inhibitor with additional serotonergic receptor effects of uncertain significance: a $5\text{-}HT_3$, $5\text{-}HT_7$ and $5\text{-}HT1_D$ receptor antagonist, $5\text{-}HT1_A$ receptor agonist, $5\text{-}HT1_B$ receptor partial agonist, and serotonin (5-HT) transporter (SERT) inhibitor. The multiple receptor effects have led to its being classified 'multimodal' [38R].

Overall, the adverse effect profile of vortioxetine appears similar to the SSRIs. In the pre-approval studies, the only side effects occurring at a rate greater than 5%, and at least twice that of placebo, were nausea, vomiting and constipation, all of which occurred in a dose-dependent fashion. Nausea was particularly evident on initiation of treatment, occurring in up to 20% of patients within 2 days of starting treatment; however, up to 10% of patients on 10–20 mg daily continued to experience nausea after 6–8 weeks. Like SSRI antidepressants, sexual dysfunction emerging during treatment (assessed via the

Arizona Sexual Experience Scale) was noted to occur in a dose-dependent manner, affecting 24% of men and 34% of women on 20 mg daily, compared to 14% of men and 20% of women taking placebo [39S]. Treatment discontinuation effects were observed in about 5% of those patients taking the higher doses (20 mg) resulting in the recommendation that the dose be reduced to 10 mg daily for a week prior to discontinuation. Vortioxetine has not been associated with QTc prolongation within the dose range of 5–20 mg. Hyponatremia may occur with the elderly, necessitating monitoring of electrolytes after commencing treatment [40R]. Short-term studies have reported that discontinuation due to adverse effects occurs in 6% of those taking vortioxetine compared with 4% of patients taking placebo [41R]. Using pooled data from 9 short-term studies, Citrome's recent meta-analysis found that, in respect of adverse events resulting in discontinuation, the number needed to harm was 36 for vortioxetine, compared to 24 for duloxetine and 10 for venlafaxine [42R].

Vilazodone

Five randomized controlled trials comparing vilazodone against placebo have been published. Hellerstein and Flaxer observed that the commonest treatment-emergent adverse events, occurring in more than 5% of patients and twice the rate for placebo, were diarrhea and nausea. The rate and onset of adverse effects were consistent across the studies examined. Adverse effects were mostly mild to moderate in nature, tended to be most evident on initiation and in the first week of treatment, and were dose dependent [43R]. In a recent meta-analysis, Zhang et al. analysed five randomized controlled trials involving 1200 patients treated with vilazodone, comparing them with 1193 patients on placebo. They found that the most common adverse events were diarrhea and nausea (diarrhea; OR 3.54, 95% CI 2.81–4.45; $P < 0.00001$; nausea 3.85, 95% CI 3.00–4.96; $P < 0.00001$). That analysis found that discontinuations due to adverse events occurred at a rate almost three times that of placebo (OR 2.71, 95% CI 1.81–4.05; $P < 0.00001$) [44R].

References

[1] Targownik LE. Are we worried enough about selective serotonin receptor inhibitors and upper gastrointestinal bleeding? Clin Gastroenterol Hepatol. 2015;13(1):51–4 [E].

[2] Cheng YL, Hu HY, Lin XH, et al. Use of SSRI, but not SNRI, increased upper and lower gastrointestinal bleeding: a nationwide population-based cohort study in Taiwan. Medicine. 2015;94(46): e2022 [C].

[3] Jiang HY, Chen HZ, Hu XJ, et al. Use of selective serotonin reuptake inhibitors and risk of upper gastrointestinal bleeding: a systematic review and meta-analysis. Clin Gastroenterol Hepatol. 2015;13(1):42–50 [M].

[4] Shin JY, Park MJ, Lee SH. Risk of intracranial haemorrhage in antidepressant users with concurrent use of non-steroidal anti-inflammatory drugs: nationwide propensity score matched study. BMJ. 2015;351:h3517 [C].

[5] Bruning AHL, Heller HM, Kieviet N, et al. Antidepressants during pregnancy and postpartum hemorrhage: a systematic review. Eur J Obstet Gynecol Reprod Biol. 2015;189:38–47 [R].

[6] Grzeskowiak LE, McBain R, Dekker GA, et al. Antidepressant use in late gestation and risk of postpartum hemorrhage: a retrospective cohort study. BJOG. 2015. http://dx.doi.org/10.1111/1471-0528.13612. [Epub ahead of print], [C].

[7] Malm H, Sourander A, Gissler M, et al. Pregnancy complications following prenatal exposure to SSRIs or maternal psychiatric disorders: results from population-based national register data. Am J Psychiatr. 2015;172(12):1224–32 [C].

[8] Johansen RL, Mortensen LH, Andersen AM, et al. Maternal use of selective serotonin reuptake inhibitors and risk of miscarriage—assessing potential biases. Paediatr Perinat Epidemiol. 2015;29(1):72–81 [C].

[9] Bérard A, Iessa N, Chaabane S, et al. The risk of major cardiac malformations associated with paroxetine use during the first trimester of pregnancy: a systematic review and meta-analysis. Br J Clin Pharmacol. 2015;81:589–604 [M].

[10] Bérard A, Zhao JP, Sheehy O. Sertraline use during pregnancy and the risk of major malformations. Am J Obstet Gynecol. 2015;212(6):795.e1–795.e12 [C].

[11] Reefhuis J, Devine O, Friedman JM, et al. Specific SSRIs and birth defects: Bayesian analysis to interpret new data in the context of previous reports. BMJ. 2015;351:h3190 [MC].

[12] Furu K, Kieler H, Haglund B, et al. Selective serotonin reuptake inhibitors and venlafaxine in early pregnancy and risk of birth defects: population based cohort study and sibling design. BMJ. 2015;350:h1798 [C].

[13] Wemakor A, Casson K, Garne E, et al. Selective serotonin reuptake inhibitor antidepressant use in first trimester pregnancy and risk of specific congenital anomalies: a European register-based study. Eur J Epidemiol. 2015;30(11): 1187–98 [MC].

[14] US Food and Drug Administration. Public health advisory: FDA Drug Safety Communication: Selective serotonin reuptake inhibitor (SSRI) antidepressant use during pregnancy and reports of a rare heart and lung condition in newborn babies, [7/19/2006] http://www.fda.gov/drugs/drugsafety/ucm283375.htm. Accessed February 28, 2015 [S].

[15] Chambers CD, Hernandez-Diaz S, Van Marter LJ, et al. Selective serotonin-reuptake inhibitors and risk of persistent pulmonary hypertension of the newborn. NEJM. 2006;354(6):579–87 [C].

[16] US Food and Drug Administration. Public health advisory: treatment challenges of depression in pregnancy and the possibility of persistent pulmonary hypertension in newborns, [12-14-2011] http://www.fda.gov/Drugs/DrugSafety/PostmarketDrugSafetyInformationforPatientsandProviders/ucm124348.htm. Accessed February 28, 2015 [S].

[17] Huybrechts KF, Bateman BT, Palmsten K, et al. Antidepressant use late in pregnancy and risk of persistent pulmonary hypertension of the newborn. JAMA. 2015;313(21):2142–51 [C].

[18] Boukhris T, Sheehy O, Mottron L, et al. Antidepressant use during pregnancy and the risk of autism spectrum disorder in children. JAMA Pediatr. 2016;170(2):117–24 [C].

[19] Man KK, Tong HH, Wong LY, et al. Exposure to selective serotonin reuptake inhibitors during pregnancy and risk of autism spectrum disorder in children: a systematic review and meta-analysis of observational studies. Neurosci Biobehav Rev. 2015;49:82–9 [M].

[20] Gebara MA, Lipsey KL, Karp JF, et al. Cause or effect? Selective serotonin reuptake inhibitors and falls in older adults: a systematic review. Am J Geriatr Psychiatry. 2015;23(10):1016–28 [S].

[21] Park H, Satoh H, Miki A, et al. Medications associated with falls in older people: systematic review of publications from a recent 5-year period. Eur J Clin Pharmacol. 2015;71(12):1429–40 [S].

[22] Williams LJ, Pasco JA, Stuart AL, et al. Psychiatric disorders, psychotropic medication use and falls among women: an observational study. BMC Psychiatry. 2015;15(1):1 [C].

[23] Sheu YH, Lanteigne A, Stürmer T, et al. SSRI use and risk of fractures among perimenopausal women without mental disorders. Inj Prev. 2015;21(6):397–403 [C].

[24] Wang CY, Fu SH, Wang CL, et al. Serotonergic antidepressant use and the risk of fracture: a population-based nested case–control study. Osteoporos Int. 2016;27(1):57–63 [C].

[25] Feuer AJ, Demmer RT, Thai A, et al. Use of selective serotonin reuptake inhibitors and bone mass in adolescents: an NHANES study. Bone. 2015;78:28–33 [C].

[26] Kvelde T, Lord SR, Close JC, et al. Depressive symptoms increase fall risk in older people, independent of antidepressant use, and reduced executive and physical functioning. Arch Gerontol Geriatr. 2015;60(1):190–5 [C].

[27] Coupland C, Hill T, Morriss R, et al. Antidepressant use and risk of suicide and attempted suicide or self harm in people aged 20 to 64: cohort study using a primary care database. BMJ. 2015;350:h517 [C].

[28] Wang MT, Chu CL, Yeh CB, et al. Antidepressant use and risk of recurrent stroke: a population-based nested case-control study. J Clin Psychiatry. 2015;76(7):e877–85 [C].

[29] Garcia Ruiz PJ, Cabo I, Bermejo PG, et al. Escitalopram-induced paroxysmal dystonia. Clin Neuropharmacol. 2007;30(2):124–6 [A].

[30] Patel OP, Simon MR. Oculogyric dystonic reaction to escitalopram with features of anaphylaxis including response to epinephrine. Int Arch Allergy Immunol. 2006;140(1):27–9 [A].

[31] Morgan RJ, Dolenc TJ. Escitalopram-induced progressive cervical dystonia. Psychosomatics. 2015;56(5):572–5 [A].

[32] Derijks HJ, Meyboom RH, Heerdink ER, et al. The association between antidepressant use and disturbances in glucose homeostasis: evidence from spontaneous reports. Eur J Clin Pharmacol. 2008;64(5):531–8 [A].

[33] Khoza S, Barner JC. Glucose dysregulation associated with antidepressant agents: an analysis of 17 published case reports. Int J Clin Pharm. 2011;33(3):484–92 [A].

[34] Francino MC, Deguigne MB, Badin J, et al. Hypoglycaemia: a little known effect of venlafaxine overdose. Clin Toxicol. 2012;50(3):215–7 [A].

[35] Meertens JH, Monteban-Kooistra WE, Ligtenberg JJ, et al. Severe hypoglycemia following venlafaxine intoxication: a case report. J Clin Psychopharmacol. 2007;27(4):414–5 [A].

[36] Brvar M, Koželj G, Mašič LP. Hypoglycemia in venlafaxine overdose: a hypothesis of increased glucose uptake. Eur J Clin Pharmacol. 2015;71(2):261–2 [A].

[37] Amoako AO, Brown C, Riley T. Syndrome of inappropriate antidiuretic hormone secretion: a story of duloxetine-induced hyponatraemia. BMJ Case Rep. 2015;2015. http://dx.doi.org/10.1136/bcr-2014-208037, pii: bcr2014208037, [R].

[38] Sanchez C, Asin KE, Artigas F. Vortioxetine, a novel antidepressant with multimodal activity: review of preclinical and clinical data. Pharmacol Ther. 2015;145:43–57 [R].

[39] Zhang J, Mathis MV, Sellers JW, et al. The US Food and Drug Administration's perspective on the new antidepressant vortioxetine. J Clin Psychiatry. 2014;76(1):1–478 [S].

[40] Keks NA, Hope J, Culhane C. Vortioxetine: a multimodal antidepressant or another selective serotonin reuptake inhibitor? Australas Psychiatry. 2015;23(3):210–3 [R].

[41] Sanchez C, Asin KE, Artigas F. Vortioxetine, a novel antidepressant with multimodal activity: review of preclinical and clinical data. Pharmacol Ther. 2015;145:43–57 [R].

[42] Citrome L. Vortioxetine for major depressive disorder: a systematic review of the efficacy and safety profile for this newly approved antidepressant—what is the number needed to treat, number needed to harm and likelihood to be helped or harmed? Int J Clin Pract. 2014;68(1):60–82 [R].

[43] Hellerstein DJ, Flaxer J. Vilazodone for the treatment of major depressive disorder: an evidence-based review of its place in therapy. Core Evid. 2015;10:49 [R].

[44] Zhang XF, Wu L, Wan DJ, et al. Evaluation of the efficacy and safety of vilazodone for treating major depressive disorder. Neuropsychiatr Dis Treat. 2015;11:1957 [R].

CHAPTER

3

Lithium

Megan E. Maroney*,1, Mei T. Liu†, Thomas Smith‡, Kelan L. Thomas§

*Rutgers University Ernest Mario School of Pharmacy, Piscataway, NJ, USA
†Jersey City Medical Center, Jersey City, NJ, USA
‡Manchester University College of Pharmacy, Fort Wayne, IN, USA
§Touro University California College of Pharmacy, Vallejo, CA, USA
1Corresponding author: mmaroney@pharmacy.rutgers.edu

GENERAL INFORMATION

Lithium continues to be a first-line option for the treatment and prevention of mood episodes associated with bipolar disorder [1R,2R,3R]. It may have neuroprotective effects, is the only mood stabilizer with evidence that it reduces the risk of suicide, and is also effective as an adjunctive treatment option for major depressive disorder (MDD) [4R,5M,6H]. Some authors argue that it is underutilized, particularly for MDD [7A].

A large meta-analysis comparing the efficacy and tolerability of medications used to augment response to antidepressants for MDD found that lithium was more effective (response OR=1.56; 95% Credible Interval [CrI] 1.05–2.55), but less tolerable (side effects discontinuation OR=2.30; 95% CrI 1.04–6.03) than placebo [8R]. In a comprehensive review of treatments for acute bipolar depression, lithium was found to be well tolerated, with a number needed to harm (NNH) of 38 for nausea. However, it appeared only marginally efficacious for this particular indication, with a number needed to treat (NNT) to achieve response of 15; authors concluded that lithium remains inadequately tested since they only used one trial to calculate NNT and NNH values [9R].

Despite its sizable evidence base, clinicians are often hesitant to prescribe lithium due to its narrow therapeutic index and concern for long-term adverse effects. To mitigate the risk of adverse effects, Malhi recently advocated for a twofold approach: avoiding prolonged periods of high lithium plasma concentrations by maintaining concentrations at the lower end of the therapeutic range (i.e. 0.6 mEq/L) and regularly assessing these lithium concentrations along with monitoring parameters such as thyroid function, renal function and calcium concentrations [10r].

℞ The potential risks of lithium need to be weighed against the potential benefits for each individual patient. Finding a way to determine who might respond to lithium without a trial and error process would be highly valuable. Mertens and colleagues recently studied the effects of lithium on hippocampal neurons derived from patients with bipolar disorder using induced pluripotent stem-cell (iPSC) technology and subsequently compared lithium responders to non-responders. Lithium was found to diminish the hyperactivity of hippocampal dentate gyrus granule cell-like neurons derived from bipolar patients who responded to lithium, possibly by reversing aberrant gene expression; the authors concluded that the findings from their bipolar disorder neuronal model may be helpful in determining who may respond to lithium and potentially useful in developing new drug treatments for bipolar disorder [11E].

ORGANS AND SYSTEMS

Cardiovascular

Lithium's cardiovascular adverse effects, including bradycardia and pro-arrhythmic activity, have been well documented. However, other cardiovascular side effects, while rare, occur as well. One recent case report has proposed that lithium may have a direct toxic effect on cardiac myocytes. A 35-year-old African American woman with bipolar disorder was brought to the emergency room unresponsive with unstable cardiac vital signs, including hypotension (90/63 mmHg), bradycardia (35 bpm) and a prolonged QTc interval (531 ms) with diffuse T-wave inversions. Upon further diagnostic workup, she was diagnosed with lithium-induced transient myocarditis due to serum cardiac marker elevation (troponins 3.14 ng/mL, CK-MB/CK relative index 5.76) and left ventricular systolic dysfunction with an ejection fraction of 15%. Her serum lithium level was supratherapeutic (3.7 mEq/L), and her serum creatinine was also elevated (1.7 mg/dL). The patient was treated with hemodialysis and inotropes. These led to her stabilization, reduced lithium levels and eventual improvement. She was discharged without further complications. While cardiac complications have been witnessed in lithium overdose, T-wave inversions, prolonged QTc intervals, and left ventricular dysfunction are rare. After ruling out other possible causes, the medical team attributed these complications to lithium, particularly because of their rapid improvement after lithium levels fell [12A].

Nervous System

LOWERING OF SEIZURE THRESHOLD

Use of lithium has been cautioned in patients undergoing electroconvulsive therapy (ECT) due to concerns of confusion and other cognitive adverse effects, as well as increased seizure duration. However, lithium dose reduction or discontinuation prior to ECT is not always a possibility in clinical practice. Galvez and colleagues analyzed data for 179 patients from three ECT research studies to examine the effect of various demographic and clinical factors, including concomitant psychotropic medications, on seizure threshold. Treatment with lithium significantly predicted lower initial seizure threshold in a multiple regression model ($R^2 = 0.043$, $P < 0.01$). The researchers suggest that lithium may lower seizure threshold by altering brain excitability through its effects on membrane ion channels and neurotransmitter systems such as glutamate, noradrenaline and serotonin. Lithium's potential to lower the seizure threshold should be taken into consideration, especially for patients undergoing ECT [13C].

DEMENTIA/COGNITIVE IMPAIRMENT

Both reversible and irreversible cases of neurotoxicity, including symptoms resembling dementia, have been reported with lithium treatment, most often in patients with elevated lithium concentrations. Two recent cases of reversible cognitive impairment have been described in patients with lithium blood levels within the normal therapeutic range (0.6–1.0 mEq/L) [14A,15A].

Riepe and colleagues reported on a 74-year-old male treated with venlafaxine and lithium (serum level 0.8 mEq/L) for recurrent depressive episodes and primidone for familial essential tremor who developed cognitive impairment in the form of short-term memory difficulties. Neuropsychological testing revealed deficits in episodic memory, cognitive flexibility, semantic fluency and attention. Positron emission tomography with fluorodeoxyglucose (FDG-PET) showed reduced glucose metabolism in the temporo-parietal areas and the posterior cingulum, which strongly resembled the pattern seen in Alzheimer's disease (AD). Lithium and primidone were both discontinued at this time as possible causes of the patient's memory impairment and reduced cerebral glucose metabolism. Approximately 1 month after discontinuing treatment with lithium and primidone, glucose utilization normalized in all brain regions and neuropsychological testing returned to normal. An amyloid-PET was also performed to further rule out AD. The authors suggested that the pattern of glucose metabolism reduction seen in this patient was most consistent with a lithium toxicity PET imaging case report. Primidone typically reduces glucose metabolism in nearly all brain regions and therefore did not match the pattern seen in this patient. The authors concluded that this was the first case report of an AD-like glucose utilization pattern when lithium serum levels were within the normal therapeutic range. The authors recommended consideration of dosage reduction or discontinuation for drugs known to impair cognition in elderly patients. They warn that due to pharmacokinetic and pharmacodynamics changes that occur with age, adverse effects normally associated with toxic lithium levels may occur even if the serum concentrations are within the normal range [14A].

Soriano-Barcelo and colleagues reported a similar case of reversible dementia with lithium in a 56-year-old male diagnosed with bipolar I disorder. At age 54, after 4 years of lithium 1200 mg/day, quetiapine 600 mg/day and clonazepam 2 mg/day, the patient had developed short- and long-term memory loss, temporal–spatial disorientation, attention difficulties and functional disability; he had mild cognitive impairment according to his 20/30 score on the Mini Mental State Examination (MMSE). All lithium levels drawn during treatment were within the normal range (less than 0.91 mEq/L). Eventually the patient became dependent on assistance for basic activities of daily living and was diagnosed with dementia. Two years later, at the age of 56, he was hospitalized for treatment of a pulmonary embolism and presented with altered consciousness and psychomotor agitation that was assumed to be delirium caused by his febrile condition. His most recent lithium level from 1 month prior to hospitalization was 0.84 mEq/L. His delirium was managed by increasing quetiapine to 1000 mg/day, adding risperidone 6 mg/day and continuing lithium 1200 mg/day. Two weeks into the hospitalization, the patient developed worsening temporal–spatial disorientation, myoclonic movements, visual hallucinations, dysarthria, bowel incontinence, ataxia and dysphagia. At this time, the patient's serum lithium level was found to be 1.94 mEq/L and an electroencephalogram (EEG) showed disorganized background activity and other findings suggestive of non-convulsive status epilepticus due to toxic encephalopathy, so lithium was discontinued. Subsequent EEGs showed progressive normalization after lithium discontinuation, but the patient's confusional state persisted until approximately 1 week after gradual discontinuation of risperidone (~4 weeks after lithium discontinuation). Two months after discharge from the hospital, his medication regimen consisted of carbamazepine 600 mg/day, quetiapine 600 mg/day and clonazepam 6 mg/day, but now the patient scored a perfect 30/30 on the MMSE and was functioning independently. Therefore, the authors attributed his previous 2 years of cognitive impairment to lithium. They caution that when dementia symptoms appear in younger patients, medications such as lithium should be considered a possible culprit, even if serum levels are within the normal therapeutic range. They also warn that patients being treated with a combination of lithium and antipsychotic medication (particularly with high dopamine receptor occupancy) may be more at risk of developing neurotoxicity, which they suggest was supported by the fact that the patient's delirium only improved after discontinuation of the risperidone. The authors also note that this case illustrates that neurotoxicity may still be reversible even after 2 years of continued treatment with lithium [15A].

Dr. David Kahn provided commentary along with this case, pointing out that penetration of lithium into brain tissue may vary from one individual to another. Also, the effectiveness of the lithium/sodium exchange pumps in neurons decreases with age, which makes older individuals more prone to neurotoxicity despite normal therapeutic plasma levels. Therefore, plasma levels may be misleading for some individuals, and each patient should also be monitored for adverse effects by direct observation and treated based on their symptoms [15A].

POSTERIOR REVERSIBLE ENCEPHALOPATHY SYNDROME (PRES)

Fitzgerald and colleagues reported two cases of posterior reversible encephalopathy syndrome (PRES) associated with supra-therapeutic lithium levels. The first case was a 50-year-old female who presented with altered mental status, hypoxia, emesis, generalized weakness, tremulousness, myoclonus and elevated blood pressure (155/64 mmHg). An EEG showed moderate generalized slowing and epileptiform sharp waves. Her home medications included clonazepam, quetiapine, gabapentin, lithium, duloxetine, levothyroxine, dicyclomine, olmesartan/hydrochlorothiazide and carisoprodol. The serum lithium level drawn on admission was >4 mEq/L and lithium was discontinued. Her mental status improved

gradually over the course of the hospitalization, but three separate tonic–clonic seizures occurred on day 10 of admission. At this time, a computed tomography (CT) of the head showed symmetric hypoattenuation of the subcortical white matter consistent with PRES. Magnetic resonance imaging (MRI) on day 14 confirmed the finding of PRES with symmetric subcortical FLAIR hyperintensities. She returned to her baseline level of functioning and was discharged home on day 33. The MRI 5 months post-discharge showed complete resolution of PRES [16A].

The second case involved a 61-year-old male being treated with amitriptyline, sertraline, levothyroxine and lithium who presented with weakness, syncope and "jerking" movements of his extremities that all worsened over 3 weeks. The patient's lithium was discontinued after the level was found to be 1.7 mEq/L on admission. An EEG showed background slowing and CT of the head was normal. The patient's mental status gradually declined and his blood pressure was elevated with systolic pressures in the 170 mmHg. On day 9, his mental status remained altered, even after blood pressure controls were initiated, and MRI of the brain showed symmetric vasogenic edema in the parieto-occipital and temporal lobes consistent with PRES. The patient's mental status never returned to baseline during the admission, and he was eventually transferred to a long-term care facility [16A].

The authors of this case series caution that lithium-associated PRES may be underrecognized due to symptom overlap with lithium toxicity, particularly seizures. PRES is often associated with hypertension, although blood pressure is normal or only mildly elevated in roughly 25% of PRES cases. Both of the patients described by the authors had some degree of hypertension, but this does not eliminate the culpability of lithium. The authors hypothesize that lithium may elicit PRES through alteration of vascular endothelial growth factor (VEGF) expression and/or by induction of matrix metalloproteinase-1 expression. As both patients displayed symptoms of PRES several days after the initial presentation of lithium toxicity (9–10 days), the authors suspect that a rebound phenomenon related to lithium withdrawal may potentially explain this delay [16A].

Neuromuscular Functioning
TREMOR

Vandewalle and colleagues reviewed the literature on drug-induced movement disorders of antidepressants and mood stabilizers published between 1966 and January 2014. They also included movement disorders reported in the database from The Netherlands Pharmacovigilance Centre Lareb, which collects data on adverse events with medications and vaccines spontaneously reported by healthcare professionals, patients and manufacturers. The authors stated that about two-thirds of lithium patients will experience tremors. The Dutch database also showed that tremor was the most commonly reported movement disorder with 29 cases, while only ≤2 cases were reported for each of the other lithium-induced motor disturbances. Tremor occurs more often in lithium-treated patients who are also being treated with carbamazepine, selective serotonin reuptake inhibitors (SSRIs), or diuretics. Slow, careful titration and the use of sustained release products may decrease the risk of lithium-induced tremor [17R].

CHOREOATHETOSIS

A 75-year-old woman who had been treated with lithium for 34 years presented to the emergency department with a serum creatinine level of 2.0 mg/dL, and a lithium level of 2.2 mEq/L along with other signs and symptoms of lithium toxicity: confusion, impaired short-term memory, word-finding difficulty, dysarthria, tremor and ataxia. Lithium was discontinued, the patient was treated with fluids, and on the second day of hospitalization, she developed severe choreoathetosis—involuntary, non-rhythmic, dance-like writhing. The movements continued for several days after the patient's renal function and lithium level normalized. The choreoathetosis and remaining cognitive dysfunction improved by hospital day 10, and the patient was discharged. The authors suggest that this case presented similar to other previously reported cases of lithium-induced choreoathetosis with complete resolution of symptoms within 1–2 weeks. When neurologic impairment persists beyond 2 months, it is called syndrome of irreversible lithium-effectuated neurotoxicity (SILENT) [18A].

OTHER MOVEMENT DISORDERS

Vandewalle and colleagues also found that lithium toxicity can be associated with chorea and orolingual dyskinesias. General risk factors for the development of motor side effects from psychotropic medications include older age, female sex, medical comorbidities such as diabetes or liver disease and personal or family history of movement disorders [17R].

Sensory Systems
DOWNBEAT NYSTAGMUS

Nystagmus is known to occur with acute lithium intoxication, but can also occur at normal blood levels. Monden and colleagues describe a case of a 52-year-old woman being treated with 800 mg/day of lithium for the past 4 years who presented with complaints of double vision and moving images, while her lithium level was measured to be 0.8 mEq/L. The neurologist diagnosed downbeat nystagmus and discontinued lithium after conducting various tests and ruling out other potential causes, such as multiple sclerosis, neoplasm, stroke, poisoning and vitamin B12 deficiency. The adverse event scored a 6 on the Naranjo nomogram, indicating that the nystagmus was likely due to lithium. The patient was then managed with a combination of quetiapine and valproic acid for her bipolar disorder and even tried clonazepam, but the nystagmus did not improve. Only 3 of the 16 reported cases of lithium-induced downbeat nystagmus that the authors found improved by lowering the dose or discontinuing lithium. Treatment options for lithium-induced nystagmus include clonazepam, baclofen, gabapentin, trihexyphenidyl, aminopyridine, dalfampridine, or, if all else fails, surgical intervention [19A].

Endocrine
THYROID

It is well documented in prescribing information that lithium can adversely affect the thyroid and parathyroid glands. The prevalence rates of hypercalcemia and hyperparathyroidism are estimated to range from 0.1% to 0.7% in the general population compared to 8.6% for hyperparathyroidism and 24.1% for hypercalcemia in lithium-treated patients [20MC,21C,22A].

Shapiro and colleagues reported a 66-year-old male patient with schizoaffective disorder who was admitted to the psychiatric unit for relapse of psychotic mania. The patient was in remission for the previous 11 years and was maintained on lithium 1200 mg/day and olanzapine 15 mg/day. A routine primary care screening 4 months prior to admission revealed an elevated serum calcium level at 11.0 mg/dL. The patient's medical records indicated that he had elevated calcium levels for the past 9 years. Three months prior to admission, his lithium level was 1.0 mEq/L, and intact parathyroid hormone (iPTH) level was 92.2 pg/mL. Lithium was discontinued due to hypercalcemia, and divalproex was initiated at 1000 mg/day, 17 days before the psychiatric admission. Upon admission, physical examination, comprehensive metabolic screen, complete blood count, toxicology screening, and thyroid stimulating hormone were within normal limits, but his serum calcium level was still elevated at 10.7 mg/dL. On day 10 of the hospitalization, the calcium level normalized to 9.8 mg/dL, but the patient had an elevated iPTH level (76.7 pg/mL), elevated urinary calcium level (362.5 mg/24 hours) and low 25-hydroxy vitamin D level (21 ng/mL). A technetium-99m sestamibi scan showed increased uptake in one parathyroid gland that was suggestive of adenoma. Bone mineral density testing by dual-energy X-ray absorptiometry (DXA) scan showed mild osteopenia in the left hip (T-score=1.4 SD). The patient was diagnosed with primary hyperparathyroidism based on hypercalciuria and enhanced localized parathyroid uptake. Lithium was restarted on hospitalization day 10, and the patient was discharged on lithium

1200 mg/day and risperidone 3 mg/day. Laboratory values at follow-up at 12 weeks after discharge revealed a serum lithium level of 0.98 mEq/L, elevated serum calcium level (10.7 mg/dL), and an elevated iPTH level (86.3 pg/mL). The authors suggest that calcium testing should be completed at baseline, 6 months and then annually along with other lithium monitoring standards [22A].

Hyperthyroidism and thyrotoxicosis are less common adverse effects associated with lithium, but the incidence is 2–3 times higher than expected in the general population. Patients with bipolar disorder with thyrotoxicosis may present with symptoms that can be mistaken for bipolar mania. De Sousa Gurgel and colleagues reported a 19-year-old male patient with schizoaffective disorder who was hospitalized due to aggressive behavior, agitation, irritability, delusional speech, and decreased need for sleep. The patient had severe psychomotor agitation that persisted despite being treated with 20 mg/day of olanzapine, 900 mg/day of lithium, and 600 mg/day of levomepromazine. Tremor of upper extremities and sinus tachycardia at rest were observed on daily physical exams during the hospitalization. Laboratory tests showed elevated creatine kinase (5092 U/L) and free thyroxine (3.13 ng/dL), but normal thyrotropin (0.61 mcIU/mL) and a serum lithium (0.61 mEq/L). Lithium was replaced by sodium valproate, and rapid improvement in agitation, tremor, and heart rate was seen. Ninety-six hours after lithium discontinuation laboratory testing showed decreased creatine kinase (976 U/L), normal free thyroxine (1.1 ng/dL) and thyrotropin (0.74 mcIU/mL), along with negative thyroid antibodies. The patient was diagnosed with lithium-associated thyrotoxicosis and subsequent spontaneous remission without requiring anti-thyroid medication [23A].

Renal/Urinary Tract

Lithium can cause various types of renal adverse effects such as acute toxic effects, nephrogenic diabetes insipidus, or chronic renal dysfunction. The risk of end-stage renal failure associated with lithium, although considered rare, has been estimated to be 0.5–1%. However, many studies are not able to detect long-term adverse renal outcomes associated with lithium due to their short duration [24MC]. Aprahamian and colleagues conducted a 2-year randomized, placebo-controlled study, with a single-blinded extension phase of up to 4 years, to determine the effect of low-dose lithium on renal function in elderly patients treated for amnestic mild cognitive impairment. The study showed that low-dose lithium treatment did not impair renal function in the elderly as measured by the abbreviated Modification of Diet in Renal Disease (aMDRD) and Chronic Kidney Disease Epidemiology Collaboration (CKD-EPI) equations [25c]. However, there are still concerns that the 4-year duration of the study may have been inadequate to fully evaluate the risk of renal toxicity, especially since other studies have suggested that developing lithium-induced nephropathy and end-stage renal failure may take more than 13 years [26r]. Despite this criticism, the researchers explained that 4 years is the longest lithium trial ever conducted involving a randomized controlled phase [27r].

Skin

Wang and colleagues performed a meta-analysis to compare the rates of rash between lamotrigine and other medications including lithium. Understanding these comparative risks is useful for selecting drug therapy, since both lamotrigine and lithium are commonly used in the treatment of bipolar disorder and known to induce dermatologic side effects. In analyzing the literature, the authors did not find a significant difference between the likelihood of rash with lamotrigine compared with lithium therapy (OR 1.12, 95% CI: 0.62–2.03) [28M].

A case of lithium-induced purpura was reported in a 51-year-old male of Han ethnicity. The patient was admitted to the psychiatric hospital due to mania symptoms and lithium carbonate was initiated. Shortly after starting lithium, his family noticed red or purple discolorations on the patient's skin that did not blanch when applying pressure. The purpura was covering much of the patient's lower extremities with scattered ecchymotic patches found throughout his physical exam. Blood work revealed normal liver and renal function, white blood cells (WBC) of 10.49×10^9/L, percentage of neutrophils was 82.4%, platelet count of 209×10^9/L, and lithium level was 1.01 mEq/L. The authors suggest that his purpura might have been immune complex mediated, since lithium is a hapten that obtains immunity by binding body protein. The body is capable of producing antigen–antibody reactions, and the purpura could have theoretically been caused by auto-antibodies acting against the platelet antigens after the patient started taking lithium. His lithium was stopped and mannitol 250 mL intravenous infusion was administered. His lithium level decreased to 0.59 mEq/L after 24 hours, and there was little purpura left on the patient's skin after 1 week [29A].

A case of lithium-induced ostraceous psoriasis, consisting of dark-brown crusty plaques on the face, scalp, chest, back and abdomen, mimicking dermatitis neglecta was reported in a 38-year-old male patient after 10 months of lithium therapy. The patient initially described the dermatologic appearances as painful and itchy "dots" during the first 2 weeks. He attempted treatment with antihistamines and topical steroids, but this was unsuccessful. After examination and biopsy, psoriasis was diagnosed, and the patient was placed on methotrexate, folic acid, and a 10% urea emollient in addition to his discontinuing lithium. This led to significant improvement after 1 month of treatment. Dermatological side effects such as psoriasis are well known with lithium, but its mechanism is unknown. Some have attributed it to lithium's effect on glycogen synthase kinase leading to keratinocyte proliferation and other changes in the upper dermis. However, Petersein and colleagues have recently developed a different theory (see Section mechanism of ADR). This is the first reported case of lithium causing a dermatitis neglecta-like appearance [30A].

Sexual Function

Up to a third of bipolar patients treated with lithium may experience sexual dysfunction as measured by the Arizona Sexual Experience Scale [31C]. Elnazer and colleagues recently sought to clarify the incidence, potential causes, and treatment of lithium-induced sexual dysfunction through a systematic review. They summarized the results of 13 preclinical and clinical studies. In preclinical studies, lithium was found to reduce testosterone and spermatogenesis in male rats, while increasing estrogen levels in females. Lithium also appears to impair nitric oxide-mediated relaxation of cavernosal tissue in rats after chronic administration [32R].

One study of 104 euthymic patients stabilized on lithium for bipolar disorder found that co-administration of a benzodiazepine may be associated with an even higher risk of sexual dysfunction than monotherapy or other concomitant psychotropic medications (49% vs 31%). However, there was no relationship between sexual dysfunction and serum lithium or prolactin concentrations in the trials reviewed [32R].

As far as treatment options, one randomized controlled trial showed that aspirin 240 mg/day may reduce overall sexual dysfunction and improve erectile function in males with lithium-induced sexual dysfunction. No other treatments were investigated in the literature [32R].

SECOND-GENERATION EFFECTS

Pregnancy

Lithium, a known teratogen, poses a risk to the fetus in pregnant women on lithium therapy, but environmental lithium exposure may also be harmful with high concentrations in drinking water. In order to analyze the potential effects of lithium on fetal growth and development, Harari and colleagues designed a prospective population-based cohort study on maternal exposure to variable lithium concentrations in drinking water during pregnancy in Northern Argentina [33C].

Their findings support the risks of lithium, even through drinking water, during pregnancy. Metrics such as head and femur fetus measurements and length at birth were inversely related to lithium levels in the blood and urine of the mother. Even more concerning was that even relatively low lithium levels, as compared to patients on lithium therapy, were found to increase these risks. These findings should be explored more in the future [33C].

Lactation

The use of lithium in breastfeeding mothers is usually concerning. With guidelines for bipolar disorder supporting the use of atypical antipsychotics, many women are switched from lithium to this class of agent during pregnancy or lactation. However, the best practice for each patient must be individualized, and some evidence suggests that serum lithium concentration may be low and well tolerated in nursing infants.

A case of a 34-year-old breastfeeding woman on lithium for bipolar disorder highlights this. The woman initially decided to continue lithium therapy during pregnancy and after delivery. While breastfeeding and taking 600 mg lithium daily, the mother's lithium level was low (0.45 mEq/L), but the infant's lithium level was 0.26 mEq/L at day 10 of life. The treating provider and patient elected to try two different atypical antipsychotics (quetiapine and aripiprazole) in place of lithium. However, the patient experienced intolerable sedation with quetiapine during the first antipsychotic trial and a marked decrease in milk supply with aripiprazole during the second antipsychotic trial. Based on these intolerable side effects, the patient eventually decided to restart lithium. The infant was closely monitored during breastfeeding, and no adverse effects were observed [34A].

SUSCEPTIBILITY FACTORS

R A retrospective cohort study using a laboratory information system was conducted by Shine and colleagues to determine the incidence of lithium-induced thyroid and parathyroid dysfunction along with any associated risk factors. The study included adult patients (≥18 years) who had at least two measurements of serum creatinine, thyrotropin, calcium, glycated hemoglobin (HbA_{1C}), or lithium levels between October 1st, 1985 and March 31st, 2014. Patients with documented lithium levels (≥2 detectable measurements) were categorized as the lithium-exposed group (n=2795), and all other patients of the same sex and age group without lithium measurements were considered non-exposed controls (n=689228). Cox proportional hazards analyses were performed and adjusted for age (< or ≥60 years), sex and diabetes covariates. Lithium exposure was significantly associated with the development of stage three chronic kidney disease (HR 1.93; 95% CI 1.76–2.12), hypothyroidism (HR 2.31; 95% CI 2.05–2.60) and high total calcium concentration (HR 1.43; 95% CI 1.21–1.69), but not the development of hyperthyroidism (HR 1.22; 95% CI 0.96–1.55) or high adjusted calcium concentration (HR 1.08; 95% CI 0.88–1.34). The effect of lithium exposure on development of hypothyroidism was seen in all four age/sex subgroups, but *the largest effect was in younger women (HR 2.37; 95% CI 2.10–2.69), who were also most susceptible to stage three chronic kidney disease (HR 2.05; 95% CI 1.86–2.25). Serum lithium concentrations higher than the median (>0.6 mEq/L) were associated with stage three chronic kidney disease (HR 1.62; 95% CI 1.41–1.85), hypothyroidism (HR 1.62; 95% CI 1.35–1.94), hyperthyroidism (HR 1.88; 95% CI 1.33–2.66) high total serum calcium (HR 1.54; 95% CI 1.22–1.95) and high adjusted serum calcium concentrations (HR 2.05; 95% CI 1.54–2.72). The study results indicated that the younger women subgroup and patients with high serum lithium concentrations were more likely to develop lithium-induced hypothyroidism and chronic kidney disease. The older women subgroup was more likely to develop lithium-induced high total serum calcium (HR 1.92; 95% CI 1.58–2.33) and high adjusted serum calcium concentrations (HR 1.39; 95% CI 1.13–1.71) [24MC].*

Bocchetta and colleagues conducted a study to evaluate the effects of glomerular filtration rate in patients who were treated with lithium for up to 33 years ($n = 953$). All lithium patients registered from 1980 to 2012 at an Italian clinic were screened for enrollment, and estimated glomerular filtration rate (eGFR) was calculated from serum creatinine concentration using the MDRD Study Group equation. In the cross-sectional data analysis, the eGFR was found to be lower in women (by 3.47 mL/min/1.73 m^2), older patients (0.73 mL/min/1.73 m^2 per year of age), and in patients with longer duration of lithium treatment (0.73 mL/min/1.73 m^2 per year). The longitudinal data showed that the median time lithium taken for patients to decline to eGFR lower than 60 mL/min/1.73 m^2 and 45 mL/min/1.73 m^2 was 25 years and 31 years, respectively. This study concluded that the duration of lithium treatment and age are risk factors for reduced renal function [35C].

MECHANISM OF ADR

The mechanisms of both the therapeutic and adverse effects of lithium are not entirely clear, despite its many years of use. Petersein and colleagues evaluated lithium with antidepressants and found lithium to enhance pro-excitatory cytokine production (IL-1β, IL-2, IL-6, IL-17 and TNF-a), a new finding previously unreported. Therefore, lithium's pro-inflammatory effects may potentially explain autoimmune adverse effects like cutaneous skin reactions and Hashimoto thyroiditis [36c].

DIAGNOSIS OF ADVERSE DRUG REACTIONS

Laboratory parameters such as serum creatinine have traditionally been used to assess patient's renal function. There is evidence that microcyst formation in the kidneys may cause the decreased glomerular filtration rate and subsequent increase in serum creatinine measured in lithium-related end-stage renal disease. The microcysts increase in number over time before the actual elevation in creatinine occurs, and there is an inverse relationship between the size of cysts and the GFR of the patient. Lithium-associated cysts tend to be equally distributed throughout the kidney, and T2-weighted MRI may be effective in detecting the presence of microcysts ≥0.9 mm. Additional research is needed to determine the optimal interval of imaging, manner of quantifying the microcyst volume or density and its quantitative relationship with GFR decline [37R].

Researchers recently reported on the use of MRI in the diagnosis of lithium-induced nephropathy. This was used in the case of a 66-year-old female on lithium therapy for bipolar disorder for 28 years. She developed renal impairment (eGFR 30 mL/min/1.73 m^2) and hypercalcemia (serum Ca = 2.86 mEq/L). Electrocardiogram and urinalysis were normal. Coronal T2-weighted MRI showed normal kidney size and 2–3 mm microcysts throughout both kidneys that were indicative of chronic lithium-induced nephropathy. The authors concluded that MRI is superior to ultrasound in diagnosing this adverse effect. Usually, symmetric uniform corticomedullary microcysts are found bilaterally, and in the presence of long-term lithium use, are indicative of lithium-related nephropathy [38A].

References

[1] Yatham LN, Kennedy SH, Parikh SV, et al. Canadian Network for Mood and Anxiety Treatments (CANMAT) and International Society for Bipolar Disorders (ISBD) collaborative update of CANMAT guidelines for the management of patients with bipolar disorder: update 2013. Bipolar Disord. 2013;15:1–44 [R].

[2] National Institute for Health and Care Excellence (NICE). Bipolar disorder: the assessment and management of bipolar disorder in adults, children and young people in primary and secondary care (CG185), Available from, https://www.nice.org.uk/guidance/cg185; 2016. Published September 2014. Updated February 2016. Accessed February 28, 2016 [R].

[3] American Psychiatric Association. Practice guideline for the treatment of patients with bipolar disorder. 2nd ed; Available from, http://psychiatryonline.org/pb/assets/raw/sitewide/practice_guidelines/guidelines/bipolar.pdf. Accessed February 28, 2016 [R].

[4] Bauer M, Adli M, Ricken R, et al. Role of lithium augmentation in the management of major depressive disorder. CNS Drugs. 2014;28:331–42 [R].

[5] Cipriani A, Hawton K, Stockton S, et al. Lithium in the prevention of suicide in mood disorders: updated systematic review and meta-analysis. BMJ. 2013;346:f3646 [M].

[6] Marmol F. Lithium: bipolar disorder and neurodegenerative diseases. Possible cellular mechanisms of the therapeutic effects of lithium. Prog Neuropsychopharmacol Biol Psychiatry. 2008;32:1761–71 [H].

[7] Jollant F. Add-on lithium for the treatment of unipolar depression: too often forgotten? J Psychiatry Neurosci. 2015;40(1):E23–4 [A].

[8] Zhou X, Ravindran AV, Qin B, et al. Comparative efficacy, acceptability, and tolerability of augmentation agents in treatment-resistant depression: systematic review and network meta-analysis. J Clin Psychiatry. 2015;76(4):e487–98 [R].

[9] Vazquez GH, Holtzman JN, Tondo L, et al. Efficacy and tolerability of treatments for bipolar depression. J Affect Disord. 2015;183:258–62 [R].

[10] Malhi GS. Lithium therapy in bipolar disorder: a balancing act? Lancet. 2015;386(9992):415–6 [r].

[11] Mertens J, Wang QW, Kim Y, et al. Differential responses to lithium in hyperexcitable neurons from patients with bipolar disorder. Nature. 2015;527(7576):95–9 [E].

[12] Narayanan MA, Haddad TM, Bansal O, et al. Acute cardiomyopathy precipitated by lithium: is there a direct toxic effect on cardiac myocytes? Am J Emerg Med. 2015;33(9):1330. e1–5 [A].

[13] Galvez V, Hadzi-Pavlovic D, Smith D, et al. Predictors of seizure threshold in right unilateral ultrabrief electroconvulsive therapy: role of concomitant medications and anaesthesia used. Brain Stimul. 2015;8(3):486–92 [C].

[14] Riepe MW, Walther B, Vonend C, et al. Drug-induced cerebral glucose metabolism resembling Alzheimer's disease: a case study. BMC Psychiatry. 2015;15:157 [A].

[15] Soriano-Barcelo J, Alonso MT, Traba MB, et al. A case with reversible neurotoxicity after 2 years of dementia secondary to maintenance lithium treatment. J Psychiatr Pract. 2015;21(2):154–9 [A].

[16] Fitzgerald RT, Fitzgerald CT, Samant RS, et al. Lithium toxicity and PRES: a novel association. J Neuroimaging. 2015;25(1):147–9 [A].

[17] Vandewalle W, Boon E, Sienaert P. Movement disorders due to modern antidepressants and mood stabilizers. Tijdschr Psychiatr. 2015;57(2):132–7 [R].

[18] Cobb A, Messerli A, Klingeman H, et al. A rare complication of lithium toxicity. Minn Med. 2015;98(8):42 [A].

[19] Monden MA, Nederkoorn PJ, Tijsma M. Downbeat nystagmus—a rare side-effect of lithium carbonate. Tijdschr Psychiatr. 2015;57(1):49–53 [A].

[20] Yeh MW, Ituarte PH, Zhou HC, et al. Incidence and prevalence of primary hyperparathyroidism in a racially mixed population. J Clin Endocrinol Metab. 2013;98:1122–9 [MC].

[21] Albert U, De Cori D, Aguglia A, et al. Lithium-associated hyperparathyroidism and hypercalcaemia: a case–control cross-sectional study. J Affect Disord. 2013;151:786–90 [C].

[22] Shapiro HI, Davis KA. Hypercalcemia and "primary" hyperparathyroidism during lithium therapy. Am J Psychiatry. 2015;172(1):12–5 [A].

[23] De Sousa GW, Dutra PE, Higa RA, et al. Hyperthyroid rage: when bipolar disorder hides the real disorder. Clin Neuropharmacol. 2015;38(1):38–9 [A].

[24] Shine B, McKnight RF, Leaver L, et al. Long-term effects of lithium on renal, thyroid, and parathyroid function: a retrospective analysis of laboratory data. Lancet. 2015;386(9992):461–8 [MC].

[25] Aprahamian I, Santos FD, dos Santos B, et al. Long-term, low-dose lithium treatment does not impair renal function in the elderly: a 2-year randomized, placebo-controlled trial followed by single-blind extension. J Clin Psychiatry. 2014;75(7):e672–8 [c].

[26] Lozano R. Renal toxicity of long-term lithium treatment for mild cognitive impairment. J Clin Psychiatry. 2015;76(2):e232 [r].

[27] Aprahamian I, Forlenza OV. Drs. Aprahamian and Forlenza reply. J Clin Psychiatry. 2015;76(2):e232–3 [r].

[28] Wang XQ, Xiong J, Xu WH, et al. Risk of a lamotrigine-related skin rash: current meta-analysis and postmarketing cohort analysis. Seizure. 2015;25:52–61 [M].

[29] Quan W, Wang H, Jia F, et al. Purpura associated with lithium intoxication. Chin Med J (Engl). 2015;128(2):284 [A].

[30] Nascimento BA, Carvalho AH, Dias CM, et al. A case of generalized ostraceous psoriasis mimicking dermatitis neglecta. An Bras Dermatol. 2015;90(Suppl 1):197–9 [A].

[31] Grover S, Ghosh A, Sarkar S, et al. Sexual dysfunction in clinically stable patients with bipolar disorder receiving lithium. J Clin Psychopharmacol. 2014;34(4):475–82 [C].

[32] Elnazer HY, Sampson A, Baldwin D. Lithium and sexual dysfunction: an under-researched area. Hum Psychopharmacol. 2015;30(2):66–9 [R].

[33] Harari F, Langeen M, Casimiro E, et al. Environmental exposure to lithium during pregnancy and fetal size: a longitudinal study in the Argentinean Andes. Environ Int. 2015;77:48–54 [C].

[34] Frew JR. Psychopharmacology of bipolar I disorder during lactation: a case report of the use of lithium and aripiprazole in a nursing mother. Arch Womens Ment Health. 2015;18(1):135–6 [A].

[35] Bocchetta A, Ardau R, Fanni T, et al. Renal function during long-term lithium treatment: a cross-sectional and longitudinal study. BMC Med. 2015;13:12 [C].

[36] Petersein C, Sack U, Mergl R, et al. Impact of lithium alone and in combination with antidepressants on cytokine production in vitro. J Neural Transm (Vienna). 2015;122(1):109–22 [c].

[37] Khan M, El-Mallakh RS. Renal microcysts and lithium. Int J Psychiatry Med. 2015;50(3):290–8 [R].

[38] Judge PK, Winearls CG. The utility of magnetic resonance imaging in the diagnosis of chronic lithium nephropathy. QJM. 2015;108(1):75–6 [A].

4

Hypnotics and Sedatives

Tina C. Lee[1]

University of the Incarnate Word Feik School of Pharmacy, San Antonio, TX, USA
[1]Corresponding author: tclee@uiwtx.edu

BENZODIAZEPINES

Midazolam

Immunologic

An anaphylactoid-like reaction to midazolam during oral and maxillofacial surgery was reported in early 2015 [1A]. A 59-year-old woman weighing 56 kg experienced hypotension, bronchoconstriction, and edema during a tumor resection of the right mandible. She has a history of allergies to several antibiotics (did not specify which antibiotics) and contrast dye for CT scans. Due to her allergy history, it was discussed and consented to not use thiopental or other histamine-releasing anesthetics. She was given a test dose of midazolam (0.01 mg/kg) prior to the anesthesia induction. Then she was given 5 mg (0.1 mg/kg) and her systolic blood pressure suddenly dropped to 65 mmHg, with widespread flushing across her body and eyelid edema. She was given 50 mcg of epinephrine and 1000 mg IV methylprednisolone. She experienced ischemic ST depression in lead II; therefore, she received continuous infusion of dopamine and nitroglycerin for 30 minutes. The surgery was postponed for 1 week where she received H_1 and H_2 antagonist using sevoflurane plus nitrous oxide, and oxygen with atropine sulfate after a test dose. This anesthetic technique was used on the patient at different hospitals for previous surgeries without any reactions.

The authors concluded that we should consider anaphylactoid reactions with midazolam in patients with a history of multiple drug allergies, but they did not discuss the possible mechanism of action of the anaphylactoid reaction.

Pediatric

A case report was published about unpredictable drug reaction in children with Cornelia de Lange Syndrome, a genetic condition that can lead to severe developmental abnormalities [2A].

A 3-year-old girl weighing 9 kg with the Cornelia de Lange Syndrome had a fundoplication and gastrostomy under general anesthesia. Prior to the procedure, all laboratory analysis was normal, and she had no allergies or reactions to medications. The only medication she received prior to the start of the procedure due to extreme anxiety was midazolam 0.5 mg/kg. Approximately 10 minutes later, she stopped breathing and had to be intubated. There were no signs of symptoms that this was an anaphylactic reaction to midazolam. The authors report of another child with Cornelia de Lange Syndrome was sedated for a different procedure but did not use midazolam due to the case reported above. This child had no adverse events during the sedation or procedure using atropine (premedication), fentanyl, propofol, and vecuronium. Children with Cornelia De Lange Syndrome have had reactions to haloperidol and chlorpromazine reported, but this is the first report for midazolam.

HYPNOSEDATIVE

Death

Previous reports have been published finding an association between increased risk of mortality and exposure to hypnotics, even after adjusting for confounders, while other studies found no association. A study using the Norwegian Pharmacy Database examined to find a confounding factor that previous studies did not account for: terminal illness, as an explanation for increased mortality and exposure to hypnotics [3c]. This cohort found that people exposed to taking hypnotics had increased risk of mortality than the control group (OR 2.3). However, there was an increased exposure to the hypnotics in older patients with closer proximity of death, where almost half of the people were exposed to hypnotics within 2 months of their death. The authors concluded that the association of hypnotics and mortality may be confounded by symptomatic treatment of terminal illness rather than a causal relationship.

Zaleplon

Psychological

A 43-year-old male with schizophrenia developed anemsic somnambulism after taking zaleplon [4A]. The patient was lost to follow up without any psychiatric medications for 4 years. He has no other medical history besides schizophrenia. When he was restarted on his risperidone and zaleplon, he experienced somnambulism with eating after taking zaleplon. After discontinuing zaleplon, somnambulism disappeared. He was later hospitalized for psychosis and was accidently given zaleplon in the hospital. A repeat of somnambulism with eating occurred in the hospital. This is the first case of somnambulism that has occurred after taking zaleplon without a prior history of somnambulism.

Zolpidem

Central Nervous System

In 2015, a study completed in Taiwan evaluated the association between zolpidem and all forms of dementia, non-Alzheimer disease, and Alzheimer disease [5C]. It was a population-based case–control study using data from the Taiwan National Health Insurance Research Database (NHIRD). The case group had to be >65 years old and diagnosed with ICD-9 codes for dementia or Alzheimer disease from 2006 to 2010. Diagnosis of Alzheimer disease came from board certified neurologists and had to meet other specific criteria for causes of declined cognitive function. The control group were people in the database without the diagnosis of dementia and matched to the case group. The biggest risk factor was zolpidem exposure. A total of 8406 patient files were identified for the case group and 16 812 for the control group. The dementia subjects had longer exposure to zolpidem compared to the control group (302.8 days vs 345.1 days, $p = 0.001$). After adjusting for confounders such as age, sex, and different comorbidities such as coronary artery disease, diabetes, and stroke, the association between zolpidem use and dementia was statistically significant (adjusted OR: 1.33, CI: 1.24–1.41; $p < 0.0001$) except not in the Alzheimer's group (adjusted OR: 1.17; CI: 0.9–1.54; $p = 0.241$). The binding of zolpidem to α1 subunit of the $GABA_A$ receptor causes cognitive function. As the brain ages, there are more of these binding units, and it is believed that this may put the elderly population at an increased risk of non-Alzheimer's dementia.

Central Nervous System

Previous studies have reported of short-term use of zolpidem improving motor symptoms in patients with Parkinson's disease. A study was conducted using the Taiwan National Health Insurance Program database to determine if zolpidem affects the risk of developing Parkinson's disease [6C]. This study had a longer follow-up period (3 months to 10 years). The database identified 2961 subjects taking zolpidem for more than 3 months in 1998–2000 and developed Parkinson's disease. When the data were stratified based on age, sex, or duration of follow-up, the subjects that used zolpidem had a higher incidence of Parkinson's disease than the control subjects (6.48 vs 2.29 per 1000 person years; incidence density rate ratio (IRR) 2.82; CI: 2.31–3.45). The incidence of Parkinson's disease was 4% higher in the zolpidem cohort than control after a 12-year follow-up period ($p < 0.0001$). However, the impact of zolpidem and the increased risk of Parkinson's disease were seen in the younger cohort (<55 years old) than the older cohort of zolpidem users. But this difference between the age groups was non-significant after 5-year follow-up. It is unclear why the difference is non-significant after 5 years. Having a psychiatric comorbidity such as depression also increased the risk of Parkinson's disease in the zolpidem cohort (HR 4.79; CI: 3.43–6.69). There also appeared to have a dose-dependent relationship with low dose (<400 mg of zolpidem per year) HR = 0.7 (CI: 0.43–1.13) vs high dose (>1600 mg of zolpidem per year) HR = 2.94 (CI: 2.14–4.05). Despite other studies that discuss the improvement of symptoms with short-term use of zolpidem, the authors wonder if larger doses may result in worse motor control, leading to an earlier diagnosis of Parkinson's disease. More studies are necessary to analyze the long-term use of zolpidem and the increased risk of Parkinson's disease.

Liver

Again in Taiwan, a population-based case–control study was completed examining the association between the use of zolpidem and pyogenic liver abscess [7C]. The Taiwan National Health Insurance Program database was used to identify inpatient claims for the first attack of pyogenic liver abscess using the ICD-9 code during 2000–2011. For each case of pyogenic liver abscess patient, four control patients without abscess were matched to be the control group. Patients with a history of a benzodiazepine prescription were included in the study, but other nonbenzodiazepine hypnotics such as zopiclone, zaleplon, and eszopiclone were excluded. Based on the pharmacokinetic properties of zolpidem, the definition of current zolpidem use was last tablet of zolpidem used less than 7 days of admission for pyogenic liver abscess while greater than 7 days was considered late zolpidem use. Logistic regression adjusted for possible confounders showed a statistically significant adjusted odds ratio of pyogenic liver abscess to be 3.89 with current zolpidem use (95% CI 2.89–5.23) when comparing to patients that never used zolpidem. There was a non-statistical significant adjusted OR when comparing late zolpidem use vs nonusers of 0.85 (95% CI 0.7–1.03). However, this study also showed that benzodiazepines, biliary stone, and diabetes also were other statistically significant factors associated with pyogenic liver abscess. Both the low dose ($\leq$10 mg) and high dose (>10 mg) of zolpidem had significant adjusted OR associated with the abscess (low dose: adjusted OR: 2.13; CI: 1.46–3.1; high dose: adjusted OR: 13.8; CI: 7.6–25.1). Due to data showing that current zolpidem users had the statistical association of pyogenic abscess compared to late users of zolpidem, the authors concluded that only in subjects, actively using zolpidem had an increased risk of developing a pyogenic liver abscess.

Pancreas

In December 2014, a study from Taiwan was published evaluating the association between zolpidem use and acute pancreatitis [8C]. Since 2001–2012, the US Food and Drug Administration (FDA) have reported 81 cases of pancreatitis in people taking zolpidem (usually within 1 month of zolpidem use). Using the Taiwan National Health Insurance Program database and ICD-9 code for acute pancreatitis, patients were identified. Results showed that 4535 cases of acute pancreatitis from 2000 to 2011 that matched with 18 140 control subjects. After adjusting for confounding factors, the adjusted OR for acute pancreatitis for zolpidem users was 7.2 (CI 5.81–8.92) compared to subjects that never used zolpidem. However, when stratifying early zolpidem use (last used zolpidem 8–14 days prior to pancreatitis diagnosis) and late use of zolpidem (last used zolpidem within 7 days of pancreatitis), there was no statistical difference. Analysis was completed looking at different comorbidities and immediate use of zolpidem. Subjects that did not have comorbidities that can cause pancreatitis (alcoholism, diabetes, biliary stones, hepatitis B and C, hypertriglyceridemia) and used zolpidem within 7 days of pancreatitis had an OR 18.04, but in subjects with at least one of these comorbidities and used zolpidem within 7 days, the OR increased to 30.32 (CI 23.71–38.79). Low ($\leq$10 mg) and high doses (>10 mg) of zolpidem showed increased risk of pancreatitis, but the high dose group had a higher OR (8.70 vs 6.76).

The authors hypothesize that zolpidem may have a direct toxic effect on the pancreas. Due to the short pharmacokinetic properties of zolpidem, subjects not taking zolpidem actively may not have seen a statistical significant risk of pancreatitis as the medication is no longer in the body. The risk also appears to be dose-dependent with daily doses >10 mg having higher risk of acute pancreatitis.

Zolpidem and Zopiclone

Nervous System

In Japan, a case report was published about a drug-induced hemichorea in a 92-year-old female after taking zolpidem (10 mg/day) and zopiclone (7.5 mg/day) every night for 2 weeks [9A]. She had an 8-day history of involuntary movement of her right-sided upper and lower extremities (unilateral). Her only past medical history was for hypertension, and no conditions involving her central nervous system. All images and laboratory studies were normal. Physical exam showed intractable right-sided unilateral hemichorea, and the rest of her exam was unremarkable. Zolpidem and zopiclone were discontinued, and the patient received tiapride for a few days. Her symptoms gradually disappeared the next few days.

SEDATIVES

Fentanyl

Pediatric

NERVOUS SYSTEM

A retrospective cohort study conducted on preterm infants born between 23 and 30 weeks gestation with the purpose to examine the association between cumulative fentanyl dose and brain injury and diameters using MRI scans [10c]. Data were collected on total exposure to all sedative and/or analgesic agents the first week of life and from birth until term equivalent age or prior to discharge from the NICU. Weight and occipitofrontal circumference were also recorded at birth and prior to the MRI to evaluate body and head growth. One hundred and thirty-three infants were identified, but thirty infants did not get an MRI due to death prior to scan, transfer to different NICU, or parental refusal. The demographic characteristics were similar between the infants. The most common sedative/analgesic medication used on the infants was fentanyl, with 78 infants (76%) receiving the medication before term equivalent age with the median cumulative dose of 3 micrograms/kg. Less than half of the infants identified survived without brain injury. There was a statistical significant of lower survival without brain injury in infants exposed with higher cumulative doses of fentanyl (OR 0.5; CI 0.4–0.7, $p < 0.001$). There was no statistical significant between the fentanyl doses and incidence of severe intraventricular hemorrhage or white matter injury. However, after correcting for covariates, there was a significant increase of cerebellar hemorrhage (OR 2.1, CI 1.1–4.1, $p = 0.002$) during the first week of life. Fentanyl dose before term equivalent age was also significant for reduction in transverse cerebellar diameter, including hemorrhage presence ($r^2 = 0.461$, $p = 0.002$). For infants that survived and adjusting for gestational age at birth, there was no significant difference seen for different developmental testing at 2 years old.

Nitrous Oxide

Pediatric

RESPIRATORY

A case report of laryngospasm with nitrous oxide on a 16-month old boy was reported in late 2015. The child had a 2 cm laceration to the left eyebrow from an unwitnessed fall [11A]. He had no medical history, no medical allergies, and no recent respiratory infections. He was fasted of food and fluids for 4 hours prior to the sedation. His baseline oxygen saturation was 99%. He went into a deep sedation using nitrous oxide at concentrations from 0% to 70%. After 7 minutes since the start of nitrous oxide, he started gagging, gulping with dry heaving without overt vomiting or stridor. His oxygen saturation dropped to 70% and had visible cyanosis. On exam, there was no air entry on auscultation with visible chest wall movement. There was no change in his status with airway realignment with jaw thrusts, chin lift, or suctioning. Doctors applied positive airway pressure with 100% oxygen, and then he started to cough and cry. Auscultation now had bilateral rales, while his O_2 sats remained at 90% with supplemental oxygen. His chest X-ray showed upper bilateral infiltrates. He received oral antibiotics and was discharged the next day. Laryngospasm has been seen with ketamine and rarely propofol, but this may be the first report from nitrous oxide.

Propofol

Respiratory

In Texas, a case report was published reporting acute pulmonary edema associated with the use of propofol [12A]. The patient was a 23-year-old male that presented to the ED after a work-related injury to his left food. He was a healthy male with no past medical history, allergies, or any medications or illicit drug use. Routine labs showed everything was in normal limits when presenting to the ED. Due to the patient's low pain tolerance, analgesia and sedation were requested prior to manipulation of the injured foot (nondisplaced proximal third metatarsal fracture). To put his foot in a splint, meperidine 75 mg and IV propofol 75 mg aliquots up to a total of 359 mg over 1 hour were used. He tolerated the procedure well and had continuous cardiopulmonary monitoring. About an hour after the procedure, the patient was awake and alert, saturating at 96% on room air. However, 10 minutes later, the patient developed an acute cough with moderate quantity hemoptysis and SpO_2 saturation dropping to 80% (HR 95 bpm, RR 18 bpm, BP: 128/70). Four liters per minute of supplemental oxygen was started to bring SpO_2 to 90%. His physical exam revealed bilateral crackles in both lung fields with normal heart sounds. His chest X-ray showed patchy bilateral infiltrates that were confirmed by CT scan. Diagnostic studies were ordered to determine the cause of his hypoxia including D-Dimer, troponin I assays, and coagulation profile. The patient was admitted to the telemetry floor and started on IV antibiotics and IV furosemide (40 mg IV every 6 hours). During his admission, he was worked up for various fungal infections, TB, HIV infections, sputum and blood cultures, that all resulted in a negative test result. His chest X-ray 2 days later showed near resolution of the infiltrates and was discharged home in stable, asymptomatic condition.

The authors ruled out other causes of the pulmonary edema. Negative pressure pulmonary edema was unlikely the cause as there was no airway compromise during propofol administration and the constant monitoring afterwards. Assays showed there was no myocardial damage or cardiac dysfunction, thus, ruing out cardiogenic pulmonary edema. There are no reports of meperidine causing pulmonary edema in the literature, although there are reports of opiate-related pulmonary edema. There are few cases of propofol-associated pulmonary edema in the literature that occurred within 30 minutes to 1 hour and had varying degrees of severity in hypoxic or hypercarbic respiratory failure. It is thought the cause of this pulmonary edema may be from the diisopropyl chain and phenol group in propofol that can cause allergic reactions. An anaphylactic reaction may have cause vasodilation to allow for significant edema in the lungs. More studies are necessary to examine the epidemiology, mechanisms, and preventive measures for propofol-associated pulmonary edema.

References

[1] Ayuse T, Kurata S, Ayuse T. Anaphylactoid-like reaction to midazolam during oral and maxillofacial surgery. Anesth Prog. 2015;62:64–5 [A].

[2] Stevic M, Milojevic I, Bokun Z, et al. Unpredictable drug reaction in a child with Cornelia de Lange syndrome. Int J Clin Pharm. 2015;37:1–3 [A].

[3] Neutel CI, Johansen HL. Association between hypnotics use and increased mortality: causation or confounding? Eur J Clin Pharmacol. 2015;71:637–42 [c].

[4] Chen YW, Tseng PT, Wu CK, et al. Zaleplon-induced anemsic somnambulism with eating behaviors under once dose. Acta Neurol Taiwan. 2014;23:143–5 [A].

[5] Shih HI, Lin CC, Tu YF, et al. An increased risk of reversible dementia may occur after zolpidem derivative use in the elderly population. Medicine. 2015;94(17):e809. http://dx.doi.org/10.1097/MD.0000000000000809 [C].

[6] Huang HC, Tsai CH, Muo CH, et al. Risk of Parkinson's disease following zolpidem use: a retrospective, population-based cohort study. J Clin Psychiatry. 2015;76(1):e104–10 [C].

[7] Liao KF, Lin CL, Lai SW, et al. Zolpidem use associated with increased risk of pyogenic liver abscess. Medicine. 2015;94(32):e1302. http://dx.doi.org/10.1097/MD.0000000000001302 [C].

[8] Lai SW, Lin CL, Liao KF. Increased relative risks of acute pancreatitis in zolpidem users. Psychopharmacology. 2015;232:2043–8 [C].

[9] Watari T, Tokuda Y. Drug-induced hemichorea. BMJ Case Rep. 2015; http://dx.doi.org/10.1136/bcr-2014-208872 [A].

[10] McPherson C, Haslam M, Pineda R, et al. Brain injury and development in preterm infants exposed to fentanyl. Ann Pharmacother. 2015;49(12):1291–7 [c].

[11] Babl FE, Grindlay J, Barrett MJ. Laryngospasm with apparent aspiration during sedation with nitrous oxide. Ann Emerg Med. 2015;66:475–8 [A].

[12] Waheed MA, Oud L. Acute pulmonary edema associated with propofol: an unusual complication. West J Emerg Med. 2014;15(7):845–8 [A].

5

Antipsychotic Drugs

P. Chue*,[1], J. Chue[†]

*University of Alberta, Edmonton, AB, Canada
[†]Clinical Trials and Research Program, Edmonton, AB, Canada
[1]Corresponding author: pchue@ualberta.ca

GENERAL [SEDA-15, 2438; SEDA-32, 83; SEDA-33, 89; SEDA-34, 51; SEDA-35, 85; SEDA-36, 59; SEDA-37, 63]

Comparative Studies

A 12-week, randomised study ($n = 198$) of first episode patients (FEP) with schizophrenia (15–40 years) comparing aripiprazole and risperidone found that there was more *akathisia* with aripiprazole; and higher *total* and *LDL-cholesterol, fasting glucose,* and *prolactin* levels with risperidone [1C].

In a 13-week study ($n = 22$) of antipsychotic (AP)-naive, FEP were treated with either risperidone long-acting injection (LAI) or flupenthixol decanoate over 13 weeks and compared to matched healthy controls [2c]. There were significant group × time interactions for the ventral diencephalon volumes that correlated bilaterally with *BMI increase* and *HDL-cholesterol reductions*, and unilaterally with *glucose elevation*.

A 14-week study ($n = 50$) of AP-naive schizophrenia patients found that olanzapine was associated with significant *glucose elevation*, in comparison to risperidone, aripiprazole, haloperidol and healthy controls [3c]. Risperidone-, aripiprazole- and haloperidol-treated groups had *glucose elevations* only in excess to healthy controls.

An 8-week, double-blind, randomised study ($n = 126$) in schizophrenia compared blonanserin (8–24 mg/day) to risperidone (2–6 mg/day) and found risperidone was associated with *elevated prolactin* and *cardiac-related abnormalities*, while blonanserin was associated with more *extra-pyramidal symptoms* (*EPS*) [4C].

A Chinese study ($n = 42$) of treatment of methamphetamine-associated psychosis found significantly *higher discontinuation* rates and *greater akathisia* and *agitation* with aripiprazole, than for risperidone [5c].

A Korean, retrospective, propensity score-matched cohort study ($n = 14\,103$) found a substantially increased risk for haloperidol in the elderly for the risk of *ischemic stroke*, compared with risperidone [6C].

Observational Studies

A 1-year, naturalistic, longitudinal study ($n = 37$) in children and adolescents (2–18 years) without prior exposure to second-generation APs (SGAs) found that mean weight increased significantly (10.8 kg for risperidone, 9.7 kg for quetiapine) [7c]. Body mass index (BMI) z scores also increased significantly for both; obesity developed in 40.0% of patients on risperidone and 50.0% on quetiapine, with a significant increase in mean levels of fasting *glucose* with risperidone and a significant increase in total *cholesterol: HDL-cholesterol* with quetiapine.

A 12-week, non randomised, prospective study ($n = 342$) of adolescents found that 15.2% developed *EPS* (quetiapine = 1.5%, olanzapine = 13.8%, risperidone = 16.1%, ziprasidone = 20.0%, and aripiprazole = 27.3%) [8C]. Rates of *EPS* were significantly lower only for quetiapine and olanzapine; *anticholinergic* initiation was most frequent with risperidone, while rates of *dyskinesia* were higher with olanzapine and ziprasidone.

A 1-year, multicentre, observational study ($n = 285$) of a naive and quasi-naive pediatric population found a higher risk of *dyskinesia* with risperidone, and *EPS* with risperidone and olanzapine, compared with quetiapine [9C].

A 12-week study ($n = 22$) in children and adolescents with bipolar disorder and conduct disorder found *BMI* and *prolactin* increased significantly with risperidone, compared with quetiapine [10c].

A retrospective, cohort study of Medicaid-enrolled youths found that the risk for incident *diabetes mellitus* (*DM*) was increased in those initiated on SGAs

($n = 107\,551$) vs. controls ($n = 1\,221\,434$) [11MC]. Compared with a risperidone reference group, *DM* risk was higher among those initiating ziprasidone and aripiprazole, but not quetiapine or olanzapine.

An effectiveness study comparing risperidone LAI to first-generation AP (FGA) LAIs (flupenthixol decanoate, haloperidol decanoate) found that there was more *anticholinergic* and *benzodiazepine* use with FGA-LAIs [12c].

A Chinese study ($n = 285$) of FEP found higher mean *UKU neurological subscores* with haloperidol than olanzapine or amisulpride; and risperidone was associated with higher mean *Barnes Akathisia Rating Scale (BARS) total scores* than olanzapine, amisulpride or sulpiride [13C].

A US database study of adults (18–79 years) treated with SGAs found that 7.7–17.0% experienced $\geq 7\%$ *weight gain* (average *weight gain* = 10 kg); olanzapine was most commonly associated with *weight gain* and ziprasidone the least [14C].

An analysis of the FDA Adverse Event Reporting System (FAERS) for children (1997–2011) found that signal scores for *neuroleptic malignant syndrome (NMS)* were greater for haloperidol and aripiprazole; *QT prolongation* for ziprasidone and risperidone; *leukopenia* for clozapine; and *suicide attempt* for haloperidol, olanzapine, quetiapine, risperidone, and aripiprazole [15MC].

Systematic Reviews

A meta-analysis of SGAs in the treatment of delirium found that SGAs (amisulpride, olanzapine, quetiapine, risperidone, ziprasidone) were associated with a lower incidence of *EPS* compared with haloperidol [16M]. Another systematic review of APs in delirium found a greater and dose-dependent risk of *akathisia* with haloperidol for the FGAs, and with paliperidone and ziprasidone for the SGAs [17M].

A meta-analysis (23 studies, $n = 5819$) of the use of SGAs (aripiprazole, risperidone, olanzapine, quetiapine) in dementia found significantly higher risks for *somnolence, urinary tract infection, edema* and *abnormal gait,* but not falls, injuries or death vs. placebo [18M].

A meta-analysis (41 studies) of children and young adults (<24 years) found APs to be associated with *adverse glucose metabolism* changes (greatest with olanzapine, followed by quetiapine, aripiprazole and risperidone) [19M]. The prevalence and incidence of *DM* were also greater with APs than in healthy and psychiatric controls. A second meta-analysis of the use of APs (risperidone, aripiprazole, haloperidol, olanzapine) in children with intellectual disability found an association with *elevated prolactin* levels and *weight gain* [20M]. A third meta-analysis (55 studies, $n = 5423$) of antipsychotics in youth <18 years found that risperidone (within group) and ziprasidone (within group and vs. placebo) significantly *increased QTc* [21M].

A systematic review of antipsychotic polypharmacy found an *increased QTc prolongation* risk with clozapine when combined with sertindole or ziprasidone [22M].

A meta-analysis of FEP found an approximately twofold greater risk of *weight gain* with AP use except with ziprasidone; olanzapine and clozapine caused the highest *weight gain* compared to placebo [23M].

A literature review of SGAs in acute bipolar depression reported that olanzapine monotherapy, quetiapine-IR, quetiapine-XR, aripiprazole, and ziprasidone had significantly increased risk for *AEs* with *NNHs* of 24, 8–14, 9, 12, and 10, respectively [24r]. For *somnolence,* quetiapine-XR had the smallest *Number Needed to Harm (NNH)* of 4. For *weight gain* ($\geq 7\%$), olanzapine monotherapy and olanzapine in combination with fluoxetine had the smallest *NNHs* of 5 for both. For *akathisia,* aripiprazole had the smallest NNH of 5.

A literature review of SGAs and *weight gain* found that clozapine and olanzapine were highest risk; amisulpride, asenapine, iloperidone, paliperidone, quetiapine, risperidone and sertindole were intermediate risk; and aripiprazole, lurasidone and ziprasidone were lowest risk [25r]. Another literature review in early onset schizophrenia found that olanzapine caused the most significant *weight gain* [26r].

CARDIOVASCULAR

A prospective study of treatment-naïve, Danish elderly ($n = 91\,774$, ≥ 70 years) initiated on APs found that compared with risperidone, the incidence rate ratios of major *adverse cardiovascular events* were higher for treatment with levomepromazine and haloperidol; and lower for treatment with flupenthixol, ziprasidone, chlorprothixene, and quetiapine (short- and long-term) [27C].

A case–crossover study ($n = 17\,718$) found that AP use (clotiapine, haloperidol, prochlorperazine, thioridazine, olanzapine, quetiapine, risperidone, and sulpiride) was associated with a 1.5 times increased risk of *ventricular arrhythmia* and/or *sudden cardiac death* [28C]. The risk was correlated with higher potency of *HERG potassium channel blockade.*

A study ($n = 3482$) of QTc *prolongation* in Asian patients with schizophrenia found that thioridazine caused QTc *prolongation* most frequently, followed by sulpiride, clozapine, and chlorpromazine [29C].

A study ($n = 454$) of AP overdoses presenting to a toxicology service found a significant risk of *QT prolongation* for overdoses with amisulpride and thioridazine (including 1 case of *Torsade des pointes [Tdp]*); and abnormal *QT intervals* (associated with *tachycardia*) for overdoses with quetiapine, olanzapine, and risperidone overdoses [30C].

A Swedish matched case–control register study of elderly patients (>65 years) found that haloperidol was associated with greater *Tdp arrhythmia* risk and *mortality* than risperidone, olanzapine or quetiapine [31C].

A meta-analysis of observational studies investigating sudden *cardiac* and *unexpected death* included two cohort (740 306 person-years) and four case–control (2557 cases; 17 670 controls) studies [32M]. Compared with non-users, the risk was increased for quetiapine, olanzapine, risperidone, haloperidol, clozapine and thioridazine; mean *hERG blockade* potency accounted for 43% of the heterogeneity.

A nested, case–control study ($n = 626$) of nursing home residents (≥ 65 years) found that the odds of *falling* were statistically greater with SGAs vs. controls [33C]. *Fall* risk was greater with high-dose (>150 mg/day) quetiapine and with high-dose (>2 mg/day) risperidone, while olanzapine (regardless of dose) was not associated with *increased fall* risk.

RESPIRATORY

A retrospective cohort study ($n = 92 234$) of elderly patients (≥ 65 years) prescribed that SGAs found an increased risk of *pneumonia* with risperidone and olanzapine, compared with the use of quetiapine [34C].

NERVOUS SYSTEM

A cross-sectional and retrospective study of non-elderly patients with schizophrenia treated with SGAs (risperidone, amisulpride, olanzapine, aripiprazole, ziprasidone, or clozapine) and unexposed to FGAs found a 35% prevalence of *tardive dyskinesia (TD)* and *tardive dystonia* [35c].

A nested, case–control study ($n = 60 121$) found that current use of medium-to-high potency FGAs was associated with a 2.5 times increased risk of *seizures* compared with non-use in patients with affective disorders; while in patients with dementia, current and past use of all APs, except amisulpride, aripiprazole, risperidone, or sulpiride, was associated with an increased risk of *seizures* [36C].

A meta-analysis (24 studies) found that aripiprazole, asenapine and lurasidone had a significantly higher risk of *akathisia* compared to placebo or other SGAs [37M]. Lurasidone having the highest individual RR; *agitation* and *anxiety* RRs were also higher with the newer SGAs compared with the older SGAs.

The propensity of SGAs (risperidone, olanzapine, aripiprazole, clozapine) to cause *EPS* was evaluated in a study ($n = 146$) of *disturbance of speech production* [38c]. Risperidone was found to significantly affect measures of *dysarthria*, compared to the other antipsychotics; duration of exposure and the presence of *EPS* also correlated with *dysarthria*.

Recurrent episodes of *oculogyric crises* were reported in 8 patients from a FEP program ($n = 452$) after 3 months to 2 years of treatment with 1 or more SGAs [39C].

R_x *NMS is a rare, severe, idiosyncratic adverse reaction to APs. While the SGAs were originally assumed to be free from* the risk of causing NMS, several cases of NMS induced by SGAs have been reported. A review (6 studies, $n = 186$) found that NMS induced by SGAs is characterized by lower incidence, lower clinical severity, and less frequent lethal outcome than NMS induced by FGAs [40c]. Furthermore, for certain APs (clozapine, aripiprazole, amisulpride), more atypical features are reported e.g. less intense EPS or high fever.

METABOLISM

An analysis of the FAERS database (2004–2013) found the *adverse hyperglycemic* reports for quetiapine, olanzapine, risperidone, aripiprazole, haloperidol, clozapine, prochlorperazine, and chlorpromazine were 12 471 (28.9%), 8423 (37.9%), 5968 (27.0%), 4045 (23.7%), 3445 (31.5%), 2614 (14.3%), 1800 (19.8%), and 1003 (35.7%), respectively (with increased reporting ratio with polypharmacy) [41C].

A sequence symmetry analysis of health insurance claims data from Japan of SGAs (risperidone, paliperidone, perospirone, blonanserin, clozapine, olanzapine, quetiapine, aripiprazole, zotepine) found an increased risk of *hyperlipidemia* only for olanzapine [42C].

A cross-sectional study ($n = 174$) found monotherapy with clozapine, olanzapine, or quetiapine was associated with *metabolic syndrome (MetS)*, compared to monotherapy with risperidone or monotherapy with aripiprazole or ziprasidone [43c].

An Australian, observational study ($n = 1155$, 18–64 years) in patients with psychosis found an increased risk of *DM* with AP treatment (clozapine, quetiapine, aripiprazole, risperidone, olanzapine) in those patients without a family history of DM [44C].

A meta-analysis found that all individual APs were associated with a significantly higher *MetS* risk compared to the antipsychotic-naïve [45M]. *MetS* risk was significantly higher with clozapine and olanzapine (except vs. clozapine) than other APs, and significantly lower with aripiprazole than other APs (except vs. amisulpride).

GASTROINTESTINAL

A database study of the comparative risk of *oral ulcerations* with APs found that olanzapine, quetiapine, and sulpiride had a higher risk, while aripiprazole had a lower risk, compared with haloperidol [46C].

TERATOGENICITY

A systematic review on first-trimester exposure and pregnancy outcome with respect to *congenital malformation* determined the relative risk (RR) estimates and 95% confidence intervals as 1.0 (0.7–1.4) for olanzapine, 1.0 (0.6–1.7) for quetiapine, 1.5 (0.9–2.2) for risperidone and 1.4 (0.5–3.1) for aripiprazole [47M].

SUSCEPTIBILITY FACTORS

In a 12-week study ($n = 100$) of FEP investigating the DRD2 s2514218, genotype C/C homozygotes had more *akathisia* than the T allele carriers for aripiprazole; while for risperidone male T allele carriers had greater *prolactin* elevations compared to male C/C homozygote [48C].

An initial, 14-week study ($n = 218$) followed by a 190-day, replication study ($n = 190$) investigated single nucleotide polymorphisms (SNPs) in orexin receptors 1 and 2 (HCRTR1 and HCRTR2) and *weight gain* [49C]. *Weight gain* was nominally associated with several SNPs in HCRTR2 in patients of European ancestry treated with either clozapine or olanzapine; two SNPs rs3134701 and rs12662510 were nominally associated in the replication analysis.

A meta-analysis (8 studies; $n = 2461$) evaluated *adiponectin* levels in patients with schizophrenia treated with different SGAs [50M]. Clozapine and olanzapine but not quetiapine were associated with significantly *lower adiponectin levels* than risperidone.

INDIVIDUAL DRUGS

Amisulpride [SEDA-32, 92; SEDA-33, 99; SEDA-34, 60; SEDA-35, 85; SEDA-36, 59; SEDA-37, 67]

Observational Studies

A prospective, open-label study of *bone turnover* found that 4 weeks of treatment with amisulpride significantly increased *prolactin levels, C-terminal peptide of type I collagen levels* and *decreased osteocalcin/C-terminal peptide of type I collagen* [51c]. No significant changes in bone turnover were observed with haloperidol or quetiapine.

CARDIOVASCULAR

A case of a 45-year-old male who developed symptomatic *bradycardia* with amisulpride (400–800 mg/day) is reported [52A].

SUSCEPTIBILITY

A 12-week, naturalistic study ($n = 185$) of Chinese patients with schizophrenia found that *prolactin elevation* was influenced by the COMT rs4680 SNP variant [53C].

Aripiprazole [SEDA-32, 93; SEDA-33, 99; SEDA-34, 60; SEDA-35, 96; SEDA-36, 59; SEDA-37, 68]

Comparative Studies

A 12-week, international, multicenter, randomised, double-blind, study ($n = 623; 18$–70 years) in schizophrenia

evaluated 2 doses of aripiprazole lauroxil LAI and placebo [54C]. The most common *AEs* were *insomnia, akathisia, headache,* and *anxiety; injection-site pain* was low and was associated with the first injection.

A randomised, double-blind study of aripiprazole or placebo added to venlafaxine in elderly patients ($n = 468; >60$ years) with treatment-resistant depression found increased *akathisia* and *parkinsonism* with aripiprazole [55C].

Observational Studies

A 48-week, open-label study ($n = 48$) found that 27% experienced an *exacerbation of psychosis* after switching to aripiprazole, which was correlated with longer duration of prior AP treatment [56c].

An 8-week study ($n = 10$) in autistic children reported mild to moderate *AEs* including *increased appetite and weight gain, sedation* and *agitation* [57c].

A *post hoc* analysis of aripiprazole LAI in obese and non obese patients found the most common *AEs* to be *insomnia, headache, injection-site pain, akathisia, upper respiratory tract infection, weight increase,* and *weight decrease* [58c].

A study of the addition of aripiprazole to patients on risperidone with hyperprolactinemia resulted in a reduction of *prolactin* and normalization of *menstrual disturbances* and improvement in *psychosis* [59c].

Systematic Reviews

A meta-analysis of the addition of aripiprazole to clozapine resulted in significant *weight reduction* but *AEs* including *moderate sinus tachycardia, psychotic disorder, auditory hallucinations, nausea, anxiety,* and *akathisia* [60M]. A meta-analysis (5 studies, $n = 684$) of RCTs comparing aripiprazole with pooled APs in Japanese patients with schizophrenia reported *decreased fatigue, prolactin, EPS, weight, total cholesterol* and *triglyceride levels* with aripiprazole [61M].

A systematic review (5 studies, $n = 688$) of aripiprazole in children with autistic disorder (6–17 years) found that the *discontinuation rate due to AEs* was greater for aripiprazole than placebo [62M]. *AEs* greater with aripiprazole than placebo included *sedation, fatigue (dose-dependent), vomiting, increased appetite, somnolence, drooling, EPS, tremor,* and *akathisia,* but were generally mild to moderate; severe *AEs* included *presyncope, aggression* and *weight gain.*

A meta-analysis (12 studies, $n = 935$) evaluating the treatment of tic disorders in children (4–18 years) found that the most common *AEs* included *drowsiness* (5.1–58.1%), *increased appetite* (3.2–25.8%), *nausea* (2–18.8%) and *headache* (2–16.1%) [63M]. Another meta-analysis (5 studies; $n = 511$) found that aripiprazole had a lower incidence of *EPS* than haloperidol [64M].

A meta-analysis found *decreased QTc interval* and *lower QTc prolongation risk* with aripiprazole compared with placebo and active controls in healthy patients [65M]. *Tdp* was reported in two case reports and sudden cardiac death was reported in one case report and one case series; epidemiological studies indicated *weak/moderate torsadogenicity*.

A meta-analysis (8 studies, $n = 604$) of the use of aripiprazole in treating AP-induced *hyperprolactinemia* reported efficacy in reducing prolactin but *increased somnolence* and *headache* [66M].

A meta-analysis of aripiprazole LAI (4 studies, $n = 1860$) found that aripiprazole had greater *weight gain* than placebo, but less than oral aripiprazole [67M].

A systematic review of aripiprazole augmentation of clozapine (4 studies, $n = 347$) found that there was a significant association with *agitation/akathisia* and *anxiety* [68M].

CARDIOVASCULAR

A case of severe *arrhythmia* in a 13-year-old female after 4 days of treatment with aripiprazole is reported [69A].

NERVOUS SYSTEM

A case of *tardive dystonia* in a 24-year-old male on aripiprazole after 3 years and successfully treated with clozapine is reported [70A]. A case of *TD* in a neuroleptic-naïve male after 6 months of treatment with aripiprazole occurring after addition of fluoxetine; and a second case of a middle-aged female with *dyskinetic movements* after stopping aripiprazole are reported [71A]. A case of *tics* in a 30-year-old male switched from olanzapine and another case of *tics* after combining aripiprazole and pimozide are reported [72A,73A]. Two cases of *NMS* in patients on aripiprazole and clozapine are reported; both with atypical features [74A].

SENSORY SYSTEMS

A case of a 47-year-old female treated with aripiprazole for 8 years who developed *retinal atrophy* is reported [75A]. A case of *acute transient myopia* in a 30-year-old female after 5 days of aripiprazole is reported [76A].

HEMATOLOGIC

A case of *transient morning pseudoneutropenia*, in an 11-year-old male is reported [77A].

MOUTH AND TEETH

A case *of nasal and gingival bleeding* with aripiprazole is reported [78A].

SALIVARY GLANDS

A case of *sialorrhea* with aripiprazole, successfully treated with diphenhydramine, is reported [79A].

GASTROINTESTINAL

A case of *hiccups* in an adolescent with aripiprazole is reported [80A]. A case series of 4 patients with *hiccups*, attributed to aripiprazole and benzodiazepines, is reported [81A].

URINARY TRACT

A case of *nocturnal enuresis* in a child with autistic disorder, successfully treated with desmopressin, is reported [82A].

DRUG–DRUG INTERACTIONS

A case of *serotonin syndrome* occurring in a 20-year-old female on aripiprazole, after discontinuation of sertraline and the addition of fluoxetine, is reported [83A]. Two cases of *akathisia* (29-year-old female, 56-year-old male) attributed to increased sensitivity due to the combination of aripiprazole, lamotrigine and an antidepressant are reported [84A].

Asenapine [SEDA-37, 69]

Comparative Studies

A study of asenapine in children with bipolar disorder ($n = 403$; 10–17 years) found that the most common *AEs* (incidence $\geq 5\%$ and at least twice placebo) were *somnolence, sedation, hypoesthesia oral, paresthesia oral*, and *increased appetite*; there was a greater incidence of *weight gain* ($\geq 7\%$), and mean adverse changes in *lipids*, fasting *insulin* and *glucose* with asenapine [85C].

In an 8-week double-blind study and a 26-week open-label extension in adolescents with schizophrenia, *weight gain* and *somnolence, sedation*, and *hypersomnia* were more common with asenapine than with placebo [86C]. *Akathisia, fasting glucose elevation*, and *EPS* were also more common with higher dose (5 mg bid), than with placebo.

Systematic Reviews

A Cochrane review (5 studies) found that there were significantly fewer incidents of *serious AEs* compared with placebo [87M]. A review of asenapine in bipolar disorder found that the most common *AE* was *somnolence*, and increases in *HbA1c, lipids and weight* were greater than placebo; the most commonly reported *EPS* was *akathisia* [88R].

CARDIAC

A case of *myocarditis* in a 52-year-old female, after 19 days treatment with asenapine, is reported [89A].

NERVOUS SYSTEM

A case of *myasthenia* with asenapine is reported [90A].

GASTROINTESTINAL

A case of *pseudo-Stauffer's syndrome* in a male in his mid-50s with asenapine is reported [91A].

EYES

A case of *paradoxical pinpoint pupils* in a 33-year-old female with asenapine and recurring on rechallenge is reported [92A].

DRUG–DRUG INTERACTIONS

A case of *sudden-onset dystonia* in a 44-year-old female on asenapine for 1.5 months, attributed to an interaction with ciprofloxacin, is reported [93A].

Blonanserin [SEDA-37, 69]

Observational Studies

An 8-week study of blonanserin compared to amisulpride (*n* = 50) found that both caused a significant increase in *weight, BMI* and *waist hip ratio* [94c].

ENDOCRINE

A case series of 6 patients followed for 12 months demonstrated a dose-dependent (>8.0 mg/day) effect on *prolactin elevation* [95c].

Brexpiprazole

Studies

A 6-week randomised, placebo-controlled study (*n* = 636) in schizophrenia found that the most common AE was *akathisia* (greater with the 4 mg dose); *weight gain* was 1.45 and 1.28 kg for the 2 and 4 mg doses, respectively [96C].

Two 6-week studies (*n* = 424, *n* = 353) in major depressive disorder found that the most common *AEs* were *akathisia, headache* and *weight gain* [97C,98C].

Cariprazine

Comparative Studies

A 3-week study (*n* = 312) in bipolar mania found that the most common (≥5% and twice the rate of placebo) *AEs* for cariprazine were *akathisia, nausea, constipation,* and *tremor* (highest doses) [99C]. Another 3-week study (*n* = 497) in bipolar mania found that the most common *AEs* for cariprazine (≥10% and twice placebo) were *akathisia, EPS, tremor, dyspepsia,* and *vomiting* [100C]. An 8-week study in bipolar depression found that the most common *AEs* (≥10%) with cariprazine were *akathisia* and *insomnia; weight gain* was slightly higher with cariprazine than with placebo [101C].

A 6-week study (*n* = 617) in acute schizophrenia found that the most common *AEs* (≥5% and twice the rate of placebo) were *akathisia, EPS,* and *tremor;* most were mild to moderate in severity [102C]. Another 6-week study

with an active comparator in acute schizophrenia found that the most common *AEs* were *insomnia* (≥10%), *akathisia,* and *headache* [103C].

Chlorpromazine [SEDA-35, 85; SEDA-36, 59; SEDA-37, 69]

Comparative Studies

An 8-week study (*n* = 83) in first episode, acute mania of chlorpromazine or olanzapine added to lithium found that both caused *weight gain* (5.6 and 7.7 kg, respectively) [104c].

NERVOUS SYSTEM

A case of *TD* in a 57-year-old male treated with chlorpromazine for hiccups for 10 days is reported [105A].

SKIN

A case of palmo-plantar *lichenoid eruptions* in a 30-year-old female with chlorpromazine, and resolving on discontinuation, is reported [106A]. Two cases of *photoallergic contact dermatitis* with chlorpromazine are reported [107A]. A third case of severe *skin pigmentation* and *corneal opacities* in a 50-year-old female on high-dose chlorpromazine over 10 years is reported [108A].

Clozapine [SEDA-32, 94; SEDA-33, 102; SEDA-34, 6; SEDA-35, 99; SEDA-36, 59; SEDA-37, 69]

Observational Studies

A retrospective, chart analysis (*n* = 355) of patients on clozapine found that older age of initiation was associated with increased risk of *cardiovascular* (except tachycardia), *HDL-cholesterol* and *fasting glucose abnormalities* [109C]. A study (*n* = 190) of patients who discontinued clozapine found *neutropenia* and other *AEs* accounted for 25.2%, and *death* for 10% (of which *respiratory infections* accounted for 25%) of *discontinuations* [110C]. A study comparing FGA polypharmacy (*n* = 21) with clozapine monotherapy (*n* = 27) found an increased rate of *MetS* and significant elevation of *triglycerides* with clozapine [111c]. A study (*n* = 56) of male, forensic patients on clozapine for at least 3 months found *nocturnal hypersalivation* (84%) and *weight gain* (57%) were the most common *AEs* [112c].

Systematic Reviews

A systematic review (15 studies, *n* = 1044) of clozapine in bipolar disorder found that *sedation, constipation, sialorrhea, weight gain,* and *body ache/pain* were the commonly reported *AEs; leukopenia, agranulocytosis,* and *seizure* were less common that in schizophrenia [113M]. A review was conducted to evaluate the uncommon *AEs* occurring with clozapine specifically; *ischemic colitis, paralytic ileus, hematemesis, gastroesophageal reflux disease, priapism, urinary incontinence, pityriasis rosea, intertriginous erythema, pulmonary thromboembolism, pseudo-pheochromocytoma, periorbital edema, parotitis* [114R]. A review of *myocarditis* found an overall incidence of 3%, and recommended investigation of *fever* given non-specific signs [115R]. A review of seizure disorder found a variety of *seizure presentations* with *tonic–clonic seizures* being the most common [116R].

CARDIOVASCULAR

A 10-year study ($n = 129$) found that the incidence of *myocarditis* and *cardiomyopathy* was 3.88% and 4.65%, respectively, and there was a significant association with SSRI use [117C]. A 4-week study ($n = 15$) of patients initiated on clozapine found *declining left ventricular (LV) diastolic* and *systolic function*, an *increase in systolic pulmonary artery pressure, A-wave velocity*, and *LV myocardial performance index* and a *decrease in the E/A ratio* [118c]. A case of *atrial fibrillation* in a 49-year-old female on clozapine after a single dose of olanzapine, which recurred with a higher dose of clozapine monotherapy, is reported [119A]. Three cases of *myocarditis* developing within 2 weeks are reported in a 17-year-old male, a 20-year-old male and a 46-year-old male [120A,121A,122A]. A case of a 33-year-old female who developed *neutropenia, agranulocytosis, venous thromboembolism*, and *allergic vasculitis* after 2 years on clozapine is reported [123A]. A case of *left ventricular thrombus* as a complication of *cardiomyopathy* in a 48-year-old male is reported [124A]. A case of *myocarditis* is reported [125A]. A case of *myocarditis* in a male in his mid-30s after 1 month on clozapine is reported [126A]. A case of *myocarditis* in a 44-year-old female after 2 weeks on clozapine is reported [127A]. Two cases of *late-onset myocarditis* with clozapine in a 62-year-old male after 18 years and a case of a 52-year-old male after 6 years are reported [128A]. A case–control study ($n = 109$) identified *eosinophilia*, and elevations in *C-reactive protein* and *troponin* occurring with clozapine-induced *myocarditis* 129C]. A case of *myocarditis* in a 27-year-old male was felt to be due to rheumatic fever [130A]. Two cases of *supra-ventricular tachycardia* in a 40-year-old and a 45-year-old male on clozapine are reported [131A,132A]. A case of *myocarditis* in a 30-year-old male after reinitiation of clozapine, despite previous treatment over 10 years, is reported [133A].

NERVOUS SYSTEM

A chart review ($n = 222$) found an overall incidence of *seizures* of 6%, with dose-dependent effect [134C]. A case of *myoclonus* preceding *seizure* is reported in a 20-year-old male on clozapine [135A]. Two cases of *negative myoclonus* are reported; one in conjunction with a urinary tract infection, the second case in a 31-year-old male after 3 months treatment [136A,137A]. A study ($n = 654$) of *stuttering* associated with clozapine found a prevalence of 0.92% [138C]. A case of *akathisia* in a 32-year-old male

after 3 weeks on clozapine is reported [139A]. A case of *oculogyric crisis* in a 25-year-old male is reported [140A].

PSYCHIATRIC

A study ($n = 65$) of *obsessive compulsive symptoms (OCS)* in patients with schizophrenia on clozapine found a prevalence of 29.2% for *OCS* and 13.8% for *obsessive compulsive disorder (OCD)*, with correlations between severity and *suicidal* and *depressive* symptoms [141c]. Another study ($n = 220$) found that 5.9% developed *OCS/OCD* on clozapine and 25% of patients with pre-existing *OCS/OCD* had worsening of symptoms [142C].

HEMATOLOGIC

A 12-month study ($n = 101$) of hematological indices found cumulative incidence rates of 48.9% for *neutrophilia*, 5.9% for *eosinophilia*, 3% for *thrombocytosis* and 3% for *thrombocytopenia*; a total of 5 patients developed *neutropenia* [143C]. Another 2-year study ($n = 94$) found a high incidence of *anemia* in patients initiated on clozapine [144c]. A study ($n = 980$) found 13 patients developed *neutropenia* and 3 developed *agranulocytosis*; the majority of patients were receiving additional psychotropics [145C]. A 6-year analysis of an Argentinian pharmacovigilance database found 378 cases of *adverse hematological events* (*leukopenia, neutropenia, agranulocytosis*) [146C]. A study ($n = 19$) of patients rechallenged after *neutropenia* found 4 patients with recurrence of *neutropenia*, of whom 2 developed *agranulocytosis* [147c]. A case of *neutropenia* and rechallenge is reported [148c]. Two cases of *rapid onset eosinophilia* in a 45-year-old male after 7 days, and in a 32-year-old male after 4 weeks on clozapine are reported [149A,150A]. Two cases of *benign eosinophilia* in a 32-year-old female and a 46-year-old female are reported [151A]. A case of *pancytopenia* and *sepsis* is reported in a 26-year-old male after 4 weeks on clozapine [152A]. A case of *eosinophilia* in a 32-year-old male after 4 weeks on clozapine followed by *parotitis* on rechallenge is reported [153A]. A case of *pulmonary eosinophila* in 16-year-old female after 2 weeks on clozapine is reported [154A]. A case of *late-onset neutropenia* in a 46-year-old female resulting in discontinuation of clozapine is reported [155A]. A case series of 5 patients who developed *lymphoma*, out of 221 patients on clozapine, is reported [156c].

GASTROINTESTINAL

A case of *fatal obstruction* in a 61-year-old male after 5 weeks of clozapine is reported [157A]. A case of *paralytic ileus* in a 60-year-old female is reported [158A].

RENAL

A review of 12 cases of *acute renal failure* resolving with discontinuation of clozapine reported that *eosinophilia* or *fever* were common presenting signs [159c]. A case of *acute interstitial nephritis* in a 29-year-old female leading to discontinuation of clozapine is reported [160A].

SEXUAL FUNCTION

A case of *priapism* in a 31-year-old male on clozapine is reported [161A].

IMMUNOLOGIC

A case of a 54-year-old male who developed *Stevens–Johnson syndrome* after 2 years was attributed to the immune modulatory effect of clozapine [162A].

BODY TEMPERATURE

A review of *fever* with clozapine reported a prevalence of 0.5–55% [163c].

FETOTOXICITY

A 6-month study of infants exposed *in utero* to clozapine (*n* = 33) vs. other Aps (*n* = 30) found that clozapine-exposed infants had *lower adaptive scores (delayed development), more disturbed sleep* and *labile mood* [164c]. A case of *decreased fetal heart rate variability* is reported in a female treated with clozapine during pregnancy [165A].

SUSCEPTIBILITY FACTORS

A study (*n* = 160) of SNPs of the GABA-A α2 gene found an association of *weight gain* and the rs279858 marker in patients homozygous for the TT genotype, taking olanzapine or clozapine [166C]. A study (*n* = 621) of SNPs of the sterol regulatory element binding transcription factor 2 (SREBF2) gene found an increased risk of *MetS* in patients with the A-allele of rs2267443 or rs1052717 h [167C]. A study (*n* = 102) of SNPs of complement 3 (C-3) found an association of *MetS* and in particular *triglycerides* with rs2277984 [168C].

DRUG–DRUG INTERACTIONS

A case of a multiple drug interaction of clozapine, antifungals and oral contraceptives resulted in *pericarditis, pericardial effusion* and *eosinophilia* in a 20-year-old female postulated to be due to increased clozapine levels [169A]. A case of a 50-year-old male on a long-term stable dose with *clozapine toxicity* as a result of smoking cessation due to chest infection is reported [170A]. The addition of pregabalin to clozapine was associated with *increased falls* and *bone fractures* in 2 cases possibly due to increased serum levels [171A]. The addition of lamotrigine to clozapine resulted in *rapid onset agranulocytosis* in a 60-year-old patient [172A]. A study (*n* = 65) found that patients receiving lamotrigine and clozapine (*n* = 10) had greater *OCS*, than patients on clozapine alone [173c].

Droperidol [SEDA-36, 59; SEDA-37, 71]

Observational Studies

A study (*n* = 1009) of the use of droperidol in the emergency department found 6 patients had an *abnormal QT* but there were no cases of *Tdp* [174C].

Reviews

A review (5 studies) of droperidol in migraine found that the most common *AEs* were *EPS* and *sedation* [175R].

CARDIOVASCULAR

A study (*n* = 63) of patients under anesthesia found that droperidol increased *QTcF* by 6.8 ms but did not affect dispersion of ventricular polarization [176c].

In a study (*n* = 62) of children undergoing single ventricle palliation droperidol was associated with significant, but transient *QT prolongation* [177c].

NERVOUS SYSTEM

A case of a 75-year-old male who developed *catatonic syndrome* after a single dose of droperidol is reported [178A].

Flupenthixol [SEDA-37, 71]

Observational Studies

A 12-month study (*n* = 107) of FEP treated with flupenthixol LAI found significant increases in *BMI, waist circumference* and *triglycerides* and decrease in *HDL-cholesterol* [179C].

Haloperidol [SEDA-35, 107; SEDA-36, 59; SEDA-37, 72]

Observational Studies

A retrospective, cohort study (*n* = 14 103) of elderly patients prescribed either haloperidol or risperidone found a significantly increased risk of *ischemic stroke* with haloperidol [180C]. A retrospective case–control study (*n* = 90 786) of elderly patients with dementia found that haloperidol had the greatest *mortality risk* [181C].

Systematic Reviews

A Cochrane review (63 studies) found that haloperidol produced significantly less *akathisia* in the medium-term compared with other FGAs [182M].

NERVOUS SYSTEM

A case of *NMS* in a 78-year-old female with dementia with haloperidol is reported [183A].

A case of worsening *tics* in a 12-year-old male on haloperidol is reported [184A].

IMMUNOLOGIC

A case of *angioedema* in a 47-year-old female after a single dose of haloperidol short-acting injection is reported [185A].

Iloperidone [SEDA-33, 103; SEDA-35, 109; SEDA-36, 59; SEDA-37, 72]

Observational Studies

A 12-week, randomised, open-label switch study (*n* = 500) found that the most common *AEs* with iloperidone were *dizziness* (particularly with rapid switch) and *dry mouth* [186C].

Levosulpiride [SEDA-37, 72]

Observational Studies

A Chinese study (*n* = 42) of oral and injectable formulations of levosulpiride in healthy volunteers found that 54.8% experienced *AEs* including *gastrointestinal disturbance, drowsiness, rash* and *EPS* [187c].

Loxapine [SEDA-35, 108; SEDA-36, 59; SEDA-37, 72]

Comparative Studies

A placebo-controlled study (*n* = 60) of inhaled loxapine in patients on a stable, oral AP regime found that the most common *AEs* were *cough, sedation,* and *dysgeusia* [188c].

Systematic Reviews

A systematic review reported common *AEs* of oral loxapine included *tremor, hypomania, rigidity, akathisia, drowsiness, dry mouth, constipation* and *weight changes*, and for inhaled loxapine was *dysgeusia* [189M].

Lurasidone [SEDA-37, 72]

Comparative Studies

A study (*n* = 150; 6–17 years) in autistic disorder found that the most common *AEs* were *vomiting* and *somnolence* [190C].

A study (*n* = 241) in acute schizophrenia found that the most common *AEs* were *sedation, dyspepsia, nausea, akathisia,* and *vomiting* [191C].

A study (*n* = 209) in MDD with mixed features found the most common *AEs* were *nausea* and *somnolence* [192C].

Observational Studies

A *post hoc* analysis (6 studies) found that mean *weight change* at 12 months was −0.4 kg with lurasidone, +2.6 kg with risperidone, and +1.2 kg with quetiapine XR, and ≥7% *weight gain* was observed in 16.0%, 25.8%, and 15.2% of patients, respectively [193C].

Reviews

Two reviews of lurasidone in bipolar depression found that most frequently occurring *AEs* were *nausea, akathisia, EPS* and *somnolence* [194R,195R].

Olanzapine [SEDA-32, 99; SEDA-33, 104; SEDA-34, 66; SEDA-35, 108; SEDA-36, 59; SEDA-37, 73]

Comparative Studies

A 2-week study (*n* = 24) found a significant increase in *weight, triglyceride, insulin* and *leptin* levels with olanzapine, compared with placebo [196c].

Observational Studies

In a 12-month study (*n* = 343), olanzapine was associated with early and significant *metabolic abnormalities*, compared with haloperidol [197C].

A 6-year study (*n* = 669) with olanzapine LAI found that 40.8% of patients experienced ≥7% *weight gain*, and there were 29 incidents of *post delirium sedation syndrome (PDSS)* [198C].

A study (*n* = 82) of olanzapine short-acting injection in elderly patients (≥65 years) found the most common *AEs* were *sedation* and *hypotension* [199c].

Systematic Reviews

A meta-analysis (13 studies) of olanzapine LAI found that there was fewer *AEs* (*anticholinergic use, akathisia, EPS, dystonia, QT prolongation*) compared with haloperidol LAI [200M]. A review of 338 *PDSS* events (0.07% of injections, 0.46–1.03% of patients) found that the most common symptoms were *sedation, confusion, dysarthria, somnolence, dizziness* and *disorientation* [201C]. The majority (91%) occurred within 1 hour, most resolved in 72 hours and none were fatal.

CARDIOVASCULAR

A case of *PDSS* in a female of low BMI after her fourth injection is reported [202A]. A case of *hypotension* in a 22-year-old female on 15 mg olanzapine is reported [203A].

A case of *pulmonary thromboembolism* with olanzapine is reported [204A].

NERVOUS SYSTEM

A case of *NMS* in a 63-year-old male 3 days after surgery is reported [205A]. A case of *NMS* in a long-term patient on olanzapine is reported [206A]. A case of *NMS* in an adolescent male with anorexia is reported [207A].

SKIN

A case of *pellagroid skin lesions* with olanzapine is reported [208A].

GASTROINTESTINAL

A case of acute *pancreatitis* in a 44-year-old male after 3 weeks on olanzapine is reported [209A]. A case of *ischemic colitis* in a 38-year-old female is reported [210A].

SUSCEPTIBILITY FACTORS

Two studies ($n=328$, 8 weeks; $n=208$, 4 weeks) of patients with schizophrenia found that SNP rs1478697 of the ataxin-2 binding protein 1 (A2BP1) gene was significantly associated with *weight gain* [211C].

A study ($n=32$) of the gastric inhibitory polypeptide receptor polymorphism, rs10423928, in olanzapine-treated patients with schizophrenia found that *BMI* change for the A/T+A/A genotypes was significantly higher than that for the T/T genotype [212c].

A case of acute *necrotizing pancreatitis* with olanzapine associated with 759C/T polymorphism of HTR2C gene is reported [213A].

IMMUNOLOGIC

A case of tender *pre-tibial edema* in a 45-year-old female after 2 weeks on olanzapine is reported [214A].

Paliperidone [SED-33, 108; SEDA-35, 85; SEDA-36, 59; SEDA-37, 74]

Comparative Studies

A 15-month, relapse prevention study ($n=334$) with paliperidone LAI in schizoaffective disorder found that the most common *AEs* (placebo, paliperidone LAI) were *increased weight* (4.7%, 8.5%), *insomnia* (7.1%, 4.9%), *schizoaffective disorder* (5.9%, 3.0%), *headache* (3.5%, 5.5%), and *nasopharyngitis* (3.5%, 5.5%) [215C]. The incidence of any *EPS* event was 7.1% for placebo and 8.5% for paliperidone LAI.

A long-term study ($n=506$) of paliperidone LAI (3-monthly) found that *headache* (9% vs. 4%), *weight increase* (9% vs 3%), *nasopharyngitis* (6% vs 1%), and *akathisia* (4% vs 1%) were more common, than with placebo [216C].

An 8-week acute phase followed by an 18-week maintenance phase in adolescents with schizophrenia ($n=228$, 12–17 years) of paliperidone ER compared with aripiprazole found that the most common (>10% patients) *AEs* for paliperidone ER were *akathisia, headache, somnolence, tremor*, and *weight gain*, and for aripiprazole were *worsening of schizophrenia* and *somnolence* [217C]. *EPS* including *dystonia* and *hyperkinesia* occurred in >2% in paliperidone ER-treated vs. aripiprazole-treated patients.

Observational Studies

A 13-week study ($n=212$) in hospitalized patients with acute exacerbation of schizophrenia and PLAI found the most common (>5%) *AEs* were *hyperprolactinemia, constipation, nasopharyngitis, insomnia, increased weight*, and *tremor* [218C]. *Worsening of schizophrenia* (3.3%) and *sinus bradycardia* (2.0%) was serious *AEs*.

A 2-year study ($n=400$; 12–17 years) of paliperidone ER in adolescents found the most common *AEs* included *somnolence, increased weight, headache, insomnia, nasopharyngitis, akathisia, schizophrenia exacerbation*, and *tremor* [219C]. There were no clinically significant mean changes in growth-adjusted z score for change in weight, height, or BMI; Tanner ratings showed normal maturation. The most frequently occurring *EPS* events were *parkinsonism* (15.5%) and *hyperkinesia* (13.8%); no cases of TD were reported. *Hyperprolactinemia* was measured in 56% of patients, and 9.3% of patients had *prolactin-related AEs*. A low percentage of patients (4.3%, $n=14$) had a shift from normal or *impaired fasting glucose* to *high*.

A 6-month study ($n=716$) of FEP treated with paliperidone ER found that the most common (>5%) *AEs* were *sleep disturbance* and *anxiety* [220C]. Another study ($n=80$) of paliperidone ER in FEP found that the most common *AEs* were *insomnia* (17.9%), *nausea* (8.3%), *akathisia* (4.8%), *anxiety* (4.8%) and *depression* (4.8%); *body weight* values at the end of the study were significantly higher [221c]. A third 8-week study ($n=294$) of paliperidone ER in FEP found that the most common *AEs* were *EPS*, and *agitation, somnolence*, and *xerostomia* [222C].

An 18-month study ($n=521$) of FEP treated with paliperidone LAI found that the most common *AEs* were *EPS, injection-site pain* and *insomnia* [223C].

A 6-month study ($n=212$) of paliperidone LAI in patients with unsuccessful response to oral APs found that the most *AEs* (≥5%) were *injection-site pain, insomnia, psychotic disorder, headache* and *anxiety* [224C].

An analysis of the Japanese Early Post-marketing Phase Vigilance reported 32 *deaths* in patients receiving paliperidone LAI (including 12 cases of *sudden death*, 7 *suicides* and 4 due to *NMS*) in approximately 11 000 patients [225MC].

A comparison of *injection-site pain* of phase 1 data with paliperidone LAI and a published study of FGA-LAIs using the same VAS scale found lower rates of *injection-site pain* with paliperidone LAI [226c].

A 15-month study ($n=442$) comparing paliperidone LAI with oral APs in both recent-onset and chronic patients with schizophrenia found that the most common *AEs* for paliperidone LAI vs. oral APs were *injection-site pain* (recent-onset, 26% vs. 0%; chronic, 17% vs. 0%); *increased weight* (14% vs. 6%; 12% vs. 6%); *akathisia* (14% vs. 9%; 10% vs. 7%); *insomnia* (12% vs. 17%; 18% vs. 10%); and *anxiety* (12% vs. 6%; 10% vs. 8%) [227C].

A study ($n = 16$) of paliperidone LAI in borderline PD found statistically significant *weight gain;* and 3 patients experienced *galactorrhea* leading to discontinuation [228c].

Systematic Reviews

A meta-analysis (50 studies) of paliperidone ER in Chinese populations found that *EPS* was lower than for risperidone, but higher than for olanzapine; *weight gain* and *somnolence* were lower than for olanzapine, but *prolactin-related AEs* were higher [229M].

PSYCHIATRIC

A case of *mania* after switch from paliperidone ER to paliperidone LAI in a 22-year-old female is reported [230A]. A case of *paroxysmal perceptual alteration* in a patient with schizophrenia in a 46-year-old female that developed with paliperidone ER and treated with biperiden is reported [231A].

ENDOCRINE

A case of a 15-year-old male who responded to paliperidone ER but developed *hyperprolactinemia, weight gain and impaired fasting glucose* was successfully treated with the addition of bromocriptine [232A].

SKIN

A case of necrotizing *infection* in the deltoid in a 26-year-old female after long-term treatment with paliperidone LAI is reported [233A].

MUSCULOSKELETAL

A case of *myalgia* and *rhabdomyolysis* with *elevated* CK in a 46-year-old female after 9 days on paliperidone ER is reported [234A].

Prochlorperazine [SEDA-35, 85; SEDA-36, 59; SEDA-37, 74]

NERVOUS SYSTEM

A case of *hemidystonia* mimicking acute stroke in a 32-year-old, pregnant female after 4 doses of prochlorperazine is reported [235A].

Quetiapine [SEDA-32, 104; SEDA-33, 110; SEDA-34, 69; SEDA-35, 85; SEDA-36, 59; SEDA-37, 74]

Observational Studies

In a 12-week study ($n = 61$) evaluating a switch to quetiapine XR, 4 patients experienced *AEs* including *headache, exacerbation of psychosis* and *dysuria* [236c]. In a 12-month study ($n = 29$) evaluating a switch to quetiapine

IR, 3 patients discontinued because of *exacerbation of psychosis* and 2 dropped out because of *somnolence* [237c].

A 12-week study ($n = 114$) comparing risperidone and quetiapine XR in the treatment of depressive symptoms in schizophrenia found that *sedation, somnolence* and *dry mouth* were more common with quetiapine, while *anxiety, insomnia, asthenia, hyperprolactinemia* (57.6% of risperidone patients and 8.1% of quetiapine patients) and *somnolence* were more common with risperidone [238C].

A chart review ($n = 55$) of quetiapine in pediatric ICU patients (2 months to 20 years) reported 3 cases of *QTc prolongation;* one requiring a dose reduction [239c].

An analysis of the Spanish Pharmacovigilance System of ADRs in Parkinson's disease found 5 cases of *NMS*; 3 with quetiapine, 1 with haloperidol and 1 with olanzapine [240c].

Reviews

A meta-analysis (15 studies) of quetiapine IR found that it caused *sedation* and clinically significant *weight gain,* but no EPS [241M].

CARDIOVASCULAR

A case of *ischemic stroke* in a 42-year-old male smoker is reported [242A]. A case of *myocarditis* in an 18-year-old male started on quetiapine in addition to regular methylphenidate is reported [243A].

NERVOUS SYSTEM

A case of *cervical dystonia* is reported in a female [244A]. A case of *restless legs* after a single dose of quetiapine is reported as well as a case series of 4 [245A,246A]. A case of *NMS* in a 60-year-old female with history of infection and catatonia is reported [247A]. A fatal case of *NMS* in a female with Parkinson's disease is reported [248A].

GASTROINTESTINAL

A case of a middle-aged male who developed *pancreatitis* due to *hypertriglyceridemia* with quetiapine is reported [249A]. A case of *ischemic colitis* with quetiapine is reported [250A]. A case of *necrotizing ischemic colitis* in a 39-year-old male after 7 days on quetiapine and an anticholinergic is reported [251A].

ENDOCRINE

A case of a 21-year-old Asian male with history of risk factors who developed *MetS* and *DKA* after 12 months on quetiapine is reported [252A].

HEMATOLOGIC

Two cases of *thrombocytopenia* are reported in a 78-year-old male and a 72-year-old female; the latter recurring on rechallenge [253A]. A case of *leucopenia* and *thrombocytopenia* in a 23-year-old, Chinese male after

3 months on quetiapine also on valproic acid, is reported [254A]. A case of *neutropenia* in a 19-year-old female on quetiapine who was successfully switched to clozapine is reported [255A].

SEXUAL

Three cases of *priapism* with quetiapine, one case in a 25-year-old male also on duloxetine, one case in a 28-year-old male also on lithium, and one recurring case in a 48-year-old male, are reported [256A,257A,258A].

IMMUNOLOGIC

A case of oral *labial edema* in a 65-year-old female requiring discontinuation of quetiapine is reported [259A].

SUSCEPTIBILITY FACTORS

A study ($n=79$) of the pharmacogenetics of quetiapine in healthy volunteers found that polymorphisms of CYP2C19 and AGT were associated with *higher prolactin levels* and polymorphisms of CYP2C19 and CYP1A1 with *somnolence* [260c].

ADVERSE DRUG REACTIONS

Data from the US Drug Abuse Warning Network (DAWN) of ED visits (67 497) involving quetiapine suggested an *increased risk of adverse drug reactions* when used without medical supervision for recreational/self-medication purposes [261MC].

Risperidone [SEDA-32, 107; SEDA-33, 111; SEDA-34, 70; SEDA-35, 85; SEDA-36, 59; SEDA-37, 75]

Comparative Studies

An 8-week, placebo-controlled study ($n=84$; 5–17 years) of risperidone in children and adolescents with autistic disorder found long-term treatment (21 months) associated with *increased appetite, weight gain,* and *enuresis,* but not neurological *AEs* [262c].

Observational Studies

A cross-sectional study ($n=108$) of ambulatory patients receiving either olanzapine or risperidone found that *movement disorders* including *tremor* and *dystonia* and *asthenia/lassitude/fatigue* were higher for olanzapine, while *gynecomastia* and *ejaculatory dysfunction* were higher for risperidone [263C].

NERVOUS SYSTEM

A case of *lower extremity motor weakness* in a 5-year-old male with intellectual disability after 3 weeks on risperidone is reported [264A].

METABOLIC

A 10-month, prospective study ($n=5$) in male children and adolescents (9–13 years) with psychiatric illness found that treatment with risperidone was associated with an *increased BMI* and a significantly *lower ratio of Bacteroidetes:Firmicutes,* compared with AP-naive psychiatric controls ($n=10$, 10–14 years) [265c]. A study ($n=73$) of children with autism spectrum disorder found that 18 weeks treatment was associated with an *increased BMI,* which was correlated with *decrease in ferritin levels* [266c].

ENDOCRINE

A case–control, cohort study ($n=401\,924$, 15–25 years) of males found that risperidone increased the risk of *gynecomastia* fourfold compared to controls, with a greater risk in ≤18 years of age [267MC].

SUSCEPTIBILITY FACTORS

A study of patients on risperidone ($n=120$; 8–20 years) and controls ($n=197$) found that 65.6% had *hyperprolactinemia,* which correlated with the presence of the C allele of the rs6318 single nucleotide polymorphisms of the 5-HT$_{2C}$ gene for both males and females [268C]. A 4-week study ($n=216$) of patients with schizophrenia found that SNPs on serotonin transporter gene (solute carrier family 6, member 4, SLC6A4) were correlated with risperidone-induced *weight gain* [269C].

Sertindole [SEDA-32, 110; SEDA-33, 114; SEDA-34, 73; SEDA-35, 85; SEDA-36, 59; SEDA-37, 75]

Comparative Studies

A 12-week study ($n=222$) compared sertindole (12–20 mg) with quetiapine (400–600 mg) in patients with schizophrenia [270C]. Sertindole was associated with moderate *QTc prolongation* and worsening of *T-wave morphology;* 9.6% of quetiapine patients had a >20 ms *QTcF prolongation,* compared with 33.3% of sertindole patients.

Observational Studies

In an observational study ($n=18$), sertindole was associated with a *QTc prolongation* of 19 ms and an increased *QT variability and heart rate variability* ratio; both these parameters can result in increased *cardiovascular mortality* [271c].

Reviews

A literature review reported that sertindole had low potential for *sedation* and *EPS,* acceptable *metabolic profile* but *cardiac safety* concerns [272r].

Ziprasidone [SEDA-32, 111; SEDA-33, 114; SEDA-34, 74; SEDA-35, 85; SEDA-36, 59; SEDA-37, 75]

Reviews

A review of ziprasidone in schizophrenia and bipolar disorder recommends caution in *arrhythmias* and with concomitant drugs that also cause *QTc prolongation* [273r].

METABOLISM

A case of 25-year-old Chinese female who developed *weight gain* and *MetS* after a switch from a combination of olanzapine, valproate and sulpiride to ziprasidone (high-dose) monotherapy is reported [274A].

HEMATOLOGIC

A case of transient *agranulocytosis* with ziprasidone in a 45-year-old man receiving hemodialysis is reported [275A].

IMMUNOLOGIC

Six cases (4 females, 20–69 years) of *Drug Reaction with Eosinophilia and Systemic symptoms (DRESS)* from FAERS are reported; in 3 cases recurrence occurred with rechallenge [276c]. A case of *systemic hypersensitivity* in a 65-year-old male after dose increase is reported [277A].

References

[1] Robinson DG, Gallego JA, John M, et al. A randomized comparison of aripiprazole and risperidone for the acute treatment of first-episode schizophrenia and related disorders: 3-month outcomes. Schizophr Bull. 2015;41(6):1227–36 [C].

[2] Emsley R, Asmal L, Chiliza B, et al. Changes in brain regions associated with food-intake regulation, body mass and metabolic profiles during acute antipsychotic treatment in first-episode schizophrenia. Psychiatry Res. 2015;233(2):186–93 [c].

[3] Wani RA, Dar MA, Margoob MA, et al. Diabetes mellitus and impaired glucose tolerance in patients with schizophrenia, before and after antipsychotic treatment. J Neurosci Rural Pract. 2015;6(1):17–22 [c].

[4] Li H, Yao C, Shi J, et al. Comparative study of the efficacy and safety between blonanserin and risperidone for the treatment of schizophrenia in Chinese patients: a double-blind, parallel-group multicenter randomized trial. J Psychiatr Res. 2015;69:102–9 [C].

[5] Wang G, Zhang Y, Zhang S, et al. Aripiprazole and risperidone for treatment of methamphetamine-associated psychosis in Chinese patients. J Subst Abuse Treat. 2016;62:84–8. pii: S0740-5472(15)00293-7. [c].

[6] Shin JY, Choi NK, Lee J, et al. A comparison of risperidone and haloperidol for the risk of ischemic stroke in the elderly: a propensity score-matched cohort analysis. J Psychopharmacol. 2015;29(8):903–9 [C].

[7] Ronsley R, Nguyen D, Davidson J, et al. Increased risk of obesity and metabolic dysregulation following 12 months of second-generation antipsychotic treatment in children: a prospective cohort study. Can J Psychiatry. 2015;60(10):441–50 [c].

[8] Carbon M, Kapoor S, Sheridan E, et al. Neuromotor adverse effects in 342 youth during 12 weeks of naturalistic treatment with 5 second-generation antipsychotics. J Am Acad Child Adolesc Psychiatry. 2015;54(9):718–27 [C].

[9] Garcia-Amador M, Merchán-Naranjo J, Tapia C, et al. Neurological adverse effects of antipsychotics in children and adolescents. J Clin Psychopharmacol. 2015;35(6):686–93 [C].

[10] Masi G, Milone A, Stawinoga A, et al. Efficacy and safety of risperidone and quetiapine in adolescents with bipolar II disorder comorbid with conduct disorder. J Clin Psychopharmacol. 2015;35(5):587–90 [c].

[11] Rubin DM, Kreider AR, Matone M, et al. Risk for incident diabetes mellitus following initiation of second-generation antipsychotics among Medicaid-enrolled youths. JAMA Pediatr. 2015;169(4): e150285 [MC].

[12] Yu HY, Hsiao CY, Chen KC, et al. A comparison of the effectiveness of risperidone, haloperidol and flupentixol long-acting injections in patients with schizophrenia-A nationwide study. Schizophr Res. 2015;169(1–3):400–5 [c].

[13] Lee EH, Hui CL, Lin JJ, et al. Quality of life and functioning in first-episode psychosis Chinese patients with different antipsychotic medications. Early Interv Psychiatry. 2015;http://dx.doi.org/10.1111/eip.12246 [C].

[14] Arterburn D, Wood GC, Theis MK, et al. Antipsychotic medications and extreme weight gain in two health systems. Obes Res Clin Pract. 2016;10(4):408–23 pii: S1871-403X(15)00126-X. [C].

[15] Kimura G, Kadoyama K, Brown JB, et al. Antipsychotics-associated serious adverse events in children: an analysis of the FAERS database. Int J Med Sci. 2015;12(2):135–40 [MC].

[16] Kishi T, Hirota T, Matsunaga S, et al. Antipsychotic medications for the treatment of delirium: a systematic review and meta-analysis of randomised controlled trials. J Neurol Neurosurg Psychiatry. 2016;87:767–74 [M].

[17] Forcen FE, Matsoukas K, Alici Y. Antipsychotic-induced akathisia in delirium: a systematic review. Palliat Support Care. 2016;14:77–84 [M].

[18] Tan L, Tan L, Wang HF, et al. Efficacy and safety of atypical antipsychotic drug treatment for dementia: a systematic review and meta-analysis. Alzheimers Res Ther. 2015;7(1):20 [M].

[19] Galling B, Correll CU. Do antipsychotics increase diabetes risk in children and adolescents? Expert Opin Drug Saf. 2015;14(2):219–41 [M].

[20] McQuire C, Hassiotis A, Harrison B, et al. Pharmacological interventions for challenging behaviour in children with intellectual disabilities: a systematic review and meta-analysis. BMC Psychiatry. 2015;15(1):303 [M].

[21] Jensen KG, Juul K, Fink-Jensen A, et al. Corrected QT changes during antipsychotic treatment of children and adolescents: a systematic review and meta-analysis of clinical trials. J Am Acad Child Adolesc Psychiatry. 2015;54(1):25–36 [M].

[22] Takeuchi H, Suzuki T, Remington G, et al. Antipsychotic polypharmacy and corrected QT interval: a systematic review. Can J Psychiatry. 2015;60(5):215–22 [M].

[23] Tek C, Kucukgoncu S, Guloksuz S, et al. Antipsychotic-induced weight gain in first-episode psychosis patients: a meta-analysis of differential effects of antipsychotic medications. Early Interv Psychiatry. 2016;10:193–202 [M].

[24] Gao K, Yuan C, Wu R, et al. Important clinical features of atypical antipsychotics in acute bipolar depression that inform routine clinical care: a review of pivotal studies with number needed to treat. Neurosci Bull. 2015;31(5):572–88 [r].

[25] Musil R, Obermeier M, Russ P, et al. Weight gain and antipsychotics: a drug safety review. Expert Opin Drug Saf. 2015;14(1):73–96 [r].

[26] Hrdlicka M, Dudova I. Atypical antipsychotics in the treatment of early-onset schizophrenia. Neuropsychiatr Dis Treat. 2015;11:907–13 [r].

[27] Sahlberg M, Holm E, Gislason GH, et al. Association of selected antipsychotic agents with major adverse cardiovascular events and noncardiovascular mortality in elderly persons. J Am Heart Assoc. 2015;4(9):e001666 [C].

[28] Wu CS, Tsai YT, Tsai HJ. Antipsychotic drugs and the risk of ventricular arrhythmia and/or sudden cardiac death: a nation-wide case-crossover study. J Am Heart Assoc. 2015;4(2). http://dx.doi.org/10.1161/JAHA.114.001568 pii: e001568 [C].

[29] Xiang YT, Chiu HF, Ungvari GS, et al. QTc prolongation in schizophrenia patients in Asia: clinical correlates and trends between 2004 and 2008/2009. Hum Psychopharmacol. 2015;30(2):94–9 [C].

[30] Berling I, Isbister GK. Prolonged QT risk assessment in antipsychotic overdose using the QT nomogram. Ann Emerg Med. 2015;66(2):154–64 [C].

[31] Danielsson B, Collin J, Jonasdottir Bergman G, et al. Antidepressants and antipsychotics classified with torsades de pointes arrhythmia risk and mortality in older adults—a Swedish nationwide study. Br J Clin Pharmacol. 2016;81(4):773–83 [C].

[32] Salvo F, Pariente A, Shakir S, et al. Sudden cardiac and sudden unexpected death related to antipsychotics: a meta-analysis of observational studies. Clin Pharmacol Ther. 2016;99(3):306–14 [M].

[33] Bozat-Emre S, Doupe M, Kozyrskyj AL, et al. Atypical antipsychotic drug use and falls among nursing home residents in Winnipeg, Canada. Int J Geriatr Psychiatry. 2015;30(8):842–50 [C].

[34] Mehta S, Pulungan Z, Jones BT, et al. Comparative safety of atypical antipsychotics and the risk of pneumonia in the elderly. Pharmacoepidemiol Drug Saf. 2015;24(12):1271–80 [C].

[35] Ryu S, Yoo JH, Kim JH, et al. Tardive dyskinesia and tardive dystonia with second-generation antipsychotics in non-elderly schizophrenic patients unexposed to first-generation antipsychotics: a cross-sectional and retrospective study. J Clin Psychopharmacol. 2015;35(1):13–21 [c].

[36] Bloechliger M, Rüegg S, Jick SS, et al. Antipsychotic drug use and the risk of seizures: follow-up study with a nested case-control analysis. CNS Drugs. 2015;29(7):591–603 [C].

[37] Thomas JE, Caballero J, Harrington CA. The incidence of akathisia in the treatment of schizophrenia with aripiprazole, asenapine and lurasidone: a meta-analysis. Curr Neuropharmacol. 2015;13(5):681–91 [M].

[38] Sinha P, Vandana VP, Lewis NV, et al. Predictors of effect of atypical antipsychotics on speech. Indian J Psychol Med. 2015;37(4):429–33 [c].

[39] Gardner DM, Abidi S, Ursuliak Z, et al. Incidence of oculogyric crisis and long-term outcomes with second-generation antipsychotics in a first-episode psychosis program. J Clin Psychopharmacol. 2015;35(6):715–8 [C].

[40] Belvederi Murri M, Guaglianone A, Bugliani M, et al. Second-generation antipsychotics and neuroleptic malignant syndrome: systematic review and case report analysis. Drugs R&D. 2015;15(1):45–62 [c].

[41] Kato Y, Umetsu R, Abe J, et al. Hyperglycemic adverse events following antipsychotic drug administration in spontaneous adverse event reports. J Pharm Health Care Sci. 2015;1:15 [C].

[42] Takeuchi Y, Kajiyama K, Ishiguro C, et al. Atypical antipsychotics and the risk of hyperlipidemia: a sequence symmetry analysis. Drug Saf. 2015;38(7):641–50 [C].

[43] Kang SH, Lee JI. Metabolic disturbances independent of body mass in patients with schizophrenia taking atypical antipsychotics. Psychiatry Investig. 2015;12(2):242–8 [c].

[44] Foley DL, Mackinnon A, Morgan VA, et al. Effect of age, family history of diabetes, and antipsychotic drug treatment on risk of diabetes in people with psychosis: a population-based cross-sectional study. Lancet Psychiatry. 2015;2(12):1092–8 [C].

[45] Vancampfort D, et al. Risk of metabolic syndrome and its components in people with schizophrenia and related psychotic disorders, bipolar disorder and major depressive disorder: a systematic review and meta-analysis. World Psychiatry. 2015;14(3):339–47 [M].

[46] Lai EC, Hsieh CY, Wong MB, et al. Comparative risk of oral ulcerations among antipsychotics users—population-based retrospective cohort study. Pharmacoepidemiol Drug Saf. 2016;25(2):123–32 [C].

[47] Ennis ZN, Damkier P. Pregnancy exposure to olanzapine, quetiapine, risperidone, aripiprazole and risk of congenital malformations. A systematic review. Basic Clin Pharmacol Toxicol. 2015;116(4):315–20 [M].

[48] Zhang JP, Robinson DG, Gallego JA, et al. Association of a schizophrenia risk variant at the DRD2 locus with antipsychotic treatment response in first-episode psychosis. Schizophr Bull. 2015;41(6):1248–55 [C].

[49] Tiwari AK, Brandl EJ, Zai CC, et al. Association of orexin receptor polymorphisms with antipsychotic-induced weight gain. World J Biol Psychiatry. 2015;8:1–9 [C].

[50] Bartoli F, Crocamo C, Clerici M, et al. Second-generation antipsychotics and adiponectin levels in schizophrenia: a comparative meta-analysis. Eur Neuropsychopharmacol. 2015;25(10):1767–74 [M].

[51] Liang Y, Su YA, Zhao ZG, et al. Acute effects of haloperidol, amisulpride, and quetiapine on bone turnover markers in patients with schizophrenia. J Clin Psychopharmacol. 2015;35(5):583–6 [c].

[52] Huang LC, Huang LY, Tseng SY, et al. Amisulpride and symptomatic bradycardia: a case report. Gen Hosp Psychiatry. 2015;37(5):497.e1–2 [A].

[53] Chen CY, Yeh YW, Kuo SC, et al. Catechol-O-methyltransferase gene variants may associate with negative symptom response and plasma concentrations of prolactin in schizophrenia after amisulpride treatment. Psychoneuroendocrinology. 2015;65:67–75 [C].

[54] Meltzer HY, Risinger R, Nasrallah HA, et al. A randomized, double-blind, placebo-controlled trial of aripiprazole lauroxil in acute exacerbation of schizophrenia. J Clin Psychiatry. 2015;76(8):1085–90 [C].

[55] Lenze EJ, Mulsant BH, Blumberger DM, et al. Efficacy, safety, and tolerability of augmentation pharmacotherapy with aripiprazole for treatment-resistant depression in late life: a randomised, double-blind, placebo-controlled trial. Lancet. 2015;386(10011):2404–12 [C].

[56] TakAEsu Y, Kishimoto T, Murakoshi A, et al. Factors associated with discontinuation of aripiprazole treatment after switching from other antipsychotics in patients with chronic schizophrenia: a prospective observational study. Psychiatry Res. 2016;236:71–4 [c].

[57] Habibi N, Dodangi N, Nazeri A. Efficacy and safety of aripiprazole for treatment of irritability in children with autistic disorder: an open-label study. Iran J Med Sci. 2015;40(6):548–9 [c].

[58] De Hert M, Eramo A, Landsberg W, et al. Efficacy and safety of aripiprazole once-monthly in obese and nonobese patients with schizophrenia: a post hoc analysis. Neuropsychiatr Dis Treat. 2015;11:1299–306 [c].

[59] Ranjbar F, Sadeghi-Bazargani H, Niari Khams P, et al. Adjunctive treatment with aripiprazole for risperidone-induced hyperprolactinemia. Neuropsychiatr Dis Treat. 2015;11:549–55 [c].

[60] Choi YJ. Efficacy of adjunctive treatments added to olanzapine or clozapine for weight control in patients with schizophrenia: a systematic review and meta-analysis. Scientific World Journal. 2015;2015:970730 [M].

[61] Kishi T, Matsuda Y, Matsunaga S, et al. Aripiprazole for the management of schizophrenia in the Japanese population: a systematic review and meta-analysis of randomized controlled trials. Neuropsychiatr Dis Treat. 2015;11:419–34 [M].

[62] Ghanizadeh A, Tordjman S, Jaafari N. Aripiprazole for treating irritability in children and adolescents with autism: a systematic review. Indian J Med Res. 2015;142(3):269–75 [M].

[63] Yang CS, Huang H, Zhang LL, et al. Aripiprazole for the treatment of tic disorders in children: a systematic review and meta-analysis. BMC Psychiatry. 2015;15:179 [M].

[64] Fang Q, Chen L, Chen QB, et al. Efficacy and safety of aripiprazole in the treatment of childhood tic disorders: a meta-analysis. Zhongguo Dang Dai Er Ke Za Zhi. 2015;17(7):715–20 [M].

[65] Polcwiartek C, Sneider B, Graff C, et al. The cardiac safety of aripiprazole treatment in patients at high risk for torsade: a systematic review with a meta-analytic approach. Psychopharmacology (Berl). 2015;232(18):3297–308 [M].

[66] Meng M, Li W, Zhang S, et al. Using aripiprazole to reduce antipsychotic-induced hyperprolactinemia: meta-analysis of currently available randomized controlled trials. Shanghai Arch Psychiatry. 2015;27(1):4–17 [M].

[67] Oya K, Kishi T, Iwata N. Efficacy and tolerability of aripiprazole once monthly for schizophrenia: a systematic review and meta-analysis of randomized controlled trials. Neuropsychiatr Dis Treat. 2015;11:2299–307 [M].

[68] Srisurapanont M, Suttajit S, Maneeton N, et al. Efficacy and safety of aripiprazole augmentation of clozapine in schizophrenia: a systematic review and meta-analysis of randomized-controlled trials. J Psychiatr Res. 2015;62:38–47 [M].

[69] Shao Q, Quan W, Jia X, et al. Severe arrhythmia induced by orally disintegrating aripiprazole tablets (Bosiqing(®)): a case report. Neuropsychiatr Dis Treat. 2015;11:3019–21 [A].

[70] Joe S, Park J, Lim J, et al. Remission of irreversible aripiprazole-induced tardive dystonia with clozapine: a case report. BMC Psychiatry. 2015;15:253 [A].

[71] Patra S. Tardive dyskinesia and covert dyskinesia with aripiprazole: a case series. Curr Drug Saf. 2016;11(1):102–3 [A].

[72] Guo X, Lu D, Jiang Y. Aripiprazole-associated tic in a schizophrenia patient. Neuropsychiatr Dis Treat. 2015;11: 873–4 [A].

[73] Mazlum B, Zaimoğlu S, Öztop DB. Exacerbation of tics after combining aripiprazole with pimozide: a case with Tourette syndrome. J Clin Psychopharmacol. 2015;35(3):350–1 [A].

[74] Tseng PT, Chang YC, Chang CH, et al. Atypical neuroleptic malignant syndrome in patients treated with aripiprazole and clozapine: a case-series study and short review. Int J Psychiatry Med. 2015;49(1):35–43 [A].

[75] Faure C, Audo I, Zeitz C, et al. Aripiprazole-induced chorioretinopathy: multimodal imaging and electrophysiological features. Doc Ophthalmol. 2015;131(1):35–41 [A].

[76] Karadağ H, Acar M, Özdel K. Aripiprazole induced acute transient bilateral myopia: a case report. Balkan Med J. 2015;32(2):230–2 [A].

[77] Pinnaka S, Roberto AJ, Giordano A, et al. Aripiprazole-induced transient morning pseudoneutropenia in an 11-year-old male. J Child Adolesc Psychopharmacol. 2015; http://dx.doi.org/10.1089/cap.2015.0128 [Epub ahead of print] [A].

[78] Hoşoğlu E, Bayram Ö, Hergüner S. Nasal and gingival bleeding during aripiprazole but not haloperidol treatment. J Child Adolesc Psychopharmacol. 2015; http://dx.doi.org/10.1089/cap.2015.0135 [Epub ahead of print] [A].

[79] Kılınç S, Hergüner A, Hergüner S. Aripiprazole-induced sialorrhea responsive to diphenhydramine treatment. J Child Adolesc Psychopharmacol. 2015; http://dx.doi.org/10.1089/cap.2015.0133 [Epub ahead of print] [A].

[80] Bilgiç A, Yılmaz S, Yılmaz E. Hiccups associated with aripiprazole in an adolescent with bipolar disorder. J Child Adolesc Psychopharmacol. 2015; http://dx.doi.org/10.1089/cap.2014.0138 [Epub ahead of print] [A].

[81] De Filippis S, Ranieri V, Cuomo I, et al. Hiccup with aripiprazole plus benzodiazepines resolving with pregabalin and/or benzodiazepine switch/discontinuation: four case reports. J Clin Psychopharmacol. 2015;35(2):195–7 [A].

[82] Karakurt MN, Süren S. Desmopressin use in the treatment of aripiprazole-induced nocturnal enuresis in a child diagnosed with autistic disorder. J Child Adolesc Psychopharmacol. 2015;25(6):518–9. http://dx.doi.org/10.1089/cap.2014.0138 [Epub ahead of print] [A].

[83] Bostankolou G, Ayhan Y, Cuhadaroglu F, et al. Serotonin syndrome with a combination of aripiprazole and fluoxetine: a case report. Ther Adv Psychopharmacol. 2015;5(2):138–40 [A].

[84] Pondé MP, Freire AC. Increased anxiety, akathisia, and suicidal thoughts in patients with mood disorder on aripiprazole and lamotrigine. Case Rep Psychiatry. 2015;2015:419746 [A].

[85] Findling RL, Landbloom RL, Szegedi A, et al. Asenapine for the acute treatment of pediatric manic or mixed episode of bipolar I disorder. J Am Acad Child Adolesc Psychiatry. 2015;54(12):1032–41 [C].

[86] Findling RL, Landbloom RP, Mackle M, et al. Safety and efficacy from an 8 week double-blind trial and a 26 week open-label extension of asenapine in adolescents with schizophrenia. J Child Adolesc Psychopharmacol. 2015;25(5):384–96 [C].

[87] Hay A, Byers A, Sereno M, et al. Asenapine versus placebo for schizophrenia. Cochrane Database Syst Rev. 2015;11:CD011458 [M].

[88] Scheidemantel T, Korobkova I, Rej S, et al. Asenapine for bipolar disorder. Neuropsychiatr Dis Treat. 2015;11:3007–17 [R].

[89] Lim X, Tibrewal P, Dhillon R, et al. Can asenapine cause myocarditis? Asian J Psychiatr. 2015;14:78–9 [A].

[90] Hategan A, Bourgeois JA. Asenapine-associated myasthenic syndrome. J Clin Psychopharmacol. 2015;35(1):107–8 [A].

[91] Schultz K, Wang L, Barr A, et al. A case of pseudo-Stauffer's syndrome related to asenapine use. Schizophr Res. 2015;169(1–3):500–1 [A].

[92] Gill JS, Jambunathan S, Wong S, et al. Paradoxical pinpoint pupils with asenapine. Asia Pac Psychiatry. 2015;7(2):230 [A].

[93] Ridout KK, Ridout SJ, Pirnie LF, et al. Sudden-onset dystonia in a patient taking asenapine: interaction between ciprofloxacin and asenapine metabolism. Am J Psychiatry. 2015;172(11):1162–3 [A].

[94] Deepak TS, Raveesh BN, Parashivamurthy BM, et al. Clinical assessment of weight gain with atypical antipsychotics—blonanserin vs amisulpride. J Clin Diagn Res. 2015;9(6):FC07–10 [c].

[95] Takahashi S, Suzuki M, Uchiyama M. One-year follow-up of serum prolactin level in schizophrenia patients treated with blonanserin: a case series. Psychiatry Investig. 2015;12(4):566–8 [c].

[96] Correll CU, Skuban A, Ouyang J, et al. Efficacy and safety of brexpiprazole for the treatment of acute schizophrenia: a 6-week randomized, double-blind, placebo-controlled trial. Am J Psychiatry. 2015;172(9):870–80 [C].

[97] Thase ME, Youakim JM, Skuban A, et al. Adjunctive brexpiprazole 1 and 3 mg for patients with major depressive disorder following inadequate response to antidepressants: a phase 3, randomized, double-blind study. J Clin Psychiatry. 2015;76(9):1232–40 [C].

[98] Thase ME, Youakim JM, Skuban A, et al. Efficacy and safety of adjunctive brexpiprazole 2 mg in major depressive disorder: a phase 3, randomized, placebo-controlled study in patients with inadequate response to antidepressants. J Clin Psychiatry. 2015;76(9):1224–31 [C].

[99] Sachs GS, Greenberg WM, Starace A, et al. Cariprazine in the treatment of acute mania in bipolar I disorder: a double-blind, placebo-controlled, phase III trial. J Affect Disord. 2015;174:296–302 [C].

[100] Calabrese JR, Keck Jr. PE, Starace A, et al. Efficacy and safety of low- and high-dose cariprazine in acute and mixed mania associated with bipolar I disorder: a double-blind, placebo-controlled study. J Clin Psychiatry. 2015;76(3):284–92 [C].

[101] Durgam S, Earley W, Lipschitz A, et al. An 8-week randomized, double-blind, placebo-controlled evaluation of the safety and efficacy of cariprazine in patients with bipolar I depression. Am J Psychiatry. 2016;173(3):271–81 [C].

[102] Kane JM, Zukin S, Wang Y, et al. Efficacy and safety of cariprazine in acute exacerbation of schizophrenia: results from an international, phase III clinical trial. J Clin Psychopharmacol. 2015;35(4):367–73 [C].

[103] Durgam S, Cutler AJ, Lu K, et al. Cariprazine in acute exacerbation of schizophrenia: a fixed-dose, phase 3, randomized, double-blind, placebo- and active-controlled trial. J Clin Psychiatry. 2015;76(12):e1574–82 [C].

[104] Conus P, Berk M, Cotton SM, et al. Olanzapine or chlorpromazine plus lithium in first episode psychotic mania: an 8-week randomised controlled trial. Eur Psychiatry. 2015;30(8):975–82 [c].

[105] Yehl JL, Sheyner I, Fasnacht KS, et al. A case of tardive dyskinesia in the last weeks of life. J Pain Palliat Care Pharmacother. 2015;29(2):144–7 [A].

[106] Kikuchi N, Yamamoto T. A probable case of chlorpromazine-induced lichenoid eruptions initially involved palmoplantar areas. Indian J Dermatol. 2015;60(6):638 [A].

[107] Esteve-Martínez A, Ninet Zaragoza V, de la Cuadra Oyanguren J, et al. Photoallergic contact dermatitis due to chlorpromazine: a report of 2 cases. Actas Dermosifiliogr. 2015;106(6):518–20 [A].

[108] Molina-Ruiz AM, Pulpillo Á, Molina-Ruiz RM, et al. Chlorpromazine-induced severe skin pigmentation and corneal opacities in a patient with schizophrenia. Int J Dermatol. 2016;55(8):909–12. http://dx.doi.org/10.1111/ijd.13085 [A].

[109] Hyde N, Dodd S, Venugopal K, et al. Prevalence of cardiovascular and metabolic events in patients prescribed clozapine: a retrospective observational, clinical cohort study. Curr Drug Saf. 2015;10(2):125–31 [C].

[110] Mustafa FA, Burke JG, Abukmeil SS, et al. "Schizophrenia past clozapine": reasons for clozapine discontinuation, mortality, and alternative antipsychotic prescribing. Pharmacopsychiatry. 2015;48(1):11–4.

[111] Softic R, Sutovic A, Avdibegovic E, et al. Metabolic syndrome in schizophrenia—who is more to blame: FGA polypharmacy or clozapine monotherapy? Psychiatr Danub. 2015;27(4):378–84 [c].

[112] Qurashi I, Stephenson P, Chu S, et al. An evaluation of subjective experiences, effects and overall satisfaction with clozapine treatment in a UK forensic service. Ther Adv Psychopharmacol. 2015;5(3):146–50 [c].

[113] Li XB, Tang YL, Wang CY, et al. Clozapine for treatment-resistant bipolar disorder: a systematic review. Bipolar Disord. 2015;17(3):235–47 [M].

[114] De Fazio P, Gaetano R, Caroleo M, et al. Rare and very rare adverse effects of clozapine. Neuropsychiatr Dis Treat. 2015;11:1995–2003 [R].

[115] Ronaldson KJ, Fitzgerald PB, McNeil JJ. Clozapine-induced myocarditis, a widely overlooked adverse reaction. Acta Psychiatr Scand. 2015;132(4):231–40 [R].

[116] Williams AM, Park SH. Seizure associated with clozapine: incidence, etiology, and management. CNS Drugs. 2015;29(2):101–11 [R].

[117] Youssef DL, Narayanan P, Gill N. Incidence and risk factors for clozapine-induced myocarditis and cardiomyopathy at a regional mental health service in Australia. Australas Psychiatry. 2016;24(2):176–80. http://dx.doi.org/10.1177/1039856215604480 [C].

[118] Curto M, Comparelli A, Ciavarella GM, et al. Impairment of left ventricular function early in treatment with clozapine: a preliminary study. Int Clin Psychopharmacol. 2015;30(5):282–9 [c].

[119] Çam B, Gülseren L, Mete L, et al. Clozapine and olanzapine associated atrial fibrillation: a case report. Turk Psikiyatri Derg. 2015;26(3):221–6 [A].

[120] Aboueid L, Toteja N. Clozapine-induced myocarditis: a case report of an adolescent boy with intellectual disability. Case Rep Psychiatry. 2015;2015:482375 [A].

[121] Cohen R, Lysenko A, Mallet T, et al. A case of clozapine-induced myocarditis in a young patient with bipolar disorder. Case Rep Cardiol. 2015;2015:283156 [A].

[122] Hatton JL, Bhat PK, Gandhi S. Clozapine-induced myocarditis: recognizing a potentially fatal adverse reaction. Tex Heart Inst J. 2015;42(2):155–7 [A].

[123] Voulgari C, Giannas R, Paterakis G, et al. Clozapine-induced late agranulocytosis and severe neutropenia complicated with streptococcus pneumonia, venous thromboembolism, and allergic vasculitis in treatment-resistant female psychosis. Case Rep Med. 2015;2015:703218 [A].

[124] Malik SA, Malik S, Dowsley TF, et al. Left ventricular thrombus as a complication of clozapine-induced cardiomyopathy: a case report and brief literature review. Case Rep Cardiol. 2015;2015:835952 [A].

[125] Molina Martín de Nicolás J, Parra Fuertes JJ, Gómez Mariscal E E, et al. Clozapine-associated myocarditis. Med Clin (Barc). 2015;145(9):e19–20.

[126] Barry AR, Windram JD, Graham MM. Clozapine-associated myocarditis: case report and literature review. Can J Hosp Pharm. 2015;68(5):427–9 [A].

[127] Cook SC, Ferguson BA, Cotes RO, et al. Clozapine-induced myocarditis: prevention and considerations in rechallenge. Psychosomatics. 2015;56(6):685–90 [A].

[128] Tan LH, Suetani S, Clark S, Wilson D. Late onset myocarditis with clozapine use. Aust N Z J Psychiatry. 2015;49(3):295 [A].

[129] Ronaldson KJ, Fitzgerald PB, McNeil JJ. Evolution of troponin, C-reactive protein and eosinophil count with the onset of clozapine-induced myocarditis. Aust N Z J Psychiatry. 2015;49(5):486–7 [C].

[130] Goodison G, Siskind D, Harcourt-Rigg C, et al. Clarifying the diagnosis of myocarditis in a patient on clozapine. Australas Psychiatry. 2015;23(3):311–3 [A].

[131] Kirpekar CV, Faye DA, Gawande S, et al. Clozapine induced supra ventricular tachycardia. Indian J Psychol Med. 2015;37(2):254–5 [A].

[132] Settem JV, Trivedi S, Kamath AG, et al. Clozapine-induced supraventricular tachycardia and its treatment with verapamil. Indian J Psychol Med. 2015;37(3):358–9 [A].

[133] Baptista T, Rojas N, Dávila DF. Heterogeneity of clozapine-associated myocarditis: an opportunity for novel preventing strategies. Aust N Z J Psychiatry. 2015;49(11):1068 [A].

[134] Grover S, Hazari N, Chakrabarti S, et al. Association of clozapine with seizures: a brief report involving 222 patients prescribed clozapine. East Asian Arch Psychiatry. 2015;25(2):73–8 [C].

[135] Osborne IJ, McIvor RJ. Clozapine-induced myoclonus: a case report and review of the literature. Ther Adv Psychopharmacol. 2015;5(6):351–6 [A].

[136] Takahashi T, Masuya Y, Ueno K, et al. Clozapine-related negative myoclonus associated with urinary tract infection: a case report. J Clin Psychopharmacol. 2015;35(2):205–6 [A].

[137] Praharaj SK, Vemanna N, Sharma PS. Knee buckling (negative myoclonus) associated with clozapine: is there a dose threshold? Clin Toxicol (Phila). 2015;53(9):918–9 [A].

[138] Murphy R, Gallagher A, Sharma K, et al. Clozapine-induced stuttering: an estimate of prevalence in the west of Ireland. Ther Adv Psychopharmacol. 2015;5(4):232–6 [C].

[139] Grover S, Sahoo S. Clozapine induced akathisia: a case report and review of the evidence. Indian J Pharmacol. 2015;47(2): 234–5 [A].

[140] Nebhinani N, Avasthi A, Modi M. Oculogyric crisis with clozapine: a case report and review of similar case reports in the literature. Indian J Psychol Med. 2015;37(3):342–4 [A].

[141] Szmulewicz AG, Smith JM, Valerio MP. Suicidality in clozapine-treated patients with schizophrenia: role of obsessive-compulsive symptoms. Psychiatry Res. 2015;230(1):50–5 [c].

[142] Grover S, Hazari N, Chakrabarti S, Avasthi A. Relationship of obsessive compulsive symptoms/disorder with clozapine: a retrospective study from a multispeciality tertiary care centre. Asian J Psychiatr. 2015;15:56–61 [C].

[143] Lee J, Takeuchi H, Fervaha G, et al. The effect of clozapine on hematological indices: a 1-year follow-up study. J Clin Psychopharmacol. 2015;35(5):510–6 [C].

[144] Lee J, Bies R, Bhaloo A, et al. Clozapine and anemia: a 2-year follow-up study. J Clin Psychiatry. 2015;76(12):1642–7 [c].

[145] Lau KL, Yim PH. Neutropenia and agranulocytosis in Chinese patients prescribed clozapine. East Asian Arch Psychiatry. 2015;25(4):164–7 [C].

[146] Balda MV, Garay OU, Papale RM, et al. Clozapine-associated neutropenia and agranulocytosis in Argentina (2007–2012). Int Clin Psychopharmacol. 2015;30(2):109–14 [C].

[147] Meyer N, Gee S, Whiskey E, et al. Optimizing outcomes in clozapine rechallenge following neutropenia: a cohort analysis. J Clin Psychiatry. 2015;76(11):e1410–6 [c].

[148] Bavle A, Vidhyavathi M. Case report of clozapine-induced neutropenia and rechallenge. J Neuropsychiatry Clin Neurosci. 2015;27(1):e61 [c].

[149] Kadiyala PK, Ahmed MA, Pinto DA, Mathai JP. Clozapine induced eosinophilia: an often neglected important adverse effect. Indian J Psychiatry. 2015;57(4):429–30 [A].

[150] Wysokiński A, Kolińska J. Rapidly developing and self-limiting eosinophilia associated with clozapine. Psychiatry Clin Neurosci. 2015;69(2):122 [A].

[151] Aneja J, Sharma N, Mahajan S, et al. Eosinophilia induced by clozapine: a report of two cases and review of the literature. J Family Med Prim Care. 2015;4(1):127–9 [A].

[152] Pushpakumara J, Karunarathna P, Sivathiran S, et al. Clozapine induced pancytopenia leading to severe sepsis: an unusual early complication. BMC Res Notes. 2015;8:792 [A].

[153] Saguem BN, Bouhlel S, Ben Salem C, et al. Eosinophilia and parotitis occurring early in clozapine treatment. Int J Clin Pharm. 2015;37(6):992–5 [A].

[154] Hashimoto N, Maeda T, Okubo R, et al. Simple pulmonary eosinophilia associated with clozapine treatment. J Clin Psychopharmacol. 2015;35(1):99–101 [A].

[155] Tatar ZB, Yeşilyurt S. Late-onset neutropenia due to clozapine. Indian J Psychiatry. 2015;57(3):325–6 [c].

[156] Meltzer M. Lymphoma developing during clozapine therapy. Aust N Z J Psychiatry. 2016;50(5):498–9. http://dx.doi.org/10.1177/0004867415621389, pii: 0004867415621389 [A].

[157] Oke V, Schmidt F, Bhattarai B, et al. Unrecognized clozapine-related constipation leading to fatal intra-abdominal sepsis—a case report. Int Med Case Rep J. 2015;8:189–92 [A].

[158] Sarac H, Henigsberg N, Bagaric-Krakan L. Clozapine-induced paralytic ileus. Psychiatr Danub. 2015;27(3):283–4 [c].

[159] Woesner ME, Kanofsky JD. Revisiting the discussion: termination of clozapine treatment due to renal failure. J Clin Psychiatry. 2015;76(12):1694 [A].

[160] Chan SY, Cheung CY, Chan PT, et al. Clozapine-induced acute interstitial nephritis. Hong Kong Med J. 2015;21(4):372–4 [A].

[161] Donizete da Costa F, Toledo da Silva Antonialli K, et al. Priapism and clozapine use in a patient with hypochondriacal delusional syndrome. Oxf Med Case Reports. 2015;2015(3):229–31 [A].

[162] Wu MK, Chung W, Wu CK, et al. The severe complication of Stevens-Johnson syndrome induced by long-term clozapine treatment in a male schizophrenia patient: a case report. Neuropsychiatr Dis Treat. 2015;11:1039–41 [c].

[163] Bruno V, Valiente-Gómez A, Alcoverro O. Clozapine and fever: a case of continued therapy with clozapine. Clin Neuropharmacol. 2015;38(4):151–3 [c].

[164] Shao P, Ou J, Peng M, et al. Effects of clozapine and other atypical antipsychotics on infants development who were exposed to as fetus: a post-hoc analysis. PLoS One. 2015;10(4):e0123373 [A].

[165] Guyon L, Auffret M, Coussemacq M, Béné J, et al. Alteration of the fetal heart rate pattern induced by the use of clozapine during pregnancy. Therapie. 2015;70(3):301–3 [C].

[166] Zai CC, Tiwari AK, Chowdhury NI, et al. Association study of GABAA α2 receptor subunit gene variants in antipsychotic-associated weight gain. J Clin Psychopharmacol. 2015;35(1):7–12 [C].

[167] Yang L, Chen J, Liu D, et al. Association between SREBF2 gene polymorphisms and metabolic syndrome in clozapine-treated patients with schizophrenia. Prog Neuropsychopharmacol Biol Psychiatry. 2015;56:136–41 [C].

[168] Zhang C, Zhang Y, Cai J, et al. Complement 3 and metabolic syndrome induced by clozapine: a cross-sectional study and retrospective cohort analysis. Pharmacogenomics J. 2015; http://dx.doi.org/10.1038/tpj.2015.68 [Epub ahead of print] [A].

[169] Cadeddu G, Deidda A, Stochino ME, et al. Clozapine toxicity due to a multiple drug interaction: a case report. J Med Case Rep. 2015;9:77 [A].

[170] ten Bokum EM, van de Oever HL, Radstake DW, et al. Clozapine intoxication due to cessation of smoking and infection. Neth J Med. 2015;73(7):345–7.

[171] Schjerning O, Lykkegaard S, Damkier P, et al. Possible drug-drug interaction between pregabalin and clozapine in patients with schizophrenia: clinical perspectives. Pharmacopsychiatry. 2015;48(1):15–8 [A].

[172] Urban AE, Wiglusz MS, Cubała WJ, et al. Rapid-onset agranulocytosis in a patient treated with clozapine and lamotrigine. Psychiatr Danub. 2015;27(Suppl 1):S459–61 [A].

[173] Szmulewicz AG, Valerio MP, Smith JM. Obsessive-compulsive symptoms in adjunctive therapy with lamotrigine in clozapine-medicated patients. Schizophr Res. 2015;166(1–3):364–5 [c].

[174] Calver L, Page CB, Downes MA, et al. The safety and effectiveness of droperidol for sedation of acute behavioral disturbance in the emergency department. Ann Emerg Med. 2015;66(3). 230–238.e1. [C].

[175] Thomas MC, Musselman ME, Shewmaker J. Droperidol for the treatment of acute migraine headaches. Ann Pharmacother. 2015;49(2):233–40 [R].

[176] Agámez Medina GL, González-Arévalo A, Gómez-Arnau JI, et al. Effects of droperidol and ondansetron on dispersion of ventricular repolarization: a randomized double-blind clinical study in anesthetized adult patients. Rev Esp Anestesiol Reanim. 2015;62(9):495–501 [c].

[177] Scott JP, Stuth EA, Stucke AG, et al. Droperidol transiently prolongs the QT interval in children undergoing single ventricle palliation. Pediatr Cardiol. 2015;36(1):196–204 [c].

[178] Brakman M, de Graaff PJ, Visser EC. Catatonic syndrome after single low dose of droperidol. Ned Tijdschr Geneeskd. 2015;160: A9712 [A].

[179] Chiliza B, Asmal L, Oosthuizen P, et al. Changes in body mass and metabolic profiles in patients with first-episode schizophrenia treated for 12 months with a first-generation antipsychotic. Eur Psychiatry. 2015;30(2):277–83 [C].

[180] Shin JY, Choi NK, Lee J, et al. A comparison of risperidone and haloperidol for the risk of ischemic stroke in the elderly: a propensityscore-matched cohort analysis. J Psychopharmacol. 2015;29(8):903–9 [C].

[181] Maust DT, Kim HM, Seyfried LS, et al. Antipsychotics, other psychotropics, and the risk of death in patients with dementia: number needed to harm. JAMA Psychiatry. 2015;72(5):438–45 [C].

[182] Dold M, Samara MT, Li C, et al. Haloperidol versus first-generation antipsychotics for the treatment of schizophrenia and other psychotic disorders. Cochrane Database Syst Rev. 2015;1: CD009831 [M].

[183] Oka M, Komasawa N, Nishihara I, et al. A case of neuroleptic malignant syndrome associated with undiagnosed dementia with lewy bodies. Masui. 2015;64(11):1190–2 [A].

[184] Nath K, Bhattacharya A, Hazarika S, et al. Paradoxical worsening of tics with haloperidol. Ther Adv Psychopharmacol. 2015;5(5):314–5 [A].

[185] AlMadhyan AB. Angioedema associated with haloperidol. Int J Health Sci (Qassim). 2015;9(1):76–8 [A].

[186] Citrome L, Weiden PJ, Alva G, et al. Switching to iloperidone: an omnibus of clinically relevant observations from a 12-week, open-label, randomized clinical trial in 500 persons with schizophrenia. Clin Schizophr Relat Psychoses. 2015;8(4):183–95 [C].

[187] Xu M, Zhou Y, Ni Y, et al. Tolerability and pharmacokinetic comparison of oral, intramuscular, and intravenous administration of levosulpiride after single and multiple dosing in healthy Chinese volunteers. Clin Ther. 2015;37(11):2458–67 [c].

[188] Spyker DA, Riesenberg RA, Cassella JV. Multiple dose pharmacokinetics of inhaled loxapine in subjects on chronic, stable antipsychotic regimens. J Clin Pharmacol. 2015;55(9):985–94 [c].

[189] Popovic D, Nuss P, Vieta E. Revisiting loxapine: a systematic review. Ann Gen Psychiatry. 2015;14:15 [M].

[190] Loebel A, Brams M, Goldman RS, et al. Lurasidone for the treatment of irritability associated with autistic disorder. J Autism Dev Disord. 2016;46(4):1153–63 [C].

[191] Potkin SG, Kimura T, Guarino J. A 6-week, double-blind, placebo- and haloperidol-controlled, phase II study of lurasidone in patients with acute schizophrenia. Ther Adv Psychopharmacol. 2015;5(6):322–31 [C].

[192] Suppes T, Silva R, Cucchiaro J, et al. Lurasidone for the treatment of major depressive disorder with mixed features: a randomized, double-blind, placebo-controlled study. Am J Psychiatry. 2016;173(4):400–7 [C].

[193] Meyer JM, Mao Y, Pikalov A, et al. Weight change during long-term treatment with lurasidone: pooled analysis of studies in patients with schizophrenia. Int Clin Psychopharmacol. 2015;30(6):342–50 [C].

[194] Sanford M, Dhillon S. Lurasidone: a review of its use in adult patients with bipolar I depression. CNS Drugs. 2015;29(3):253–63 [R].

[195] Franklin R, Zorowitz S, Corse AK, et al. Lurasidone for the treatment of bipolar depression: an evidence-based review. Neuropsychiatr Dis Treat. 2015;11:2143–52 [R].

[196] Daurignac E, Leonard KE, Dubovsky SL. Increased lean body mass as an early indicator of olanzapine-induced weight gain in healthy men. Int Clin Psychopharmacol. 2015;30(1):23–8 [c].

[197] Fabrazzo M, Monteleone P, Prisco V, et al. Olanzapine is faster than haloperidol in inducing metabolic abnormalities in schizophrenic and bipolar patients. Neuropsychobiology. 2015;72(1):29–36 [C].

[198] Anand E, Berggren L, Deix C, et al. A 6-year open-label study of the efficacy and safety of olanzapine long-acting injection in patients with schizophrenia: a post hoc analysis based on the European label recommendation. Neuropsychiatr Dis Treat. 2015;11:1349–57 [C].

[199] Duong S, Yeung KT, Chang F. Intramuscular olanzapine in the management of behavioral and psychological symptoms in hospitalized older adults: a retrospective descriptive study. J Aging Res. 2015;2015:570410 [c].

[200] Bushe CJ, Falk D, Anand E, et al. Olanzapine long-acting injection: a review of first experiences of post-injection delirium/sedation syndrome in routine clinical practice. BMC Psychiatry. 2015;15:65 [M].

[201] Kishi T, Matsunaga S, Iwata N. Intramuscular olanzapine for agitated patients: a systematic review and meta-analysis of randomized controlled trials. J Psychiatr Res. 2015;68: 198–209 [C].

[202] Luedecke D, Schöttle D, Karow A, et al. Post-injection delirium/sedation syndrome in patients treated with olanzapine pamoate: mechanism, incidence, and management. CNS Drugs. 2015;29(1):41–6 [A].

[203] Jana AK, Praharaj SK, Roy N. Olanzapine-induced orthostatic hypotension. Clin Psychopharmacol Neurosci. 2015;13(1):113–4 [A].

[204] Wang Q, Guan L, Li RM, et al. Pulmonary thromboembolism associated with olanzapine treatment. Chin Med J (Engl). 2015;128(3):419–20 [A].

[205] Zhao Z, Zhang H, Wang S, et al. Sudden discontinuation and reinstitution of olanzapine-associated atypical neuroleptic malignant syndrome in a patient undergoing lung surgery. Int J Clin Exp Med. 2015;8(7):11639–41 [A].

[206] Kouparanis A, Bozikas A, Spilioti M, et al. Neuroleptic malignant syndrome in a patient on long-term olanzapine treatment at a stable dose: successful treatment with dantrolene. Brain Inj. 2015;29(5):658–60 [A].

[207] Ayyıldız H, Turan Ş, Gülcü D, et al. Olanzapine-induced atypical neuroleptic malignant syndrome in an adolescent man with anorexia nervosa. Eat Weight Disord. 2016;21(2):309–11. http://dx.doi.org/10.1007/s40519-015-0247-3 [A].

[208] Singh LK, Sahu M, Praharaj SK. Olanzapine-induced reversible pellagroid skin lesion. Curr Drug Saf. 2015;10(3):251–3 [A].

[209] Baysal B, Kayar Y, Özmen A, et al. Olanzapine-induced acute pancreatitis. Turk J Gastroenterol. 2015;26(3):289–90 [A].

[210] Sáez González E, Díaz Jaime FC, Blázquez Martínez MT, et al. Olanzapine-induced ischemic colitis. Rev Esp Enferm Dig. 2016;108(8):507–9. http://dx.doi.org/10.17235/reed.2015.3856/2015 [A].

[211] Dong L, Yan H, Huang X, et al. A2BP1 gene polymorphisms association with olanzapine-induced weight gain. Pharmacol Res. 2015;99:155–61 [C].

[212] Ono S, Suzuki Y, Fukui N, et al. GIPR gene polymorphism and weight gain in patients with schizophrenia treated with olanzapine. J Neuropsychiatry Clin Neurosci. 2015;27(2):162–4 [c].

[213] Rizos E, Tournikioti K, Alevyzakis E, et al. Acute necrotizing pancreatitis following olanzapine treatment and 759C/T polymorphism of HTR2C gene: a case report. In Vivo. 2015;29(5):529–31 [A].

[214] Mathan K, Muthukrishnan V, Menon V. Olanzapine-induced tender pitting pre-tibial edema. J Pharmacol Pharmacother. 2015;6(2):114–5 [A].

[215] Fu DJ, Turkoz I, Simonson RB, et al. Paliperidone palmitate once-monthly reduces risk of relapse of psychotic, depressive, and manic symptoms and maintains functioning in a double-blind, randomized study of schizoaffective disorder. J Clin Psychiatry. 2015;76(3):253–62 [C].

[216] Berwaerts J, Liu Y, Gopal S, et al. Efficacy and safety of the 3-month formulation of paliperidone palmitate vs placebo for relapse prevention of schizophrenia: a randomized clinical trial. JAMA Psychiatry. 2015;72(8):830–9 [C].

[217] Savitz AJ, Lane R, Nuamah I, et al. Efficacy and safety of paliperidone extended release in adolescents with schizophrenia: a randomized, double-blind study. J Am Acad Child Adolesc Psychiatry. 2015;54(2). 126–137.e1. [C].

[218] Li H, Turkoz I, Zhang F. Efficacy and safety of once-monthly injection of paliperidone palmitate in hospitalized Asian patients with acute exacerbated schizophrenia: an open-label, prospective, noncomparative study. Neuropsychiatr Dis Treat. 2015;12:15–24 [C].

[219] Savitz A, Lane R, Nuamah I, et al. Long-term safety of paliperidone extended release in adolescents with schizophrenia: an open-label, flexible dose study. J Child Adolesc Psychopharmacol. 2015;25(7):548–57 [C].

[220] Helldin L, Peuskens J, Vauth R, et al. Treatment response, safety, and tolerability of paliperidone extended release treatment in patients recently diagnosed with schizophrenia. Ther Adv Psychopharmacol. 2015;5(4):194–207 [C].

[221] Üçok A, Saka MC, Bilici M. Effects of paliperidone extended release on functioning level and symptoms of patients with recent onset schizophrenia: an open-label, single-arm, flexible-dose, 12-months follow-up study. Nord J Psychiatry. 2015;69(6):426–32 [c].

[222] Si T, Tan Q, Zhang K, et al. An open-label, flexible-dose study of paliperidone extended-release in Chinese patients with first-onset psychosis. Neuropsychiatr Dis Treat. 2015;11:87–95 [C].

[223] Zhang F, Si T, Chiou CF, et al. Efficacy, safety, and impact on hospitalizations of paliperidone palmitate in recent-onset schizophrenia. Neuropsychiatr Dis Treat. 2015;11:657–68 [C].

[224] Hargarter L, Cherubin P, Bergmans P, et al. Intramuscular long-acting paliperidone palmitate in acute patients with schizophrenia unsuccessfully treated with oral antipsychotics. Prog Neuropsychopharmacol Biol Psychiatry. 2015;58:1–7 [C].

[225] Fujii Y. What lessons should we learn from the death of patients on Xeplion? Seishin Shinkeigaku Zasshi. 2015;117(2):132–45 [MC].

[226] Gopal S, Palermo T, Sliwa JK, et al. Comparing injection site pain with paliperidone palmitate versus first-generation depot antipsychotics in subjects with schizophrenia. Innov Clin Neurosci. 2015;12(5–6):10–1 [c].

[227] Alphs L, Bossie C, Mao L, et al. Treatment effect with paliperidone palmitate compared with oral antipsychotics in patients with recent-onset versus more chronic schizophrenia and a history of criminal justice system involvement. Early Interv Psychiatry. 2015; http://dx.doi.org/10.1111/eip.12271 [Epub ahead of print] [C].

[228] Palomares N, Montes A, Díaz-Marsá M, et al. Effectiveness of long-acting paliperidone palmitate in borderline personality disorder. Int Clin Psychopharmacol. 2015;30(6):338–41 [c].

[229] Cai S, Lu H, Bai Z, et al. Paliperidone extended-release tablets in Chinese patients with schizophrenia: meta-analysis of randomized controlled trials. Neuropsychiatr Dis Treat. 2015;11:1817–34 [M].

[230] Demirci K, Keleş S, Demirdaş A, et al. Manic symptoms during a switch from paliperidone ER to paliperidone palmitate in a patient with schizophrenia. Case Rep Psychiatry. 2015;2015:528370 [A].

[231] Benna P, Rubino E, Marino C, et al. Paroxysmal perceptual alteration in a schizophrenic patient treated with paliperidone: a case report. Ann Clin Psychiatry. 2015;27(3):223–4 [A].

[232] Naguy A, Al-Tajali A. Bromocriptine mitigated paliperidone metabolic and neuro-hormonal side effects and improved negative domain in a case of early onset schizophrenia. Nord J Psychiatry. 2016;70:318–9 [A].

[233] Leung JG, Kooda KJ, Frazee EN, et al. Paliperidone palmitate associated with necrotizing deep tissue infection and sepsis requiring surgical intervention. Case Rep Psychiatry. 2015;2015:364325 [A].

[234] Fernández-Macho JG, Espárrago-Llorca G, Morales-Gómez GR, et al. Paliperidone-induced rhabdomyolysis: a case report. Actas Esp Psiquiatr. 2015;43(2):66–8 [A].

[235] Coralic Z, Kim AS, Vinson DR. Prochlorperazine-induced hemidystonia mimicking acute stroke. West J Emerg Med. 2015;16(4):572–4 [A].

[236] Pan PY, Lee MS, Yeh CB. The efficacy and safety of once-daily quetiapine extended release in patients with schizophrenia switched from other antipsychotics: an open-label study in Chinese population. BMC Psychiatry. 2015;15:1 [c].

[237] Hashimoto N, Toyomaki A, Honda M, et al. Long-term efficacy and tolerability of quetiapine in patients with schizophrenia who switched from other antipsychotics because of inadequate therapeutic response—a prospective open-label study. Ann Gen Psychiatry. 2015;14(1):1 [c].

[238] Kasper S, Montagnani G, Trespi G, et al. Treatment of depressive symptoms in patients with schizophrenia: a randomized, open-label, parallel-group, flexible-dose subgroup analysis of patients treated with extended-release quetiapine fumarate or risperidone. Int Clin Psychopharmacol. 2015;30(1):14–22 [C].

[239] Joyce C, Witcher R, Herrup E, et al. Evaluation of the safety of quetiapine in treating delirium in critically ill children: a retrospective review. J Child Adolesc Psychopharmacol. 2015;25(9):666–70 [c].

[240] Lertxundi U, Ruiz AI, Aspiazu MÁ, et al. Adverse reactions to antipsychotics in Parkinson disease: an analysis of the Spanish pharmacovigilance database. Clin Neuropharmacol. 2015;38(3):69–84 [c].

[241] Hutton P, Taylor PJ, Mulligan L, et al. Quetiapine immediate release vs. placebo for schizophrenia: systematic review, meta-analysis and reappraisal. Br J Psychiatry. 2015;206(5):360–70 [M].

[242] BozkurtZincir S, Ozdilek BF, Zincir S. Association of quetiapine with ischemic brain stem stroke: a case report and discussion. Ther Adv Psychopharmacol. 2015;5(4):246–9 [A].

[243] Wassef N, Khan N, Munir S. Quetiapine-induced myocarditis presenting as acute STEMI. BMJ Case Rep. 2015;2015. http://dx.doi.org/10.1136/bcr-2014-207151 pii: bcr2014207151. [A].

[244] Tso G, Kolur U. Quetiapine-induced cervical dystonia. Australas Psychiatry. 2015. pii: 1039856215618526 [Epub ahead of print] [A].

[245] Soyata AZ, Çelebi F, Yargıç LI. Restless legs syndrome after single low dose quetiapine administration. Curr Drug Saf. 2016;11:172–3 [A].

[246] Vohra A. Quetiapine induced restless legs syndrome: a series of four cases. Asian J Psychiatr. 2015;16:73–4 [A].

[247] Chiou YJ, Lee Y, Lin CC, et al. A case report of catatonia and neuroleptic malignant syndrome with multiple treatment modalities: short communication and literature review. Medicine (Baltimore). 2015;94(43):e1752 [A].

[248] Schattner A, Kitroser E, Cohen JD. Fatal neuroleptic malignant syndrome associated with quetiapine. Am J Ther. 2016;23(5):e1209–10 [Epub ahead of print] [A].

[249] Franco JM, Vallabhajosyula S, Griffin TJ. Quetiapine-induced hypertriglyceridaemia causing acute pancreatitis. BMJ Case Rep. 2015;2015. http://dx.doi.org/10.1136/bcr-2015-209571, pii: bcr2015209571 [A].

[250] Vernay J. Quetiapine-induced ischemic colitis. A case report. Presse Med. 2015;44(5):538–41 [A].

[251] de Beaurepaire R, Trinh I, Guirao S, et al. Colitis possibly induced by quetiapine. BMJ Case Rep. 2015;2015. http://dx.doi.org/10.1136/bcr-2014-207912, pii: bcr2014207912. [A].

[252] Jalota R, Bond C, José RJ. Quetiapine and the development of the metabolic syndrome. QJM. 2015;108(3):245–7 [A].

[253] Lalli A, Michel B, Georget S, et al. Thrombocytopenia with quetiapine: two case reports, one with positive rechallenge. Rev Bras Psiquiatr. 2015;37(4):351–2 [A].

[254] Fan KY, Chen WY, Huang MC. Quetiapine-associated leucopenia and thrombocytopenia: a case report. BMC Psychiatry. 2015;15:110 [A].

[255] Crépeau-Gendron G, L'Heureux S. Quetiapine XR-induced neutropenia: is a clozapine trial still possible for treatment-resistant schizophrenia? A case report. Early Interv Psychiatry. 2015;9(2):151–5 [A].

[256] Koloth R, John AP. Occurrence of stuttering priapism on low dose of quetiapine. Aust N Z J Psychiatry. 2015;49(8):757 [A].

[257] Wysokiński A. Persistent penile erection (priapism) associated with quetiapine and lithium. J Neuropsychiatry Clin Neurosci. 2015;27(1):e77 [A].

[258] Jackson JC, Torrence CL. Quetiapine-induced priapism requiring frequent emergency admissions: a case report. Urol Case Rep. 2014;3(1):1–2 [A].

[259] Aguglia A, Maina G. Can quetiapine extended release (ER) induce labial edema in a female patient with treatment-resistant major depressive episode? Aging Clin Exp Res. 2016;28(4):791–3 [A].

[260] Cabaleiro T, López-Rodríguez R, Román M, et al. Pharmacogenetics of quetiapine in healthy volunteers: association with pharmacokinetics, pharmacodynamics, and adverse effects. Int Clin Psychopharmacol. 2015;30(2):82–8 [c].

[261] Mattson ME, Albright VA, Yoon J, et al. Emergency department visits involving misuse and abuse of the antipsychotic quetiapine: results from the Drug Abuse Warning Network (DAWN). Subst Abuse. 2015;9:39–46 [MC].

[262] Aman M, Rettiganti M, Nagaraja HN, et al. Tolerability, safety, and benefits of risperidone in children and adolescents with autism: 21-month follow-up after 8-week placebo-controlled trial. J Child Adolesc Psychopharmacol. 2015;25(6):482–93 [c].

[263] de Araújo AA, Ribeiro SB, Dos Santos AC, et al. Quality of life and hormonal, biochemical, and anthropometric profile between olanzapine and risperidone users. Psychiatr Q. 2016;87(2):293–304 [C].

[264] Kiliçaslan F, Bayazit H, Kandemir H, et al. Motor weakness related to risperidone. J Child Adolesc Psychopharmacol. 2015;25(6):520 [A].

[265] Bahr SM, Tyler BC, Wooldridge N, et al. Use of the second-generation antipsychotic, risperidone, and secondary weight gain are associated with an altered gut microbiota in children. Transl Psychiatry. 2015;5:e652 [c].

[266] Calarge CA, Ziegler EE, Del Castillo N, et al. Iron homeostasis during risperidone treatment in children and adolescents. J Clin Psychiatry. 2015;76(11):1500–5 [c].

[267] Etminan M, Carleton B, Brophy JM. Risperidone and risk of gynecomastia in young men. J Child Adolesc Psychopharmacol. 2015;25(9):671–3 [MC].

[268] Dos Santos Júnior A, Henriques TB, de Mello MP, et al. Hyperprolactinemia in children and adolescents with use of risperidone: clinical and molecular genetics aspects. J Child Adolesc Psychopharmacol. 2015;25(10):738–48 [C].

[269] Wang F, Mi W, Ma W, et al. A pharmacogenomic study revealed an association between SLC6A4 and risperidone-induced weight gain in Chinese Han population. Pharmacogenomics. 2015;16(17):1943–9 [C].

[270] Nielsen J, Matz J, Mittoux A, et al. Cardiac effects of sertindole and quetiapine: analysis of ECGs from a randomized double-blind study in patients with schizophrenia. Eur Neuropsychopharmacol. 2015;25(3):303–11 [C].

[271] Nielsen J, Wang F, Graff C, Kanters JK. QT dynamics during treatment with sertindole. Ther Adv Psychopharmacol. 2015;5(1):26–31 [c].

[272] Zoccali RA, Bruno A, Muscatello MR. Efficacy and safety of sertindole in schizophrenia: a clinical review. J Clin Psychopharmacol. 2015;35(3):286–95 [r].

[273] Mandrioli R, Protti M, Mercolini L. Evaluation of the pharmacokinetics, safety and clinical efficacy of ziprasidone for the treatment of schizophrenia and bipolar disorder. Expert Opin Drug Metab Toxicol. 2015;1:149–74 [r].

[274] Lee CP, Chen AP, Juang YY. Weight gain while switching from polypharmacy to ziprasidone: a case report. Clin Schizophr Relat Psychoses. 2015;9(3):141–4 [A].

[275] Iskandar JW, Vance JE, Kablinger A, et al. Transient agranulocytosis associated with ziprasidone in a 45-year-old man on hemodialysis. J Clin Psychopharmacol. 2015;35(3):347–8 [A].

[276] Chan VC, La Grenade L, Diak IL, et al. US Food and Drug Administration warning about the risk of drug reaction with eosinophilia and systemic symptoms with ziprasidone. J Clin Psychiatry. 2015;76(9):e1138–9 [c].

[277] Lister JF, Voinov B, Thimothy L, et al. Drug-induced systemic hypersensitivity reaction associated with ziprasidone: an atypical occurrence. J Clin Psychopharmacol. 2015;35(4):478–80 [A].

6

Antiepileptics

Brian Spoelhof*,[1], Lynn Frendak*, Nicole Kiehle*, Ashley Martinelli*,
Lucia Rivera Lara[†]

*Department of Pharmacy, Johns Hopkins Bayview Medical Center, Baltimore, MD, USA
[†]Departments of Neurology, Anesthesiology, and Critical Care Medicine, Johns Hopkins Medicine,
Baltimore, MD, USA
[1]Corresponding author: brian.spoelhof@jhmi.edu

BARBITURATES

Nervous System

A case of pseudoseizure was reported in a 38-year-old female who had been taking phenytoin 100 mg and phenobarbital 30 mg for 5 years for treatment of idiopathic generalized tonic–clonic seizures. Serum levels of phenytoin were found to be 28.79 µg/mL and phenobarbital 42 µg/mL. Both drugs were discontinued and the patient's symptoms improved [1A].

Pregnancy

An observational study evaluating maternal antiepileptic use and intrauterine death found that exposure to phenobarbital resulted in an 8.5 percent rate of spontaneous abortion or stillbirths. Rates were higher with exposure to phenobarbital in combination with another antiepileptic [2C].

BRIVARACETAM

Meta-Analysis

A meta-analysis of 5 randomized studies determined that brivaracetam was associated with a 3.0- to 5.98-fold increase in fatigue and nasopharyngitis at 20 mg, a 2.38- to 2.95-fold increase in fatigue and irritability at 50 mg, and a 2.21-fold increase in somnolence at 150 mg. This results are consistent with levetiracetam and may describe a class-wide effect [3M].

Observational Studies

A small open-label study evaluated switching from levetiracetam to brivaracetam. One-third of patients experiences drug-related adverse effects. Headache, fatigue, and back pain were the most reported adverse effects [4c].

Drug Interactions

An open-label pharmacokinetic study in 14 healthy patients evaluated the effect of brivaracetam and carbamazepine coadministration on drug levels. Carbamazepine decreased brivaracetam and the hydroxyl metabolite AUC by 29% and 17%, respectively. Furthermore, the AUC of a carbamazepine active metabolite, carbamazepine epoxide was increased twofold [5c].

Nervous System

A patient developed myoclonic epilepsy following conversation from levetiracetam to brivaracetam in a small open-label study [4c].

Psychiatric

A patient with history of mood and morbid thoughts developed suicidal ideation and attempted suicide in a small open-label trial [4c]. Despite patient history, emotional lability cannot be ruled out as a potential adverse effect.

CARBAMAZEPINE

Observational Trial

A pooled analysis evaluated the tolerability of intravenous carbamazepine demonstrated dizziness, somnolence, headache, and blurred vision. There were no differences in reported adverse effects between oral and IV carbamazepine [6c].

Cardiovascular

A 56-year-old male had been treated with carbamazepine 400 mg per day for at least 1 year presented with recurrent attacks of dizziness and syncope. Symptoms had persisted for 1 month. The patient has a heart rate of 52 bpm and an ECG demonstrated a 2:1 AV nodal block. Carbamazepine levels were obtained and were normal (7 mg/dL, range: 6–12 mg/dL). Carbamazepine was switched to valproic acid and all symptoms resolved [7A].

Nutrition

A study of 160 individuals evaluated antiepileptic withdrawal in patients who had been controlled on monotherapy for greater than 2 years. A total of 47 patients on carbamazepine withdrew therapy and 37 on carbamazepine did not withdraw. Those that withdrew carbamazepine therapy had favorable changes in their lipid profile. Decreases in total cholesterol, LDL and Apoprotien B were noted [8c].

Skin

A 38-year-old woman had been taking carbamazepine for 3 month when she developed a scattered rash with target-like lessions. The patient had a 1-week history of worsening fever, malaise, and itchy eruptions. Laboratory examination revealed eosinophilia (24%), and elevated AST (103 U/L), ALLT (187 U/L), Alkaline phosphates (1098 U/L), y-glutamyl transferase (670 U/L). Carbamazepine therapy was ceased, and the patient was treated with prednisone. Symptoms resolved within 2 weeks [9A].

Drug Interaction

An *in vitro* study analyzed the effect of carbamazepine and sertraline coadministration in human fetal brain and kidney tissue. Neurocytotoxicity was noted 15 min following infusion. Cytotoxic effect correlated with carbamazepine conversion to 2-hydroxycarbamazepine [10H]. Results may indicated potential interaction between sertraline and carbamazepine through CYP 3A4 inhibition. Case reports demonstrating a clinical effect have been limited.

Monitoring Therapy

A study evaluated the need for carbamazepine epoxide serum concentrations in addition to carbamazepine serum concentrations. The study evaluated concentrations in 107 individuals. The results demonstrated low levels of the epoxide metabolite in most individuals, and only two cases that exceeded the therapeutic window [11h].

A study demonstrated the cost-effectiveness of pharmacogenomic testing to prevent cutaneous reactions [12h].

Pharmacogenomics

A case control, observation trial in a Vietnamese cohort evaluated 38 confirmed cases of carbamazepine-induced severe cutaneous adverse drug reactions. The presence of HLA-B*1502 was associated with an OR of 33.78 (95% CI, 7.55–151.03) [13c]. Several studies have confirmed the effects of HLA-B*1502 in Asian populations on the risk of cutaneous reactions with carbamazepine.

ESLICARBAZEPINE

Multicenter Study

A multicenter, double-blind, randomized, control trial to evaluate eslicarbazepine for acute mania found the most common side effects reported were mild and included dizziness, headache, vomiting, nausea, and diarrhea. Several side effects that were deemed serious occurred infrequently: 2 cases of mania with eslicarbazepine 300 mg, 1 case of anemia and oesophageal stenosis with eslicarbazepine 900 mg, 1 case of pneumonia with eslicarbazepine 900 mg, 1 case of bronchitis with eslicarbazepine 1800 mg, 1 case of depression with eslicarbazepine 1800 mg, and 1 case of gastrointestinal disorder with 1800 mg [14C].

GABAPENTIN

Meta-Analysis

A meta-analysis of 133 randomized controlled trials examining gabapentin for postoperative pain found that while gabapentin reduced the incidence of nausea, vomiting, and pruritus, it was associated with an increased incidence of sedation compared to control in this patient population [15M].

A meta-analysis of 10 publications evaluating the use of gabapentin in alcohol withdrawal found no severe adverse effects. The most common adverse effects reported were similar to those reported in gabapentin used for other indications and included vertigo, nausea, dizziness, ataxia, insomnia, sleepiness, euphoria, headache, and fatigue [16M].

Observational Studies

A small pharmacovigilance study compared the safety and efficacy of gabapentin to pregabalin in palliative patients. Pain scores were not significantly different between the two groups; however, gabapentin doses were approximately half that of pregabalin doses, and patients treated with gabapentin were almost three times more likely to experience adverse effects. Most common adverse effects were somnolence, ataxia, nausea, tremor, and nystagmus [17c].

Nervous System

A randomized controlled trial examining the efficacy of gabapentin 600 mg preoperatively followed by 200 mg q8h for pain following cesarean delivery found a 16 percent increased incidence of sedation in the gabapentin group compared to control at 24 hours [18c].

A retrospective cohort study evaluated the efficacy and safety of gabapentin for uremic pruritus and restless leg syndrome in patients with chronic kidney disease. Drowsiness was the most commonly reported adverse effect followed by dizziness, fatigue, blurred vision, unsteadiness, and confusion. Almost half (47%) of patients reported more than one adverse effect, and 17% of patients discontinued gabapentin due to adverse effects [19c].

A randomized crossover study to evaluate pharmacokinetics, pharmacodynamics, safety, and tolerability of gabapentin enacarbil, a prodrug of gabapentin, in combination with morphine found an increased incidence of dizziness in patients treated with gabapentin enacarbil. This adverse effect of the prodrug is consistent with gabapentin [20E].

A case of gabapentin-induced encephalopathy was described in an 85-year-old female. The patient presented with symptoms of confusion, memory deterioration, and time disorientation 5 days after beginning gabapentin for partial seizures. A dose of 300 mg on day 1 followed by 900 mg daily was administered [21A].

LACOSAMIDE

Cardiovascular

Data from three multicenter, randomized, double-blind, placebo-controlled trials of lacosamide in 1308 patients with partial onset seizures were pooled to assess for cardiac-related adverse events. Lacosamide was titrated to effect with patients receiving 200 mg/day, 400 mg/day, 600 mg/day or placebo. PR interval prolongation, +4.4 ms, occurred in patients receiving 400 mg/day, but no patients had symptomatic arrhythmias or adverse events requiring cessation of lacosamide [22M].

Intensive care unit patients received a 400 mg intravenous loading dose and found the PR interval to be prolonged following infusion. The change was not consistent with the longest PR interval at 240 ms [23A].

To assess whether lacosamide prolongs the corrected QT interval (QTc), 247 healthy volunteers were randomized to receive lacosamide 400 mg/day (6 days), lacosamide 800 mg/day (6 days), placebo (6 days), or moxifloxacin as a positive control (3 days). Lacosamide did not prolong the Qtc even at supratherapeutic dosing. Additionally, no relationship was found between peak plasma concentration and QTc values. Common adverse events include dizziness, nausea, headache, vomiting. One patient experienced a spontaneous abortion, and two patients withdrew from the study due to neck pain or feeling drunk with nausea, ear discomfort, and moderate syncope [24A].

Nervous System

Lacosamide 300 mg/day was administered to 27 healthy adult patients with good sleep hygiene to assess the impact on sleep parameters. No sleep disturbances were found although patients noted common adverse events of affect lability, headache, somnolence, and dizziness [25c].

In patients with Lenox–Gastaut syndrome, lacosamide was evaluated as combination therapy in a retrospective analysis of 19 adult patients after multiple antiepileptic drugs, corpus callostomy surgery, or vagal nerve stimulation failures and experiencing a least four seizures per month during the month prior to lacosamide introduction. Two patients experienced greater than 50% reduction in seizures, and one patient experienced less than 50% reduction; however, 16 patients had an increase in tonic seizures. Seven of 18 patients also reported an increase in astatic seizures. At this time, addition of lacosamide for patients with Lennox–Gastaut syndrome must be carefully decided as it has the potential to increase seizure frequency [26A].

Sexual Function

A 27-year-old male receiving oxcarbazine 2000 mg/day for posttraumatic epilepsy. Due to continued simple and complex partial seizures, he was initiated on lacosamide and titrated to 400 mg/day. A few days after achieving the target dose, he experienced new-onset severe reduction in libido with erectile dysfunction with denial of any new medications or substance abuse. Lacosamide was titrated off, and topiramate was initiated with complete resolution of symptoms [27A].

LAMOTRIGINE

Skin

Rash is one of the most frequent adverse effects of lamotrigine. The incidence of rash is seen in up to 10% of patients and can be mild urticarial to severe reactions such as Stevens–Johnson syndrome (SJS) and toxic epidermal necrolysis (TEN) [28r]. A review of the Spanish Pharmacovigilance database found that over the reporting period from 1980 to 2009, lamotrigine was one of the most commonly reported drugs associated with SJS and TEN with 37 and 20 reports of each, respectively [29r].

Cosmetic side effects can lead to changes or discontinuation of antiepileptic drugs. In a retrospective review of adult patients started on antiepileptic drugs, researchers found that lamotrigine had a lower incidence of cosmetic adverse effects compared to other therapies. It was found that lamotrigine had a higher incidence of acne compared to other therapies (0.6%) [30C].

A 4-year-old male started on lamotrigine presented 3 weeks later with toxic epidermal necrolysis (TEN). He had fever, headache, pruritus and dermal eruption on the face, trunk, limbs and genitals that involved 70% of his body surface area [31r].

Immunologic

A case report of a 59-year-old female found that she was experiencing fever and systemic rash. She had been started on lamotrigine 3 weeks prior to the rash which was desquamating erythematous over her face, lips, torso and extremities. She had peripheral eosinophilia, elevation of transaminases and was diagnosed with Drug Reaction with Eosinophilia and Systemic Symptoms (DRESS). The medication was discontinued and her symptoms resolved [32c].

Second-Generation Effects

A prospective review of pregnant women on various antiepileptic drugs monitored intrauterine death. Patients exposed to lamotrigine monotherapy found a combined rate of spontaneous abortions and stillbirth of 7.8% ($n = 1910$). This was not dose dependent as the highest rate of events was found in dose range between 180 and 325 mg [2C].

A controlled cohort study of children exposed to maternal antiepileptic drugs looked at IQ at 6 years old after in utero exposure. Children exposed to lamotrigine had similar IQ or verbal, nonverbal and spatial abilities compared to the controls [33C].

A review of treatments for bipolar disorder during pregnancy reported that lamotrigine monotherapy does not increase the risk of major congenital malformations. Rates of malformation were similar to the rates found in the general public estimated at 2–3% [34M]. The risk of malformation seems to be increased as doses greater than 300 mg/day [35r].

Susceptibility Factors

A single center study looked at Korean patients who experienced maculopapular eruption after use of lamotrigine. When compared to patients who tolerated lamotrigine therapy, it was found that the frequency of the HLA-A*2402 allele was significantly higher in the group that did not tolerate lamotrigine. Patients with concomitant HLA*2402 and Cw*0102 alleles were more significantly more frequent in the group that did not tolerate lamotrigine therapy compared with the patients that did tolerate. The A*3303 allele frequency was significantly lower in the group who experience rash than in the general population suggesting a protective effect for this allele [36c].

A review of Chinese articles looking for lamotrigine-induced SJS/TEN found that the HLA-B*1502 allele was significantly associated with the risk of developing SJS/TEN. Patients using lamotrigine with allele were nearly five times more likely to develop SJS/TEN [37M].

A single center review of Japanese patients with skin eruptions treated with lamotrigine looked at allele frequencies between patients with cutaneous reactions and those that were tolerant of lamotrigine therapy. The group with the reactions found significantly higher incidence of HLA-DRB1*0405 and DQB1*0401 [38c].

LEVETIRACETAM

Nervous System

The most common adverse effects reported with levetiracetam are neurologic including dizziness, headache and fatigue. A randomized, double-blind, parallel group trial conducted in elderly patients with new-onset focal epilepsy found this to be true with greater than 25% of patients in the levetiracetam group reporting these symptoms [39C].

A retrospective review looking at efficacy of levetiracetam and serum levels in children at a single center found mainly neurological effects. Of the 50 patients enrolled, 30% of patients reported violent behavior as the most common adverse effect ($n = 8$). This was the only adverse effect that significantly correlated with levetiracetam serum concentrations; however, it was the patients lower serum concentrations that demonstrated violent behavior [40c].

Another case reported obsessive–compulsive behavior induced by levetiracetam. A 14-year-old female with history of generalized tonic–clonic seizures was started on levetiracetam and found to have compulsive behaviors after 2 months of therapy. After this therapy was identified as a possible cause, it was discontinued and the obsessive–compulsive behaviors completely disappeared [41c].

In a prospective, open-label, randomized study comparing carbamazepine and levetiracetam as monotherapy in partial seizures, it was found that aggressive behavior was more common in the levetiracetam group. Adverse effects were more common in the levetiracetam group with behavioral changes being most common included increased aggressive behavior, increased anxiety and suicidal tendency [42c].

A retrospective, long-term observational study looking at monotherapy options for partial epilepsy in China found that patients treated with levetiracetam most commonly experienced neurological adverse effects. These included drowsiness, memory problems and anxiety/irritability/nervousness. Only three patients over the 7-year study period reported intolerable adverse effects of rash, dizziness and anxiety/irritability/nervousness [43c].

Electrolyte Balance

Two patients with severe hypokalemia associated with levetiracetam were reported. Serum potassium in both patients decreased to 2.43 and 2.44 mmol/L, respectively. The second patient was reported to have normal serum potassium prior to initiation up to 4.5 mmol/L. Upon discontinuation of levetiracetam, the hypokalemia subsided within 3 days in both patients. Both of these patients also experienced hypomagnesemia with levels reaching 1.35 mg/dL and 0.58 mmol/L [44r].

Hematological

A case report of a 79-year-old female started on levetiracetam after a temporal craniotomy with resection experienced anemia on the fifth postoperative day. She also was noted to have thrombocytopenia and leukopenia. Medications that could have caused these were discontinued and other causes ruled out. On the 10th postoperative day, levetiracetam was discontinued and within 24 hours, platelet counts improved and other cell lines began to improve over the following 5 days [45r].

Skin

A 35-year-old woman presenting with new-onset generalized tonic–clonic convulsions was initiated on levetiracetam 500 mg daily. This dose was gradually increased to 1000 mg daily. After 10 days of therapy, the patient presented with erythematous skin lesions on her knees and elbows. She was on no other medications at the time. She diagnosed with psoriasiform drug eruption due to

levetiracetam which began to disappear a few weeks after discontinuation of the offending agent [46r].

Immunologic

A case report of unexplained fever and eosinophilia was reported in a 24-year-old male who was initiated on levetiracetam upon admission for seizure activity and acute mental status changes. The patient had normal absolute eosinophil count of 0.24 K/μL and was afebrile upon admission. The patient became persistently febrile on day 3 of admission with T_{max} of 103.4 °F. The absolute eosinophil count began to rise on day 8 and peaked on day 18 despite discontinuation of levetiracetam on day 14. The authors attributed this probability to levetiracetam as probable with the Naranjo scale [47r].

A separate case report of a 53-year-old man who developed DRESS syndrome after receiving levetiracetam. The patient experienced fever, significant leukocytosis up to 28000 mm³ and eosinophilia up to 50%. He developed a severe skin rash on the face, back, upper arms and abdomen. The rash resolved 10 days after discontinuing levetiracetam and receiving steroids [48r].

Second Generation

An observational international cohort study reviewed major congenital malformations after prenatal anti-epileptic drug exposure. Patients were included if the pregnancy was exposed to medications at the time of conception and no later than 16 weeks of gestation and included 7055 pregnancies. Among patients on monotherapy with anti-epileptics, women on levetiracetam had the highest rate of spontaneous abortions and stillbirths ($n=28$) of the six therapies reviewed [2C].

OXCARBAZEPINE

Sensory Systems

59-year-old male with systemic lupus erythematosus, lupus neuropathy, focal epilepsy, and left thalamic stroke with central neuropathic pain and right hemiataxia was admitted to the emergency department due to daily dizziness and unsteady gait lasting 3–5 hours every afternoon. Home medications include amitriptyline 50 mg/day, phenytoin 350 mg/day divided, levetiracetam 2500 mg/day divided, and oxcarbazepine 1800 mg/day divided. Exam was positive for somnolence and appendicular and trunk ataxia and nystagmus in the direction of the gaze with rotation component and spontaneous eyelid nystagmus in the primary direction of gaze. Attacks occurred 30 min following oxcarbazepine afternoon dosing and were correlated with high plasma levels. Reduced dosing of oxcarbazepine resolved symptoms and should be considered in patient presenting with nystagmus on oxcarbazepine therapy [49A].

Psychiatric

Depression is common among epilepsy patients and can decrease quality of life more than frequent seizures alone. The prevalence of depression among 289 Polish epileptic patients was assessed to evaluate risk factors for depression. Multivariate analysis revealed independent variables associated with depression diagnosis including frequent seizures (OR=2.43), use of depression-inducing medications (OR=3.33), age (OR=1.03 for every year more), and use of oxcarbazepine (OR=2.26). Use of oxcarbazepine likely reflects patients on several agents with frequent seizures as it is not first line therapy. Additionally patients on oxcarbazepine were more likely to live alone, a risk factor for depression. Oxcarbazepine cannot be directly linked as a cause of depression, but general risk for depression should be assessed if multiple agents are utilized to control epilepsy [50C].

Skin

Oxcarbazepine is known for having a lower incidence of allergic reactions, such as Stevens–Johnson syndrome (SJS) and toxic epidermal necrolysis (TEN), and enzyme induction compared to carbamazepine. A 60-year-old man on losartan for hypertension presented with a hemorrhagic stroke with initiation of phenytoin for seizure management. Phenytoin was changed to oxcarbazepine due to poor control. After 2 weeks of therapy, the patient developed generalized rash, ulcers, and hyperemic conjunctivae with an elevated C-reactive protein and positive skin biopsy confirming TEN. Patient improved within a week of oxcarbazepine discontinuation and was maintained on levetiracetam without breakthrough seizures [51A].

A second case report of a 40-year-old Indian male on pantoprazole 40 mg/day and lorazepam 0.5 mg/day was initiated on oxcarbazepine 300 mg twice daily, for convulsions and a space occupying lesion in the left inferior parietal lobe. Due to concern for a tuberculoma, isoniazid 300 mg, rifampicin 450 mg, ethambutol 1000 mg, pyrazinamide 1500 mg, and vitamin B6 40 mg and streptomycin 750 mg injection. The following day the patient experienced an extensive maculopapular rash covering his whole body except his face, palms, and sole. Oxcarbazepine was replaced with levetiracetam with rash resolution. It is likely due to the drug–drug interaction of isoniazid, a CYP3A4 inhibitor, and oxcarbazepine, a CPY3A4 inducer that may have led to increased levels of oxcarbazepine [52A].

Musculoskeletal

Patients with epilepsy have a higher rate of fractures than the general population. A study assessing 48 adult patients with epilepsy on either levetiracetam (n=21) or oxcarbazepine (n=27) monotherapy for at least 6 months found that patients receiving AEDs and the control group (n=42) had low levels of 25-OH vitamin D3. Levels of calcium and ionized calcium were normal in patients using oxcarbazepine, but they were significantly lower than the control group (8.94±0.53, 9.32±0.36 mg/dL, p=0.003) and (4.25±0.19, 4.46±0.20 mg/dL, p=0.006). Levels of 25-OH vitamin D3 levels were also significantly lower in the oxcarbazepine group (7.29±3.95, 12.25± 9.07 ng/mL, p=0.011). No overall trends could be identified based on length of therapy [53c].

Sex

Seventy-nine patients on carbamazepine (n=26) or oxcarbazepine (n=49) for trigeminal neuralgia and neuralgiform headaches completed an adverse events profile during an office visit to identify the frequency of adverse events associated with their medication therapy. Dose and female gender were positive predictors of adverse events in multivariate analysis. Patients on carbamazepine versus oxcarbazepine had a lower adverse event score. Females had a 50% probability of experiencing an adverse event if the dose is four times the standard dose of at doses of 1200 mg oxcarbazepine and 800 mg of carbamazepine versus a 20% probability for males at doses of 1800 mg of oxcarbazine and 1200 mg carbamazepine. Common adverse events included tiredness (31.3%), sleepiness (18.2%), memory problems (22.7%), disturbed sleep (14.1%), and difficulty concentrating or unsteadiness (both 11.6%). It appears that lower doses in females produce a higher rate of adverse events. Consider toxicities at lower dosing ranges for female patients as they may require conversion to another antiepileptic therapy [54C].

Drug–Drug Interactions

An 8-year-old Caucasian male with autism spectrum disorder (ASD) was initiated on oxcarbazepine 450 mg twice daily due to aggressive behaviors and failure of several other agents. Current medications included clonidine 0.1 mg twice daily, quetiapine 200 mg twice daily and 300 mg at bedtime. He presented for an acute psychiatric admission, oxcarbazepine was tapered and therapeutic drug monitoring of quetiapine performed. Prior to initiation of oxcarbazepine, quetiapine levels were 62 ng/mL; however, they decreased significantly to 24 ng/mL during admission. Following a 2 week taper off oxcarbazepine and increasing quetiapine to 300 mg three times daily, the patient recovered and did not require subsequent psychiatric admissions over the next 2 months. Oxcarbazepine appears to reduce concentrations of quetiapine through the CYP3A4 enzyme. Patients should be monitored closely for their psychiatric conditions if oxcarbazepine is initiated [55A].

Oxcarbazepine and verapamil are substrates of *p*-glycoprotein and verapamil also inhibits the transporter leading to possible drug interactions. Twelve healthy volunteers approximately 30 years of age received oxcarbazepine monotherapy 300 mg every 12 hours or oxcarbazepine plus verapamil 80 mg every 8 hours for 5 days to assess the influence of verapamil on oxcarbazepine. Verapamil increased the AUC of both oxcarbazepine enantiomers in 10% of volunteers. It is possible that dose reductions may be necessary with this drug combination, consider monitoring [56c].

A 33-year-old female on long-term oxcarbazepine (1200 mg/day) for epilepsy was initiated on rifampicin 600 mg daily and clindamycin 300 mg twice day for treatment-resistant acne vulgaris with therapeutic drug monitoring of oxcarbazepine and 10-monohydroxy-carbazepine (MHD), the active metabolite. Rifampicin significantly reduced the MHD concentration by 49% on day 7, without a reduction in oxcarbazepine levels. A 75% dose increase in oxcarbazepine dosing to 2100 mg achieved pre-rifampicin levels. Discontinuation of rifampicin led to increased levels of MHD and gradual titration of oxcarbazepine to the pre-rifampicin dose. Oxcarbazepine levels must be monitored if rifampicin is co-administered [57A].

PERAMPANEL

Observational Studies

An retrospective observational trial of 310 patients found patients experienced sedation (23.8%), behavioral and mood disturbance (22.6%), dizziness (13.5%), unsteadiness (11.3%) [58C].

A pooled analysis of phase II trials evaluating the rate of adverse events over time demonstrated adverse *effects* were most common at the initiation of therapy and following dose titration. This result was most common with somnolence, dizziness, and fatigue [59C]. These results indicate that the adverse events of perampanel are transient and should be discussed with patients at dose increases.

Cardiovascular

A double-blind parallel controlled trial was conducted to assess the effects of perampanel on cardiac repolarization and QTc prolongation. Compared with placebo doses of perampanel less than 12 mg had no effect on QTc [60c].

Nervous System

An observational review of perampanel use found 11% or patients developed neuropsychiatric symptoms severe enough to precipitate discontinuation. Reactions included depression, irritability, and aggression [61c].

A separate post-marketing observational trial found irritability and fatigue in 36.4% and 22.7% of patients, respectively [62c].

Liver

A prospective open-label study evaluated the effect of perampanel on liver function compared to placebo. Laboratory analysis included alanine aminotransferase, alkaline phosphatase, aspartate aminotransferase, gamma-glutamyl transpeptidase, and total bilirubin. No appreciable differences were noted [63C].

Susceptibility Factors

A pooled analysis of 3 phase 3 trials evaluated efficacy, safety, and pharmacokinetics, difference between male and female sex. There was a consistent rate of treatment emergent adverse effects between males and females. However, there was a 17% decrease in clearance or perampanel in females. This is likely due to changes in body weight and composition [64r].

An observational trial found no difference in reports of adverse events between adults with and without learning disabilities. However, mood and behavioral disturbances were higher in those with learning disability [58C]. This may not be a reflection of the perampanel, rather the patient population.

A sub group analysis of phase III clinical trials demonstrated a potential risk of perampanel in elderly patients. Falls, dizziness, and fatigue were higher in elderly patients [65c]. Due to the severity of these adverse events in the elderly population caution should be used in elderly patients.

Interactions

A pharmcokinetic study demonstrated that carbamazepine, oxcarbazepine, topiramte, and phenytoin reduced perampanel concentrations by 69%, 37%, 18%, and 13%, respectively [66E].

A small observational study compared perampanel use in those taking enzyme-inducing antiepileptics to those who do were taking non-enzyme-inducing antiepileptics confirmed pharmacokinetic data. The use of enzyme-inducing antiepileptics had lower response rates. Overall treatment emergent adverse events were similar between the groups, but fatigue, somnolence, dizziness, and irritability were lower in those taking enzyme-inducing antiepileptics [67c]. Furthermore, a *post-hoc* analysis of a phase III trial predicted a lower response rate in patients taking multiple antiepileptics [68C]. However, this may be an effect of refractory epilepsy or an enzyme-inducing interaction.

PHENYTOIN

Nervous System

A small observational study investigating the efficacy and safety of fosphenytoin use for acute encephalopathy in children found one case of apnea and oral dyskinesia. The patient was found to have an elevated serum phenytoin level of 27.8 mcg/mL following a loading dose of 22.5 mg/kg and 3 maintenance doses of 7.5 mg/kg [69c].

Immunologic

A hypersensitivity reaction was reported in a 49-year-old male who was taking phenytoin with diazepam and ranitidine for generalized tonic–clonic seizures. The patient developed skin rash, bullae, and fever 3 days after beginning therapy. It was thought that this reaction was due to a CYP2C19 drug–drug interaction with diazepam or a cytochrome P450 interaction with ranitidine [70A].

A case of purple glove syndrome was reported in a 35-year-old male 20 days after beginning oral phenytoin 300 mg/day. Previously, purple glove syndrome has been associated with IV administration of phenytoin [71A].

Musculoskeletal

A case of osteopathy was reported in a 29-year-old female taking phenytoin 300 mg daily for 10 years for seizure disorder. The patient initially presented with bilateral hip pain and movement restriction and was found to have vitamin D deficiency, osteomalacia, and secondary hyperparathyroidism. After treatment with parathormone and high doses of vitamin D, she continued to have pain and new hypervitaminosis D. She improved over 6 months, and vitamin D normalized after phenytoin was discontinued [72A].

Drug–Drug Interactions

A case of phenytoin toxicity was reported in a 48-year-old female taking a combination of capecitabine for breast cancer treatment and prophylactic phenytoin for brain metastases. The interaction is thought to be due to a CYP2C9 metabolism interaction [73A].

PREGABALIN

Meta-Analysis

A meta-analysis of 9 trials evaluating the efficacy and safety of pregabalin for diabetic peripheral neuropathy determined that pregabalin was associated with dizziness, somnolence, peripheral edema, weight gain, asthenia, euphoria, and gait disturbances. Dizziness and somnolence are dose related and occur more frequently with 600 mg compared to 300 mg doses. A fixed-effect model found higher rates of constipation and dry mouth in the pregabalin group compared with placebo; however, the same was not found with a random-effect model so no definitive conclusions could be drawn. In addition, pregabalin was associated with higher dose related withdrawal rates due to adverse effects [74M].

Gastrointestinal

A small randomized controlled trial comparing pregabalin to diazepam for tonsillectomy pain control found a small increase in the frequency of nausea and vomiting in the pregabalin group. The difference was not significant [75c].

Nervous System

The most common adverse effects of pregabalin reported are dizziness and somnolence. This was confirmed by multiple randomized and comparative studies:

A comparative study looking at pregabalin for postoperative shoulder pain after thoracotomy in patients with lung cancer found a higher incidence of somnolence in the pregabalin group compared to the control group [76c].

A prospective, randomized, placebo-controlled double-blind study comparing pregabalin to placebo in prevention of catheter-related bladder discomfort found higher sedation scores in the pregabalin group compared to the control group [77c].

A double-blind, randomized, placebo-controlled, multidose trial comparing pregabalin to placebo for pain after total knee arthroplasty found an increase in dose-dependent drowsiness in the pregabalin group [78c].

A prospective, randomized, double-blind study compared pregabalin to ondansetron for the treatment of uraemic pruritus in dialysis patients. Of the 62 patients in the pregabalin group 5 discontinued therapy due to adverse effects: somnolence ($n=3$) and severe dizziness and loss of balance ($n=2$) [79C].

RETIGABINE

Observational Trial

A retrospective observational trial of approximately 200 patients was conducted at 4 tertiary referral German hospitals. Three-fourths of patients experienced adverse events. The most common reactions were neuropsychiatric in nature, consisting of problems with alertness, wakefulness, concentration and fatigue in 27.2% of patients. Furthermore patients experience speech impairment, gait disorders, impaired cognition, and behavioral disorders. Mildly elevated liver functions tests and urinary issues were reported in 12.85% and 14.4% of patients [80C].

Nervous System

A small observational study found dizziness, somnolence, vertigo, fatigue and asthenia has treatment emergent adverse effects occurring in greater than 5% of patients [81c].

Psychiatric

A 21-year-old male with no significant past medical history developed several psychiatric complications 1 week after an increased dose from 600 to 700 mg/day. He developed a feeling that his furniture was moving and leading to him "jumping wildly" to reduce the effect. Furthermore, he also developed coenesthesia and the feeling of small stones entering his mouth. He returned to baseline days after reducing the retigabine dose [82A].

Mouth and Teeth

A 70-year-old male on retigabine 300 mg three times daily presented with purple/blue lesion on the roof of his mouth. Further examination noted similar discoloration of the nail beds. Time of onset was unable to be determined due to the infrequency of monitoring the roof of the mouth [83A].

Skin

A short letter described the risk of blue-gray skin discoloration after the United States Food and Drug Administration updated retigabine's approved labeling [84r].

Diagnosis of Adverse Effects

Two surveys were conducted to assess provider and pharmacist [85H] knowledge of the risks of retigabine, one in the United States, the other in Europe. The results demonstrated mixed levels of knowledge on the uses and risks of retigabine [85H,86H].

RUFINAMIDE

Gastrointestinal

A retrospective cohort study of patients with refractory epilepsy syndromes found that patients on rufinamide most commonly experienced gastrointestinal adverse effects. There were 3 patients out of 133 that discontinued therapy due to intolerable vomiting and gastritis and 21% of all patients experienced some type of GI adverse effect [87c].

TOPIRAMATE

Sensory Systems

A case of bilateral acute angle closure was reported in a 39-year-old female 1 week after beginning phentermine 3.75 mg/topiramate 23 mg for weight loss. The patient presented with symptoms of acute bilateral vision loss and eye pain and was found to have bilateral acute angle closure, chorodial thickening measured by enhanced depth optical coherence tomography imaging, bilateral suprachoroidal effusions, and induced myopia. She was treated with IV methylprednisolone, mannitol, difluprednate ophthalmic emulsion, atropine sulfate, and brimonidine and timolol [88A].

Psychological

An observational study evaluating the use of topiramate for epilepsy in patients with intellectual disability found reduced cognitive speed, verbal short-term memory, verbal working memory, and semantic verbal fluency while taking topiramate compared to off-therapy [89c]. This is similar to previously reported adverse effects with topiramate use in patients without intellectual disability [90c].

A double-blind, placebo-controlled study comparing the efficacy and safety of topiramate, zonisamide, and levetiracetam in alcohol use disorders found that the topiramate group had increased mental slowing, reduced verbal fluency, reduced working memory, and increased irritability compared to placebo. In addition, 19% of patient treated with topiramate reported paresthesias and 14% reported erectile dysfunction [91c].

Psychiatric

A case series of 7 adolescent females with eating disorders related to topiramate use was reported. All patients received topiramate ranging from 25 to 150 mg for headache. Three patients had no previous history of eating disorders and 4 patients reported worsening or reoccurring disorders [92c].

Acid–Base Balance

A retrospective study conducted in veterans found a statistically significant decrease of 2.7 mEq/L in sodium bicarbonate after initiation of topiramate. However, the study did not find that sodium bicarbonate levels <17 mEq/L or a decrease in sodium bicarbonate levels ≥5 mEq/L correlated with side effects. Side effects reported were fatigue, mood changes, kidney stones, and a single case of metabolic acidosis [93C].

Urinary Tract

A case of calcium phosphate kidney stones was reported in a 40-year-old female taking topiramate 100 mg daily for chronic migraine. The patient had previously been stable on topiramate therapy for 2 years without adverse effects and had never before experienced kidney stones [94A]. In a response related to the same case, the authors noted that in some cases of chronic migraine and idiopathic intracranial hypertension refractory to other treatments, the use of topiramate may outweigh the risk of recurrent stones [95r].

VALPROIC ACID

Psychiatric

Hyperammonemia due to valproic acid therapy is well documented in the literature. A new case report highlights how important it is to check serum ammonia levels in patients with new altered mental status on valproic acid therapy. A 31-year-old with newly diagnosed mania and bipolar disorder was initiated on divalproex sodium 500 mg twice daily and olanzapine 5 mg daily with some improvement. Topiramate was added for vascular headaches which caused disorientation, confusion, gait instability, and subsequent discontinuation. Repeat labs including electrolytes, liver function tests, and CPK were within normal limits. Due to persistent mania symptoms, he was planned for electroconvulsive therapy (ECT) on day 29. Divalproex was tapered to 250 mg twice daily to prevent interference with ECT. The patient improved after two sessions, and slowly the divalproex dose was increased to 1500 mg divided with return of manic symptoms and

discontinuation of ECT at day 46. Again labs were assessed and serum valproate levels were 65 mg/L, and ammonia was 98 µmol/L. Divalproex was discontinued, and the patient was stabilized on oxcarbazine and aripiprazole and discharged on day 70 [96A].

Liver

An 18-month-old girl with Lennox–Gastaut syndrome was started on a 3:1, 1050-calorie classic ketogenic diet after multiple antiepileptic drug failures. Prior to the diet, she was receiving stable doses of topiramate 2.5 mg/kg/day, valproic acid 20 mg/kg/day, and clobazam 0.75 mg/kg/day, all in divided doses with normal LFTs. The evening of hospital discharge, she was febrile and received amoxicillin–clavulanate at an outside emergency department yet returned to the hospital the following morning with lethargy, hypotonia, and cyanotic extremities. Labs were significant for AST 924 IU/L, glucose 47 mg/dL, anion gap 16 meq/L, WBC 17000 K/mm^3 and ammonia 57 µmol/L with positive parainfluenza. Ketogenic diet and valproic acid were discontinued. Liver enzymes resolved over the subsequent 9 days, and ketogenic diet was reinstated and maintained for the next 12 months without further liver enzyme abnormalities. It is likely that this patient had several risk factors for developing liver injury due to medications, diet, and illness; however, stopping valproic acid therapy allowed for maintenance of the ketogenic diet and improved seizure control [97A].

Urinary Tract

Enuresis is common in children and has been linked to patients receiving valproic acid therapy. Seventy-two children were enrolled from an ongoing prospective trial, mean age 8 years 7 months, who were initiated and maintained on valproate for at least 1 month to assess the characteristics and risk factors for the development of valproate-induced enuresis. 17 patients experienced enuresis. Ten resolved while on valproate therapy, six required discontinuation. The mean dose was 13.6 mg/kg/day, and patients with enuresis had a mean dose 21.6 mg/kg/day and experienced enuresis within 14 days of starting therapy. This data show a small link between valproate therapy and the development on enuresis. As this can be a challenging adverse event for caregivers, this should be monitored; however, due to the lack of strong data, valproate therapy may not need to be discontinued [98c].

Skin

A 12-year-old boy achieved control of his absence seizures with 15 mg/kg/day of valproic acid. Two weeks after treatment, he developed a pruritic, maculopapular rash without mucosal involvement leading to discontinuation of therapy and resolution of rash. He was trialed on several agents including levetiracetam, ethosuximide, lamotrigine, and amantadine; however, all resulted in emergence of intolerable adverse events and poor seizure control. A desensitization protocol was initiated for valproic acid, starting at 0.05 mg/day and doubling every 2 days over a 1-month period to achieve the target dose of 400 mg twice daily by day 29. The patient tolerated the desensitization protocol well with no adverse events noted at 6-month follow-up [99A].

Teratogenicity

Valproic acid is known to cause teratogenicity and major congenital malformations (MCMs) especially at higher doses. A new observational study examined the occurrence of MCMs in the children of 1588 women taking valproic acid monotherapy or combination therapy in 42 countries. Enrolled women were taking AEDs at the time of conception and enrolled before gestation week 16 and before fetal outcome are known. The frequency of MCM at 1 year after birth was 10% for the monotherapy group and 11.3% for valproic acid + lamotrigine, and 11.7% for valproic acid + another AED. Mean valproic acid dosing at conception was significantly higher for the combination therapy group. The doses associated with cardiac malformations were 1001 ± 515 mg/day, 1108 ± 511 mg/day for hypospadias, 1258 ± 492 mg/day for neural tube defects, and 1382 ± 625 mg/day for multiple MCMs which are consistent with prior literature. Valproic acid teratogenicity appears to primarily be dose related [100C].

Drug–Drug Interactions

Carbapenem Therapy

A study of 28 children receiving concomitant treatment with valproic acid and a carbapenen was conducted to analyze the causes of simultaneous prescriptions, the consequence of coadministration, and the clinical outcomes associated with the therapy. 17 patients were already receiving valproic acid at the time of carbapenem initiation, with 64% reporting good seizure control. The other 11 patients received the combination simultaneously for the first time. Overall 78.6% of patients received therapy in the intensive care unit with meropenem (one patient with intramuscular ertapenem). Indications included nosocomial infection (25%), respiratory tract infection (25%), and resistant organism infection (25%) with median treatment duration of 3 days (1–9). Only 53% of patients received levels before starting carbapenem therapy, and drug levels were monitored at 24 hours for 17 patients.

At 24 hours, all but two patients were below the therapeutic range. Beyond 24 hours, all patients were below therapeutic range. Thirteen patients experienced clinical seizures with low valproic acid levels. This is the largest study in a pediatric patient population. It demonstrates the importance of avoiding this therapy combination when appropriate and the importance of close therapeutic drug level monitoring [101c].

This carbapenem interaction was also noted in an adult patient. An 80-year-old man with bipolar disorder was hospitalized for radiation after pathological rib fracture and adenocarcinoma with unknown primary. He was controlled on divalproex ER 750 mg twice daily for 16 years with trough serum levels between 75 and 105 mcg/mL. Additional medications included alpraxolam, hydromorphone, benzonatate, and omeprazole. On hospital day 25, he developed thrombocytopenia (nadir 43000/μL), and divalproex was reduced to 500 mg twice daily and treated with prednisone for idiopathic thrombocytopenia purpura with subsequent platelet recovery. Valproic acid levels measured 50 and 54 μg/mL. On day 67, he developed ESBL-positive *Escherichia coli* urinary tract infection and ertapenem 1000 mg daily was initiated. Two days later, he became excessively manic with pressured speech, demandingness, profanity, and irritability with decreased sleep. Valproic acid levels measured 22 and 19 μg/mL on days 69 and 71, respectively. Ertapenem was discontinued after 3 doses and serum levels returned to baseline by day 75. The likely mechanism for this interaction is carbapenem inhibition of acylpeptide hydrolase which hydrolyzes the inactive and renally cleared phase II product, valproic acid glucuronide back to the parent compound. This is a critical drug–drug interaction. For patients on valproic acid and requiring a carbapenem, consider drug level monitoring to ensure therapeutic levels for the duration of antimicrobial therapy [102A].

VIGABATRIN

Meta-Analysis

A systematic review and meta-analysis was conducted of trials comparing vigabatrin to carbamazepine. Vigabatrin demonstrated a 2.18-fold increase risk of 2.18 for weight gain, 2.00 for insomnia, 2.22 for depression, 5.37 for visual disturbances, and 15.68 for visual disturbances. There was a decrease in skin rash and leucopenia [103M].

Observational Studies

A large observational cohort reviewed 5 years of vigabatrin used. 4.1–4.8% of patients discontinued therapy due to unspecified adverse events [104C].

Nervous System

An 8-month-old female on vigabatrin 600 min twice daily for 4 weeks underwent a routine MRI of the brain. Imaging demonstrated extensive bilateral T2 hyperintensity and reduced diffusion signal of the basal ganglia, thalami, midbrain, dorsal pons, and dentate nuclei. The patient was asymptomatic despite concern for hypoxic-ischemic injury [105A]. A similar case of a 7-month-old female on 135 mg/kg/day of vigabatrin for 6 weeks was reported. The patient demonstrated restricted diffusion of the globi pallidi, thalami, and dorsal brainstem. The patient was asymptomatic. Repeat MRI demonstrated resolution of symptoms following 8 weeks after withdrawal of therapy [106A].

Sensory System

A commentary on vigabatrin-induced retinal disease recommended routine monitoring of children with electroretinograms. They further determined that 21% of patient demonstrated disease with 5.3% at 6 months and 13.3% at 12 months [107c]. Results were confirmed with a large observational trail [108c]. Another large observational trial demonstrated that 1% of patients developed a visual field defects [104C].

A small trial confirmed that one-third of children developed visual field defects. This risk ranged from 9% to 63% based on length of vigabatrin therapy [109c].

Genotoxicity

A trial of genotoxicty reported DNA damage at doses of 100 and 250 mg/kg in rats. Results were limited and not observed after 14 days of treatment [110E].

ZONISAMIDE

Sensory Systems

The first case of zonisamide-induced angle closure was reported in a patient initiated on the therapy for migraines. A 39-year-old Hispanic female presented with significantly narrowed observed angles compared with previous exams. She reported a 2-day history of sudden onset and progressive worsening of blurred vision in both eyes. The patient's vision returned to baseline 10 days after discontinuation of the zonisamide [111c].

Nervous System

The most common adverse effects of zonisamide reported are somnolence.

A retrospective study looking at zonisamide use in pediatric patients found somnolence as the most common adverse effect which diminished over time ($n = 24$) [112c].

An observational study of 151 patients assessed tolerability of zonisamide as adjunctive treatment for difficult-to-treat epilepsy confirmed most common adverse events were fatigue followed by headache. Most of the adverse effects were reported as mild to moderate in severity. Dizziness was the most common adverse effect that leads to discontinuation of zonisamide (5.3%) [113c].

Gastrointestinal

A retrospective study in which patients were administered a loading dose of zonisamide found 9.4% of patients reported nausea and vomiting ($n = 32$). These side effects were less common at follow-up visits [114c].

References

[1] Garekar H, Dhiman V. A case of pseudoseizures precipitated by anticonvulsant toxicity. Gen Hosp Psychiatry. 2015;37:372.e1–2. http://dx.doi.org/10.1016/j.genhosppsych.2015.03.010 [A].

[2] Tomson T, Battino D, Bonizzoni E, et al. Antiepileptic drugs and intrauterine death: a prospective observational study from EURAP. Neurology. 2015;85:580–8. http://dx.doi.org/10.1212/WNL.0000000000001840 [C].

[3] Tian X, Yuan M, Zhou Q, et al. The efficacy and safety of brivaracetam at different doses for partial-onset epilepsy: a meta-analysis of placebo-controlled studies. Expert Opin Pharmacother. 2015;16:1755–67. http://dx.doi.org/10.1517/14656566.2015.1058360[M] [M].

[4] Yates SL, Fakhoury T, Liang W, et al. An open-label, prospective, exploratory study of patients with epilepsy switching from levetiracetam to brivaracetam. Epilepsy Behav. 2015;52:165–8. http://dx.doi.org/10.1016/j.yebeh.2015.09.005 [c].

[5] Stockis A, Chanteux H, Rosa M, et al. Brivaracetam and carbamazepine interaction in healthy subjects and in vitro. Epilepsy Res. 2015;113:19–27. http://dx.doi.org/10.1016/j.eplepsyres.2015.03.003 [c].

[6] Tolbert D, Cloyd J, Biton V, et al. Bioequivalence of oral and intravenous carbamazepine formulations in adult patients with epilepsy. Epilepsia. 2015;56:915–23. http://dx.doi.org/10.1111/epi.13012 [c].

[7] Celik IE, Akyel A, Colgecen M, et al. A rare cause of 2:1 atrioventricular block: carbamazepine. Am J Emerg Med. 2015;33:1541.e3–4. http://dx.doi.org/10.1016/j.ajem.2015.07.055 [A].

[8] Lossius MI, Nakken KO, Mowinckel P, et al. Favorable change of lipid profile after carbamazepine withdrawal. Acta Neurol Scand. 2015;134:219–23. http://dx.doi.org/10.1111/ane.12534 [c].

[9] Hoshina D, Furuya K, Okita I. Erythema multiforme-like drug reaction with eosinophilia and systemic symptoms (DRESS). Clin Exp Dermatol. 2015;40:455–6. http://dx.doi.org/10.1111/ced.12541 [A].

[10] Ghosh C, Hossain M, Spriggs A, et al. Sertraline-induced potentiation of the CYP3A4-dependent neurotoxicity of carbamazepine: an in vitro study. Epilepsia. 2015;56:439–49. http://dx.doi.org/10.1111/epi.12923 [H].

[11] Burianová I, Bořecká K. Routine therapeutic monitoring of the active metabolite of carbamazepine: is it really necessary? Clin

Biochem. 2015;48:866–9. http://dx.doi.org/10.1016/j.
clinbiochem.2015.05.014 [h].

[12] Plumpton CO, Yip VLM, Alfirevic A, et al. Cost-effectiveness of screening for HLA-HLA-A*31:01 prior to initiation of carbamazepine in epilepsy. Epilepsia. 2015;56:556–63. http://dx.doi.org/10.1111/epi.12937 [h].

[13] Van Nguyen D, Chu HC, Van Nguyen D, et al. HLA-B*1502 and carbamazepine-induced severe cutaneous adverse drug reactions in Vietnamese. Asia Pac Allergy. 2015;5:68–77. http://dx.doi.org/10.5415/apallergy.2015.5.2.68 [c].

[14] Grunze H, Kotlik E, Costa R, et al. Assessment of the efficacy and safety of eslicarbazepine acetate in acute mania and prevention of recurrence: experience from multicentre, double-blind, randomised phase II clinical studies in patients with bipolar disorder I. J Affect Disord. 2014;174C:70–82. http://dx.doi.org/10.1016/j.jad.2014.11.013 [C].

[15] Doleman B, Heinink TP, Read DJ, et al. A systematic review and meta-regression analysis of prophylactic gabapentin for postoperative pain. Anaesthesia. 2015;70:1186–204. http://dx.doi.org/10.1111/anae.13179 [M].

[16] Leung JG, Hall-Flavin D, Nelson S, et al. The role of gabapentin in the management of alcohol withdrawal and dependence. Ann Pharmacother. 2015;49:897–906. http://dx.doi.org/10.1177/1060028015585849 [M].

[17] Clark K, Quinn SJ, Doogue M, et al. Routine prescribing of gabapentin or pregabalin in supportive and palliative care: what are the comparative performances of the medications in a palliative care population? Support Care Cancer. 2015;23:2517–20. http://dx.doi.org/10.1007/s00520-015-2837-z [c].

[18] Monks DT, Hoppe DW, Downey K, et al. A perioperative course of gabapentin does not produce a clinically meaningful improvement in analgesia after cesarean delivery. Anesthesiology. 2015;123:320–6. http://dx.doi.org/10.1097/ALN.0000000000000722 [c].

[19] Cheikh Hassan HI, Brennan F, Collett G, et al. Efficacy and safety of gabapentin for uremic pruritus and restless legs syndrome in conservatively managed patients with chronic kidney disease. J Pain Symptom Manage. 2015;49:782–9. http://dx.doi.org/10.1016/j.jpainsymman.2014.08.010 [c].

[20] Chen C, Upward J, Arumugham T, et al. Gabapentin enacarbil and morphine administered in combination versus alone: a double-blind, randomized, pharmacokinetic, and tolerability comparison. Clin Ther. 2015;37:349–57. http://dx.doi.org/10.1016/j.clinthera.2014.10.015 [E].

[21] Beauvais K, Disson-Dautriche A, Jacquin A, et al. Gabapentin-induced encephalopathy. Clin Neurophysiol. 2015;126:845–6. http://dx.doi.org/10.1016/j.clinph.2014.07.016 [A].

[22] Rudd GD, Haverkamp W, Mason JW, et al. Lacosamide cardiac safety: clinical trials in patients with partial-onset seizures. Acta Neurol Scand. 2015;132:355–63. http://dx.doi.org/10.1111/ane.12414 [M].

[23] Ramsay RE, Sabharwal V, Khan F, et al. Safety & pK of IV loading dose of lacosamide in the ICU. Epilepsy Behav. 2015;49:340–2. http://dx.doi.org/10.1016/j.yebeh.2015.06.032 [A].

[24] Kropeit D, Johnson M, Cawello W, et al. Lacosamide cardiac safety: a thorough QT/QTc trial in healthy volunteers. Acta Neurol Scand. 2015;132:346–54. http://dx.doi.org/10.1111/ane.12416 [A].

[25] Hudson JD, Guptill JT, Byrnes W, et al. Assessment of the effects of lacosamide on sleep parameters in healthy subjects. Seizure. 2015;25:155–9. http://dx.doi.org/10.1016/j.seizure.2014.10.012 [c].

[26] Andrade-Machado R, Luque-Navarro-de Los Reyes J, Benjumea-Cuartas V, et al. Efficacy and tolerability of add-on lacosamide treatment in adults with Lennox-Gastaut syndrome: an observational study. Seizure. 2015;33:81–7. http://dx.doi.org/10.1016/j.seizure.2015.10.009 [A].

[27] Calabrò RS, Magaudda A, Nibali VC, et al. Sexual dysfunction induced by lacosamide: an underreported side effect? Epilepsy Behav. 2015;46:252–3. http://dx.doi.org/10.1016/j.yebeh.2015.01.031 [A].

[28] Murru A, Popovic D, Pacchiarotti I, et al. Management of adverse effects of mood stabilizers. Curr Psychiatry Rep. 2015;17:603. http://dx.doi.org/10.1007/s11920-015-0603-z [r].

[29] Ordoñez L, Salgueiro E, Jimeno FJ, et al. Spontaneous reporting of Stevens-Johnson syndrome and toxic epidermal necrolysis associated with antiepileptic drugs. Eur Rev Med Pharmacol Sci. 2015;19:2732–7 [r].

[30] Chen B, Choi H, Hirsch LJ, et al. Cosmetic side effects of antiepileptic drugs in adults with epilepsy. Epilepsy Behav. 2015;42:129–37. http://dx.doi.org/10.1016/j.yebeh.2014.10.021 [C].

[31] Romero-Tapia SJ, Cámara-Combaluzier HH, Baeza-Bacab MA, et al. Use of intravenous immunoglobulin for Stevens-Johnson syndrome and toxic epidermal necrolysis in children: report of two cases secondary to anticonvulsants. Allergol Immunopathol (Madr). 2015;43:227–9. http://dx.doi.org/10.1016/j.aller.2013.12.008 [r].

[32] Nathan K, Agarwal A, Gable B, et al. Lamotrigine-induced drug reaction with eosinophilia and systemic symptoms (DRESS). BMJ Case Rep. 2015;2015:1–2. http://dx.doi.org/10.1136/bcr-2014-209170 [c].

[33] Baker GA, Bromley RL, Briggs M, et al. IQ at 6 years after in utero exposure to antiepileptic drugs: a controlled cohort study. Neurology. 2015;84:382–90. http://dx.doi.org/10.1212/WNL.0000000000001182 [C].

[34] Epstein RA, Moore KM, Bobo WV. Treatment of bipolar disorders during pregnancy: maternal and fetal safety and challenges. Drug Healthc Patient Saf. 2015;7:7–29. http://dx.doi.org/10.2147/DHPS.S50556 [M].

[35] Damkier P, Videbech P, Larsen ER. Use of psychotropic drugs during pregnancy and breast-feeding. Acta Psychiatr Scand. 2016;133:429–30. http://dx.doi.org/10.1111/acps.12546 [r].

[36] Moon J, Park H-K, Chu K, et al. The HLA-A*2402/Cw*0102 haplotype is associated with lamotrigine-induced maculopapular eruption in the Korean population. Epilepsia. 2015;56:e161–7. http://dx.doi.org/10.1111/epi.13087 [c].

[37] Zeng T, Long Y-S, Min F-L, et al. Association of HLA-B*1502 allele with lamotrigine-induced Stevens-Johnson syndrome and toxic epidermal necrolysis in Han Chinese subjects: a meta-analysis. Int J Dermatol. 2015;54:488–93. http://dx.doi.org/10.1111/ijd.12570 [M].

[38] Ito A, Shimada H, Ishikawa K, et al. Association between HLA-DRB1*0405, −DQB1*0401 and -DQA1*0303 alleles and lamotrigine-induced cutaneous adverse drug reactions. A pilot case-control study from Japan. J Affect Disord. 2015;179:47–50. http://dx.doi.org/10.1016/j.jad.2015.03.018 [c].

[39] Werhahn KJ, Trinka E, Dobesberger J, et al. A randomized, double-blind comparison of antiepileptic drug treatment in the elderly with new-onset focal epilepsy. Epilepsia. 2015;56:450–9. http://dx.doi.org/10.1111/epi.12926 [C].

[40] Sheinberg R, Heyman E, Dagan Z, et al. Correlation between efficacy of levetiracetam and serum levels among children with refractory epilepsy. Pediatr Neurol. 2015;52:624–8. http://dx.doi.org/10.1016/j.pediatrneurol.2015.01.012 [c].

[41] Fujikawa M, Kishimoto Y, Kakisaka Y, et al. Obsessive-compulsive behavior induced by levetiracetam. J Child Neurol. 2015;30:942–4. http://dx.doi.org/10.1177/0883073814541471 [c].

[42] Suresh SH, Chakraborty A, Virupakshaiah A, et al. Efficacy and safety of levetiracetam and carbamazepine as monotherapy in partial seizures. Epilepsy Res Treat. 2015;2015:415082. http://dx.doi.org/10.1155/2015/415082 [c].

[43] Zhu F, Lang S-Y, Wang X-Q, et al. Long-term effectiveness of antiepileptic drug monotherapy in partial epileptic patients: a 7-year study in an epilepsy center in China. Chin Med J (Engl). 2015;128:3015–22. http://dx.doi.org/10.4103/0366-6999.168968 [c].

[44] Vallianou NG, Geladari E, Chroni P, et al. Levetiracetam-associated hypokalemia and hypomagnesaemia among two patients treated for seizures. CNS Neurosci Ther. 2015;21:539. http://dx.doi.org/10.1111/cns.12398 [r].

[45] Alzahrani T, Kay D, Alqahtani SA, et al. Levetiracetam-induced pancytopenia. Epilepsy Behav Case Rep. 2015;4:45–7. http://dx.doi.org/10.1016/j.ebcr.2015.06.001 [r].

[46] Gencler OS, Gencler B, Altunel CT, et al. Levetiracetam induced psoriasiform drug eruption: a rare case report. Saudi Pharm J. 2015;23:720–2. http://dx.doi.org/10.1016/j.jsps.2015.02.010 [r].

[47] Flannery AH, Willey MD, Thompson Bastin ML, et al. Eosinophilia and fever with levetiracetam: a case report. Pharmacotherapy. 2015;35:e131–5. http://dx.doi.org/10.1002/phar.1617 [r].

[48] Eleni K. Dress syndrome induced by levetiracetam. J Eur Acad Dermatol Venereol. 2015;29:377–8. http://dx.doi.org/10.1111/jdv.12346 [r].

[49] Matarazzo M, Galán Sánchez-Seco V, Méndez-Guerrero AJ, et al. Drug-related eyelid nystagmus: two cases of a rare clinical phenomenon related to carbamazepine and derivatives. Clin Neuropharmacol. 2016;39:49–50. http://dx.doi.org/10.1097/WNF.0000000000000125 [A].

[50] Bosak M, Turaj W, Dudek D, et al. Depressogenic medications and other risk factors for depression among Polish patients with epilepsy. Neuropsychiatr Dis Treat. 2015;11:2509–17. http://dx.doi.org/10.2147/NDT.S91538 [C].

[51] Guleria VS, Sharda C, Rana T, et al. Oxcarbazepine induced toxic epidermal necrolysis—a rare case report. Indian J Pharmacol. 2015;47:459–61. http://dx.doi.org/10.4103/0253-7613.161279 [A].

[52] Biswas A, Mitra R, Sen S, et al. Oxcarbazepine induced maculopapular rash—a case report. J Clin Diagn Res. 2015;9:FD01–2. http://dx.doi.org/10.7860/JCDR/2015/10744.5375 [A].

[53] Güveli BT, Aksoy D, Ak PD, et al. Effects of oxcarbazepine and levetiracetam on calcium, ionized calcium, and 25-OH vitamin-D3 levels in patients with epilepsy. Clin Psychopharmacol Neurosci. 2016;14:74–8. http://dx.doi.org/10.9758/cpn.2016.14.1.74 [c].

[54] Besi E, Boniface DR, Cregg R, et al. Comparison of tolerability and adverse symptoms in oxcarbazepine and carbamazepine in the treatment of trigeminal neuralgia and neuralgiform headaches using the liverpool adverse events profile (AEP). J Headache Pain. 2011;16:563. http://dx.doi.org/10.1186/s10194-015-0563-z [C].

[55] Mcgrane IR, Loveland JG, Zaluski HJ, et al. Serum quetiapine concentration changes with concomitant oxcarbazepine therapy in a boy with autism spectrum disorder. J Child Adolesc Psychopharmacol. 2015;25:729–30. http://dx.doi.org/10.1089/cap.2015.0117 [A].

[56] Antunes Nde J, Wichert-Ana L, Coelho EB, et al. Influence of verapamil on the pharmacokinetics of oxcarbazepine and of the enantiomers of its 10-hydroxy metabolite in healthy volunteers. Eur J Clin Pharmacol. 2016;72:195–201. http://dx.doi.org/10.1007/s00228-015-1970-4 [c].

[57] Sigaroudi A, Kullak-Ublick GA, Weiler S. Concomitant administration of rifampicin and oxcarbazepine results in a significant decrease of the active MHD metabolite of oxcarbazepine. Eur J Clin Pharmacol. 2016;72:377–8. http://dx.doi.org/10.1007/s00228-015-1991-z [A].

[58] Shah E, Reuber M, Goulding P, et al. Clinical experience with adjunctive perampanel in adult patients with uncontrolled epilepsy: a UK and Ireland multicentre study. Seizure. 2016;34:1–5. http://dx.doi.org/10.1016/j.seizure.2015.10.017 [C].

[59] Ko D, Yang H, Williams B, et al. Perampanel in the treatment of partial seizures: time to onset and duration of most common adverse events from pooled Phase III and extension studies. Epilepsy Behav. 2015;48:45–52. http://dx.doi.org/10.1016/j.yebeh.2015.05.020 [C].

[60] Yang H, Laurenza A, Williams B, et al. Lack of effect of perampanel on QT interval duration: results from a thorough QT analysis and pooled partial seizure phase III clinical trials. Epilepsy Res. 2015;114:122–30. http://dx.doi.org/10.1016/j.eplepsyres.2015.04.010 [c].

[61] Brodie MJ, Stephen LJ. Prospective audit with adjunctive perampanel: preliminary observations in focal epilepsy. Epilepsy Behav. 2016;54:100–3. http://dx.doi.org/10.1016/j.yebeh.2015.11.002 [c].

[62] Juhl S, Rubboli G. Perampanel as add-on treatment in refractory focal epilepsy. The Dianalund experience. Acta Neurol Scand. 2016. Epub ahead of print. http://dx.doi.org/10.1111/ane.12558 [c].

[63] Laurenza A, Yang H, Williams B, et al. Absence of liver toxicity in perampanel-treated subjects: pooled results from partial seizure phase III perampanel clinical studies. Epilepsy Res. 2015;113:76–85. http://dx.doi.org/10.1016/j.eplepsyres.2015.03.005 [C].

[64] Vazquez B, Yang H, Williams B, et al. Perampanel efficacy and safety by gender: subanalysis of phase III randomized clinical studies in subjects with partial seizures. Epilepsia. 2015;56:e90–4. http://dx.doi.org/10.1111/epi.13019 [r].

[65] Leppik IE, Wechsler RT, Williams B, et al. Efficacy and safety of perampanel in the subgroup of elderly patients included in the phase III epilepsy clinical trials. Epilepsy Res. 2015;110:216–20. http://dx.doi.org/10.1016/j.eplepsyres.2014.11.015 [c].

[66] Patsalos PN, Gougoulaki M, Sander JW. Perampanel serum concentrations in adults with epilepsy. Ther Drug Monit. 2016;38:358–64. http://dx.doi.org/10.1097/FTD.0000000000000274 [E].

[67] Gidal BE, Laurenza A, Hussein Z, et al. Perampanel efficacy and tolerability with enzyme-inducing AEDs in patients with epilepsy. Neurology. 2015;84:1972–80. http://dx.doi.org/10.1212/WNL.0000000000001558 [c].

[68] Glauser T, Laurenza A, Yang H, et al. Efficacy and tolerability of adjunct perampanel based on number of antiepileptic drugs at baseline and baseline predictors of efficacy: a phase III post-hoc analysis. Epilepsy Res. 2016;119:34–40. http://dx.doi.org/10.1016/j.eplepsyres.2015.11.014 [C].

[69] Nakazawa M, Akasaka M, Hasegawa T, et al. Efficacy and safety of fosphenytoin for acute encephalopathy in children. Brain Dev. 2015;37:418–22. http://dx.doi.org/10.1016/j.braindev.2014.06.009 [c].

[70] Indu T, Basutkar R. Hypersensitivity reaction associated with phenytoin. J Basic Clin Pharm. 2015;6:119. http://dx.doi.org/10.4103/0976-0105.168054 [A].

[71] Jain RS, Nagpal K, Kumar S, et al. Purple glove syndrome occurring after oral administration of phenytoin in therapeutic doses: mechanism still a dilemma. Am J Emerg Med. 2015;33:123.e5–6. http://dx.doi.org/10.1016/j.ajem.2014.05.039 [A].

[72] Patil MM, Sahoo J, Kamalanathan S, et al. Phenytoin induced osteopathy—too common to be neglected. J Clin Diagn Res.

2015;9:OD11–2. http://dx.doi.org/10.7860/JCDR/ 2015/15224.6820 [A].

[73] Ciftci R, Tas F, Karabulut S, et al. Combination of capecitabine and phenytoin may cause phenytoin intoxication: a case report. Am J Ther. 2013;19:2013–5. http://dx.doi.org/10.1097/MJT.0b013e318293b10a [A].

[74] Zhang S-S, Wu Z, Zhang L-C, et al. Efficacy and safety of pregabalin for treating painful diabetic peripheral neuropathy: a meta-analysis. Acta Anaesthesiol Scand. 2015;59:147–59. http://dx.doi.org/10.1111/aas.12420 [M].

[75] Park SS, Kim D-H, Nam I-C, et al. The effectiveness of pregabalin for post-tonsillectomy pain control: a randomized controlled trial. PLoS One. 2015;10:e0117161. http://dx.doi.org/10.1371/journal.pone.0117161 [c].

[76] Imai Y, Imai K, Kimura T, et al. Evaluation of postoperative pregabalin for attenuation of postoperative shoulder pain after thoracotomy in patients with lung cancer, a preliminary result. Gen Thorac Cardiovasc Surg. 2015;63:99–104. http://dx.doi.org/10.1007/s11748-014-0466-y [c].

[77] Srivastava VK, Agrawal S, Kadiyala VN, et al. The efficacy of pregabalin for prevention of catheter-related bladder discomfort: a prospective, randomized, placebo-controlled double-blind study. J Anesth. 2014;29:212–6. http://dx.doi.org/10.1007/s00540-014-1911-x [c].

[78] YaDeau JT, Lin Y, Mayman DJ, et al. Pregabalin and pain after total knee arthroplasty: a double-blind, randomized, placebo-controlled, multidose trial. Br J Anaesth. 2015;115:285–93. http://dx.doi.org/10.1093/bja/aev217 [c].

[79] Yue J, Jiao S, Xiao Y, et al. Comparison of pregabalin with ondansetron in treatment of uraemic pruritus in dialysis patients: a prospective, randomized, double-blind study. Int Urol Nephrol. 2015;47:161–7. http://dx.doi.org/10.1007/s11255-014-0795-x [C].

[80] Nass RD, Kurth C, Kull A, et al. Adjunctive retigabine in refractory focal epilepsy: postmarketing experience at four tertiary epilepsy care centers in Germany. Epilepsy Behav. 2016;56:54–8. http://dx.doi.org/10.1016/j.yebeh.2015.12.034 [C].

[81] Lerche H, Daniluk J, Lotay N, et al. Efficacy and safety of ezogabine/retigabine as adjunctive therapy to specified single antiepileptic medications in an open-label study of adults with partial-onset seizures. Seizure. 2015;30:93–100. http://dx.doi.org/10.1016/j.seizure.2015.06.002 [c].

[82] Huber B, Bocchicchio M. A retrospective evaluation of retigabine in patients with cognitive impairment with highly drug-resistant epilepsy. Epilepsy Behav. 2015;44:234–7. http://dx.doi.org/10.1016/j.yebeh.2015.02.008 [A].

[83] Beacher NG, Brodie MJ, Goodall C. A case report: retigabine induced oral mucosal dyspigmentation of the hard palate. BMC Oral Health. 2015;15:122. http://dx.doi.org/10.1186/s12903-015-0102-y [A].

[84] Clark S, Antell A, Kaufman K. New antiepileptic medication linked to blue discoloration of the skin and eyes. Ther Adv Drug Saf. 2015;6:15–9. http://dx.doi.org/10.1177/2042098614560736 [r].

[85] Ishihara L, Beck M, Travis S, et al. Physician and pharmacist understanding of the risk of urinary retention with retigabine (ezogabine): a REMS assessment survey. Drugs Real World Outcomes. 2015;2:335–44. http://dx.doi.org/10.1007/s40801-015-0042-5 [H].

[86] Ishihara L, Lewis A, Kolli S, et al. European survey of prescriber understanding of risks associated with retigabine. Drugs Real World Outcomes. 2015;2:345–53. http://dx.doi.org/10.1007/s40801-015-0044-3 [H].

[87] Kessler SK, McCarthy A, Cnaan A, et al. Retention rates of rufinamide in pediatric epilepsy patients with and without

[88] Lennox-Gastaut syndrome. Epilepsy Res. 2015;112:18–26. http://dx.doi.org/10.1016/j.eplepsyres.2015.02.003 [c].

Grewal DS, Goldstein D a, Khatana AK, et al. Bilateral angle closure following use of a weight loss combination agent containing topiramate. J Glaucoma. 2015;24:e132–6. http://dx.doi.org/10.1097/IJG.0000000000000157 [A].

[89] Brandt C, Lahr D, May TW. Cognitive adverse events of topiramate in patients with epilepsy and intellectual disability. Epilepsy Behav. 2015;45:261–4. http://dx.doi.org/10.1016/j.yebeh.2014.12.043 [c].

[90] Sommer BR, Mitchell EL, Wroolie TE. Topiramate: effects on cognition in patients with epilepsy, migraine headache and obesity. Ther Adv Neurol Disord. 2013;6:211–27. http://dx.doi.org/10.1177/1756285613481257 [c].

[91] Knapp CM, Ciraulo DA, Sarid-Segal O, et al. Zonisamide, topiramate, and levetiracetam. J Clin Psychopharmacol. 2015;35:34–42. http://dx.doi.org/10.1097/JCP.0000000000000246 [c].

[92] Lebow J, Chuy JA, Cedermark K, et al. The development or exacerbation of eating disorder symptoms after topiramate initiation. Pediatrics. 2015;135:e1312–6. http://dx.doi.org/10.1542/peds.2014-3413 [c].

[93] Sciegienka A, Argo T, Cantrell M, et al. Association between topiramate use and serum bicarbonate levels in a veteran population. Ann Pharmacother. 2015;49:670–3. http://dx.doi.org/10.1177/1060028015579197 [C].

[94] Jion YI, Raff A, Grosberg BM, et al. The risk and management of kidney stones from the use of topiramate and zonisamide in migraine and idiopathic intracranial hypertension. Headache. 2015;55:161–6. http://dx.doi.org/10.1111/head.12480 [A].

[95] Raff A, Jion YI, Grosberg BM, et al. Topiramate and nephrolithiasis: a response. Headache J Head Face Pain. 2015;55:701–2. http://dx.doi.org/10.1111/head.12565 [r].

[96] Dixit S, Namdeo M, Azad S. Valproate induced delirium due to hyperammonemia in a case of acute mania: a diagnostic dilemma. J Clin Diagn Res. 2015;9:VD01–2. http://dx.doi.org/10.7860/JCDR/2015/11830.5758 [A].

[97] Stevens CE, Turner Z, Kossoff EH. Hepatic dysfunction as a complication of combined valproate and ketogenic diet. Pediatr Neurol. 2016;54:82–4. http://dx.doi.org/10.1016/j.pediatrneurol.2015.10.006 [A].

[98] Yamak WR, Hmaimess G, Makke Y, et al. Valproate-induced enuresis: a prospective study. Dev Med Child Neurol. 2015;57:737–41. http://dx.doi.org/10.1111/dmcn.12737 [c].

[99] Toker O, Tal Y, Horev L, et al. Valproic acid hypersensitivity and desensitization. Dev Med Child Neurol. 2015;57:1076–8. http://dx.doi.org/10.1111/dmcn.12835 [A].

[100] Tomson T, Marson A, Boon P, et al. Valproate in the treatment of epilepsy in girls and women of childbearing potential. Epilepsia. 2015;56:1006–19. http://dx.doi.org/10.1111/epi.13021 [C].

[101] Miranda Herrero MC, Alcaraz Romero AJ, Escudero Vilaplana V, et al. Pharmacological interaction between valproic acid and carbapenem: what about levels in pediatrics? Eur J Paediatr Neurol. 2015;19:155–61. http://dx.doi.org/10.1016/j.ejpn.2014.12.010 [c].

[102] Molnar GP, Stephens KJ, George LV, et al. A critical interaction between ertapenem and valproic acid. J Clin Psychopharmacol. 2015;35:348–50. http://dx.doi.org/10.1097/JCP.0000000000000325 [A].

[103] Xiao Y, Gan L, Wang J, et al. Vigabatrin versus carbamazepine monotherapy for epilepsy. Cochrane Database Syst Rev. 2012;1:CD008781. http://dx.doi.org/10.1002/14651858.CD008781.pub2 [M].

[104] Krauss G, Faught E, Foroozan R, et al. Sabril® registry 5-year results: characteristics of adult patients treated with vigabatrin. Epilepsy Behav. 2016;56:15–9. http://dx.doi.org/10.1016/j.yebeh.2015.12.004 [C].

[105] Hussain K, Walsh TJ, Chazen JL. Brain MRI findings with vigabatrin therapy: case report and literature review. Clin Imaging. 2016;40:180–2. http://dx.doi.org/10.1016/j.clinimag.2015.07.016 [A].

[106] Goyal C, Kapadia TH, Gadgil P, et al. Vigabatrin-induced reversible changes on magnetic resonance imaging of the brain. Neurol India. 2015;63:430–1. http://dx.doi.org/10.4103/0028-3886.158237 [A].

[107] Kotagal P. Limiting retinal toxicity of vigabatrin in children with infantile spasms. Epilepsy Curr. 2015;15:327–9. http://dx.doi.org/10.5698/1535-7511-15.6.327 [c].

[108] Westall CA, Wright T, Cortese F, et al. Vigabatrin retinal toxicity in children with infantile spasms: an observational cohort study. Neurology. 2015;83:2262–8. http://dx.doi.org/10.1212/01.wnl.0000471111.65017.4f [c].

[109] Riikonen R, Rener-Primec Z, Carmant L, et al. Does vigabatrin treatment for infantile spasms cause visual field defects? An international multicentre study. Dev Med Child Neurol. 2015;57:60–7. http://dx.doi.org/10.1111/dmcn.12573 [c].

[110] Coelho VR, Sousa K, Pires TR, et al. Genotoxic and mutagenic effects of vigabatrin, a γ-aminobutyric acid transaminase inhibitor, in Wistar rats submitted to rotarod task. Hum Exp Toxicol. 2015;35:358–65. http://dx.doi.org/10.1177/0960327115611970 [E].

[111] Case C. Zonisamide-induced angle closure and myopic shift. Optom Vis Sci. 2015;92:46–51 [c].

[112] Thampratankul L, Khongkhatithum C, Visudtibhan A. Efficacy and safety of zonisamide in Thai children and adolescents with intractable seizures. J Child Neurol. 2015;30:527–31. http://dx.doi.org/10.1177/0883073814549246 [c].

[113] Nakken KO, Lindstrøm P, Andersen H. Retention rate of zonisamide in intractable epilepsy. Acta Neurol Scand. 2015;131:268–74. http://dx.doi.org/10.1111/ane.12379 [c].

[114] Jongeling AC, Richins RJ, Bazil CW. Safety and tolerability of an oral zonisamide loading dose. Seizure. 2015;32:69–71. http://dx.doi.org/10.1016/j.seizure.2015.09.012 [c].

7

Opioid Analgesics and Narcotic Antagonists

Michael G. O'Neil[*,1], *Justin G. Kullgren*[†]

*Department of Pharmacy Practice, Drug Diversion, Pain Management and Substance Abuse Specialist, South College School of Pharmacy, Knoxville, TN, USA
†Department of Pharmacy, The Ohio State University Wexner Medical Center, Columbus, OH, USA
[1]Corresponding author: moneil@southcollegetn.edu

ORAL OPIOID ANTAGONISTS FOR OPIOID-RELATED CONSTIPATION, IBD ASSOCIATED CONSTIPATION AND PROLONGED POST-SURGICAL ILEUS

Increased opioid prescribing for malignant and nonmalignant pain, the need for new treatment options in patients with irritable bowel disease-associated constipation (IBD-C) and the lack of treatment options for prolonged postsurgical ileus has warranted development of new pharmacological agents or innovative uses of traditional ones. Opioid-induced bowel dysfunction (OBD) is broad term for a variety of gastrointestinal adverse effects induced by opioids that includes: nausea, vomiting, constipation, abdominal cramping, bloating and abdominal pain [1S]. Opioid-induced constipation (OIC) is one of the most common adverse effects found in patients diagnosed with OBD [1S]. For patients requiring long-term opioid management, OIC may impact patient quality of life to a greater extent than the pain the opioids are prescribed to minimize [2C]. Some patients with constipation associated with IBD have gained improvement in gastrointestinal symptoms when opioid antagonists have been administered to block endogenous opiate receptors in the intestinal tract [3c,4c]. Postoperative ileus is a common complication of various types of abdominal surgeries [5]. Utilization of opioid antagonists to facilitate improvement in gastrointestinal motility following abdominal surgery has proven to be effective in decreasing the duration of postoperative ileus and length of stay in postsurgical patients [6M].

The pathways of OIC, IBD-associated constipation and postsurgical ileus involve both the central and peripheral nervous systems [3c,7–10]. Opioid peptide receptors have been identified throughout the intestinal tract [9,10].

Mu (μ)-opioid receptors exert inhibitor effects on intestinal motility and secretion [10,11E]. Pathways include inhibition of acetylcholine (Ach) release through μ-opioid receptors on cholinergic ascending excitatory neurons in the gastrointestinal tract resulting in inhibition of peristalsis, while mu-opioid receptors in descending neurons inhibit the release of vasoactive intestinal peptide (VIP) and nitric oxide (NO) that prevents relaxation during peristalsis [9,10]. Cellular mechanisms of GI motility dysfunction effected by opioids include but are not limited to complex cascades of cellular processes in the gastrointestinal tract involving 3 G coupled receptors, cyclic AMP, protein kinases, calcium channels and potassium channels [7,9,10,11E,12].

Although oral administration of the opioid antagonist naloxone has been shown to be effective in the treatment of OIC when combined with opioids, oral naloxone doses required to achieve an adequate response in OIC patients may induce physiologic withdrawal or reduce desired analgesic effects. [3c,4c,13c,14,15c,16C,17c]. The oral opioid antagonist naltrexone has significant oral bioavailability but also has had limited use in treating OIC due to its ability to penetrate into the central nervous system (CNS), induce physiologic opioid withdrawal and block desired analgesic effects [12,18]. The need for more localized gastrointestinal opioid antagonism in patients with OIC, IBD-C or postsurgical ileus has prompted development of newer opioid antagonists with less penetration into the CNS.

Opioid antagonists with limited CNS penetration have been developed and evaluated for OIC, IBD-C or postsurgical ileus. Methylnaltrexone (Relistor® Valeant Pharmaceuticals) was approved for subcutaneous injection for OIC in 2008 [19]. More recently, the Food and Drug Administration (FDA) approved methylnaltrexone for noncancer-related OIC as well as a new oral formulation [19]. Reported adverse effects of oral methylnaltrexone include abdominal pain, nausea, diarrhea, and hyperhidrosis [20C]. In 2014, naloxegol (Movantik® Astra Zeneca Pharmaceuticals) was approved by the FDA for OIC [21]. Diarrhea, nausea, vomiting, and flatulence have been reported with naloxegol [22]. Alvimopan (Entereg® Merck Pharmaceuticals) was initially approved in 2008 for acceleration of GI motility following partial large or small-bowel resection with primary anastomosis in gastrointestinal surgeries in hospitalized patients [23]. The FDA expanded the indication in 2013 to include acceleration of the time for upper and lower GI recovery following surgeries that include partial bowel resection with primary anastomosis [23]. Alvimopan has demonstrated significant efficacy minimizing postoperative ileus and decreasing hospital length of stay [24M]. Common adverse effects reported with alvimopan include constipation, dyspepsia, and flatulence [25].

OPIOID RECEPTOR AGONISTS

Opioid Class

Death

The Center for Disease Control (CDC) evaluated trends in multiple causes of death in patients to assess trends associated with drug overdose deaths. They reported in 2014 alone a total of 47 055 drug overdose deaths in the United States, representing a 1-year increase of 6.5%, from 13.8 per 100 000 persons in 2013 to 14.7 per 100 000 persons in 2014. Of note was the increase in the synthetic opioid fentanyl when compared to previous years [26S].

Drug Interaction

The US Food and Drug Administration (FDA) required addition of a boxed warning to prescription opioid painkillers and cough medicines, and benzodiazepines following evidence the two drug classes are increasingly being prescribed together. The FDA review determined the number of patients being prescribed an opioid and benzodiazepine concurrently increased by 41% between 2002 and 2014, equating to an additional 2.5 million people per year receiving both drug classes together. Consequences of concurrent prescribing have been associated with accidental overdose resulting in death [27S].

Infection

A self-controlled case series analysis on a retrospective cohort of 13 796 patients with rheumatoid arthritis (RA) enrolled in Tennessee Medicaid in 1995–2009 was evaluated. Within-person comparisons of the risk of hospitalization for serious infection during periods of opioid use versus non-use were evaluated. Risks associated with new opioid use, use of opioids known to have immunosuppressive properties, use of long-acting opioids, and different opioid dosages were assessed. Researchers concluded based on within-person comparisons of patients with RA, opioid use was associated with an increased risk of hospitalization for serious infection. This is the first large study reporting opioid-associated immunosuppression [28M].

Codeine

Pharmacogenetics

Researchers investigated 98 women that received codeine following cesarean section. Participants were genotyped for specific genetic variations of catechol-O-methyltransferase (COMT). Participants assessed their own pain control after surgery. Researchers concluded there were significant differences in mean dose consumption between the various genotypes. The variations were found to be associated with the amount of codeine used. Researchers concluded that early assessment of these determinants of polymorphisms could help optimize postsurgical pain control following the procedure [29c].

Diamorphine

Neurological

A case report describes cerebral infarctions in the setting of heroin-induced hypereosinophilia. Investigators concluded that hypereosinophilia syndrome should be considered when evaluating drug-induced cerebral infarctions [30A].

Dextromethorphan

Analgesia

A Cochrane Central Register of Controlled Trials, Pubget, and comprehensive database search evaluated total consumption of IV or intramuscular opioids. Pain score comparisons were performed postoperatively in groups that received dextromethorphan peri-operatively. Researchers suggested dextromethorphan use peri-operatively reduces the postoperative opioid consumption [31M].

Dihydrocodeine

Dermatological

This is a case report of a woman in her 60s presenting with diffuse erythema, nonfollicular pustules, and fever diagnosed with acute generalized exanthematous pustulosis (AGEP). Diagnosis was confirmed using histopathologic findings and use of a dihydrocodeine phosphate drug test. This is the first reported case of dihydrocodeine-associated AGEP [32A].

Fentanyl

Neurological

Eighty patients requesting analgesia during labor were randomly assigned to receive pethidine or fentanyl for pain relief. Pethidine was associated with more nausea and vomiting in the mother. Patients receiving fentanyl had newborns with lower Apgar scores and required more resuscitative measures such as naloxone [33c].

Researchers performed a comprehensive retrospective evaluation of 103 infants that were reported to be born less than 30 weeks gestation (mean gestational age 26.9 ± 1.8 weeks). Data collected including demographics, pre- and post-delivery histories, cerebral magnetic resonance imaging and fentanyl exposure. Cerebral Magnetic Resonance Images (MRI) was evaluated. Childhood development was also assessed. Researchers concluded that higher total fentanyl doses might be associated with a cerebellar injury and lower cerebellar diameter [34M].

A case report describes a 7 year old with symptoms consistent with serotonin syndrome following surgery for an intracranial hemorrhage and use of intraoperative fentanyl. Symptoms included shivering, tremor, hypertonia, hyperreflexia, clonus, bilateral mydriasis, and intracranial hypertension. Pediatric reports of serotonin syndrome are generally considered to be rare [35A].

Drug Interaction

Researchers retrospectively evaluated 112 045 patients that were receiving a serotonergic agent, and 4538 of these patients that concomitantly received fentanyl. Researchers concluded that the risk of serotonin syndrome with concurrent use of fentanyl and serotonergic agents is very low [36M].

A 36-year-old male admitted to the burn unit for severe burns was treated with multiple agents that included high dose fentanyl, methadone and voriconazole. The patient subsequently developed symptoms consistent with serotonin syndrome that later resolved following discontinuation of all suspected agents. The authors concluded that opioids alone might be associated with serotonin syndrome [37A].

Analgesia

Researchers retrospectively evaluated six studies for fentanyl-induced hyperalgesia from October 1995 through January 2015. Two studies do not support the association of hyperalgesia induced by prior fentanyl use while four studies do [38M].

Death

This is a case report of an accidental death of a 2 year old. The child had received an abrasion on her knee and her grandmother inadvertently placed a fentanyl patch as a bandage over the abrasion. The grandmother admitted mistaking the patch for a bandage. The child was found deceased the morning after placing the patch [39A].

Dermatological

This is a case report of a 19-year-old male who applied an unauthorized transdermal fentanyl patch to alleviate symptoms of his eczema. The patient was suspected of having anaphylaxis based on a recent prescription of flucloxacillin, poor respiratory response and the presence of a diffuse erythematous rash. Standard treatment for anaphylaxis failed to revive the patient. However, the patient recovered following immediate administration of naloxone. The authors concluded the patient's eczema likely contributed to accelerated absorption of fentanyl [40A].

Morphine

Metabolic

This is a case report of a 29-year-old female that developed clinically significant hypothermia following intrathecal morphine for cesarean section administered as a subarachnoid block. Temperatures declined to rectal temps as low as 34.4°C. During this same time period, the patient complained of feeling hot, nauseous and dizzy. The patient also began vomiting during this time. The patient failed to respond to traditional warming methods. The patient was treated with a total of 80 mcg IV naloxone with resolution of hypothermia and other symptoms over the next 2 hours [41A].

Neurological

This is an observational study involving 230 preterm infants as part of the Victorian Infant Brain Study cohort. Patients were all admitted to the neonatal intensive care unit. Regional brain volumes at term and 7 years were assessed. Multiple behavioral, motor, communication, cognitive and emotional evaluations were completed at ages 2 and 7 years. Twenty-five percent of participants received morphine while in the neonatal intensive care unit. Patients receiving low dose morphine during this time had significant differences in neurostructure and behavior alterations that did not last into later childhood years [42M].

Respiratory

This is a retrospective, a population-based nested case–control study. Data were extracted from a Longitudinal Health Insurance Database in Taiwan from 1998 to 2010. A DVT cohort of 3668 patients without a prior history of pulmonary embolism (PE) was compared to 174 patients who developed PE. Patients were evaluated for morphine dosages within 30 days prior to development of PE. Analysis revealed that patients with DVT who received morphine within 30 days had a 4.54 increase of developing a PE. Risk of developing a PE was also correlated with morphine dosage [43M].

Oxycodone

Neurological

This is a case report of a 42-year-old female with end stage renal disease (ESRD) on hemodialysis that developed profound sedation and respiratory depression requiring reversal with naloxone. The patient had also been on chronic methadone and was initiated on hydromorphone post-surgery for analgesia. This incident developed after the patient was converted from hydromorphone to oxycodone. The authors concluded that altered oxycodone elimination due to ESRD contributed to the toxicity. The use of oxycodone in hemodialysis patients requires further evaluation [44A].

Tapentadol

Neurological

The National Poison Center Data System database was retrospectively evaluated from November 2008 to December 31, 2013 for all patients 0–17 years of age reported to have ingested tapentadol. Ninety-three of the 104 exposures were unintentional. There were no deaths reported. Reported symptoms were consistent with those found in adult patients including nausea, vomiting, tachycardia, slurred speech, itching, miosis, hallucinations and respiratory depression. This is the first toxicity report in pediatric patients [45M].

Tramadol

Metabolic

This was prospective cross-sectional study evaluating the blood glucose effects in patients that overdosed on tramadol from February to June 2013 in Tehran, Iran. Blood glucoses were assessed at 0, 8 and 12 hours after admission. Patients with hypoglycemia were treated with hypertonic dextrose infusions until patients' blood glucoses were stable. A total of 128 patients were

evaluated. Seizure was noted in 59.4% of patients. Fourteen patients experienced hypoglycemia within the first 12 hours of admission. Hyperglycemia was experienced in 8 patients (6.25%) on admission day. Dosages of tramadol did not correlate with likelihood of glucose abnormalities. Patients with known or suspected tramadol overdose should have careful monitoring of blood glucoses [46M].

Researchers utilizing the United Kingdom Clinical Practice Research Datalink Statistics database performed a case–control analysis between 1998 and 2012 of all patients initiated on tramadol or codeine for noncancer pain to assess risk of hypoglycemia associated with tramadol. The study included 334 034 patients. Hypoglycemia requiring hospital admission was reported in 1105 patients taking tramadol. Researchers concluded when compared to codeine tramadol was associated with a higher incidence of hypoglycemia requiring hospitalization [47M].

This is a population-based study comparing the incidence of hospitalizations due to hyponatremia associated with tramadol compared to codeine. The UK Clinical Practice Research Datalink and Hospital Episodes Statistics database were searched from 1998 through 2012. A cohort of 332 880 patients taking tramadol within 30 days was evaluated. Researchers concluded there was a threefold greater risk of hospitalization of hyponatremia secondary to tramadol when compared to codeine [48M].

Psychiatric

This is a case report of 59-year-old female that developed acute persecutory symptoms following initiation of tramadol/acetaminophen 1-month prior for joint pain. She had a history of bipolar disorder previously stabilized with lithium. The patient required acute risperidone treatment in addition to her lithium. She required only the previous monotherapy with lithium after the tramadol was discontinued [49A].

Cardiovascular

This is a case report of a 7-year old that developed cardiogenic shock after accidental overdose of tramadol. Cardiogenic shock was confirmed by physical exam, chest X-ray and echocardiogram showing an ejection fracture less than 30%. Cardiac function normalized after 2 days [50A].

PARTIAL OPIOID RECEPTOR AGONISTS

No Information for the current year.
No additional information to add.

OPIOID RECEPTOR ANTAGONISTS

No Information for the current year.
No additional information to add.

References

[1] Chou R, Fanciullo G, Fine P, et al. Clinical guidelines for the use of chronic opioid therapy in chronic noncancer pain. J Pain. 2009;10:113–30 [S].

[2] Bell T, Annunziata K, Leslie J. Opioid-induced constipation negatively impacts pain management, productivity, and health-related quality of life: findings from the National Health and Wellness Survey. J Opioid Manag. 2009;5(3):137–44 [C].

[3] Hawkes N, Rhodes J, Evans B, et al. Naloxone treatment for irritable bowel syndrome—a randomized controlled trial with an oral formulation. Aliment Pharmacol Ther. 2002;16(9):1649–54 [c].

[4] Sanders M, Jones S, Löwenstein O, et al. New formulation of sustained release naloxone can reverse opioid induced constipation without compromising the desired opioid effects. Pain Med. 2015;16(8):1540–50 [c].

[5] Senagore AJ. Pathogenesis and clinical and economic consequences of postoperative ileus. Am J Health Syst Pharm. 2007;64(20 Suppl 13):S3–7.

[6] Drake T, Ward A. Pharmacological management to prevent ileus in major abdominal surgery: a systematic review and meta-analysis. J Gastrointest Surg. 2016;20(6):1253–64 [M].

[7] Shook J, Pelton J, Hruby V, et al. Peptide opioid antagonist separates peripheral and central opioid anti-transit effects. J Pharmacol Exp Ther. 1987;243:492–500.

[8] Philippe D, Dubuquoy L, Groux H, et al. Anti-inflammatory properties of the μ opioid receptor support its use in the treatment of colon inflammation. J Clin Invest. 2003;111(9):1329–38.

[9] Sternini C, Patierno S, Selmer I, et al. The opioid system in the gastrointestinal tract. Neurogastroenterol Motil. 2004;16(Suppl 2):3–16.

[10] Sternini C. Receptors and transmission in the brain-gut axis: potential for novel therapies. III. Mu-opioid receptors in the enteric nervous system. Am J Physiol Gastrointest Liver Physiol. 2001;281:G8–G15.

[11] Valle L, Puig M, Pol O. Effects of mu-opioid receptor agonists on intestinal secretion and permeability during acute intestinal inflammation in mice. Eur J Pharmacol. 2000;389:235–42 [E].

[12] Nelson A, Camilleri M. Chronic opioid induced constipation in patients with nonmalignant pain: challenges and opportunities. Therap Adv Gastroenterol. 2015;8(4):206–20.

[13] Meissnera W, Schmidta U, Hartmann M. Oral naloxone reverses opioid-associated constipation. Pain. 2000;84(1):105–9 [c].

[14] Yuan C, Foss J. Antagonism of gastrointestinal opioid effects. Reg Anesth Pain Med. 2000;25:639–42.

[15] Culpepper-Morgan J, Inturrisi C, Portenoy R, et al. Treatment of opioid-induced constipation with oral naloxone: a pilot study. Clin Pharmacol Ther. 1992;52(1):90–5 [c].

[16] Löwenstein O, Leyendecker P, Hopp M, et al. Combined prolonged-release oxycodone and naloxone improves bowel function in patients receiving opioids for moderate-to-severe non-malignant chronic pain: a randomized controlled trial. Expert Opin Pharmacother. 2009;10(4):531–43 [C].

[17] Smith K, Hopp M, Mundin G, et al. Low absolute bioavailability of oral naloxone in healthy subjects. Int J Clin Pharmacol Ther. 2012;50(5):360–7 [c].

[18] Pappagallo M. Recent advances in the treatment of opioid bowel dysfunction and postoperative ileus. Am J Surg. 2001;182(5, Suppl 1):S11–8.

[19] Anderson P. FDA Okays oral relistor for opioid-induced constipation. Medscape. 2016;.

[20] Michna E, Weil A, Duerden M, et al. Efficacy of subcutaneous methylnaltrexone in the treatment of opioid-induced constipation: a responder post hoc analysis. Pain Med. 2015;15(6):564–71 [C].

[21] Anderson P. FDA Okays naloxegol (movantik) in opioid-induced constipation. Medscape. 2014;.

[22] Leppert W, Woron J. The role of naloxegol in the management of opioid-induced bowel dysfunction. Therap Adv Gastroenterol. 2016;9(5):736–46.

[23] Brooks M. FDA OKs expanded use of alvimopan (entereg). Medscape. 2013;.

[24] Xu L, Zhou X, Yi P, et al. Alvimopan combined with enhanced recovery strategy for managing postoperative ileus after open abdominal surgery: a systematic review and meta-analysis. J Surg Res. 2016;203(1):211–21 [M].

[25] Kraft M, MacLaren R, Du W, et al. Alvimopan (Entereg) for the management of postoperative ileus in patients undergoing bowel resection. PT. Proc Natl Acad Sci USA. 2010;35(1):44–9.

[26] Rudd R, Aleshire N, Zibbell J, et al. Increases in drug and opioid overdose deaths in the United States, 2000–2014. MMWR Morb Mortal Wkly Rep. 2016;64(50–51):1378–82 [S].

[27] The Pharmaceutical Journal 297 (7893), Online, http://dx.doi.org/10.1211/PJ.2016.20201656.

[28] Wiese A, Griffin M, Stein C, et al. Opioid analgesics and the risk of serious infections among patients with rheumatoid arthritis: a self-controlled case series study. Arthritis Rheumatol. 2016;68(2):323–31 [M].

[29] Baber M, Chaudhry S, Kelly L, et al. The pharmacogenetics of codeine pain relief in the postpartum period. Pharmacogenomics J. 2015;15(5):430–5 [c].

[30] Bolz J, Meves S, Kara K, et al. Multiple cerebral infarctions in a young patient with heroin-induced hypereosinophilic syndrome. Neurol Sci. 2015;356(1–2):193–5 [A].

[31] King M, Ladha K, Gelineau A, et al. Perioperative dextromethorphan as an adjunct for postoperative pain: a meta-analysis of randomized controlled trials. Anesthesiology. 2016;124(3):696–705 [M].

[32] Nakai N, Sugiura K, Akiyama M, et al. Acute generalized exanthematous pustulosis caused by dihydrocodeine phosphate in a patient with psoriasis vulgaris and a heterozygous IL36RN mutation. JAMA Dermatol. 2015;151(3):311–5 [A].

[33] Rezk M, El-Shamy E, Massod A, et al. The safety and acceptability of intravenous fentanyl versus intramuscular pethidine for pain relief during labor. Clin Exp Obstet Gynecol. 2015;42(6):781–4 [c].

[34] McPherson C, Haslam M, Pineda R, et al. Brain injury and development in preterm infants exposed to fentanyl. Ann Pharmacother. 2015;49(12):1291–7 [M].

[35] Robles L. Serotonin syndrome induced by fentanyl in a child: case report. Clin Neuropharmacol. 2015;38(5):206–8 [A].

[36] Koury K, Tsui B, Gulur P. Incidence of serotonin syndrome in patients treated with fentanyl on serotonergic agents. Pain Physician. 2015;18(1):E27–30 [M].

[37] Hillman A, Witenko C, Sultan S, et al. Serotonin syndrome caused by fentanyl and methadone in a burn injury. Pharmacotherapy. 2015;35(1):112–7 [A].

[38] Lyons P, Rivosecchi R, Nery J, et al. Fentanyl-induced hyperalgesia in acute pain management. J Pain Palliat Care Pharmacother. 2015;29(2):153–60 [M].

[39] Bakovic M, Nestic M, Mayer D. Death by band-aid: fatal misuse of transdermal fentanyl patch. Int J Legal Med. 2015;129(6):1247–52 [A].

[40] Doris M, Sandilands E. Life-threatening opioid toxicity from a fentanyl patch applied to eczematous skin. Reactions Weekly. 2015;1559(1):78 [A].

[41] Mach J, Van Havel T, Gadwood J, et al. Intrathecal opioid-induced hypothermia following subarachnoid block with morphine injection for elective cesarean delivery: a case report. AANA J. 2016;84(1):23–6 [A].

[42] Steinhorn R, McPherson C, Anderson PJ, et al. Neonatal morphine exposure in very preterm infants-cerebral development and outcomes. J Pediatr. 2015;166(5):1200–7 [M].

[43] Lee C, Muo C, Liang J, et al. Pulmonary embolism is associated with current morphine treatment in patients with deep vein thrombosis. Clin Respir J. 2015;9(2):233–7 [M].

[44] Tran B, Kohan L, Vorenkamp K. Postoperative oxycodone toxicity in a patient with chronic pain and end-stage renal disease. A A Case Rep. 2015;4(4):44–6 [A].

[45] Borys D, Stanton M, Gummin D, et al. Tapentadol toxicity in children. Pediatrics. 2015;135(2):e392–6 [M].

[46] Nasouhi S, Talaie H, Pajoumand A, et al. Hypo and hyperglycemia among tramadol overdose patients in Loghman Hakim Hospital, Tehran, Iran. Pak J Pharm Sci. 2015;28(6): 1959–63 [M].

[47] Fournier J, Azoulay L, Yin H, et al. Tramadol use and the risk of hospitalization for hypoglycemia in patients with noncancer pain. JAMA Intern Med. 2015;175(2):186–93 [M].

[48] Fournier JP, Yin H, Nessim S, et al. Tramadol for noncancer pain and the risk of hyponatremia. Am J Med. 2015;128(4). 418-25.e5. [M].

[49] Chen K, Lu M, Shen W. Tramadol-related psychosis in a patient with bipolar I disorder. Acta Neuropsychiatr. 2015;27(2): 126–8 [A].

[50] Perdreau E, Iriart X, Mouton J, et al. Cardiogenic shock due to acute tramadol intoxication. Cardiovasc Toxicol. 2015;15(1): 100–3 [A].

8

Anti-Inflammatory and Antipyretic Analgesics and Drugs Used in Gout

Hanna Raber[*,1], *Kirk Evoy*[†,‡], *Linda Lim*[†,‡]

*College of Pharmacy, The University of Utah, Salt Lake City, UT, USA
†College of Pharmacy, The University of Texas at Austin, Austin, TX, USA
‡School of Medicine, University of Texas Health Science Center San Antonio, Pharmacotherapy Education and Research Center, San Antonio, TX, USA
[1]Corresponding author: hanna.raber@gmail.com

ANILINE DERIVATIVES [SEDA-35, 197; SEDA-37, 115]

Paracetamol [SEDA-35, 197; SEDA-37, 115]

Breast

A recently published meta-analysis examined the association between NSAID use and breast cancer [1M]. There were a total of 8 case–control studies and 3 cohort studies identified that assessed the risk of breast cancer with acetaminophen use specifically. Results indicated that acetaminophen use reduced invasive breast cancer risk in both the case–control group (RR 0.95; 95% CI 0.88–1.01) and cohort studies (RR 0.92; 95% CI 0.95–1.00). The postulated mechanism of reduced breast cancer incidence with the use of NSAIDS is through COX-2 blockade. As acetaminophen is not typically strongly connected with COX-2, the association found with acetaminophen will require further investigation.

Drug–Drug Interaction

A prospective, randomized, controlled, double-blind parallel group trial found a suggested interaction between acetaminophen and ondansetron [2c]. Patients aged between 2 and 7 years scheduled for a tonsillectomy or adenoidectomy were evaluated post-procedure for a pain score after receiving acetaminophen with ondansetron or droperidol. Patients who received acetaminophen and ondansetron used significantly more morphine, in μg, than the droperidol and acetaminophen group (322.5 IQR and 0 IQR, respectively, $p = 0.01$). However,

pain scores in the two groups were similar. This increased morphine dose could indicate that ondansetron blocks the analgesic effects of acetaminophen.

Drug Overdose

In a retrospective cohort study, the association between acetaminophen poisoning and acute pancreatitis was examined [3C]. A total of 2958 patients who experienced acetaminophen poisoning were included. A risk of acute pancreatitis was 3.11-fold higher in the acetaminophen cohort than in the comparison cohort.

The AST/ALT may be a helpful tool to identify patients with resolving transaminases after acute paracetamol poisoning [4c]. A study identified 37 patients who received acetylcysteine after severe acetaminophen poisoning. The study found an AST/ALT ratio less than or equal to 0.4 was 99% sensitive for identifying patients with resolving transaminases. This finding may be beneficial to identify patients that have passed the peak AST concentrations and have resolving hepatic injury.

It was concluded in a published cohort study, that early measurement of plasma kidney injury molecule 1 (KIM-1) represents a more sensitive predictor of patient outcomes than serum creatinine concentration post-APAP overdose [5c]. Currently, serum creatinine is the primary lab used to predict renal function, and overall prognosis, however, is not very specific in the setting of acetaminophen-induced acute liver injury. A total of 74 patients with acetaminophen overdose were included in the study. Subjects were separated into cohorts based on the presence or absence of liver injury. Serum KIM-1

ISSN: 0378-6080
http://dx.doi.org/10.1016/bs.seda.2016.08.007

was assessed on day 1 of admission for acetaminophen overdose. Plasma KIM-1 was elevated in patients that died or required liver transplant ($p < 0.005$). Plasma KIM-1 was also superior to serum creatinine for reaching the King's College Criteria, a scoring system used for prognosis prediction (KIM-1: AUC, 0.87; 95% CI: 0.78–0.95; Creatinine: AUC, 0.76; 95% CI: 0.64–0.88). The clinical utility of KIM-1 will need to be assessed further; however, its regular use in this patient population would represent a change in current practice.

Acetaminophen-induced liver injury was also indicated by microRNAs in human serum [6c]. Blood samples from 6 healthy subjects and 6 acetaminophen-overdosed subjects were compared for the presence of microRNAs. The study identified 3 novel microRNAs that were elevated in the serum of acetaminophen-overdosed subjects and returned to normal after the administration of N-acetyl cysteine.

Musculoskeletal

Long-term acetaminophen use was associated with psoriasis and psoriatic arthritis in a recently published cohort study [7C]. Data were based on self-reported biannual questionnaires. Regular acetaminophen users were at higher risk of developing psoriasis (HR 1.29; 95% CI 1.08–1.54) and psoriasis with concomitant psoriatic arthritis (HR 2.23; 95% CI 1.63–3.07) when compared with to non-regular users.

Pregnancy

A large ($n = 1490$), longitudinal, prebirth, cohort study explored the association between wheeze, asthma, and allergen sensitization during early childhood (3–5 years old) and midchildhood (7–10 years) with maternal and early infant (up to 1 year of age) acetaminophen and ibuprofen use [8MC]. Infant acetaminophen exposure was associated with higher asthma (OR 1.21, 95% CI 1.04–1.41) and recurrent wheeze (OR 1.29, 95% CI 1.06–1.56) risk during early childhood and increased asthma risk (but not persistent wheeze) during midchildhood (OR 1.27, 95% CI 1.05–1.54). When adjusting for infant respiratory or ear infections as a potential confounder, only the risk of asthma at midchildhood was still significantly increased (OR 1.27, 95% CI 1.00–1.48). Ibuprofen use during infancy led to an increased risk of recurrent wheeze (OR 1.38, 95% CI 1.19–1.60) and asthma (OR 1.35, 95% CI 1.19–1.52) during early childhood but did not increase the risk of wheeze, asthma or allergen sensitization during midchildhood. When adjusting for respiratory or ear infections, only early childhood asthma risk was increased with ibuprofen exposure (OR 1.19, 95% CI 1.05–1.36).

Prenatal acetaminophen exposure was associated with significantly higher rates of recurrent wheeze (OR 1.53,

95% CI 1.23–1.90) and asthma (OR 1.36, 95% CI 1.14–1.61) during early childhood, with both remaining significantly higher after adjustment for confounders (OR 1.41, 95% CI 1.06–1.89 and OR 1.26, 95% CI 1.02–1.58 for wheeze and asthma, respectively). Prenatal ibuprofen exposure was associated only with a significantly higher risk of asthma in early childhood (OR 1.55, 95% CI 1.12–2.14), though this risk did not remain significantly elevated after adjustment for confounders. Neither prenatal acetaminophen nor ibuprofen use was associated with higher risks of wheeze, asthma, or allergen sensitization during midchildhood.

While a number of studies have been published identifying a possible increased risk of asthma with acetaminophen use or prenatal exposure to acetaminophen, this study significantly contributed to the current literature due to its inclusion of both ibuprofen as a comparator and its analysis of respiratory and ear infections as a potential confounder, both features that many previous studies have not adequately addressed. Based on this research displaying significantly diminished associations between prenatal and infant acetaminophen and ibuprofen exposure when controlling for ear and respiratory tract infections, the authors concluded that such infections may represent a significant, unaddressed confounder in a number of previous studies on this topic.

The potential association between paracetamol use during the first 12 months of life and the previous 12 months of childhood and body mass index was studied in a cross-sectional study [9C]. Parents of a total of 76 216 children aged 6–7 years and 188 469 adolescents aged 13–14 from 71 centers in 35 countries were asked to complete questionnaires on paracetamol use, height, weight, and parental smoking. A weak association between paracetamol use among children and an increased body mass index was found but only in affluent countries. Paracetamol use during the first 12 months of life resulted in a $0.07 \, \text{kg/m}^2$ higher body mass index for children in affluent countries. Recent paracetamol use within the previous 12 months was associated with a $0.17 \, \text{kg/m}^2$ higher body mass index among adolescents in affluent countries. The significance of the observed difference between affluent and non-affluent countries is unclear.

A review article examined the potential association between paracetamol use during pregnancy and child neurological development [10R]. This article reviewed the results of two cohort studies and one sibling-controlled study. Results of these studies conclude that exposure to paracetamol during pregnancy is associated with a weak to moderate statistically significant increased risk of ADHD/HKD disorders or neurodevelopmental detrimental effects.

ARYLALKANOIC ACID DERIVATIVES [SEDA-35, 200; SEDA-36, 119–120; SEDA-37, 116]

Diclofenac [SEDA-35, 200; SEDA-36, 119; SEDA-37, 116]

Drug Formulations

SoluMatrix® diclofenac is a low-dose diclofenac drug product that produces 10–20 times smaller particles to enhance the dissolution rate of diclofenac. One study evaluated safety in 300 patients for at least 6 months of therapy and 100 patients treated for 12 months [11C]. Adverse effects occurring most frequently (≥3%) were upper respiratory tract infection, headache, urinary tract infection, diarrhea, nasopharyngitis, and nausea. The most common serious adverse effect was osteoarthritis pain flare, which was reported in three patients (0.5%). Myocardial infarction was reported in two patients. Additional adverse effects that led to discontinuation from the study included increased alanine aminotransferase (ALT) (1.7%), increased aspartate aminotransferase (AST) (1%), increased serum creatinine (0.8%), increased blood pressure (0.5%), gastrointestinal disorders (4.7%), and increased hepatic enzymes (0.3%).

Ibuprofen [SEDA-35, 200; SEDA-36, 119; SEDA-37, 117]

Drug Dose Regimens

Intravenous (IV) ibuprofen was approved by the U.S. Food and Drug Administration in 2009. This Phase IV multicenter trial assessed the safety and efficacy profile of IV ibuprofen infusions given over 5–10 minutes [12C]. Adverse events occurring 6 hours after administration were assessed. The most common adverse event was infusion site pain/discomfort, which occurred in 24 of 150 patients (16%). Other reactions that occurred at ≥3% included flatulence (5%), nausea (3%), abnormal breath sounds (3%), and hyperglycemia (3%).

In the second part of this Phase IV trial, safety of IV ibuprofen given over 5–10 minutes was assessed in adult patients undergoing surgical procedures in the hospital [13C]. Adverse events were assessed 6 hours after administration. Similarly to the first part of the trial, the most common adverse event was pain or discomfort at the infusion site in 42 of the 300 patients (14%). Other adverse events include nausea (3%), flatulence (3%), anemia (3%), and bradycardia (3%). In the investigators opinion, bradycardia was unrelated to IV ibuprofen.

Respiratory

A study analyzed the pooled safety results from the REDUCE-1 and REDUCE-2 trials to determine the safety of ibuprofen alone versus ibuprofen and famotidine [14M]. Laryngitis, lower respiratory tract infections, and rib fracture were not reported in the ibuprofen and famotidine group; however, they were reported in 4.3% of patients in the ibuprofen group ($p = 0.0163$ for laryngitis and lower respiratory tract infections, $p = 0.0206$ for rib fracture).

Comparative Study

In a meta-analysis, intravenous (IV) ibuprofen used for treatment of patent ductus arteriosus in preterm, low birth weight, or both infants was studied [15M]. Early versus expectant administration of IV ibuprofen was compared. There was a statistically significant difference between the number of days on supplemental oxygen during the first 2 days. The mean difference between 105 infants was 2 days (95% CI 0.04–3.96; p-value 0.05).

INDOLEACETIC ACIDS [SEDA-37, 121]

Indomethacin [SEDA-37, 121]

Pregnancy

In a systematic review and meta-analysis assessing 2 observational studies, 8454 infants were assessed overall [16M]. In this analysis, 1731 infants were exposed to antenatal indomethacin, and 6723 were not exposed. This analysis was conducted to determine the effects of indomethacin exposure to neonates. Indomethacin is often used as a first-line tocolytic agent, but there has been an increasing concern about the safety of indomethacin crossing the placenta and inhibiting prostaglandin synthesis in fetal organs. Severe intraventricular hemorrhage (IVH) was defined as Papile's classification stage III and IV. Severe IVH was found to be higher among infants who received tocolysis with indomethacin compared to those infants who received no tocolytics or tocolysis with other agents (RR 1.29; 95% CI 1.06–1.56). The number needed to harm was 26. The incidence of necrotizing enterocolitis (NEC) was also increased among infants exposed to indomethacin than those who were not exposed (RR 1.36, 5% CI 1.08–1.71). The number needed to harm for NEC was 30. Similarly, the incidence of periventricular leukomalacia (PVL) also increased with antenatal exposure to indomethacin (RR 1.59, 95% CI 1.17–2.17). The number needed to harm was 28.

OXICAMS [SEDA-36, 126; SEDA-37, 121]

Lornoxicam [SEDA-36, 127]

Skin

An otherwise healthy 25-year-old male diagnosed with perforated acute retrocaecal subhepatic appendicitis status post appendectomy was readmitted to the hospital due to potential fluid collection in the retrocolic space with abdominal pain, nausea, tachycardia, and mood changes [17A]. In addition, the patient was noted to have a large skin erythema on one leg. After discontinuation of lornoxicam, all symptoms, surgical site infection, and questionable abdominal collection resolved.

PROPIONIC ACID DERIVATIVES
[SEDA-35, 200; SEDA-36, 127; SEDA-37, 121]

Naproxen [SEDA-35, 200; SEDA-36, 127; SEDA-37, 121]

Nervous System

A 28-year-old male ingested approximately 320 tablets of naproxen 220 mg (70.4 g) with an unknown quantity of alcohol about 90 minutes prior to presenting to the emergency department [18c]. At 90 minutes, the patient's peak naproxen serum concentration was 1580 mg/L. The patient experienced two generalized tonic–clonic seizures for which he was given lorazepam, phenytoin, and sedated with midazolam and propofol in order to be intubated endotracheally. The mechanism behind these seizures is not known. In animals, there is evidence that cyclooxygenase (COX) inhibitors lead to excitatory effects of the hippocampus, which is associated with seizures.

SALICYLATES [SEDA-35, 202; SEDA-36, 127, SEDA-37, 122]

Acetylsalicylic Acid (Aspirin) [SEDA-35, 202; SEDA-36, 127; SEDA-37, 122]

Bleeding

A case of spontaneous chest wall hematoma in a 41-year-old man taking aspirin 100 mg/day for cerebrovascular disease was reported [19A]. The man was not taking any other antiplatelet or anticoagulant agents and no precipitating factor was identified. With aspirin discontinuation, the hematoma resolved.

Overdose

A 20-year-old female presented to the hospital after ingestion of 66 g of acetylsalicylic acid [20A]. While vital signs and hepatic and renal function labs were normal and the patient was alert on admission, she subsequently developed acute liver failure with hepatic coma, as well as acute renal failure and pancreatitis. An emergency living donor liver transplantation was performed. Examination of the resected liver displayed pathologic findings indicating the acute liver failure was aspirin induced. Following surgery, the patient's symptoms slowly improved, eventually leading to full recovery and hospital discharge 53 days post aspirin ingestion.

MISCELLANEOUS DRUGS

Benzydamine [SEDA-35, 207]

Pregnancy

A series of three cases of premature constriction of the ductus arteriosus after maternal use of 3 mg benzydamine hydrochloride lozenges during the third trimester of pregnancy was reported [21A]. The women were 26, 27, and 29 years old and were not taking any concomitant medications. In each case, the child was successfully delivered and healthy. While fetal ductus arteriosus is a known adverse effect of NSAID use during pregnancy, the authors report these to be the first published cases linked to benzydamine therapy.

Flupirtine

Pharmacogenomics

A study to assess the impact of genetic polymorphisms of NAT2, UGT1A1, and GSTP1 on the generation of terminal mercapturic acid derivatives, and thus a potentially increased risk for hepatotoxicity with flupirtine, was conducted in 36 healthy subjects [22E]. In this study, these polymorphisms did not influence this hepatotoxic pathway.

Nefopam [SEDA-35, 207; SEDA-36, 128; SEDA-37, 123]

Post-Surgery Use

Three randomized, controlled trials assessed short-term nefopam use for post-surgery pain, including: 120 patients randomized following gynecologic surgery to pain management with bolus nefopam or ketorolac added to oxycodone patient-controlled analgesia (PCA) [23C]; ninety-four patients randomized following laparoscopic gynecologic surgery to pain management with either fentanyl or nefopam PCA [20A]; and forty-two patients randomized to nefopam intravenous infusion or saline following bimaxillary osteotomy. Adverse effects were mild and similar between treatment groups in each trial.

DRUGS USED IN THE TREATMENT OF GOUT

Allopurinol [SEDA-35, 207; SEDA-36, 129; SEDA-37, 123]

Hypersensitivity

A retrospective nationwide population study utilizing the Taiwan National Health Insurance Research Database to investigate the incidence of, risk factors for, and mortality associated with allopurinol hypersensitivity in the 495 863 identified new users of allopurinol [24R]. The incidence of allopurinol hypersensitivity, related hospitalizations, and related mortality was 4.68, 2.02, and 0.39 per 1000 new users. Risk factors associated with allopurinol hypersensitivity were female sex, age sixty or older, initial allopurinol dose exceeding 100 mg/day, renal or cardiovascular comorbidities, and use for treating asymptomatic hyperuricemia. Limitations of this study include the potential for missing data within the registry, retrospective design, and exclusively Taiwanese study population.

A case of acute generalized exanthematous pustulosis (AGEP) as a rare manifestation of allopurinol hypersensitivity syndrome (AHS) in a 67-year-old male was reported [25A]. The patient presented to the hospital 10 days after developing a widespread skin eruption and 8 weeks after beginning therapy with allopurinol 200 mg daily. Upon presentation, the patient was febrile, exhibited diffuse maculopapular eruptions on the trunk, arms, legs, follicular and nonfollicular pustules on the face and trunk, and an edematous superficial dermis with mixed inflammatory infiltration consistent with AGEP. Laboratory analysis displayed a white blood cell count of 13.2×10^9/L with atypical lymphocytes and hypereosinophilia, and mildly elevated liver enzymes, while renal function was normal. The EuroSCAR AGEP score was 5, indicating a probable case, with a late onset, prolonged course, and multi-organ involvement differentiating this from a case of drug rash with eosinophilia and systemic symptoms (DRESS), according to the authors. The patient's other medications at the time were aspirin and candesartan, which he had been taking for multiple years. Discontinuation of allopurinol and prednisone therapy (30 mg daily for 2 weeks followed by an extended taper) led to significant improvement within 72 hours and resolution of skin manifestations and fever within a few days.

A case series was published describing 21 patients with mild allopurinol hypersensitivity reactions who subsequently underwent a desensitization protocol in an attempt to allow for continued use of the medication [26c]. Though previous reports of allopurinol desensitization have been published, this series was unique in that they compared a traditional "slow" protocol (starting with 10 micrograms titrated up to 100 or 300 mg after 16 days) as well as a less commonly used "fast" protocol (starting with 50 micrograms and titrating to 100 mg within 5 days). Desensitization was successful in 64% of cases following the slow protocol (7/11), but only 40% (4/10) with the fast protocol, indicating that the slow protocol may be more effective, though the sample size is limited.

Pharmacogenomics

Allopurinol-induced severe cutaneous adverse reactions (SCARs) have recently been linked to the presence of the HLA-B*58:01 allele, and as a result, some clinicians have called for genomic testing prior to initiation of allopurinol [27MC]. To evaluate the effectiveness in reducing SCARs through genomic screening, a prospective cohort study, consisting exclusively of Han Chinese patients, was conducted in Taiwan, in which 2926 previously allopurinol-naïve patients with an indication for allopurinol were screened for HLA-B*58:01 prior to starting the medication. 571 patients (19.6%) tested positive and were treated with an alternative medication to allopurinol, while the remaining 2339 were prescribed allopurinol. Based on historical studies regarding the incidence of allopurinol-induced SCARs in Taiwan, seven patients (0.3% per year) were expected to develop SCARs. However, in this study population in which only patients testing negative for the HLA-B*58:01 allele were administered allopurinol, 0 patients developed SCARs (95% CI 0.28–0.31%; $p = 0.0026$ compared to the historical estimate). Based on these findings, and previous studies indicating that routine genomic screening of Thai or Korean populations prior to allopurinol initiation would be more cost-effective than a global substitution of febuxostat for allopurinol, the authors deemed that this may be a viable option to significantly reduce the incidence of SCARs, though these findings should be evaluated further, particularly in patients of other ethnic groups.

Additionally, a report of two cases of allopurinol-induced exfoliative dermatitis (less severe than SCARs) in which both patients, 49- and 73-year-old males from China, tested positive for the HLA-B*58:01 allele was published [28A]. Both patients responded to discontinuation of allopurinol and initiation of 40 mg/day methylprednisolone injections, with symptom resolution within 1–2 weeks.

Acute Gout

To assess whether initiating allopurinol during an acute gout attack would prolong the time to symptom resolution, a randomized, double-blind, placebo-controlled trial compared 17 patients receiving placebo to 14 patients receiving allopurinol 100 mg daily for 14 days followed by 200 mg daily [29c]. In addition to allopurinol or placebo, all patients received colchicine or NSAID therapy. Patients were included if they presented to the clinic with an acute gout attack within 72 hours of initial therapy and were excluded if they exhibited a glomerular filtration rate of less than 50 mg/dL or liver function tests more than 1.25 times the upper limit of normal. Time to resolution was 15.4 days in the allopurinol group versus 13.4 days in the placebo group ($p = 0.5$). Thus, this trial concluded that there was not a significant difference in symptom resolution between groups. However, with the small sample size limiting the ability to detect a statistical difference among the groups and the trend towards longer time to resolution, the results of this trial should be cautiously applied to clinical practice.

Other

A randomized, controlled trial was conducted in which 128 patients with hyperuricemic heart failure received allopurinol 600 mg daily [30C]. Allopurinol was well tolerated with the rate of overall adverse events and serious adverse events comparable to placebo. The adverse event profile was similar to previous studies including allopurinol, and no previously unreported adverse events emerged.

Colchicine [SEDA-35, 208; SEDA-37, 124]

Breastfeeding

A small prospective observational cohort study was conducted in Israel to assess the risk of infants exposed to colchicine during lactation [31c]. Outcomes of 38 infants breastfed from a mother taking colchicine were assessed for up to 3 years after exposure and compared to 76 infants whose mother took amoxicillin (a medication known to be safe during breastfeeding), matched with study group for year of birth, gestational age, and maternal age. Resulting data displayed no increase in adverse neonatal symptoms (3/38 versus 4/76, $p = 0.68$) or delayed development or neurological abnormalities (2/38 versus 2/76, $p = 0.60$).

Overdose

A case was presented regarding a 6-year-old girl who overdosed with approximately 0.9 mg/kg of colchicine, above the 0.8 mg/kg dose that is typically fatal, per the study authors [32A]. The patient presented to the hospital 12 hours after ingestion with encephalopathy, dehydration, and respiratory distress, and received gastric lavage, activated charcoal (1 g/kg every 6 hours) and intravenous fluids. Her symptoms worsened, resulting in multi-organ failure, including circulatory failure and acute respiratory distress syndrome requiring intubation and mechanical ventilation. At this time, plasma exchange (PE) was initiated. After two PE sessions, organ failures resolved, and the patient was discharged after 11 days in the hospital. This was one of the first reported cases of PE for colchicine overdose.

Additionally, a report of severe poisoning of a 68-year-old woman due to *Colchicum autumnale*, a plant whose stems contain colchicine, was reported [33A]. Three days after ingestion, the woman presented to the hospital with hypotension, severe dehydration, nausea, metabolic acidosis, leukocytosis, thrombocytopenia, rhabdomyolysis, and acute renal, liver, and cardiac failure. Bowel irrigation and continuous dobutamine infusions were administered without significant

improvement. Venous-arterial extracorporeal life support (ECLS) was initiated along with mechanical ventilation, hemodialysis, and transfusion of multiple blood products. This led to cardiac function improvement by day 9 and ECLS discontinuation at day 10. Despite cardiac arrhythmias following removal of ECLS, including a cardiac arrest on day 12, the patient progressively improved over a long hospitalization, finally being discharged from the intensive care unit 24 days after ingestion. This case led the authors to conclude that ECLS may be indicated for refractory cardiogenic shock in such patients suffering from severe colchicine poisoning.

Other

A small ($n = 59$), randomized, controlled trial of colchicine 0.5 mg twice daily in patients before and after coronary artery bypass graft was conducted [34c]. Adverse effects were limited to minor gastrointestinal complaints.

Febuxostat [SEDA-35, 209; SEDA-36, 129; SEDA-37, 125]

A case of possible febuxostat-induced rhabdomyolysis in a 68-year-old man with stage three chronic kidney disease (glomerular filtration rate 35 mL/minute/1.73 m²) was published [35A]. One month prior to hospitalization, the man began taking febuxostat 40 mg daily in addition to previously prescribed aspirin, simvastatin, gemfibrozil, furosemide, metoprolol, moxonidine, insulin, and omeprazole. Notably, the patient had been discharged from the hospital 4 days prior after an 8-day hospitalization due to pneumonia. With discontinuation of febuxostat (in addition to simvastatin and gemfibrozil) and initiation of hemodialysis for concomitant acute kidney failure, the patient recovered and was discharged from the hospital 23 days later. The authors of this case note that in the only other published report of rhabdomyolysis linked to febuxostat, the patient was also taking a statin in the setting of chronic kidney disease, and thus the combination may represent an increased risk of febuxostat-induced rhabdomyolysis.

Leflunomide [SEDA-36, 151; SEDA-37, 125]

Miscellaneous

A small ($n = 32$) observational study assessing the impact of adding leflunomide to failed methotrexate therapy in children with juvenile idiopathic arthritis was conducted [36c]. Mean follow-up was 1.61 years. Overall, the treatment was well tolerated, with only three patients reporting adverse effects. However, one patient developed macrophage activation syndrome (MAS) 5 months after starting leflunomide, which was ultimately fatal. Unfortunately, this case was not discussed in detail, and the likely attribution of this adverse effect to leflunomide was not specified in this article. While it is not listed as a possible adverse effect in the leflunomide prescribing information, rare reports of leflunomide-induced MAS have been published.

A 168-patient trial of IgA nephropathy patients randomized to either valsartan, valsartan and leflunomide, valsartan and clopidogrel, or all three medications was conducted [37C]. Little could be gleaned from this trial in terms of leflunomide adverse effects, as it was only studied in combination. However, the combinations were well tolerated, and no unique adverse effects were reported.

Rasburicase [SEDA-35, 209; SEDA-36, 131]

Hematologic

Three case reports of rasburicase-induced methemoglobinemia and one report of rasburicase-induced Heinz body hemolytic anemia were published in 2015 [38A,39A,40A]. Two case reports found rasburicase-induced methemoglobinemia in African-American females who received rasburicase for tumor lysis syndrome [38A]. Only one of these patients had confirmed G6PD deficiency. Previously published case reports have been limited to only male patients.

An additional case of rasburicase-induced methemoglobinemia was reported after a 56-year-old Hispanic male received rasburicase for the prevention of tumor lysis syndrome [39A]. The patient's symptoms resolved; however, it was later confirmed that the patient had G6PD deficiency.

The final case report was a 58-year-old male with rasburicase-induced Heinz body hemolytic anemia [40A]. This patient was also receiving rasburicase to prevent tumor lysis syndrome and had confirmed G6PD deficiency. The hemolysis presented within 24 hours of administration and resolved upon discontinuation of rasburicase.

Immunologic

Rasburicase-induced anaphylaxis was found to have a higher incidence after the second exposure [41c]. In a retrospective chart review of 97 patients who received rasburicase for hyperuricemia, six patients experienced anaphylaxis following a subsequent exposure to rasburicase. No patients experienced anaphylaxis after the initial course of rasburicase. In the patients who experienced anaphylaxis, the mean time between first and second exposure to rasburicase was 257 days, and the time from exposure to symptoms of anaphylaxis was 2 hours in five of the six patients. This finding represents a higher rate of anaphylaxis with rasburicase than was previously reported in the package insert.

Special Review

℞ : New Drug Approval: Lesinurad

In December 2015, lesinurad, a novel uric acid transporter 1 (URAT1) inhibitor for the treatment of hyperuricemia associated with gout in combination with a xanthine oxidase inhibitor, received United States Food and Drug Administration approval [42S]. This medication acts through inhibition of transporter proteins involved in uric acid reabsorption in the kidney, namely, URAT1 which is responsible for most of the reabsorption of renally filtered uric acid and organic anion transporter 4 (OAT4) which is linked to diuretic-induced hyperuricemia. Lesinurad is intended for patients who have not achieved target serum uric acid levels with a xanthine oxidase inhibitor alone.

At the time of writing, full manuscripts of only one Phase II and two Phase I trials had been published [43C,44c,45c]. In the Phase II trial, 227 patients were randomized to 2:1 to lesinurad (200, 400, or 600 mg) in combination with allopurinol versus allopurinol alone for 4 weeks [43C]. At least one adverse effect was observed in 46%, 48%, 54%, and 46% of the patients receiving lesinurad 200, 400, and 600 mg and placebo, respectively. Gout flares were the most common adverse effect categorized as possibly related to study treatment, with increased lipase the only other adverse effect deemed possibly related to treatment and occurring in more than 1 patient. For the 200 mg dose, 10.9% experienced gout flares necessitating treatment compared to 6.9% of placebo patients. No serious adverse effects were reported. Elevations in serum creatinine above the reference range were seen more commonly in patients receiving lesinurad than placebo (2.5%, 10%, 7.5%, and 1.6% for lesinurad 200, 400, and 600 mg and placebo, respectively).

However, the full prescribing information provides additional data regarding the adverse effects observed in the pivotal Phase III trials [42S]. In three randomized, placebo-controlled trials of lesinurad in combination with a xanthine oxidase inhibitor (two with allopurinol and one with febuxostat), 511 patients received lesinurad 200 mg and 510 patients received lesinurad 400 mg versus 516 patients administered placebo, with a maximum follow-up of 12 months. Adverse effects were significantly more frequent with 400 mg doses, including increases in renal effects and cardiovascular events, leading to approval of only the 200 mg dose. The United States prescribing information carries a warning for both renal adverse effects, with mention that these events were more common with 400 mg doses, and cardiovascular events, with mention that a causal relationship has not been established.

In the pooled data, elevated serum creatinine was more common with lesinurad 200 mg than placebo (4.3% versus 2.3%) [42S]. However, renal failure (1.2% versus 2.1%) and nephrolithiasis (0.6% versus 1.7%) were less common with lesinurad 200 mg than placebo, with no serious renal-related adverse reactions occurring with lesinurad 200 mg. Other adverse effects occurring in greater than 2% of patients taking lesinurad 200 mg with at least a 1% increase compared to placebo *included headache (5.3% versus 4.1%), influenza (5.1% versus 2.7%) and gastroesophageal reflux disease (0.8% versus 2.7%). There was a statistically significant increase in the incidence of a composite cardiovascular endpoint of cardiovascular death, fatal myocardial infarction, and non-fatal stroke in one Phase III study of lesinurad 200 mg versus placebo, but the overall incidence was quite low (0.96% versus 0.71%; incidence rate ratio 1.36, 95% CI 0.23–9.25).*

Currently, the FDA recommends no dosage adjustment in elderly patients or those with reduced hepatic function. In patients with an estimated creatinine clearance greater than 45 mL/minute, no dosage adjustment is necessary, but use is not recommended in those with an estimated creatinine clearance less than 45 mL/minute. The drug is also contraindicated in kidney transplant recipients and in the setting of tumor lysis syndrome or Lesch–Nyhan syndrome.

Lesinurad offers an exciting new therapeutic option for patients with gout unable to achieve goal serum uric acid levels with a xanthine oxidase inhibitor alone. The approved 200 mg dose appears to be well tolerated with only mild-to-moderate adverse effects observed. Ongoing clinical trials and post-marketing surveillance will be important to assess for the possibility of other rare adverse events.

References

[1] Pedro M, Baeza S, Escudero M, et al. Effect of COX-2 inhibitors and other non-steroidal inflammatory drugs on breast cancer risk: a meta-analysis. Breast Cancer Res Treat. 2015;149(2):525–36 [M].

[2] Ramirez L, Cros J, Marin B, et al. Analgesic interaction between ondansetron and acetaminophen after tonsillectomy in children: the Paratron randomized, controlled trial. Eur J Pain. 2015;19(5):661–8 [c].

[3] Chen A, Lin C, Hsu C, et al. Acetaminophen poisoning and risk of acute pancreatitis. Medicine (Baltimore). 2015;94(29):e1195 [C].

[4] McGovern A, Vitkovitsky I, Jones D, et al. Can AST/ALT ratio indicate recovery after acute paracetamol poisoning? Clin Toxicol (Phila). 2015;53(3):164–7 [c].

[5] Antoine D, Sabbisetti V, Francis B, et al. Circulating kidney injury molecule 1 predicts prognosis with poor outcome in patients with acetaminophen-induced liver injury. Hepatology. 2015;62(2):591–9 [c].

[6] Krauskopf J, Caiment F, Claessen S, et al. Application of high-throughput sequencing to circulating microRNAs reveals novel biomarkers for drug-induced liver injury. Toxicol Sci. 2015;143(2):268–76 [c].

[7] Wu S, Han J, Qureshi A, et al. Use of aspirin, non-steroidal anti-inflammatory drugs, and acetaminophen (paracetamol), and risk of psoriasis and psoriatic arthritis: a cohort study. Acta Derm Venereol. 2015;95(2):217–23 [C].

[8] Sordillo JE, Scirica CV, Rifas-Shiman SL, et al. Prenatal and infant exposure to acetaminophen and ibuprofen and the risk for wheeze and asthma in children. J Allergy Clin Immunol. 2015;135(2):441–8 [MC].

[9] Krauskopf J, Caiment F, Claessen S, et al. Application of high-throughput sequencing to circulating microRNAs reveals novel biomarkers for drug-induced liver injury. Toxicol Sci. 2015;143(2):268–76 [C].

[10] De Fays L, Van Malderen K, De Smet K, et al. Use of paracetamol during pregnancy and child neurological development. Dev Med Child Neurol. 2015;57(8):718–24 [R].

[11] Altman RD, Strand V, Hochberg MC, et al. Low-dose SoluMatrix diclofenac in the treatment of osteoarthritis: a 1-year, open-label, Phase III safety study. Postgrad Med. 2015;127:517–28. http://dx.doi.org/10.1080/00325481.2015.1040716 [C].

[12] Bergese SD, Candiotti K, Ayad SS, et al. The shortened infusion time of intravenous ibuprofen part 1: a multicenter, open-label, surveillance trial to evaluate safety and efficacy. Clin Ther. 2015;37:360–7 [C].

[13] Gan TJ, Candiotti Turan A, et al. The shortened infusion time of intravenous ibuprofen, part 2: a multicenter, open-label, surgical surveillance trial to evaluate safety. Clin Ther. 2015;37:368–75 [C].

[14] Bello AE, Grahn AY, Ball J, et al. One-year safety of ibuprofen/famotidine fixed combination versus ibuprofen alone: pooled analyses of two 24-week randomized, double-blind trials and a follow-on extension. Curr Med Res Opin. 2015;31:407–20. http://dx.doi.org/10.1185/03007995.2014.1000086 [M].

[15] Ohlsson A, Walia R, Shah SS. Ibuprofen for the treatment of patent ductus arteriosus in preterm or low birth weight (or both) infants. Cochrane Database Syst Rev. 2015;2:CD003481. http://dx.doi.org/10.1002/14651858.CD003481.pub.6 [M].

[16] Hammers AL, Sanchez-Ramos L, Kaunitz AM. Antenatal exposure to indomethacin increases the risk of severe intraventricular hemorrhage, necrotizing enterocolitis, and periventricular leukomalacia: a systematic review with meta-analysis. Am J Obstet Gynecol. 2015;212:505.e1–505.e13 [M].

[17] Alharbi MB. Lornoxicam side effects may lead to surgical mismanagement, in case of postoperative intra-abdominal collection: a case report and literature review. Case Rep Surg. 2015;2015:245807. http://dx.doi.org/10.1155/2015/545807 [A].

[18] Al-Abri SA, Anderson IB, Pedram F, et al. Massive naproxen overdose with serial serum levels. J Med Toxicol. 2015;11:102–5. http://dx.doi.org/10.1007/s13181-014-0396-1 [c].

[19] Shirota T, Ikegami T, Sugiyama S, et al. Successful living donor liver transplantation for acute liver failure after acetylsalicylic acid overdose. Clin J Gastroenterol. 2015;8:97–102 [A].

[20] Krzezowski W, Wilczynski J, Grzesiak M, et al. Prenatal sonographic diagnosis of premature constriction of the fetal ductus arteriosus after maternal self-medication with benzydamine hydrochloride. J Ultrasound Med. 2015;34:531–5 [A].

[21] Ghosh D, McGann PM, Furlong TJ, et al. Febuxostat-associated rhabdomyolysis in chronic renal failure. Med J Aust. 2015;203(2):107–9 [A].

[22] Siegmund W, Modess C, Scheuch E, et al. Metabolic activation and analgesic effect of flupirtine in healthy subjects, influence of the polymorphic NAT2, UGT1A1, and GSTP1. Br J Clin Pharmacol. 2014;79(3):501–13 [E].

[23] Hwang B, Kwon J, Lee D, et al. A randomized clinical trial of nefopam versus ketorolac combined with oxycodone in patient controlled analgesia after gynecologic surgery. Int J Med Sci. 2015;12(8):64–649 [C].

[24] Yang C, Chen C, Deng S, et al. Allopurinol use and risk of fatal hypersensitivity reactions a nationwide population based study in Taiwan. JAMA Intern Med. 2015;175(9):1550–7 [R].

[25] Salem CB, Saidi W, Larif S, et al. Pustular drug hypersensitivity syndrome due to allopurinol. Indian J Pharmacol. 2015;47(1):123–4 [A].

[26] Bruno Soares J, Caiado J, Lopes A, et al. Allopurinol desensitization: a fast or slow protocol? J Investig Allergol Clin Immunol. 2015;25(4):295–315 [c].

[27] Ko T, Tsai C, Chen S, et al. Use of HLA-B*58:01 genotyping to prevent allopurinol induced severe cutaneous adverse reactions in

Taiwan: national prospective cohort study. BMJ. 2015;351:h4848. http://dx.doi.org/10.1136/bmj.h4848 [MC].

[28] Zeng M, Zhang M, Liu F, et al. Drug eruptions induced by allopurinol associated with HLA-B*5801. Indian J Dermatol Venereol Leprol. 2015;81:43–5 [A].

[29] Hill EM, Sky K, Sit M, et al. Does starting allopurinol prolong acute treated gout? A randomized clinical trial. J Clin Rheumatol. 2015;21:120–5 [c].

[30] Givertz MM, Anstrom KJ, Redfield MM, et al. Effects of xanthine oxidase inhibition in hyperuricemic heart failure patients the xanthine oxidase inhibition for hyperuricemic heart failure patients (EXACT-HF) study. Circulation. 2015;131:1763–71. http://dx.doi.org/10.1161/CIRCULATIONHA. 114.014536 [C].

[31] Herscovici T, Merlob P, Stahl B, et al. Colchicine use during breastfeeding. Breastfeed Med. 2015;10(2):92–5. http://dx.doi.org/10.1089/bfm.2014.0086 [c].

[32] Demirkol D, Karacabey BN, Aygun F. Plasma exchange treatment in a case of colchicine intoxication. Ther Apher Dial. 2015;19(1):95–6 [A].

[33] Boisrame-Helms J, Rahmani H, Stiel L, et al. Extracorporeal life support in the treatment of colchicine poisoning. Clin Toxicol. 2015;53(8):827–9 [A].

[34] Giannopoulos G, Angelidis C, Kouritas VK, et al. Usefulness of colchicine to reduce perioperative myocardial damage in patients who underwent on-pump coronary artery bypass grafting. Am J Cardiol. 2015;115:1376–81 [c].

[35] Yazkan R, Ceviker K, Camas HE. Whatever will be, will be: spontaneous chest wall hematoma with regular use of low-dose acetylsalicylic acid. Can J Cardiol. 2015;31:820.e7–8 [A].

[36] Chickermane PR, Khubchandani RP. Evaluation of the benefits of sequential addition of leflunomide in patients with polyarticular

course juvenile idiopathic arthritis failing standard dose methotrexate. Clin Exp Rheumatol. 2015;33:287–92 [c].

[37] Cheng G, Liu D, Margetts P, et al. Valsartan combined with clopidogrel and/or leflunomide for the treatment of progressive immunoglobulin A nephropathy. Nephrology. 2015;20:77–84 [C].

[38] Roberts D, Freed J. Rasburicase-induced methemoglobinemia in two African-American female patients: an under-recognized and continued problem. Eur J Haematol. 2015;94(1):83–5 [A].

[39] Oluwasanjo A, Alese O, Swierczynski S, et al. Rasburicase-induced methaemoglobinaemia and G6PD deficiency in an unusual suspect. Br J Haematol. 2015;170(5):595 [A].

[40] Hrisinko A, Chen Y. Rasburicase-induced Heinz body hemolytic anemia in a patient with chronic lymphocytic leukemia. Blood. 2015;126(6):826 [A].

[41] Allen K, Champlain A, Cotliar J, et al. Risk of anaphylaxis with repeated courses of rasburicase: a research on adverse drug events and reports (RADAR) project. Drug Saf. 2015;38(2):183–7 [c].

[42] Zurampic® [package insert]. Wilmington, DE: AstraZeneca Pharmaceuticals LP; 2015. [S].

[43] Perez-Ruiz F, Sundy JS, Minder JN, et al. Lesinurad in combination with allopurinol: results of a phase 2, randomized, double-blind study in patients with gout with an inadequate response to allopurinol. Ann Rheum Dis. 2016;75:1074–80. http://dx.doi.org/10.1136/annrheumdis-2015-207919 [C].

[44] Fleischmann R, Kerr B, Yeh L, et al. Pharmacodynamic, pharmacokinetic, and tolerability evaluation of concomitant administration of lesinurad and febuxostat in gout patients with hyperuricemia. Rheumatology. 2014;53:2167–74 [c].

[45] Zancong S, Rowlings C, Kerr B, et al. Pharmacokinetics, pharmacodynamics, and safety of lesinurad, a selective uric acid reabsorption inhibitor, in healthy adult males. Drug Des Devel Ther. 2015;9:3423–34 [c].

9

General Anaesthetics and Therapeutic Gases

Abhishek Jha, Elizabeth Flockton[1]

Royal Liverpool Hospital, Liverpool, United Kingdom
[1]Corresponding author: elizabeth.flockton@rlbuht.nhs.uk

ANAESTHETIC VAPOURS

Halogenated Vapours

Comparative Studies

Volatile anaesthetic agents exert a cardioprotective effect with a reduced incidence of peri-operative myocardial ischaemia during off-pump coronary artery bypass surgeries. A small study ($n = 40$) compared the pharmacological myocardial effects of sevoflurane and desflurane in the early post-operative period (1–8 h) using troponin T and CKMB levels, and in the late post-operative period (third post-operative day) using echocardiographic measurements to obtain a myocardial performance index [1c]. Sevoflurane and desflurane were comparable in cardioprotective effects in the early post-operative period. Desflurane demonstrated superior cardioprotection in the late post-operative period ($p = 0.013$).

The neuroprotective effects of desflurane, isoflurane, and sevoflurane are compared in a retrospective study of 90 patients undergoing neurosurgical procedures [2c]. Blood from the radial artery and jugular bulb were extracted at fixed time points and analysed for haemoglobin content, oxygen saturation, oxygen partial pressure, oxygen content, glucose concentration, and lactate concentration to provide data on cerebral oxygen and glucose metabolism. Intra-operative haemodynamics and emergence times were also measured. The investigators report superiority of sevoflurane based on onset and recovery profile (data not provided), more stable haemodynamics, and cerebral homeostasis (raw data but no statistical analysis provided).

A small study compared the awakening properties of desflurane, isoflurane, and sevoflurane following craniotomy for resection of supratentorial tumour in the paediatric population [3c]. Tracheal extubation time and emergence time were significantly longer in the isoflurane group. The incidence of brain swelling, haemodynamic instability and post-operative adverse events was similar in all groups.

Meta-Analysis

The rates of upper airway adverse events and emergence times in patients undergoing laryngeal mask airway (LMA) anaesthesia using desflurane, sevoflurane, isoflurane, or propofol are compared in a meta-analysis [4M]. The rates of upper airway adverse events were comparable between all agents. Emergence time (time to eye-opening, time to LMA removal, time to respond to command, and time to state date of birth) was significantly faster in the desflurane group. It should be noted that the meta-analysis was limited by small scale studies and heterogeneity between studies.

Emergence profiles and post-operative events in paediatric patients receiving desflurane and sevoflurane anaesthesia are compared [5M]. Eleven randomised controlled trials in 1273 patients were included and suggest desflurane is the superior agent with shorter times to extubation ($p < 0.01$), eye-opening ($p < 0.01$), and awakening ($p < 0.01$) and was associated with a lower incidence of emergence agitation ($p = 0.02$). No differences in oculocardiac reflex, nausea and vomiting, or severe pain were detected.

Desflurane [SEDA-35, 217; SEDA-36, 139; SEDA-37, 129]

Comparative Studies

The effects of desflurane and propofol on post-operative spirometry, emergence time, and post-operative pain in elderly patients undergoing knee surgery are compared [6c]. Emergence time was more rapid in the desflurane group. Post-operative FEV1 values were significantly reduced compared to pre-operative baseline for 24 h after surgery in both groups ($p < 0.001$). No difference in FEV1, FVC, FEV1/FVC, or post-operative pain between the two groups was detected.

Isoflurane [SEDA-35, 217; SEDA-36, 139; SEDA-37, 129]

Comparative Studies

The immediate recovery time and post-operative respiratory complications in patients undergoing laparotomy for bariatric surgery with two anaesthetic protocols have been compared [7c]. A short-acting protocol of sevoflurane, remifentanil, rocuronium with ropivacaine epidural ($n = 200$) was compared with a long-acting protocol of isoflurane, sufentanil, atracurium with levo-bupivacaine epidural ($n = 152$). The isoflurane (long-acting group) had a longer time to extubation (30.4 ± 7.9 min vs. 18.2 ± 9.6 min, $p < 0.0001$) and a slightly higher rate of post-operative respiratory complications (6.58% vs. 2.5%, $p = 0.048$). Irrespective of treatment group, an extubation time of greater than 20 min was associated with a 4.5-fold increased risk of post-operative respiratory complications.

Musculoskeletal

The incidence of post-operative shivering associated with isoflurane or propofol general anaesthesia for elective general and orthopaedic surgeries has been compared—the incidence of shivering was comparable between the two groups [8C].

Sevoflurane [SEDA-35, 217; SEDA-36, 139; SEDA-37, 129]

Comparative Studies

Cardiovascular stability and adverse respiratory events during LMA insertion with sevoflurane induction and maintenance of anaesthesia are compared with propofol total intravenous anaesthesia [9c]. The sevoflurane group received 8% sevoflurane until loss of eyelash reflex and the propofol group received propofol to achieve an effect-site concentration of 8 μcg/mL. Both groups demonstrated hypotension (decrease >20% of baseline), but the incidence was lower in the sevoflurane group. No difference in respiratory adverse events (cough during LMA insertion) was detected between the two groups.

The provision of acceptable (excellent or good) intubating conditions by sevoflurane (1.0 age-adjusted MAC) is compared with rocuronium (0.45–0.6 mg/kg to achieve maximal neuromuscular block) [10c]. Both study groups received remifentanil and propofol intravenous

anaesthesia. Overall intubating conditions, assessed using GRCP guidelines, were comparable between the two groups. Acceptable intubating conditions were significantly more common in the rocuronium group ($p = 0.029$), as was lack of response to tube insertion and cuff inflation ($p = 0.02$). The sevoflurane had a non-significant increased incidence of vocal cord erythema. The incidence of hoarseness and sore throat was similar.

The effect of sevoflurane and propofol on post-operative cognitive dysfunction (POCD) is compared in patients pre-operatively identified to have decreased cerebral oxygenation (SjvO2 < 50%) undergoing elective abdominal surgery [11C]. Both groups received remifentanil and then propofol or sevoflurane to keep a BIS value of 40–60. Cognitive function assessed using MMSE or MoCA at baseline, day 1, and day 7 following surgery was comparable between the two groups at the different time points. Levels of S100β protein were similarly elevated at extubation and day 1 following surgery in both groups. SjvO2, as a marker of cerebral oxygenation, increased during induction, at 1 h, 2 h, and end of surgery in both groups. In the sevoflurane group, SjvO2 also increased at extubation. Cerebral blood flow/cerebral metabolic rate of oxygen consumption (CBF/CMRO2), as a measurement of cerebral oxygenation, was higher in the sevoflurane group at induction, 1 h, 2 h, and end of surgery.

The quality of anaesthesia provided by sevoflurane and propofol to patients undergoing anterior cervical discectomy and fusion surgery is compared [12c]. There were no differences in duration of anaesthesia, duration of surgery, time to extubation, or post-operative complications (PONV, sore throat, dizziness). The propofol group required significantly more opioid ($p = 0.005$) and had a greater intra-operative blood loss ($p = 0.019$).

Short-term sedation using sevoflurane or propofol to facilitate injection of local anaesthesia for oculoplastic surgery is compared [13C]. Patients were randomised to receive 8% sevoflurane ($n = 124$) or bolus of propofol 0.5 mg/kg ($n = 124$), or placebo ($n = 123$). Pain tolerance, patient satisfaction, and complications were measured. Propofol and sevoflurane had comparable pain scores and patient satisfaction, and both were superior to placebo ($p < 0.001$). Significantly more patients in the sevoflurane group required restraint during periocular injections than propofol or placebo ($p < 0.001$). Three patients in the sevoflurane group experienced emergence agitation and a further 3 experienced severe PONV.

Liver

The effect of volatile anaesthesia on acute graft injury in patients undergoing cadaveric liver transplant surgery is assessed [14c]. Patients were randomised to receive maintenance anesthesia with propofol ($n = 48$) or sevoflurane ($n = 50$). There was no difference in the primary endpoint—peak aspartate transaminase (AST). In addition, no differences in any of the measured biochemical markers of acute liver injury or clinical outcome (ICU and hospital length of stay, hospital mortality, and complications) were observed. Sevoflurane did not offer any additional protective effect to propofol on ischaemia/reperfusion injury during cadaveric liver transplant surgery.

Reproductive System

The effect of sevoflurane on intrauterine bleeding during dilation and evacuation procedures performed between 18 and 24 weeks gestation has been studied [15c]. Patients receiving sevoflurane were more likely to receive an intervention for excess bleeding and to have a measured blood loss in excess of 300 mL than the standard treatment group (no volatile agent). The study is underpowered to detect clinically or statistically significant results.

Immunologic

A sub-study of a prospective randomised controlled trial of patients undergoing elective open abdominal aortic surgery was undertaken to compare the effects of sevoflurane and propofol anaesthesia on inflammatory response (and thus a possible cardioprotective effect) [16c]. A short-term difference was observed at 30 min post-operatively with lower levels of monocyte chemotactic protein-1 and interleukin-8 ($p < 0.001$), and higher levels of interleukin-6 and matrix metalloproteinase-9 ($p = 0.003$) in the sevoflurane group. The results were deemed to be statistically but not clinically significant.

OTHER VAPOURS

Nitrous Oxide [SEDA-35, 217; SEDA-36, 139; SEDA-37, 129]

Comparative Studies

Continuous entonox (mixture 50% nitrous oxide: 50% oxygen) is compared to as-required entonox to manage pain in patients undergoing colonoscopy [17c]. Patients ($n = 100$) rated their overall pain and experience of pain during the procedure. There was no placebo group. No difference in overall pain or procedural pain was detected between groups. Light headedness was reported more frequently in the continuous use group (48% vs. 21%, $p = 0.009$).

The analgesic efficacy of 30-min inhaled entonox versus intramuscular morphine sulphate 0.1 mg/kg on pain scores in patients presenting with renal colic is reported [18c]. Both groups received the same dose of diclofenac. Pain scores in the two groups were comparable at baseline

but thereafter were significantly lower at 3-, 5-, 10-, and 30-min after treatment. The need for rescue analgesia after 30 min was similar. The difference in onset time between the two treatments does not appear to have been accounted for.

The anxiolytic effect of nitrous oxide is compared with cognitive behavioural therapy (CBT) and placebo for the reduction of anxiety during dental procedures in preschool children [19c]. Nitrous oxide and CBT were equally effective, and both were superior to placebo.

Combination Studies

Conscious sedation for dental treatment using propofol with or without 40% nitrous oxide is assessed [20C]. The propofol plus nitrous oxide group required less propofol (249.8 ± 121.7 mg vs. 310.3 ± 122.4 mg, $p = 0.022$), experienced less reduction in mean blood pressure (11.0 ± 8.0 mmHg vs. 15.8 ± 10.2 mmHg, $p = 0.034$), and reported less recall of the procedure.

Meta-Analysis

The outcomes of patients undergoing general anaesthesia with or without nitrous oxide have been assessed in a meta-analysis [21M]. Thirty-five randomised controlled studies involving 13 872 adult patients were included. Pulmonary atelectasis was significantly increased in the nitrous oxide group (OR 1.57, 95% CI 1.18–2.10, $p = 0.002$) but had no effect on morbidity or mortality. Further analysis of high quality studies suggested a potential increased risk of pneumonia and severe nausea and vomiting associated with nitrous oxide.

Nervous System

A case of severe motor neuropathy resulting from nitrous oxide toxicity is reported [22A]. The patient presented with predominantly sensory symptoms and signs following 2 months of nitrous oxide misuse. The sensory symptoms fully resolved after correction of vitamin B12 deficiency and abstinence from nitrous oxide. The case report is unusual in that the subject then represented with severe motor axonal neuropathy despite normal B12, homocysteine, and methylmalonic acid levels as well as the exclusion of metabolic diseases associated with motor neuropathy. Nitrous oxide toxicity occurring independently of vitamin B12 has been suggested.

The efficacy of nitrous oxide in the management of procedural pain is again reported [23c,24c,25c]. Entonox or oxygen was administered to nulliparous women undergoing intrauterine device insertion. Procedural pain scores were comparable between the two groups, but patient satisfaction was higher in the entonox group [25c]. The analgesic efficacy of nitrous oxide compared to paracervical infiltration with lidocaine or placebo for hysteroscopic polypectomy showed superior analgesia in the nitrous oxide group [23c]. A study assessing the analgesic efficacy of entonox compared to placebo for bone marrow aspiration and/or biopsy showed no reduction in procedural pain or increase in patient satisfaction in the entonox group [24c].

Psychiatric

The potential role of nitrous oxide as a therapeutic agent in the management of treatment-resistant major depression is explored as is the possible mechanism of action by which NMDA receptor antagonism occurs [26H].

Long-Term Effects: Genotoxicity

A review of the potential carcinogenicity and genotoxic effect of nitrous oxide is reported [27R]. The authors conclude that the evidence does not support a carcinogenic effect but that there may be a weak genotoxic effect with DNA damage comparable to that reported for isoflurane and sevoflurane.

INTRAVENOUS AGENTS

Comparative Studies

The cardiovascular stability, seizure duration and post-procedure cognitive function following electroconvulsive therapy (ECT) after anaesthesia with thiopental, etomidate, or propofol have been compared [28C]. The efficacy and safety profiles were comparable between the three groups.

Meta-Analysis

The safety and efficacy of anaesthetic agents as procedural sedatives for cardioversion have been assessed in a meta-analysis [29C]. Twenty-three studies with 1250 patients were included in the analysis. Propofol, etomidate, thiopentone, sevoflurane (2 studies), and midazolam have been utilised resulting in few studies using the same comparator drugs. The quality of evidence in the studies included in the analysis was low with limited information on patient selection, treatment allocation, and blinding of anaesthetists and outcome assessors. No agent was deemed to be inadequate for use in cardioversion.

A meta-analysis comparing seizure duration during ECT with induction agents etomidate ($n=704$), propofol ($n=258$), thiopental ($n=2491$), or methohexital ($n=84$) is reported [30C]. Seventeen studies were analysed and pooled data on EEG seizure duration and motor seizure duration compared. Longer EEG seizure duration was seen in the etomidate group (by 2.23 s), but the wide CI (-3.62 to 8.01) and the non-statistically significant p-value ($p=0.46$) should be noted. Pooled data on motor seizure activity showed longer duration in the etomidate

group when compared to the other agents. The wide range of numbers in the various agent groups should be noted. No data on inter-study variability or specific detail of ECT are provided.

NON-BARBITURATE ANAESTHETICS

Etomidate [SEDA-35, 217; SEDA-36,139; SEDA-37, 129]

Comparative Studies

The efficacy and safety of etomidate and propofol as procedural sedatives for elective cardioversion in ASA I–III patients with ejection fraction >35% are compared [31c]. The etomidate group were shown to have superior cardiovascular stability (incidence of hypotension of 16.65% vs. 33.3% in the propofol group, $p<0.05$), and a more rapid recovery time (435.7 s in the etomidate group vs. 659.1 s in the propofol group, $p<0.001$). The number of shocks delivered and the time to discharge were similar in the two groups.

The cardiovascular stability of etomidate and propofol given by intermittent bolus injection to achieve deep sedation in autistic children undergoing intrathecal stem cell transplantation has been assessed [32c]. The propofol group ($n=30$) received an initial bolus dose of 2 mg/kg with supplemental increments of 1 mg/kg. The etomidate group ($n=30$) received initial bolus of 0.2 mg/kg with supplemental doses of 0.1 mg/kg. The etomidate group demonstrated less change in blood pressure and heart rate from baseline values at every 5-min observation until 30 min after initial bolus ($p<0.05$). The incidence of pain on injection was higher in the propofol group (5 vs. 0 patients), whilst the etomidate group had a higher incidence of myoclonus (8 vs. 0 patients).

Propofol [SEDA-35, 217; SEDA-36, 139; SEDA-37, 129]

Comparative Studies

A small study of procedural sedation with propofol plus fentanyl or propofol plus midazolam to facilitate relocation of anterior shoulder dislocations has been performed [33c]. No information on methods for randomisation or blinding has been provided, and the study is underpowered to detect any significant results.

The theory that intra-operative opioid use is associated with hyperalgesia and increased analgesic use postoperatively is assessed in patients undergoing laparoscopic cholecystectomy [34c]. Patients received an opioid-free anaesthetic regimen (dexmedetomidine, lidocaine, and propofol infusions) or opioid-based anaesthesia (fentanyl bolus followed by remifentanil and propofol infusions). The opioid-free group had lower post-operative fentanyl consumption until 2 h, but thereafter, fentanyl consumption was similar. The opioid-free group required less rescue analgesia and had a lower incidence of nausea and vomiting.

Meta-Analysis

An analysis of the Pediatric Research Consortium Database assessing the safety and efficacy of propofol administered by paediatric critical care physicians has been undertaken [35R]. Propofol-based procedural sedation was given by critical care physicians to 91 189 children. Adjuncts were used in 41.7% of cases. 99.9% of cases were completed successfully. Adverse events were predominantly of respiratory aetiology—airway obstruction (1.6%), desaturation (1.5%), coughing (1%), and emergency airway intervention (0.7%). No deaths were reported. Risk factors for adverse events were identified and included: location of sedation; number of adjuncts co-administered with propofol; upper and lower respiratory tract disease; premature birth; and ASA status.

A meta-analysis of propofol with or without adjunct, given to patients of all ages, as a procedural sedative in the emergency department has been undertaken [36M]. Ten studies involving 813 patients were identified but small study numbers, study heterogeneity, and differing comparator interventions mean that no reliable conclusions can be drawn.

Nervous System

A meta-analysis of the efficacy of propofol in the management of emergence agitation following sevoflurane and desflurane anaesthesia in children is reported [37M]. The studies included in the analysis were heterogeneous and had a high risk of bias. The meta-analysis concludes that adjunctive treatment with propofol is effective in preventing emergence agitation and does not delay discharge from the post-anaesthesia care unit.

A small study has compared the efficacy of propofol and sumatriptan in the treatment of acute migraine presenting to the emergency department [38c]. The propofol treatment group had lower pain scores at 30 min, but the two groups were similar thereafter. The possibility of propofol-related sedation affecting pain scores should be considered.

Propofol-related pain on injection has been assessed in two studies [39c,40M]. A meta-analysis of 5 heterogeneous studies involving small patient numbers ($n = 545$) suggests magnesium sulphate may attenuate the pain associated with propofol injection [40M]. A study of 100 patients randomised to receive 20 μcg nitroglycerine or placebo via a cannula sited in the dorsum of the hand prior to propofol injection found a reduction in severity of pain experienced upon injection of propofol [39c].

Metabolism

A case of grass-green urine secondary to propofol infusion is reported [41A]. The patient was receiving propofol via infusion to facilitate the management of his traumatic brain injury (intracranial bleeding and cerebral oedema) in the intensive care unit. The patient received propofol at a peak infusion rate of 550 mg/h. The green discolouration of the urine resolved on cessation of propofol.

Gastrointestinal

The efficacy and safety of intra-operative low-dose propofol infusion are compared to intravenous bolus of dexamethasone at induction of anaesthesia or placebo in the prevention of post-operative nausea and vomiting following laparoscopic cholecystectomy [42c]. The incidence of PONV (irrespective of severity) at post-operative time intervals 0–6 h, 6–12 h, and 12–24 h was significantly lower in the propofol and dexamethasone groups compared to placebo. Propofol and dexamethasone were equally effective in the prevention of PONV.

Special Treatment Note: "The Use of Propofol as a Sedative for Endoscopic Procedures"

Over the last few years, there has been increasing interest in the role of propofol for sedation and anaesthesia with or without adjuncts to facilitate endoscopic procedures. This year the efficacy and safety of propofol for different endoscopic procedures are reviewed.

Oesophagogastroduodenoscopy (OGD)

Age: Children aged between 1 and 12 years ($n = 179$) underwent OGD facilitated by general anaesthesia [43c]. They received either intubation with sevoflurane maintenance anaesthesia, intubation with propofol maintenance anaesthesia, or native airway with propofol maintenance anaesthesia. The native airway with propofol group had a statistically significant increased rate of respiratory complications ($p < 0.0001$) including minor (SpO2 85–94%) and severe (SpO2 < 85%) desaturation, aspiration, and airway obstruction. Operating room efficiency was comparable between all groups. Patients aged 60–80 years undergoing OGD received either etomidate or propofol sedation [44c]. Both groups received 0.4–0.6 μcg/kg remifentanil over 60s followed by either 0.1–0.15 mg/kg etomidate plus an additional bolus of 4–6 mg if required ($n = 360$) or 1–2 mg/kg propofol plus an additional bolus of 20–40 mg if required ($n = 360$). The etomidate group demonstrated superior cardiovascular stability (SBP, DBP, and HR, $p < 0.05$) and more stable oxygen saturation levels ($p < 0.05$). Duration of procedure, recovery time and time to discharge were similar as were physician, anaesthetist, and patient satisfaction scores.

Personnel administering: The safety of non-anaesthetist administered sedation using propofol target controlled infusion (TCI) guided by BIS is reported [45C]. Patients undergoing endoscopic submucosal dissection for oesophageal and gastric cancer (n = 250) received propofol TCI to achieve an initial blood concentration of 1.2 μcg/mL and to target BIS value 60–80. Propofol was adjusted in 0.2 μcg/mL blood concentration increments in response to the BIS value or patient movement. The median upper and lower bound blood concentrations were 1.2 and 1.4 μcg/mL, respectively, and the mean procedure time was 89 ± 59 min. There were relatively few adverse events—hypotension (SBP < 90 mmHg) in 10.8%, oxygen desaturation (SpO2 < 90%) in 3.6%, and severe desaturation (SpO2 < 85%) in 0.8%. Anaesthetist versus non-anaesthetist administered propofol sedation for OGD, colonoscopy, or both procedures is compared [46c]. Both treatment groups received 0.5 mg/kg propofol with 10–20 mg increments as-required plus fentanyl at the discretion of the sedation provider. The anaesthetist-administered group received a higher mean dose of propofol (257.02 ± 78.44 mg vs. 188.4 ± 78.87 mg, p < 0.05), had a higher incidence of deep sedation (66.1% vs. 44.7%, p < 0.05), and had a lower incidence of hypotension (17.8% vs. 26.1%, p < 0.05). The incidence of hypoxia was comparable, but the duration of hypoxia was shorter in the anaesthetist-administered sedation group (4.22 ± 13.07 s vs. 7.26 ± 17.69 s, p < 0.05).

Dexmedetomidine vs. propofol: Patients undergoing OGD received propofol 0.6 mg/kg with additional increments of 10–20 mg or dexmedetomidine 1 μcg/kg over 15 min followed by 0.5 μcg/kg infusion to achieve a target sedation score [47c]. The propofol group had a higher incidence of deep sedation but similar recovery time to dexmedetomidine, and a higher incidence of decreased mean blood pressure. Three patients in the dexmedetomidine group experienced dizziness, bradycardia, and nausea. Patient satisfaction was higher in the propofol group.

In another study, 40 patients undergoing drug-induced sleep endoscopy (sedation induced somnolence to localise pathology causing obstructive sleep apnoea syndrome) received either propofol (0.7 mg/kg infusion for 10 min then 0.5 mg/kg/h) or dexmedetomidine (1 μcg/kg infusion for 10 min then 0.3 μcg/kg/h) [48c]. Propofol was the superior agent in achieving a rapid time to adequate sedation as well as maintaining haemodynamic stability. Dexmedetomidine was associated with more stable respiratory parameters (RR and SpO2), although there were no episodes of severe desaturation in the propofol group.

Systematic reviews: Two meta-analyses assessing propofol compared to other agents in the context of sedation and analgesia for endoscopy procedures are reported [49M,50M]. The first meta-analysis (27 studies) compared the incidence of adverse events (hypoxia, hypotension, apnoea, and arrhythmia) in patients receiving propofol (n = 1324) to midazolam or opioids (n = 1194) [50M]. Propofol had a similar incidence of adverse events to the comparator agents irrespective of procedure duration. OGD in cirrhotic patients using sedation with propofol or midazolam is compared in the second meta-analysis [49M]. Five studies involving 433 patients were analysed. Propofol achieved a more rapid time to target sedation and had a faster recovery time without an increase in adverse cardiorespiratory events.

Endoscopic Retrograde Cholangiopancreatography (ERCP)

Combination studies: Two studies have assessed the effect of adjuncts on propofol consumption and pain during ERCP [51c,52c]. One study (n = 90) compared propofol to propofol–remifentanil and propofol–fentanyl [52c]. All groups received propofol loading dose 1.5 mg/kg and then infusion of 1 mg/kg/h with additional increments of 0.5 mg/kg to achieve target sedation score. The remifentanil group received an infusion of 0.05 μcg/kg/min, and the fentanyl group received a bolus of 1 μcg/kg at induction and then increments as-required during the procedure. Both remifentanil and fentanyl groups required significantly less propofol than the control group. The remifentanil group also required significantly less propofol than the fentanyl group and less pain than the control group. The second study (n = 60) compared dexmedetomidine (loading 1 μcg/kg over 15 min and infusion at 0.5 μcg/kg/h) to ketamine (loading 1 mg/kg and infusion at 0.5 mg/kg/h) [51c,52c]. Both groups received propofol loading dose 2 mg/kg and infusion at 5 mg/kg/h with as-required increments of 0.5 mg/kg. Propofol consumption between the two groups was similar as were the reported pain scores. The dexmedetomidine group demonstrated superior cardiovascular stability and no incidence of post-operative cognitive dysfunction.

Colonoscopy

Comparative studies: Propofol infusion is compared to etomidate infusion for colonoscopy [53c]. Both groups received fentanyl bolus 1 μcg/kg. The doses of propofol and etomidate are unclear. The propofol group had a higher sedation score. Otherwise, no difference between the groups was found. In another study, propofol was compared to sevoflurane in patients aged ≥ 60 years [54c]. Both groups received 0.5 mg/kg propofol, and then sedation was maintained with 1% sevoflurane delivered via semi-closed circuit with as-required increases in sevoflurane concentration or 0.25 mg/kg incremental doses of propofol were given to maintain target sedation score. Patients in the propofol group were more likely to have an episode of apnoea, require airway intervention, and to reach deep sedation or general anaesthesia than those in the sevoflurane group.

Musculoskeletal

A pilot study of 30 patients was undertaken to assess whether morbidly obese patients receiving propofol-based anaesthesia had a higher incidence of rhabdomyolysis than those receiving inhalational anesthesia [55c]. An increased incidence of rhabdomyolysis in the propofol group was not detected in this small pilot study.

Immunologic

The potential effects of propofol intravenous anaesthesia compared to inhalational anaesthesia on proinflammatory cytokine levels in bronchoalveolar lavage (BAL) and clinical outcomes following one-lung ventilation are assessed in a meta-analysis [56M]. The cytokines studies were TNF-α, IL-1β, IL-6, and IL-8. Clinical outcomes were incidence of atelectasis, pneumonia, total number of respiratory complications, duration of ICU and hospital stay. Eight randomised controlled trials were included—the outcome measures varied between studies, study sample sizes were small ($n = 365$), and 7 trials had an unclear risk of bias. All the proinflammatory cytokines were significantly reduced in the inhalational group, with the exception of IL-1β which was non-significantly reduced. Individual respiratory complications were comparable between groups but total respiratory complications and hospital length of stay were significantly lower in the inhalational group.

Death

A large meta-analysis comparing mortality for patients receiving propofol infusion to any anaesthetic agent has been undertaken [57M]. One hundred and thirty-seven studies were included in the final analysis. Overall there was no mortality difference between propofol and non-propofol groups. Sub-analyses performed for the cardiac surgery population and for volatile anaesthesia as the comparator group also failed to show an increase in mortality associated with propofol.

BARBITURATE ANAESTHETICS

Thiopentone Sodium [SEDA-35, 217; SEDA-36, 139; SEDA-37, 129]

Comparative Studies

The effect of induction doses of thiopentone 5 mg/kg and etomidate 0.3 mg/kg on cardiorespiratory stability is compared in a small study ($n = 60$) [58M]. In-line with previous studies, the thiopentone group experienced more instability in systolic blood pressure and heart rate, and a higher incidence of apnoea [58M].

References

[1] Sivanna U, Joshi S, Babu B, et al. A comparative study of pharmacological myocardial protection between sevoflurane and desflurane at anaesthetic doses in patients undergoing off pump coronary bypass graftin surgery. Indian J Anaesth. 2015;59(5):282–6 [c].

[2] Shan J, Sun L, Wang D, et al. Comparison of the neuroprotective effects and recovery profiles of isoflurane, sevoflurane and desflurane as neurosurgical pre-conditioning on ischaemia/reperfusion cerebral injury. Int J Clin Exp Pathol. 2015;8(2):2001–9 [c].

[3] Ghoneim AA, Azer MS, Ghobrial HZ, et al. Awakening properties of isoflurane, sevoflurane, and desflurane in pediatric patients after craniotomy for supratentorial tumours. J Neurosurg Anesthesiol. 2015;27(1):1–6 [c].

[4] Stevanovic A, Rossaint R, Fritz HG, et al. Airway reactions and emergence times in general laryngeal mask anaesthesia. Eur J Anaesthesiol. 2015;32:106–16 [M].

[5] He J, Zhang Y, Xue R, et al. Effect of desflurane versus sevoflurane in pediatric anesthesia: a meta-analysis. J Pharm Pharm Sci. 2015;18(2):199–206 [M].

[6] Kim Y-S, Lim B-G, Kim H, et al. Effects of propofol or desflurane on post-operative spirometry in elderly after knee surgery: a double-blind randomised study. Acta Anaesthesiol Scand. 2015;59(6):788–95 [c].

[7] Sudré EC, de Batista PR, Castiglia YM. Longer immediate recovery time after anesthesia increases risk of respiratory complications after laparotomy for bariatric surgery: a randomized clinical trial and a cohort study. Obes Surg. 2015;25(11):2205–12 [c].

[8] Khalighi E, Arghavani H, Yarnazari R, et al. Comparing the effects of using isoflurane and propofol on shivering after general anesthesia in patients undergoing elective general and orthopaedic surgeries. J Isfahan Med Sch. 2015;33(348) [C].

[9] Sukhupragarn W, Leurcharusmee P, Sotthisopha T. Cardiovascular effects of volatile induction and maintenance of anesthesia (VIMA) and total intravenous anesthesia (TIVA) for laryngeal mask airway (LMA) anesthesia: a comparison study. J Med Assoc Thai. 2015;98(4):388–93 [c].

[10] Mencke T, Jacobs RF, Machmueller S, et al. Intubating conditions and side effects of propofol, remifentanil and sevoflurane compared with propofol, remifentanil and rocuronium: a randomised, prospective, clinical trial. BMC Anesthesiol. 2014;14:39–46 [c].

[11] Guo J-Y, Fang J-Y, Xu S-R, et al. Effects of propofol versus sevoflurane on cerebral oxygenation and cognitive outcome in patients with impaired cerebral oxygenation. Ther Clin Risk Manag. 2016;12:81–5 [C].

[12] Lin C-K, Feng Y-T, Hwang S-L, et al. A comparison of propofol target controlled infusion-based and sevoflurane-based anesthesia in adults undergoing elective anterior cervical discectomy and fusion. Kaohsiung J Med Sci. 2015;31:150–5 [c].

[13] Tawfik HA, Mostafa M. Sevoflurane versus propofol sedation during periocular anesthetic injections in oculoplastic procedures: an open-label randomized comparison. Saudi J Ophthalmol. 2015;29:126–9 [C].

[14] Beck-Schimmer B. Conditioning with sevoflurane in liver transplantation: results of a multicenter randomized controlled trial. Transplantation. 2015;99:1606–12 [c].

[15] Micks E, Edelman A, Botha R, et al. The effect of sevoflurane on interventions for blood loss during dilation and evacuation procedures at 18-24 weeks gestation: a randomized controlled trial. Contraception. 2015;91(6):488–94 [c].

[16] Lindholm EE, Aune E, Seljeflot I, et al. Biomarkers of inflammation in major vascular surgery: a prospective randomised trial. Acta Anaesthesiol Scand. 2015;59:773–87 [c].

[17] Ball AJ. A randomized controlled trial comparing continuous and as-required nitrous oxide use during screening endoscopy. Eur J Gastroenterol Hepatol. 2015;27(3):271–8 [c].

[18] Kariman H, Majidi A, Taheri S, et al. Analgesic effects of inhalation of nitric oxide (entonox) and parenteral morphine sulfate in patients with renal colic; a randomized clinical trial. Bull Emerg Trauma. 2015;3(2):46–52 [c].

[19] Kebriaee F, Sarraf Shirazi A, Fani K, et al. Comparison of the effects of cognitive behavioural therapy and inhalation sedation on child dental anxiety. Eur Arch Paediatr Dent. 2015;16(2):173–9 [c].

[20] Yokoe C, Hanamoto H, Sugimura M, et al. A prospective, randomized controlled trial of conscious sedation using propofol combined with inhaled nitrous oxide for dental treatment. J Oral Maxillofac Surg. 2015;73(3):402–9 [C].

[21] Sun R, Jia WQ, Zhang P, et al. Nitrous oxide-based techniques versus nitrous oxide-free techniques for general anaesthesia. Cochrane Database Syst Rev. 2015;11:CD008984 [M].

[22] Morris N, Lynch K, Greenberg SA. Severe motor neuropathy or neuronopathy due to nitrous oxide toxicity after correction of vitamin B12 deficiency. Muscle Nerve. 2015;51:614–6 [A].

[23] Del Valle RC, Solano CJA, Rodríguez MA, et al. Inhalation analgesia with nitrous oxide versus other analgesic techniques in hysteroscopic polypectomy: a pilot study. J Minim Invasive Gynecol. 2015;22(4):595–600 [c].

[24] Kuivalainen A-M, Ebeling F, Poikonen E, et al. Nitrous oxide analgesia for bone marrow aspiration and biopsy—a randomized, controlled and patient blinded study. Scand J Pain. 2015;7:28–34 [c].

[25] Singh RH, Thaxton LD, Carr S, et al. Nitrous oxide for intrauterine device insertion in nulliparous women: a randomized controlled trial. Obstet Gynecol. 2015;125(Suppl 1) [c].

[26] Zorumski CF, Nagele P, Mennerick S, et al. Treatment-resistant major depression: rationale for NMDA receptors as targets and nitrous oxide as therapy. Front Psychiatry. 2015;6:172–95 [H].

[27] O'Donovan MR, Hammond TG. Is nitrous oxide a genotoxic carcinogen? Mutagenesis. 2015;30(4):459–62 [R].

[28] Ozge C, Ipekcoglu D, Menges OO, et al. Comparison of propofol, etomidate, and thiopental in anesthesia for electroconvulsive therapy: a randomized double-blind clinical trial. J ECT. 2015;31(2):91–7 [C].

[29] Lewis SR, Nicholson A, Reed SS, et al. Anaesthetic and sedative agents used for electrical cardioversion (Review). Cochrane Database Syst Rev. 2015;3:CD010824 [C].

[30] Singh PM. Evaluation of etomidate for seizure duration in electroconvulsive therapy: a systematic review and meta-analysis. J ECT. 2015;31(4):213–25 [C].

[31] Desai PM, Kane D, Sarkar MS. Cardioversion: what to choose? Etomidate or propofol. Ann Card Anaesth. 2015;18(3):306–11 [c].

[32] Ma Y-H, Li Y-W, Ma L, et al. Anesthesia for stem cell transplantation in autistic children: a prospective, randomized, double-blind comparison of propofol and etomidate following sevoflurane induction. Exp Ther Med. 2015;9:1035–9 [c].

[33] Hatamabadi HR, Dolatabadi AA, Derakhshanfar H, et al. Propofol versus midazolam for procedural sedation of anterior shoulder dislocation in emergency department: a randomized clinical trial. Trauma Mon. 2015;20(2):e13530 [c].

[34] Bakan M, Umutoglu T, Topuz U, et al. Opioid-free total intravenous anesthesia with propofol, dexmedetomidine and lidocaine infusions for laparoscopic cholecystectomy: a prospective randomized double-blinded study. Rev Bras Anestesiol. 2015;65(3):191–9 [c].

[35] Kamat PP, McCracken CE, Gillespie SE, et al. Pediatric critical care physician-administered procedural sedation using propofol: a report from the Pediatric Sedation Research Consortium Database. Pediatr Crit Care Med. 2015;16(1):11–20 [R].

[36] Wakai A, Blackburn C, McCabe A, et al. The use of propofol for procedural sedation in emergency departments (Review). Cochrane Database Syst Rev. 2015;7:CD007399 [M].

[37] Jiang S, Liu J, Li M, et al. The efficacy of propofol on emergence agitation—a meta-analysis of randomized controlled trials. Acta Anaesthesiol Scand. 2015;59(10):1232–45 [M].

[38] Moshtaghion H, Heiranizadeh N, Rahimdel A, et al. The efficacy of propofol vs. subcutaneous sumatriptan for treatment of acute migraine headaches in the emergency department: a double-blinded clinical trial. Pain Pract. 2015;15:701–5 [c].

[39] Derakhshan P, Karbasy SH, Bahador R. The effects of nitroglycerine on pain control during the propofol injection; a controlled, double-blinded, randomized clinical trial. Anesth Pain Med. 2015;5(3):e26141 [c].

[40] Li M, Zhao X, Zhang L, et al. Effects and safety of magnesium sulfate on propofol-induced injection pain, a meta-analysis of randomized controlled trials. Int J Clin Exp Med. 2015;8(5):6813–21 [M].

[41] Pedersen AB, Kobborg TK, Larsen JR. Grass-green urine from propofol infusion. Acta Anaesthesiol Scand. 2015;59:265–7 [A].

[42] Celik M, Dostbil A, Aksoy M, et al. Is infusion of subhypnotic propofol as effective as dexamethasone in prevention of postoperative nausea and vomiting related to laparoscopic chloecystectomy? A randomized controlled trial. BioMed Res Int. 2015;2015. Article ID 349806. [c].

[43] Patino M, Glynn S, Soberano M, et al. Comparison of different anesthesia techniques during esophagogastroduedenoscopy in children: a randomized trial. Paediatr Anaesth. 2015;25(10):1013–9 [c].

[44] Shen X-C, Ao X, Cao Y, et al. Etomidate-remifentanil is more suitable for monitored anesthesia care during gastroscopy in older patients than propofol-remifentanil. Med Sci Monit. 2015;21:1–8 [c].

[45] Imagawa A, Hata H, Nakatsu M, et al. A target-controlled infusion system with bispectral index monitoring of propofol sedation during endoscopic submucosal dissection. Endosc Int Open. 2015;3:E2–6 [c].

[46] de Paulo GA, Martins FPB, Macedo EP, et al. Sedation in gastrointestinal endoscopy: a prospective study comparing nonanesthesiologist-administered propofol and monitored anesthesia care. Endosc Int Open. 2015;3:E7–E13 [c].

[47] Wu Y, Zhang Y, Hu X, et al. A comparison of propofol vs. dexmedetomidine for sedation, haemodynamic control and satisfaction, during esophagogastroduodenscopy under conscious sedation. J Clin Pharm Ther. 2015;40(4):419–25 [c].

[48] Kuyrukluildiz U, Binici O, Onk D, et al. Comparison of dexmedetomidine and propofol used for drug-induced sleep endoscopy in patients with obstructive sleep apnea syndrome. Int J Clin Exp Med. 2015;8(4):5691–8 [c].

[49] Tsai H-C, Lin Y-C, Ko C-L, et al. Propofol versus midazolam for upper gastrointestinal endoscopy in cirrhotic patients: a met-analysis of randomized controlled trials. PLoS One. 2015;10(2):e0117585 [M].

[50] Wadhwa V, Issa D, Lopez R, et al. Propofol versus traditional sedative agents for gastrointestinal endoscopy: a systematic review and meta-analysis. Gastrointest Endosc. 2015;81(Suppl 5):AB309–10 [M].

[51] Abdalla MW, El Shal SM, El Sombaty AI, et al. Propofol dexmedetomidine versus propofol ketamine for anesthesia of endoscopic retrograde cholangiopancreatography (ERCP) (a randomized comparative study). Eg J Anaesth. 2015;31(2):97–105 [c].

[52] Haytual C, Aydinli B, Demir B, et al. Comparison of propofol, propofol-remifentanil, and propofol-fentanyl administrations with each other used for the sedation of patients to undergo ERCP. BioMed Res Int. 2015;2015. Article ID 465465. [c].

[53] Banihashem N, Alijanpour E, Basirat M, et al. Sedation with etomidate-fentanyl versus propofol-fentanyl in colonoscopies: a prospective randomized study. Caspian J Intern Med. 2015;6(1):15–9 [c].

[54] El Ahl MIS. Modified sevoflurane-based sedation technique versus propofol sedation technique: a randomized-controlled study. Saudi J Anaesth. 2015;9:19–22 [c].

[55] Lehavi A, Sandler O, Mahajna A, et al. Comparison of rhabdomyolysis markers in patients undergoing bariatric surgery

with propofol and inhalation-based anesthesia. Obes Surg. 2015;25(10):1923–7 [c].

[56] Sun B, Wang J, Lulong B, et al. Effects of volatile vs. propofol-based intravenous anesthetics on the alveolar inflammatory response to one-lung ventilation: a meta-analysis of randomized controlled trials. J Anesth. 2015;29:570–9 [M].

[57] Pasin L, Landoni G, Cabrini L, et al. Propofol and survival: a meta-analysis of randomized clinical trials. Acta Anaesthesiol Scand. 2015;59:17–24 [M].

[58] Shilpashri AM, Anitha Hanji S, Gayathri G, et al. Etomidate is rapid acting and has good cardiovascular and respiratory stability than thiopentone sodium. Indian J Public Health. 2015;6(3):172 [M].

10

Local Anesthetics

Sujana Dontukurthy, Allison Kalstein, Joel Yarmush[1]

New York Methodist Hospital, Brooklyn, NY, USA

[1]Corresponding author: joelyarmush@gmail.com

GENERAL INFORMATION

Adverse events of local anesthetics are usually seen when a topically administered medication reveals hypersensitivity, or when the administered (topical, tissue, vascular, etc.) medication is absorbed systemically and exceeds safe drug levels. Local anesthetic systemic toxicity (LAST) is usually caused by blockade of inhibitory pathways in the cerebral cortex, resulting in excitatory cell preponderance and thus enhanced nerve activity. LAST usually manifests initially as neurotoxicity, including perioral tingling, change in sensorium and if severe, seizure activity. Cardiac toxicity symptoms are seen if the toxicity progresses. Cardiovascular symptoms manifest first as hypotension and tachycardia, followed by cardiovascular collapse.

Para-aminobenzoic acid is a metabolite of ester local anesthetic metabolism. It is often indicted in hypersensitivity reactions seen when ester local anesthetics are used and our survey of the literature demonstrates this. Some ester local anesthetics (e.g., benzocaine) are only available for topical administration, and adverse reactions are limited to dermatologic hypersensitivity and anaphylaxis.

Ultrasound has facilitated the widespread use of regional anesthetic blocks. This has led to more precise blocks, often with less volume of local anesthetic needed. However, certain (e.g., transversus abdominus plane, TAP) blocks continue to use large volumes of local anesthetic and are now more prevalent leading to more cases of LAST.

Certainly, LAST is talked about more often, if not actually seen more often, then prior to the onset of ultrasound-guided peripheral nerve blocks. Our survey reveals many reviews of LAST and its treatment with lipid emulsions.

COMBINED OR NONSPECIFIC LOCAL ANESTHETICS

Cardiovascular and Central Nervous System Toxicity

LAST and Its Treatment

Several reviews of LAST and its treatment with lipid emulsions (i.e., intralipids) were surveyed. Some articles examined at least some aspects of the history, causes, mechanism and/or treatment of LAST in general [1M,2M,3M,4M,5M]. Some covered LAST and its treatment from a gynecologic [6M] or emergency medicine [7R] or pediatric regional anesthesia [8R] perspective. Others were more involved.

One article [9R] reviewed LAST seen with regional anesthesia. Much of the world's literature on case reports of LAST associated with regional anesthesia from March 2010 to March 2014 was reviewed. Sixty-seven cases of LAST were discovered. Fifty of them involved a single injection of local anesthetic (LA), while eight involved a continuous infusion. Seven occurred after topical administration, and two were seen after inadvertent direct venous administration.

Regional anesthesia block by anesthesia personnel was performed in 78% of the 50 patients receiving a single injection of LA. The most common blocks were interscalene (23%), followed by epidural/caudal (16%) and dorsal penile block (13%). The remaining 22% were field blocks performed by non-anesthesia personnel. Cardiovascular and neurologic toxicity was found to be the most common adverse event from LAST.

One article [10R] described a retrospective review of LAST following peripheral nerve blocks (PNB) performed at a single institution from 2009 to 2014. Over 80 000 blocks were reviewed and no cardiac arrests and three seizures were identified as being caused by LAST.

There were three cardiac arrests with PNB, but the causes of the arrests were attributed to concomitant neuraxial anesthetics and hemodynamic instability. The seizures all resolved without sequela. The cases involving seizures revealed administration of (a) 50 ml of 1.5% mepivacaine plus 10 ml of 0.75% bupivacaine plus 1:200 000 epinephrine given for an interscalene block in a 76-year-old, 99.6 kg, woman with nerve stimulator guidance, (b) 30 ml of 0.5% bupivacaine given for a popliteal block in a 70-year-old, 62 kg, woman with ultrasound guidance and (c) 30 ml of 1.5% mepivacaine plus 10 ml of 0.75% bupivacaine plus 1:200 000 epinephrine given for an infraclavicular block in a 53-year-old, 57 kg, woman with ultrasound guidance.

The authors state that the average total volume for upper extremity blocks was 40 ml of local anesthetic, down from a prior prospective study [11c], which used 50 ml per block. They suggest that given the rarity of cardiac arrest, vigilance and careful administration is what is most needed, regardless of total volume, to prevent adverse events of LAST.

One article [12H] looked at awareness of LAST. A questionnaire-based study assessed the level of understanding and treatment of LAST among 200 postgraduate residents (anesthesia residents were excluded), in a tertiary care hospital in India. The majority of responders were unaware of the toxic dose of local anesthetics. Just 70% of responders believed that local anesthetics could be toxic, and of these believers, only 81% correctly identified the signs and symptoms of cardiotoxicity. Furthermore, only 2% of the responders were cognizant of the fact that lipid emulsion is part of the treatment for LAST. One can infer from the responses that increased awareness about detection and treatment of LAST is needed.

As LAST is not often seen, two articles described how simulation or hypothetical scenarios could aid in identifying and ultimately treating LAST. The first article [13H] demonstrated how LAST can occur in the operating room if local anesthetics are used without strict adherence to protocols and vigilance. The second article [14H] described a program, which uses simulated cases to assist in recognition and treatment of LAST in a non-operative location.

One article [15R] highlighted the different theories on how lipid emulsions actually work in treating LAST. The article discusses case reports of LAST in the adult and pediatric population and their successful resuscitation with lipid emulsion. The mechanism by which lipids reverse LAST may be increased clearance from cardiac tissue or by counteracting local anesthetic inhibition of myocardial fatty acid oxidation, enabling energy production and reversal of cardiac depression. Suggested doses for using 20% intralipid call for administration of 1.5 ml/kg as an initial bolus followed by 1–2 repeated doses for persistent asystole.

Inadvertent Subarachnoid Block During a Lumbar Paravertebral Block

A 60-year-old woman was undergoing a paravertebral block in a private pain management clinic. The block was performed bilaterally at the L5-S1 space, apparently without the aid of fluoroscopy or ultrasound guidance. A solution of 10 mg of lidocaine, 10 mg levobupivacaine and 40 mg depomedrol was injected according to the authors. The patient immediately noted pain in the lower limbs followed by hypotension and nausea with subsequent cardiac arrest and eventual death 40 minutes later despite resuscitative efforts [16A].

An autopsy was performed 48 hours after death, and high levels of lidocaine and bupivacaine were found in the CSF. Blood levels ruled out an intravascular injection.

The authors recommend that the blocks should be performed under ultrasound guidance, with proper training of personnel, in an area with proper resuscitative equipment. Intralipid should be considered as a first line therapy when toxicity is suspected after a peripheral nerve block, as well as early intubation and resuscitation if high spinal is suspected.

We agree with the recommendations and further point out that the stated dose of lidocaine and levobupivacaine injected intrathecally does not seem that excessive and would not usually cause cardiovascular collapse if treated properly.

Lipid Emulsion for Local Anesthetic Toxicity in Rat Aorta

This paper [17E] looked at attenuation of vasodilatation by lipid emulsion caused by toxic doses of local anesthetic on isolated endothelium denuded rat aorta. They found that the vasodilatation caused by bupivacaine was attenuated in a dose-dependent manner by inhibition of the Rho kinase–myosin phosphatase pathway, and the vasodilatation caused by mepivacaine was not attenuated at all.

Cell Toxicity

Chondrocyte Toxicity from a Combination of Local Anesthetics and Corticosteroids

An *in vivo* study [18E] was conducted in canine shoulder joints. A couple of local anesthetics (i.e., 1% lidocaine, 0.0625% bupivacaine) in various combinations with a couple of corticosteroids (i.e., methylprednisolone and triamcinolone) were injected into canine shoulder joints. The dogs were euthanatized after 24 hours. The injected shoulder joints were aseptically disarticulated to harvest joint capsule and full thickness articular cartilage sections from the humeral head. Tissue metabolism and cell viability were assessed after 24 hours and after 7 days.

The study showed that even a single intraarticular injection of a clinically relevant dose of local anesthetic and corticosteroid might have detrimental effects on articular cartilage. Compared with the saline injection control, almost all local anesthetic–corticosteroid combination groups were associated with a significant decrease in chondrocyte and synoviocyte viability and metabolism. The single exception was that low dose bupivacaine (0.0625%) with triamcinolone did not show any detrimental effects.

Chondrocyte Toxicity Decreased by Vitamin C

An *in vitro* study [19E] of human chondrocytes showed toxicity with local anesthetics. Toxicity was greatest for 1% lidocaine followed by 0.5% bupivacaine followed by 0.75% ropivacaine. Vitamin C, when added to the local anesthetics, raised viability percentage with decreased apoptotic cell counts. Vitamin C at 500 mcM concentration was more potent than at 250 mcM which was more potent than at 125 mcM.

The authors postulate that the antioxidant properties of vitamin C may have been responsible for these results.

This *in vitro* study [20E] was conducted in human articular chondrocytes. The chondrocytes were exposed to 0.5% levobupivacaine, 0.5% bupivacaine and 0.9% normal saline for 15, 30 or 60 minutes. The cell viability was assessed using flow cytometry analysis and trypan blue exclusion assay.

The study showed that levobupivacaine and bupivacaine showed more cell death than normal saline after 60 minutes of exposure but not with 15 or 30 minutes of exposure. Cell death was greater for levobupivacaine than bupivacaine but was not significant.

Neurotoxic Effects of Local Anesthetics on Neuroblastoma Cells

Local anesthetics (LAs) were found to cause toxicity in mouse neuroblastoma cells [21E]. At low concentrations of LAs, toxicity was seen via neurite inhibition. At high concentrations of LAs, toxicity was seen via apoptosis. The level of toxic potential of LAs was tetracaine > prilocaine > lidocaine > procaine. The authors felt that as procaine is short acting and least toxic, it should be the preferred local anesthetic drug used.

An *in vitro* study [22E] was performed looking at cell death comparing articaine, lidocaine, mepivacaine, bupivacaine, prilocaine and ropivacaine in human neuroblastoma cells. Undifferentiated SH-SY5Y cells were exposed for 20 minutes to different concentrations of each local anesthetic.

The authors reported less toxicity with ropivacaine and articaine, medium toxicity with mepivacaine, prilocaine and lidocaine, and high toxicity with bupivacaine.

Thus, the authors felt that articaine and ropivacaine should be the preferred local anesthetics used.

Genotoxicity of Levobupivacaine and Bupivacaine in Drosophila

Levobupivacaine has been cited as having less cardiovascular and nervous system toxicity than comparable doses of bupivacaine [23E]. To examine this further, the somatic wing mutation and recombination test in the *Drosophila melanogaster* was used to determine genotoxicity of the anesthetics. Testing revealed that bupivacaine and levobupivacaine did not exhibit mutagenic or recombinogenic activity until toxic doses were reached at the larval stage. At high concentrations of drug in the high-bioactivation (HB) cross, bupivacaine (500 mcg/ml) did not exhibit any genotoxicity but the levobupivacaine (1000 mcg/ml) did.

Nervous System

Neurologic Complications Associated with Regional Anesthesia and Pain Medicine

The authors present a comprehensive, if not exhaustive, review and advisory of neurologic injuries after neuraxial and peripheral nerve blocks with local anesthetics [24R]. They reveal that neurologic complications are still rare. Many factors for the injuries are discussed, but local anesthetics themselves are usually not found to be the prime causative factor. While the incidence (2–4/10 000 blocks) of peripheral nerve injury has not changed with the advance from the peripheral nerve stimulator-assisted block to the ultrasound-guided block, the very rare (1:3600 to 1:200 000) but often catastrophic neuraxial complications associated with regional anesthetic and pain blocks seem to be rising. A suggestion is made that the rise in complications is because neuraxial, and pain blocks are now more common and that the patients who get these blocks are both sicker and more fragile.

Local anesthetic toxicity after spinal blocks manifested as transient neurologic symptoms (TNS) was also discussed. The cause of the neurologic symptoms remains controversial but seems to be directly related to the concentration of local anesthetic. It can be seen after administration of most of the various local anesthetics. Of note, is that intrathecal chloroprocaine does not seem to be associated with TNS.

Lipid Emulsion Lessens Neurotoxicity in Rats

This paper [25E] demonstrated that lipid emulsion decreased the local anesthetic-induced CNS toxicity in rats. The relative toxicities were found to be as follows: lidocaine > levobupivacaine > ropivacaine.

BENZOCAINE

Dermatologic

Allergic Contact Dermatitis of the Vagina and Perineum

This paper [26M] reviews causes of contact dermatitis of the vagina and perineum. It indicts the ester local anesthetics in general amongst other drugs, but singles out benzocaine, which is found in many commercial products as an offending agent. The paper describes a cycle, which starts with vaginal or perineal itching. A benzocaine containing anti-itch medication provides temporary relief with subsequent return of itching caused by the benzocaine-induced contact dermatitis. More itching is followed by more benzocaine containing anti-itch medication.

Benzocaine as a Cause of Orodynia

Primary orodynia (i.e., burning mouth syndrome) is seen where there is no identifiable underlying cause. Secondary orodynia is seen when there may be an underlying cause. This paper [27A] presents two cases of orodynia where 20% benzocaine was used orally and may be the underlying causative agent.

Two healthy women (52 and 58 years old) were treated for painful oral rashes with oral gel, which contained 20% benzocaine. Despite apparent resolution of the rashes and normal oral mucosa, both patients developed painful burning in the mouth. Testing for contact dermatitis revealed sensitivity to benzocaine in both patients.

BUPIVACAINE

Cardiovascular

Treatment of Bupivacaine Toxicity with Two Different Lipid Emulsions

Bupivacaine was deliberately injected intravascularly into swine to simulate LAST [28E]. The dose injected caused hypotension and other deleterious hemodynamic changes but was not enough to cause cardiac arrest.

A lipid emulsion made up of long-chain triglycerides proved to be as effective in treating the cardiovascular effects as a lipid emulsion made up of a mixture of long- and medium-chain triglycerides.

Anaphylaxis to Bupivacaine

Hypotension from spinal anesthesia is not uncommon and usually resolves with either fluids or administration of small doses of vasopressors such as ephedrine or phenylephrine. This case [29A] involved sustained hypotension caused by an anaphylactic reaction to bupivacaine.

The authors suggest that anaphylaxis can be added to the differential diagnosis of LAST, and epinephrine can be considered if hypotension does not immediately respond to conventional treatment.

Cell Toxicity

Bupivacaine Myotoxicity

This *in vitro* study [30E] suggests a new mechanism of bupivacaine-induced myotoxicity. After a bupivacaine local anesthetic challenge in mouse myoblasts, autophagosome formation was induced as a stress response. However, the clearance of autophagosome was impaired, suggesting that this is the cause of the myotoxicity.

Nervous System

Local Anesthetic Toxicity Under General Anesthesia

A 25-year-old man presented with signs and symptoms of acute duodenal perforation and was scheduled for an emergent exploratory laparotomy with combined general and epidural anesthesia [31A]. Before the induction of general anesthesia, an epidural catheter was inserted at the L1–L2 level. A test dose was given to confirm that the catheter was neither intravascular nor intrathecal. The patient was then induced with propofol. Intubation was facilitated with vecuronium. Maintenance included oxygen, nitrous oxide and desflurane. Before surgical incision, 12 ml of 0.5% bupivacaine with 50 mcg fentanyl was given via the epidural catheter in divided boluses over 20 minutes.

Approximately 1 hour after incision, during a period with only minimal paralysis, the patient had tonic–clonic movements, which resolved with 100 mg IV thiopental. Approximately 15 minutes later, the patient again had tonic–clonic type movements, which resolved with midazolam and phenytoin. Surgery lasted approximately 2 hours. He was extubated after complete neuromuscular blockade reversal. (Aside: Presumably this occurred after the patient met extubation criteria, including being awake and following commands.) Approximately 15 minutes after extubation, he once again displayed tonic–clonic movements, which resolved with lorazepam. The patient was monitored in the intensive care unit in the postoperative period where no further episodes were observed. All laboratory tests were within normal limits, and he was discharged home 1 week later.

The authors postulate that the patient had LAST despite a negative test dose and negative aspiration probably due to inadvertent intravascular administration of local anesthetics or due to systemic absorption from the epidural space.

We feel that this was a very unusual presentation of LAST as the total dose of drug and the time from drug administration to symptoms seem inconsistent with inadvertent intravenous administration of local anesthetics or due to systemic absorption from the epidural space. The exact mechanism for the seizure still has to be elucidated.

Convulsions During Interscalene Block

A 67-year-old woman had an interscalene block under nerve stimulator guidance [32A]. She was given 0.375% bupivacaine in 5 ml aliquots after negative aspiration. At the very tail of the fifth injection, the patient suddenly became unresponsive and had a sudden tonic–clonic seizure. General anesthesia was induced with thiopental with resolution of the seizure followed by intubation. Maintenance of anesthesia was with propofol and remifentanil infusions. Blood levels of bupivacaine were 1.664 mcg/ml (i.e., below toxic threshold) immediately after intubation and not measurable after 135 minutes of surgery.

The authors hypothesize that the seizure was caused by inadvertent intra-arterial injection because of the suddenness of the events and the subthreshold intravascular level of bupivacaine. Thiopental given for sedation and propofol given for maintenance of anesthesia have antiepileptic properties. Propofol is delivered as a lipid emulsion, and the authors further hypothesized that the propofol infusion acted as lipid emulsion therapy reducing the bupivacaine intravascular level. However, further studies would be needed, as propofol is not currently recommended as an alternative to intralipid therapy.

Intralipid Therapy for LAST

A 51-year-old woman with a history of asthma had a posterior colpoperineorrhaphy and transobturator sling insertion under general anesthesia [33A]. Shortly prior to the conclusion of the procedure, 80 ml of 0.5% bupivacaine with epinephrine was injected into the surgical site by the surgeon for postoperative analgesia.

In the post-anesthesia care unit (PACU), the patient presented with dizziness, agitation, oculogyric crisis, posturing and left lower extremity weakness and numbness. Neurology was consulted and approximately 20 minutes after the symptoms, the patient was treated with a bolus of intralipid emulsion repeated 20 minutes later with a second bolus followed by continuous infusion. The patient had resolution of her systemic symptoms with gradual recovery of motor and sensory symptoms upon completion of the infusion. The patient was hemodynamically stable throughout the course of events, with only a single episode of hypotension in the PACU, which responded to a bolus of phenylephrine 100 mcg.

This patient received twice the maximum recommended dose of local anesthetic. The gradual and partial systemic absorption led to signs and symptoms of LAST without overt cardiac symptoms. Both systemic symptoms and peripheral nervous system blockade were resolved with intralipid emulsion.

This case report emphasizes the fact that intralipid emulsion not only reverses LAST but also lessens the peripheral nervous system blockade.

CINCHOCAINE

Dermatologic

Sensitivity to Cinchocaine

A 60-year-old woman was found to have a maculopapular rash seemingly after taking ibuprofen and rabeprazole [34A]. Subsequent skin testing revealed sensitivity to cinchocaine, an ester local anesthetic, and not ibuprofen and rabeprazole. Upon further questioning, the patient revealed that she had used an antihemorrhoidal cream containing cinchocaine (i.e., dibucaine). She was not sensitive to benzocaine, tetracaine, procaine or lidocaine.

The authors point out that cinchocaine is not always included in skin sensitivity panels of local anesthetics and the causative agent may have been missed.

LIDOCAINE

Cardiovascular and Central Nervous System Toxicity

Intralipid for Treatment of LAST

A 35-year-old, 65 kg, woman with a history of DM, ESRD and CAD presented to the emergency department with a labial abscess [35A]. She was hemodynamically stable. Her medications included amlodipine and carvedilol.

The gynecologic consultant drained the labial abscess using 50 ml of 2% lidocaine. About 15 minutes after the procedure, the patient started vomiting and demonstrated seizure activity with eventual loss of consciousness. The airway was immediately secured. Before any intralipid emulsion could be administered, the patient suffered pulseless electrical activity cardiac arrest.

The patient was successfully resuscitated using intralipid emulsion and the ACLS algorithm. The authors postulate that while the recommended maximum dose of lidocaine may have been exceeded, the concomitant intake of nodal blocking agents such as calcium channel blockers and beta-blockers may have caused an increase in sensitivity to bupivacaine thereby enhancing drug toxicity.

LAST After a Circumcision

A 4-month-old healthy child was circumcised in a doctor's office utilizing a bilateral dorsal penile nerve block with 16 mg/kg of lidocaine [36A]. Fifteen minutes later, the infant experienced a tonic–clonic seizure, which was treated with rectal diazepam 2 mg/kg given over a 5-minute period. The child stopped breathing and suffered a cardiac arrest necessitating cardiopulmonary resuscitation. An ambulance arrived after a period of time, and the cardiac monitor revealed ventricular tachycardia with spontaneous reversion to sinus rhythm. The infant was intubated and taken to the hospital, where the diagnosis of lidocaine toxicity was entertained. The infant was give intralipids 2 ml/kg and was able to be extubated after 24 hours with no occurrence of any other adverse events. A blood lidocaine concentration of 4 mg/l was measured 4 hours after administration of the medication.

The authors admit that too much lidocaine and diazepam were administered. The authors further state that the proper setting for peripheral nerve blocks is in the hospital, which has trained personnel to treat adverse events.

Cell Toxicity

Lidocaine Causes Chondrocyte Toxicity

An *in vitro* study [37E] was conducted in rabbit chondrocytes derived from full thickness articular cartilage taken from the knee, hip and shoulder joints. The chondrocytes were exposed to different concentrations of lidocaine (i.e., 1, 3, 10 and 30 mM) and were monitored with live microscopy. The study demonstrated that lidocaine acutely causes membrane blebbing in articular chondrocytes and subsequent cell death at clinically relevant concentrations. The mean percentage of blebbing cells was significantly higher at 30 mM compared to 1 mM and the control group. Rho kinase (ROCK) inhibitors prevented the lidocaine-induced blebbing suggesting that ROCK induction is what causes the cell damage.

MEPIVACAINE

Cardiovascular

Concentration, Dose and Volume Effects of Mepivacaine on Axillary Blocks

This double-blind prospective study [38c] showed no adverse events when mepivacaine (i.e., 20 ml of 1.5% mepivacaine or 30 ml of 1.0% mepivacaine or 30 ml of 1.5% mepivacaine) was used for axillary block in three groups of 15 patients, each. It did demonstrate that dose and concentration and not volume prolonged the block. One could infer from the authors' conclusions that good

practice would increase the concentration of drug administered (to a reasonable level) while simultaneously decreasing the volume and limiting toxicity.

LAST in Pediatrics

An 8-year-old, 50-pound, girl was sedated with oral promethazine, inhalational oxygen/nitrous oxide and intramuscular meperidine for multiple tooth extractions [39A]. She was then injected with 6 cartridges of 3% mepivacaine (54 mg/cartridge). She suffered seizures and had respiratory difficulty. Resuscitative efforts (for presumed arrest) were unsuccessful, and the girl died from anoxic encephalopathy. No mention is made of intralipid therapy in the child.

The authors acknowledge that an overdose of drug was given. They review LAST in the child and give detailed information on how to calculate and hopefully avoid potential toxic doses.

Dermatologic

Fixed Drug Eruptions with Mepivacaine

Two cases of cytotoxic T cell-mediated Fixed Drug Eruptions (FDE) are discussed [40A]. Only the first case demonstrated a cutaneous hypersensitivity to local anesthetics. Mepivacaine was used as a local anesthetic for a minor procedure, and the patients had lesions distant from the actual injection. The lesion location was fixed and reproducible with testing. Testing revealed sensitivity to mepivacaine and lidocaine but not bupivacaine.

PRAMOCAINE

Dermatologic

Contact Dermatitis with Pramocaine

Pramocaine, also known as Pramoxine, is a topical ester local anesthetic used commercially that is usually tolerated well. Contact dermatitis has been reported previously, but this paper [41A] claims to be the first paper to report actual anaphylaxis.

A 47-year-old man reported to the ER with symptoms of acute anaphylaxis. After treatment and resolution of his symptoms, history revealed that he recently applied a topical antibiotic compound that contained pramocaine on a small cut in the hand. His symptoms began after the application. He further revealed that he had used this topical antibiotic in times past without any problems, until the penultimate application where he had swelling which resolved spontaneously.

Testing revealed sensitivity to the pramocaine. Anaphylaxis was presumably caused by repeated exposure of the drug with systemic entry. As with any topical local anesthetic, caution should be exercised when applying the medication to a compromised (i.e., cut or deeply abraded) area.

ROPIVACAINE

Cardiovascular

Absorption of Ropivacaine After TAP Block

This study [42c] confirmed that there is considerable absorption of ropivacaine after transversus abdominis plane block and rectus sheath block. The total volume of drug used was 30 ml, and blood levels did not reach classic standard levels of toxicity and no LAST was seen.

Cell Toxicity

Chondrocyte Toxicity of Ropivacaine and Triamcinolone in Rats

An *in vivo* study [43E] was conducted in rats using high and low concentrations of ropivacaine and triamcinolone. The chondrocyte viability was studied at 1 week and 5 months after injection into the knee joint. Viability at 1 week was significantly lower when higher concentration of drugs was used compared to the lower concentration of drugs. After 1 week, there was no difference in viability between high and low concentration of ropivacaine. However, there was significant difference between high and low concentration of triamcinolone.

Nervous System

LAST with Peripheral Nerve Block Continuous Infusions

A 20-year-old patient status post heart transplant for a complex congenital heart disease had a postoperative course complicated by respiratory failure, renal failure and multiple fasciotomies of the lower extremities for compartment syndrome [44A]. The patient presented for a left knee amputation. Due to the condition of the patient, the operation was performed under peripheral nerve block with a continuous catheter left *in situ* for postoperative analgesia. The patient tolerated the surgery well and had good postoperative pain relief. Subsequently, he was scheduled for a right knee amputation. The operation was performed with single shot sciatic and saphenous nerve blocks with 0.5% ropivacaine. As the patient had severe postoperative pain, a peripheral nerve catheter was inserted and a continuous infusion of ropivacaine 0.2% was started. As the patient had unrelenting pain, boluses were given everyday, and the infusion rate was gradually increased. The patient had excellent pain relief but on postoperative day 5, he had

vision changes. A day later, he complained that his food tasted bad. The regional anesthesia team evaluated the nerve catheter with negative aspiration for blood. The tip of the catheter could not be located on ultrasound, and the catheter was removed and blood for ropivacaine levels was obtained. Ophthalmological evaluation was normal, and serum ropivacaine concentrations came back as 10 mcg/ml. Maximum tolerable levels for total serum ropivacaine are 1–2 mcg/ml with neurologic symptoms reported at levels as low as 2–3 mcg/ml.

The authors state that the patient had LAST, even though the infusions were adjusted to a safe dosage. The authors postulated serum ropivacaine concentration was high as the patient had low albumin, acidosis and decreased peripheral circulation. Also around 20% of local anesthetic is cleared in the lungs, and the patient had months of lung injury and respiratory issues that may have inhibited this clearance mechanism. Further, the patient was taking voriconazole, a known cytochrome P450 3A4 inhibitor, which may have inhibited hepatic ropivacaine metabolism. In addition, the patient had acute renal failure contributing to increased drug levels.

The authors state that the dose of local anesthetics should be block specific, site specific and patient specific. Caution is warranted when dosing local anesthetics in medically complex patients.

TETRACAINE

Dermatologic

A 51-year-old woman presented with erythematous bullous eruption in the interbuttock groove after wearing new panties [45A]. It was revealed that the patient had applied an anesthetic ointment containing tetracaine to the area. The bullous appearance was unusual as an initial presentation but may be caused by rubbing of the buttocks according to the authors.

The authors felt that a careful history and patch testing before administering any drug. Also, one should be prudent when considering topical anesthetics for off-label use.

References

[1] Dickerson DM, Apfelbaum JL. Anesthetic systemic toxicity. Aesthet Surg J. 2014;34(7):1111–9 [M].
[2] Fencl JL. Local anesthetic systemic toxicity: perioperative implications. AORN J. 2015;101(6):697–700 [M].
[3] Fettiplace MR, Weinberg G. Past, present, and future of lipid resuscitation therapy. J Parenter Enteral Nutr. 2015;39(1 Suppl):72S–83S [M].
[4] Muller SH, Diaz JH, Kaye AD. Clinical applications of intravenous lipid emulsion therapy. J Anesth. 2015;29(6):920–6 [M].

[5] Noble KA. Local anesthetic toxicity and lipid rescue. J Perianesth Nurs. 2015;30(4):321–35 [M].

[6] Sobolewski B, Doman P, Stetkiewicz T, et al. The toxic impact of local anaesthetics in menopausal women: causes, prevention and treatment after local anaesthetic overdose. Local anaesthetic systemic toxicity syndrome. Prz Menopauzalny. 2015;14(1):65–70 [M].

[7] Cao D, Heard K, Foran M, et al. Intravenous lipid emulsion in the emergency department: a systematic review of recent literature. J Emerg Med. 2015;48(3):387–97 [R].

[8] Walker BJ, Long JB, De Oliveira GS, et al. Peripheral nerve catheters in children: an analysis of safety and practice patterns from the pediatric regional anesthesia network (PRAN). Br J Anaesth. 2015;115(3):457–62 [R].

[9] Vasques F, Behr AU, Weinberg G, et al. A review of local anesthetic systemic toxicity cases since publication of the American Society of Regional Anesthesia recommendations: to whom it may concern. Reg Anesth Pain Med. 2015;40(6):698–705 [R].

[10] Liu SS, Ortolan S, Sandoval MV, et al. Cardiac arrest and seizures caused by local anesthetic systemic toxicity after peripheral nerve blocks: should we still fear the reaper? Reg Anesth Pain Med. 2016;41(1):5–21 [R].

[11] Liu SS, Gordon MA, Shaw PM, et al. A prospective clinical registry of ultrasound-guided regional anesthesia for ambulatory shoulder surgery. Anesth Analg. 2010;111(3):617–23 [c].

[12] Sagir A, Goyal R. An assessment of the awareness of local anesthetic systemic toxicity among multi-specialty postgraduate residents. J Anesth. 2015;29(2):299–302 [H].

[13] Fencl JL. Guideline implementation: local anesthesia. AORN J. 2015;101(6):682–92 [H].

[14] Cropsey CL, McEvoy MD. Local anesthetic systemic toxicity in a nonoperative location. Simul Healthc. 2015;10(5):326–8 [H].

[15] Collins S, Neubrander J, Vorst Z, et al. Lipid emulsion in treatment of local anesthetic toxicity. J Perianesth Nurs. 2015;30(4):308–20 [R].

[16] Busardò FP, Tritapepe L, Montana A, et al. A fatal accidental subarachnoid injection of lidocaine and levobupivacaine during a lumbar paravertebral block. Forensic Sci Int. 2015;256:17–20 [A].

[17] Ok SH, Byon HJ, Kwon SC, et al. Lipid emulsion inhibits vasodilation induced by a toxic dose of bupivacaine via attenuated dephosphorylation of myosin phosphatase target subunit 1 in isolated rat aorta. Int J Med Sci. 2015;12(12):958–67 [E].

[18] Sherman SL, Khazai RS, James CH, et al. In vivo toxicity of local anesthetics and corticosteroids of chondrocyte and synoviocyte viability and metabolism. Cartilage. 2015;6(2):106–12 [E].

[19] Tian J, Li Y. Comparative effects of vitamin C on the effects of local anesthetics ropivacaine, bupivacaine, and lidocaine on human chondrocytes. Rev Bras Anestesiol. 2016;66(1):29–36 [E].

[20] Cobo-Molinos J, Poncela-Garcia M, Marchal-Corrales JA, et al. Effect of levobupivacaine on articular chondrocytes: an in-vitro investigation. Eur J Anaesthesiol. 2014;31(11):635–9 [E].

[21] Mete M, Aydemir I, Tuglu IM, et al. Neurotoxic effects of local anesthetics on the mouse neuroblastoma NB2a cell line. Biotech Histochem. 2015;90(3):216–22 [E].

[22] Malet A, Faure MO, Deletage N, et al. The comparative cytotoxic effects of different local anesthetics on a human neuroblastoma cell line. Anesth Analg. 2015;120(3):589–96 [E].

[23] Gurbuzel M, Karaca U, Karayilan N. Genotoxic evaluation of bupivacaine and levobupivacaine in the Drosophila wing spot test. Cytotechnology. 2016;68(4):979–86. Epub ahead of print: Feb 19, 2015 [E].

[24] Neal JM, Barrington MJ, Brull R, et al. The second ASRA practice advisory on neurologic complications associated with regional anesthesia and pain medicine: executive summary 2015. Reg Anesth Pain Med. 2015;40(5):401–30 [R].

[25] Wu G, Sun B, Liu LI, et al. Lipid emulsion mitigates local anesthesia-induced central nervous system toxicity in rats. Exp Ther Med. 2015;10(3):1133–8 [E].

[26] Harper J, Zirwas M. Allergic contact dermatitis of the vagina and perineum: causes, incidence of, and differentiating factors. Clin Obstet Gynecol. 2015;58(1):153–7 [M].

[27] Arshdeep, De D, Handa S. Does contact allergy to benzocaine cause orodynia? Indian J Dermatol Venereol Leprol. 2015;81(1):84–6 [A].

[28] Udelsmann A, Melo MdeS. Hemodynamic changes with two lipid emulsions for treatment of bupivacaine toxicity in swines. Acta Cir Bras. 2015;30(2):87–93 [E].

[29] Iwasaki M, Tachibana K, Mitsuda N, et al. Bupivacaine-induced anaphylaxis in a parturient undergoing cesarean section. Masui. 2015;64(2):200–4 [A].

[30] Li R, Ma H, Zhang X, et al. Impaired autophagosome clearance contributes to local anesthetic bupivacaine-induced myotoxicity in mouse myoblasts. Anesthesiology. 2015;122(3):595–605 [E].

[31] Prakash R, Gautam S, Kumar S, et al. Local anaesthetic systemic toxicity in a patient under general anaesthesia: a diagnostic challenge. J Clin Diagn Res. 2015;9(2):UD03–4 [A].

[32] Güngör İ, Akbaş B, Kaya K, et al. Sudden developing convulsion during interscalene block: does propofol anesthesia diminish plasma bupivacaine level? Agri. 2015;27(1):54–7 [A].

[33] Kamel I, Trehan G, Barnette R. Intralipid therapy for inadvertent peripheral nervous system blockade resulting from local anesthetic overdose. Case Rep Anesthesiol. 2015;2015:486543 [A].

[34] Matos D, Serrano P, Brandão FM. Maculopapular rash of unsuspected cause: systemic contact dermatitis to cinchocaine. Cutan Ocul Toxicol. 2015;34(3):260–1 [A].

[35] Tierney KJ, Murano T, Natal B. Lidocaine induced cardiac arrest in the emergency department: effectiveness of lipid therapy. J Emerg Med. 2016;50(1):47–50 [A].

[36] Doye E, Desgranges FP, Stamm D, et al. Severe local anesthetic intoxication in an infant undergoing circumcision. Arch Pediatr. 2015;22(3):303–5 [A].

[37] Maeda T, Toyoda F, Imai S, et al. Lidocaine induces ROCK-dependent membrane blebbing and subsequent cell death in rabbit articular chondrocytes. J Orthop Res. 2016;34(5):754–62. Epub ahead of print: Nov 25, 2015 [E].

[38] Fenten MG, Schoenmakers KP, Heesterbeek PJ, et al. Effect of local anesthetic concentration, dose and volume on the duration of single-injection ultrasound-guided axillary brachial plexus block with mepivacaine: a randomized controlled trial. BMC Anesthesiol. 2015;15(130):1–8 [c].

[39] Saraghi M, Moore PA, Hersh EV. Local anesthetic calculations: avoiding trouble with pediatric patients. Gen Dent. 2015;63(1):48–52 [A].

[40] Barbarroja-Escudero J, Sanchez-Gonzalez MJ, Rodriguez-Rodriguez M, et al. Fixed drug urticaria: a report of two patients. Allergol Int. 2015;64(1):101–3 [A].

[41] Kim SJ, Goldberg BJ. Anaphylaxis due to topical pramoxine. Ann Allergy Asthma Immunol. 2015;114(1):72–3 [A].

[42] Murouchi T, Iwasaki S, Yamakage M. Chronological changes in ropivacaine concentration and analgesic effects between transversus abdominis plane block and rectus sheath block. Reg Anesth Pain Med. 2015;40(5):568–71 [c].

[43] Sola M, Dahners L, Weinfold P, et al. The viability of chondrocytes after an in vivo injection of local anaesthetic and/or corticosteroid: a laboratory study using a rat model. Bone Joint J. 2015;97-B(7):933–8 [E].

[44] Grigg E, Anderson C, Pankovich M, et al. Systemic ropivacaine toxicity from a peripheral nerve infusion in a medically complex patient. J Clin Anesth. 2015;27(4):338–40 [A].

[45] Bruscino N, Corradini D, Francalanci S, et al. A case of allergic contact dermatitis due to tetracaine with unusual presentation. G Ital Dermatol Venereol. 2015;150(2):266–7 [A].

11

Neuromuscular Blocking Agents and Skeletal Muscle Relaxants

Mona U. Shah[1]

Department of Pharmacy, Falls Church, VA, USA
[1]Corresponding author: mona.shah@inova.org

NEUROMUSCULAR BLOCKING AGENTS

General

Neuromuscular blocking agents (NMBAs) are hydrophilic drugs that are commonly used in clinical practice for paralysis in rapid sequence intubation, tracheostomy, to facilitate mechanical ventilation in patients with acute lung injury (ALI) or acute respiratory distress syndrome (ARDS), and to prevent and treat shivering in patients undergoing therapeutic hypothermia. However, NMBAs are not benign drugs. Their routine use is avoided in patients with elevated intracranial pressure (ICP) from traumatic brain injury (TBI) due to masking of seizures and higher incidence of pneumonia. A recent systematic review of seven clinical trials investigated the usefulness of NMBAs in patients with TBI and/or increased ICP. The results showed that NMBA boluses prevented stimulation-related ICP surges and that paralysis was effective during tracheal suctioning and physiotherapy but not during bronchoscopy. Succinylcholine increased ICP in two of three clinical studies and one of six animal studies, thus leaving a degree of uncertainty about its effects on ICP. There are more consistent safety reports related to ICP when non-depolarizing NMBAs in patients with TBI. Hence, the positive effects of NMBAs on facilitating mechanical ventilation in TBI patients must be carefully weighed against the potential for harm with continuous paralysis [1M].

Succinylcholine is a depolarizing NMBA that is mainly used during endotracheal intubation. The non-depolarizing NMBAs are divided into two classes: aminosteroidals (rocuronium, vecuronium, pancuronium) and benzylisoquinolines (atracurium, cisatracurium). Response to NMBA varies based on receptor types—immature (fetal) and mature nicotinic acetylcholine (ACh) receptors. Immature ACh receptors are synthesized in response to the loss of nerve function during spinal cord injury, burn, prolonged immobility, or Guillian–Barre syndrome. The immature receptors demonstrate increased response to succinylcholine than non-depolarizing NMBAs. Upregulation of the immature ACh receptors can cause tachyphylaxis, when NMBAs are used for a prolonged period. Isolated cases of tachyphylaxis in TBI and cross resistance between steroidal and benzylisoquinolines NMBAs have been reported [1M].

DEPOLARIZING NEUROMUSCULAR BLOCKING AGENTS

Succinylcholine (Suxamethonium) (SEDA-36; SEDA-37)

Susceptibility Factors

GENETIC FACTORS

The duration of neuromuscular blockade (NMB) following succinylcholine administration is highly variable and dependent on dosage. Succinylcholine's duration of action may be prolonged by genetic variants of butyrylcholinesterase enzyme (BChE). Pregnancy, malnutrition, metoclopramide, and certain $\beta2$ agonists are known to decrease BChE activity. Clinical factors such as age, health status, sex, medication, concomitant disease or genetic variants on duration of NMB after succinylcholine 1 mg/kg was assessed in a prospective, observational study of 1630 surgical patients undergoing rapid sequence intubation (RSI). The duration of NMB varied from 80 seconds to 44 minutes with a median (IQR) duration of 7.3 (5.8–9.3) minutes. Sixteen percent of patients had NMB duration greater than 10 minutes where higher American Society of Anesthesiologists (ASA) health class, increased age, male sex, pregnancy, cancer, hepatic disease, use of etomidate and metoclopramide were identified as independent risk factors. Of these, higher ASA class had the greatest influence on NMB duration. The authors concluded that in patients with molecular genetic variants of BChE or those with clinical risk factors for a prolonged neuromuscular blockade, an alternative to succinylcholine for RSI should be considered [2c].

PHARMACOGENETICS

In a review of pharmacogenetics of adverse drug reactions, Turner and colleague describe a strong genetic predisposition in patients diagnosed with malignant hyperthermia (MH). All halogenated anesthetics have been implicated in precipitating MH in individuals with RYR1 mutation on chromosome 19 in skeletal muscle. Succinylcholine augments the adverse reactions to these anesthetics, but its role in precipitating fulminant MH remains controversial. While ~75% of MH events occur in patients with no family history, genetic screening for MH is untenable, and approximately 30% of MH cases are not associated with RYR1 mutation [3r].

The genetic variants of succinylcholine that contribute to the differences seen in efficacy, pharmacokinetics, and adverse effects experienced by patients during the perioperative period are listed in the table below [4R]:

Drug	Gene(s) affected by polymorphism	Genetic variant	Phenotypic effect of polymorphism
Succinylcholine	BChE RYR1	293A > G, 1699G > A, 695T > A Multiple at 19q13.1	Reduced hydrolysis, increased duration leading to prolonged blockade and apnea Malignant hyperthermia

NON-DEPOLARIZING NEUROMUSCULAR BLOCKERS

Organs and Systems

CARDIOVASCULAR (SEDA-37)

Atracurium causes dose-dependent histamine release, resulting in tachycardia and hypotension, whereas pancuronium's vagal blockade leads to an increase in heart rate, blood pressure and cardiac output. Cisatracurium, a stereoisomer of atracurium, does not cause clinically significant histamine release and has organ-independent metabolism, which makes it an ideal drug for ICU, but not RSI due to its slow onset of action. With so many NMBAs in the armamentarium, there is not a single agent that is ideal in terms of potency, rapid onset of action, and hemodynamic stability [5r]. Non-depolarizing, cysteine-reversible NMBAs such as gantacurium and CW002 may just be the answer.

RESPIRATORY

The NMBAs used during anesthesia are potent, and patients require adequate gas exchange during prolonged procedures to prevent accidental awareness under general anesthesia. There is a significant and unpredictable risk for residual neuromuscular blockade (RNMB) that may result in respiratory complications, muscular weakness, increased length of hospital stay, and delayed extubation. Many studies have found a high incidence of RNMB (failure to return to train-of-four, TOF ratio > 0.9) after anesthesia and surgery, with a range of 4–64% [6r]. The potential causes of post-operative respiratory complications include underlying comorbidities, intraoperative mechanical ventilation, surgical trauma, fluid resuscitation, anesthetic agents as well as higher doses of NMBAs. Objective quantitative monitoring of neuromuscular transmission is the only reliable method to exclude RNMB; however, this approach is not used consistently in clinical practice. A survey of anesthesiologists reported that neuromuscular transmission monitoring was only used by 17–50% of providers. Most anesthesiologists use subjective assessment of TOF count in response to TOF stimulation, which alone is not enough to decrease the dose-dependent risk of respiratory complications associated with NMBAs. The dose-dependent relationship between intermediate NMBAs and post-operative complications was validated by McLean and colleagues in a large cohort of 48 499 patients, where high doses of NMBAs increased postoperative respiratory complications compared to low doses (OR 1.28; 95% CI; 1.04–1.57; $p = 0.02$). This was yet another study that supported the quantitative monitoring of the depth of NMB during the intraoperative period and before tracheal extubation [7C].

IMMUNOLOGIC

One of the causes of anaphylactic reaction during anesthesia is thought to be NMBA. In a review of case histories of 85 patients between 2000 and 2010, there were 6 patients who underwent skin testing due to a prior history of an allergic reaction to a NMBA. The NMBA that induced a negative skin test was successfully used as an alternative during surgery. Four of the six patients reported allergies to rocuronium, pancuronium, or vecuronium but did not experience an adverse reaction with cisatracurium, which was safely used during anesthesia [8C]. Cisatracurium has been shown to have the lowest risk of hypersensitivity reactions in large cohort studies, and reportedly has the lowest rate of cross-sensitization with other NMBAs in allergic patients [9r].

Rocuronium

Susceptibility Factors

AGE

Maturation of neuromuscular transmission continues to occur after birth for the first 2 months. Succinylcholine is not recommended for prolonged paralysis in ventilated babies due to its short duration of action. It is contraindicated in neonates with hyperkalemia, neuromuscular disease, muscle injury, trauma, burn, renal failure, pneumothorax, glaucoma, intestinal obstruction, and increased intracranial pressure. As a substitute to succinylcholine, non-depolarizing NMBAs are used to maintain paralysis in infants who are not breathing in synchrony with the ventilator and may be at risk for pneumothorax or higher intrapulmonary pressures. All studies included in the systemic review of neuromuscular paralysis in ventilated patients used pancuronium, a long-acting agent with adverse effects of tachycardia and hypertension. Comparison of vecuronium with cisatracurium in neonates after cardiac surgery suggested a prolonged recovery time of 4 hours in one-third of the patients receiving vecuronium. Hence, a short acting non-depolarizing agent such as rocuronium may be considered in infants undergoing tracheal intubation, when succinylcholine is contraindicated; however, there is insufficient data to suggest the same in neonates [10R].

GENETIC FACTORS

Prior studies have shown that rocuronium pharmacokinetics varies in patients due to the inter-individual differences in metabolism, excretion, or target-site sensitivity. Rocuronium is a quaternary ammonium muscle relaxant that is cleared via liver uptake and biliary excretion through organic anion transporter, OATP 1B1, which is encoded by SLCO1B1 gene. Previous reports have indicated that alterations in SLCO1B1 gene variant can impact drug metabolism. Mei and colleagues conducted a study to explore the role of SLCO1B1, ABCB1, and CHRNA1 gene polymorphisms on the efficacy of rocuronium in Chinese patients that were scheduled to undergo elective surgery. Two hundred patients completed genotyping and anesthesia. There were no significant differences in age, body mass index, medications received and duration of surgery among patients in different genotypes of the same gene ($p > 0.05$). The authors found that the clinical duration and recovery time of rocuronium were prolonged in patients with SLCO1B1 and ABCB1 gene variants and that ABCB1 rs1128503 C > T genotype may be an important factor for different clinical actions of rocuronium. Pharmacogenomics is necessary in guiding the optimal use of rocuronium [11c]. The genetic variants of rocuronium are also described in the table below [4R]:

Drug	Gene(s) affected by polymorphism	Genetic variant	Phenotypic effect of polymorphism
Rocuronium	SLCO1B1 ABCB1	rs2306283 A > G rs1128503 C > T	Reduced elimination, increased duration of action and recovery time

Gantacurium

GENERAL INFORMATION

The benzylisoquinoline compound, gantacurium, is an ultra-short acting non-depolarizing NMBA whose duration is determined by the rapid rate at with exogenous L-cysteine binds to and permanently inactivates the molecule. In humans, gantacurium has modest potency with rapid onset of action. Maximum NMB occurs within 90 seconds or within a minute with larger doses. Gantacurium's kinetic profile is similar to succinylcholine. When tested in humans, there was a transient increase in cardiovascular effects at gantacurium dose of 3xED$_{95}$ and histamine release at dose of 4xED$_{95}$, but the propensity of these adverse effects was less than that observed with mivacurium (removed from the market due to economic reasons) [13r]. The NMB with gantacurium can be reduced from 10 minutes with spontaneous recovery to 3 minutes by adding 10 mg/kg L-cysteine [13r]. Despite rapid onset, ultra-short duration, gantacurium's clinical development has been hampered by modest histamine release. The gantacurium derivative CW002 is an intermediate acting, cysteine-inactivated, non-depolarizing NMBA currently in clinical trial. The phase 1, dose escalation (range 0.02–0.14 mg/kg), pharmacodynamic/pharmacokinetic study in volunteers is completed. Preliminary analysis indicate an ED$_{95}$ of ~0.07 mg/kg, a duration at 1.5–2 × ED$_{95}$ of ~55 minutes with an onset time of ~2.9 minutes, and mean terminal half-life of 26 minutes. There were no hemodynamic changes or evidence of histamine release or bronchoconstriction with CW002 [12R].

NEUROMUSCULAR BLOCKERS: REVERSAL AGENTS

℞

SPECIAL REVIEW

There is a dose-dependent relationship between NMBAs and risk of post-operative RNMB, which is associated with increased respiratory morbidity. Hence, RNMB should be monitored and reversed when indicated. Two pharmacological methods are approved: acetylcholinesterase (AChE) inhibitors (neostigmine) and molecular encapsulating agents (sugammadex and calabadions). Neostigmine increases AChE concentration at both nicotinic and muscarinic sites resulting in muscarinic adverse effects such as nausea, vomiting, miosis, bradycardia, and bronchospasm. As a result, AChE inhibitor is always used in combination with glycopyrrolate or atropine. Since neostigmine has a ceiling effect, it can only be used to reverse shallow levels of NMB. On the other hand, encapsulating agents rapidly reverse all levels of RNMB, and complete recovery of muscle strength is achieved almost immediately after administration.

Sugammadex (Bridion) was approved by the U.S. Food and Drug Administration on December 15, 2015, for the reversal of steroidal NMBAs (rocuronium and vecuronium). Sugammadex is highly water soluble; urinary excretion is the main route of elimination for sugammadex and sugammadex–rocuronium complex. The efficacy and safety of sugammadex 2 mg/kg for the reversal of rocuronium 0.6 mg/kg in patients with end-stage renal disease (ESRD; CrCl < 30 mL/min) in 13 adult patients undergoing elective surgery was performed by Staals et al. [15C]. The clearance and half-life of sugammadex was increased 17-fold and 15-fold, respectively. Due to reduced speed of sugammadex reversal of NMBA, the use of sugammadex in patients with severe renal impairment (CrCl < 30 mL/min) is not recommended [16R]. In such cases, neostigmine may be used as an alternative but should be monitored closely as 50–75% plasma clearance of neostigmine depends on renal excretion. In liver cirrhosis, the volume of distribution is increased and so is the half-life of NMBAs. Sugammadex is not metabolized or excreted by the liver and may be safely used in patients with liver dysfunction, but caution is advised if hepatic impairment is accompanied by coagulopathy or severe edema. Adverse effects of sugammadex include dose-dependent prolongation of aPTT and PT/INR. The potential drug–drug interaction with sugammadex includes flucloxacillin, fusidic acid, and toremifene.

Calabadions are broad-spectrum reversal agents currently in preclinical development. Based on preclinical data, calabadions facilitate the recovery of NMBAs, ketamine and etomidate-induced respiratory depression. With almost 100-fold binding ability of encapsulating agents to NMBAs, the minimal effective dose of these agents should be used to maintain neuromuscular transmission (TOF > 0.9) [14R]. Calabadion 1, first-generation calabadion, has a higher affinity to steroidal NMBA than benzylisoquinoline. It reverses cisatracurium and rocuronium without affecting heart rate, blood pressure, pH, or arterial blood gas. Calabadion 2, a second-generation calabadion, has an 89-fold stronger affinity toward rocuronium than sugammadex, and in-vivo experiments show faster reversal of RNMB with calabadion 2 compared with calabadion 1. In living rats, the molar potency of calabadion 2 to reverse vecuronium and rocuronium was higher compared with that of sugammadex. Calabadion 2 is renally eliminated and does not affect blood pressure or heart rate [17E]. Moreover, lower doses of calabadion 2 are required to reverse non-depolarizing NMBAs due to its high selectivity to the target agent, potentially leading to even less dose-dependent side effects compared to calabadion 1 [14R].

Sugammadex

Partownavid and colleagues provide a comprehensive review of clinical trials related to sugammadex. Sugammadex causes a rapid and dose-dependent reversal of profound NMB induced by high-dose rocuronium 1–1.2 mg/kg or vecuronium 0.1 mg/kg. Sugammadex doses up to 32 mg/kg have been safely used for reversal of NMBAs in healthy individuals. Adverse events thought to be related to sugammadex include headache, nausea, vomiting, increased AST, dry mouth, movement, bradycardia, and QTc prolongation (does not appear to be dose dependent). When sugammadex was studied in patients with underlying pulmonary disease, 2.6% of patients experienced bronchospasm, which may be related to the underlying disease or a hypersensitivity reaction from sugammadex administration [16R].

Abad-Gurumeta and colleagues compared the efficacy and safety of sugammadex versus neostigmine in a systematic review of 14 randomized controlled trials of 1553 patients. The primary outcome was the rate of post-operative RNMB. Secondary outcomes were the rates of drug-related adverse effects, including nausea or vomiting. Sugammadex reduced all signs of RNMB (RR 0.46; $p = 0.0004$) and minor respiratory events (RR 0.51; $p = 0.0034$). However, there was no difference in critical respiratory events (RR 0.13; $p = 0.06$) or the rate of post-operative nausea and vomiting (PONV) [18M].

A single, prospective, randomized, double-blinded study compared the incidence of PONV in 100 patients that underwent general anesthesia for extremity surgery (tendon repair and skin graft). Patients were randomly assigned to receive 2 mg/kg sugammadex or neostigmine 70 mcg/kg and atropine 0.4 mg per mg of neostigmine. Rocuronium 0.6 mg/kg was given for tracheal intubation with additional boluses of 0.15 mg/kg to maintain TOF 2/4. Antiemetic medications were not administered preoperatively. PONV was treated with ondansetron 4 mg IV, and if persistent, with metoclopramide 10 mg IV. The nausea and vomiting scores were significantly lower in the sugammadex group upon arrival in the recovery room, but similar during the remaining initial 24 hours (60% vs 58%). Extubation, first eye opening, and head lift times were also shorter in the sugammadex group ($p \leq 0.001$ for each). Patients in the neostigmine group experienced significant bradycardia, whereas patients in the sugammadex group had more coughing. One patient in the sugammadex group experienced respiratory depression, but did not require re-intubation [19C].

Second-Generation Effects

PREGNANCY

• A 19-year-old, who is a 27-week gestation pregnant patient, was admitted to the emergency department for ovarian torsion. Rocuronium 50 mg (0.9 mg/kg), fentanyl, and propofol were administered, and laparoscopic surgery was performed without incident. The surgery lasted 120 minutes and TOF was 1/4. The authors did not find any information on the use of sugammadex in pregnancy, and the company's medical liaison also discouraged the use of sugammadex in pregnancy due to potential for harm to the patient and fetus. The TOF increased to 4/4 (21%), so neostigmine 2 mg and atropine 0.5 mg were used for reversal. Patient was successfully extubated and discharged without adverse event. Until more information becomes available, risk versus benefit of sugammadex in pregnancy must be considered [20A].

Susceptibility Factors

DISEASE

A 42-year-old woman (BMI: 30.4; weight 74 kg) with history of multiple sclerosis (on glatiramer therapy for 3 years and attack free) presented to the hospital for evaluation of severe abdominal pain and nausea. Patient was diagnosed with acute pancreatitis and prepared for an emergent laparotomy. Anesthesia was induced with propofol, fentanyl and maintained with sevoflurane and nitrous oxide. Rocuronium 45 mg was given for tracheal intubation. Another dose of rocuronium 10 mg was administered after 30 minutes for TOF of 50%. After laparotomy, acute necrotizing pancreatitis was diagnosed and 66 minutes into the procedure, sevoflurane was stopped and 150 mg (2 mg/kg) sugammadex was administered to reverse TOF of 50%. Approximately 2 minutes later, TOF was 90%. Patient was successfully extubated without signs of residual blockade in the post recovery period. Three days later, the patient underwent an open abdominal surgery due to abdominal cavity infection with general anesthesia. The patient received similar doses of rocuronium and sugammadex. Thereafter, the patient's abdominal cavity was cleaned under

general anesthesia four more times at 3-day intervals. Sugammadex was successfully used to reverse rocuronium's RNMB without precipitating multiple sclerosis attacks after each operation [21A].

Drug Administration

DRUG DOSAGE REGIMEN

In a single center, randomized, double-blind study involving 50 patients, pipecuronium was used as the NMBA during routine elective surgery and sugammadex doses of 1–4 mg/kg or placebo were administered to reverse moderate NMB. Sugammadex adequately reversed pipecuronium-induced moderate NMB during sevoflurane anesthesia. When TOF returned to 2/4, sugammadex dose of 2 mg/kg was sufficient to reverse pipecuronium-induced NMB [23c].

SKELETAL MUSCLE RELAXANTS

General Information

The choice of skeletal muscle relaxants depends on symptom relief, side effect profile, and tolerability. There is no clear evidence that one agent is superior to another, so medications are usually tailored to patient-specific situations. Somnolence, sedation, and anticholinergic symptoms are some of the common adverse effects of all skeletal muscle relaxants.

℞ *The role of muscle relaxants in the treatment of pain was reviewed by Cohen and Warfield [22M]. Muscle relaxants have poor evidence for the treatment of acute low back pain and when compared to placebo, patients taking active drug are 50% more likely to experience side effects such as drowsiness, dizziness, or dry mouth. In majority of cases, long-term use of muscle relaxants for chronic back pain is not recommended due to their high side effect profile unless there is ongoing benefit without significant side effects. Cyclobenzaprine is the most widely prescribed muscle relaxant for conditions such as myofascial pain or fibromyalgia. When compared with ibuprofen 800 mg TID, cyclobenzaprine 5 mg TID was no better than ibuprofen in the treatment of acute cervical pain but the degree of pain intensity relief and onset of effect was greater with cyclobenzaprine. In clinical practice, cyclobenzaprine 10 mg TID is commonly prescribed for muscle spasms and is associated with high incidence of side effects (drowsiness and xerostomia); however, in an industry-funded study, 5 mg TID dose was equally efficacious and produced fewer side effects. While cyclobenzaprine is chemically related to tricyclic antidepressant, amitriptyline, carisoprodol is a non-tricyclic antidepressant muscle relaxant. Carisoprodol is efficacious at a dose of 250 mg QID, although it is prescribed at a higher dose of 350 mg QID, which translates to increased adverse effects. Carisoprodol is metabolized to meprobamate via the CYP2C19 variant of cytochrome P450-CYP2C19 gene in the liver, so an individual with two CYP2C19 alleles could make more meprobamate, an anxiolytic and hypnotic with potential for mental impairment. Baclofen is the main stay of treatment for upper motor neuron spasticity such as tetanus, stiff man syndrome, cerebral palsy, and multiple sclerosis. Abrupt withdrawal of baclofen can cause seizures, respiratory depression, and delirium that may require ICU admission. While baclofen and tizanidine have similar efficacy for the treatment of spasm, tizanidine causes hepatotoxicity and hypotension, but not baclofen. Dantrolene too has adverse effects that include cardiovascular and pulmonary toxicity, hepatotoxicity, visual disturbances, hallucinations, seizures, and depression [22M].*

Baclofen

Baclofen, a gamma-amino butyric acid (GABA) receptor agonist, is a centrally acting agent that is commonly used to treat spasticity. Baclofen is also used off-label for the treatment of alcohol dependence. A recent review by Warren and Davis describe the evidence for baclofen in the treatment of gastroesophageal reflux disease (GERD). Increase in transient lower esophageal sphincter relaxation (TLESR) contributes to GERD symptoms. Baclofen inhibits TLESR by stimulating $GABA_B$ receptors in the alpha-motor neurons. Nine trials were included in the literature review, of which, six examined reflux symptoms and lower esophageal sphincter (LES) function after single dose or short course (less than 2 days) of baclofen. Three trials followed patients with GERD for 14 days or longer. All trials showed reduction in TLESRs and reflux episodes with baclofen and subsequent improvement in quality of life. Drowsiness and dizziness were the most common adverse events reported. Following diagnostic evaluation, baclofen (40–60 mg/day) may be a considered for refractory GERD in patients that have failed previous therapies with histamine-2 receptor antagonists (H_2RA), proton pump inhibitors (PPI), and metoclopramide. Larger long-term tolerability and efficacy trials are needed to add baclofen in the armamentarium for the treatment of refractory GERD [24R].

Long-Term Effects
DRUG DEPENDENCE
- 76-year-old woman with past medical history of multiple sclerosis (MS) was admitted to the hospital with diarrhea and bright-red-blood-per-rectum. Colon biopsy was positive for ischemic colitis. During hospitalization, patient experienced spasticity, urinary retention, tachycardia, altered mental status, and respiratory failure requiring intubation. Methylprednisolone was started due to suspicion of

MS flare, but there was no improvement in symptoms. After negative diagnostic work-up, it was concluded that the patient may be experiencing withdrawal from oral baclofen due to poor absorption secondary to colitis. Oral baclofen was transitioned to intravenous diazepam, with gradual resolution of symptoms. Withdrawal from oral baclofen secondary to malabsorption should be considered in symptomatic patients with gastrointestinal dysfunction [25r].

Botulinum Toxin

General Information

Botulinum toxin (BTX), a.k.a. Botox or Dysport, is produced by Gram-positive anaerobic bacterium, *Clostridium botulinum*. BTX is typically associated with cosmetic procedures, but it is also used for the treatment of pain.

MECHANISM

BTX blocks the release of acetylcholine from nerve endings and helps to alleviate pain. Due to its long lasting effect up to 5 months after initial injection, BTX makes an excellent drug for chronic pain and is FDA approved for the treatment of migraines. Besides hypersensitivity reaction, there are no known adverse events or drug interactions with BTX.

USES

BTX types A (considered first-line) and B are used to treat spasticity related to traumatic brain injury, stroke, cerebral palsy, multiple sclerosis, and spinal cord injury. It is also used to treat non-dystonic disorders of involuntary muscle activity (tremor, tics, myoclonus, trismus, tinnitus, hemifacial spasm, and nocturnal bruxism); focal dystonias (blepharospasm; cervical, laryngeal, limb, oromandibular, truncal dystonias); strabismus (nystagmus, conjugate eye movement); chronic pain and disorders of localized muscle spasms; sweating, salivary, and allergic disorders; and smooth muscle hyperactive disorders [26R].

Sunil and colleagues conducted a literature review of studies related to BTX in the treatment of muscle-specific oro-facial pain and found BTX A to be an effective agent for the treatment of tempomandibular disorders (TMD), and depending on the target muscle, BTX A dose of 10–50 units per site with a total dose of 200 units in the masticatory system may be used. The most common side effect was adjacent muscle weakness due to diffusion of the solution [27c].

ADVERSE REACTIONS

Systemic adverse reactions from BTX injection have occurred as a result of intravascular spread or migration through facial planes. Life-threatening cases of dysphagia, dyspnea, botulism, as well as blurred vision, diplopia, dysarthria, dysphonia, generalized muscle weakness, ptosis, and urinary incontinence are also reported. When BTX was used for 24-week period in patients with chronic migraines, there were no serious adverse events. While BTX's long-term effects help to decrease prescription pain medications for chronic pain and also improve quality of life, the cost of drug and denial of prior authorization from insurance companies for off-label use has prevented its wide-spread use in chronic pain management [26R].

Wu and colleagues conducted a systematic review of trials to evaluate the evidence behind effectiveness of BTX for lower limb spasticity after stroke. Seven randomized controlled trials (603 patients) comparing BTX to placebo or conventional therapy were included in the meta-analysis. The authors concluded that there was a statistical significant decrease in muscle tone at week 4 ($p=0.001$) and 12 ($p=0.02$) after BTX injection and BTX showed more persistent clinical benefits in lower limb spasticity compared to placebo after stroke. Common adverse events reported were myalgia, injection site pain, erythema, convulsions, and incoordination ($p=0.43$) [28M].

Drug Administration

DRUG–DRUG AND DRUG–DISEASE INTERACTION

BTX should be used with extreme caution in patients taking aminoglycosides, penicillamine, quinine, calcium channel blockers; pregnancy and lactation as well as in patients with neuromuscular disorders such as myasthenia gravis and Eaton–Lambert syndrome. The mechanism is unclear, but some patients develop antibodies to BTX due to unknown predisposing factors. This risk can be mitigated by administering appropriate doses and avoiding frequent and higher dose BTX injections [27c].

Carisoprodol and Meprobamate

General Information

Carisoprodol is often used for the acute treatment of severe muscle spasm. It is metabolized to an active metabolite, meprobamate, which is highly addictive due to its effect on $GABA_A$ receptors in the brain. Carisoprodol is used for short-term management of acute spasm due to its potential for abuse; however, when used long-term, dose must be tapered slowly to avoid withdrawal symptoms (insomnia, restlessness, anorexia, upset stomach, anxiety, and seizures). Depending on patient's needs, carisoprodol may be used for 2–3 weeks at doses up to 1400 mg/day [29r].

Second-Generation Effects

PREGNANCY

There is limited information regarding safety of carisoprodol in pregnancy. There are 16 case reports of human pregnancies with normal outcomes after carisoprodol exposure; however, no consistent patterns of congenital anomalies with in-utero exposure to meprobamate have been reported [30r].

LACTATION

Carisoprodol is excreted in breast milk, but two case reports found no adverse effects from carisoprodol ingestion via breast milk. If carisoprodol is necessary during lactation, the infant should be monitored for signs of sedation and difficulty with feeding [30r].

Cyclobenzaprine

General Information

Cyclobenzaprine can be used for acute or chronic pain associated with muscle strain that limits activities of daily living. When compared to placebo, cyclobenzaprine reduced pain and improved global function in 1 of every 3–9 patients during the first week of treatment [31r]. In a randomized, double-blind study comparing cyclobenzaprine 5–10 mg every 8 hours or placebo in combination with naproxen 500 mg twice daily for the management of lower back pain in adults showed that addition of naproxen to cyclobenzaprine did not improve functional outcomes [32C].

Cyclobenzaprine is structurally similar to tricyclic antidepressants (TCAs) and has similar anticholinergic side effects such as sedation, dizziness, tachycardia, arrhythmias and may worsen heart failure, cardiac conduction abnormalities, and benign prostatic hyperplasia [29r].

Second-Generation Effects

LACTATION

It is unknown whether cyclobenzaprine is excreted in breast milk [30r].

Drug Administration

DRUG OVERDOSE

• A 22-year-old male was found unresponsive with shallow breathing after an accidental overdose of cyclobenzaprine. Emergency medical services (EMS) gave him 2 mg intranasal naloxone. About 15 minutes into transport, the patient went into ventricular fibrillation (VF) and CPR and ACLS protocols were initiated. Patient was cold, but rectal temperature was unreadable. Hence, a core temperature of 23.3 °C (74 °F) was obtained by inserting the target temperature management system (IVTTMs). Patient continued to be in VF arrest in the emergency department. When patient's family reported that the patient may have ingested 30 pills of 10 mg cyclobenzaprine, sodium bicarbonate drip and intravenous intralipid emulsion (ILE) were initiated. Patient remained hypothermic (despite warm fluids) and pulseless (organized QRS rhythm on the monitor). Patient was taken to the operating room for cardiopulmonary bypass and pulse returned ~30 minutes into rewarming on bypass. Patient recovered completely by day 3 except residual weakness in his legs. Aggressive rewarming via IVTTMs, intralipid emulsion therapy and sodium bicarbonate for widened QRS are important modalities to consider in severe cyclobenzaprine overdose [33A].

- Chua-Tuan and colleagues describe a case of a 16-year-old female with seizure disorder who was found unresponsive in pulseless ventricular tachycardia after intentional overdose of 4.5 g lacosamide, 120 mg cyclobenzaprine, and unknown amount of levetiracetam. After one unsynchronized defibrillation attempt, patient went into sinus tachycardia. She subsequently experienced tonic–clonic seizure and became bradycardic, for which she received treatment. In the emergency department, patient had a blood pressure of 151/97 mmHg, pulse of 162 bpm, and respiratory rate of 24 breaths/minute. After intubation, patient became bradycardic and went into asystole but soon recovered after CPR and 1 mg of IV atropine and 1 mg of IV epinephrine. Patient received 150 mEq of sodium bicarbonate for possible sodium channel blockade. Nine hours after initial presentation, patient's lacosamide level was elevated at 22.8 mcg/mL (normal range: 1–16.3 mcg/mL); cyclobenzaprine and levetiracetam levels were therapeutic. Patient was discharged to a psychiatric facility after her neurologic status returned to baseline. The sodium channel blockade from co-ingestion of high dose of lacosamide and therapeutic cyclobenzaprine may have contributed to cardiac conduction delay and cardiac arrest in this patient [34A].

Metaxalone (Skelaxin®)

General Information

Metaxalone is a water-soluble, centrally acting skeletal muscle relaxant that has no direct effect on the muscle tissue. It is generally prescribed for the treatment of acute, chronic, traumatic, and inflammatory musculoskeletal disorders at a dose range of 800–3200 mg/day. Adverse reactions from metaxalone use are related to CNS depression (drowsiness, dizziness, headache, nausea, and vomiting); hence, the potential for abuse is higher with this agent. Other adverse effects include hepatotoxicity and hemolytic anemia [29r].

Organs and Systems
DEATH

- A 32-year-old woman was treated in the emergency department after being found unresponsive at home for an unspecified time period. Clinical history included depression and recent muscle strain. Prescription medications included metaxalone, alprazolam, and duloxetine. Despite cardiopulmonary resuscitative efforts, patient was declared brain dead 27 hours after admission. Postmortem specimen and toxicology testing revealed markedly elevated metaxalone levels in blood, serum, vitreous humor, brain, and liver. There were higher concentrations of metaxalone in the tissues and brain compared to vitreous humor, which suggested greater fat solubility and higher volume of distribution of metaxalone. Cause of death was opined to be complications from circulatory shock due to acute overdose of metaxalone [35A].

Methocarbamol

Patients that are sensitive to metaxalone can be prescribed methocarbamol, which is an indirect CNS depressant. Adverse effects include anaphylactic reactions, drowsiness, dizziness, nausea, vomiting, dyspepsia, jaundice, leucopenia, metallic taste, and vertigo [29r].

Orphenadrine (Norflex)

Orphenadrine is mostly used as an adjuvant for joint pain, muscle pain, neuropathic pain. It blocks histamine and cholinergic receptors, similar to diphenhydramine, and also antagonizes NMDA receptors. Common side effects include anticholinergic symptoms and rarely aplastic anemia [29r].

Tizanidine (Zanaflex)

Tizanidine is used for the treatment of muscle spasticity and as an adjuvant for insomnia. Since it stimulates α_2-adrenergic receptors, the common side effects are hypotension and sedation. It also causes hallucinations, dry mouth, asthenia, weakness and liver injury (monitor liver enzymes every 6 months and symptoms of jaundice) [29r].

References

[1] Sanfilippo F, Santonocito C, Veenith T, et al. The role of neuromuscular blockade in patients with traumatic brain injury: a systematic review. Neurocrit Care. 2015;22:325–34 [M].

[2] Dell-Kuster S, Levano S, Burkhart CS, et al. Predictors of the variability in neuromuscular block duration following succinylcholine: a prospective, observational study. Eur J Anaesthesiol. 2015;32:687–96 [c].

[3] Turner RM, Pirmohamed M. Pharmacogenetics of adverse drug reactions. In: Grech G, Grossman I, editors. Preventative and predictive genetics: towards personalized medicine, advances in predictive, preventative and personalized medicine. Switzerland: Springer International Publishing; 2015. p. 109–56 [r].

[4] Behrooz A. Pharmacogenetics and anaesthetic drugs: implications for perioperative practice. Ann Med Surg. 2015;4:470–4 [R].

[5] Johnson JS, Loushin MK. The effects of anesthetic agents on cardiac function. In: Iaizzo PA, editor. Handbook of cardiac anatomy, physiology, and devices. Switzerland: Springer International Publishing; 2015. p. 295–305 [r].

[6] Rodney G, Raju PK, Ball DR. Not just monitoring: a strategy for managing neuromuscular blockade. Anaesthesia. 2015;70:1105–9 [r].

[7] McLean DJ, Diaz-Gill D, Farhan HN, et al. Dose-dependent association between intermediate-acting neuromuscular blocking agents and postoperative respiratory complications. Anesthesiology. 2015;122:1201–13 [C].

[8] Audicana MT, Lobera T, Gonzáles I, et al. Allergic reactions in anesthesia: do diagnostic studies ensure safety of reoperation? J Investig Allergol Clin Immunol. 2015;25(6):441–3 [C].

[9] Mertes PM, Volcheck GW. Anaphylaxis to neuromuscular-blocking drugs. Anesthesiology. 2015;122:5–7 [r].

[10] Boyle EM, Anand KJS. Sedation, analgesia and neuromuscular blockade in the neonatal ICU. In: Rimensberger PC, editor. Pediatric and neonatal mechanical ventilation. Berlin/Heidelberg: Springer-Verlag; 2015. p. 1019–29 [R].

[11] Mei Y, Wang SY, Li Y, et al. Role of SLCO1B1, ABCB1, and CHRNA1 gene polymorphisms on the efficacy of rocuronium in Chinese patients. J Clin Pharmacol. 2015;55(3):261–8 [c].

[12] Heerdt PM, Sunaga H, Savarese JJ. Novel neuromuscular blocking drugs and antagonists. Curr Opin Anaesthesiol. 2015;28:403–10 [R].

[13] Murrell MT, Savarese JJ. New vistas in neuromuscular blockers. In: Kaye AD, Kaye AM, Urman RD, editors. Essentials of pharmacology for anesthesia, pain medicine, and critical care. New York: Springer Science and Business Media; 2015. p. 827–35 [r].

[14] Haerter F, Eikermann M. Reversing neuromuscular blockade: inhibitors of the acetylcholinesterase versus the encapsulating agents sugammadex and calabadion. Expert Opin Pharmacother. 2016;17(6):819–33 [R].

[15] Staals LM, Snoeck MMJ, Driessen JJ, et al. Reduced clearance of rocuronium and sugammadex in patients with severe to end-stage renal failure: a pharmacokinetic study. Br J Anaesth. 2010;104:31–9 [C].

[16] Partownavid P, Romito BT, Ching W, et al. Sugammadex: a comprehensive review of published human science, including renal studies. Am J Ther. 2015;22:298–317 [R].

[17] Haerter F, Simons JC, Foerster U, et al. Comparative effectiveness of calabadion and sugammadex to reverse non-depolarizing neuromuscular-blocking agents. Anesthesiology. 2015;123(6):1337–49 [E].

[18] Abad-Gurumeta A, Ripollés-Melchor J, Casans-Francés R, et al. A systematic review of sugammadex vs neostigmine for reversal of neuromuscular blockade. Anaesthesia. 2015;70:1441–52 [M].

[19] Koyuncu O, Turhanoglu S, Akkurt CO, et al. Comparison of sugammadex and conventional reversal on postoperative nausea and vomiting: a randomized, blinded trial. J Clin Anesth. 2015;27:51–6 [C].

[20] Varela N, Lobato F. Sugammadex and pregnancy, is it safe? J Clin Anesth. 2015;27(2):183–4 [A].

[21] Sinikoglu N, Totoz T, Gumus F, et al. Repeated sugammadex usage in a patient with multiple sclerosis: a case report. Wien Klin Wochenschr. 2016;128:71–3 [A].

[22] Cohen RI, Warfield CA. Role of muscle relaxants in the treatment of pain. In: Deer TR, Leong MS, Gordin V, editors. Treatment of chronic pain by medical approaches: the American academy of pain medicine textbook on patient management. New York: Springer; 2015. p. 67–75.

[23] Tassonyi E, Pongracz A, Nemes R, et al. Reversal of pipecuronium-induced moderate neuromuscular block with sugammadex in the presence of a sevoflurane anesthetic: a randomized trial. Anesth Analg. 2015;121(2):373–80 [c].

[24] Warren RL, Davis SM. The role of baclofen in the treatment of gastroesophageal reflux disease. J Pharm Technol. 2015;31(6):258–61 [R].

[25] Valimahomed A, Padro-Guzman J. Baclofen withdrawal secondary to gastrointestinal malabsorption in a patient with colitis. Am J Phys Med Rehabil. 2016;95(3):a24 [r].

[26] Patil S, Willett O, Thompkins T, et al. Botulinum toxin: pharmacology and therapeutic roles in pain states. Curr Pain Headache Rep. 2016;20(15):1–8 [R].

[27] Dutt SC, Ramnani P, Thakur D, et al. Botulinum toxin in the treatment of muscle specific oro-facial pain: a literature review. J Maxillofac Oral Surg. 2015;14(2):171–5 [c].

[28] Wu T, Li JH, Song HX, et al. Effectiveness of botulinum toxin for lower limbs spasticity after stroke: a systematic review and meta-analysis. Top Stroke Rehabil. 2016;23(3):217–23 [M].

[29] Kaye AD, Daste LE. Muscle relaxants and antispasticity medications. In: Sackheim KA, editor. Pain management and palliative care: a comprehensive guide. New York: Springer Science & Business Media; 2015. p. 71–4 [r].

[30] Kim J, Hébert MF. Pharmacological treatment of musculoskeletal conditions during pregnancy and lactation. In: Fitzgerald CM, Segal NA, editors. Musculoskeletal health in pregnancy and postpartum. Switzerland: Springer International Publishing; 2015. p. 227–42 [r].

[31] Braschi E, Garrison S, Allan GM. Cyclobenzaprine for acute back pain. Can Fam Physician. 2015;61:1074 [r].

[32] Friedman BW, Dym AA, Davitt M, et al. Naproxen with cyclobenzaprine, oxycodone/acetaminophen, or placebo for treating acute low back pain: a randomized clinical trial. JAMA. 2015;314(15):1572–80 [C].

[33] Westrol MS, Awad NI, Bridgeman PJ, et al. Use of intravascular heat exchange catheter and intravenous lipid emulsion for hypothermic cardiac arrest after cyclobenzaprine overdose. Ther Hypothermia Temp Manag. 2015;5(3):171–6 [A].

[34] Chua-Tuan JL, Cao D, Iwanicki JL, et al. Cardiac sodium channel blockade after an intentional ingestion of lacosamide, cyclobenzaprine, and levetiracetam: case report. Clin Toxicol. 2015;53(6):565–8 [A].

[35] Curtis B, Jenkins C, Wiens AL. A rare fatality attributed solely to metaxalone. J Anal Toxicol. 2015;39(4):321–3 [A].

12

Drugs That Affect Autonomic Functions or the Extrapyramidal System

T. Nakaki[1]

Department of Pharmacology, Teikyo University School of Medicine, Tokyo, Japan
[1]Corresponding author: nakaki@med.teikyo-u.ac.jp

DRUGS THAT STIMULATE BOTH ALPHA-AND BETA-ADRENOCEPTORS [SEDA-33, 313; SEDA-34, 233; SEDA-35, 255; SEDA-36, 179; SEDA-37, 163]

Adrenaline (Adrenaline) and Noradrenaline (noradrenaline) [SEDA-32, 281; SEDA-33, 259; SEDA-34, 233; SEDA-35, 255; SEDA-36, 179; SEDA-37, 163]

Review

Anaphylactic shock is a life-threatening condition which needs detailed and meticulous clinical assessment and thoughtful treatment. Adrenaline can aggravate myocardial ischemia, prolong QTc interval, and induce coronary vasospasm and arrhythmias. Elderly patients, especially with a history of hypertension and coronary artery disease, are prone to these side effects. In patients who may have received β-blockers in the initial management of the acute coronary syndrome, the usual dose of adrenaline may be ineffective. It may also promote more vasospasm due to unopposed alpha adrenergic effect. Furthermore, commercially available preparations of adrenaline usually contain as a preservative, sodium metabisulfite. This substance is commonly used as an antioxidant in the food and pharmaceutical preparations. There are reports of hypersensitivity, anaphylaxis, and even death from Kounis syndrome from sulfite administration. Anaphylactoid shock has been reported during epidural anesthesia for cesarean section, in which the responsible agent was metabisulfite, as additive agent of adrenaline-containing local anesthetic. This situation poses a therapeutic dilemma in the sulfite-sensitized patients who suffer from anaphylactic shock. Physicians dealing with anaphylactic shock should be aware of this treacherous association [1A].

Cardiovascular

Patients resuscitated from cardiac arrest who have received adrenaline may have neurological problems during the post-resuscitation period, and intact survival is associated with the dose of adrenaline, and the time of its administration. Cardiac arrest is known to be associated with a heightened activity of the autonomic adrenergic nervous system, and the literature is replete of cases of patients who suffered Takotsubo syndrome after receiving only 1 mg of adrenaline. The author proposes several analytical points of the underlying mechanism(s) of the poor outcome of the patients who received adrenaline: (1) the causes of death after resuscitation (heart failure?); (2) angiographic appearance at cardiac catheterization or echocardiography, of the patients who underwent such procedures, for evidence of left apical and/or mid-ventricular ventricular "ballooning"; (3) evidence of reversibility of such changes in possible subsequent echocardiography interrogation; and (4) any evidence of regional wall motion abnormalities in myocardial territories, not perfused by the culprit vessel, which had led to a possible acute myocardial infarction, (atypical forms of Takotsubo syndrome) [2A].

Administration of adrenaline may cause cardiac complications, one of which could be Takotsubo cardiomyopathy or myocardial ischaemia. The use of adrenaline includes topical application as well as systemic administration. Lacrimal system probing and syringing is a useful procedure to assess the anatomy and functional status of the lacrimal drainage system and is used in cases of epiphora. The procedure may be accompanied by the administration of local anaesthetics together with adrenaline to reduce pain during the procedure.

Case study 1

A 23-month-old girl who presented with bilateral epiphora underwent bilateral lacrimal probing and syringing, during which a cocaine adrenaline solution was used. Two hours after the procedure, she developed acute pulmonary oedema secondary to myocardial ischaemia. The patient was treated with intravenous glyceryl trinitrate and milrinone infusions; cardiac enzymes and left ventricular function normalised over the subsequent 72 hours. Topical administration of cocaine and adrenaline solution may have dangerous systemic cardiac effects and should always be used judiciously [3A]. Cardiopulmonary resuscitation guidelines recommend the use of adrenaline during cardiopulmonary arrest. However, it should be noted that the use of adrenaline could be harmful in the event of cardiac arrest caused by coronary artery spasm [4A].

Case study 2

Intravenous adrenaline was administered during resuscitation of two cases who had witnessed cardiac arrest due to ventricular fibrillation and complete heart block. Emergent coronary angiography revealed of spasm of the entire right and left coronary artery systems. One patient's coronary artery spasm was successfully reversed immediately with administration of intracoronary boluses of nitroglycerin. The other patient's hemodynamic instability persisted, requiring temporary mechanical circulatory support with an intra-aortic balloon pump. His hemodynamics finally improved with administration of intravenous diltiazem and nitroglycerin under the intraaortic balloon pump support. They both were discharged from the hospital without any other complications.

Hematologic

A prospective observational study was aimed to determine the link between catecholamine use and dose with enterocyte damage. Sixty critically ill patients receiving catecholamines and 27 not receiving catecholamines were included. Plasma intestinal fatty acid-binding protein, a erythrocyte damage marker, was higher among patients receiving catecholamine than in controls, suggesting that enterocyte damage reflects possibly an adverse effect of catecholamines [5c].

Ephedrine [SEDA-32, 282; SEDA-33, 317; SEDA-34, 235; SEDA-35, 256; SEDA-37, 163]

Cardiovascular

The various cardiovascular adverse effects may occur with both oral and nasal administration of ephedrine and pseudoephedrine and after a single dose or prolonged (5 days) treatment, without dose–effect relationship and independently of vascular status and age. This effect may induce hypertension episodes, myocardial infarction, stroke and various neurological symptoms. Cases of unexpected death in children taking common cold treatments in were also reported. The adrenergic effect of these amines also induces hypolipidemia by reducing blood lipid concentrations [6R].

Ephedrine action is similar to amphetamine, which acts as sympathomimetic and increases mental concentration, and one of ephedrine misuse is doping problem of athletes. The adverse effects of ephedrine include myocardial damage, which is reported in two cases, in which two competitive athletes induced ventricular arrhythmias by abuse of ephedrine. Endomyocardial biopsies guided by electroanatomic mapping revealed contraction-band necrosis, a myocardial injury frequently observed in cases of catecholamine excess. The study suggests that long-term abuse of ephedrine may result in myocardial damage and that these structural alterations may promote areas of slow conduction favoring re-entrant ventricular tachyarrhythmias and a long-lasting risk of ventricular arrhythmias [7A].

Case study 1

A 38-year-old cyclist presented with rapid sustained ventricular tachycardia during an electrocardiogram stress test performed because of dizziness.

A 34-year-old boxer complained of palpitations, and resting electrocardiogram revealed ventricular bigeminy. Both patients denied cocaine abuse at first but it turned out the first patient had been taking one capsule of an ephedrine compound (containing 10 mg of ephedra alkaloids and 100 mg of caffeine) two times a day for 1 year. The second had been consuming three 500 g bottles of an ephedrine compound (containing 20 mg of ephedra alkaloids and 100 mg of caffeine) per day for 3 months. Two-dimensional echocardiography revealed a left ventricular wall thickness of 10 mm in the first case and 11 mm in the second case. Late gadolinium enhancement imaging showed a region, consistent with a focal fibrosis area, in accord with the lateral-basal portion of the right ventricle outflow tract. The origin of ventricular arrhythmias from the basis of the right ventricular outflow tract lateral wall was confirmed, and radiofrequency pulses were successfully delivered in the first patient. In the second patient, the focus of premature ventricular beats was identified in the right ventricular outflow tract posterolateral wall. Radiofrequency pulses were delivered, obtaining a long-lasting abolition of ventricular premature beats. In the follow-up period, both patients were free from arrhythmia recurrences.

Droxidopa (New Listing)

Droxidopa is a prodrug which is metabolized by aromatic L-amino acid decarboxylase to noradrenaline in neuronal cells. Droxidopa is used in place of noradrenaline itself to increase the concentration of brain noradrenaline because noradrenaline penetrates poorly the blood–brain barrier. It is indicated for the treatment of orthostatic dizziness, lightheadedness in adult patients with symptomatic neurogenic orthostatic hypotension caused by primary autonomic failure (Parkinson's disease, multiple system atrophy, and pure autonomic failure), dopamine beta-hydroxylase deficiency, and non-diabetic autonomic neuropathy. It is formulated as a once-daily transdermal patch which provides a slow and constant supply of the drug over the course of 24 hours. Adverse effects include headache, dizziness, nausea, hypertension, and fatigue.

Psychiatric

Patients with neurogenic orthostatic hypotension underwent up to 2 weeks of double-blind titration of droxidopa or placebo, followed by 8 weeks of double-blind maintenance treatment (100–600 mg thrice-daily). Adverse-event incidence was similar across groups, but 12.4% of droxidopa and 6.1% of placebo subjects withdrew because of adverse events. The most common adverse events on droxidopa (vs. placebo) were headache (13.5% vs. 7.3%) and dizziness (10.1% vs. 4.9%) [8c].

DRUGS THAT PREDOMINANTLY STIMULATE ALPHA-1-ADRENOCEPTORS [SEDA-33, 318; SEDA-34,236; SEDA-35, 257; SEDA-36, 186; SEDA-37, 163]

Phenylephrine [SEDA-15, 2808; SEDA-32, 283; SEDA-33, 318; SEDA-34, 236]

Systematic Review

A meta-analysis of cardiovascular adverse effects of topical phenylephrine was reported. Eight randomized controlled studies with a total of 916 participants were included. Phenylephrine, 2.5%, leads to no clinically relevant change in blood pressure or heart rate, and the changes in blood pressure and heart rate seen with phenylephrine, 10%, are short lived. Thus, phenylephrine, 2.5%, is safe to use in clinical routine [9M].

Review

A report evaluated subjective nasal congestion symptom relief and safety of 4 different doses of phenylephrine hydrochloride 10-mg tablets and placebo in adults with seasonal allergic rhinitis. At least one treatment-emergent adverse event was experienced by 18.4% of the participants, the most common being headache (3.0%) [10MC].

Systematic Review

Increased bioavailability of phenylephrine is reported when combined with paracetamol for the symptomatic treatment of the common cold and influenza. Such formulations could increase phenylephrine-related cardiovascular adverse events particularly in susceptible individuals. Criteria-fulfilled 47 articles of 1172 literature search revealed that blood pressure and heart rate changes are potentiated by phenylephrine with paracetamol in patients with underlying hypertension. Combination paracetamol phenylephrine oral therapy has potential to increase blood pressure more than phenylephrine alone in those with cardiovascular compromise [11M].

Genetic Factors

A study was performed to investigate whether the β2-adrenoceptor genotype affected phenylephrine dose requirements during cesarean delivery. Women undergoing elective cesarean delivery were studied. Spinal anesthesia was initiated with hyperbaric bupivacaine. Hypotension was treated with a phenylephrine infusion using a standardized algorithm for 15 minutes after the administration of spinal anesthesia. Ninety-six women completed the protocol with full data available for analysis. When adjusted for covariates, there was an increase of 200 μg (95% CI, 4–396; $P = 0.04$) in phenylephrine administered to Arg16 homozygous genotype subjects compared with Gly16 homozygous genotype subjects. Phenylephrine stimulates predominantly α1-adrenoceptors, but it does β2-adrenoceptor with clinical significance [12c].

DRUGS THAT STIMULATE α1-ADRENOCEPTORS [SEDA-33, 265; SEDA-34, 285; SEDA-35, 257; SEDA-36, 187; SEDA-37]

Dobutamine [SEDA-33, 319; SEDA-34,285; SEDA-35, 257; SEDA-36, 187; SEDA-37, 164]

Management of Adverse Drug Reactions

This study population consisted of 58 acute decompensated heart failure patients requiring inotropic support, who were randomized to ivabradine ($n = 29$) or control ($n=29$). Dobutamine was administered at incremental doses of 5, 10 and 15 µg/kg/min, with 6-h steps. Holter recording was continued during dobutamine infusion. Ivabradine 7.5 mg was given at the initiation of dobutamine and readministered at 12 h of infusion. Also, a nonrandomized beta-blocker group with 15 patients receiving beta-blocker was included in the analysis. Control and beta-blocker groups did not receive ivabradine. In the control group, mean heart rate gradually and significantly increased at each step of dobutamine infusion, whereas no significant increase in heart rate was observed in the ivabradine group. The median increase in heart rate from baseline was significantly higher in the control group compared to those in the ivabradine group [13c].

Cardiovascular

Dobutamine stress testing is commonly used in detecting and estimating the prognosis in coronary artery disease. Transient wall motion abnormalities due to stress cardiomyopathy can occur in the absence of obstructive coronary artery disease. This case could be related to Takotsubo syndrome.

Case study 1

A 48-year-old female with intermittent chest pain underwent dobutamine stress echocardiogram to rule out obstructive coronary artery disease. Her physical exam, cardiac enzymes and transthoracic echocardiogram were unremarkable. After 40 µg/kg/min and 0.5 mg atropine, she complained of intense chest pain and became hypertensive. Stress echocardiogram demonstrated mid-anterior and mid-septal hypokinesis. Emergent coronary angiogram demonstrated normal coronaries. Left ventricular angiogram in the right anterior oblique projection revealed mid-ventricular ballooning during systole with apical and basal hypercontractility. Patient demonstrated excellent recovery with expectant management [14A].

DRUGS THAT STIMULATE β2-ADRENOCEPTORS

Indacaterol [SEDA-33, 361–2; SEDA-34, 318; SEDA-36, 188; SEDA-37, 165]

Systematic Review

A study was performed to compare the safety of indacaterol versus placebo and alternative twice-daily long-acting salmeterol, formoterol and eformoterol for the treatment of patients with stable COPD. Significant adverse events, mortality and dyspnoea were included as secondary outcomes, but data were insufficient for analysis of differences in exacerbation rates for both placebo and twice-daily β2-agonist comparisons [15M].

Indacaterol vs Tiotropium

A systematic review was performed to compare the clinical efficacy and safety between indacaterol and tiotropium in patients with moderate-to-severe COPD. The incidences of nasopharyngitis, serious cardiovascular events, and serious adverse events were not different between indacaterol and tiotropium, while those of cough (OR=1.68, $P<0.001$, and RR=1.63) and COPD worsening (OR=1.18, $P=0.003$, and RR=1.12) were higher for indacaterol than tiotropium. However, when one study with only severe COPD patients was removed from the meta-analysis, the difference in the incidence of COPD worsening between indacaterol and tiotropium became non-significant (OR=1.13, $P=0.204$, and RR=1.09). The clinical efficacy and serious adverse events between indacaterol and tiotropium were equivocal in patients with moderate-to-severe COPD. Cough is a common complaint associated with indacaterol, and COPD worsening needs to be carefully monitored in severe COPD patients when treated with indacaterol [16M].

DRUGS THAT STIMULATE DOPAMINE RECEPTORS [SEDA-33, 266; SEDA-34, 283; SEDA-35, 262; SEDA-36, 190; SEDA-37, 167]

Cabergoline [SEDA-17, 169; SEDA-35, 262; SEDA-36, 190; SEDA-37, 167]

Management of Adverse Drug Reactions

Dopamine agonists such as cabergoline, which are a standard treatment for microprolactinomas, can have serious adverse effects such as psychosis or valvular heart disease. The following case report demonstrates how a partial dopamine agonist aripiprazole, in doses ranging from 2 to 10 mg/day, was effective in suppressing prolactin in a woman with a microprolactinoma who developed psychiatric side effects from cabergoline [17A].

Case study 1

A 32-year-old woman developed cyclical mood swings after being prescribed cabergoline for a pituitary microprolactinoma. These mood swings persisted for over 2 years, at which point she developed an acute manic episode with psychotic features and was admitted to a psychiatry unit. Cabergoline was discontinued and replaced with aripiprazole 10 mg/day. Her manic episode quickly resolved, and she was discharged within 6 days of admission. The aripiprazole suppressed her prolactin levels for over 18 months of follow-up, even after the dose was lowered to 2 mg/day. There was no significant change in tumor size over 15 months, treatment was well tolerated, and the woman remained psychiatrically stable.

Ropinirole [SEDA-36, 199]

Nervous System

An open-label extension study evaluated the safety profile of ropinirole prolonged release administered for 24 weeks as adjunctive to levodopa in Chinese patients with advanced Parkinson's disease. Of the 295 enrolled patients, 282 completed the study. The most common reason for withdrawal was adverse events ($n = 9$, 3.1%). Overall, 114 (38.6%) patients experienced on-treatment adverse events; the most frequent reported adverse events ($\geq 2\%$) were dyskinesia (6.1%), dizziness (4.1%), nausea (3.4%), hallucinations (3.4%), somnolence (2.7%) and decreased weight (2.4%). Sixty-eight patients (23.1%) experienced treatment-related adverse events. Six patients experienced serious adverse events, of which hallucination was determined to be a treatment-related serious adverse event. Results on safety support the long-term use of ropinirole prolonged release as an adjunctive to levodopa in Chinese patients with advanced Parkinson's disease [18c].

Rotigotine [SEDA-35, 264; SEDA-37, 167]

Systematic Review

The most common adverse events of rotigotine in the treatment of primary restless legs syndrome included application site reactions, nausea, headache and fatigue [19M].

Pramipexole, Ropinirole vs Rotigotine

An open-label study in patients with advanced-stage Parkinson's disease receiving levodopa, and experiencing sleep disturbance or early-morning motor impairment. Pramipexole/ropinirole was switched to equivalent dose rotigotine overnight or in two stages. During the 4-week treatment period, rotigotine dose adjustments were permitted (up to 16 mg/24 h). In the study, 79/87 (91%) patients completed and 2 (2%) withdrew due to adverse events. Most (84; 97%) had adverse events occurring $\geq 5\%$: application site pruritus (10%), application site erythema (7%), dizziness (7%), dyskinesia (7%), erythema (6%), pruritus (6%). Switch from pramipexole or ropinirole to rotigotine (up to 14 mg/24 h) was feasible and possibly associated with some benefit [19M].

DOPAMINE RECEPTOR AGONISTS
[SEDA-34, 242; SEDA-35, 261; SEDA-36, 191; SEDA-37, 169]

Piribedil [SEDA-35, 263; SEDA-37, 169]

℞

SPECIAL REVIEW

Piribedil and Impulse Control Disorders Recent studies suggest that impulse control disorders in Parkinson's disease are not uncommon, and antiparkinsonian therapy, mainly the use of dopaminergic agonists, plays a causal role in the development of these symptoms [20R,21R,22R]. Four patients with Parkinson's disease and one with multisystem atrophy who presented a history of pathological gambling, hyper sexuality, punding, and pathological use of the Internet secondary to piribedil, which is a dopaminergic agonist and had not been aware of this adverse events. This previously undescribed association suggests that the development of these disorders might be related to piribedil administration. It is also the first report of a patient with multisystem atrophy developing such adverse effects [23].

A 49-year-old woman complained of a 2-year history of tremor in her right hand that progressively involved her right lower limb. On examination, she presented severe resting, postural, and action tremors, as well as rigidity and mild bradykinesia. Initial treatment with levodopa led to partial symptom amelioration, but progressively, tremor became severe and could not be controlled even with high doses of levodopa. A year later, a thalamotomy was performed with an excellent response. She developed tremor in her left hand, and treatment was switched to piribedil (200 mg/day) with a further increase to the dosage of 250 mg/day. Her family stated that they were very worried because she had developed some behavioral disorders. They reported that the patient often went to bingo halls where she would spend the whole night. Once, she even betted her salary, also asked for loans, and even took money from her children. As she evaluated other compulsive behavior, she described sexual disorders, including hyper sexuality and compulsive Internet use. These disorders had appeared when she started treatment with levodopa and had worsened in the last year together with the increased dose of piribedil. She started both psychiatric and psychological therapies. At present, this behavior persists, although it is slightly less severe.

A 71-year-old man complained of a 5-year history of tremor in his right hand, gait disorders, bradykinesia, and rigidity. On examination, tremor at rest in his right hand; rigidity in his 4 limbs, mainly in his upper limbs; bradykinesia; and slow gait were observed. The brain magnetic resonance image showed brain atrophy. The patient had been on levodopa and cabergoline for several years. Three years ago, he developed behavioral disorders and pathological gambling. He went to the casino almost every day. Later, cabergoline was discontinued and piribedil (200 mg/day) was started. Since then, the patient developed exacerbated pathological gambling, hyper sexuality, *and compulsive overeating. Piribedil was then gradually tapered to be on 50 mg/day; however, the compulsive disorders persist.*

A 69-year-old man developed rest tremor in his left hand and associated mild rigidity and bradykinesia led diagnosis of Parkinson's disease. He was successfully treated with 100 mg levodopa/benserazide four times a day. Because of progressive worsening, a year later, 50 mg piribedil was prescribed, and because of visual hallucinations and confusion, 10 mg/day memantine was added. On the first examination, he was markedly hypomimic and hypophonic. Bilateral rest tremor associated to rigidity and bradykinesia more severe on the left side was evident. His gait was short stepped, and his postural reflexes were slightly abnormal. At that time, piribedil dose was increased to 150 mg/day. Two months later, his motor status was much better. However, a pattern of bizarre conducts became evident. He spent several hours working on the television and wall clock with purposeless movements and obsessive conducts. Because of the persistence of hallucinations, 5 mg/day donepezil was started, and piribedil was discontinued; a marked amelioration of the abnormal behavior and hallucinations was observed.

A 61-year-old man with a 5-year history of Parkinson's disease and alcohol abuse but had given up drinking a year ago. He was on levodopa–carbidopa at 100:25 mg two times a day and complained of progressive wearing off for the past 2 years. At examination, moderate asymmetric rigidity and bradykinesia predominant in his right hemibody were evident in the on-state with marked worsening in the off-state. Levodopa doses were increased up to 100:25 mg three times a day, and a piribedil dosage of 50 mg three times a day was added. Two months later, the parkinsonian symptoms had markedly improved, but sleep/rapid eye movement behavior disorders became evident, and he began to eat sweets compulsively. In addition to pathological eating, his wife reported that he had become extremely jealous. Piribedil doses were decreased, and psychiatric treatment started with partial control of both symptoms.

A 68-year-old woman developed postural instability and gait abnormalities 2 years ago, leading to repetitive falls a few months after onset. Within the next year, significant rigidity and bradykinesia became evident. She also complained of micrography and, 2 years after, hypophonia and dysarthria that rapidly became severe. Her medical history was unremarkable except for the sleep disorder and hypothyroidism treated with levothyroxine. A diagnosis of Parkinson's disease was considered, but a trial with levodopa showed no significant improvement. She was then treated with pramipexole without response either. On examination, she presented a moderate-to-severe asymmetric and akinetic parkinsonian syndrome with severe hypophonia and dysarthria. She required assistance for most of her daily activities. Urinary urge incontinence had developed, and a violet reddish color on her palms was evident. Symmetric soft edema on her legs had developed since she started pramipexole therapy. A brain magnetic resonance imaging

disclosed mild diffuse atrophy and leucoaraiosis. An autonomic evaluation (Ewing test) showed both parasympathetic and sympathetic dysfunctions. A polysomnogram showed mild obstructive hypo apneas and sleep/rapid eye movement behavior disorders. An apomorphine test failed to improve the symptom. A diagnosis of probable multiple-system atrophy type P was made, and Pramipexole was withdrawn. A trial with levodopa was performed with mild improvement in motor scores. Motor and phono audiologic rehabilitation therapies were encouraged. After a few months of levodopa treatment, the patient referred symptoms that were consistent with wearing-off phenomena, so levodopa dosages were initially increased to a final dosage of 850 mg/day. Wearing off improved but did not resolve, and piribedil was added progressively, reaching a total daily dose of 150 mg. Significant improvements in bradykinesia, rigidity, and hypophonia were observed. Two months after, she complained of sporadic visual hallucinations. Her relatives were also concerned because of changes they had observed in her behavior, as she was eating compulsively and asked for extra meals at any time. She also developed hyper sexuality. Piribedil was withdrawn, and the compulsive disorder improved significantly but not completely. Quetiapine at 25 mg/day led to disappearance of such symptoms.

A 73-year-old female patient with Parkinson's disease developed impulse control disorders and dopamine dysregulation syndrome owing to piribedil overdose. She was initially put on piribedil 150 mg, and owing to disease progression, levodopa was added 4 years later. Three years later, piribedil was raised to 200 mg, but presumably owing to a misunderstanding, she took 400 mg/day, which was well tolerated and produced an improvement in her parkinsonian symptoms. However, over the next few weeks, she started shopping compulsively, buying unnecessary clothes and food. In addition, she visited her dog's veterinarian several times a day with nonsense queries. During an examination, mild dyskinesia was evident. We diagnosed impulse control disorders and most likely dopamine dysregulation syndrome dopamine dysregulation syndrome. Piribedil doses were decreased to 200 mg/day, and levodopa increased up to 750 mg/day, with a clear improvement in compulsive behavior without worsening of the dyskinesia. Our case shows that even in cases in which regular doses of dopamine agonists are harmless; dose increments can often induce these unwanted effects [24A].

PIRIBEDIL-INDUCED IMPULSE CONTROL DISORDERS WERE ALSO DESCRIBED IN THE FOLLOWING SIX CASE REPORTS [25A]

Case study 1

This study involved a 67-year-old man suffering from Parkinson's disease for 8 years and a long history of depression. He was initially administered low doses of pramipexole, which were eventually increased to 4.5 mg/day. After 2 years of treatment, he developed pathological gambling. Pramipexole was discontinued, and carbidopa/

levodopa 500 mg/day was initiated in association with paroxetine 20 mg/day. As the response was poor, quetiapine 25 mg/day was added with complete control of the pathological gambling. Due to progressive worsening of the rigidity and walking difficulties, piribedil 150 mg/day was added. He presented considerable motor improvement, but he developed severe pathological gambling after 23 months of treatment, and piribedil had to be withdrawn. After discontinuation, pathological gambling disappeared, and carbidopa/levodopa had to be increased up to 1250 mg/day to control his motor symptoms.

Case study 2

A 48-year-old woman suffering from Parkinson's disease for 5 years was first put on pramipexole 3 mg/day. As she developed compulsive shopping and eating disorders with a weight increase of 15 kg, pramipexole was discontinued and ropinirole started at 6 mg/day associated with paroxetine at 20 mg/day and psychotherapy. As there was no improvement of the impulse control disorders, ropinirole had to be stopped. He was put on piribedil 200 mg/day and quetiapine 50 mg/day. However, despite initial improvement after 3 months of treatment she developed pathological gambling and hyper sexuality. Piribedil was completely stopped and carbidopa/levodopa at 250 mg/day started, while quetiapine was kept at the same dose. The patient improved her impulse control disorders.

Case study 3

A 49-year-old man with Parkinson's disease initially treated with piribedil at 150 mg/day developed pathological gambling after 24 months of exposure causing him severe social and familial problems. Piribedil was switched to ropinirole 8 mg/day and psychotherapy was initiated. As his pathological gambling did not improve, the dopamine agonist was stopped and carbidopa/levodopa was prescribed at a dose of 1000 mg/day to control his motor symptoms. The patient experienced little improvement in pathological gambling.

Case study 4

A 65-year-old man suffering from Parkinson's disease for 9 years was initially treated with piribedil at 150 mg/day for 30 months when he developed pathological gambling. Piribedil was discontinued and carbidopa/levodopa/entacapone 50 mg/tid was added. Carbidopa/levodopa/entacapone regimen was changed later for carbidopa/levodopa at 500 mg/day resulting in good control of his motor symptoms, without pathological gambling.

Case study 5

A 67-year-old man suffering from Parkinson's disease for 10 years was initially treated with pramipexole 1.75 mg/day. Five years later, due to progressive worsening, pramipexole was increased to 4.5 mg/day,

and carbidopa/levodopa/entacapone 50 mg four times/day was added. A year later, he developed irritability, compulsive eating and pathological gambling, and pramipexole had to be progressively withdrawn. Paroxetine at 20 mg/day and quetiapine at 25 mg/day were introduced with the resolution of his pathological gambling. As his motor function worsened, piribedil up to 200 mg/day was added with carbidopa/levodopa/entacapone 100 mg/tid, carbidopa/levodopa/entacapone 50 mg/qid, levodopa/benserazide in the fast release formulation 100/25 mg/tid and paroxetine 20 mg/day. The patient stopped quetiapine by himself. Two years later, he developed compulsive eating and pathological gambling; piribedil was then stopped with complete resolution of the impulse control disorders. Carbidopa/levodopa/entacapone, levodopa/benserazide and paroxetine were increased due to worsening of motor symptoms and depression.

Case study 6

A 50-year-old woman suffering from Parkinson's disease for 11 years was treated with pramipexole in low doses with progressive increases reaching 4 mg/day and levodopa/benserazide, up to 600 mg/day with good control of her symptoms, except for her right hand resting tremor. Three years after the diagnosis was made and while on pramipexole, she developed compulsive eating and shopping disorders. Pramipexole was discontinued, and she was put on piribedil at 200 mg/day. However, she developed pathological gambling, along with hyper sexuality, binge eating and compulsive shopping. At the time piribedil was reduced to 100 mg/day and amantadine 300 mg/day was added with no control of the impulse control disorders. A left thalamotomy was performed for the severe right hand resting tremor. As she continued presenting impulse control disorders, piribedil was stopped, and she was put on levodopa/benserazide 500 mg/day, and levodopa/benserazide in the fast release formulation 100/25 mg qid, with a marked improvement in the impulse control disorders.

MANAGEMENT OF ADVERSE EVENTS

There is a lack of high quality evidence available to guide the management of impulse control disorders. Another review summarized management strategies, before concentrating on the concept of dopamine agonist withdrawal syndrome and its implications for the management of impulse control disorders. Further, This article refers to controversies including the role of more recently available antiparkinsonian drugs, and potential future approaches involving routes of drug delivery, nonpharmacological treatments (such as cognitive behavioral therapy and deep brain stimulation), and other as yet experimental strategies [26R] (Figure 1).

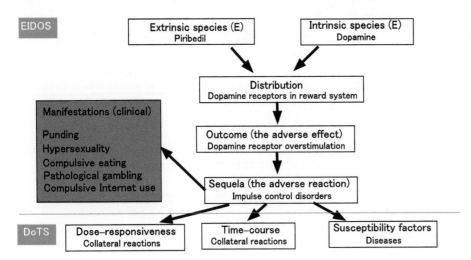

FIG. 1 The EIDOS and DoTS descriptions of impulse control disorders.

Levodopa [SEDA-32, 285; SEDA-33, 320; SEDA-34, 286–8; SEDA-35, 259; SEDA-36, 192; SEDA-37, 169]

Polyneuropathy is an adverse event, which is accompanied by levodopa/carbidopa intestinal gel treatment. The management of this adverse effect has not been established. A case record provides some insights into the pathogenesis of the event.

Case study

An acute case of polyneuropathy during levodopa/carbidopa intestinal gel treatment was reported. Based on literature investigation and the case presented by the authors, they discussed the possible role of high-levodopa dosage, vitamin B12, B6 and folate deficiency and accumulation of homocysteine and methylmalonic acid in the pathogenesis to conclude that there are several lines of circumstantial evidence that alterations of 1-carbon pathway are implicated in acute and subacute polyneuropathy during levodopa/carbidopa intestinal gel treatment [27A].

Route of Drug Administration

The cessation of levodopa administration may cause the malignant syndrome, which is a life-threatening adverse event. Perioperative periods pose a problem regarding the administration of levodopa. One solution of this issue may be the changes in administration route of levodopa and a case study reports a successful management of Parkinson's disease by perioperative levodopa administration.

Case study

A 70-year-old man with severe Parkinson's disease was scheduled for thoracic aortic aneurysm resection and aortic valve replacement. The authors administered levodopa intravenously during the perioperative period to avoid the malignant syndrome which is reported to arise with abrupt cessation of anti-Parkinson's drugs. The dose of intravenous administration was tapered with the resumption of oral intake. No manifestation of malignant syndrome was observed. Blood concentrations of levodopa were measured several times during the perioperative period. The concentration of levodopa during the surgery was relatively high; however, no adverse events of overdose (e.g. dyskinesis) occurred.

In the postoperative period, administration of levodopa was changed to the oral route and serum levels of levodopa showed a notable decrease, the cause of which may be poor absorption through the digestive system during the perioperative period. Therefore, in the peri- and post-operative periods, it may be necessary to take great care when reducing the infusion dose [28A].

Skin

Continuous infusion of levodopa/carbidopa intestinal gel is an effective treatment for patients with advanced Parkinson's disease that cannot be further improved by oral therapy. To evaluate the safety and tolerability of a device (T-Port®) for the intestinal infusion of levodopa/carbidopa gel in patients with 24 advanced Parkinson's disease. Post-operative complications were similar to endoscopic gastrojejunostomy placement (four peritoneal irritation, one pocket pain). Eight patients with prior experience with the endoscopic gastrojejunostomy preferred the intestinal infusion of levodopa/carbidopa gel. The total device experience was 83.6 years, and the average survival time was 3.6 (range 1.1–5.2) years. Two patients had died due to non-device-related reasons. Sixteen devices had been explanted due to 15 stoma reactions (14 inflammations and one infection) and one tilting of the device. The number of adverse device effects proved to be significantly lower as compared to the endoscopic gastrojejunostomy literature data [29c].

Gastrointestinal

Adverse effects were in general minor but one case of intestinal perforation and one of abdominal cellulite among 72 patients were observed [30c].

Systematic Reviews

PubMed, Google scholar, Cochrane Central Register of Controlled Trials and the Web of Science were searched for randomized, placebo-controlled trials on the long-term use of levodopa alone vs levodopa-sparing therapy as initial treatment for Parkinson's disease. Eleven RCTs were included. The author found greater number of patients on a levodopa-sparing therapy as it is three times more likely to discontinue treatment prematurely due to adverse events than levodopa treatment patients (43.7% vs 15.8%). Levodopa alone is the most effective medication available for treating the motor symptoms of Parkinson's disease patients, despite the greater incidence of involuntary movements. Meanwhile, more patients on dopamine agonists or MAOB inhibitors were more likely to discontinue treatment prematurely than levodopa alone treatment patients within the long follow-up period [31c].

Drug Administration Route

Levodopa–carbidopa intestinal gel is delivered continuously by percutaneous endoscopic gastrojejunostomy tube, which reduces levodopa-plasma-level fluctuations and can translate to reduced motor complications. Parkinson's disease patients with severe motor fluctuations despite optimized therapy received levodopa–carbidopa intestinal gel monotherapy. Additional Parkinson's disease medications were allowed >28 days post-levodopa–carbidopa intestinal gel initiation. Most adverse events were mild/moderate and transient; complication of device insertion (34.9%) was the most common. Serious adverse events occurred in 105 (32.4%), most commonly complication of device insertion (6.5%). Levodopa–carbidopa intestinal gel was generally well tolerated over 54 weeks [32c].

Drug–Drug Interactions

Parkinsonism is one of the most common extrapyramidal side effects of haloperidol. It is well established that haloperidol may impair the antiparkinsonian effect of levodopa. The following case is a drug interaction of haloperidol with levodopa in a parkinsonism patient [33A].

Case study

A 60-year-old female weighing 52 kg was admitted to the hospital with the complaints of involuntary movements. Ten years back, she was diagnosed to have parkinsonism disease and initiated on antiparkinsonian drugs. She was on tablet carbidopa/levodopa 110 mg tid and tablet trihexyphenidyl 1 mg tid. for past 3 years. There was no past history of illicit substance or alcohol abuse. There was no family history of movement disorders. Four months ago, she had consulted a local doctor for decreased sleep and headache and was prescribed tablet haloperidol 5 mg tid. After 4 weeks of initiation of haloperidol, her symptoms of Parkinsonism worsened. She increased the dose of carbidopa/levodopa and trihexyphenidyl, but the symptoms persisted. A month later, she visited another hospital and was admitted to the inpatient psychiatric unit with an additional diagnosis of neuroleptic-induced parkinsonism. On physical examination, she was found to have bradykinesia, lip smacking, flexed posture, and cogwheel rigidity. Based on detailed review of the patient medical history, haloperidol was suspected to be the causative agent for current episode in this patient and was replaced with tablet risperidone 1 mg bd. She continued to receive carbidopa/levodopa (110 mg bd) and trihexyphenidyl (2 mg in the morning) during the remaining 11 days of her hospital stay. Eight days after the withdrawal of haloperidol, her symptoms improved significantly.

Placebo-Controlled Studies

A 9-month open-label extension study assessed the long-term safety and clinical utility of a multiparticulate extended-release formulation of carbidopa–levodopa in early and advanced Parkinson's disease. Among 268 early Parkinson's disease patients, 53.4% reported adverse events; the most frequent adverse events were nausea (5.6%) and insomnia (5.6%). Among 349 advanced patients, 60.2% reported adverse events; the most frequent adverse events were dyskinesia (6.9%) and fall (6.6%). At month 9 (or early termination), 78.3% of early patients were taking the formulation three times daily (median: 720 mg/day) and 87.7% of advanced patients were taking the formulation three or four times daily (median: 1450 mg/day). Adjusting for 70% bioavailability relative to immediate-release carbidopa–levodopa, the median dosages correspond to ~500 and ~1015 mg/day of immediate-release levodopa in early and advanced Parkinson's disease, respectively. [34c].

Management of Adverse Reactions

Single oral treatment with placebo or eltoprazine, at 2.5, 5 and 7.5 mg, was tested in combination with a suprathreshold dose of levodopa. Following levodopa challenge, 5 mg eltoprazine caused a significant reduction of levodopa-induced dyskinesias on area under the curves of Clinical Dyskinesia Rating Scale and Rush Dyskinesia Rating Scale, and maximum Clinical Dyskinesia Rating Scale score. It was concluded that a single dose, oral treatment with eltoprazine has beneficial antidyskinetic effects without altering normal motor responses to L-DOPA. All doses of eltoprazine were well tolerated, with no major adverse effects [35c].

Mechanisms

A meta-analysis was conducted to evaluate the association between the polymorphism of the dopamine receptor D2 (DRD2)/kinase domain containing 1 gene and common illicit drug dependence risk including stimulants, opioid and marijuana. The DRD2/ANKK1 TaqIA polymorphism was significantly associated with increased risk of opioid dependence, but not associated with stimulants or marijuana dependence [36R].

Pramipexole

Randomized Controlled Trial

A study aimed to evaluate the efficacy and adverse events of pramipexole for the treatment of 204 adult, Chinese people with primary restless leg syndrome. The most frequent adverse events in pramipexole and placebo groups were a headache (14.7% vs 12.8%), nausea (15.7% vs 6.8%), insomnia (9.8% vs 8.8%), dizziness (7.8% vs 7.8%), fatigue (5.9% vs 4.9%). No deaths were recorded [37c].

MISCELLANEOUS OTHER DRUGS THAT INCREASE DOPAMINE ACTIVITY

Amantadine

Entacapone [SEDA-15, 1219; SEDA-32, 289; SEDA-33, 324; SEDA-34, 246]

RANDOMIZED CONTROLLED TRIAL

A pooled analysis was performed at three randomized, double-blind, 6-month, phase III studies to compare the treatment effects of entacapone (compared to placebo) in Parkinson's disease patients receiving levodopa/carbidopa or levodopa/benserazide. A total of 551 Parkinson's disease patients experiencing wearing-off were included in the analysis; 300 patients were on levodopa/benserazide and 251 on levodopa/carbidopa at baseline. Reported adverse events were comparable between levodopa/carbidopa and levodopa/benserazide users [38M].

DRUGS THAT AFFECT THE CHOLINERGIC SYSTEM [SEDA-31, 272; SEDA-32, 290; SEDA-33, 324; SEDA-34, 290, 318, SEDA-35, 266; SEDA-36, 199; SEDA-37, 172]

Anticholinergic Drugs [SEDA-31, 273; SEDA-32, 290; SEDA-33, 324; SEDA-34, 290, 318; SEDA-35, 266; SEDA-36, 199; SEDA-37, 172]

Ipratropium [SEDA-35, 266; SEDA-36, 247; SEDA-37, 198]

RANDOMIZED CONTROLLED TRIAL

A prospective, single-blinded, randomized, controlled, equivalence trial in a tertiary paediatric emergency department. Patients aged 2–15 years with acute, moderate asthma were randomized to two groups, one receiving salbutamol, prednisolone and ipratropium bromide (ipratropium group), the other receiving only salbutamol and prednisolone (control group). Three-hundred forty-seven subjects were analyzed. Adverse effects were more prevalent in the ipratropium group (13.2% vs 4.6%), a relative risk of 2.86 (95% CI 1.31–6.21) [39c].

Glycopyrronium [SEDA-36, 249; SEDA-37, 199]

RANDOMIZED CONTROLLED TRIAL

In a 26-week, multi-center, double-blind, placebo-controlled, parallel-group study, patients with moderate-to-severe COPD were randomized to glycopyrronium 50 µg od or placebo (2:1). Of the 460 patients randomized, 459 were included in the full analysis set (glycopyrronium, $n = 306$; placebo, $n = 154$; mean age 64.7 years; 425 (92.4%)) completed the study. Overall incidence of adverse events (43.6% vs 47.4%) including chronic obstructive pulmonary disease (19% vs 25.3%), nasopharyngitis (5.9% vs 7.8%), cough (1.6% vs 1.9%), benign prostatic hyperplasia (1.3% vs 0.6%), viral upper respiratory tract infection (1.3% vs 0.6%) and serious adverse events (5.6% vs 9.1%) including death (1.3% vs 0.6%) were similar [40MC].

Tiotropium [SEDA-35, 319; SEDA-36, 247; SEDA-37, 199]

RANDOMIZED CONTROLLED TRIAL

A randomised, blinded, placebo-controlled trial in 773 moderate/severe COPD patients compared once-daily glycopyrronium 50 µg, once-daily tiotropium 18 µg or placebo, when combined with salmeterol/fluticasone propionate 50/500 µg twice daily. Serious adverse events were small intestinal obstruction in glycopyrronium + salmeterol/fluticasone group (0.8%, $P > 0.05$) and atrial fibrillation in tiotropium + salmeterol/fluticasone group (0.8%, $P > 0.05$) [41C].

SYSTEMATIC REVIEW

An analysis provides an updated comprehensive safety evaluation of tiotropium using data from placebo-controlled HandiHaler(®) and Respimat(®) trials. Pooled analysis of adverse event data from tiotropium HandiHaler(®) 18 μg and Respimat(®) 5 μg randomized, double-blind, parallel-group, placebo-controlled, clinical trials in patients with COPD (treatment duration ≥4 weeks). In the study, 11 626 patients were included with placebo and 12 929 with tiotropium, totaling 14 909 (12 469 with HandiHaler®); 2440 with Respimat(®) patient-years of tiotropium exposure. The risk [RR (95% CI)] of adverse effects [0.90 (0.87, 0.930)] and of serious adverse effects [0.94 (0.89, 0.99)] was significantly lower in the tiotropium than in the placebo group HandiHaler® and Respimat® pooled results, and there was a numerically lower risk of fatal adverse effects [0.90 (0.79, 1.01)]. Incidences of typical anticholinergic adverse effects, but not serious adverse effects, were higher with tiotropium. Analyzed separately by inhaler, the risks of adverse effects and serious adverse effects in the tiotropium groups remained lower than in placebo and similarly for fatal adverse effects [42M].

TIOTROPIUM VS GLYCOPYRRONIUM

A randomised, blinded, placebo-controlled trial in moderate/severe COPD patients compared once-daily glycopyrronium 50 μg, once-daily tiotropium 18 μg or placebo, when combined with salmeterol/fluticasone propionate 50/500 μg twice daily. Serious adverse events were similar for glycopyrronium+salmeterol/fluticasone propionate, tiotropium+salmeterol/fluticasone propionate and placebo+salmeterol/fluticasone propionate with an incidence of 5.8%, 8.5% and 5.8%, respectively [41C].

Oxybutynin [SEDA-32, 266]
RANDOMIZED CONTROLLED TRIAL

Nine boys and 19 girls (6.4 ± 2.18 years old) were randomly divided into parasacral transcutaneous electrical stimulation with placebo drug (group 1) and oxybutynin with sham scapular electrical therapy (group 2). Group 1 showed no side effects while dry mouth, hyperthermia and hyperemia developed in 58%, 25% and 50% of group 2 patients (P = 0.002, 0.096 and 0.005, respectively). Treatment was discontinued by 13.3% of patients in group 2 [43c].

A phase 3 study was performed in 626 patients with urinary incontinence. Patients were randomized 1:1:1 to receive 12 weeks of oxybutynin transdermal gel 3% 84 mg, oxybutynin transdermal gel 3% 56 mg, or placebo gel applied once daily. Dry mouth was the most common treatment-related adverse events, occurred more often with oxybutynin transdermal gel 3% 84 mg/day (12.1%) vs. placebo (5.0%) (P = 0.028); Application site erythema occurred more often with oxybutynin transdermal gel 3% 84 mg/day (3.7%) versus placebo (1.0%) (P = NS); No serious treatment-related adverse events occurred [44C].

Imidafenacin

Imidafenacin is an antagonist of muscarinic cholinergic receptors and used for treatments of overactive bladder in many countries worldwide except for the United States.

SYSTEMATIC REVIEW

A systematic review was performed to assess the efficacy and safety of imidafenacin for treating overactive bladder in adult. A total of 1428 patients were included in the analysis, which compared imidafenacin with propiverine and solifenacin. Imidafenacin was better tolerated than propiverine in the safety, indicated by dry mouth (OR 0.73, 95% CI 0.54–0.98, P = 0.04) and any adverse events (OR 0.63, 95% CI 0.46–0.88, P = 0.006) and was also better tolerated than solifenacin in the safety, indicated by constipation (OR 0.21, 95% CI 0.08–0.53, P = 0.001) and any adverse events (OR 0.33, 95% CI 0.15–0.71, P = 0.004) [45M].

Solifenacin [SEDA-35, 266]
RANDOMIZED CONTROLLED TRIAL

A multicenter, randomized, double-blind study evaluating solifenacin vs placebo on return to continence in patients who were still incontinent 7–21 days after catheter removal after robot-assisted radical prostatectomy. Overall 640 patients were randomized to solifenacin vs placebo and 17 failed to take medication. There was no difference in time to continence (P = 0.17). Continence was achieved by study end in 91 of 313 (29%) vs 66 of 309 (21%), respectively (P = 0.04). Pads per day change from baseline was −3.2 and −2.9, respectively (P = 0.03). Dry mouth was the only common adverse event seen in 6.1% and 0.6%, respectively. Constipation rates were similar [46C].

GASTROINTESTINAL

A multicentre, open-label, phase IV study enrolled patients aged ≥20 years with overactive bladder, as determined by an overactive bladder symptom score. Patients meeting eligibility criteria continued to receive solifenacin (2.5 or 5 mg once daily) and additional mirabegron (25 mg once daily) for 16 weeks. The most common treatment-emergent adverse events was constipation, with similar incidence in the groups receiving a dose increase to that observed in the groups maintained on the original dose [47c].

Choline Esterase Inhibitors

Rivastigmine **[SEDA-35, 12; SEDA-36, 5; SEDA-37, 9]***Donepezil* **[SEDA-35, 13; SEDA-36, 6; SEDA-37, 10]***Galantamine* **[SEDA-35, 14; SEDA-36, 7; SEDA-37, 11]**

SYSTEMATIC REVIEWS

A systematic review of prospective, randomised controlled trials were performed in order to assess the efficacy and safety of choline esterase inhibitors compared with placebo in patients with Parkinson's disease. From 945 references identified and screened, 19 were assessed for eligibility, and 4 trials were included for a total of 941 patients with Parkinson's disease. The choline esterase inhibitors included rivastigmine, donepezil, and galantamine. Adverse drug reactions were significantly higher than the placebo group. In this systematic review, however, the adverse drug reactions were not specifically defined. A significantly reduced death rate was observed in the treated cohort as compared with placebo [48M].

References

[1] Kounis NG, Soufras GD, Davlouros P, et al. Combined etiology of anaphylactic cardiogenic shock: amiodarone, epinephrine, cardioverter defibrillator, left ventricular assist devices and the Kounis syndrome. Ann Card Anaesth. 2015;18(2):261–4 [A].

[2] Madias JE. Is the worse outcome associated with epinephrine in resuscitated patients due to Takotsubo syndrome? Int J Cardiol. 2015;182:223 [A].

[3] McGovern E, Moylett E, McMahon CJ. Myocardial ischaemia following cocaine and adrenaline exposure in a child during an ophthalmological procedure. Ir Med J. 2015;108(3):89–90 [A].

[4] Zhang ZP, Su X, Yang YC, et al. Cardiac arrest with coronary artery spasm: does the use of epinephrine during cardiopulmonary arrest exacerbate the spasm? Am J Emerg Med. 2015;33(3):479.e5–6 [A].

[5] Piton G, Cypriani B, Regnard J, et al. Catecholamine use is associated with enterocyte damage in critically ill patients. Shock. 2015;43(5):437–42 [c].

[6] Laccourreye O, Werner A, Giroud JP, et al. Benefits, limits and danger of ephedrine and pseudoephedrine as nasal decongestants. Eur Ann Otorhinolaryngol Head Neck Dis. 2015;132(1):31–4 [R].

[7] Casella M, Dello Russo A, Izzo G, et al. Ventricular arrhythmias induced by long-term use of ephedrine in two competitive athletes. Heart Vessels. 2015;30(2):280–3 [A].

[8] Hauser RA, Isaacson S, Lisk JP, et al. Droxidopa for the short-term treatment of symptomatic neurogenic orthostatic hypotension in Parkinson's disease (nOH306B). Mov Disord. 2015;30(5):646–54 [c].

[9] Stavert B, McGuinness MB, Harper CA, et al. Cardiovascular adverse effects of phenylephrine eyedrops: a systematic review and meta-analysis. JAMA Ophthalmol. 2015;133(6):647–52 [M].

[10] Meltzer EO, Ratner PH, McGraw T. Oral phenylephrine HCL for nasal congestion in seasonal allergic rhinitis: a randomized, open-label, placebo-controlled study. J Allergy Clin Immunol Pract. 2015;3(5):702–8 [MC].

[11] Atkinson HC, Potts AL, Anderson BJ. Potential cardiovascular adverse events when phenylephrine is combined with paracetamol: simulation and narrative review. Eur J Clin Pharmacol. 2015;71(8):931–8 [M].

[12] Odekon L, Landau R, Blouin JL, et al. The effect of beta2-adrenoceptor genotype on phenylephrine dose administered during spinal anesthesia for cesarean delivery. Anesth Analg. 2015;120(6):1309–16 [c].

[13] Cavusoglu Y, Mert U, Nadir A, et al. Ivabradine treatment prevents dobutamine-induced increase in heart rate in patients with acute decompensated heart failure. J Cardiovasc Med (Hagerstown). 2015;16(9):603–9 [c].

[14] Chandraprakasam S, Kanuri S, Hunter C. Mid-ventricular variant of dobutamine-induced stress cardiomyopathy. Res Cardiovasc Med. 2015;4(2):e25223 [A].

[15] Geake JB, Dabscheck EJ, Wood-Bake R, et al. Indacaterol, a once-daily beta2-agonist, versus twice-daily beta(2)-agonists or placebo for chronic obstructive pulmonary disease. Cochrane Database Syst Rev. 2015;1:Cd010139 [M].

[16] Kim JS, Park J, Lim SY, et al. Comparison of clinical efficacy and safety between indacaterol and tiotropium in |COPD: meta-analysis of randomized controlled trials. PLoS One. 2015;10(3): e0119948 [M].

[17] Burback L. Management of a microprolactinoma with aripiprazole in a woman with cabergoline-induced mania. Endocrinol Diabetes Metab Case Rep. 2015;2015:150100 [A].

[18] Zhang Z, Wang J, Zhang X, et al. An open-label extension study to evaluate the safety of ropinirole prolonged release in Chinese patients with advanced Parkinson's disease. Curr Med Res Opin. 2015;31(4):723–30 [c].

[19] Ding J, Fan W, Chen HH, et al. Rotigotine in the treatment of primary restless legs syndrome: a meta-analysis of randomized placebo-controlled trials. J Huazhong Univ Sci Technolog Med Sci. 2015;35(2):169–75 [M].

[20] Seeman P. Parkinson's disease treatment may cause impulse-control disorder via dopamine D3 receptors. Synapse. 2015;69(4):183–9 [R].

[21] Napier TC, Corvol JC, Grace AA, et al. Linking neuroscience with modern concepts of impulse control disorders in Parkinson's disease. Mov Disord. 2015;30(2):141–9 [R].

[22] Weintraub D, David AS, Evans AH, et al. Clinical spectrum of impulse control disorders in Parkinson's disease. Mov Disord. 2015;30(2):121–7 [R].

[23] Tschopp L, Salazar Z, Gomez Botello MT, et al. Impulse control disorder and piribedil: report of 5 cases. Clin Neuropharmacol. 2010;33(1):11–3.

[24] Giugni JC, Tschopp L, Escalante V, et al. Dose-dependent impulse control disorders in piribedil overdose. Clin Neuropharmacol. 2012;35(1):49–50 [A].

[25] Micheli FE, Giugni JC, Espinosa ME, et al. Piribedil and pathological gambling in six parkinsonian patients. Arq Neuropsiquiatr. 2015;73(2):115–8 [A].

[26] Samuel M, Rodriguez-Oroz M, Antonini A, et al. Management of impulse control disorders in Parkinson's disease: controversies and future approaches. Mov Disord. 2015;30(2):150–9 [R].

[27] Uncini A, Eleopra R, Onofrj M. Polyneuropathy associated with duodenal infusion of levodopa in Parkinson's disease: features, pathogenesis and management. J Neurol Neurosurg Psychiatry. 2015;86(5):490–5 [A].

[28] Terashima S, Yanagido Y, Watabe A, et al. Perioperative management of a patient with severe Parkinson's disease with intravenous levodopa administration. Masui. 2015;64(8): 845–848 [A].

[29] van Laar T, Nyholm D, Nyman R. Transcutaneous port for levodopa/carbidopa intestinal gel administration in Parkinson's disease. Acta Neurol Scand. 2016;133(3):208–15 [c].

[30] Buongiorno M, Antonelli F, Camara A, et al. Long-term response to continuous duodenal infusion of levodopa/carbidopa gel in patients with advanced Parkinson disease: the Barcelona registry. Parkinsonism Relat Disord. 2015;21(8):871–6 [c].

[31] Xie CL, Zhang YY, Wang XD, et al. Levodopa alone compared with levodopa-sparing therapy as initial treatment for Parkinson's disease: a meta-analysis. Neurol Sci. 2015;36(8):1319–29 [c].

[32] Fernandez HH, Standaert DG, Hauser RA, et al. Levodopa-carbidopa intestinal gel in advanced Parkinson's disease: final 12-month, open-label results. Mov Disord. 2015;30(4):500–9 [c].

[33] Lucca JM, Ramesh M, Parthasarathi G, et al. An adverse drug interaction of haloperidol with levodopa. Indian J Psychol Med. 2015;37(2):220–2 [A].

[34] Waters CH, Nausieda P, Dzyak L, et al. Long-term treatment with extended-release carbidopa-levodopa (IPX066) in early and advanced Parkinson's disease: a 9-month open-label extension trial. CNS Drugs. 2015;29(4):341–50 [c].

[35] Svenningsson P, Rosenblad C, Af Edholm Arvidsson K, et al. Eltoprazine counteracts l-dopa-induced dyskinesias in Parkinson's disease: a dose-finding study. Brain. 2015;138(Pt 4):963–73 [c].

[36] Deng XD, Jiang H, Ma Y, et al. Association between DRD2/ANKK1 TaqIA polymorphism and common illicit drug dependence: evidence from a meta-analysis. Hum Immunol. 2015;76(1):42–51 [R].

[37] Zhang J, Liu B, Zheng Y, et al. Pramipexole for Chinese people with primary restless legs syndrome: a 12-week multicenter, randomized, double-blind study. Sleep Med. 2015;16(1):181–5 [c].

[38] Kuoppamaki M, Leinonen M, Poewe W. Efficacy and safety of entacapone in levodopa/carbidopa versus levodopa/benserazide treated Parkinson's disease patients with wearing-off. J Neural Transm (Vienna). 2015;122(12):1709–14 [M].

[39] Wyatt EL, Borland ML, Doyle SK, et al. Metered-dose inhaler ipratropium bromide in moderate acute asthma in children: a single-blinded randomised controlled trial. J Paediatr Child Health. 2015;51(2):192–8 [c].

[40] Wang C, Sun T, Huang Y, et al. Efficacy and safety of once-daily glycopyrronium in predominantly Chinese patients with moderate-to-severe chronic obstructive pulmonary disease: the GLOW7 study. Int J Chron Obstruct Pulmon Dis. 2015;10:57–68 [MC].

[41] Frith PA, Thompson PJ, Ratnavadivel R, et al. Glycopyrronium once-daily significantly improves lung function and health status when combined with salmeterol/fluticasone in patients with COPD: the GLISTEN study, a randomised controlled trial. Thorax. 2015;70(6):519–27 [C].

[42] Halpin DM, Dahl R, Hallmann C, et al. Tiotropium Handihaler(®) and Respimat(®) in COPD: a pooled safety analysis. Int J Chron Obstruct Pulmon Dis. 2015;10:239–59 [M].

[43] Quintiliano F, Veiga ML, Moraes M, et al. Transcutaneous parasacral electrical stimulation vs oxybutynin for the treatment of overactive bladder in children: a randomized clinical trial. J Urol. 2015;193(5 Suppl):1749–53 [c].

[44] Goldfischer ER, Sand PK, Thomas H, et al. Efficacy and safety of oxybutynin topical gel 3% in patients with urgency and/or mixed urinary incontinence: a randomized, double-blind, placebo-controlled study. Neurourol Urodyn. 2015;34(1):37–43 [C].

[45] Huang W, Zong H, Zhou X, et al. Efficacy and safety of imidafenacin for overactive bladder in adult: a systematic review and meta-analysis. Int Urol Nephrol. 2015;47(3):457–64 [M].

[46] Bianco FJ, Albala DM, Belkoff LH, et al. A randomized, double-blind, solifenacin succinate versus placebo control, phase 4, multicenter study evaluating urinary continence after robotic assisted radical prostatectomy. J Urol. 2015;193(4):1305–10 [C].

[47] Yamaguchi O, Kakizaki H, Homma Y, et al. Safety and efficacy of mirabegron as 'add-on' therapy in patients with overactive bladder treated with solifenacin: a post-marketing, open-label study in Japan (MILAI study). BJU Int. 2015;116(4):612–22 [c].

[48] Pagano G, Rengo G, Pasqualetti G, et al. Cholinesterase inhibitors for Parkinson's disease: a systematic review and meta-analysis. J Neurol Neurosurg Psychiatry. 2015;86(7):767–73 [M].

13

Dermatological Drugs, Topical Agents, and Cosmetics

Adrienne T. Black[1]

3E Company, Warrenton, VA, USA
[1]Corresponding author: adrienne159@gmail.com

INTRODUCTION

This chapter provides a concise overview of drug-induced skin reactions or side effects reported in the literature from January 2015 to December 2015. The effects include those resulting from medications used to treat dermal disorders such as acne and psoriasis as well as drug-associated cutaneous reactions by antivirals, neurological treatments and chemotherapy. The information presented includes case reports, clinical trial results, pooled clinical trial analyses and literature reviews.

ACNE

Clindamycin Phosphate and Benzoyl Peroxide

A clinical trial was conducted in Japan to evaluate the efficacy and safety of topical clindamycin phosphate and benzoyl peroxide combination gel for the treatment of acne vulgaris. A total of 800 patients were randomized into 3 treatment groups: clindamycin phosphate (1.2%) and benzoyl peroxide (3.0%) combination gel once daily, twice daily or clindamycin phosphate (1.2%) alone twice daily. All treatments were topical and applied for 12 weeks. The majority of adverse events were mild or moderate; a higher incidence occurred with the combination gel (once daily, 24.0%; twice daily, 35.1%) versus clindamycin phosphate alone (9.0%) [1C].

Tretinoin

A prospective, randomized, open-label, active-controlled, parallel-group, multicenter, phase 4 clinical trial compared the safety and efficacy of a tretinoin

(0.025%) nanogel with the standard tretinoin (0.025%) formulation for treatment of facial acne vulgaris. A total of 207 patients with facial acne vulgaris applied the nanogel ($n = 207$) or the standard formulation ($n = 98$) to the face once daily for 12 weeks. Most adverse events were mild in nature and occurred less frequently with the nanogel as compared to the standard treatment (13.3% versus 24.7%, respectively). The most common adverse event was dryness (nanogel, 4.8%; standard gel, 8.2%); peeling of skin, burning sensation and photosensitivity occurred only with the standard treatment [2C].

ACTINIC KERATOSIS

Ingenol Mebutate

A phase 3b study (NCT01787383) was conducted to evaluate the use of ingenol mebutate to treat actinic keratosis. A total of 199 adult patients with non-hyperkeratotic actinic keratoses on two separate body regions (face/scalp and trunk/extremities) were treated with 0.015% or 0.05% ingenol mebutate gel for 3 days as either simultaneously ($n = 101$, applied at the same time but each to separate body areas) or sequentially ($n = 98$, 0.015% first and then 0.05%, each to separate body areas). The frequency of adverse events was similar with both medication concentrations; the most common side effect was pruritus and pain at the application site [3C].

5-Fluorouracil and Ingenol Mebutate

The standard treatment of actinic keratosis is administration of 5-fluorouracil cream. An open-label, prospective, randomized, controlled clinical trial was conducted to compare the safety of 5-fluorouracil cream with ingenol mebutate gel, a new topical treatment for facial actinic keratosis. A total of 100 patients with facial actinic keratosis applied the ingenol gel (0.015%) once daily for 3 consecutive days or 5-fluorouracil (5.0%) cream twice daily for 4 weeks. Adverse effects were generally similar between the treatments and included pruritus, pain, tearing, conjunctival hyperemia and headaches. In contrast, eyelid edema occurred more frequently with ingenol mebutate application [4c].

5-Fluorouracil Plus Salicylic Acid

The safety of 5-fluorouracil plus salicylic acid as a treatment for actinic keratosis was assessed in an exploratory, open, randomized study in Germany (NCT01358851). A total of 66 adult patients with moderate or severe grade 2 or 3 hyperkeratotic actinic keratoses on the face or scalp received topical 5-fluorouracil (5%) with salicylic acid (10%) ($n=33$) once daily for 6 weeks or up to 2 cryosurgery treatments ($n=33$) 3 weeks apart. Drug-related adverse events were reported in both treatment groups: combination ($n=63$) and cryosurgery ($n=2$). The most common 5-fluorouracil plus salicylic acid-related adverse effects were burning sensation ($n=3$) and application site erythema ($n=3$); these effects were considered serious and lead to either an interruption ($n=3$) or discontinuation ($n=3$) of treatment [5c].

ANTIFUNGALS

Voriconazole

A retrospective analysis was performed to determine the prevalence of phototoxic reactions associated with voriconazole, an antifungal agent, in 430 pediatric patients receiving treatment between 2003 and 2013. Phototoxicity occurred in 20% of all patients but was more likely in patients with treatment of at least 6 months (47%) and in all nonmelanoma skin cancer patients (100%). The phototoxic reactions were managed by discontinuation of voriconazole (5%), dermatology referral (6%) and sun protection advising from their primary physician (26%) [6R].

Isavuconazole

An open-label, multicenter, sequential-cohort, phase 2 study assessed the safety of isavuconazole, a triazole molecule with broad-spectrum antifungal activity, as a prophylaxic treatment in neutropenic patients in Germany (NCT00413439). A total of 20 adult patients with acute myeloid leukemia and neutropenia who had undergone chemotherapy were divided into 2 study groups, low-

and high-dose isavuconazole, administered intravenously until 2 days after resolution of the neutropenia up to a maximum of 28 days. The low-dose group ($n=11$) received 3 initial doses of isavuconazole (400, 200, and 200 mg) on day 1, the 200 mg twice daily on day 2, and then 200 mg once from day 3 to the end of treatment. The doses for the high-dose group ($n=12$) were double that for the low-dose group: 3 initial doses of isavuconazole (800, 400, and 400 mg) on day 1, then 400 mg twice daily on day 2, and then 400 mg once daily from day 3 to the end of treatment. Drug-related adverse events occurred in both treatment groups, low-dose ($n=5$) and high-dose ($n=8$), and included headache and rash ($n=3$ for each group). Isavuconazole treatment was discontinued due to hypersensitivity reactions in each group ($n=1$ each); no other serious drug-related adverse events occurred [7c].

Isavuconazole and Voriconazole

The safety of isavuconazole was compared to that of the current standard voriconazole medication in a phase 3, double-blind, global multicenter, comparative-group study (NCT00412893). Patients ($n=527$ total; 258 per treatment group) with invasive mold disease received isavuconazole (200 mg) intravenously 3 times daily on days 1 and 2 and then 200 mg either intravenously or orally once daily; or voriconazole (6 mg/kg) intravenously twice daily on day 1, 4 mg/kg intravenously twice daily on day 2 and then intravenously 4 mg/kg twice daily or orally. Adverse events occurred in both treatment groups: isavuconazole ($n=247$) and voriconazole ($n=255$). The most common of these effects were gastrointestinal disorders (isavuconazole, $n=174$; voriconazole, $n=180$) and infections and infestations (isavuconazole, $n=152$; voriconazole, $n=158$). When compared to voriconazole, isavuconazole treatment had a lower rate of hepatobiliary disorders ($n=42$ versus $n=23$, respectively), eye disorders ($n=69$ versus $n=39$, respectively), and general skin or subcutaneous tissue disorders ($n=110$ versus $n=86$, respectively) [8C].

ATOPIC DERMATITIS

Azathioprine and Betamethasone

A prospective, single-blind, randomized trial compared the efficacy and occurrence of side effects of a topical azathioprine (4%) and betamethasone (0.05%) combination versus topical betamethasone (0.05%) alone for the treatment of atopic dermatitis. A total of 70 patients (2–18 years) with moderate to severe atopic dermatitis received treatments twice daily for 8 weeks. The frequency of adverse effects was similar in both treatment groups; the betamethasone alone group reported irritation ($n = 3$) and itching ($n = 2$) which subsided within 2 weeks [9c].

Crisaborole

Crisaborole, a recently developed phosphodiesterase-4 inhibitor, was evaluated for the treatment of atopic dermatitis in a randomized, double-blind phase 2a study (NCT01301508) in 25 adults with mild to moderate atopic dermatitis and two distinct lesions. Patients received 2% topical crisaborole ointment or vehicle twice daily for 6 weeks (one treatment per lesion). Adverse events ($n = 29$) occurred in 11 patients and included localized application site reactions in 3 patients. No serious adverse events were reported; the majority of adverse events (90%) were considered mild and not treatment related [10c].

In a second randomized, double-blind, dose-ranging, phase 2 study, crisaborole treatment was assessed in 96 adolescents (12–17 years old) with mild to moderate atopic dermatitis and having two distinct lesions. Treatments included 0.5% or 2% topical crisaborole applied once ($n = 44$) or twice ($n = 42$) daily for 29 days. No serious adverse effects were reported in either group with only 4 mild application site reactions occurring (once daily, $n = 3$; twice daily, $n = 1$) [11c].

JNJ-39758979

A phase 2a, randomized, double-blind, placebo-controlled, multicenter, parallel-group clinical study was conducted to evaluate the safety and efficacy of JNJ-39758979, a H4 R-antagonist, in adult Japanese patients with moderate atopic dermatitis. Patients were to receive JNJ-39758979 (100 or 300 mg) or placebo once daily for 6 weeks. However, the study was stopped prior to completing the planned enrollment number (88 patients enrolled versus 105 patients planned) and unblinded due the development of adverse effects. The occurrence of adverse events was similar for JNJ-39758979 and placebo except for 2 patients treated with 300 mg JNJ-39758979 who developed neutropenia. The authors state that administration of JNJ-39758979 is associated with drug-induced agranulocytosis [12c].

UR-1505 and Tacrolimus

UR-1505 is designed for treatment of inflammatory skin diseases by modulating immune responses. A randomized, double-blind controlled phase 2 exploratory trial was conducted in 25 patients with atopic dermatitis lesions on two symmetrical areas received either 0.5%, 1%, or 2% UR-1505 or 0.1% tacrolimus ointment ($n = 13$ for vehicle, $n = 8$ for UR-1505 0.5%, $n = 9$ for 1% UR-1505, $n = 8$ for 2% UR-1505, and $n = 12$ for tacrolimus) once daily for 28 days. No adverse reactions were reported; however, frequent local symptoms were reported after medication application such as itching, tingling, tightness, and heat/burning sensations. These symptoms occurred at similar rates for vehicle, 1% UR-1505, and 2% UR-1505 but occurred more frequently with 0.5% UR-1505 and tacrolimus treatment [13c].

BASAL CELL CARCINOMA

Vismodegib

A multicenter, open-label trial to determine the safety of vismodegib, a Hedgehog pathway inhibitor, for treatment of advanced basal cell carcinoma is currently underway in 1227 patients (18 years and older) with local or metastatic advanced basal cell carcinoma and who are ineligible for surgery (NCT01367665). All patients received oral vismodegib (150 mg) once daily in 28-day treatment cycles with a median 36.4 weeks of treatment duration. This report describes the interim analysis results, conducted of 500 patients with 1 year of follow-up. Adverse events (grade 1 or 2) occurred in 491 patients and included muscle spasms ($n = 317$), alopecia ($n = 307$), dysgeusia ($n = 269$), weight loss ($n = 162$), asthenia ($n = 141$), decreased appetite ($n = 126$), ageusia ($n = 112$), diarrhea ($n = 83$), nausea ($n = 80$), and fatigue ($n = 80$). Serious adverse events occurred in 108 of 499 patients including 21 deaths [14C].

A second nonrandomized, multicenter, open-label, phase 2 trial (NCT01201915) was conducted in 74 patients with new, operable, nodular basal cell carcinoma. All patients received vismodegib (150 mg/day) followed by lesion excision; the treatment groups were vismodegib for 12 weeks ($n = 24$), vismodegib for 12 weeks followed by 24 weeks of observation before excision ($n = 25$), and vismodegib for 8 weeks on followed by 4 weeks off and treatment again for 8 weeks ($n = 25$). Adverse events were reported in 73 patients with the most commonly were muscle spasms (76%), alopecia (58%), and dysgeusia (50%). Study discontinuation occurred with 5 patients due to dysgeusia ($n = 3$), muscle spasm ($n = 2$) and alopecia ($n = 2$). Serious adverse events ($n = 6$) included atrial fibrillation, hemorrhoidal hemorrhage, small intestinal hemorrhage, hepatitis, bladder cancer, liposarcoma, and ischemic stroke; most of these events were considered non-treatment related. One case of hepatitis was drug related and resolved with 2 months of vismodegib discontinuation. Of note, the majority of the adverse effects fully resolved within 6–12 weeks of end of treatment [15c].

MELANOMA

BRAF Inhibitors: Vemurafenib and Dabrafenib

A retrospective cohort study compared the adverse effects of a BRAF inhibitor (vemurafenib or dabrafenib) monotherapy versus a BRAF-kinase inhibitor combination (dabrafenib with trametinib dimethyl sulfoxide, a kinase inhibitor) as treatment for metastatic melanoma. The study included 185 patients in Australia with stage 3 or 4 melanoma treated with dabrafenib ($n=119$), vemurafenib ($n=36$) or the combination therapy ($n=30$). Adverse events occurred more frequently with dabrafenib and vemurafenib as compared to the combination therapy and included Grover disease (dabrafenib, $n=51$, and vemurafenib, $n=14$), plantar hyperkeratosis (dabrafenib, $n=47$, and vemurafenib, $n=14$), verrucal keratosis (dabrafenib, $n=79$, and vemurafenib, $n=26$) and photosensitivity (dabrafenib, $n=1$ and vemurafenib, $n=14$). Severe adverse events including the development of cutaneous squamous cell carcinoma were also reported with the monotreatments (dabrafenib, $n=31$; vemurafenib, $n=13$). No cases of squamous cell carcinoma, verrucal keratosis, Grover disease were reported with the combination therapy, although folliculitis occurred more frequently with the combination treatment ($n=12$) as compared to dabrafenib alone ($n=8$) [16C].

A similar clinical trial in Australian patients with metastatic melanoma extended the BRAF inhibitors vemurafenib or dabrafenib or combination BRAF inhibitor/kinase inhibitor treatment duration for at least 1 year. Although it was thought that adverse skin effects generally occur in the first 8–26 weeks of treatment with BRAF inhibitors, this study showed that these effects (Grover disease (45%), plantar hyperkeratosis (45%), verrucal keratosis (18%) and cutaneous squamous cell carcinoma (16%)) were still evident after 52 weeks of continuous monotherapy. In contrast, the most common adverse event after 52 weeks with the combination treatment was an acneiform eruption (40%) [17C].

An open-label, phase 3 trial with the same treatments for metastatic melanoma (vemurafenib and dabrafenib monotreatment or a combination of BRAF inhibitor with trametinib) showed similar results (NCT01597908). A total of 704 patients with metastatic melanoma with a BRAF V600 mutation were treated with either the combination therapy (dabrafenib, 150 mg twice daily, and trametinib, 2 mg once daily; $n=352$) or vemurafenib (960 mg twice daily; $n=352$). Severe adverse events (grade 3 or 4) and patient discontinuations occurred at similar rate across all treatments (combination therapy, 52%; vemurafenib, 63%). Pyrexia was the most common effect leading to dose reduction or discontinuation in the combination group, and rash was the most common cause of dose reduction in the vemurafenib group. Of note, cutaneous squamous cell carcinoma and keratoacanthomas occurred more frequently with vemurafenib treatment as with the combination treatment (18% versus 1%, respectively) [18C].

The adverse cutaneous effects of vemurafenib treatment for 2–52 weeks in 20 patients with a BRAF mutant (V600E, V600K, V600R) metastatic malignant melanoma were assessed in a prospective study. Adverse skin events occurred in 11 patients; these events occurred between 2 and 16 weeks after starting treatment in 10 patients and more than 1 event reported in each patient. The effects included verrucous papillomas ($n=8$), squamous cell carcinoma ($n=2$), keratoacanthomas ($n=4$), hyperkeratotic, folliculocentric eruption ($n=7$), facial erythema ($n=4$), seborrhoeic dermatitis-like eczema on the scalp ($n=11$), cystic lesions ($n=3$), hand–foot skin reaction ($n=3$), alopecia ($n=2$) and phototoxic reactions after UV exposure ($n=5$) [19c].

Ipilimumab

The safety and efficacy of ipilimumab for treatment of metastatic melanoma were assessed in an open-label, multicenter, phase 2, single-arm trial in Germany (NCT01355120). A total of 103 adult patients with unresectable stage III or stage IV metastatic melanoma who had received at least one dose of chemotherapy or immunotherapy were included; no patients had received ipilimumab. All patients received 4 intravenous infusions of ipilimumab (3 mg/kg) in weeks 1, 4, 7 and 10. Adverse events occurred in 51 patients; of these, 35 events were considered treatment related. The cutaneous adverse reactions (dermatitis, pruritus, rash and erythema) were grade 1 or 2, while 20 events were grade 3–4 and included colitis, diarrhea, gastric perforation. One possible treatment-related death occurred (pancytopenia with following cerebral hemorrhage and respiratory insufficiency) [20C].

Nivolumab

A randomized, double-blind, multicenter, phase 3 study assessed the efficacy and safety of nivolumab, a programmed death 1 (PD-1) checkpoint inhibitor, ipilimumab alone or a combination nivolumab and ipilimumab for treatment of metastatic melanoma (NCT01844505). Patients ($n=314$) received either nivolumab (3 mg/kg) every 2 weeks ($n=316$), the combination nivolumab (1 mg/kg) plus ipilimumab (3 mg/kg) every 3 weeks and then nivolumab only (3 mg/kg) every 2 weeks, or 3 mg of ipilimumab alone (3 mg/kg) every 3 weeks ($n=315$). All treatments were administered intravenously until disease progression or study discontinuation. Adverse events occurred in all groups: nivolumab

(82.1%), nivolumab plus ipilimumab (95.5%) and ipilimumab (86.2%), and included diarrhea, fatigue and pruritus. Serious adverse events lead to study discontinuation with nivolumab (7.7%), the combination treatment (36.4%) and ipilimumab (14.8%); these effects included diarrhea and colitis with 2 deaths (nivolumab, 1 case of neutropenia; and ipilimumab, 1 case of cardiac arrest) [21C].

Pembrolizumab

The efficacy and safety of pembrolizumab, a programmed cell death-1 (PD-1) antibody, were compared with ipilimumab for the treatment of advanced melanoma in a randomized, controlled, phase 3 trial in 16 countries. A total of 834 patients with advanced melanoma received pembrolizumab (10 mg/kg) intravenously every 2 weeks ($n=279$) or 3 weeks ($n=277$), or 4 intravenous doses of ipilimumab (3 mg/kg, $n=278$) every 3 weeks. Adverse events of grades 3–5 occurred in all groups: 13.3% with pembrolizumab, 2 weeks; 10.1% with pembrolizumab, 3 weeks; 19.9% with the ipilimumab group. The rates of study discontinuation due to adverse events for the 3 treatment groups were 4.0%, 6.9%, and 9.4%, respectively. One ipilimumab-related fatality was reported due to cardiac arrest in a diabetic patient brought on by drug-induced diarrhea and metabolic changes [22C].

A multicenter, randomized phase 2 trial from 73 centers in 12 countries evaluated the efficacy and safety of pembrolizumab versus the standard chemotherapy for treatment of ipilimumab-refractory melanoma (NCT01704287). Patients ($n=540$) with ipilimumab-refractory or BRAF (V600) mutant-positive melanoma received pembrolizumab (2 mg/kg, $n=180$; or 10 mg/kg, $n=181$) intravenously every 3 weeks or a chemotherapeutic agent selected by the investigators (paclitaxel plus carboplatin, paclitaxel, carboplatin, dacarbazine, or oral temozolomide, $n=179$). Adverse events (grade 3–4) occurred in all groups, and the most common overall effect was fatigue: 2 mg/kg pembrolizumab ($n=2$), 10 mg/kg pembrolizumab ($n=1$), and chemotherapy ($n=8$). Other grade 3–4 effects were edema and myalgia (2 cases with 2 mg/kg pembrolizumab), and hypopituitarism, colitis, diarrhea, hyponatremia, and pneumonitis (2 cases for each effect with 10 mg/kg pembrolizumab). The chemotherapy group reported 9 cases of anemia, 8 cases of fatigue, 6 cases of neutropenia and 6 cases of leukopenia [23C].

A case report described a 75-year-old man with metastatic melanoma who developed spongiotic dermatitis after 3 cycles of pembrolizumab (10 mg/kg every 3 weeks). Pembrolizumab treatment was stopped after cycle 6 due to disease progression. The patient presented with extensive erythematous papules and plaques with intact and ruptured vesicles and bullae at the 30-day follow-up after drug discontinuation. A diagnosis of bullous pemphigoid was confirmed by skin biopsy. The symptoms improved rapidly after 1 week with administration of a tapering dose of oral prednisone [24A].

PSORIASIS

Methotrexate

This report described a 57-year-old man with psoriasis vulgaris being treated with oral methotrexate presented with unstable psoriasis. Upon hospitalization, an injection of methotrexate (10 mg) was given for treatment of the unstable psoriasis symptoms. Within 24 hours, erythematous lesions developed with neutropenic blood counts. The symptoms resolved with administration of intravenous folinic acid, and cyclosporine (100 mg) twice daily was then given for management of the unstable psoriasis. However, the patient developed thrombocytosis 1 week after starting cyclosporine treatment; the symptoms fully resolved with discontinuation of cyclosporine. The patient was then given acitretin (50 mg) once daily for treatment of unstable psoriasis and is in remission at the time of this report [25A].

Apremilast

The efficacy and safety of apremilast, a phosphodiesterase 4 inhibitor, for treatment of severe plaque psoriasis were assessed in a phase 3, multicenter, double-blind, placebo-controlled trial (ESTEEM 1) (NCT01194219). A total of 844 patients initially received oral 30 mg apremilast ($n=562$) or placebo ($n=282$) twice daily for 16 weeks. From weeks 16–32, patients who had received the placebo in the first phase were switched to apremilast. In the final phase (weeks 32–52), patients who received apremilast in the first phase and who had a 75% reduction from their PASI score continued to receive apremilast or were switched to placebo. The majority of adverse events with apremilast treatment or placebo were mild or moderate (39.5% and 31.2%, respectively) and included diarrhea, nausea, respiratory tract infection, nasopharyngitis, and headache. Serious adverse events occurred with apremilast ($n=34$) and placebo ($n=8$); the apremilast group reported 3 cases each of coronary artery disease and nephrolithiasis and 2 cases each of urinary tract infection, acute myocardial infarction and chronic obstructive pulmonary disease. Discontinuation due to adverse events occurred in 59 cases with apremilast and 9 cases with placebo [26C].

A second phase 3, double-blind, placebo-controlled trial (ESTEEM 2) with the same study design also assessed the efficacy and safety of apremilast in 411 patients with moderate to severe plaque psoriasis. The most common adverse events in the apremilast groups were nausea, diarrhea, nasopharyngitis and upper respiratory tract infection. The incidence of adverse effects did not change throughout the 52 weeks of apremilast treatment [27C].

BI 655066

A single-rising-dose, multicenter, randomized, double-blind, placebo-controlled, within-dose cohort phase 1 trial was conducted to determine the safety of BI 655066, a human IgG1 monoclonal antibody to the IL-23 p19 subunit, for treatment of moderate to severe plaque psoriasis. Patients with psoriasis were divided into 3 treatment groups: BI 655066 (0.01, 0.05, 0.25, 1, 3, or 5 mg/kg) intravenously ($n=18$); BI 655066 (0.25 or 1 mg/kg) subcutaneously ($n=13$); or a matched placebo ($n=8$). Adverse events occurred at similar rates with both BI 655066 and placebo. Serious adverse events (4 cases) were reported with BI 655066, but these effects were not considered related to the treatment [28c].

Calcipotriol Plus Betamethasone

A newly developed aerosol foam combination formulation of calcipotriol (50 µg/g) and betamethasone (0.5 mg/g) was compared to the standard calcipotriol/betamethasone combination ointment in a phase 2a, single-center, investigator-blinded, exploratory study for treatment of plaque psoriasis. A total of 24 patients with psoriasis vulgaris were treated with the combination foam, combination ointment, or vehicle. All treatments were applied by study personnel once daily, 6 days/week for 4 weeks. Adverse events ($n=17$) occurred in 11 patients in all groups with the most common being headache and arthralgia. No serious adverse events were reported, and no study discontinuations occurred [29c].

Etanercept

The safety of etanercept treatment for chronic moderate to severe plaque psoriasis was evaluated in a 5-year postmarketing, surveillance registry of 2510 patients with psoriasis. All patients had received at least 1 dose of etanercept and greater than 80% of patients remained on etanercept treatment throughout the study. The incidence of reported serious adverse effects was 22.2% including 6.5% for serious infections, 3.2% for malignancies except for nonmelanoma skin cancer, 3.6% for nonmelanoma skin cancer, 2.8% for coronary artery disease, 0.7% for psoriasis degeneration, 0.2% for central nervous system demyelination disorders, 0.1% each for lymphoma, tuberculosis, opportunistic infections and lupus [30MC].

Infliximab

A report described a 50-year-old male patient receiving infliximab treatment for chronic plaque psoriasis. A pruritic symmetrical macular erythematous rash developed 2 days after administration of 10 infliximab infusions and resolved 1 week later. However, the symptoms reappeared following subsequent infusions; the lesions were more widespread and of longer duration with each successive infusion. Clinical examination and skin biopsy confirmed the diagnosis of symmetrical drug-related intertriginous and flexural exanthema (SDRIFE or Baboon syndrome). The symptoms resolved within 2 weeks after discontinuation of infliximab and application of topical steroids. Adalimumab was then used to treat the psoriasis, and no further reactions were reported [31A].

VITILIGO

Afamelanotide and UVB Therapy

A randomized multicenter study to determine the efficacy and safety of a combination treatment of afamelanotide and UVB phototherapy for vitiligo was conducted in adults (18 years and older) with nonsegmental vitiligo on 15–50% of the body (NCT01430195). Patients received either the combination therapy ($n=28$) or the UVB treatment alone ($n=27$). For the combination therapy group, UVB therapy was initially administered alone for 1 month, followed by the addition of subcutaneous afamelanotide (16 mg) administration; this combination treatment continued for an additional 4 months. The other group received UVB therapy alone for the entire duration of the study. Adverse events included erythema with both treatments and minor infections and nausea in the combination therapy group [32c].

CUTANEOUS SIDE EFFECTS FROM ANTIBIOTIC MEDICATIONS

Ciprofloxacin

This report describes 3 cases of patients (all males, 53, 41 and 22 years) who presented with multiple well-defined erythematous and hyperpigmented patches with bullous lesions within 1 week of receiving oral ciprofloxacin. The symptoms were resolved with oral prednisolone (tapering regimen starting with 40 mg/day), oral antihistamines, local soframycin and topical steroids for the hyperpigmented lesions. The patients were advised to avoid ciprofloxacin in the future [33A].

Daptomycin

A non-interventional, multicenter, retrospective registry (European Cubicin® Outcome Registry and Experience; EU-CORE(SM)) evaluated the outcome and safety of daptomycin treatment in patients with complicated skin and soft tissues infection. All patients ($n = 6075$ total; $n = 1972$ with complicated skin and soft tissues infection) received one of 3 doses of daptomycin (≤ 6, >6 to <8, or ≥ 8 mg/kg/day) for a median treatment duration of 10 days; the most frequently administered doses were 4 mg/kg/day (38.9%) and 6 mg/kg/day (35.2%). Adverse events were reported in 203 patients; 46 cases of these events were potentially associated with daptomycin treatment. Serious adverse events occurred in 12 patients, and discontinuation of daptomycin due to adverse events (primarily musculoskeletal and connective tissue disorders) occurred in 47 patients [34MC].

Delafloxacin with Tigecycline

A randomized, double-blind, multicenter, phase 2 trial in the United States assessed the safety of delafloxacin versus tigecycline in patients with various complicated skin and skin structure infections (NCT 0719810). Adult patients received delafloxacin (300 mg, $n = 49$) intravenously every 12 hours, delafloxacin (450 mg, $n = 51$) intravenously every 12 hours, or tigecycline ($n = 50$) intravenously 100 mg, 1 dose and then 50 mg every 12 hours. All treatments were administered over 5–14 days. Adverse events occurred in all treatment groups (delafloxacin 300 mg, $n = 22$; delafloxacin 450 mg, $n = 32$; tigecycline, $n = 36$). The most common adverse effect was nausea (delafloxacin 300 mg, $n = 6$; delafloxacin 450 mg, $n = 13$; tigecycline, $n = 23$) with vomiting and rash occurring only with the high doses of delafloxacin and tigecycline. The presence of adverse events also lead to study discontinuation in the 450 mg delafloxacin ($n = 2$) and tigecycline ($n = 3$) groups, while no discontinuations occurred with 300 mg delafloxacin [35c].

Oritavancin and Vancomycin

A phase 3, multicenter, global, randomized, double-blind, comparative efficacy and safety study evaluated the use of oritavancin, a lipoglycopeptide antibiotic with activity against Gram-positive bacteria, versus vancomycin for treatment of acute bacterial skin and skin structure infections (NCT01252732). Patients received one of the following treatments: a single intravenous 1200 mg dose of oritavancin ($n = 503$) every 12 hours; intravenous doses of 15 mg/kg or 1 g/kg vancomycin ($n = 502$) every 12 hours; or an intravenous placebo. The treatment duration for all groups was 7–10 days. The majority of adverse effects were similar between the treatments and included nausea, headache, vomiting, cellulitis, increased alanine aminotransferase and phlebitis at infusion site. Study discontinuation due to adverse effects was reported with oritavancin ($n = 18$; cellulitis, infection, osteomyelitis) and vancomycin ($n = 13$) [36C].

CUTANEOUS SIDE EFFECTS FROM ANTIVIRAL MEDICATIONS

Telaprevir

Telaprevir, a protease inhibitor antiviral agent, has been the treatment of choice for hepatitis C virus (HCV) genotype-1 infected patients but is associated with an increased frequency of severe adverse cutaneous reactions. A 50-year-old woman received a triple therapy (telaprevir, 2250 mg/day; PEG-interferon-alpha-2a, 180 µg/week; and ribavirin, 1000 mg/day) for treatment of HCV-related chronic hepatitis. After 8 weeks, eczematous lesions (grade 1) developed on 18% of her body. Topical steroid and oral antihistamines were ineffective, and the eruptions spread to 36% of the body and progressed to grade 2. After 2 more days, the reaction developed to grade 3, a fever was present and the patient was hospitalized and telaprevir was discontinued. Symptom resolution occurred with once daily intravenous methyl prednisolone (40 mg) and chlorpheniramine maleate (20 mg). The diagnosis of a telaprevir-induced T-cell-dependent immune reaction was confirmed by a lymphocyte transformation test [37A].

Similar results were found in an observational post-marketing study of 3563 patients in Japan who received the combination drug (telaprevir, PEG-interferon and ribavirin) therapy for treatment of chronic hepatitis C. The triple therapy was administered for 12 weeks, followed by PEG-interferon and ribavirin for an additional 12 weeks. Serious adverse reactions, including skin disorders, occurred in the first 12 weeks (96.5%) and in the second 12 weeks (35.7%) [38MC].

CUTANEOUS SIDE EFFECTS FROM CANCER MEDICATIONS

Afatinib and Methotrexate

An open-label, multicenter, phase 3, randomized controlled trial in 19 countries compared the safety of afatinib, a human epidermal growth factor receptor 2 and epidermal growth factor receptor kinase inhibitor, to methotrexate for metastatic squamous cell carcinoma of the head and neck (NCT01345682). Adults ($n = 483$) with recurrent or metastatic squamous cell carcinoma of the head and neck or who had received first-line platinum-based therapy and were not suitable for salvage surgery or radiotherapy were included in the study. The treatments were oral afatinib ($n = 322$, initial dose of 40 mg up to a maximum dose of 50 mg) once daily or intravenous methotrexate ($n = 161$, initial dose of 40 mg/m^2 up to a maximum dose of 50 mg/m^2) weekly injection; administration was in 28-day cycles with a maximum of 29 months. The most common serious adverse events (grade 3 or 4) occurred with afatinib ($n = 44$) as compared methotrexate ($n = 18$). These effects included rash or acne (afatinib, $n = 31$; methotrexate, $n = 0$), diarrhea (afatinib, $n = 3$; methotrexate, $n = 3$), stomatitis (afatinib, $n = 20$; methotrexate, $n = 13$), fatigue (afatinib, $n = 18$; methotrexate, $n = 5$), and neutropenia (afatinib, $n = 1$; methotrexate, $n = 11$) [39C].

Bendamustine

This report described 3 cases of hypersensitivity reactions resulting from administration of bendamustine for treatment of B-cell non-Hodgkin lymphoma. The patients had initially received bendamustine without reaction in the first treatment cycle but developed pruritus, erythema, edema, maculopapular exanthema, hives, and a high fever within 1 week after beginning the second cycle. In one case, the reaction began within 3 hours of administration. It was determined that 2 of the 3 patients had bendamustine-induced immediate and delayed cutaneous hypersensitivity reactions, while the third patient experienced a bendamustine-induced fever [40A].

Bevacizumab and Erlotinib

The safety of bevacizumab alone versus a combination bevacizumab and erlotinib for inoperable metastatic colorectal cancer was assessed in an open-label, multicenter, international, randomized, phase 3 study. Patients ($n = 700$) with metastatic colorectal cancer received intravenous bevacizumab only (7.5 mg/kg) every 3 weeks or the combination of intravenous bevacizumab (7.5 mg/kg) every 3 weeks plus oral erlotinib (150 mg) once daily. A grade 3–4 skin rash was reported with the bevacizumab plus erlotinib combination ($n = 47$), while no events occurred with bevacizumab alone [41C].

Brentuximab

An open-label, phase 2 trial evaluated the safety and efficacy of brentuximab vedotin, a monoclonal antibody, for treatment of CD30(+) cutaneous T-cell lymphoma. A total of 48 patients with CD30(+) lymphoproliferative disorders or mycosis fungoides (MF) received an infusion of brentuximab (1.8 mg/kg) every 21 days. Adverse events (grade 3 or 4) included neutropenia ($n = 5$), nausea ($n = 2$), chest pain ($n = 2$), deep vein thrombosis ($n = 1$), transaminitis ($n = 1$) and dehydration ($n = 1$). Serious adverse events included grade 1–2 peripheral neuropathy ($n = 31$) which was resolved in 14 patients but still ongoing in 17 patients at the time of this report [42c].

Cetuximab

A meta-analysis of 13 phase 1, 2 and 3 trials of patients with solid tumors treated with cetuximab showed that a cetuximab-induced rash was significantly correlated with improved progression-free survival as compared to patients without rash. The results also indicated that the cetuximab-induced skin rash was associated with favorable outcomes in these patients [43M].

Sorafenib

Sorafenib, an oral multitargeted kinase inhibitor with activity against tyrosine protein kinases, is frequently used for the treatment of hepatocellular and metastatic renal cell carcinomas. However, sorafenib treatment (average dose of 400–800 mg) has been directly linked to drug-induced cutaneous reactions as described in multiple clinical trials and postmarketing surveillance studies conducted in multiple countries [44MC,45C,46C,47MC, 48c,49c]. The most common adverse events were hand–foot skin reactions (approximately 20–60%) and rash (approximately 20–25%) with other cutaneous effects (alopecia, pruritus, erythema) occurring less frequently. In many instances, the hand–foot skin reactions and rashes were considered serious adverse effects and lead to a high rate of sorafenib discontinuation. Several case reports describe additional sorafenib-induced cutaneous reactions including facial acneiform eruption [50A], Stevens–Johnson syndrome, erythema multiforme and generalized maculopapular eruptions [51A].

Sym004

A proof of concept clinical trial was conducted to assess the efficacy and safety of Sym004, a 1:1 mixture of 2 anti-epidermal growth factor receptor monoclonal antibodies (992 and 1024), for treatment of squamous cell carcinoma of the head and neck. A total of 26 patients with incurable, recurrent and/or metastatic squamous cell carcinoma of the head and neck and with acquired resistance to other anti-epidermal growth factor receptor monoclonal antibody-containing treatments received Sym004 (12 mg/kg) via weekly infusions until disease progression or toxicity. Epidermal growth factor receptor-related adverse events occurred in all patients and included grade 3 skin reactions ($n = 13$) and grade ≥ 3 hypomagnesemia ($n = 10$) [52c].

Trastuzumab

A case report described the development of flagellate erythema with pruritus and skin lesions in a 64-year-old woman with metastatic breast cancer. The symptoms began 3 days after starting trastuzumab and flagellate erythema was confirmed through skin biopsy. This report is similar to those describing the development of flagellate erythema following treatment of other chemotherapeutics including bleomycin, bendamustine, docetaxel, and peplomycin [53A].

CUTANEOUS SIDE EFFECTS FROM NEUROLOGICAL MEDICATIONS

Avagacestat

The safety of avagacestat, a γ-secretase inhibitor, for treatment of Alzheimer disease was evaluated using a multicenter global population in a randomized, placebo-controlled phase 2 clinical trial with a parallel, untreated, nonrandomized observational cohort (NCT00890890). A total of 263 patients received oral avagacestat (50 or 125 mg, $n = 132$) daily or placebo ($n = 131$); an additional 102 patients formed the untreated observational cohort. Discontinuation of avagacestat treatment occurred primarily due to gastrointestinal effects (19.6% with 50 mg and 43% with 125 mg). Serious adverse events included the development of nonmelanoma skin cancer with avagacestat ($n = 49$) versus placebo ($n = 31$) [54C].

Phenytoin

Phenytoin, an anti-convulsant, is used in conjunction with cranial radiation therapy for treatment of brain tumors; erythema multiforme has been reported to develop in patients receiving such a treatment combination. A report described a 41-year-old woman who received whole brain radiation therapy and chemotherapy following surgery for removal of a brain tumor. Phenytoin was administered prior to surgery and throughout the subsequent radiation therapy. Minor skin reactions occurred 24 days after starting phenytoin treatment and developed rapidly to a generalized erythematous and maculopapular rash with significant periorbital and perioral edema and painful mucosal oral lesions. Discontinuation of phenytoin and administration of intravenous corticosteroids and topical steroids resulted in complete recovery within 3 weeks [55A].

INDIVIDUAL MEDICATIONS

General Drug-Induced Skin Reactions

A prospective, observational study was conducted in a tertiary care hospital to determine the cause and severity of cutaneous adverse drug reactions. Suspected skin drug reactions in 90 patients following systemic drug treatment were analyzed for morphological pattern, causality and severity based on the World Health Organization-Uppsala Monitoring Centre causality assessment system. Reported adverse events were maculopapular rash (76.7%), urticaria (8.89%), Stevens–Johnson syndrome (4.4%) and fixed dose eruptions (3.33%). Antiretrovirals were the most common drug category associated with adverse reactions (75.56% or 68/90 of the reported reactions). Other drug categories included antimicrobials, antiepileptics and non-steroidal anti-inflammatory drugs (NSAIDs). Nevirapine, in particular, was associated with 52/90 (57.8%) cases of adverse cutaneous events and included maculopapular rash ($n = 39$), urticaria ($n = 5$), Stevens–Johnson syndrome ($n = 4$), and pustular rash and angioedema ($n = 2$ each). Antimicrobials, antiepileptics and non-steroidal anti-inflammatory drugs (NSAIDs) were additional categories implicated in causing adverse skin drug reactions. The authors also noted that female patients were twice as likely to experience adverse cutaneous drug reactions as were males [56M].

Apremilast

A phase 2, multicenter, placebo-controlled study assessed the efficacy and safety of apremilast for treatment of oral ulcers in Behçet's syndrome (NCT00866359). Patients ($n = 111$) with Behçet's syndrome and 2 or more oral ulcers received apremilast (30 mg) twice daily or placebo for 12 weeks. After 12 weeks, the placebo group was switched to apremilast for an additional 28 days. Adverse events included nausea, vomiting, and diarrhea and were more common with apremilast (22, 9, and 12 events, respectively) than with the placebo (10, 1, and 2 events, respectively). Serious adverse events occurred with apremilast ($n = 2$) and placebo ($n = 1$); the 2 apremilast cases were worsening of a preexisting anal fissure due to diarrhea and transient paralysis of both legs, while the placebo patient had fever [57C].

Interferon Beta-1b (IFN-β)

A case of multiple cutaneous necrotic ulcers following treatment with interferon-beta-1b (IFN-β, 8 million IU) by subcutaneous injection was reported in a 49-year-old woman with relapsing-remitting multiple sclerosis. After 3 months, erythematous patches and plaques were evident at the injection sites and developed into indurated erythema with necrotic lesions. A skin confirmed the diagnosis of cutaneous necrotic ulcerations. The IFN-β-1b injections were switched from subcutaneous to intramuscular, and the skin lesions were treated with routine wound care, surgical debridement, and skin grafting [58A].

Isoniazid and Ethionamide

Isoniazid and ethionamide are common anti-tuberculosis drugs; ethionamide is a structural analogue of isoniazid. As a result, these two drugs have a similar metabolism, toxicity and molecular targets, causing concern for potential cross-reactivity reactions. This concern was addressed in a study with 69 patients on isoniazid treatment who developed adverse skin reactions; serious adverse reactions in 25 patients included drug rash with eosinophilia and systemic symptoms (DRESS), Stevens–Johnson syndrome or toxic epidermal necrolysis. Isoniazid was discontinued in these cases and ethionamide treatment started when the initial symptoms had subsided. These 25 patients then underwent rechallenge with isoniazid; a rechallenge reaction occurred in 20 patients. At the same time, 5 patients from the same group reacted to ethionamide. It was noted that none of the patients who reacted to isoniazid or ethionamide showed cross-reactivity to the other drug [59c].

Lamotrigine

A literature search identified published reports of induced drug-induced hypersensitivity syndrome or drug reaction with eosinophilia and systemic symptoms (DRESS) associated with lamotrigine administration. The reported cases included 57 patients (38 female and 19 male) with reactions between January 1999 and April 2014. Initial symptoms included fever, skin rash, liver involvement, hypereosinophilia, and lymphadenopathy. The latency period between start of lamotrigine therapy and the onset of symptoms ranged from 9 to 120 days with an average of 27 days. Many patients ($n = 37$) experienced multisystem involvement. The majority of patients fully recovered, although 3 severe outcomes occurred: liver failure requiring transplant (1 case) and 2 deaths (septic shock and multiple organ failure, 1 each) [60M].

Nilotinib

An open-label, single-center, pilot trial evaluated the safety and tolerability of nilotinib, a novel tyrosine kinase inhibitor, in patients with diffuse cutaneous systemic sclerosis (NCT01166139). Adults ($n = 10$) received oral nilotinib (200 mg) once daily for 7 days, then 200 mg twice daily for 3 weeks and finally 400 mg twice daily. Nilotinib treatment occurred for at least 12 months in 7 patients; 2 patients withdrew from treatment due to grade 1 or 2 QTc elongation and 1 patient discontinued after 3 months due to progression of preexisting coronary artery disease. A total of 71 adverse events occurred with 92% being grade 1 or 2; 75% of these events were considered potentially related to nilotinib treatment. The most common effect was abnormal liver function values which

were asymptomatic in the patients. Serious adverse events included the 2 cases of study discontinuation due to prolonged QTc times and were considered treatment related [61c].

Sodium Nitrite

A multicenter, randomized, controlled, dose-ranging clinical trial was conducted in 40 European genitourinary medicine clinics to determine the efficacy and safety of acidified nitrite creams for the treatment of anogenital warts (NCT02015260). A total of 299 subjects (18 years and older) with 2–50 external anogenital warts received treatment for 12 weeks. Follow-up visits extended an additional 12 weeks. Treatments included sodium nitrite (3%) plus citric acid (4.5%) twice daily, sodium nitrite (6%) plus citric acid (9%) twice daily, and sodium nitrite (6%) plus citric acid (9%) once daily at night with placebo applied in the morning. The control group applied the placebo cream twice daily. No serious adverse events occurred, although a dose-dependent increase in itching, pain, edema, and staining of the anogenital skin was associated with increasing concentrations of the nitrite–citric acid treatment. These adverse effects resulted in 21 patients withdrawing from the study, while no withdrawals occurred in the placebo group [62C].

Sulfasalazine

A report described a case of a Stevens–Johnson syndrome and toxic epidermal necrolysis resulting from sulfasalazine treatment. A 33-year-old woman was hospitalized for symptoms (epidermal detachment over 18% of the body, blisters and red macular and papular lesions) occurring 15 days after administration of sulfasalazine. The diagnosis of Stevens–Johnson Syndrome and toxic epidermal necrolysis was confirmed by skin biopsy; the epidermal detachment of 10–30% met the criteria of a Stevens–Johnson Syndrome/Toxic Epidermal Necrolysis overlap. Sulfasalazine treatment was discontinued, symptomatic treatment was started and recovery was observed within 17 days [63A].

Vildagliptin

A case report described 3 patients who developed bullous pemphigoid following administration of vildagliptin, a treatment for type 2 diabetes mellitus. Symptoms were evident from 1 to 37 months after starting vildagliptin treatment. In 2 of the 3 patients, the symptoms were temporarily resolved with the addition of clobetasol treatment, although vildagliptin administration was continued. In both cases, however, the bullous lesions reappeared 3 months later. In all 3 cases, full resolution of the symptoms occurred with discontinuation of vildagliptin. These cases are similar to previous reports of suspected vildagliptin-induced bullous pemphigoid [64A].

Zoledronic Acid

A case report described the development of dermatomyositis following administration of zoledronic acid, a common treatment for postmenopausal osteoporosis. A 62-year-old woman exhibited diffuse, erythematous scaly plaques 12 hours after intravenous administration of zoledronic acid. A skin biopsy indicated interface dermatitis with a patchy scale crust containing neutrophils and inspissated serum, necrotic keratinocytes, and a lymphocytic infiltrate [65A].

References

[1] Kawashima M, Hashimoto H, Alió Sáenz AB, et al. Clindamycin phosphate 1.2%-benzoyl peroxide 3.0% fixed-dose combination gel has an effective and acceptable safety and tolerability profile for the treatment of acne vulgaris in Japanese patients: a phase III, multicentre, randomised, single-blinded, active-controlled, parallel-group study. Br J Dermatol. 2015;172(2):494–503 [C].

[2] Chandrashekhar BS, Anitha M, Ruparelia M, et al. Tretinoin nanogel 0.025% versus conventional gel 0.025% in patients with acne vulgaris: a randomized, active controlled, multicentre, parallel group, Phase IV clinical trial. J Clin Diagn Res. 2015;9(1): WC04–9 [C].

[3] Pellacani G, Peris K, Guillen C, et al. A randomized trial comparing simultaneous vs. sequential field treatment of actinic keratosis with ingenol mebutate on two separate areas of the head and body. J Eur Acad Dermatol Venereol. 2015;29(11):2192–8 [C].

[4] Samorano LP, Torezan LA, Sanches JA. Evaluation of the tolerability and safety of a 0.015% ingenol mebutate gel compared to 5% 5-fluorouracil cream for the treatment of facial actinic keratosis: a prospective randomized trial. J Eur Acad Dermatol Venereol. 2015;29(9):1822–7 [c].

[5] Simon JC, Dominicus R, Karl L, et al. A prospective randomized exploratory study comparing the efficacy of once-daily topical 0.5% 5-fluorouracil in combination with 10.0% salicylic acid (5-FU/SA) vs. cryosurgery for the treatment of hyperkeratotic actinic keratosis. J Eur Acad Dermatol Venereol. 2015;29(5):881–9 [c].

[6] Sheu J, Hawryluk EB, Guo D, et al. Voriconazole phototoxicity in children: a retrospective review. J Am Acad Dermatol. 2015;72(2):314–20 [R].

[7] Cornely OA, Böhme A, Schmitt-Hoffmann A, et al. Safety and pharmacokinetics of isavuconazole as antifungal prophylaxis in acute myeloid leukemia patients with neutropenia: results of a phase 2, dose escalation study. Antimicrob Agents Chemother. 2015;59(4):2078–85 [c].

[8] Maertens JA, Raad II, Marr KA, et al. Isavuconazole versus voriconazole for primary treatment of invasive mould disease caused by Aspergillus and other filamentous fungi (SECURE): a phase 3, randomised-controlled, non-inferiority trial. Lancet. 2016;387:760–9. S0140-6736(15)01159-9 [pii] [C].

[9] Iraji F, Farhadi S, Faghihi G, et al. Efficacy of topical azathioprine and betamethasone versus betamethasone-only emollient cream in 2–18 years old patients with moderate-to-severe atopic dermatitis: a randomized controlled trial. Adv Biomed Res. 2015;4:228 [c].

[10] Murrell DF, Gebauer K, Spelman L, et al. Crisaborole topical ointment, 2% in adults with atopic dermatitis: a Phase 2a, vehicle-controlled, proof-of-concept study. J Drugs Dermatol. 2015;14(10):1108–12 [c].

[11] Stein Gold LF, Spelman L, Spellman MC, et al. A Phase 2, randomized, controlled, dose-ranging study evaluating crisaborole topical ointment, 0.5% and 2% in adolescents with mild to moderate atopic dermatitis. J Drugs Dermatol. 2015;14(12):1394–9 [c].

[12] Murata Y, Song M, Kikuchi H, et al. Phase 2a, randomized, double-blind, placebo-controlled, multicenter, parallel-group study of a H4 R-antagonist (JNJ-39758979) in Japanese adults with moderate atopic dermatitis. J Dermatol. 2015;42(2):129–39 [c].

[13] Vives R, Pontes C, Sarasa M, et al. Safety and activity of UR-1505 in atopic dermatitis: a randomized, double-blind Phase II exploratory trial. Clin Ther. 2015;37(9):1955–65 [c].

[14] Basset-Seguin N, Hauschild A, Grob JJ, et al. Vismodegib in patients with advanced basal cell carcinoma (STEVIE): a pre-planned interim analysis of an international, open-label trial. Lancet Oncol. 2015;16(6):729–36 [C].

[15] Sofen H, Gross KG, Goldberg LH, et al. A phase II, multicenter, open-label, 3-cohort trial evaluating the efficacy and safety of vismodegib in operable basal cell carcinoma. J Am Acad Dermatol. 2015;73(1):99–105 [c].

[16] Carlos G, Anforth R, Clements A, et al. Cutaneous toxic effects of BRAF inhibitors alone and in combination with MEK inhibitors for metastatic melanoma. JAMA Dermatol. 2015;151(10):1103–9 [C].

[17] Anforth R, Carlos G, Clements A, et al. Cutaneous adverse events in patients treated with BRAF inhibitor-based therapies for metastatic melanoma for longer than 52 weeks. Br J Dermatol. 2015;172(1):239–43 [C].

[18] Robert C, Karaszewska B, Schachter J, et al. Improved overall survival in melanoma with combined dabrafenib and trametinib. N Engl J Med. 2015;372(1):30–9 [C].

[19] Vanneste L, Wolter P, Van den Oord JJ, et al. Cutaneous adverse effects of BRAF inhibitors in metastatic malignant melanoma, a prospective study in 20 patients. J Eur Acad Dermatol Venereol. 2015;29(1):61–8 [c].

[20] Zimmer L, Eigentler TK, Kiecker F, et al. Open-label, multicenter, single-arm phase II DeCOG-study of ipilimumab in pretreated patients with different subtypes of metastatic melanoma. J Transl Med. 2015;13:351 [C].

[21] Larkin J, Chiarion-Sileni V, Gonzalez R, et al. Combined nivolumab and ipilimumab or monotherapy in untreated melanoma. N Engl J Med. 2015;373(1):23–34 [C].

[22] Robert C, Schachter J, Long GV, et al. Pembrolizumab versus ipilimumab in advanced melanoma. N Engl J Med. 2015;372(26):2521–32 [C].

[23] Ribas A, Puzanov I, Dummer R, et al. Pembrolizumab versus investigator-choice chemotherapy for ipilimumab-refractory melanoma (KEYNOTE-002): a randomised, controlled, phase 2 trial. Lancet Oncol. 2015;16(8):908–18 [C].

[24] Carlos G, Anforth R, Chou S, et al. A case of bullous pemphigoid in a patient with metastatic melanoma treated with pembrolizumab. Melanoma Res. 2015;25(3):265–8 [A].

[25] Tejaswi C, Mohanan S, Murugaiyan R, et al. Double trouble: cyclosporine-induced thrombocytosis in a patient with methotrexate toxicity: are they related? J Pharmacol Pharmacother. 2015;6(3):160–2 [A].

[26] Papp K, Reich K, Leonardi CL, et al. Apremilast, an oral phosphodiesterase 4 (PDE4) inhibitor, in patients with moderate to severe plaque psoriasis: results of a phase III, randomized, controlled trial (Efficacy and Safety Trial Evaluating the Effects of Apremilast in Psoriasis [ESTEEM] 1). J Am Acad Dermatol. 2015;73(1):37–49 [C].

[27] Paul C, Cather J, Gooderham M, et al. Efficacy and safety of apremilast, an oral phosphodiesterase 4 inhibitor, in patients with moderate-to-severe plaque psoriasis over 52 weeks: a phase III, randomized controlled trial (ESTEEM 2). Br J Dermatol. 2015;173(6):1387–99 [C].

[28] Krueger JG, Ferris LK, Menter A, et al. Anti-IL-23A mAb BI 655066 for treatment of moderate-to-severe psoriasis: safety, efficacy, pharmacokinetics, and biomarker results of a single-rising-dose, randomized, double-blind, placebo-controlled trial. J Allergy Clin Immunol. 2015;136(1):116–124.e7 [c].

[29] Queille-Roussel C, Olesen M, Villumsen J, et al. Efficacy of an innovative aerosol foam formulation of fixed combination calcipotriol plus betamethasone dipropionate in patients with psoriasis vulgaris. Clin Drug Investig. 2015;35(4):239–45 [c].

[30] Kimball AB, Rothman KJ, Kricorian G, et al. OBSERVE-5: observational postmarketing safety surveillance registry of etanercept for the treatment of psoriasis final 5-year results. J Am Acad Dermatol. 2015;72(1):115–22 [MC].

[31] Bulur I, Keseroglu HO, Saracoglu ZN, et al. Symmetrical drug-related intertriginous and flexural exanthema (Baboon syndrome) associated with infliximab. J Dermatol Case Rep. 2015;9(1):12–4 [A].

[32] Lim HW, Grimes PE, Agbai O, et al. Afamelanotide and narrowband UV-B phototherapy for the treatment of vitiligo: a randomized multicenter trial. JAMA Dermatol. 2015;151(1):42–50 [c].

[33] Nair PA. Ciprofloxacin induced bullous fixed drug reaction: three case reports. J Family Med Prim Care. 2015;4(2):269–72 [A].

[34] Cogo A, Gonzalez-Ruiz A, Pathan R, et al. Real-world treatment of complicated skin and soft tissue infections with daptomycin: results from a large European registry (EU-CORE). Infect Dis Ther. 2015;4(3):273–82 [MC].

[35] O'Riordan W, Mehra P, Manos P, et al. A randomized phase 2 study comparing two doses of delafloxacin with tigecycline in adults with complicated skin and skin-structure infections. Int J Infect Dis. 2015;30:67–73 [c].

[36] Corey GR, Good S, Jiang H, et al. Single-dose oritavancin versus 7–10 days of vancomycin in the treatment of Gram-positive acute bacterial skin and skin structure infections: the SOLO II noninferiority study. Clin Infect Dis. 2015;60(2):254–62 [C].

[37] Federico A, Aitella E, Sgambato D, et al. Telaprevir may induce adverse cutaneous reactions by a T cell immune-mediated mechanism. Ann Hepatol. 2015;14(3):420–4 [A].

[38] Shiraishi M, Umebayashi I, Matsuda H, et al. Postmarketing surveillance of telaprevir-based triple therapy for chronic hepatitis C in Japan. Hepatol Res. 2015;45(13):1267–75 [MC].

[39] Machiels JP, Haddad RI, Fayette J, et al. Afatinib versus methotrexate as second-line treatment in patients with recurrent or metastatic squamous-cell carcinoma of the head and neck progressing on or after platinum-based therapy (LUX-Head & Neck 1): an open-label, randomised phase 3 trial. Lancet Oncol. 2015;16(5):583–94 [C].

[40] Barbarroja-Escudero J, Sanchez-Gonzalez MJ, Antolin-Amerigo D, et al. Hypersensitivity reactions and drug fever by bendamustine: a case report of three patients. Allergol Int. 2015;64(1):109–11 [A].

[41] Tournigand C, Chibaudel B, Samson B, et al. Bevacizumab with or without erlotinib as maintenance therapy in patients with metastatic colorectal cancer (GERCOR DREAM; OPTIMOX3): a randomised, open-label, phase 3 trial. Lancet Oncol. 2015;16(15):1493–505 [C].

[42] Duvic M, Tetzlaff MT, Gangar P, et al. Results of a Phase II trial of brentuximab vedotin for CD30+ cutaneous T-cell lymphoma and lymphomatoid papulosis. J Clin Oncol. 2015;33(32):3759–65 [c].

[43] Abdel-Rahman O, Fouad M. Correlation of cetuximab-induced skin rash and outcomes of solid tumor patients treated with cetuximab: a systematic review and meta-analysis. Crit Rev Oncol Hematol. 2015;93(2):127–35 [M].

[44] Akaza H, Oya M, Iijima M, et al. A large-scale prospective registration study of the safety and efficacy of sorafenib tosylate in unresectable or metastatic renal cell carcinoma in Japan: results of over 3200 consecutive cases in post-marketing all-patient surveillance. Jpn J Clin Oncol. 2015;45(10):953–62 [MC].

[45] Bruix J, Takayama T, Mazzaferro V, et al. Adjuvant sorafenib for hepatocellular carcinoma after resection or ablation (STORM): a phase 3, randomised, double-blind, placebo-controlled trial. Lancet Oncol. 2015;16(13):1344–54 [C].

[46] Chao Y, Chung YH, Han G, et al. The combination of transcatheter arterial chemoembolization and sorafenib is well tolerated and effective in Asian patients with hepatocellular carcinoma: final results of the START trial. Int J Cancer. 2015;136(6):1458–67 [C].

[47] Jäger D, Ma JH, Mardiak J, et al. Sorafenib treatment of advanced renal cell carcinoma patients in daily practice: the large international PREDICT study. Clin Genitourin Cancer. 2015;13(2):156–64 [MC].

[48] Worden F, Fassnacht M, Shi Y, et al. Safety and tolerability of sorafenib in patients with radioiodine-refractory thyroid cancer. Endocr Relat Cancer. 2015;22(6):877–87 [c].

[49] Zhang HL, Qin XJ, Wang HK, et al. Clinicopathological and prognostic factors for long-term survival in Chinese patients with metastatic renal cell carcinoma treated with sorafenib: a single-center retrospective study. Oncotarget. 2015;6(34):36870–83 [c].

[50] Cohen PR. Sorafenib-associated facial acneiform eruption. Dermatol Ther (Heidelb). 2015;5(1):77–86 [A].

[51] Sohn KH, Oh SY, Lim KW, et al. Sorafenib induces delayed-onset cutaneous hypersensitivity: a case series. Allergy Asthma Immunol Res. 2015;7(3):304–7 [A].

[52] Machiels JP, Specenier P, Krauss J, et al. A proof of concept trial of the anti-EGFR antibody mixture Sym004 in patients with squamous cell carcinoma of the head and neck. Cancer Chemother Pharmacol. 2015;76(1):13–20 [c].

[53] Cohen PR. Trastuzumab-associated flagellate erythema: report in a woman with metastatic breast cancer and review of antineoplastic therapy-induced flagellate dermatoses. Dermatol Ther (Heidelb). 2015;5(4):253–64 [A].

[54] Coric V, Salloway S, van Dyck CH, et al. Targeting prodromal Alzheimer disease with avagacestat: a randomized clinical trial. JAMA Neurol. 2015;72(11):1324–33 [C].

[55] Kazanci A, Tekkök İH. Phenytoin induced erythema multiforme after cranial radiation therapy. J Korean Neurosurg Soc. 2015;58(2):163–6 [A].

[56] Pawar MP, Pore SM, Pradhan SN, et al. Nevirapine: most common cause of cutaneous adverse drug reactions in an outpatient department of a tertiary care hospital. J Clin Diagn Res. 2015;9(11):FC17–20 [M].

[57] Hatemi G, Melikoglu M, Tunc R, et al. Apremilast for Behçet's syndrome—a phase 2, placebo-controlled study. N Engl J Med. 2015;372(16):1510–8 [C].

[58] Faghihi G, Basiri A, Pourazizi M, et al. Multiple cutaneous necrotic lesions associated with interferon beta-1b injection for multiple sclerosis treatment: a case report and literature review. J Res Pharm Pract. 2015;4(2):99–103 [A].

[59] Lehloenya RJ, Muloiwa R, Dlamini S, et al. Lack of cross-toxicity between isoniazid and ethionamide in severe cutaneous adverse drug reactions: a series of 25 consecutive confirmed cases. J Antimicrob Chemother. 2015;70(9):2648–51 [c].

[60] Wang XQ, Lv B, Wang HF, et al. Lamotrigine induced DIHS/DRESS: manifestations, treatment, and outcome in 57 patients. Clin Neurol Neurosurg. 2015;138:1–7 [M].

[61] Gordon JK, Martyanov V, Magro C, et al. Nilotinib (Tasigna™) in the treatment of early diffuse systemic sclerosis: an open-label, pilot clinical trial. Arthritis Res Ther. 2015;17:213 [c].

[62] Ormerod AD, van Voorst Vader PC, Majewski S, et al. Evaluation of the efficacy, safety, and tolerability of 3 dose regimens of topical sodium nitrite with citric acid in patients with anogenital warts: a randomized clinical trial. JAMA Dermatol. 2015;151(8):854–61 [C].

[63] Zizi N, Elmrahi A, Dikhaye S, et al. Stevens Johnson syndrome-toxic epidermal necrolysis overlap induced by sulfasalazine treatment: a case report. Tunis Med. 2015;93(7):413–5 [A].

[64] Béné J, Jacobsoone A, Coupe P, et al. Bullous pemphigoid induced by vildagliptin: a report of three cases. Fundam Clin Pharmacol. 2015;29(1):112–4 [A].

[65] Succaria F, Collier M, Mahalingam M. Zoledronic acid-induced interface dermatitis. Am J Dermatopathol. 2015;37(12):933–5 [A].

14

Antihistamines (H1 Receptor Antagonists)

Alan Polnariev[1]

College of Pharmacy, University of Florida, Gainesville, FL, USA

[1]Corresponding author: apolnariev@gmail.com

GENERAL

Regarding their effects on the central nervous system (CNS), antihistamines can be classified into one of three categories. Those that markedly impair cognitive and psychomotor function by crossing the blood–brain barrier; those that despite crossing into the brain, do not cause significant impairment at low therapeutic doses; and those that do not cross into the brain and therefore, do not possess intrinsic potential for diminishing CNS function. The first-generation antihistamines have well-documented sedative, anticholinergic and dysrhythmogenic effects; there are also concerns regarding carry-over effects in terms of next-day somnolence and psychomotor responses following their use. These effects on movement dysfunction have been linked to altered neurotransmission in cholinergic and histaminergic pathways [1R]. One randomized, double-blind, crossover study was conducted to evaluate the effects of zolpidem (10 mg), diphenhydramine (50 mg), ketotifen (1 mg) or placebo on next-day sleepiness and psychomotor performance in 22 healthy male participants. The drugs were administered in four separate sessions before sleep with a greater than 1-week washout period. Participants were evaluated for subjective sleepiness, objective sleepiness and psychomotor performance, the morning and afternoon after administration. Ketotifen had the strongest carry-over effect followed by diphenhydramine, with no effect seen for zolpidem or placebo [2c]. The authors recommended that consideration be given to the risks associated with first-generation antihistamine use for the treatment of insomnia secondary to allergies.

There are few reports that directly compare the antihistaminic efficacy and impairment of psychomotor functions of first-generation and second-generation drugs. A double-blind, placebo-controlled, crossover study in 24 healthy subjects compared promethazine, a first-generation antihistamine, with the second-generation antihistamines fexofenadine and olopatadine. The study was done to measure their potency as peripheral inhibitors of histamine-induced wheal and flare together with examination of their sedative effects on the CNS using a battery of psychomotor tests. Compared with fexofenadine and promethazine, olopatadine showed the most rapid inhibitory effect on the histamine-induced wheal and flare test. In a battery of psychomotor assessments, promethazine significantly impaired psychomotor function while fexofenadine and olopatadine had no significant effect in any of the tests used. Promethazine, fexofenadine and olopatadine did not affect behavioral activity, as measured by wrist actigraphy. These results suggest that at therapeutic doses, olopatadine has greater inhibitory effect on the histamine-induced wheal and flare test compared with promethazine and that neither olopatadine nor fexofenadine cause significant cognitive or psychomotor impairment in healthy subjects [3c].

Recent studies compared the sedative effects of first and second-generation antihistamines, i.e., hydroxyzine and bilastine, respectively, under different conditions. The first study evaluated the psychomotor and subjective sedative effects of bilastine, hydroxyzine, and cetirizine, all in combination with alcohol in 24 volunteers. This randomized, double-blind, double-dummy, crossover, positive-controlled and placebo-controlled clinical trial assessed psychomotor performance tests (e.g., fine motor, finger tapping and simple reaction time) and subjective self-reports (drunkenness, drowsiness, and mental slowness) at 1-week intervals. The results showed that the most pronounced level of impairment was observed in the group receiving hydroxyzine 25 mg plus alcohol. In contrast, objective measures showed less impairment in groups that received bilastine 20 mg plus alcohol or alcohol alone, both to a similar extent. The authors concluded that concomitant administration of bilastine (at therapeutic dose) and alcohol does not induce central nervous system depressant effects greater than alcohol alone [4c]. The second study used positron emission tomography (PET) to determine histamine H1-receptor occupancy (H1RO) incidence of subjective sedation and objective psychomotor performance after a single oral dose of bilastine 20 mg, hydroxyzine 25 mg, or placebo. H1RO served as a marker of psychometric function since a level of H1RO greater than 50% has been clearly linked with a high rate of sleepiness and cognitive decline. While some subjects reported accounts of sleepiness and/or sedation with hydroxyzine, there were no such reported events with bilastine. It was therefore concluded that a single dose of bilastine 20 mg was not associated with subjective sedation or objective impairment of psychomotor performance and thus lacks clinically significant sedative side effects [5c]. In another study analyzing H1RO, the subjective sleepiness stemming from levocetirizine was compared to that of fexofenadine. Eight healthy volunteers underwent positron emission tomography (PET) imaging after a single oral administration of levocetirizine (5 mg), fexofenadine (60 mg) or placebo in a double-blind crossover study. Researchers found no significant difference between subjective sleepiness and the mean brain H1RO after levocetirizine administration and fexofenadine administration leading researchers to conclude that neither subjective sleepiness nor plasma concentrations was significantly correlated with the brain H1RO of the two antihistamines [6a].

Generally, second-generation antihistamines (AH) have fewer sedative effects than their first-generation counterparts. However, significant inter-drug variances remain in the degree of cognitive and/or psychomotor impairment within the therapeutic class. Recently, researchers reviewed 45 studies and compared these differences in cognitive disruption by using the Proportional Impairment Ratio (PIR). Results from studies involving cetirizine, desloratadine, ebastine, fexofenadine, levocetirizine, loratadine, mequitazine, and/or olopatadine were included in the PIR calculations. The authors found that fexofenadine was the least impairing AH compared to all other drugs assessed in this review. Desloratadine and levocetirizine have a favorable ranking in terms of their relatively low cognitive and psychomotor impairment, while olopatadine was found to be, on average, up to eight times more impairing than the other second-generation AHs. Ebastine was found to be comparatively as favorable, clinically, as fexofenadine. Loratadine and cetirizine showed dose-dependent impairment, which meant that neither would satisfy the Consensus Group on New Generation Antihistamines (CONGA) requirements for classification as a non-impairing AH. The authors concluded that the results suggest noticeable inter-drug differences in the extent of the objectively determined sedative effects produced by second-generation AHs [7R].

RX

Special Review

Pharmacogenetics

Pharmacogenetics is being used to develop personalized therapies tailored to a patient's distinct genetic composition of allele variations in the genes implicated with drug metabolizing processes, medication effectiveness, and clinical outcomes for conditions related to histamine pathways [8R,9R]. Several polymorphisms found in the genetic coding of enzymes such as CYP2D6 and CYP3A5 have been associated with the therapeutic efficacy and/or side effects of antihistamines. With expanding research in the field of pharmacogenetics, clinicians are beginning to better understand how to apply the science of genetic variances to clinical practice [8R,10M,11R, 12M,13R,14R,15R].

Genetic polymorphisms in histamine-related genes, such as FCERI and HNMT, are theorized to influence mast cell activation and histamine metabolism. Mast cells are the major effector cell type that release histamine, cytokines and chemical mediators involved in the pathology of histamine-related conditions such as atopic dermatitis, chronic urticaria, and asthma [16c]. In a study conducted to better understand the association between HNMT polymorphisms and atopic dermatitis, researchers genotyped 763 Korean children for allelic determinants at four polymorphic sites in the HNMT gene. The researchers found that certain specific polymorphisms of the HNMT gene appear to incline susceptible individuals to develop nonatopic eczema and eczema (namely, HNMT 314C>T and 939A>G polymorphisms, respectively). This association between the 939A>G genotype and eczema is speculated to be related to raised serum IgE levels—a central element to the phenomenon of allergy and a diagnostic feature of atopic dermatitis [17c]. In another study examining histamine-related genes, researchers enrolled 93 children and adults to evaluate known single nucleotide polymorphisms (SNPs) in genes along the histamine biotransformation of the H1 receptor and the histamine response pathway. The researchers sought to determine how differences in the allele, genotype and haplotype frequency of subjects with and without asthma relate to HRH1 mRNA expression relative to genotype. While no differences in genetic expression and asthma were detected between subjects in the genotype/allele frequency for the SNPs, there were observed genetic differences relative to subjects' race and gender. Histamine pathway haplotype was associated with a diagnosis of asthma but genotype and allele were not [18c].

Pharmacogenetics is rapidly growing in its use to help researchers better understand the effects of genetic factors on clinical outcomes. Recent studies have shown how genetic polymorphisms can affect the gene expression of drug metabolizing enzymes, minimum effective drug dose and disease pathology. The following three studies examine how genetic polymorphisms can serve as pharmacodynamic predictors of antihistamine efficacy in patients with histamine-related conditions namely, chronic urticaria (CU) and chronic spontaneous utricaria (CSU). The term chronic spontaneous urticaria (CSU) is increasingly used instead of CU. CSU refers to CU in which appearance of lesions is not triggered by consistent or identifiable factors, and it specifically excludes the physical urticaria syndromes [19S]. Some CU patients are relatively refractory to antihistamines and the underlying mechanism of inter-individual variation in their physiological reactivity is still unknown. In the following three studies, three different genetic polymorphisms were assessed to compare the therapeutic effectiveness of antihistamines in CU/CSU patients. In the first study, 384 patients with chronic utricaria (CU) were compared to 231 other patients as normal controls to assess the effect of the CRTH2 gene polymorphism. No significant differences were noted between the two groups in respect to the genotype and allele frequencies of the CRTH2 polymorphisms. Furthermore, no significant associations were observed within the clinical parameters examined by the researchers such as atopy status, serum total IgE, prevalence of autoantibodies and duration of CU. However, the patients with CU required higher doses of antihistamines to control their clinical symptoms than those in the control group. The authors concluded that although gene expression may not have had a direct observable effect on CU, it may have contributed to the higher dose of the antihistamines needed to treat patients with the condition [20c].

In a recent study, researchers investigated whether FCER1A polymorphisms are associated with the risk of CSU, and to determine whether these polymorphisms influence the therapeutic efficacy of non-sedating H1-antihistamines. 191 CSU patients treated with non-sedating H1-antihistamine monotherapy (namely desloratadine, mizolastine or fexofenadine) and were then assigned an urticaria activity score (UAS7) upon clinical assessment after 4 weeks of treatment. The FCER1A, rs2298805, rs10908703 and rs2494262 genotypes were evaluated in this study and most notably, significant differences in the allele frequency of rs2298805A were found between CSU patients and healthy subjects as well as treatment effective and ineffective groups. From these findings, researchers concluded that the genotype rs2298805 may be associated with risk for CSU and the therapeutic efficacy of non-sedating H1-antihistamines for patients with CSU [21c]. In another study examining the polymorphisms effecting chronic spontaneous utricaria (CSU) of the C5AR1 −1330 T/G gene and antihistamine therapy, 191 patients with CSU and 102 healthy controls were treated with various non-sedating antihistamines (i.e.,

desloratadine, mizolastine, and fexofenadine) as monotherapy for 4 weeks. In their research, the authors found for the first time that a genetic polymorphism of C5AR1 −1330GT could impact the therapeutic efficacy of desloratadine for a particular subset of patients with CSU. Specifically, it was observed that patients with −1330GT heterozygotes had the least clinical effect from desloratadine. To their surprise, the authors did not find a substantial clinical difference among −1330T/G genotypes when treated with mizolastine. The researchers concluded that the C5AR1 −1330T/G gene may serve as a useful pharmacodynamic predictor of the efficacy of non-sedating H1-antihistamines in patients with chronic spontaneous utricaria [22C].

The significant inter-individual variations of genetic expression often cause differences in the pharmacokinetics, bioavailability and thus the therapeutic effect of antihistamines. In one study, researchers gave 12 healthy young males and 12 non-pregnant females a dose of combination doxylamine–pyridoxine which is indicated for treatment of nausea and vomiting in pregnancy. After a 21-day washout period, dose administration and blood samplings were repeated to measure the concentrations of doxylamine, pyridoxine and its metabolites. The differences between the two sexes were assessed and researchers found a higher maximum concentration for doxylamine in females and a higher maximum concentration for pyridoxal-5′-phosphate in males. As a result of the pharmacokinetic differences found in this study, namely between both genders, the authors concluded that bioequivalence studies for drugs, namely antihistamines, targeted specifically for women should not be conducted in males because they poorly predict empirical treatment outcomes [23c]. Another study aimed to evaluate the effect on plasma concentrations of genetic polymorphisms, i.e., CYP3A5 and MDR1 after a single, oral dose of 10 mg rupatadine (RUP) was done using 36 healthy male Chinese volunteers as subjects. Researchers collected, assessed and compared rupatadine plasma concentrations and several pharmacokinetic parameters (e.g., Mean C_{max}, $AUC_{(0-t)}$ and $AUC_{(0-\infty)}$) among the various polymorphic alleles of CYP3A5 and MDR1. The results indicate statistically significant correlations between the varying polymorphisms of the alleles and their respective values observed. The authors speculate that CYP3A5 and MDR1 polymorphisms may be the main causative factor in explaining the pharmacokinetic differences and plasma concentrations of RUP. This study can therefore provide a rationale for the safe and effective use of the medication [24c].

Special Review Rupatadine

Several recently published articles in the literature spotlight the favorable safety, efficacy and side effect profile of rupatadine, and thus a special review on this relatively new, second-generation, selective oral H1-antihistamine is warranted. In a prospective, non-interventional, observational, study conducted in multiple centers in Belgium, 2838 adults were evaluated for symptoms of their moderate to severe allergic rhinitis while on 6 weeks of treatment with rupatadine (10 mg, once daily). With only a few minor adverse effects reported, 21% of participants experienced "complete relief" from their symptoms and 62% experienced "strong relief" [25C]. In a two-center, randomized, double-blind, 3-way crossover, placebo-controlled study of 23 patients with chronic cold urticaria, researchers assessed the effects of up-dosing rupatadine. Patients were randomized to receive placebo, rupatadine 20 mg/day, or rupatadine 40 mg/day for 1 week. Both 20 and 40 mg rupatadine were highly effective in reducing the development of chronic cold urticaria symptom without any increase in dose-dependent adverse events [26c]. In a trial of 70 patients with CSU, patients receiving rupatadine were compared to those receiving cetirizine to assess: (i) mean number of wheals; (ii) pruritus; (iii) mean total symptom score (MTSS); (iv) size of wheal; (v) interference of wheals with sleep; and (vi) sedation. Patients with CSU were divided randomly into two treatment groups. By week 3, evaluations in all clinical parameters revealed a statistically significant treatment response to rupatadine versus the cetirizine group [27c]. In a prospective, open, randomized study of 100 patients, 50 patients were treated with levocetirizine and 50 were treated with rupatadine. Although symptoms improved in both groups, patients in the levocetirizine group showed greater improvement. A significant reduction in the mean quality of life index scores used to evaluate patients were observed in both groups, but the decrease was statistically significant in the levocetirizine group. Somnolence was the most common side effect in both groups but patients in the levocetirizine group showed greater psychomotor impairment [28c]. Researchers studied rupatadine's effects in children aged 2–11 years with CSU in a double-blind, randomized, parallel group, multicenter, placebo-controlled trial. They found rupatadine to have a statistically and clinically significant improvement, over placebo, in the relief of urticaria symptoms and quality of life in children with chronic spontaneous urticarial without significant incidence of adverse effects [29C].

OTHER ANTIHISTAMINES

Cetirizine [SEDA-35; SEDA-36, 235; SEDA-37, 188]

In a recently reported case of cetirizine induced, acute generalized exanthematous pustulosis (AGEP), the first of its kind reported in the literature, an 11-year-old girl with a history of seasonal allergic rhinitis and type 1 diabetes mellitus presented with a worsening pruritic eruption, 4 days in duration, associated with emesis and malaise. The eruption started on the face and subsequently spread to the chest, arms, and bilateral axilla, sparing the abdomen. The erythematous macules developed pustules within 48 hours. Two days prior to the eruption, the patient began taking 5 mg of cetirizine daily. The patient denied fever and joint pain. Laboratory testing revealed neutrophilia of 9770/μL (normal, 1800–7000/μL), normal eosinophil count of 30/μL (normal, <650/μL), elevated erythrocyte sedimentation rate of 18 mm/h (normal, 0–10 mm/h), and an elevated C-reactive protein of 6.31 mg/dL (normal, <1.0 mg/dL). Bacterial culture of the pustule was negative. A cutaneous shave biopsy was performed and demonstrated non-follicular subcorneal pustules comprised of neutrophils with rare eosinophils and mild papillary edema consistent with AGEP. Hydrocortisone cream, calamine lotion, triple antibiotic ointment, and oral diphenhydramine failed to provide any relief. No other medications or supplements were started within 2 months prior to the development of the eruption. Cetirizine was discontinued and the patient was started on systemic loratadine and locally applied triamcinolone 0.1% ointment. Systemic steroids were avoided due to her history of diabetes. On follow-up, the patient reported complete resolution of erythema and pustules after 14 days. The authors underline the importance of noting this reaction because of the extensive clinical use of cetirizine and because other pustular cutaneous reactions may present similarly, identifying and immediately discontinuing the drug, once the reaction is identified is essential [30A].

A 39-year-old woman complained of evanescent skin eruptions following the intake of a number of oral medications including cetirizine. There was no history of spontaneous urticaria or angioedema, systemic symptoms, atopy or any other drug allergies prior to the six episodes over the course of the previous 8 months which lead to her admission with a generalized eruption of itchy wheals within 8–10 hours of taking cetirizine. All clinical exams, labs and tests were within normal limits. The patient was admitted and subjected to a patient blinded, placebo-controlled oral drug provocation test. Four hours after taking a tablet of cetirizine 10 mg, she developed generalized, discrete to confluent, wheals (associated with pruritus but not angioedema) which subsided spontaneously after 7–8 hours. She developed wheals after taking a tablet of diclofenac 25 mg, which she had previously used for occasional pain relief, and mild pruritus following intake of a dose of fexofenadine 120 mg. Oral levocetirizine provocation could not be performed as she declined any further oral drug provocation. Intradermal testing done with injections pheniramine maleate (22.75 mg/mL) and hydroxyzine hydrochloride

(25 mg/mL) was negative. An injectable formulation of cetirizine was not available and was hence not tested. She was advised to avoid cetirizine in the future and to take diclofenac and/or fexofenadine with caution, as needed, as they demonstrated the safest results (i.e., least severe effects) for this patient during testing. The authors of the case report state that upon follow-up spanning an 18-month period, the patient avoided cetirizine and levocetirizine, has taken fexofenadine on and off for non-dermatological indications and had not reported any recurrence of urticarial lesions [31A].

Chlorpheniramine [SEDA-34, 272; SEDA-36, 235; SEDA-37, 188]

In a rare case of chlorpheniramine-induced anaphylaxis, diagnosed by skin tests and basophil activation test (BAT), a 33-year-old female with underlying chronic urticaria developed anaphylaxis 10 minutes after being administered with intravenous chlorpheniramine. She had suddenly developed abdominal discomfort, urticarial aggravation, dizziness and hypotension (blood pressure, 72/44 mm Hg). The reactions resolved after treatments with epinephrine, corticosteroids and saline hydration. The diagnosis was made on the basis of recurrent history, and supplemented by skin tests and BAT and the authors claim the utility of these tests for diagnosing drug hypersensitivity reactions [32a].

A 37-year-old woman was admitted to the allergy and immunology clinic 3 weeks after a systemic reaction composed of widespread pruritus, redness of the neck, palpitation, and dyspnea. Her symptoms emerged within minutes after intravenous administration of chlorpheniramine maleate. She had a medical history of ischemic heart disease and hyperlipidemia an unverified history of allergy to penicillin since childhood. As per the authors of this case report, she was scheduled for a coronary angiography by the cardiology clinic and because of her possible penicillin allergy, a premedication was planned to avoid a potential allergy to radiocontrast media. An ampoule of chlorpheniramine maleate was administered intravenously before the coronary angiography process, and then the reaction in question occurred. Physical examination revealed neck and facial erythema and edema of the uvula. The patient had a heart rate of 120/min, a blood pressure of 190/120 mm Hg, and a respiratory rate of 16/min. This was considered an anaphylactic reaction, and she was treated with 40 mg of methylprednisolone intravenously and 4 L/min of oxygen by mask immediately. Within 15 minutes, her symptoms gradually decreased, and 45 minutes later her physical and vital findings returned to normal. At the allergy clinic, the intradermal test with 1/100 dilution of chlorpheniramine maleate confirmed a positive result

(a wheal of 3.3 mm and a flare of 8–10 mm). Additionally, the patient's systemic symptoms including excessive fatigue, blurred vision, palpitations, burning and itching on the neck and face, and numbness in the hands and arms, occurred within minutes [33A].

Diphenhydramine [SEDA-34, 272; SEDA-35; SEDA-36, 235; SEDA-37, 189]

Diphenhydramine toxicity commonly manifests with antimuscarinic features, including dry mucous membranes, tachycardia, urinary retention, mydriasis, tachycardia, and encephalopathy. Many of these manifestations parallel the signs of anticholinergic toxicity; therapy is generally supportive as described in the following two similar case reports. Upon ingestion of an excessive amount of diphenhydramine, a 30-year-old woman presented with seizures and a wide complex tachycardia due to sodium channel blockade and cardiovascular collapse. Treatment with several typical modalities proved unsuccessful (sodium bicarbonate, lidocaine and hypertonic saline). Although intravenous fat emulsion (IFE) therapy is recommended as *adjunctive* therapy, due to the lipophilicity of diphenhydramine (octanol/water partition coefficient of 3.3), the patient rapidly improved after IFE administration [34A]. A second report involves a 23-year-old male who presented to the emergency department with recurrent seizures, hypotension and wide complex tachycardia (blood pressure of 73/32 mm Hg, heart rate of 145 beats per minute, QRS width of 172 ms) after ingesting 2000–2500 mg of DPH and despite treatment with sodium bicarbonate, the patient experienced worsening toxicity (serum DPH level of 4100 ng/mL). The patient was eventually and ultimately treated with multiple intravenous fat emulsion bolus infusions that were temporally associated with improvement in the QRS duration (106 ms) and discontinuation of the wide complex tachycardia, which narrowed to a sinus rhythm with a rate of 115 beats per minute [35A].

In a review of toxicology reports, autopsy reports, and death investigator narratives, authors cite reports of fatal overdoses involving DPH blood concentrations reportedly as high as 21 263 ng/mL. One such case describes a rare occurrence of DPH abuse via documented intravenous administration leading to death. The authors conclude that as people continue to seek legal alternative drugs to abuse and the ease of obtaining information via online forums, there is a potential to see an increase in the number of cases involving excessive use of DPH [36A].

Doxylamine [SEDA-32, 307; SEDA-34, 273; SEDA-36, 235; SEDA-37, 189]

Researchers performed an observational case series with data collected retrospectively from a poison system database for all single-substance, pediatric (5 years old and younger), doxylamine ingestions for the period of 1997–2012. A total of 140 cases were identified; 74 (53%) involved males. Ages ranged from 6 months to 5 years. In 30 cases (21%), the exact amount ingested was documented and ranged from 6.25 to 50 mg with a maximum weight-based dose of 6.2 mg/kg. In 76 cases, the estimated maximum dose ranged from 12.5 to 375 mg with a maximum weight-based dose of 37 mg/kg. All symptoms were mild and self-limiting. The only documented intervention was the administration of activated charcoal in 13 cases. Unintentional isolated pediatric doxylamine ingestions did not result in significant toxicity in the 140 reported cases. Doses of up to 6.2 mg/kg resulted in only transient drowsiness and tachycardia [37A].

Ebastine

A 21-year-old man was treated with ebastine 10 mg twice a day for the prevention of his diagnosed idiopathic anaphylaxis developed gynecomastia after 3 months of therapy. Ultrasound revealed abnormally proliferated subareolar glandular tissue in both of his breasts. The prolactin level was 74 ng/mL (normal reference, 1.61–18.77 ng/mL); testosterone was 5.78 ng/mL (normal reference, 2.41–8.27 ng/mL); estradiol was 37.44 pg/mL (normal reference, 5–4300 pg/mL); thyroid-stimulating hormone was 1.45 μIU/mL (normal reference, 0.55–4.78 μIU/mL); luteinizing hormone was 2 IU/L (normal reference, 2–12 IU/L). Initially, clinicians changed the class of H1-antihistamine that was provided to the patient, i.e., ebastine (a class of piperidine) was switched to cetirizine (a class of piperazine). One month later, the gynecomastia had progressed further despite the new H1-antihistamine (cetirizine). H1-antihistamine was then discontinued because anaphylaxis had not occurred at any point during the preventive therapy with H1-antihistamine. A few weeks later, the patient's dyspnea, cough, wheezing, and urticarial/lip angioedema had relapsed and was worsening. His breasts, however, had only somewhat regressed. Omalizumab (150 mg every 4 weeks) was then initiated as a new preventative treatment for anaphylaxis and the patient's symptoms gradually subsided. His breasts also showed gradual regression. By approximately 6 months later, his gynecomastia had completely disappeared and prolactin level had decreased to 8.91 ng/mL [38A].

Hydroxyzine [SEDA-36, 236; SEDA-37, 190]

A 47-year-old woman developed shortness of breath and generalized pruritus after taking a 25 mg tablet of hydroxyzine which necessitated treatment in the emergency department. Her physical examination was unremarkable except for mild eczema on her arms and hands and nasal mucosal edema. Her total IgE was 271 IU/mL (normal range: 150–1000 IU/mL) and complete blood count showed eosinophilia of 910/μL (normal range: 30–350). When subjected to a blinded oral challenge to hydroxyzine, the placebo (5 mL of water sweetened with sugar) caused no reaction. However, within 3 minutes after ingesting the hydroxyzine syrup the patient developed generalized pruritus and severe bronchospasm with little air movement on chest auscultation. She was treated with 0.3 mg of intramuscular epinephrine and required oxygen at 5 L by nasal cannula to bring her O_2 saturation to 95%. She was subsequently treated with nebulized albuterol. Within 30 minutes, her acute condition markedly improved. She was instructed to avoid hydroxyzine and its derivatives, cetirizine, and levocetirizine. She was prescribed fexofenadine for treatment of her allergic rhinitis and doxepin for itching from eczema, both of which she tolerated well in the past. At another visit, a skin prick test (SPT) was performed with diphenhydramine (12.5 mg/5 mL), hydroxyzine (10 mg/mL), cetirizine (1 mg/mL), levocetirizine (2.5 mg/mL), fexofenadine (30 mg/mL), doxepin (10 mg/mL), and loratadine (5 mg/mL). A few minutes later the patient complained of pruritus, shortness of breath, and developed severe repetitive cough. Her vital signs showed blood pressure of 141/60 mm Hg, heart rate of 96 beats per minute, and O_2 saturation of 100% on room air. Her oropharynx appeared normal, lungs were clear, and skin was clear except for marks of severe scratching. Because of the severity of her cough, she was given 0.3 mg of intramuscular epinephrine and 30 mg of fexofenadine for itching. Her symptoms significantly improved within 20 minutes [39A].

A 70-year-old woman whose medical history included lichen planus, developed a bilateral highly pruritic palmar erythema that evolved to a generalized morbilliform rash with subsequent complete desquamation after 4 days treatment with prednisone and hydroxyzine. At a later time, she took cetirizine for a cold, and developed a similar reaction of palmar erythema and desquamation. Cetirizine is the primary active metabolite of hydroxyzine. Skin tests (prick and intradermal tests) were performed with steroids and patch tests (read after 48 and 96 hours) with corticosteroids and antihistamines. Controlled oral challenge tests were performed with prednisone and with an alternative antihistamine. Skin tests were negative for all corticosteroids but the antihistamine test was positive for hydroxyzine. Oral challenge with prednisone and dexchlorpheniramine was negative. The patient was diagnosed with cutaneous drug eruption from hydroxyzine and cetirizine. The authors report that while rare, systemic administration of antihistamines may induce allergic hypersensitivity, which is mainly linked to phenothiazine- and piperazine-derived compounds [40A].

A 48-year-old woman with a history of psoriasis presented to a walk-in clinic complaining of generalized pruritus. She was prescribed oral hydroxyzine. Twenty-four hours after hydroxyzine ingestion, a burning erythematous eruption developed on her trunk, extremities, and genitalia. She discontinued the hydroxyzine on day 4. Two days after discontinuing hydroxyzine, fever developed and skin eruption worsened. Skin examination revealed widespread small non-follicular pustules on an erythematous background. Biopsies showed features of acute generalized exanthematous pustulosis (AGEP). AGEP is described as a significant cutaneous reaction with a sudden onset of multiple, disseminated, nonfollicular, sterile pustules on an erythematous background and usually, intertriginous accentuation is associated with fever (temperature greater than 38 °C) and neutrophilia ($>7 \times 10^9$/L). The patient was treated with prednisone and betamethasone valerate 0.1% ointment. She was later tested in the Patch Test Clinic and a 3+++ local reaction developed in response to 10% hydroxyzine at 48 and 120 hours. Biopsy of the test site showed a neutrophilic dermatosis supporting AGEP. This is the third known case of its kind involving hydroxyzine [41A].

A 72-year-old patient was admitted to the emergency department with a 3-day history of pruritus without fever. Examination revealed an obstruction of the bile duct with a mixed increase in total and conjugated bilirubin. His past medical history was positive for: diabetes, chronic pancreatitis and ischemic cardiomyopathy and was negative for any renal failure (GFR = 91 mL/min; 1.73 m^2 Cockcroft Gault formula). Prior to the initiation of hydroxyzine treatment, the patient's QTc interval was calculated at 450 ms. At day 1 of treatment for pruritus, hydroxyzine was introduced at 100 mg/day and then 175 mg/day for the next 2 days. Starting on day 4, the patient presented with several syncopal events combined with a QTc prolongation of 590 and 582 ms measured on days 6 and 10, respectively, acute renal and liver failures, a 45/min sinus bradycardia and hypokalemia (3.3 mmol/L). Hydroxyzine blood levels at days 6 and 10 were 96 and 506 ng/mL respectively (usual therapeutic concentration is 50–100 ng/mL). Torsades de Pointes was not recorded (no ECG performed during syncope) but was highly suspected. Hydroxyzine was discontinued and hypokalemia was corrected. QTc returned to normal value and syncope did not reoccur after hydroxyzine was discontinued. According to the authors, while there was one other previously published case of hydroxyzine-induced QTc prolongation, this is the first case of hydroxyzine associated QT prolongation with drug dosage data [42A].

Ketotifen

Ketotifen is a fast acting non-competitive, second-generation H1 histamine receptor antagonist and mast cell stabilizer which demonstrates greater permeability across the blood–brain barrier than newer agents in the therapeutic class [43A]. Nocturnal bruxism is a common oromandibular movement disorder highly prevalent in children, yet its pathophysiological mechanism has not been fully explained. Iatrogenic sleep bruxism has been described following treatment with several psychotropic medications but the first documented case of antihistamine-induced bruxism occurred recently in a 4-year-old child. The child experienced nocturnal bruxism during treatment for bronchospasm and rhinitis with ketotifen. Drug rechallenge was performed and confirmed the findings [44E].

Levocetirizine [SEDA-37, 191]

An otherwise healthy 8-year-old girl with a history of allergic rhinitis (maintained on levocetirizine and fluticasone nasal spray) began suffering short-lasting stabbing headache attacks. The headaches began 1 month before her hospitalization and were usually preceded by physical activity (e.g., dancing, running). The pain, which was located in the right supraorbital region, lasted for only 1 s but occurred several times throughout the day. Upon physical examination, no other associated symptoms were observed and her brain MRI was normal. Based on the patient's clinical course and laboratory results, the proposed diagnosis was primary headache. The patient was discharged and it was suggested that she keep a headache diary; this is how she made the association between the headache attacks and use of levocetirizine and thus subsequently discontinued use of the antihistamine. Six months later, the girl remained headache free further signifying that the headaches were most likely drug induced [45A].

A woman in her 60s presented with a nonproductive, progressive cough and shortness of breath. She was otherwise healthy (nonsmoker) except for seasonal allergic rhinorrhitis and had been taking levocetirizine 5 mg for 2 months prior to admission. A chest radiograph showed patchy infiltrations on both lower lung fields. High-resolution computed tomography (CT) scan findings were consistent with non-specific interstitial pneumonia. Serum markers associated with interstitial pneumonias were elevated. Room air arterial blood gas analysis revealed hypoxemia. Restrictive ventilatory impairment was noted with reduced diffusing capacity. Transbronchial lung biopsy specimens demonstrated unclassifiable alveolitis. Steroid pulse therapy was introduced to treat her respiratory distress, but the initial response to treatment was poor. A drug lymphocyte stimulation test was positive for levocetirizine. The interstitial pneumonia improved following withdrawal of levocetirizine and her illness had not recurred under steroid therapy and discontinuation of levocetirizine. The diagnosis of drug-induced lung injury (DLI) was made according to several criteria: the patient had a history of exposure to levocetirizine, the clinical manifestations were in line with DLI, all other causes of interstitial pneumonias were eliminated and lastly, the interstitial pneumonia improved following drug discontinuation. The authors admit that uncertainty remains over whether levocetirizine was unquestionably responsible for the patient's DLI but suspect that the antihistamine may have potentiated the risk for developing (DLI). The authors explain that exposure to a drug can induce DLI with some latency, ranging from a few weeks to months. Levocetirizine was assumed to cause DLI within 2 months in this case and while the outcome was relatively good, the DLI had a progressive nature only partially reversible by steroids. This is the first reported case of levocetirizine-induced lung injury [46A].

Promethazine [SEDA-36, 237; SEDA-37, 192]

Many medical textbooks recommend the use of parenteral H1 and H2 antagonists in anaphylaxis, particularly in those hypotensive patients who are resistant to adrenaline [47R]. However, a systematic review did not identify any studies to support antihistamine administration as a first-line therapy for anaphylaxis [48R]. In this regard, an epidemiological study of 490 patients with anaphylaxis reported in a sub-study that three patients with anaphylaxis intravenously treated with promethazine 25 mg subsequently developed hypotension [49R]. All were then successfully treated with epinephrine. Although the authors accept that these observations do not prove causality, they do demonstrate the potential risk of using parenteral antihistamines in patients with anaphylaxis.

References

[1] Uesawa Y, Hishinuma S, Shoji M. Molecular determinants responsible for sedative and non-sedative properties of histamine H₁-receptor antagonists. J Pharmacol Sci. 2014;124(2):160–8 [R].
[2] Katayose Y, Aritake S, Kitamura S, et al. Carry over effect on next-day sleepiness and psychomotor performance of night time administered antihistaminic drugs: a randomized controlled trial. Hum Psychopharmacol Clin Exp. 2012;27:428–36 [c].
[3] Kamei H, Isaji A, Noda Y, et al. Effects of single therapeutic doses of promethazine, fexofenadine and olopatadine on psychomotor function and histamine-induced wheal- and flare-responses: a randomized double-blind, placebo-controlled study in healthy volunteers. Arch Dermatol Res. 2012;304:263–72 [c].
[4] García-Gea C, Martínez J, Ballester MR, et al. Psychomotor and subjective effects of bilastine, hydroxyzine, and cetirizine, in combination with alcohol: a randomized, double-blind, crossover, and positive-controlled and placebo-controlled Phase I clinical trials. Hum Psychopharmacol. 2014;29(2):120–32 [c].
[5] Farré M, Pérez-Mañá C, Papaseit E, et al. Bilastine vs. hydroxyzine: occupation of brain histamine H1-receptors evaluated by positron emission tomography in healthy volunteers. Br J Clin Pharmacol. 2014;78(5):970–80 [c].
[6] Hiraoka K, Tashiro M, Grobosch T, et al. Brain histamine H1 receptor occupancy measured by PET after oral administration of levocetirizine, a non-sedating antihistamine. Expert Opin Drug Saf. 2015;14(2):199–206. http://dx.doi.org/10.1517/14740338.2015.989831. Epub 2014 Dec 3 [a].
[7] Isomura T, Kono T, Hindmarch I, et al. Central nervous system effects of the second-generation antihistamines marketed in Japan—review of inter-drug differences using the proportional impairment ratio (PIR). PLoS One. 2014;9(12):e114336. http://dx.doi.org/10.1371/journal.pone.0114336. eCollection 2014 [R].
[8] Szalai C, Tölgyesi G, Nagy A, et al. Pharmacogenomics of asthma: present and perspective. Orv Hetil. 2006;147(4):159–69. Review, Hungarian [R].
[9] Losol P, Yoo HS, Park HS. Molecular genetic mechanisms of chronic urticaria. Allergy, Asthma Immunol Res. 2014;6:13–21 [R].
[10] Cordova-Sintjago TC, Fang L, Bruysters M, et al. Molecular determinants of ligand binding at the human histamine H₁ receptor: site-directed mutagenesis results analyzed with ligand docking and molecular dynamics studies at H₁ homology and crystal structure models. J Chem Pharm Res. 2012;4(6):2937–51 [M].
[11] Saruwatari J, Matsunaga M, Ikeda K, et al. Impact of CYP2D6*10 on H1-antihistamine-induced hypersomnia. Eur J Clin Pharmacol. 2006;62(12):995–1001 [R].
[12] Morris AP, Zeggini E. An evaluation of statistical approaches to rare variant analysis in genetic association studies. Genet Epidemiol. 2010;34:188–93 [M].
[13] Hlavica P. N-oxidative transformation of free and N-substituted amine functions by cytochrome P450 as means of bioactivation and detoxication. Drug Metab Rev. 2002;34(3):451–77 [R].
[14] Hishinuma S, Sugawara K, Uesawa Y, et al. Differential thermodynamic driving force of first- and second-generation antihistamines to determine their binding affinity for human H1 receptors. Biochem Pharmacol. 2014;91(2):231–41 [R].
[15] Xu M, Ju W, Hao H, et al. Cytochrome P450 2J2: distribution, function, regulation, genetic polymorphisms and clinical significance. Drug Metab Rev. 2013;45(3):311–52 [R].
[16] Luquin E, Kaplan AP, Ferrer M. Increased responsiveness of basophils of patients with chronic urticaria to sera but hypo-responsiveness to other stimuli. Clin Exp Allergy. 2005;35:456–60 [c].
[17] Lee HS, Kim SH, Kim KW, et al. Involvement of human histamine N-methyltransferase gene polymorphisms in susceptibility to atopic dermatitis in Korean children. Allergy, Asthma Immunol Res. 2012;4(1):31–6 [c].
[18] Raje N, Vyhlidal CA, Dai H, et al. Genetic variation within the histamine pathway among patients with asthma. J Asthma. 2015;52(4):353–62 [c].
[19] Zuberbier T, Asero R, Bindslev-Jensen C, et al. EAACI/GA(2) LEN/EDF/WAO guideline: definition, classification and diagnosis of urticaria. Allergy. 2009;64:1417 [S].
[20] Palikhe NS, Kim SH, Ye YM, et al. Association of CRTH2 gene polymorphisms with the required dose of antihistamines in patients with chronic urticaria. Pharmacogenomics. 2009;10(3):375–83 [c].
[21] Guo A, Zhu W, Zhang C, et al. Association of FCER1A genetic polymorphisms with risk for chronic spontaneous urticaria and efficacy of nonsedating H1-antihistamines in Chinese patients. Arch Dermatol Res. 2015;307(2):183–90. http://dx.doi.org/10.1007/s00403-014-1525-z. Epub 2014 Nov 21 [c].
[22] Yan S, et al. Influence of component 5a receptor 1 (C5AR1)—1330 T/G polymorphism on nonsedating H1-antihistamines

therapy in Chinese patients with chronic spontaneous urticaria. J Dermatol Sci. 2014;76(3):240–5 [C].

[23] Koren G, Vranderick M, Gill S, et al. Sex differences in pharmacokinetics of doxylamine-pyridoxine combination: implications for pregnancy. Obstet Gynecol. 2014;123(Suppl 1):151S [c].

[24] Xiong Y, Yuan Z, Yang J, et al. CYP3A5*3 and MDR1 C3435T are influencing factors of inter-subject variability in rupatadine pharmacokinetics in healthy Chinese volunteers. Eur J Drug Metab Pharmacokinet. 2016;41(2):117–24 [c].

[25] Eloy P, Tobback L, Imschoot J. Rupatadine relieves allergic rhinitis: a prospective observational study. B-ENT. 2015;11(1):11–8 [C].

[26] Abajian M, Curto-Barredo L, Krause K, et al. Rupatadine 20 mg and 40 mg are effective in reducing the symptoms of chronic cold urticaria. Acta Derm Venereol. 2016;96:56–9. http://dx.doi.org/10.2340/00015555-2150 [c].

[27] Dakhale GN, Shinde AT, Mahatme MS, et al. Clinical effectiveness and safety of cetirizine versus rupatadine in chronic spontaneous urticaria: a randomized, double-blind, 6-week trial. Int J Dermatol. 2014;53(5):643–9. http://dx.doi.org/10.1111/ijd.12250. Epub 2013 Dec 10 [c].

[28] Johnson M, Kwatra G, Badyal DK, et al. Levocetirizine and rupatadine in chronic idiopathic urticaria. Int J Dermatol. 2015;54(10):1199–204. http://dx.doi.org/10.1111/ijd.12733. Epub 2014 Dec 17 [c].

[29] Potter P, Mitha E, Barkai L, et al. Rupatadine is effective in the treatment of chronic spontaneous urticaria in children aged 2–11 years. Pediatr Allergy Immunol. 2016;27:55–61. http://dx.doi.org/10.1111/pai.12460 [C].

[30] Badawi AH, Tefft K, Fraga GR, et al. Cetirizine-induced acute generalized exanthematous pustulosis: a serious reaction to a commonly used drug. Dermatol Online J. 2014;20(5):22613 [A].

[31] Singh S, Kumar P, Sharma VK. Cetirizine-induced urticaria masquerading as multiple drug intolerance syndrome. Indian J Dermatol Venereol Leprol. 2015;81:537–9 [A].

[32] Lee H-S, Song W-J, Lee J-W, et al. Chlorpheniramine-induced anaphylaxis diagnosed by basophil activation test. Asia Pac Allergy. 2015;5(3):177–80 [a].

[33] Demirel F, Gulec M, Kartal O, et al. Allergic reaction to chlorpheniramine maleate. Ann Allergy Asthma Immunol. 2015;115(2):150–2. http://dx.doi.org/10.1016/j.anai.2015.05.009 [A].

[34] Abdelmalek D, Schwarz ES, Sampson C, et al. Life-threatening diphenhydramine toxicity presenting with seizures and a wide complex tachycardia improved with intravenous fat emulsion. Am J Ther. 2014;21(6):542–4. http://dx.doi.org/10.1097/MJT.0b013e318281191b [A].

[35] Abdi A, Rose E, Levine M. Diphenhydramine overdose with intraventricular conduction delay treated with hypertonic sodium bicarbonate and i.v. lipid emulsion. West J Emerg Med.

2014;15(7):855–8. http://dx.doi.org/10.5811/westjem.2014.8.23407 [A].

[36] Botch-Jones SR, Johnson R, Kleinschmidt K, et al. Diphenhydramine's role in death investigations: an examination of diphenhydramine prevalence in 2 US geographical areas. Am J Forensic Med Pathol. 2014;35(3):181–5 [A].

[37] Cantrell FL, Clark AK, McKinley M, et al. Retrospective review of unintentional pediatric ingestions of doxylamine. Clin Toxicol (Phila). 2015;53(3):178–80. http://dx.doi.org/10.3109/15563650.2015.1006400 Epub 2015 Feb 8 [A].

[38] Sik Jung H, Park C-H, Tae Park Y, et al. Gynecomastia induced by H1-antihistamine (ebastine) in a patient with idiopathic anaphylaxis. Asia Pac Allergy. 2015;5(3):187–90 [A].

[39] Shakouri AA, Bahna SL. Hypersensitivity to antihistamines. Allergy Asthma Proc. 2013;34(6):488–96 [A].

[40] Viñas M, Castillo MJ, Hernández N, et al. Cutaneous drug eruption induced by antihistamines. Clin Exp Dermatol. 2014;39(8):918–20. http://dx.doi.org/10.1111/ced.12445 [A].

[41] O'Toole A, Lacroix J, Pratt M, et al. Acute generalized exanthematous pustulosis associated with 2 common medications: hydroxyzine and benzocaine. J Am Acad Dermatol. 2014;71(4):e147–9. http://dx.doi.org/10.1016/j.jaad.2014.05.041 [A].

[42] Vigne J, Alexandre J, Fobe F, et al. QT prolongation induced by hydroxyzine: a pharmacovigilance case report. Eur J Clin Pharmacol. 2015;71(3):379–81. http://dx.doi.org/10.1007/s00228-014-1804-9. Epub 2015 Jan 28 [A].

[43] Unno K, Ozaki T, Mohammad S, et al. First and second generation H₁ histamine receptor antagonists produce different sleep-inducing profiles in rats. Eur J Pharmacol. 2012;683(1–3):179–85. http://dx.doi.org/10.1016/j.ejphar.2012.03.017. Epub 2012 Mar 16 [A].

[44] Italiano D, Bramanti P, Militi D, et al. Ketotifen-induced nocturnal bruxism. Eur J Pediatr. 2014;173(12):1585–6. http://dx.doi.org/10.1007/s00431-013-2138-9. Epub 2013 Aug 16 [A].

[45] Biedroń A, Kaciński M, Skowronek-Bała B. Stabbing headache in an 8-year-old girl: primary or drug induced headache? Pediatrics. 2014;133(4):e1068–71. http://dx.doi.org/10.1542/peds.2013-0655 [A].

[46] Endo S, Yamamoto Y, Minami Y, et al. Histamine H1 antagonist levocetirizine as a potential cause of lung injury. Respirol Case Rep. 2015;3(2):64–7. http://dx.doi.org/10.1002/rcr2.101 [A].

[47] Tintinalli J, Stapczynski J, John Ma O, et al., Tintinalli's emergency medicine: a comprehensive study guide. 7th ed. New York: McGraw Hill; 2013. ISBN-13: 978-0071484800.

[48] Sheikh A, Ten Broek V, Brown SG, et al. H1-antihistamines for the treatment of anaphylaxis: Cochrane systematic review. Allergy. 2007;62(8):830–7 [R].

[49] Ellis BC, Brown SG. Parenteral antihistamines cause hypotension in anaphylaxis. Emerg Med Australas. 2013;25(1):92–3 [R].

15

Drugs That Act on the Respiratory Tract

Bryony Coupe[1], Andrew L. Griffiths, Gwyneth A. Davies

Asthma & Allergy Group, Swansea University Medical School, Institute of Life Science 1, Swansea University, Swansea, United Kingdom

[1]Corresponding author: coupeb@cardiff.ac.uk

INHALED GLUCOCORTICOIDS [SEDA-35, 309; SEDA-36, 241; SEDA-37, 195]

Inhaled corticosteroids (ICS) are among the most frequently recommended medications in both asthma and COPD but have a well-documented potential significant adverse event (AE)profile, including pneumonia, diabetes, increased bone fracture risk, cataracts, dysphonia and oropharyngeal candidiasis, covered in previous annuals (SEDA-35, 309; SEDA-36, 241; SEDA-37, 195).

Respiratory

PNEUMONIA

The risk of pneumonia in patients with COPD using ICS continues to be studied and much of the new literature focuses on fluticasone (see Section "Fluticasone"). A major review paper examined 27 RCTs and 9 observational studies involving patient use of ICS in general (including beclomethasone, budesonide, fluticasone, and mometasone) and mortality risk [1R]. Their goal was to contrast the well-documented increased risk of pneumonia with the lack of increased risk of pneumonia related or overall mortality. They found no difference, or a reduction, in pneumonia related and overall mortality associated with ICS use. The authors suggest that either ICS decrease the severity of pneumonia or that there is an unknown mitigating effect of ICS decreasing the risk of mortality.

TUBERCULOSIS AND INFLUENZA

In a systematic review and meta-analysis, the risk of tuberculosis and influenza with ICS and non-ICS treatment was investigated in patients with COPD treated for at least 6 months [2MC]. 25 trials for TB (22 898 subjects) and 26 trials for influenza (23 616 subjects) were included (5 involving budesonide use, 19 involving fluticasone, and 2 involving mometasone). ICS treatment was associated with a significantly higher risk of TB (OR, 2.29; 95% CI, 1.04–5.03) but not influenza (Peto OR, 1.24; 95% CI, 0.94–1.63).

Endocrine

The risk of adrenal insufficiency in patients treated with ICS continues to be investigated. A retrospective analysis of 2773 patients having a short Synacthen test (SST) at large secondary/tertiary centers in the UK between 2008 and 2013 investigated the prevalence of adrenal suppression due to treatment with glucocorticoids [3C]. Of 166 patients taking ICS (mainly beclomethasone and fluticasone), 34 (20.5%) failed the SST, defined as a 30-minute cortisol <550 nmol/L. Furthermore, adrenal suppression increased in a dose-dependent manner. The researchers also found that a basal serum cortisol level was helpful to screen which patients taking ICS would benefit from SST; a basal cortisol ≥348 nmol/L provided 100% specificity for passing the SST.

The concern regarding endocrine AEs of ICS in children has been covered previously (SEDA-37, 195; SEDA-36, 243) and has prompted several reviews in leading journals and position statements in the past year. The Canadian Society of Allergy and Clinical Immunology made the recommendation that all children receiving a high dose of ICS (≥500 mcg/day of Fluticasone Propionate or equivalent; ≥400 mcg/day under age 12) for 6 months or more should be screened for adrenal suppression using morning serum cortisol [4R]. They further requested that children should have paediatric endocrinology input if adrenal suppression is confirmed. The Drugs and Therapeutics Committee of the Paediatric Endocrine Society presented a thorough review covering the effects on HPA axis, linear growth and bone mineral density [5R]. They felt that risks to linear growth and bone mineral density were outweighed by the respiratory benefits of ICS. However, because of the potential for life-threatening HPA suppression, they recommend increased monitoring. They suggest adrenal function be tested in any symptomatic patients, those with growth velocity reduction, and high-risk asymptomatic patients. Meanwhile, hair cortisol was presented as a novel biomarker of HPA suppression [6c]. In 18 asthmatic children, median hair cortisol levels were twice as high when using ICS compared to hair samples taken from the same children prior to ICS use.

Musculoskeletal

A systematic review and meta-analysis assessed the association between long-term ICS use and bone AEs in asthmatic patients [7M]. 7 RCTs and 11 observational studies comparing ICS use (beclomethasone, budesonide, flunisolide, fluticasone and mometasone) for over 1 year to non-ICS use in patients with asthma were included. No significant association between ICS and fractures in children (pooled OR 1.02, 95% CI 0.94–1.10, two studies) or adults (pooled OR 1.09, 95% CI 0.45–2.62, four studies) was demonstrated. No reductions in bone mineral density were associated with ICS use.

Budesonide [SEDA-35, 309; SEDA-36, 241; SEDA-37, 195]

A small clinical trial compared the efficacy and side effect profile of inhaled budesonide to systemic methylprednisolone in 30 patients experiencing acute COPD exacerbation [8c]. The researchers considered the two treatments to have a similar efficacy with inhaled budesonide having a significantly lower incidence of AEs (23.8% vs. 42.9%, $P < 0.05$) such as palpitations, hypertension, hyperglycemia and gastrointestinal symptoms.

Ear, Nose, Throat

The effects on voice parameters of short-term budesonide used for persistent cough were investigated [9c]. 46 patients were administered inhaled budesonide 400 mcg twice daily for 1 month; no negative effects on voice parameters were found.

Fluticasone [SEDA-35, 309; SEDA-36, 241; SEDA-37, 195]

General AEs associated with fluticasone were examined in several clinical trials. Two major RCTs assessed the efficacy and safety of inhaled fluticasone furoate in combination with vilanterol (FF/VI). In one study, FF/VI was compared with tiotropium (TIO) for patients with moderate-to-severe COPD and high risk of cardiovascular comorbidity [10C]. The study had a 12-week treatment period and 623 subjects. Pneumonia was more frequently reported in the FF/VI group (3/310 compared

to 0/313 in the tiotropium group), which is consistent with other studies [11MC]. There were no significant effects on cardiovascular safety from either treatment, and there were no clinically significant differences in urinary cortisol ratio.

A second multicenter RCT compared different dose combinations of FF/VI (50/25, 100/25, 200/25 mcg) to placebo in 643 patients over 6 months [12C]. The incidence of AEs in the FF/VI 200/25 mcg was 48% (77/160) compared to 37–40% in the other treatment arms, most notably nasopharyngitis (19/160 (12%) compared to 7/162 (4%) in the placebo arm) and local steroid effects such as candida infection (6/160 (4%) compared to 1/162 (<1%) in the placebo arm). However, the authors concluded this was an acceptable safety profile.

Two smaller trials also examined the AEs and pharmacokinetics of inhaled FF in healthy subjects. Triple therapy of FF/VI and the anticholinergic umeclidinium (UMEC) were compared with dual therapies in a study involving 88 subjects [13c]. They found no clinically relevant differences in systemic exposure or safety between the approved dual therapies and the triple therapy. Secondly, the safety and pharmacokinetics of FF 100 mcg and UMEC 125 mcg alone or in combination were compared in a RCT with 18 healthy subjects [14c]. No clinical significant effects on ECG, vital sign values or laboratory parameters were found.

In a review of FF/VI in COPD, the authors confirmed the most frequently reported AEs of FF/VI— nasopharyngitis, headache, upper respiratory tract infection and oropharyngeal candidiasis—as consistent with other ICS/LABA class drugs and also emphasized that no head-to-head trials actually establish superiority of FF compared to other ICS [15R].

In a major review, a non-systematic analysis of published studies compared the new fluticasone propionate/formoterol (FP/F) combination in a single inhaler to other combined ICS/LABA for asthmatic patients [16R]. The authors explored long-term AEs, noting the most common to be nasopharyngitis, dyspnea and headache, but felt the rate of AEs to be low. They concluded that the safety profile of the FP/F combination extends over a longer time span than seen in other studies.

Respiratory
PNEUMONIA

In an investigation of whether blood eosinophil counts were a useful biomarker for the long-term effects of ICS, the incidence of pneumonia in treatment groups was also considered [17MC]. Researchers analysed data from two replicate, double-blind, RCTs of 12 months, in which 3177 patients with moderate-to-severe COPD were treated with VI 25 mcg alone or with the addition of FF 50, 100 or 200 mcg. They compared incidences of pneumonia in the treatment groups according to their baseline eosinophil cell count (<2% and ≥2%) and confirmed that cases of pneumonia were higher in patients treated with FF/VI than those treated with VI alone. However, the rates were similar for both eosinophil strata. Patients receiving FF/VI 100/25 mcg with an eosinophil count ≥2% had almost double the incidence of serious pneumonia (19/527) than those with an eosinophil count of <2% (5/264). This study is useful because it may guide clinicians in assessing which patients with COPD have a higher risk of pneumonia when treated with ICS, but more data are needed.

In a large observational study, the incidence of *radiologically* confirmed pneumonia in patients with COPD using ICS was investigated [18MC]. In all previous studies, pneumonia has been *clinically* diagnosed. Data were analyzed from two replicate, 1-year, double-blind trials comparing FF/VI 50/25, 100/25, 200/25 mcg and VI 25 mcg alone including a total of 3255 subjects. The incidence of radiologically confirmed pneumonia was higher in the FF groups (6% (48/820), 6% (51/806) and 7% (55/811) for FF 50, 100 and 200 mcg, respectively, compared to 3% (27/818) for VI alone), but as hypothesized, this incidence was less than the incidence of clinically diagnosed pneumonia.

The LANTERN study, a large double-blind, RCT, compared dual treatment with LABA/LAMA combination indacaterol/glycopyrronium 110/50 mcg to salmeterol/fluticasone (SFC) 50/500 mcg in 744 patients with moderate-to-severe COPD [19C]. SFC showed a threefold higher incidence of pneumonia (2.7% (10/369) compared to 0.8% (3/372) in the indacaterol/glycopyrronium arm) and a higher rate of upper respiratory tract infections (7.0% (26/369) compared to 3.5% (13/372)).

Two observational studies further investigated the association between ICS such as fluticasone and pneumonia. A cohort study, with the goal of minimizing the bias associated with case–control studies, compared pneumonia events in COPD patients who were either new users of ICS (1155 patients) or long-acting bronchodilator (LABD) monotherapies (6492 patients) [20MC]. New use of ICS was associated with a statistically significantly increased risk of pneumonia compared to new use of LABD (HR=1.49, 95% CI: 1.22–1.83) in a population-based COPD cohort. Secondly, a cluster analysis of two replicate 1-year RCTs in which FF/VI was compared to VI alone was performed [21MC]. The researchers identified clusters defined by established pneumonia risk factors such as increased airflow obstruction and multiple comorbidities. 3255 cases were analyzed, and the researchers found a nearly threefold increase in the relative risk of serious pneumonia in subjects treated with FF/VI compared with VI alone (HR=2.92, 95% CI: 1.40–6.01). Through the cluster analysis the authors determined that patients with significantly decreased lung function and BMI <19 were at most risk of pneumonia. Other risk factors included co-morbidity, previous history of pneumonia and the use of anti-depressants.

Endocrine

A double-blind, placebo-controlled RCT with 16 healthy Chinese volunteers compared different dose combinations of FF/VI (50/25, 100/25, 200/25 mcg) and placebo over a period of 7 weeks [22c]. Relative to placebo, FF/VI 100/25 and 200/25 mcg produced statistically significant dose-related decreases in serum cortisol following 7-day repeat dosing. Of note, the systemic exposure of FF in the Chinese study participants was 50% greater than levels observed in healthy Caucasian subjects, attributable to differences in lung absorption. However, the researchers note that based on their calculations, therapeutic FF doses should not produce any clinically significant HPA axis suppression.

BETA$_2$-ADRENOCEPTOR AGONISTS [SEDA-35, 315; SEDA-36, 245; SEDA-37, 197]

The safety of beta$_2$-adrenocepter agonists has been reviewed in previous annuals, with systemic effects such as tachycardia, increased blood pressure, prolonged QT interval, hyperglycemia and hypokalemia mediated by beta$_2$-adrenergic receptors in the cardiovascular system [SEDA-35, 315; SEDA-36, 245; SEDA-37, 197]. Four recent Cochrane meta-analyses and one large clinical trial have looked at the safety and efficacy of the class of drugs in general in patients with asthma and COPD.

One meta-analysis compared long-acting beta$_2$-adrenocepter agonists (LABA) plus tiotropium to tiotropium alone in patients with COPD [23M]. Ten RCTs lasting 3 months or longer were included with a total of 10 894 participants, mostly with moderate or severe COPD. Four studies used olodaterol, three used indacaterol, two used formoterol and one used salmeterol. The authors found no significant differences in hospital admissions or mortality, and there was no statistically significant difference in AEs between study groups.

There have been concerns regarding the use of LABA in patients with asthma and association with increased hospital admissions. This has resulted in US and UK regulators making the recommendation that LABA be used "for the shortest duration of time required to achieve control of symptoms" [24S]. In this vein, a Cochrane meta-analysis assessed the safety and efficacy of adding LABA to ICS in children and adolescents with asthma [25M]. They included 33 RCTs lasting at least 4 weeks in children and adolescents with asthma, totaling 6381 participants. They found no statistically significant differences in hospital admissions (RR 1.74, 95% CI 0.90–3.36) or in serious adverse events (SAEs) (RR 1.17, 95% CI 0.75–1.85).

A further Cochrane meta-analysis investigated the safety of stopping LABA in stable asthma compared to continued use of LABA/ICS [26M]. Five double-blind RCTs between 12 and 24 weeks duration with a total of 2781 patients were included. The investigators found that stopping LABA might increase the number of people having exacerbations, but the confidence intervals did not exclude the possibility that stopping LABA was beneficial (OR 1.74, 95% CI 0.83–3.65). There were too few AEs to determine whether stopping LABA had a greater effect on SAEs compared to continuing with LABA/ICS (OR 0.82, 95% CI 0.28–2.42).

The efficacy and safety of adding a LABA to ICS were compared with adding a LAMA to ICS in patients with asthma not well controlled on ICS alone in another meta-analysis [27M]. 8 parallel and cross-over RCTs of at least 12 weeks duration were included. There were very few SAEs from which the authors concluded they could not compare the treatments in terms of AEs.

Finally, the BELT RCT compared the safety and efficacy of LABA + ICS to TIO + ICS in 1070 black adults with asthma [28MC]. The investigators found that asthma-related and non-asthma-related AEs and SAEs did not differ between treatments (11/538 (2%) of LABA + ICS patients compared to 16/532 (3%) of TIO + ICS patients, $P = 0.16$). There were less asthma-related hospitalizations in the LABA + ICS group compared to the TIO + ICS group (10/538 versus 19/532, respectively). Furthermore, there were a total of 67 hospitalizations in the TIO + ICS group compared to 58 in the LABA + ICS group. Three deaths occurred, all in the TIO + ICS group; 2 of those deaths were asthma related.

Formoterol [SEDA-35, 317; SEDA-36, 245; SEDA-37, 197]

One non-systematic analysis of published studies looked at the new fluticasone propionate/formoterol (FP/F) combination in a single inhaler for asthmatic patients [16R]. As discussed previously (see Section "Inhaled Glucocorticoids"), this demonstrated comparable efficacy and encouraging side effect profile. The authors note that the different dose combinations (50/5, 125/5, 210/10 and 500/20 mcg) allow tailoring to asthma severity, and in particular that their research shows that concerns regarding the higher dose of formoterol is unsubstantiated, as the rate of AEs in studies was similar for higher and lower doses.

Indacaterol [SEDA-35, 317; SEDA-36, 246; SEDA-37, 198]

The safety of the ultra-LABA indacaterol has been reviewed previously [SEDA-36, 246; SEDA-37, 198].

Recent studies support previous conclusions that this drug has a good AE profile. A recent Cochrane meta-analysis compared the efficacy and safety of indacaterol to placebo and to other LABA to treat patients with stable COPD [29M]. 13 RCTs of at least 12 weeks duration were included with a total of 9961 participants. 10 trials compared indacaterol to placebo, while 5 trials compared indacaterol to other LABA (salmeterol, formoterol and eformoterol). The investigators found that the use of indacaterol compared to both placebo and other LABA was not associated with any increase in AEs (OR 0.89, 95% CI 0.73–1.08; and OR 1.02, 95% CI 0.79–1.32, respectively); however, the confidence intervals are too wide to rule out important differences.

A small trial investigating the pharmacokinetics of 2 doses of indacaterol (150 and 300 mcg, $n = 12$ and $n = 12$) compared to placebo ($n = 8$) in 32 healthy Chinese volunteers over 14 days found the most frequently reported AE to be cough (150 mcg, $n = 6$; 300 mcg, $n = 8$, placebo, $n = 1$) [30c]. They found dose-dependent increases in heart rate and Fridericia's corrected QT interval (QTcF) in the indacaterol groups as compared to placebo, but did not consider these to be clinically meaningful. They found no clinically significant differences in serum potassium (K^+) or serum glucose compared to placebo.

Indacaterol is also combined with the LAMA glycopyrronium bromide in a once-daily dual-bronchodilator therapy also known as QVA149. A systematic review investigated this therapy, looking at 14 RCTs [31M]. The authors also performed meta-analysis using data from the ILLUMINATE [32MC] and LANTERN [19C] trials which compared this combination to SFC in patients with COPD over a period of 26 weeks, including a total of 1263 people. They found that patients treated with QVA149 had less AEs (OR 0.77; 95% CI: 0.62–0.97) and less pneumonia (OR 0.24; 95% CI: 0.07–0.77).

The QUANTIFY multicenter RCT compared QVA149 110/50 mcg to TIO + formoterol 18/12 mcg in 934 patients with COPD over a period of 26 weeks [33MC]. The incidence of AEs was comparable between treatments (43.7% for QVA149, 42.6% for TIO + FOR). Finally, two major reviews updated the previous evidence, again supporting the good side effect profile of this combination. Ridolo et al. looked at the evidence from all RCTs comparing QVA149 to other bronchodilators and placebo and finding incidence of AEs was similar to tiotropium, salmeterol/fluticasone and placebo [34R]. They also confirmed cardiovascular safety. Prakash et al. reviewed the literature to conclude the safety profile of QVA139 was similar to that of placebo and indacaterol or glycopyrronium as monotherapies and that there was no increased risk of cardiocerebral vascular events with QVA149 versus all comparators [35R].

℞

Olodaterol

Olodaterol is a once-daily inhaled ultra long-acting beta$_2$-adrenocepter agonist approved in the USA and Europe for maintenance bronchodilator treatment of COPD. It is a highly selective agonist of beta$_2$ adrenergic receptors on airway smooth muscle, resulting in bronchodilation [36E]. Moreover, it is a nearly complete agonist, with 88% intrinsic activity, and it has an estimated bioavailability of ≈30% with a plasma protein binding of ≈60% in vitro [37E].

In four phase III trials assessing the efficacy and safety of olodaterol over 6–48 weeks in adults with COPD, it was found to be generally well tolerated with only mild or moderate AEs [38C,39C,40C,41MC]. Two smaller, shorter studies each involved two replicate RCTs in patients with moderate-to-severe COPD. The first compared olodaterol 5 and 10 mcg, formoterol 12 mcg BD or placebo in 199 patients for 6 weeks [38C]. All treatments were well tolerated with comparable incidence of AEs across treatment groups. COPD exacerbation was the most commonly reported AE, more common in the placebo group (6.3% (12/190) compared to 5.3% (10/188) in the olodaterol 5 mcg group and 4.8% (9/187) in the olodaterol 10 mcg group). The second compared olodaterol 5 and 10 mcg, tiotropium 18 mcg or placebo in 230 patients [39C]. Again, incidence of AEs was similar across groups. The most frequent AEs were nasopharyngitis (5.7% (12/211) in the placebo group, 6.5% (14/216) in the olodaterol 5 mcg group, 3.7% (8/214) in the olodaterol 10 mcg group and 5.1% (11/214) in the tiotropium group) and COPD exacerbation (4.7% (10/211) in the placebo group, 6.5% (14/216) in the olodaterol 5 mcg group, 4.2% (9/214) in the olodaterol 10 mcg group and 2.8% (6/214) in the tiotropium group). In one case, a patient discontinued treatment with olodaterol 10 mcg due to atrial fibrillation, judged to be likely due to the treatment.

Two larger, longer multicenter studies each involved two replicate RCTs in patients with moderate to very severe COPD. Firstly, olodaterol 5 mcg, 10 mcg and placebo were compared in 624 patients over 48 weeks [40C]. The incidence of AEs was similar in olodaterol to placebo, and no safety concerns were identified. The most common AE was COPD exacerbation, more common in the placebo group (34% (71/209) compared to 24% (50/208) in the olodaterol 5 mcg group, and 32.4% (67/207) in the olodaterol 10 mcg group). The authors point out their inclusion of patients with very severe COPD, often excluded from COPD studies. One laboratory parameter anomaly was observed; there was an increase in creatine phosphokinase in the olodaterol groups compared with placebo. The investigators hypothesized a pharmacologic effect of olodaterol but note that it was associated with mild or no symptoms and no increase in AEs. Secondly, 1838 patients received olodaterol 5 or 10 mcg, formoterol 12 mcg, or placebo [41MC]. Again, incidence of AEs was similar across

treatment groups with most being mild to moderate, and the majority of treatment-related AEs were respiratory events such as COPD, cough and dyspnea. No abnormalities in vital signs, laboratory parameters, or electrocardiogram results were observed.

In a multicenter dose-finding RCT [42C], olodaterol doses (2, 5, 10 and 20 mcg once daily) were compared to placebo in 405 patients with COPD. The researchers found a clear dose–response relationship regarding pulmonary function, with the plateau of the curve formed by the two higher doses. The 5 and 10 mcg were selected for phase III clinical trials. The drug was well tolerated, with no dose-dependent safety effects observed. The most common AEs included nasopharyngitis, upper respiratory tract infection, bronchitis, headache, dyspnea, cough and COPD exacerbation. Of note, there were small but statistically significant reductions in serum potassium for 20 mcg olodaterol compared to placebo at both 1 and 3 h post-dose. However, after 4 weeks of treatment, there were no statistically significant differences in serum potassium levels at any dose versus placebo.

Recently, a pooled data analysis was performed using the final results from phase III clinical trials, including 3104 patients [43MC]. The investigators concluded that the safety profiles of both olodaterol 5 mcg (the marketed and registered dose) and 10 mcg are comparable to placebo. Crucially, given the properties of LABAs, no cardiovascular concerns were indentified.

Olodaterol can also be given in combination with tiotropium; in a recent review of the literature, the authors highlighted additional improvements in lung function greater than monotherapy with each drug alone, and that the synergistic effect does not increase AEs [44R]. Two large trials recently compared olodaterol + tiotropium with the drugs as monotherapy and placebo. Firstly, two replicate RCTs investigated olodaterol + tiotropium 5/2.5 and 5/5 mcg, tiotropium 5 mcg or placebo in 1621 patients with moderate-to-severe COPD over 12 weeks [45MC]. AE incidence was similar across treatment groups, with a higher incidence of AEs leading to treatment discontinuation in the placebo group. Cardiovascular AEs were 0–3% for the olodaterol + tiotropium group, 1–1.5% for tiotropium and 2–3.9% with placebo. A second RCT compared olodaterol + tiotropium 5/2.5 and 5/5 mcg, olodaterol 5 mcg, tiotropium 5 and 2.5 mcg and placebo in 219 patients with COPD [46C]. Again, AE incidence was similar between treatment groups; according to the investigators, there was no difference between the different doses of olodaterol + tiotropium, the monotherapies or placebo. The most common AEs were nasopharyngitis (between 6.5% (9/139 in the olodaterol + tiotropium 5/5 mcg group) and 10.1% (14/138 in the placebo group)) and COPD exacerbation (between 5.1% (7/1398 in the olodaterol 5 mcg group) and 12.3% (17/138 in the placebo group)). No safety concerns were identified in vital sign measurements. The authors do point out that the short study duration limits the safety information but conclude that olodaterol + tiotropium give greater *lung function improvement than monotherapy with either drug with no apparent difference in AEs.*

Salbutamol [SEDA-35, 318; SEDA-36, 246; SEDA-37, 197]

Endocrine

A retrospective observational study studied the incidence of hypokalemia in 279 children treated for acute asthma with nebulized salbutamol [47C]. They found the incidence of hypokalemia ($[K^+] < 3.5$ mmol/L) to be 23.7% (66/279) with 4.7% (13/279) children developing moderate hypokalemia ($[K^+] < 3.0$ mmol/L). Children who developed hypokalemia received higher doses of salbutamol were nebulized more frequently or were treated with $MgSO_4$. While recognizing the limits of a retrospective study, the authors pointed out that given the small proportion of children developing clinically relevant hypokalemia ($[K^+] < 3.0$ mmol/L), probably only children nebulized frequently or receiving $MgSO_4$ require $[K^+]$ monitoring.

Salmeterol [SEDA-35, 317; SEDA-36, 246; SEDA-37, 197]

Two recent articles consider salmeterol when combined with FP. A small RCT including 52 patients with COPD compared SFC 50/250 mcg to placebo over a period of 12 weeks [48c]. In the treatment group, 25% (7/28) of subjects reported AEs, compared to no subjects in the placebo group. Dysphonia (5 subjects) and oral candidiasis (2 subjects) were the most frequently reported; oropharyngeal discomfort, pharyngitis and stomatitis were also reported.

A large review looked at the efficacy and safety of this combination compared to other treatments with a focus on studies performed in the People's Republic of China, where SFC has become a mainstay for management of both COPD and asthma [49R]. The authors concluded that SFC has similar efficacy to that in western populations but that AEs such as oral candidiasis and pneumonia were infrequently reported in Chinese populations.

Vilanterol [SEDA-36, 247; SEDA-37, 198]

The AEs associated with the combination of vilanterol with FF were covered in Section "ICS" [10C,12C,13c,15R,22c]. However, in their study, Chen et al. specifically focused on the beta2-adrenergic pharmacodynamic effects, namely, increased QTcF and reduced serum potassium [22c]. In this RCT including 16 healthy Chinese volunteers, different dose combinations of FF/VI were compared to placebo. The researchers did find evidence of statistically significant increase in QTcF

(<10 msec) and decrease in serum potassium (0.118 mmol/L); however, they were considered to be small effects which would not be clinically important.

Two major reviews considered the literature focusing on vilanterol in combination with LAMA umeclidinium (UM/VI). Albertson et al. pointed out that these agents are well tolerated because they are poorly absorbed systemically, noting that the side effects of LABA agents including cardiovascular symptoms, hypokalemia and hyperglycemia occur rarely or not at all and that the most common AEs are headaches, nasopharyngitis, upper respiratory tract infections, dry mouth, dyspnea, and cough [50R]. Blair and Deeks confirmed that amongst all studies, there were no differences in heart rate, blood pressure, QTcF or serum potassium in comparison with placebo [51R].

Susceptibility Factors

In a single-blind, nonrandomized study, UM/VI was given to 9 patients with severe renal impairment (creatinine clearance < 30 mL/min) and 9 matched healthy volunteers [52c]. No clinically relevant increases in plasma vilanterol or umeclidinium were observed. The authors concluded that no dose adjustment for UM/VI is warranted in patients with severe renal impairment.

ANTICHOLINERGIC DRUGS [SEDA-35, 318; SEDA-36, 247; SEDA-37, 198]

Inhaled anti-cholinergic drugs inhibit the parasympathetic nervous system, mediating their action via muscarinic acetylcholine receptors, and tend to be known as long-acting muscarinic antagonists (LAMA). Two recent Cochrane meta-analyses considered the safety and efficacy of the class of drugs in general in poorly controlled asthma. Anderson et al. investigated LAMA added to any dose of ICS compared to ICS alone [53M]. 5 studies lasting between 12 and 52 weeks with a total of 2563 participants were included. SAEs were rare but suggested that LAMA add-on may be associated with less SAEs compared to ICS alone (OR 0.60, 95% CI 0.23–1.57). Kew et al. compared adding a LABA to ICS with adding a LAMA to ICS (see Section "Beta2-Adrenoceptor Agonists") [27M]. The authors reported very few SAEs and concluded they could not compare the treatments in terms of AEs.

Aclidinium Bromide [SEDA-36, 249; SEDA-37, 199]

Approved in 2012, the safety of aclidinium bromide has been reviewed in two previous annuals. However, two recent multicenter studies have further assessed the safety and efficacy of this drug. One RCT compared aclidinium 400 mcg BD to placebo in 263 Korean patients with moderate-to-severe COPD [54C]. COPD exacerbation was the most common AE in both groups (placebo, 15.5% (20/128); aclidinium, 6.8% (9/133)). Anticholinergic AEs such as thirst, dry mouth and dysuria were reported in the aclidinium group only (1.5% (2/133)). A multicenter, prospective, non-interventional study looked at the effects of newly initiated aclidinium bromide treatment (400 mcg BD) in 795 patients with COPD [55C]. AEs were reported in 55 (6.9%) patients, the most frequent AEs being of the anticholinergic type: product taste abnormal (12 cases; 1.5%), cough (10 cases; 1.3%), dry mouth (6 cases; 0.8%), and headache (4 cases; 0.5%).

In a recent review looking at all trials and meta-analyses evaluating aclidinium to-date, the author confirmed the good safety and tolerability profile of aclidinium, reporting the data supporting low incidence of anticholinergic AEs and adverse cardiac events [56R].

Glycopyrronium Bromide [SEDA-36, 249; SEDA-37, 199]

Glycopyrronium as a dual-bronchodilator therapy combined with indacaterol is discussed in Section "LABA". Two large trials also investigated glycopyrronium in combination with other inhaled drugs in patients with moderate-to-severe COPD. The GLISTEN study compared once-daily glycopyrronium 50 mcg to once-daily tiotropium 18 mcg and to placebo, all combined with SFC twice daily over 12 weeks [57C]. 773 patients took part in this RCT. Compared to placebo, there were more cases of upper respiratory tract infection (6.6% (17/257) compared to 4.3% (11/257)), oral candidiasis (4.7% (12/257) compared to 3.5% (9/257)) and cough (6.2% (16/257) compared to 4.3% (11/257)). There were fewer cardiac-related AEs in the glycopyrronium arm (1.2% (3/257) compared to 3.9% (10/258; TIO) and 2.7% (7/257; placebo)). Pneumonia was not reported in the glycopyrronium arm but did occur in two patients in each of the TIO and placebo arms.

In the GLOW7 multicenter RCT, glycopyrronium was compared to placebo in 459 predominantly Chinese patients over 26 weeks [58C]. The percentage of patients experiencing at least one AE was similar between glycopyrronium (43.6%) and placebo (47.4%). A greater proportion of patients in the placebo group suffered from SAEs (9.1% (14/154) compared to 5.6% (17/305) in the glycopyrronium group). There were four deaths in the glycopyrronium group and no deaths in the placebo group. Two were due to cardiovascular causes (sudden death and hemorrhagic stroke; patients had no cardiovascular risk factors at baseline), and two were due to respiratory causes (COPD exacerbation with and without

pneumonia, considered due to underlying COPD and not related to the study). The authors felt that overall, the small imbalance of the death cases was not considered clinically meaningful, and none of the deaths were related to the treatments.

A small trial investigated the efficacy and safety of nebulized glycopyrronium compared to placebo in a RCT in which 42 patients with COPD took part [59c]. The treatment was well tolerated, and there were no clinically relevant changes in heart rate, systolic and diastolic blood pressure or in ECG parameters including QTc interval.

A review of the literature concluded that glycopyrronium is generally well tolerated with a low-incidence of anti-muscarinic side effects [35R].

Tiotropium Bromide [SEDA-35, 319; SEDA-36, 247; SEDA-37, 199]

The combination of tiotropium with olodaterol was covered in Section "LABA".

Two recent meta-analyses considered the safety of tiotropium in COPD. A Cochrane meta-analysis compared tiotropium to ipratropium, including 2 trials with a total of 1073 participants [60M]. There were fewer people experiencing one or more non-fatal SAEs on tiotropium compared to ipratropium (OR 0.5; 95% CI 0.34–0.73) and fewer hospital admissions in the tiotropium group (OR 0.34; 95% CI 0.15–0.70). There was no significant difference in mortality between the treatments (OR 1.39; 95% CI 0.44–4.39). The authors concluded it is reasonable to choose tiotropium over ipratropium. Another meta-analysis comparing tiotropium to placebo in patients with COPD made similar conclusions [61M]. 24 555 patients in 28 trials were included, and the risk of AEs and SAEs was significantly lower in the tiotropium group than the placebo group (RR 0.90 [0.87, 0.93] and RR 0.94 [0.89, 0.99], respectively). The risk of cardiac AEs (0.93 [0.85, 1.02]) was numerically lower in the tiotropium group. Incidences of typical anticholinergic AEs were higher with tiotropium.

A further meta-analysis looked at the use of tiotropium compared to placebo for the treatment of asthma in adolescents [62M]. Three studies with approximately 1000 patients were included. No significant differences were found in AEs (27.3% vs 27.1% in placebo), and SAEs (6.5% vs 7.1% in placebo). The authors note that tiotropium in doses of 2.5 mcg once daily or 5.0 mcg once daily resulted in equivalent effects and thus suggest no advantage of the higher 5 mcg once-daily dose used in adults.

BELT, the large multisite RCT discussed in Section "LABA", compared the safety and efficacy of LABA + ICS to tiotropium + ICS in 1070 black adults with asthma [28MC]. There were a total of 67 hospitalizations in the tiotropium + ICS group ($n = 532$) compared to 58 in the LABA + ICS ($n = 538$) group. Three deaths occurred, all in the tiotropium + ICS group; 2 of those deaths were asthma related.

The MATHS observational study observed the early effects of maintenance treatment with tiotropium in 1332 patients with COPD [63MC]. 1% of patients reported AEs; most commonly dry mouth and nausea. No SAEs were reported. The authors note that this supports the good side effect profile of tiotropium, but point out that underreporting, a weakness of non-interventional observational studies, cannot be excluded as a reason for low number of AEs.

Cardiovascular

A small trial investigated whether decreased heart rate variability (HRV) was associated with tiotropium use in patients with COPD [64c]. 70 patients with moderate-to-severe COPD were treated with 5 mcg tiotropium once daily with no significant change in HRV found.

Umeclidinium Bromide [SEDA-37, 200]

Umeclidinium (UMEC) is also a relatively new LAMA discussed previously [SEDA-37, 200]. Recently, two large trials have examined the efficacy and safety of this drug in patients with asthma. A multicenter RCT investigated the dose–response to UMEC (15.6, 31.25, 62.5, 125 mcg OD, 15.6 or 31.25 BD) and placebo in 350 subjects with asthma not receiving ICS over a period of 14 days [65C]. This was the first study to evaluate LAMA monotherapy in asthma. The incidence of on-treatment AEs was 9–21% for UMEC (12/131 UMEC 15.6 mcg OD and 28/135 UMEC 250 mcg OD, respectively) and 12% (15/126) for placebo. The most frequently reported AEs were headache (UMEC 2–5% (2/126 UMEC 15.6 mcg BD and 6/133 UMEC 31.25 BD, respectively), PLAC 2% (2/126)) and abnormal product taste, which was more frequent at higher UMEC doses. There was no indication of treatment- or dose-related changes in biochemistry, hematology, urinalysis parameters or liver function tests. Cardiovascular safety was closely monitored, and overall, there was no indication of effects on ECG or Holter monitor findings. The authors note that their findings do not support a therapeutic benefit of UMEC monotherapy in patients with asthma not requiring ICS.

Secondly, a study randomized 421 patients with asthma, symptomatic on ICS, to compare FF with FF/UMEC (15.6, 31.25, 62.5, 125 or 250 mcg OD) and vilanterol 25 mcg OD [66C]. The highest incidence of AEs was 25%, for FF/VI (43/172), and the lowest was 13%, for FF/UMEC 31.25 mcg (23/179). Headache was the only AE reported in more than 3% of patients in any treatment arm. Again, abnormal product taste occurred in 2% of patients in each

of the FF/UMEC 31.25 ($n = 179$) and 125 mcg ($n = 176$) treatment groups, and there was no treatment effect on clinical chemistry and hematology parameters. There were no statistically significant differences for any vital sign parameters, and cardiovascular AEs occurred with a low frequency across all treatment groups.

Small trials of umeclidinium in combination with FF [14c] and FF/VI [13c] were discussed in Section "ICS".

LEUKOTRIENE MODIFIERS [SEDA-35, 320; SEDA-36, 251; SEDA-37, 200]

One recent meta-analysis examined the benefits and harms of leukotriene receptor antagonists (LTRAs) in general, as monotherapy or in combination with ICS, compared with placebo in adults and adolescents with asthma [67M]. 50 trials were included in the systematic review, 34 in the meta-analysis, and 6 trials in the random-effects meta-analysis for LRTA monotherapy. LRTAs included were montelukast, zafirlukast and pranlukast. AEs were found to be similar throughout all groups, and across all trials, and no SAEs were reported. The authors concluded that LRTAs may be efficacious and safe both as an alternative to ICS or add-on treatment.

A large retrospective observational study evaluated the side effects of LRTAs (mainly montelukast and zafirlukast) in children with asthma [68MC]. 1024 patients treated only with LRTAs were included in the study over a 5-year period. 41 patients (4%) suffered from side effects: of these, 58.5% (24 patients) were classified as neuropsychiatric, including hyperactivity, excessive sleepiness, nervousness and agitation. Non-psychiatric side effects were observed in 41.5% (17 patients), most commonly abdominal pain and headache. The researchers note that when drugs were discontinued, the side effects disappeared, reappearing when the drugs were restarted. Moreover, they pointed out that since side effects of LRTAs appear to be common in children, patients must be informed and regularly evaluated.

Neuropsychiatric

Converse conclusions were drawn from a large observational study exploring the association between neuropsychiatric AEs and montelukast treatment in children with asthma [69MC]. Using a matched nested case–control design, 1920 cases were identified and matched with controls from a similar population. Subjects exposed to montelukast during the prior year had an unadjusted OR of 1.09 (95% CI [0.96–1.22]) and adjusted OR of 1.01 (95% CI [0.88–1.14]) for experiencing a neuropsychiatric event; therefore, the authors concluded that no consistent positive association was found between montelukast use and neuropsychiatric AEs across a range of definitions.

PHOSPHODIESTERASE INHIBITORS [SEDA-35, 321; SEDA-36, 252; SEDA-37, 201]

Roflumilast [SEDA-35, 321; SEDA-36, 252; SEDA-37, 201]

Three multisite studies and 2 smaller observational studies investigated the AE profile of roflumilast in treating COPD and asthma. The REACT study, a large RCT, examined the effect of roflumilast on patients with COPD uncontrolled on combination therapy over a period of 12 months [70MC]. 1945 participants were randomized to receive either 500 mcg roflumilast OD or placebo, along with ICS/LABA combination. AEs such as COPD exacerbation, diarrhea, and weight loss were reported in 648 of 968 (67%) patients receiving roflumilast and by 572 of 967 (59%) patients in the placebo group. Deaths occurred in 2% of both groups: 17 in the roflumilast group and 18 in the placebo group. The number of major cardiovascular AEs did not differ between groups. Weight loss as an AE was reported by 88 (9%) patients who received roflumilast compared with 27 (3%) in the placebo group. Patients receiving roflumilast lost a mean of 2.65 kg (SD 4.37), compared to 0.15 kg (SD 3.69) in the placebo group. During the 3-month follow-up period, patients who discontinued roflumilast reported increased bodyweight. The mechanism for the weight loss has not yet been explained but has been seen in previous studies [71MC].

A large retrospective observational study investigating hospital readmission rates for patients hospitalized for COPD and treated with roflumilast found that among 15755 patients, treatment with roflumilast was associated with a lower rate of hospital readmission [72MC]. Using conditional logistic regression, the authors found there was significantly lower chance of readmission to hospital for patients treated with roflumilast in comparison to those who were not (OR 0.59, 95% CI 0.37–0.93).

A multisite RCT evaluated the efficacy of roflumilast (250, 500 or 1000 mcg) compared to placebo in 197 patients with asthma [73C]. The majority of AEs were mild to moderate in intensity; the most frequent AEs included nausea, headache and diarrhea. Weight loss was *not* seen as an AE.

Two small retrospective observational studies investigated the AEs of roflumilast in patients with COPD. Hwang et al. evaluated whether starting at a lower dose of roflumilast, 250 mcg, then increasing it to 500 mcg, resulted in less AEs than starting at the higher dose [74c]. 85 patients with COPD treated with roflumilast were investigated. AEs were reported in 26% of patients, most commonly diarrhea, weight loss and nausea; in the dose-escalated group, AEs were reported in 24%; in the control group, AEs were reported in 27%. Of the patients who had increased their dose of roflumilast, 17% discontinued due to AEs, compared to 27% of patients who started with 500 mcg roflumilast. This difference was not found to be significant, however.

Finally, Muñoz-Esquerre et al. evaluated the safety of roflumilast in 55 COPD patients already receiving triple therapy (ICS/LABA/LAMA) [75c]. They found that 69% of roflumilast patients suffered with side effects during treatment, most commonly diarrhea, abdominal pain, nausea and weight loss. 49% of the total population of patients treated with roflumilast did not continue with the treatment due to the AEs.

Ɍ Monoclonal Antibodies in the Treatment of Asthma

Novel treatments are emerging which target the mediators of airway inflammation in allergic asthma, particularly interleukin response, chemotaxis and B cell activation [76R]. These biologic agents have a role in treating poorly controlled severe atopic asthma [77R,78R,79R,80R,81R]. Omalizumab is an established therapy that targets IgE [82R]. Recently approved mepolizumab inhibits interleukin-5 [83C]. The role of established anti-tumour necrosis factor drugs used in the treatment of other inflammatory conditions remains under investigation in asthma. These biotherapies are generally well tolerated [84R]; however, safety concerns include anaphylaxis, immunogenicity, infection and developing cancers, particularly lymphoma.

Omalizumab (Xolair©) is a monoclonal anti-IgE antibody that binds to the Fc portion of IgE, thus reducing circulating levels of free IgE. A Cochrane meta-analysis published in 2014 assessed omalizumab in adults and children over the age of 6 years [85M] and reviewed in SEDA-37 [p. 202]. No significant difference in mortality was reported between subcutaneous omalizumab and placebo in 9 studies with a total of 4245 participants (OR = 0.19, 95% CI 0.02– 1.67). All four deaths reported were in placebo arms. SAEs occurred less frequently in the omalizumab group compared to placebo (OR = 0.72, 95% CI 0.57–0.91), with an absolute reduction from 6% in those receiving placebo to 4% in the treatment group. A subsequent systematic review of the long-term safety of omalizumab reflected these findings [86M].

Limited data exist for the safety of omalizumab in pregnancy. The EXPECT registry is a prospective, observational study of pregnant women exposed to one or more doses of omalizumab within 8 weeks prior to conception or at any time during pregnancy [87C]. It reported that the proportion of congenital defects, pregnancy and neonatal outcomes of its 169 pregnancies to date were similar to those expected. This study is limited by its small sample size, voluntary enrolment and lack of internal comparators.

Mepolizumab (Nucala©) is a monoclonal antibody that inactivates interleukin-5 (IL-5) by blocking it from binding to the α-chain of the IL-5 receptor complex on the eosinophil cell surface [88R]. IL-5 is the main cytokine involved in eosinophil activation that mediates airway eosinophil recruitment and hyperresponsiveness. The incidence of AEs was similar in intravenous mepolizumab (N=161, 84%), subcutaneous mepolizumab (N=152, 78%) and placebo (N=158, 83%) groups in a phase 3 trial [89C]. SAEs were reported in 27 subjects (14%) in the placebo group compared to 14 (7%) in the intravenous group and 16 (8%) in the subcutaneous group. Nasopharyngitis, headache and upper respiratory tract infection were the most common AEs. Injection-site reaction was more common with subcutaneous administration (9%) than in intravenous administration and placebo (both 3%).

In summary, current evidence suggests that the two monoclonal antibodies approved for the treatment of moderate-to-severe asthma demonstrate fewer SAEs than placebo comparison. Long-term safety remains unclear. A prospective observational study with a median follow-up of 5 years (N=7857) concluded that omalizumab is not associated with an increased risk of malignancy in omalizumab vs non-omalizumab groups (HR 1.09, 95% CI, 0.87–1.38) [90MC]; however, this study has been criticised because of its design limitations, particularly its potential for selection bias, initial exclusion of those with a history of malignancy or pre-malignant condition, and high discontinuation rates [91r].

References

[1] Festic E, Scanlon PD. Incident pneumonia and mortality in patients with chronic obstructive pulmonary disease. A double effect of inhaled corticosteroids? Am J Respir Crit Care Med. 2015;191(2):141–8 [R].

[2] Dong YH, Chang CH, Wu FL, et al. Use of inhaled corticosteroids in patients with COPD and the risk of TB and influenza: a systematic review and meta-analysis of randomized controlled trials. Chest. 2014;145(6):1286–97 [MC].

[3] Woods CP, Argese N, Chapman M, et al. Adrenal suppression in patients taking inhaled glucocorticoids is highly prevalent and management can be guided by morning cortisol. Eur J Endocrinol. 2015;173(5):633–42 [C].

[4] Issa-El-Khoury K, Kim H, Chan ES, et al. CSACI position statement: systemic effect of inhaled corticosteroids on adrenal suppression in the management of pediatric asthma. Allergy Asthma Clin Immunol. 2015;11(1):9 [R].

[5] Kapadia CR, Nebesio TD, Myers SE, et al. Endocrine effects of inhaled corticosteroids in children. JAMA Pediatr. 2015;21:1–9 [R].

[6] Smy L, Shaw K, Smith A, et al. Hair cortisol as a novel biomarker of HPA suppression by inhaled corticosteroids in children. Pediatr Res. 2015;78(1):44–7 [c].

[7] Loke YK, Gilbert D, Thavarajah M, et al. Bone mineral density and fracture risk with long-term use of inhaled corticosteroids in patients with asthma: systematic review and meta-analysis. BMJ Open. 2015;5(11):e008554 [M].

[8] Sun X, He Z, Zhang J, et al. Compare the efficacy of inhaled budesonide and systemic methylprednisolone on systemic inflammation of AECOPD. Pulm Pharmacol Ther. 2015;31:111–6 [c].

[9] Tuzuner A, Demirci S, Bilgin G, et al. Voice assessment after treatment of subacute and chronic cough with inhaled steroids. J Voice. 2015;29(4):484–9 [c].

[10] Covelli H, Pek B, Schenkenberger I, et al. Efficacy and safety of fluticasone furoate/vilanterol or tiotropium in subjects with COPD at cardiovascular risk. Int J Chron Obstruct Pulmon Dis. 2016;11:1–12 [C].

[11] Dransfield MT, Bourbeau J, Jones PW, et al. Once-daily inhaled fluticasone furoate and vilanterol versus vilanterol only for prevention of exacerbations of COPD: two replicate double-blind, parallel-group, randomised controlled trials. Lancet Respir Med. 2013;1(3):210–23 [MC].

[12] Zheng J, de Guia T, Wang-Jairaj J, et al. Efficacy and safety of fluticasone furoate/vilanterol (50/25 mcg; 100/25 mcg; 200/25 mcg) in Asian patients with chronic obstructive pulmonary disease: a randomized placebo-controlled trial. Curr Med Res Opin. 2015;31(6):1191–200 [C].

[13] Brealey N, Gupta A, Renaux J, et al. Pharmacokinetics of fluticasone furoate, umeclidinium, and vilanterol as a triple therapy in healthy volunteers. Int J Clin Pharmacol Ther. 2015;53(9):753–64 [c].

[14] Yang S, Lee L, Mallett S, et al. A randomized, crossover study to investigate the pharmacokinetics and safety of inhaled fluticasone furoate and umeclidinium, administered separately and in combination via dry powder inhaler in healthy adult volunteers. Adv Ther. 2015;32(2):157–71 [c].

[15] Matera MG, Capuano A, Cazzola M. Fluticasone furoate and vilanterol inhalation powder for the treatment of chronic obstructive pulmonary disease. Expert Rev Resp Med. 2015;9(1):5–12 [R].

[16] Latorre M, Paggiaro P, Canonica W, et al. A valid option for asthma control: clinical evidence on efficacy and safety of fluticasone propionate/formoterol combination in a single inhaler. Pulm Pharmacol Ther. 2015;34:31–6 [R].

[17] Pascoe S, Locantore N, Dransfield MT, et al. Blood eosinophil counts, exacerbations, and response to the addition of inhaled fluticasone furoate to vilanterol in patients with chronic obstructive pulmonary disease: a secondary analysis of data from two parallel randomised controlled trials. Lancet Respir Med. 2015;3(6):435–42 [MC].

[18] Crim C, Dransfield MT, Bourbeau J, et al. Pneumonia risk with inhaled fluticasone furoate and vilanterol compared with vilanterol alone in patients with COPD. Ann Am Thorac Soc. 2015;12(1):27–34 [MC].

[19] Zhong N, Wang C, Zhou X, et al. LANTERN: a randomized study of QVA149 versus salmeterol/fluticasone combination in patients with COPD. Int J Chron Obstruct Pulmon Dis. 2015;10:1015 [C].

[20] DiSantostefano RL, Sampson T, Le HV, et al. Risk of pneumonia with inhaled corticosteroid versus long-acting bronchodilator regimens in chronic obstructive pulmonary disease: a new-user cohort study. PLoS One. 2014;9(5):e97149 [MC].

[21] DiSantostefano RL, Li H, Hinds D, et al. Risk of pneumonia with inhaled corticosteroid/long-acting $\beta2$ agonist therapy in chronic obstructive pulmonary disease: a cluster analysis. Int J Chron Obstruct Pulmon Dis. 2013;9:457–68 [MC].

[22] Chen X, Zheng X, Jiang J, et al. Pharmacodynamics and pharmacokinetics of fluticasone furoate/vilanterol in healthy Chinese subjects. Pharmacotherapy. 2015;35(6):586–99 [c].

[23] Farne HA, Cates CJ. Long-acting beta2-agonist in addition to tiotropium versus either tiotropium or long-acting beta2-agonist alone for chronic obstructive pulmonary disease. Cochrane Database Syst Rev. 2015;10:CD008989 [M].

[24] US Food and Drug Administration. FDA announces new safety controls for long-acting beta agonists, medications used to treat asthma. Silver Spring, MD: USFDA; 2010 [S].

[25] Chauhan BF, Chartrand C, Ni Chroinin M, et al. Addition of long-acting beta2-agonists to inhaled corticosteroids for chronic

asthma in children. Cochrane Database Syst Rev. 2015;11: CD007949 [M].

[26] Ahmad S, Kew KM, Normansell R. Stopping long-acting beta2-agonists (LABA) for adults with asthma well controlled by LABA and inhaled corticosteroids. Cochrane Database Syst Rev. 2015;6: CD011306 [M].

[27] Kew KM, Evans DJ, Allison DE, et al. Long-acting muscarinic antagonists (LAMA) added to inhaled corticosteroids (ICS) versus addition of long-acting beta2-agonists (LABA) for adults with asthma. Cochrane Database Syst Rev. 2015;6:CD011438 [M].

[28] Wechsler ME, Yawn BP, Fuhlbrigge AL, et al. Anticholinergic vs long-acting β-agonist in combination with inhaled corticosteroids in black adults with asthma: the BELT randomized clinical trial. JAMA. 2015;314(16):1720–30 [MC].

[29] Geake JB, Dabscheck EJ, Wood-Baker R, et al. Indacaterol, a once-daily beta$_2$-agonist, versus twice-daily beta$_2$-agonists or placebo for chronic obstructive pulmonary disease. Cochrane Database Syst Rev. 2015;1:CD010139 [M].

[30] Jiang J, Li L, Yin H, et al. Single-and multiple-dose pharmacokinetics of inhaled indacaterol in healthy Chinese volunteers. Eur J Drug Metab Pharmacokinet. 2015;40(2):203–8 [c].

[31] Horita N, Kaneko T. Role of combined indacaterol and glycopyrronium bromide (QVA149) for the treatment of COPD in Japan. Int J Chron Obstruct Pulmon Dis. 2015;10:813 [M].

[32] Vogelmeier CF, Bateman ED, Pallante J, et al. Efficacy and safety of once-daily QVA149 compared with twice-daily salmeterol–fluticasone in patients with chronic obstructive pulmonary disease (ILLUMINATE): a randomised, double-blind, parallel group study. Lancet Respir Med. 2013;1(1):51–60 [MC].

[33] Buhl R, Gessner C, Schuermann W, et al. Efficacy and safety of once-daily QVA149 compared with the free combination of once-daily tiotropium plus twice-daily formoterol in patients with moderate-to-severe COPD (QUANTIFY): a randomised, non-inferiority study. Thorax. 2015;70(4):311–9 [MC].

[34] Ridolo E, Montagni M, Riario-Sforza GG, et al. Combination therapy with indacaterol and glycopyrronium bromide in the management of COPD: an update on the evidence for efficacy and safety. Ther Adv Respir Dis. 2015;9(2):49–55 [R].

[35] Prakash A, Babu KS, Morjaria JB. Profile of inhaled glycopyrronium bromide as monotherapy and in fixed-dose combination with indacaterol maleate for the treatment of COPD. Int J Chron Obstruct Pulmon Dis. 2015;10:111–23 [R].

[36] Casarosa P, Kollak I, Kiechle T, et al. Functional and biochemical rationales for the 24-hour-long duration of action of olodaterol. J Pharmacol Exp Ther. 2011;337(3):600–9 [E].

[37] Bouyssou T, Casarosa P, Naline E, et al. Pharmacological characterization of olodaterol, a novel inhaled β2-adrenoceptor agonist exerting a 24-hour-long duration of action in preclinical models. J Pharmacol Exp Ther. 2010;334(1):53–62 [E].

[38] Feldman GJ, Bernstein JA, Hamilton A, et al. The 24-h FEV1 time profile of olodaterol once daily via Respimat® and formoterol twice daily via Aerolizer® in patients with GOLD 2–4 COPD: results from two 6-week crossover studies. Springerplus. 2014;3:419 [C].

[39] Lange P, Aumann JL, Hamilton A, et al. The 24 hour lung function time profile of olodaterol once daily versus placebo and tiotropium in patients with moderate to very severe chronic obstructive pulmonary disease. J Pulm Respir Med. 2014;4(4):196 [C].

[40] Ferguson GT, Feldman GJ, Hofbauer P, et al. Efficacy and safety of olodaterol once daily delivered via Respimat® in patients with GOLD 2–4 COPD: results from two replicate 48-week studies. Int J Chron Obstruct Pulmon Dis. 2014;9:629–45 [C].

[41] Koch A, Pizzichini E, Hamilton A, et al. Lung function efficacy and symptomatic benefit of olodaterol once daily delivered via Respimat® versus placebo and formoterol twice daily in patients

with GOLD 2–4 COPD: results from two replicate 48-week studies. Int J Chron Obstruct Pulmon Dis. 2014;9:697–714 [MC].

[42] Maleki-Yazdi MR, Beck E, Hamilton AL, et al. A randomised, placebo-controlled, Phase II, dose-ranging trial of once-daily treatment with olodaterol, a novel long-acting β2-agonist, for 4 weeks in patients with chronic obstructive pulmonary disease. Respir Med. 2015;109(5):596–605 [C].

[43] McGarvey L, Niewoehner D, Magder S, et al. One-year safety of olodaterol once daily via Respimat® in patients with GOLD 2–4 chronic obstructive pulmonary disease: results of a pre-specified pooled analysis. COPD. 2015;12(5):484–93 [MC].

[44] Ramadan WH, Kabbara WK, El Khoury GM, et al. Combined bronchodilators (tiotropium plus olodaterol) for patients with chronic obstructive pulmonary disease. Int J Chron Obstruct Pulmon Dis. 2015;10:2347–56 [R].

[45] Singh D, Ferguson GT, Bolitschek J, et al. Tiotropium + olodaterol shows clinically meaningful improvements in quality of life. Respir Med. 2015;109(10):1312–9 [MC].

[46] Beeh KM, Westerman J, Kirsten AM, et al. The 24-h lung-function profile of once-daily tiotropium and olodaterol fixed-dose combination in chronic obstructive pulmonary disease. Pulm Pharmacol Ther. 2015;32:53–9 [C].

[47] Hartman S, Merkus P, Maseland M, et al. Hypokalaemia in children with asthma treated with nebulised salbutamol. Arch Dis Child. 2015;100(10):970–2 [C].

[48] Asai K, Kobayashi A, Makihara Y, et al. Anti-inflammatory effects of salmeterol/fluticasone propionate 50/250 mcg combination therapy in Japanese patients with chronic obstructive pulmonary disease. Int J Chron Obstruct Pulmon Dis. 2015;10:803–11 [c].

[49] Gao J, Pleasants RA. Role of the fixed combination of fluticasone and salmeterol in adult Chinese patients with asthma and COPD. Int J Chron Obstruct Pulmon Dis. 2015;10:775–89 [R].

[50] Albertson TE, Harper R, Murin S, et al. Patient considerations in the treatment of COPD: focus on the new combination inhaler umeclidinium/vilanterol. Patient Prefer Adherence. 2015;9:235–42 [R].

[51] Blair HA, Deeks ED. Umeclidinium/vilanterol: a review of its use as maintenance therapy in adults with chronic obstructive pulmonary disease. Drugs. 2015;75(1):61–74 [R].

[52] Mehta R, Hardes K, Brealey N, et al. Effect of severe renal impairment on umeclidinium and umeclidinium/vilanterol pharmacokinetics and safety: a single-blind, nonrandomized study. Int J Chron Obstruct Pulmon Dis. 2015;10:15–23 [c].

[53] Anderson DE, Kew KM, Boyter AC. Long-acting muscarinic antagonists (LAMA) added to inhaled corticosteroids (ICS) versus the same dose of ICS alone for adults with asthma. Cochrane Database Syst Rev. 2015;8:CD011397 [M].

[54] Lee SH, Lee J, Yoo KH, et al. Efficacy and safety of aclidinium bromide in patients with COPD: a phase 3 randomized clinical trial in a Korean population. Respirology. 2015;20(8):1222–8 [C].

[55] Marth K, Schuller E, Pohl W. Improvements in patient-reported outcomes: a prospective, non-interventional study with aclidinium bromide for treatment of COPD. Respir Med. 2015;109(5):616–24 [C].

[56] Jones PW. Clinical potential of aclidinium bromide in chronic obstructive pulmonary disease. Int J Chron Obstruct Pulmon Dis. 2015;10:677–87 [R].

[57] Frith PA, Thompson PJ, Ratnavadivel R, et al. Glycopyrronium once-daily significantly improves lung function and health status when combined with salmeterol/fluticasone in patients with COPD: the GLISTEN study—a randomised controlled trial. Thorax. 2015;70(6):519–27 [C].

[58] Wang C, Sun T, Huang Y, et al. Efficacy and safety of once-daily glycopyrronium in predominantly Chinese patients with

moderate-to-severe chronic obstructive pulmonary disease: the GLOW7 study. Int J Chron Obstruct Pulmon Dis. 2015;10:57–68 [C].

[59] Leaker BR, Barnes PJ, Jones CR, et al. Efficacy and safety of nebulized glycopyrrolate for administration using a high efficiency nebulizer in patients with chronic obstructive pulmonary disease. Br J Clin Pharmacol. 2015;79(3):492–500 [c].

[60] Cheyne L, Irvin-Sellers MJ, White J. Tiotropium versus ipratropium bromide for chronic obstructive pulmonary disease. Cochrane Database Syst Rev. 2015;9:CD009552 [M].

[61] Halpin DM, Dahl R, Hallmann C, et al. Tiotropium HandiHaler® and Respimat® in COPD: a pooled safety analysis. Int J Chron Obstruct Pulmon Dis. 2015;10:239–59 [M].

[62] Rodrigo GJ, Castro-Rodríguez JA. Tiotropium for the treatment of adolescents with moderate to severe symptomatic asthma: a systematic review with meta-analysis. Ann Allergy Asthma Immunol. 2015;115(3):211–6 [M].

[63] Jahnz-Różyk K, Szepiel P. Early impact of treatment with tiotropium, long-acting anticholinergic preparation, in patients with COPD–real-life experience from an observational study. Int J Chron Obstruct Pulmon Dis. 2015;10:613–23 [MC].

[64] Wu YK, Huang CY, Yang MC, et al. Effect of tiotropium on heart rate variability in stable chronic obstructive pulmonary disease patients. J Aerosol Med Pulm Drug Deliv. 2015;28(2):100–5 [c].

[65] Lee LA, Briggs A, Edwards LD, et al. A randomized, three-period crossover study of umeclidinium as monotherapy in adult patients with asthma. Respir Med. 2015;109(1):63–73 [C].

[66] Lee LA, Yang S, Kerwin E, et al. The effect of fluticasone furoate/ umeclidinium in adult patients with asthma: a randomized, dose-ranging study. Respir Med. 2015;109(1):54–62 [C].

[67] Miligkos M, Bannuru RR, Alkofide H, et al. Leukotriene-receptor antagonists versus placebo in the treatment of asthma in adults and adolescents: a systematic review and meta-analysis. Ann Intern Med. 2015;163(10):756–67 [M].

[68] Erdem SB, Nacaroglu HT, Karkiner CS, et al. Side effects of leukotriene receptor antagonists in asthmatic children. Iran J Pediatr. 2015;25(5):e3313 [MC].

[69] Ali MM, O'Brien CE, Cleves MA, et al. Exploring the possible association between montelukast and neuropsychiatric events among children with asthma: a matched nested case-control study. Pharmacoepidemiol Drug Saf. 2015;24(4):435–45 [MC].

[70] Martinez FJ, Calverley PM, Goehring UM, et al. Effect of roflumilast on exacerbations in patients with severe chronic obstructive pulmonary disease uncontrolled by combination therapy (REACT): a multicentre randomised controlled trial. Lancet. 2015;385(9971):857–66 [MC].

[71] Calverley PM, Rabe KF, Goehring UM, et al. Roflumilast in symptomatic chronic obstructive pulmonary disease: two randomised clinical trials. Lancet. 2009;374(9691):685–94 [MC].

[72] Fu AZ, Sun SX, Huang X, et al. Lower 30-day readmission rates with roflumilast treatment among patients hospitalized for chronic obstructive pulmonary disease. Int J Chron Obstruct Pulmon Dis. 2015;10:909–15 [MC].

[73] Bardin P, Kanniess F, Gauvreau G, et al. Roflumilast for asthma: efficacy findings in mechanism of action studies. Pulm Pharmacol Ther. 2015;35:S4–S10 [C].

[74] Hwang H, Shin JY, Park KR, et al. Effect of a dose-escalation regimen for improving adherence to roflumilast in patients with chronic obstructive pulmonary disease. Tuberc Respir Dis. 2015;78(4):321–5 [c].

[75] Muñoz-Esquerre M, Diez-Ferrer M, Montón C, et al. Roflumilast added to triple therapy in patients with severe COPD: a real life study. Pulm Pharmacol Ther. 2015;30:16–21 [c].

[76] Pelaia G, Vatrella A, Maselli R. The potential of biologics for the treatment of asthma. Nat Rev Drug Discov. 2012;11(12): 958–72 [R].

[77] Menzella F, Lusuardi M, Galeone C, et al. Tailored therapy for severe asthma. Multidiscip Respir Med. 2015;10(1):1 [R].

[78] Al Efraij K, FitzGerald J. Current and emerging treatments for severe asthma. J Thorac Dis. 2015;7(11):E522–5 [R].

[79] Kane B, Fowler S, Niven R. Refractory asthma—beyond step 5, the role of new and emerging adjuvant therapies. Chron Respir Dis. 2014;12(1):69–77 [R].

[80] Hambly N, Nair P. Monoclonal antibodies for the treatment of refractory asthma. Curr Opin Pulm Med. 2014;20(1): 87–94 [R].

[81] Long A. Monoclonal antibodies and other biologic agents in the treatment of asthma. MAbs. 2009;1(3):237–46 [R].

[82] Caminati M, Senna G, Guerriero M, et al. Omalizumab for severe allergic asthma in clinical trials and real-life studies: what we know and what we should address. Pulm Pharmacol Ther. 2015;31:28–35 [R].

[83] Ortega H, Liu M, Pavord I, et al. Mepolizumab treatment in patients with severe eosinophilic asthma. N Engl J Med. 2014;371(13):1198–207 [C].

[84] Cox L. How safe are the biologicals in treating asthma and rhinitis? Allergy Asthma Clin Immunol. 2009;5(1):4 [R].

[85] Normansell R, Walker S, Milan S, et al. Omalizumab for asthma in adults and children. Cochrane Database Syst Rev. 2014;1: CD003559 [M].

[86] Lai T, Wang S, Xu Z, et al. Long-term efficacy and safety of omalizumab in patients with persistent uncontrolled allergic asthma: a systematic review and meta-analysis. Sci Rep. 2015;5:8191 [M].

[87] Namazy J, Cabana M, Scheuerle A, et al. The xolair pregnancy registry (EXPECT): the safety of omalizumab use during pregnancy. J Allergy Clin Immunol. 2015;135(2):407–12 [C].

[88] Smith D, Minthorn E, Beerahee M. Pharmacokinetics and pharmacodynamics of mepolizumab, an anti-interleukin-5 monoclonal antibody. Clin Pharmacokinet. 2011;50(4): 215–27 [R].

[89] Ortega H, Liu M, Pavord I, et al. Mepolizumab treatment in patients with severe eosinophilic asthma. N Engl J Med. 2014;371(13):1198–207 [C].

[90] Long A, Rahmaoui A, Rothman K, et al. Incidence of malignancy in patients with moderate-to-severe asthma treated with or without omalizumab. J Allergy Clin Immunol. 2014;134(3):560–7 [MC].

[91] Li J, Goulding M, Seymour S, et al. EXCELS study results do not rule out potential cancer risk with omalizumab. J Allergy Clin Immunol. 2015;135(1):289 [r].

16

Positive Inotropic Drugs and Drugs Used in Dysrhythmias

Cassandra Maynard[1], Jingyang Fan

Department of Pharmacy Practice, SIUE School of Pharmacy, Edwardsville, IL, USA

[1]Corresponding author: cmaynar@siue.edu

CARDIAC GLYCOSIDES [SED-15, 648; SEDA-35, 327; SEDA-36, 257; SEDA-37, 205]

Digoxin

Sensory System

- A 91-year-old female presented to the hospital complaining of nausea, vomiting and vision abnormalities. She had been prescribed digoxin 0.25 mg daily and diltiazem 90 mg daily 1 month prior for the treatment of her atrial fibrillation. Her visual disturbances included blurred vision, seeing blue and purple spots, and hallucinations of seeing little human beings. The patient's digoxin level was found to be 5.7 ng/mL. Ten days after discontinuing digoxin, the level was within goal at 1.1 ng/mL. All other work-up to identify an alternate cause for the patient's symptoms was negative. She continued to have reduced visual acuity at 6 months. Of note, the patient had started to experience generalized symptoms of potential toxicity after only 5 days of therapy. Symptoms progressed leading the patient to seek an emergency eye exam on day 21 of treatment which revealed decreased visual acuity. However, digoxin was not discontinued at that time and the patient's symptoms persisted until she presented to the hospital as described above [1A].

Elderly patients are more susceptible to the potential for digoxin toxicity, particularly females and those with reduced renal function. There is the possibility that diltiazem may have interacted with digoxin and resulted in an increase in digoxin levels [2c]. It is critical to be keenly aware of the potential for drug–drug interactions and the signs and symptoms of digoxin toxicity in order to seek prompt treatment. This case reinforces the need for close monitoring of digoxin therapy.

Pancreas

Patients between the ages of 20 and 84 with an initial case of acute pancreatitis were identified through The Taiwan National Health Insurance Program and labeled as the case group. Patients without pancreatitis were identified and matched to the case group based on age, gender and year of acute pancreatitis diagnosis. Various comorbidities affecting the development of acute pancreatitis were also identified and occurred at a higher rate in the case group. However, once adjusted for these factors, digoxin use did appear to be associated with an increased risk of acute pancreatitis. There were 419 patients who had an active prescription for digoxin and developed acute pancreatitis out of a total of 6116 patients with acute pancreatitis (6.85%). Whereas 966 patients in the control group prescribed digoxin, out of 24 464 patients, did not develop acute pancreatitis (3.94%). More studies are warranted to determine if there is a true cause and effect present in the development of pancreatitis with digoxin use or if this was simply a correlation [3C].

Death

Digoxin use has increasingly been associated with morbidity and mortality [4C,5C,6C]. Additional studies continue to be published which add to the growing body of evidence suggesting caution should be used when prescribing digoxin particularly for the management of rate control in atrial fibrillation. Two recent studies addressed this very same issue. A cohort of digoxin users in the ORBIT-AF registry was analyzed to determine if there was a difference in all-cause mortality compared to the

ISSN: 0378-6080
http://dx.doi.org/10.1016/bs.seda.2016.07.009

other study participants. Additional outcomes of interest included all-cause hospitalization and the composite of all-cause hospitalization and death. Of patients initiated on digoxin during the study period who did not have heart failure, an increase in death and cardiovascular hospitalization was found when compared to placebo. There was no difference in outcomes for those either with heart failure or patients who had heart failure but were initiated on digoxin at study enrollment [7C]. The ATRIA-CVRN trial focused on adults 21 years of age and older newly prescribed digoxin therapy for atrial fibrillation in the absence of heart failure. Over a median follow-up period of 1.17 years, 473 out of 4231 digoxin users died compared to 667 out of 10556 non-digoxin users ($p < 0.001$). Additionally, digoxin users experienced a higher rate of all-cause hospitalization; 3411 hospitalizations in the digoxin group compared to 5045 hospitalizations in the non-digoxin user group [8C].

Although a high quality randomized trial is needed to truly assess the effect of digoxin on mortality, literature continues to suggest an association between digoxin and an increased risk of mortality in atrial fibrillation patients, particularly those without concomitant heart failure.

ANTIDYSRHYTHMIC DRUGS

Amiodarone [SED-15, 148; SEDA-35, 332; SEDA-36, 259; SEDA-37, 208]

Cardiovascular

Amiodarone possesses antiarrhythmic as well as beta-blocking effects. It is the most commonly used antiarrhythmic agent and is often used in the acute setting for life-threatening arrhythmias. However, intravenous amiodarone has been associated with hypotension, usually thought to be due to polysorbate 80 or benzyl alcohol in the parenteral formulation.

- A 70-year-old male, with history of paroxysmal atrial fibrillation, apical hypertrophic cardiomyopathy, hypertension, and dyslipidemia, presented to the emergency department with rapid atrial fibrillation but was hemodynamically stable. Amiodarone 300 mg intravenous bolus was started after oral bisoprolol failed to lower his heart rate. Within minutes, patient's systolic blood pressure dropped below 90 mm Hg which did not respond to fluid resuscitation. He further deteriorated clinically and required intubation and inotropic support with norepinephrine and dobutamine. Bedside echocardiogram revealed severely depressed left ventricular function. Unlike previously reported cases, this patient did not have any other symptoms of anaphylaxis. Therefore,

cardiogenic shock was thought to be the most likely cause of his severe hypotension. He was stabilized and his left ventricular function recovered in the week following the event [9A].

Nervous System

A population-based cohort study was conducted in Taiwan, using claim data from the National Health Insurance Program, to investigate the association between the risk of ischemic stroke and amiodarone among patients with nonvalvular atrial fibrillation. This study showed that amiodarone use was associated with a hazard ratio (HR) of 1.8 (95% CI 1.51–2.15) after adjusting for confounding variables. Although advanced age, comorbid conditions such as diabetes and hypertension, and higher CHA_2DS_2VASc score were all independently associated with higher risk of stroke, the demographically stratified analysis showed that the risk of stroke was the highest in amiodarone users who were younger than 65, with no comorbidity, with CHA_2DS_2VASc score of 0–1 or were also taking digoxin. The authors explained that this observation may suggest that the stroke risk with amiodarone is more pronounced in patients with lower stroke risk, and the effect of amiodarone on stroke risk is weaker in those who are already at very high risk. The authors also cautioned against the combined use of amiodarone and digoxin [10MC].

Sensory Systems

Although amiodarone is well known for causing corneal micro-deposits, vortex keratopathy, a condition in which corneal deposits form a golden-brown whorl pattern in the basal epithelium of the eyes, is relatively rare. At this time, there is no literature available to suggest that this adverse event is reversible.

- A patient of unknown age complained of halos and glare in both eyes, after taking an unknown dose of amiodarone for 6 months. Ocular exam showed deep epithelial golden-brown whorl pattern of corneal deposits [11A]. It is unclear whether the patient could have had other conditions, e.g., Fabry disease or received other medications, e.g., chloroquine, nonsteroidal anti-inflammatory drugs, which have been shown to also induce vortex keratopathy [12r].
- A 50-year-old female developed halos around lights and a whorl-like pattern of corneal deposits in both eyes after taking amiodarone for 2 years. Her ocular exam was otherwise normal [13A].

Immunologic

Amiodarone-induced lupus is an uncommon adverse event that has been reported in a few case reports. In most cases, drug-induced lupus takes years to develop.

A 37-year-old Hispanic male had been receiving amiodarone 200 mg twice daily for 3 weeks for atrial fibrillation, when he presented with arthralgia, low-grade fever, malaise, joint pain, and a malar rash. His antinuclear antibody (ANA) titer was positive (1:640). His symptoms resolved with discontinuation of amiodarone and no other treatments. Three months later, the patient remained symptom free, although his ANA titer remained positive (1:80) [14A].

The proposed mechanism for drug-induced lupus is that the drug metabolites illicit T-cell response by acting as haptens. Toxicities from amiodarone usually result from high drug levels and tissue accumulation of the drug and its metabolites, seen in prolonged use of amiodarone. Unlike the previous reports of amiodarone-induced lupus, however, this patient developed symptoms and positive ANA titer shortly after the initiation of amiodarone.

Anaphylaxis due to amiodarone has also been previously reported. Patients usually responded to discontinuation of amiodarone with or without steroid treatment. However, severe anaphylaxis may result in hemodynamic instability.

• A 15-year-old boy, with a history of cardiac rhabdomyoma in the left ventricular and tumor-associated ventricular tachycardia, presented with stable ventricular tachycardia. He did not respond to adenosine or diltiazem, therefore amiodarone was given (unknown dose or duration). The patient immediately developed facial and tongue swelling, hypotension, and altered mental status, then further progressed to cardiac arrest with pulseless electrical activity. He was successfully resuscitated but continued to be hypotensive and epinephrine resistant. A bedside echocardiogram showed severe biventricular dysfunction and his electrocardiogram showed myocardial ischemia with ST elevation. He eventually required a temporary left ventricular assist device to maintain his hemodynamics. He was treated with a 5-day course of methylprednisolone and recovered completely. Interestingly, his repeated echocardiogram showed normal left ventricular function upon discharge. It is also noteworthy that this patient previously tolerated amiodarone [15A].

The exact mechanism of anaphylaxis-induced ventricular dysfunction is unknown, but a phenomenon called Kounis syndrome was proposed to be a potential cause. Kounis syndrome, also known as "allergic angina", is a hypersensitivity-associated acute coronary syndrome that could cause vasospastic angina and coronary thrombosis. Epinephrine has also been implicated in vasospasm, myocardial stunning, and platelet aggregation [16r].

Musculoskeletal

Several cases of acute back pain have been reported with intravenous infusion of amiodarone, mostly with the first dose but it could also occur with subsequent doses.

• A 45-year-old Japanese male with paroxysmal atrial fibrillation (AF) received amiodarone intravenous infusion at 1 mg/min for rapid AF and palpitation. Within 10 minutes of infusion, patient complained of severe back pain that radiated to his whole body and was described as "burning" sensation. Patient's vital signs were stable, and labs were within normal limits. The pain completely resolved within 5 minutes of discontinuation [17A].

A previous report of amiodarone-induced epigastric and lower back pain hypothesized that the polysorbate-80, an excipient in the parenteral amiodarone formulation, causes a hypotensive response following initiation of amiodarone that resulted in mesenteric ischemia and resultant lower back pain [18A]. However, the patient presented above did not have hypotension during the severe back pain. The authors speculated that the back pain may be due to an allergic reaction to amiodarone, although the patient did not have any specific immunoallergic phenomena.

Although amiodarone has been linked to myopathy, muscle toxicity in the form of diaphragm paralysis had not been reported previously.

• A 12-year-old male received 72 hours of intravenous amiodarone for ventricular tachycardia. Then it became evident that he could not be weaned off the ventilator, and diaphragm paralysis was confirmed. All of his electrolyte levels and thyroid hormone levels were normal. The medications he received included ceftriaxone, intravenous fluids, pantoprazole, dopamine, and midazolam, but no neuromuscular blockers. He also developed limb muscle weakness with a creatine phosphokinase level of 431 U/L on the 18th day. He was extubated on the 50th day and eventually recovered completely on the 64th day [19A].

Although the mechanism by which amiodarone causes myopathy is unclear, biopsies have shown muscle inflammation and necrosis [20A] as well as accumulation of lipid-like inclusion bodies [21A]. These amiodarone-induced myopathy could develop within 12 hours of initiation [22A] and improve 1–6 months after discontinuation [19A,20A].

Respiratory

Pulmonary toxicity is a well-known adverse effect that occurs in approximately 5–8% of patients receiving amiodarone. While higher dose and longer duration of amiodarone treatment are risk factors for pulmonary toxicity, it has also been reported in the acute setting, particularly with large loading doses.

- A 62-year-old male received intravenous amiodarone for postoperative atrial fibrillation (150 mg bolus followed by 1 mg/min infusion for 48 hours) and developed acute respiratory distress, necessitating noninvasive positive pressure ventilation. Chest X-ray showed bilateral alveolar–interstitial infiltrate, while CT angiogram of the chest revealed multifocal pulmonary ground-glass opacities and foci of consolidation. A bronchoscopy confirmed the diagnosis of amiodarone-induced pulmonary toxicity based on the presence of foamy macrophages. The patient's outcome was not reported [23A].
- A 78-year-old male was treated with amiodarone 200 mg four times daily for 5 days per week for 8 months when he presented with dyspnea, dry cough and low-grade fever that did not respond to antibiotic treatment. He was initially diagnosed with pleural and parenchymal asbestos-related lesions on chest CT. However, a bronchoalveolar lavage did not show any asbestos bodies, and the lung biopsy revealed a pattern consistent with acute fibrinous and organizing pneumonia. The patient was treated with methylprednisolone 40 mg twice daily in addition to discontinuation of amiodarone. He had a complete resolution of pleural effusion and alveolar consolidations on chest CT 3 months later [24A].

Endocrine

A nested case–control study, using insurance claim data, showed that there is an increased risk of acute pancreatitis associated with amiodarone use in patients with nonvalvular atrial fibrillation, adjusted odds ratio=1.53 (95% CI 1.24–1.88). This risk is significantly higher within 12 months of amiodarone initiation (odds ratio=1.86 [95% CI 1.41–2.45]), compared to the risk after 12 months of initiation (odds ratio=1.21 [95% CI 0.89–1.64]), $p=0.04$. This study supports the previous case reports of acute pancreatitis associated with amiodarone use. Although the mechanism by which amiodarone causes pancreatitis is unknown, it is thought to be related to direct cytotoxicity or immune-mediated pathway as seen in amiodarone-induced pulmonary toxicity [25MC].

Amiodarone is also well known for causing thyroid dysfunction. A recent review [26R] described two common types of thyroid dysfunction, amiodarone-induced thyrotoxicosis (AIT) and amiodarone-induced hypothyroidism (AIH). AIT is further divided into type 1 AIT, in which iodine-rich amiodarone leads to excessive production of thyroid hormones, and type 2 AIT, in which amiodarone causes thyroiditis thus releasing preformed thyroid hormones. AIH, on the other hand, involves inhibition of iodide oxidation by amiodarone. Amiodarone can also inhibit 5′-monodeiodinase which is responsible for conversion of T_4–T_3, resulting in low T_3 syndrome. Another study reported that amiodarone, instead of the iodine component of amiodarone as previously thought, increases endoplasmic reticulum stress which leads to destructive thyroiditis [27E].

Liver

Although hepatotoxicity from amiodarone has been previously reported, few systematic analyses have been conducted to evaluate this risk. A population-based case–control study was conducted to evaluate the risk of malignant neoplasm of liver and intrahepatic bile ducts (MNLIHD) associated with antiarrhythmic agents, using data from the National Health Insurance program in Taiwan. Among the five antiarrhythmic agents studied (amiodarone, mexiletine, propafenone, quinidine, and procainamide), only amiodarone was associated with a higher risk of MNLIHD (adjusted odds ratio=1.6 [95% CI 1.45–1.77]). This risk in amiodarone users was further increased with comorbidities such as chronic liver disease and cirrhosis, HBV infection, HCV infection, and alcoholism (adjusted odds ratio=18.0 [95% CI 15.7–20.5]). The risk of developing of MNLIHD is dose dependent and is more likely to occur within the first year of amiodarone use [28MC].

Most reported cases of hepatotoxicity associated with amiodarone were in the form of acute hepatitis exclusively with the intravenous formulation and reversible with discontinuation of amiodarone. Although poorly understood, the mechanism is theorized to be either due to alteration of cell membrane structure and function or an allergic process induced by polysorbate 80 in the diluent, not amiodarone itself.

- An 80-year-old male received amiodarone 150 mg IV bolus followed by 1 mg/min for 6 hours, then 0.5 mg/min for 18 hours for stable ventricular tachycardia on day 7 after an uneventful coronary artery bypass surgery. The day after amiodarone was initiated, his AST increased from 47 to 7500 units/L, ALT from 44 to 3969 units/L, total bilirubin from 0.5 to 1.6 mg/dL. He received 1300 mg of acetaminophen and atorvastatin (unknown dose) in the preceding 24 hours. Doppler was negative for bile duct dilation or obstruction, and viral serologies for hepatitis B and C were negative as well. Within 48 hours of amiodarone discontinuation, his aminotransferase levels rapidly declined. Throughout the whole event, he did not have any hypotensive episodes or shock. The patient expired on postoperative day 30, even though his liver enzymes normalized [29A].

The authors reviewed literature and found 25 cases of hepatotoxicity associated with amiodarone. Only 10 were conclusive cases of acute hepatotoxicity associated with intravenous amiodarone between 1986 and 2012 [29A]. Although the case presented above provided evidence to support amiodarone-induced hepatotoxicity, it is important to exclude ischemia as a potential cause given the similarities in clinical presentations between amiodarone-induced hepatitis and ischemic hepatitis.

- A 65-year-old female with newly diagnosed left ventricular dysfunction and community acquired pneumonia was treated for mixed cardiogenic and septic shock. Her liver enzymes were elevated, but increased dramatically after amiodarone 150 mg intravenous bolus was given to treat new onset of atrial fibrillation. Amiodarone was stopped due to hypotension and the transaminases improved. Thirteen days later, patient was started on amiodarone infusion at 0.5 mg/min after cardioversion. After 1500 mg total dose was given, her transaminases again rose quickly and steadily, even though her blood pressure remained stable. Intravenous N-acetylcysteine (NAC) 300 mg/kg was administered over 21 hours using the acetaminophen toxicity protocol. AST dropped by 50% by 12 hours of NAC and 80% by 24 hours. Although liver enzymes continued to improve, the patient eventually expired [30A].

The author argued that in this case, patient was re-challenged with amiodarone without hypotensive episodes. Therefore, amiodarone is more likely the culprit for the liver injury instead of ischemia. In addition, NAC is often used to treat drug-induced liver injury. The drastic improvement in the patient's liver enzymes after NAC treatment further supports that it was amiodarone-induced hepatitis. Although these are reasonable arguments, it was difficult to conclusively identify amiodarone as the cause in this critically ill patient.

Skin

Amiodarone is an iodine-rich compound, which contains approximately 37% iodine by weight. Some of the adverse effects of amiodarone, such as thyroid dysfunction, are thought to be caused by its iodine content.

- A 72-year-old male, with history of atrial fibrillation, type 2 diabetes, heart failure, hypertension, and chronic kidney disease, presented with pruritic scaly erythematous papules on both forearms. He was receiving amiodarone at an unknown dose for an unknown duration, in addition to furosemide, nifedipine, insulin glargine, and allopurinol. He was found to have an elevated serum creatinine of 3.79 mg/dL and iodine level of 42305 ng/mL.

A diagnosis of iododerma secondary to amiodarone was made based on the skin biopsy and markedly elevated serum iodine level. The patient's skin lesions significantly improved within 2 weeks after amiodarone discontinuation and completely resolved within 4 weeks with topical corticosteroid cream [31A].

Although the exact mechanism of iododerma is unknown, it is postulated that iodine serves as a hapten that binds to serum proteins. In this case, due to the patient's underlying kidney disease, a decreased iodine clearance led to accumulation of iodine and potentially the iododerma.

Hair

Although amiodarone is associated with a wide range of adverse effects, hair loss is a very rare side effect.

- An 85-year-old male, with history of dilated cardiomyopathy, permanent atrial fibrillation, and sustained ventricular tachycardia, was placed on amiodarone (200 mg three times daily for 3 weeks then 200 mg daily) along with implantation of an implantable cardioverter defibrillator. He was also receiving bisoprolol, quinapril, simvastatin and dabigatran. Six months after initiation of amiodarone, the patient reported significant scalp hair loss. His laboratory values were within normal limits. The patient's hair density was restored with no further hair loss 3 months after amiodarone was stopped [32A].

The mechanism by which amiodarone causes hair loss is unknown; in all reported cases, hair was completely restored after discontinuation of amiodarone.

Multiorgan

Toxicities that involve more than one organ may occur in patients receiving amiodarone.

- A 54-year-old female was receiving amiodarone 200 mg daily for paroxysmal atrial fibrillation. Seven months after the initiation of amiodarone, she presented with blue-gray discoloration on her nose and cheeks, as well as general malaise and cold intolerance which was later attributed to low T4 and high TSH consistent with hypothyroidism. She also had moderately increased liver function test. An ophthalmologic exam revealed vortex keratopathy in both eyes, worse in the left than right, with normal vision. Five months after discontinuation of amiodarone, liver function test returned to normal, and skin discoloration and vortex keratopathy improved but did not resolve completely [33A].
- A 60-year-old male has received amiodarone 400 mg daily for 8 years when he presented with shortness of breath. He was found to have grayish discoloration of

the face, diffuse alveolar and interstitial infiltrates confirmed by a chest CT and bronchoscopy, and increased liver density. No further information was available regarding the patient's recovery [34A].

These two cases demonstrated that amiodarone could cause multi-organ toxicities with low to moderate dose regardless of treatment duration.

Drug–Drug Interaction

Cytochrome P450 3A4 (CYP3A4) is a major enzyme that metabolizes many medications. P-glycoprotein (P-gp) is an efflux pump in the luminal side of the intestine, hepatocytes and renal tubule cells. Amiodarone is a known CYP3A4 and P-glycoprotein inhibitor. Medications known to be substrates of CYP3A4 or P-glycoprotein or both should be used with caution in combination with amiodarone.

RIVAROXABAN

- A 75-year-old male, with history of lobectomy secondary to bronchiectasis, presented with hemoptysis 2 weeks after amiodarone 200 mg daily was initiated. The patient had also been taking rivaroxaban 20 mg daily for a year for venous thromboembolism and atrial fibrillation. A chest computed tomography revealed left lower lobe pulmonary infiltrates with ground-glass opacities. The patient's symptoms improved after discontinuation of both rivaroxaban and amiodarone. He was later re-challenged with rivaroxaban 15 mg daily without any further complications. Although he had previously tolerated amiodarone years ago, it was not reinitiated [35A].

Rivaroxaban is a substrate for both CYP3A4 and P-glycoprotein. This case illustrates the importance of monitoring this rivaroxaban–amiodarone drug interaction, especially in patients with history of pulmonary disease.

Dofetilide [SED-15, 1173; SEDA-35, 338; SEDA-37, 209]

Nervous System

- A 71-year-old woman with atrial fibrillation was prescribed dofetilide in an attempt to achieve normal sinus rhythm, after other treatments were unsuccessful. The patient complained of sharp, increasing right-sided facial pain within 5 hours of her first dose of 250 mcg. Additionally, the patient experienced mild facial swelling, severe tenderness and an inability to open her mouth or smile. No rash

was noted, vital signs were unchanged, and the pain was unrelieved by morphine. Work-up was negative as to the cause and the patient received two more doses of dofetilide before it was stopped. Within 12 hours, the facial pain improved, and within 1 day, the patient's pain resolved [36A].

Facial paralysis is identified as an adverse effect occurring in less than 2% of users; however, it should still be considered when patients experience any form of facial pain and/or neuralgia upon initiation of dofetilide [37S].

Dronedarone [SEDA-35, 338; SEDA-36, 262; SEDA-37, 209]

Dronedarone was introduced as an alternative to amiodarone. Through the removal of iodine and the addition of a methylsulfonyl group, it was believed that the toxicities associated with amiodarone use would be eliminated. There appears to be growing evidence, from ocular to pulmonary side effects, that dronedarone may be more similar to amiodarone than we are aware.

Cardiovascular

- A 76-year-old woman was admitted to the hospital for acute congestive heart failure (ejection fraction was normal) and started on dronedarone 400 mg by mouth twice daily following direct current cardioversion for the treatment of recurrent atrial tachycardia. Prior to initiation, the patient's QTc interval was 469 msec. During a hospitalization several months later the QTc was noted to be 512 msec. The patient then experienced torsade de pointes (TdP), received amiodarone 150 mg intravenously in error and subsequently had a QTc of 743 msec. All labs with the exception of an elevated SCr of 1.4 were within normal limits. A follow-up echocardiogram revealed an ejection fraction of 25% with global hypokinesis [38A].

Dronedarone carries with it a black box warning advising against its use in patients with symptomatic heart failure with recent decompensation requiring hospitalization or New York Heart Association Class IV symptoms. This warning is based upon the findings of the ANDROMEDA trial which enrolled patients with an ejection fraction of 40% or less. The trial was stopped early due to an increase in mortality in those taking dronedarone compared to placebo [39C]. While some practitioners may think that it is acceptable to use dronedarone in those with diastolic heart failure, this case illustrates that caution should still be exercised when using this agent in all forms of heart failure.

In addition to the concern regarding its use in heart failure, extreme caution should be used to avoid concomitant medications which may potentiate the risk of developing torsade de pointes.

Respiratory

- A 68-year-old woman was prescribed dronedarone for management of paroxysmal atrial fibrillation. After 1 month of treatment, the patient developed a dry cough and dyspnea which progressively worsened over a 5-month period, at which point the patient presented to a hospital with respiratory failure. Dronedarone was discontinued and a CT scan revealed diffuse bilateral ground-glass opacities whereas a lung biopsy identified diffuse interstitial alveolar damage. The patient improved with steroid treatment and was able to be released home on oxygen. While the patient did have a remote smoking history, this was felt not to contribute to her disease. Additionally, other potential causes were also ruled out [40A].

Urinary Tract

An increase in serum creatinine without a noted decline in glomerular filtration rate has long been known as a side effect of dronedarone. Due to a growing number of reports implicating dronedarone in the development of renal failure, data from the Spanish Pharmacovigilance System were collected to identify cases of renal failure associated with the use of dronedarone. Ten case reports matching search criteria were found. While dronedarone was identified as the possible cause of the renal failure, in eight cases, the patient was on other agents known to cause renal dysfunction (e.g. angiotensin receptor blockers, loop diuretics, aldosterone antagonists, etc.). In the remaining two cases, no concomitant medications were listed. It is unknown if the patients were indeed not on any other medications or if the reporting individuals failed to submit this information [41C].

Due to the limited information available, it is difficult to ascertain whether dronedarone was the cause of the renal failure as opposed to a correlation to the event. Dronedarone use may have indirectly contributed to the acute kidney injury by causing dehydration due to nausea and vomiting and increasing the likelihood of renal injury in patients with predisposing conditions (diabetes, hypertension). More studies are required to determine if dronedarone does indeed have a direct nephrotoxic effect.

Flecainide [SED-15, 1370; SEDA-35, 339; SEDA-36, 262]

Cardiovascular

- A 24-year-old woman reported to have accidentally ingested three to four tablets of flecainide presented to the hospital unresponsive and hypotensive. Her EKG

showed wide complex bradydysrhythmia which progressed to pulseless electrical activity cardiac arrest. Venoarterial extracorporeal membrane oxygenation was initiated as a form of treatment, and the patient survived to hospital discharge on day 19 [42A].

- A 74-year-old woman with atrial fibrillation and a QTc interval of 472 msec was started on flecainide 100 mg by mouth twice daily and later increased to 150 mg twice daily. Within a few weeks, she experienced syncope which revealed a QTc interval of 561 msec with sinus bradycardia and first degree atrioventricular block. She subsequently was found to have 1:1 atrial flutter with wide QRS complex and eventually deteriorated into torsade de pointes with a QTc of 601 msec. Resolution occurred with magnesium sulfate, lidocaine and isoproterenol and discontinuation of flecainide. Lab values were normal, and genetic testing was negative [43A].

While the use of flecainide has decreased significantly with the development of newer antiarrhythmics, it is still used today. It is critical to remember the heightened risk of cardiac dysrhythmias, when this medication is taken.

References

[1] Renard D, Rubli E, Voide N, et al. Spectrum of digoxin-induced ocular toxicity: a case report and literature review. BMC Res Notes. 2015;8:368 [A].

[2] Rameis H, Magometschnigg D, Ganzinger U. The diltiazem-digoxin interaction. Clin Pharmacol Ther. 1984;36:183–9 [c].

[3] Lai S-W, Lin C-L, Liao K-F. Digoxin use may increase the relative risk of acute pancreatitis: a population-based case–control study in Taiwan. Int J Cardiol. 2015;181:235–8 [C].

[4] Corley S, Epstein AE, DiMarco JP, et al. Relationships between sinus rhythm, treatment, and survival in the Atrial Fibrillation Follow-Up Investigation of Rhythm Management (AFFIRM) Study. Circulation. 2004;109:1509–13 [C].

[5] Gjesdal K, Feyzi JOS. Digitalis: a dangerous drug in atrial fibrillation? An analysis of the SPORTIF III and V data. Heart. 2008;94:191–6 [C].

[6] Turakhia MP, Santangeli P, Winkelmayer WC, et al. Increased mortality associated with digoxin in contemporary patients with atrial fibrillation: findings from the TREAT-AF study. J Am Coll Cardiol. 2014;64:660–8 [C].

[7] Allen LA, Fonarow GC, Simon DN, et al. Digoxin use and subsequent outcomes among patients in a contemporary atrial fibrillation cohort. J Am Coll Cardiol. 2015;65:2691–8 [C].

[8] Freeman JV, Reynolds K, Fang M, et al. Digoxin and risk of death in adults with atrial fibrillation: the ATRIA-CVRN study. Circ Arrhythm Electrophysiol. 2015;8:49–58 [C].

[9] Doshi D, Jayawardana R. Amiodarone-induced life-threatening refractory hypotension. Am J Case Rep. 2015;16:617–20 [A].

[10] Chen W-C, Chen W-C, Chen C-Y, et al. Amiodarone use is associated with increased risk of stroke in patients with nonvalvular atrial fibrillation: a nationwide population-based cohort study. Medicine (Baltimore). 2015;94:e849 [MC].

[11] Altun S, Yolcu U, Ilhan A, et al. Vortex keratopathy associated with long term use of amiodarone. Am J Cardiol. 2015;115:S148 [A].

[12] Alp A, Akdam H. Vortex keratopathy: Fabry related or amiodarone induced? Am J Cardiol. 2015;116:826 [r].

[13] Chan TCY, Jhanji V. Amiodarone-induced vortex keratopathy. N Engl J Med. 2015;372:1656 [A].

[14] Yachoui R, Saad W. Amiodarone-induced lupus-like syndrome. Am J Ther. 2015;22:e20–1 [A].

[15] Averin K, Lorts A, Connor C. Anaphylactic shock after amiodarone infusion resulting in haemodynamic collapse requiring a temporary ventricular assist device. Cardiol Young. 2015;25:164–6 [A].

[16] Kounis NG, Soufras GD, Davlouros P, et al. Combined etiology of anaphylactic cardiogenic shock: amiodarone, epinephrine, cardioverter defibrillator, left ventricular assist devices and the Kounis syndrome. Ann Card Anaesth. 2015;18:261–4 [r].

[17] Yan Y, Shen H. Acute severe back pain radiating to the whole body during intravenous administration of amiodarone. Int J Clin Pharmacol Ther. 2015;53:561–2 [A].

[18] Petrou E, Lakovou I, Boutsikou M, et al. Acute epigastric and low back pain during amiodarone infusion; is it the drug or the vehicle to blame? Heart Lung. 2014;43:60–1 [A].

[19] Chandelia S, Kundal M, Dubey NK, et al. Acute diaphragm paralysis caused by intravenous administration of amiodarone. Ann Pharmacother. 2015;49:1173–4 [A].

[20] Pulipaka U, Lacomis D, Omalu B. Amiodarone-induced neuromyopathy: three cases and a review of the literature. J Clin Neuromuscul Dis. 2002;3:97–105 [A].

[21] Clouston PD, Donnelly PE. Acute necrotising myopathy associated with amiodarone therapy. Aust N Z J Med. 1989;19:483–5 [A].

[22] Saha SA. Severe muscle cramps after intravenous administration of amiodarone—a novel, potentially dose-dependent adverse effect. Br J Clin Pharmacol. 2011;71:624–5 [A].

[23] Oh E, Siddiqui N, Worringer E, et al. Acute amiodarone-induced lung toxicity. Am J Med Sci. 2015;349:89 [A].

[24] Piciucchi S, Dubini A, Tomassetti S, et al. A case of amiodarone-induced acute fibrinous and organizing pneumonia mimicking mesothelioma. Am J Respir Crit Care Med. 2015;191:104–6 [A].

[25] Alonso A, MacLehose RF, Lutsey PL, et al. Association of amiodarone use with acute pancreatitis in patients with atrial fibrillation: a nested case-control study. JAMA Intern Med. 2015;175:449–50 [MC].

[26] Danzi S, Klein I. Amiodarone-induced thyroid dysfunction. J Intensive Care Med. 2015;30:179–85 [R].

[27] Lombardi A, Inabnet WB, Owen R, et al. Endoplasmic reticulum stress as a novel mechanism in amiodarone-induced destructive thyroiditis. J Clin Endocrinol Metab. 2015;100:E1–E10 [E].

[28] Lim Y-P, Lin C-L, Lin Y-N, et al. Antiarrhythmic agents and the risk of malignant neoplasm of liver and intrahepatic bile ducts. PLoS One. 2015;10:e0116960 [MC].

[29] Stratton A, Fenderson J, Kenny P, et al. Severe acute hepatitis following intravenous amiodarone: a case report and review of the literature. Acta Gastroenterol Belg. 2015;78:233–9 [A].

[30] Mudalel ML, Dave KP, Hummel JP, et al. N-acetylcysteine treats intravenous amiodarone induced liver injury. World J Gastroenterol. 2015;21:2816–9 [A].

[31] Khetarpal S, Kovalyshyn I, Fernandez AP. Erythematous papules on the forearms. JAMA Dermatol. 2015;151:891–2 [A].

[32] Korantzopoulos P, Kyrlas K, Goudevenos JA. Amiodarone-induced hair loss: case report and review of the literature. Q J Med. 2015;108:325–7 [A].

[33] Turk U, Turk BG, Yılmaz SG, et al. Amiodarone-induced multiorgan toxicity with ocular findings on confocal microscopy. Middle East Afr J Ophthalmol. 2015;22:258–60 [A].

[34] Rehman SU, Siddiqui N, Khan NS, et al. Multisystem side effects of amiodarone. Am J Med Sci. 2015;349:454 [A].

[35] Elikowski W, Małek M, Skowroński M, et al. Hemoptysis during concomitant treatment with rivaroxaban and amiodarone in a patient with a history of pulmonary disease. Pol Merkur Lekarski. 2015;39:227–30 [A].

[36] Maluli HA. Dofetilide induced trigeminal neuralgia. Indian J Pharmacol. 2015;47:336–7 [A].

[37] Tikosyn® [package insert]. New York, NY: Pfizer Inc.; 2016, [S].

[38] Huemer M, Sarganas G, Bronder E, et al. Torsade de pointes tachycardia in a patient on dronedarone therapy. Pharmacotherapy. 2015;35:e61–5 [A].

[39] Kober L, Torp-Pedersen C, McMurray JJV, et al. Increased mortality after dronedarone therapy for severe heart failure. N Engl J Med. 2008;358:2678–87 [C].

[40] Stack S, Nguyen DV, Casto A, et al. Diffuse alveolar damage in a patient receiving dronedarone. Chest. 2015;147:e131–3 [A].

[41] Tarapues M, Cereza G, Figueras A. Dronedarone and renal impairment: evaluation of Spanish postmarketing reports and review of literature. Expert Opin Drug Saf. 2015;14:807–13 [C].

[42] Reynolds JC, Judge BS. Successful treatment of flecainide-induced cardiac arrest with extracorporeal membrane oxygenation in the ED. Am J Emerg Med. 2015;33:1542.e1–2 [A].

[43] Nasser M, Idris S, Marinelli K, et al. Flecainide-induced torsades de pointes: case report and review of literature. Rev Cardiovasc Med. 2015;16:214–20 [A].

17

Beta-Adrenoceptor Antagonists and Antianginal Drugs

Eric J. Ip[*,1], *Punam B. Patel*[*], *I-Kuan Hsu*[*], *Bonnie Lau*[*,†,‡]

[*]Department of Clinical Sciences, Touro University California College of Pharmacy, Vallejo, CA, USA
[†]Department of Emergency Medicine, Kaiser Permanente Santa Clara Medical Center, Santa Clara, CA, USA
[‡]Department of Emergency Medicine, Stanford University School of Medicine, Palo Alto, CA, USA
[1]Corresponding author: eric.ip@tu.edu

BETA-ADRENOCEPTOR ANTAGONISTS [SED-15, 452; SEDA-32, 363; SEDA-33, 397; SEDA-34, 303; SEDA-35, 351; SEDA-36, 267; SEDA-37, 215]

Atenolol

Dermatological

PITYRIASIS ROSEA-LIKE REACTION ASSOCIATED WITH ATENOLOL

A first case of atenolol-induced pityriasis rosea-like reaction has been reported. A 56-year-old female with hypertension presented to an outpatient clinic with 1 week of flat, round, and oval scaly patches that were pruritic and bright red to violet in appearance on her neck, abdomen, axilla, and upper extremities. She had no fever or other systemic symptoms. A skin biopsy revealed a perivascular lymphocytic infiltrate with eosinophils, mild spongiosis, and edema of the upper dermis. The eruptions started approximately 3 weeks after initiating oral atenolol. The patient was diagnosed with atenolol-induced pityriasis rosea-like eruption. Atenolol was discontinued, and topical corticosteroids and anti-histamines were prescribed. Clinical symptoms and itching resolved approximately 1 week later. An oral calcium channel blocker was alternatively prescribed to treat her hypertension [1A].

Labetalol

Dermatological

ACUTE GENERALIZED EXANTHEMATOUS PUSTULOSIS ASSOCIATED WITH LABETALOL

A first case of labetalol-induced acute generalized exanthematous pustulosis has been reported. A 31-year-old third-trimester pregnant female with hypertension was treated with oral labetalol 18 days prior to admission and hydralazine, methyldopa, and metamizole 3 days prior to admission. During her hospitalization, erythematous micropapular lesions presented on her face and neck that progressed 4–5 days later to become more diffuse, specifically to her flexures. She had a low-grade fever (38.7 °C) and leukocytosis (90% neutrophils). Despite discontinuation of hydralazine, methyldopa, and metamizole on the second day of the eruption, new lesions continued to appear. After 5 days of discontinuing labetalol, no new skin lesions appeared. Subsequent follow-up 1 month later included a patch test, which confirmed labetalol to be the only previously administered medication to have a positive test of pustule formation. A biopsy of the pustules confirmed the diagnosis of acute generalized exanthematous pustulosis. Of note, during patch testing to find an alternative to labetalol for the patient, it was found she also had a cross-reactivity reaction to atenolol [2A].

Metoprolol

Psychiatric

PSYCHOSIS ASSOCIATED WITH METOPROLOL IN A PATIENT HETEROZYGOUS FOR THE CYP2D6*4 ALLELE

A first case of an association between metoprolol and psychosis has been reported. A 44-year-old male with hypertension and no psychiatric history on no medications experienced confusion and insomnia 2 weeks after initiating metoprolol 50 mg oral therapy. He self-discontinued metoprolol, and symptoms diminished quickly thereafter. After restarting metoprolol several days later, he experienced chaotic thinking and delusional thoughts. The patient was admitted to the psychiatric ward for psychotic symptoms. Workup, including a physical and neurological examination and lab tests, excluded other causes of psychosis. It was felt his psychotic symptoms were due to metoprolol. The patient was found to be heterozygous for the CYP2D6*4 allele (reduced CYP2D6 activity) which may increase the side effects of metoprolol (CYP2D6 substrate). The patient was treated with olanzapine 20 mg/day, and metoprolol was discontinued. After a few days, his psychotic symptoms diminished. The patient was discharged with an olanzapine taper over 3 weeks. The patient remained symptom free. The Naranjo Adverse Drug Reaction Probability Scale suggested a "definite" relationship (score = 9) between metoprolol and psychosis. It was also discovered that the patient's mother and brother have variation in the CYP2D6 genotype and also experienced psychosis with metoprolol in the past [3A].

Nebivolol

Gynecomastia

GYNECOMASTIA ASSOCIATED WITH NEBIVOLOL

A first case of an association between nebivolol and gynecomastia has been reported. A 42-year-old male with hypertension only on nebivolol presented to the outpatient clinic reporting bilateral painful breast swelling 2 months after initiating nebivolol 5 mg oral therapy. After ruling out other causes of gynecomastia via clinical history (including inquiry on drug/herbal use), lab tests, and imaging, the patient was diagnosed with grade II gynecomastia secondary to nebivolol. Nebivolol was discontinued, and the patient was alternatively treated with amlodipine 10 mg/day. Three months later, symptoms resolved and there was no presence of breast swelling or pain. The Naranjo Adverse Drug Reaction Probability Scale suggested a "probable" relationship (score = 6) between nebivolol and gynecomastia [4A].

Propranolol

Drug–Drug Interaction

FATAL HYPERKALEMIA ASSOCIATED WITH CONCOMITANT SUCCINYLCHOLINE AND PROPRANOLOL IN A PEDIATRIC PATIENT WITH CHRONIC LIVER DISEASE

A first reported fatal case of hyperkalemia after concomitant use of succinylcholine and oral propranolol has been reported. A 14-year-old female with a history of extra hepatic portal vein obstruction (EHPVO) taking oral propranolol 40 mg/day the past 2 years was scheduled for elective esophagogastroduodenoscopy and sclerotherapy.

The patient received IV thiopentone sodium 5 mg/kg, fentanyl 1.5 mcg/kg, and succinylcholine 1.5 mg/kg at the induction of the procedure. The patient was intubated and mechanically ventilated. Fifteen minutes after starting the procedure, changes to the patient's EKG (tall T waves with widening of QRS complexes) were observed, and a clinical diagnosis of hyperkalemia was made. Calcium gluconate 500 mg with sodium bicarbonate 10 mL of 7.5% was administered, and a small decrease in amplitude of T waves was noticed. The patient's condition worsened, and her EKG showed persistent bradycardia progressing to asystole. Cardiopulmonary resuscitation was initiated immediately; an hour of resuscitation, including administration of calcium gluconate, epinephrine, and sodium bicarbonate, was unsuccessful. Her potassium level was confirmed at 7.7 mEq/L. Succinylcholine and beta-blockers independently have been known to cause hyperkalemia. The combined use of succinylcholine and propranolol (a non-selective beta blocker that is primarily hepatically cleared) in a pediatric patient with chronic liver disease likely led to the fatal hyperkalemia [5A].

Timolol

Psychiatric

PSYCHOSIS ASSOCIATED WITH TOPICAL TIMOLOL OPHTHALMIC SOLUTION

A case of topical timolol-induced simultaneous hypoglycemia, bradyarrhythmia, and psychosis has been reported. An 84-year-old male with a past medical history of hypertension, hypercholesterolemia, type 2 diabetes mellitus, and open angle glaucoma was admitted for syncope and altered mental status. Medication history included topical timolol maleate 0.5% ophthalmic solution (a non-selective beta-blocker) started 35 days prior to admission, atorvastatin 10 mg/day, enalapril 10 mg/day, and metformin 1000 mg/day. Upon admission, the patient's blood glucose was 34 mg/dL, heart rate 34 bpm, and blood pressure 58/43 mmHg. The patient was intubated and given dextrose 50% 100 mL and 0.5 mg atropine. Though his heart rate and blood pressure improved briefly, they quickly trended downward and was transferred to the ICU.

A temporary transvenous pacemaker was inserted, and he was started on an IV infusion of 10% dextrose. He was ultimately extubated 16 hours after admission, and the pacemaker was able to be turned off after 26 hours of no bradycardic events. A repeat examination still found the patient to be confused, but with no focal deficits. Ophthalmic timolol was the suspected cause of the patient's hypoglycemia, confusion, and bradyarrhythmia. The timolol ophthalmic was switched to travoprost, a prostaglandin F2 analogue, after consultation with ophthalmology. His bradycardia resolved and the patient's confusion gradually improved over the next 3 days [6A].

CALCIUM CHANNEL BLOCKERS [SED-15, 598; SEDA-32, 366; SEDA-33, 401; SEDA-34, 306; SEDA-35, 354; SEDA-36, 270; SEDA-37, 219]

Nifedipine

Cardiovascular

LOWER VASODILATORY SIDE EFFECTS AND HEADACHE WITH COMBINATION NIFEDIPINE GITS–CANDESARTAN COMPARED TO NIFEDIPINE GITS MONOTHERAPY

The DISTINCT study (reDefining Intervention with Studies Testing Innovative Nifedipine GITS–Candesartan Therapy) was a multinational, multicenter, randomized double-blinded study evaluating systolic/diastolic blood pressure and vasodilatory side effects of nifedipine GITS (an extended release form of nifedipine), candesartan, and combination nifedipine GITS–candesartan therapy. A total of 1381 patients were randomized to receive combination or monotherapy with nifedipine GITS (20, 30, or 60 mg), candesartan cilexetil (4, 8, 16, or 32 mg), or placebo. The combination nifedipine GITS–candesartan group had a lower incidence of vasodilatory side effects (18.3% vs. 23.6%) and headaches (5.5% vs. 11.0%, $P = 0.003$) versus the nifedipine GITS monotherapy group. No significant differences were seen in peripheral edema (3.6% vs. 5.8%, $P = $n.s.) between the combination nifedipine GITS–candesartan group versus the nifedipine GITS monotherapy group [7C].

Drug–Drug Interactions

Non-Dihydropyridine and Dihydropyridine Calcium Channel Blockers

LACK OF INCREASED FRACTURE RISK IN OLDER PATIENTS ON CALCIUM CHANNEL BLOCKERS COPRESCRIBED CLARITHROMYCIN VERSUS AZITHROMYCIN

A population-level retrospective cohort study among elderly patients over 66 years old taking chronic calcium channel blockers (CCBs; CYP3A4 substrate) was performed to determine whether coprescription with clarithromycin (CYP3A4 inhibitor) resulted in a higher fracture risk than azithromycin (does not inhibit CYP3A4). The population consisted of 96,226 patients coprescribed clarithromycin and 94,083 coprescribed azithromycin while taking a CCB (amlodipine, nifedipine,

felodipine, verapamil, or diltiazem). Among older adults on CCB therapy, a coprescription with clarithromycin was not associated with a higher 30-day risk of non-vertebral fracture than azithromycin (0.13% vs. 0.10%; OR $= 1.23$; 95% CI $= 0.94$–1.60; $P = 0.134$) [8c].

Amlodipine [SED-15, 175; SEDA-32, 367; SEDA-33, 401; SEDA-34, 307; SEDA-35, 354; SEDA-36, 270; SEDA-37, 219]

Dermatological

SCHAMBERG'S DISEASE ASSOCIATED WITH AMLODIPINE

A first case of an association between amlodipine and Schamberg's disease has been reported. A 31-year-old male with hypertension on lisinopril 20 mg/day was later started on amlodipine 10 mg/day to provide additional blood pressure control. After 3 months of continued use, the patient developed purpuric skin eruptions around the ankle region along with ankle edema. The edema resolved after a few days, but the skin lesions progressively worsened over 2 months. The patient presented with Schamberg's-like irregular distribution of rust-colored spots from the ankles to the knees on the outer side of the tibia. The patient did not have systemic symptoms and pertinent labs (CBC, ESR, prothrombin, partial prothrombin time) did not change significantly. Amlodipine was discontinued, and over the next 3 months, the skin changes were lessened and became brown. The skin lesions disappeared completely after another 4 months.

The patient was re-challenged with amlodipine 6 months later, and the same adverse skin reactions appeared after 1 month. A skin biopsy demonstrated perivascular inflammatory T-cell lymphocytic infiltrate and extravasation of blood cells, characteristic of Schamberg's disease. The Naranjo Adverse Drug Reaction Probability Scale suggested a "probable" relationship (score $= 8$) between amlodipine and Schamberg's disease [9A].

Amlodipine and Nitrendipine

Mouth and Teeth

GINGIVAL OVERGROWTH ASSOCIATED WITH AMLODIPINE AND NITRENDIPINE

Calcium channel blockers have been associated with gingival enlargement or overgrowth in the literature. Two additional case reports of gingival enlargement in hypertensive patients on long-term amlodipine therapy (14 years) and nitrendipine (duration not specified) were described. Treatment involved changing antihypertensive drugs, oral hygiene, antibiotic therapy, and dental prosthetics [10A].

POTASSIUM CHANNEL ACTIVATORS

Nicorandil [SED-15, 2505; SEDA-32, 365; SEDA-33, 400; SEDA-34, 305; SEDA-35, 353; SEDA-36, 270; SEDA-37, 219]

Electrolyte Balance

INTRACTABLE HYPERKALEMIA ASSOCIATED WITH NICORANDIL IN A PATIENT WITH RENAL DYSFUNCTION

A case of intractable hyperkalemia due to nicorandil use has been reported. A 68-year-old male with diabetic nephropathy was admitted with unstable angina. On admission, his serum creatinine was 1.6 mg/dL (was 2.8 mg/dL 4 months prior), and serum potassium was 5.1–5.3 mEq/L. The patient was taking cilnidipine 10 mg once daily and nicorandil (exact dose not specified) twice daily orally prior to admission. During his hospitalization, he had a coronary angiography and subsequent coronary artery bypass surgery. Post-operatively, the patient was started on a nicorandil infusion along with low-dose aspirin. His serum potassium levels trended higher and remained persistently elevated (peaked at 6.4 mEq) despite treatment with insulin with dextrose, intermittent furosemide, and potassium binding resins. Only after discontinuing the nicorandil infusion did the serum potassium level decrease. The patient's potassium decreased to 4.8 mEq/L 24 hours post-nicorandil discontinuation. Nicorandil was suspected to have caused the hyperkalemia as the patient's serum potassium decreased within a few hours after discontinuing the nicorandil infusion and other potential causes of hyperkalemia were ruled out (e.g. low cardiac output, acidosis, potassium-containing medications, and drugs known to cause hyperkalemia) [11A].

NITRATES, ORGANIC

Nitroglycerin [SED-15, 2529; SEDA-32, 366; SEDA-33, 400; SEDA-34, 305; SEDA-35, 354]

Cardiovascular

NO INCREASED HYPOTENSION IN AORTIC STENOSIS PATIENTS RECEIVING NITROGLYCERIN

Caution is advised with the use of nitroglycerin in patients with aortic stenosis, as they may be more susceptible to hypotension. A retrospective cohort study investigated the risk for clinical hypotension in patients with aortic stenosis receiving nitroglycerin for acute cardiogenic pulmonary edema. The study population consisted of 195 patients with acute pulmonary edema divided evenly into three groups: severe aortic stenosis, moderate aortic stenosis, and no evidence of aortic stenosis. After adjusting for confounders, moderate and severe aortic stenosis patients were not associated with increased risk of clinically relevant hypotension after receiving nitroglycerin (OR=0.97; 95% CI=0.40–2.37 for moderate aortic stenosis and OR=0.99; 95% CI=0.41–2.41 for severe aortic stenosis) [12c].

LATE SODIUM CHANNEL (I_{NA}) INHIBITORS

Ranolazine

Cardiovascular

T-WAVE INVERSIONS ASSOCIATED WITH RANOLAZINE

A first case of ranolazine-induced T-wave inversions has been reported. A 64-year-old female with coronary artery disease presented to the emergency room with 2 hours of chest discomfort. An initial EKG showed sinus bradycardia with a 2-mm ST-elevation in lead V2 with elevated troponin-T and CPK levels. Cardiac catheterization found non-obstructive coronary artery disease and akinesis of the apical diaphragmatic wall. These findings were consistent with Takotsubo cardiomyopathy. The patient was given one dose of ranolazine 500 mg as treatment of chronic anginal symptoms. A repeat EKG performed a few hours after ranolazine administration showed deep T-wave inversions in the inferolateral leads as well as a new QTc prolongation (505 msec vs. 416 msec). Troponin-T and CPK levels trended down and an echocardiogram showed complete resolution of the initial apical wall akinesis. After ranolazine was discontinued, a repeat EKG 24 hours later showed persistent, though decreased in amplitude, T-wave inversions and the QTc interval returned to baseline (412 msec). This case report documents ranolazine-induced T-wave inversions presumably from inhibition of the IKr potassium channel [13A].

REBUTTAL OF T-WAVE INVERSIONS WITH RANOLAZINE

A rebuttal of the case report by Kumthekar et al. [13A] has been published questioning the T-wave inversion being solely attributed to ranolazine administration. It is possible the EKG findings are consistent with Takotsubo cardiomyopathy, a stress-induced cardiomyopathy known to have EKG findings of global T-wave inversions and QTc prolongation [14r].

References

[1] Gulec A, Albayrak H, Kayapinar O, et al. Pityriasis rosea-like adverse reaction to atenolol. Hum Exp Toxicol. 2016;35(3):229–31 [A].
[2] Gomez Torrijos E, Garcia Rodriguez C, Sanchez Caminero MP, et al. First case report of acute generalized exanthematous

pustulosis due to labetalol. J Investig Allergol Clin Immunol. 2015;25(2):148–9 [A].

[3] Rietveld L, van der Hoek T, van Beek MH, et al. Familial liability for metoprolol-induced psychosis. Gen Hosp Psychiatry. 2015;37(6):620. e625–626 [A].

[4] Koklu E, Arslan S, Yuksel IO, et al. Nebivolol-induced gynecomastia. J Pharmacol Pharmacother. 2015;6(3):166–8 [A].

[5] Ganigara A, Ravishankar C, Ramavakoda C, et al. Fatal hyperkalemia following succinylcholine administration in a child on oral propranolol. Drug Metab Pers Ther. 2015;30(1):69–71 [A].

[6] Rana MA, Mady AF, Rehman BA, et al. From eye drops to ICU, a case report of three side effects of ophthalmic timolol maleate in the same patient. Case Rep Crit Care. 2015;2015:714919 [A].

[7] Kjeldsen SE, Sica D, Haller H, et al. Nifedipine plus candesartan combination increases blood pressure control regardless of race and improves the side effect profile: DISTINCT randomized trial results. J Hypertens. 2014;32(12):2488–98 discussion 2498 [C].

[8] Fraser LA, Shariff SZ, McArthur E, et al. Calcium channel blocker-clarithromycin drug interaction did not increase the risk of

nonvertebral fracture: a population-based study. Ann Pharmacother. 2015;49(2):185–8 [c].

[9] Schetz D, Kocic I. A new adverse drug reaction—Schamberg's disease caused by amlodipine administration—a case report. Br J Clin Pharmacol. 2015;80(6):1477–8 [A].

[10] Straka M, Varga I, Erdelsky I, et al. Drug-induced gingival enlargement. Neuro Endocrinol Lett. 2014;35(7):567–76 [A].

[11] Chowdhry V, Mohanty BB. Intractable hyperkalemia due to nicorandil induced potassium channel syndrome. Ann Card Anaesth. 2015;18(1):101–3 [A].

[12] Claveau D, Piha-Gossack A, Friedland SN, et al. Complications associated with nitrate use in patients presenting with acute pulmonary edema and concomitant moderate or severe aortic stenosis. Ann Emerg Med. 2015;66(4):355–62. e351 [c].

[13] Kumthekar A, Cossarini F, Shih JC, et al. Ranolazine-induced repolarization changes: a case report. Am J Med. 2015;128(7):e3–5 [A].

[14] Littmann L. Electrocardiogram changes from ranolazine or from Takotsubo? Am J Med. 2015;128(12):e37 [r].

18

Antihypertensives

Teresa DeLellis*, Sipan Keshishyan[†], Vladlena Kovalevskaya[†],
Kalee Swanson[†], Kaitlin Montagano[†], Sidhartha D. Ray[†,1]

*Department of Pharmacy Practice, College of Pharmacy, Natural and Health Sciences,
Manchester University, Fort Wayne, IN, USA

[†]Department of Pharmaceutical Sciences, Manchester University College of Pharmacy, Natural and Health Sciences,
Fort Wayne, IN, USA

[1]Corresponding author: sdray@manchester.edu

ANGIOTENSIN-CONVERTING ENZYME INHIBITORS

Captopril

Mouth

A 39-year-old female with a history of angioedema at age 9 was started on sublingual captopril for arterial hypertension. Later she presented with complaints of oral lesions for 4 months, which were diagnosed as pemphigus vulgaris. Captopril was discontinued and the lesions treated with doxycycline, niacinamide, cetirizine, and cyclosporine mouth wash. While the direct mechanism of this established adverse reaction is unknown, given the patient's history of angioedema, the authors hypothesized this case to have an autoimmune component [1A].

Enalapril

Cardiovascular

Upper-airway angioedema is a well known complication of angiotensin-converting enzyme inhibitor (ACEI) therapy; visceral angioedema is less common and frequently unrecognized. A 60-year-old female on enalapril for hypertension was diagnosed with visceral angioedema after presenting with a 2-day history of abdominal pain and diarrhea. She was found to be hypotensive with elevated serum creatinine, leukocytosis, and small bowel wall thickening by computed tomography (CT) scan. Forty-eight hours after enalapril withdrawal and supportive care, the patient's symptoms improved. CT appearance improved within 72 hours. One year later she remained symptom free [2A].

Fosinopril

Immunologic

A 51-year-old male on fosinopril and combination metoprolol/hydrochlorothiazide presented with erythroderma and palmoplantar keratoderma. He was diagnosed with Pseudo-Sezary syndrome based on skin biopsy and flow cytometry. Flow Cytometry was performed which showed a population of 2500 "Sezary-like" CD4726 T-cells/µL in the blood. All antihypertensive medications were discontinued and the condition resolved completely [3A].

Lisinopril

Alopecia

A 53-year-old male on lisinopril for heart failure presented with new alopecia. Alopecia is a known adverse effect of ACEIs, causality was determined by Naranjo Adverse Drug Reaction Probability Scale-a total score of 6 was achieved and thus identified the adverse drug reaction as probable. Lisinopril was discontinued and changed to the angiotensin receptor blocker losartan. Four weeks later the alopecia resolved [4A].

Respiratory/Mouth

ACEI-induced upper-airway angioedema can recur months after discontinuation of ACEI therapy. A 67-year-old Caucasian male on lisinopril for several years presented with three angioedema episodes recurring over several months. His past medical history was significant for type II diabetes, hypertension, hyperlipidemia, and obesity. His daily medications included aspirin, amlodipine, metoprolol, metformin, glipizide, insulin glargine, and cholecalciferol. The first episode of moderate tongue angioedema without urticarial or pruritis was attributed to amoxicillin therapy and resolved with intravenous diphenhydramine and corticosteroid treatment. The next month he presented with the same symptoms, was no longer taking amoxicillin, and the episode was attributed to lisinopril. His symptoms resolved after overnight observation in an intensive care unit, and lisinopril was permanently discontinued. Two months later the symptoms recurred with less severity shortly after initiating niacin and resolved several hours after taking two diphenhydramine tablets. Niacin was discontinued. Later, based on negative penicillin skin test and oral graded niacin challenge performed at an allergy clinic, all three episodes were attributed to the lisinopril. Niacin was resumed, and at 2-year follow-up no further episodes had occurred [5A].

Two cases have been reported of ACEI therapy likely worsening symptoms of Pollen Food Allergy Syndrome (PFAS) reactions involving angioedema. The first was a 65-year-old male with a history of seasonal allergic rhinoconjunctivitis on lisinopril for 10 years for hypertension. He presented with two episodes of tongue and lip angioedema and mouth itching within 10 minutes of apple consumption. The second episode required treatment with antihistamine, epinephrine, and corticosteroids. Lisinopril therapy was changed to losartan. At 3-year follow-up, no further episodes had occurred [6A].

The second case was a 45-year-old male, also with a history of seasonal allergic rhinoconjunctivitis, on lisinopril for 1 year for hypertension. He experienced three episodes of tongue angioedema and mouth itching several minutes after jackfruit and cashew nut consumption; the third episode required antihistamine and prednisone treatment. Lisinopril was changed to losartan, and at 1-year follow-up no further episodes had occurred [6A].

Immunologic

One case report exists for lisinopril-induced eosinophilic pleural effusions. The effusions resolved after lisinopril was discontinued and reoccurred after lisinopril re-challenge [7A].

ANGIOTENSIN RECEPTOR BLOCKERS

Eprosartan

Gastrointestinal

An 83-year-old female taking eprosartan for 10 years for hypertension presented with sudden-onset diarrhea 6 months after her daily dose was doubled to 600 mg. Celiac serology was negative despite celiac disease-like biopsy results. Symptoms resolved after changing eprosartan to amlodipine. Control biopsies at three and 6 months after the diagnosis yielded slightly improved mucosal layer, thus indicating a delayed regeneration of the duodenal mucosa after treatment with eprosartan. While similar reactions have been reported with other angiotensin receptor blockers (ARBs), this is the first case study involving eposartan [8A].

Losartan

Gastrointestinal

A 31-year-old African American female on losartan for 1 year for hypertension and end-stage renal disease on dialysis presented to the emergency department with severe abdominal pain, diarrhea, nausea, and vomiting. She had a 6-year history of abdominal pain coinciding with the start of lisinopril. One year prior to arrival in the emergency department, lisinopril was changed to losartan for resolution of a cough. All laboratory studies were normal, while CT scans revealed perihepatic fluid and small bowel wall edema. Symptoms resolved after discontinuation of losartan. After 1 year without ACEI or ARB therapy, no further symptoms had occurred [9A].

Hyponatremia

A 73-year-old type 2 diabetic male was initiated on losartan 50 mg daily for newly diagnosed moderate hypertension. After taking losartan for 3½ months, he presented to the emergency department in a drowsy state, with weakness and occasional palpitations. The patient was diagnosed with type 2 diabetes 3 years ago and was well controlled only by oral metformin 500 mg twice daily. Other than being a diabetic, patient was well. Laboratory examinations revealed that his serum sodium level was 123 mEq/L. His pulse was 90 bpm, and his blood pressure 134/88 mmHg. No evidence was found that might have indicated any metabolic, infective, organic or other pathologic causes of the current symptoms, other than the use of losartan. Losartan was discontinued. The patient was managed with sodium repletion and dietary water restriction. Water loss was promoted with furosemide 40 mg twice daily given intravenously for 5 days. Patient was discharged 1 week later in a stable condition. He was prescribed hydrochlorothiazide 25 mg daily for blood pressure control [10A].

Olmesartan

Gastrointestinal

An 84-year-old Asian female on olmesartan suffered from severe, chronic, diarrhea for 15 months despite multiple empiric treatments. After an extensive workup, she was diagnosed with ARB-induced sprue-like enteropathy. Both her symptoms and histological findings improved after olmesartan was discontinued [11A].

Two females, 82 and 76 years old, on 2 consecutive days were admitted with severe diarrhea lasting approximately 8 months. Both women presented with significant weight loss of 16 and 20 kg, respectively. Patient work-up revealed identical results for both patients and led to identical diagnosis of refractory seronegative sprue. Subtotal villous atrophy with an increased number of intraepithelial lymphocytes was the result of duodenal biopsy. Human leukocyte antigen DQ2+ and DQ8− genotyping was consistent with celiac disease. Trial of antibiotic and strict gluten free diet was ineffective. Oral budesonide was initiated which brought some relief. All of the possible causes of villous atrophy were evaluated. Both patients had been taking olmesartan 40 mg daily for 6 and 4 months, respectively. Olmesartan was discontinued which lead to complete cessation of diarrhea within a 2-week period period. Biopsy 8 weeks later showed complete recovery of villous atrophy [12A].

Telmisartan

Skin

A 53-year-old male on telmisartan and hydrochlorothiazide combination for 2 weeks for hypertension presented to the hospital with cutaneous urticarial vasculitis. Red ecchymotic lesions of variable size and shape were spread over abdomen, flanks, groin, buttocks, and extremities. Emogram showed mild leukocytosis (total leukocyte count—12,800/cmm) and neutrophilia; all other laboratory tests were normal. Symptoms resolved after treatment with prednisolone and cetirizine. Despite medical advice to the contrary, the patient resumed telmisartan and hydrochlorothiazide, resulting in lesion recurrence. The lesions responded to treatment as with the first occurrence. Later, re-challenge with similar doses of telmisartan monotherapy and hydrochlorothiazide monotherapy resulted in recurrence with telmisartan but not with hydrochlorothiazide [13A].

BETA-BLOCKERS

Carvedilol

Hyperkalemia

A 69-year-old male with chronic kidney disease stage III on carvedilol 3.125 mg twice daily was hospitalized for abdominal pain, nausea, and vomiting. During the hospitalization his serum potassium increased from 4.8 to 6.7 mEq/L when carvedilol dose was increased to 6.25 mg twice daily. Patient's hyperkalemia was unresponsive to sodium polystyrene sulfonate but normalized to 4.4 mEq/L following adjustment of carvedilol back to 3.125 mg twice daily. Although a rare, known effect of beta-blockers, this is the first case report specifically with carvedilol [14A].

Labetalol

Skin

A 31-year old patient in her third trimester with twins was treated with labetalol for 18 days and hydralazine, alpha-methyldopa, and metamizole for 3 days prior to admission for cesarean section. Before the operation she developed acute generalized exanthematous pustulosis (AGEP) on her face and neck, which became more generalized over the next 4–5 days despite withdrawal of hydralazine, alpha-methyldopa, and metamizole on day 2. No new lesions appeared after labetalol discontinuation on day 5. Patch tests performed 1 month later were negative for hydralazine, alpha-methyldopa, metamizole, and atenolol but positive for labetolol. However, she did develop recurrence 1 hour after taking atenolol 25 mg, which persisted for 48 hours despite methylprednisolone treatment [15A].

Metoprolol

Drug–Drug Interaction

A 63-year-old Caucasian male on metoprolol 200 mg daily, for stable coronary artery disease presented to the emergency room with symptomatic bradycardia (confusion and falls; heart rate 37 beats per minute). The patient was on terbinafine 250 mg daily for onychomycosis but unfortunately developed bradycardia on 49th day of a 90-day treatment regimen. The bradycardia was hypothesized to be a result of terbinafine inhibition of cytochrome P450 2D6, decreasing metoprolol clearance. A score of 7 on the Naranjo adverse drug reaction probability scale suggested a probable relationship between the patient's sinus bradycardia and the drug interaction between metoprolol and terbinafine. Heart rate increased with a decrease in metoprolol dose and returned to normal when metoprolol was changed to bisoprolol, a beta blocker that does not interact with terbinafine [16A].

Psychological

A 44-year-old Caucasian male on metoprolol 50 mg daily was admitted to a psychiatric ward due to psychotic symptoms. Metoprolol was initiated 2 weeks earlier by his general practitioner for primary hypertension. After starting metoprolol he felt confused, restless and had difficulty falling asleep. He stopped taking metoprolol and all symptoms diminished. Upon re-initiation of metoprolol, he reported chaotic thinking and delusional thoughts. His general practitioner prescribed oxazepam 10 mg three times daily and mirtazapine 15 mg daily. All physical and laboratory tests were normal. Upon admission, he was confused with vivid visual hallucinations. Patient had no medical or psychiatric history, no history of substance abuse, and other than metoprolol, he was not on any other medications. Psychiatric examination revealed delusional content of his thoughts without any signs of cognitive impairment. I was deemed that his psychotic symptoms were caused by metoprolol. Olanzapine 10 mg twice daily was initiated and metoprolol was discontinued. A few days later, his psychosis gradually disappeared. He was initiated on nifidepine 30 mg for primary hypertension. Patient was discharged 2 weeks later free of any psychiatric symptoms. Olanzapine was tapered off over the following 3 weeks [17A].

CALCIUM CHANNEL BLOCKERS

Amlodipine

Mouth and Teeth

Drug-induced gingival overgrowth (DIGO) is a well-established effect of calcium channel blockers (CCB), most commonly with nifedipine and less frequently with amlodipine. In Dublin, a 63-year-old male on amlodipine 10 mg daily for hypertension presented to a dental clinic with 2-year history DIGO that had recently become severe. The DIGO was attributed to both amlodipine and poor plaque control based on histopathological analysis. The patient was treated successfully with oral hygiene education and local debridement [18A].

Liver

A 34-year-old Caucasian male presented to the emergency department 100 days post allogenic stem cell transplant for gastrointestinal graft versus host disease (GVHD) and was treated with high-dose steroids. Three days later amlodipine 5 mg daily was started for steroid-induced hypertension. On day 3 of amlodipine therapy alanine aminotransferase (ALT) levels doubled and continued to rise, peaking on day 11 at 630 IU/L. Aspartate aminotransferase (AST) also peaked on day 11, at 421 IU/L; total bilirubin and alkaline phosphatase remained normal throughout. Amlodipine was changed to carvedilol based on results of a liver biopsy, resulting in an ALT and AST drop which trended down to normal within 2 weeks [19A].

Diltiazem

Mouth and Teeth

A 48-year-old male on diltiazem for hypertension presented with drug-induced gingival hyperplasia. Rather than starting with periodontal treatment, the patient's physician was asked to change antihypertensive therapy. With this change to a non-calcium channel blocker antihypertensive, the gingival hyperplasia improved significantly over the next 3 months without periodontal intervention [20A].

DIRECT VASODILATORS

Doxazosin

Urinary

A 70-year-old male status-post radical prostatectomy followed by salvage radiotherapy 3 years later, on doxazosin for hypertension, developed urinary incontinence after radiotherapy. While being considered for artificial urinary sphincter placement, doxazosin was discontinued. After discontinuation, his urinary symptoms resolved and did not require further intervention. This was attributed to the relaxant effects of doxazosin on the internal sphincter [21A].

Terazosin

Cardiovascular

A 71-year-old male on terazosin 5 mg daily for benign prostatic hyperplasia presented to the emergency department with acute myocardial infarction (MI). Earlier that day, he had self-medicated with an additional 5 mg terazosin dose for a blood pressure of 220/110 mmHg. An hour later he experienced angina following a syncopal episode and presented to the emergency department. Workup revealed chronic occlusion of the left anterior descending artery, as well as terazosin-induced obstruction of the left ventricular outflow tract resulting in a hemodynamically produced MI. Intravenous atenolol resulted in clinical and symptomatic improvement within minutes [22A].

Clonidine

Cardiovascular

A 30-year-old male presenting with status epilepticus being treated in the intensive care unit developed withdrawal syndrome associated with substance misuse and was treated with a clonidine infusion. Two hours after clonidine was stopped abruptly, he developed severe hypertension, tachycardia, high-grade fever, profound sweating and lacrimation, and acute pulmonary edema resulting in respiratory distress syndrome. A low-dose clonidine infusion resolved symptoms; clonidine was then slowly discontinued by slow dose taper of intravenous followed by oral clonidine. This slow discontinuation did not result in further complications, and the patient was discharged from the intensive care unit [23A].

DIURETICS

Diazoxide

Hematologic

A 24-year-old female admitted for hypoglycemia was diagnosed with an insulinoma and started on diazoxide 250 mg daily for hypoglycemia prevention. On day 5 diazoxide was increased to 500 mg daily, and to 600 mg daily on day 6. On day 10 she developed chills, a temperature of 38.0 °C, and a 4.6 kg weight gain from edema. By day 13 her platelet count had decreased from $186\,000/\mu L$ to $28\,000/\mu L$, and she developed epistaxis and purpura in her lower extremities. When platelets fell to $12\,000/\mu L$ the next day, diazoxide was discontinued, prednisolone was started at 30 mg/day, and she received 2 days of consecutive platelet transfusions. Thrombocytopenia and weight gain reversed within 8 days of diazoxide discontinuation [24A].

Furosemide

Survival

A retrospective study was performed on 173 clinically stable heart failure patients comparing 3-year composite endpoint-free survival rates (all-cause mortality, heart transplantation, and mechanical-assist device implantation) among patients on high-dose furosemide (>80 mg daily; $n=70$) to low dose furosemide (≤ 80 mg daily; $n=103$). Baseline characteristics did not differ between groups with the exception of a higher estimated glomerular filtration rate in low-dose group (72.9 ± 19.4 vs 60.8 ± 22.0 mL/min/m^2, $p<0.001$). Rates of 3-year survival free from the composite endpoint were significantly higher in the low-dose group (93.1% vs 60.0%, $p<0.001$). The high-dose furosemide group also had higher rates of renal function decline and hypokalemia (73.2% vs 48.3%, $p=0.003$, and 43.1% vs 6.5%, $p=0.001$, respectively) [25c].

Hydrochlorothiazide

Hyponatremia

A 69-year-old male on hydrochlorothiazide for 2 weeks presented to the emergency department complaining of generalized weakness for the past week, which coincided with a hydrochlorothiazide dose increase from 12.5 mg daily to 25 mg daily. Upon workup he was found to have serum sodium 120 mmol/L. Hydrochlorothiazide was discontinued, and free water restriction initiated. By day 2, symptoms considerably improved; serum sodium level showed 128 mmol/L, and the patient was ready for discharge. Hyponatremia and symptoms were completely resolved 3 days later at outpatient follow-up, and he was started on hydralazine for hypertension and instructed to discontinue further hydrochlorothiazide use [26A].

Eye

A 67-year-old female on hydrochlorothiazide presented with acute bilateral angle closure glaucoma associated with profound hyponatremia and bilateral ciliary effusions. Both the effusions and hyponatremia resolved with discontinuation of hydrochlorothiazide and free water restriction [27A].

Skin

A 32-year-old male presented 24 days after his antihypertensive was changed from losartan 50 mg daily to losartan–hydrochlorothiazide 50/12.5 mg combination, complaining of flu-like symptoms. He returned 3 days later with wide-spread bullous and vesicular lesions with an erythematous base and was sent to the emergency department for further diagnosis and treatment. A punch biopsy of a prebullous lesion demonstrated spongiotic dermatitis with clefting at the dermoepidermal junction. Inflammatory infiltrate, eosinophils and neutrophils were found in the papillary dermis. He was eventually diagnosed with bullous pemphigoid and treated with prednisone and mycophenolate mofetil. With this treatment and discontinuation of hydrochlorothiazide, the rash resolved; prednisone and mycophenolate were tapered off over 8 and 20 weeks, respectively, without recurrence of symptoms [28A].

Pancreatitis

A 31-year-old female presented to the hospital with a 2-day history of epigastric pain radiating to the back associated with nausea and vomiting. Her medical history included hypertension for which she was started on hydrochlorothiazide 25 mg 5 days prior to presentation. Her other medications included metformin for polycystic ovarian syndrome and omeprazole for heartburn. She appeared to be in moderate pain and afebrile with a heart rate of 105 bpm. Her body mass index was 39. Physical examination showed epigastric tenderness. Laboratory findings yielded leukocytosis of $18\,600/\mu L$. Liver chemistry was normal; amylase and lipase levels were 35 and 35 U/L, respectively. The patient was treated supportively with bowel rest, opiate analgesia, and intravenous fluids. She improved without complications and was discharged the next day. Hydrochlorothiazide was discontinued [29A].

Eplerenone

A single-center, prospective, open-label study evaluated 31 kidney transplant patients with impaired renal function (30 and 50 mL/min/1.73 m^2). All patients received eplerenone 25 mg/day for 8 weeks. Patients were closely monitored for changes in renal function and serum potassium.

Eight patients experienced mild hyperkalemia (>5 mmol/L), one moderate hyperkalemia (>5.5 mmol/L) and had to receive potassium-exchange resin. No instances of sever hyperkalemia (>6 mmol/L) were reported. One case of acute kidney injury occurred, after further analysis it was deemed secondary to diarrhea. It was determined that basal serum potassium and bicarbonate were independently associated with a significantly higher risk of developing mild hyperkalemia while being treated with eplerenone (OR 6.5, $p = 0.003$ and 0.7, $p = 0.007$, respectively). Furthermore, a value of 4.35 mmol/L for basal serum potassium was the best factor to predict the risk of developing hyperkalemia [30c].

References

[1] Gornowicz-Porowska J, Dmochowski M, Pietkiewicz P, et al. Mucosal-dominant pemphigus vulgaris in a captopril-taking woman with angioedema. An Bras Dermatol. 2015;90(5):748–51 [A].

[2] Mutnuri S, Khan A, Variyam EP. Visceral angioedema: an under-recognized complication of angiotensin-converting enzyme inhibitors. Postgrad Med. 2015;127(2):215–7 [A].

[3] Reeder MJ, Wood GS. Drug-induced pseudo-Seazary syndrome: a case report and literature review. Am J Dermatopathol. 2015;37(1):83–6 [A].

[4] Kataria V, Wang H, Wald JW, et al. Lisinopril-induced alopecia: a case report. J Pharm Pract. 2016. Jun 6; pii: 0897190016652554. [Epub ahead of print] [A].

[5] Pham A, Hariri S, Yusin J. Timing isn't everything: a case of recurrent angio-oedema. Allergol Immunopathol (Madr). 2015;43(2):230–1 [A].

[6] Ferastraoaru D, Rosenstreich D, Jariwala S. Severe angioedema associated with angiotensin-converting enzyme inhibitor therapy in two patients with pollen-food allergy syndrome. J Clin Hypertens. 2015;17(6):493–4 [A].

[7] Zouak A, Bongrain E, Launois C, et al. Eosinophilic pleuritic: an unusual complication of treatment with an angiotensin converting enzyme inhibitor. Rev Mal Respir. 2015;32(7):737–41 [A].

[8] Maier H, Hehemann K, Vieth M. Celiac disease-like enteropathy due to antihypertensive therapy with angiotensin-II receptor type 1 inhibitor eprosartan. Cesk Patol. 2015;51(2):87–8 [A].

[9] Muthukrishnan T, Fajt ML, Birnie KM, et al. Angiotensin receptor blocker-induced visceral angioedema. J Investig Allergol Clin Immunol. 2015;25(1):63–4 [A].

[10] Das S, Bandyopadhyay S, Ramasamy A, et al. A case of losartan-induced severe hyponatremia. J Pharmacol Pharmacother. 2015;6(4):219–21 [A].

[11] Naik DK, Martelli MG, Gonzalo DH, et al. An atypical case of chronic diarrhea: olmesartan-induced sprue-like enteropathy. BMJ Case Rep. 2015;2015. http://dx.doi.org/10.1136/bcr-2015-212318, pii: bcr2015212318 [A].

[12] Schiller D, Ziachehabi A, Silye R, et al. Two coincident cases of easily curable 'refractory sprue'. Gut. 2015;64:1773 [A].

[13] Bahajan VK, Singh R, Gupta M, et al. Telmisartan induced urticarial vasculitis. Indian J Pharmacol. 2015;47(5):560–2 [A].

[14] Hahn L, Hahn M. Carvedilol-induced hyperkalemia in a patient with chronic kidney disease. J Pharm Pract. 2015;28(1):107–11 [A].

[15] Gomez-Torrijos E, Garcia-Rodriquez C, Sancehz-Caminero MP, et al. First case report of acute generalized exanthematous pustulosis due to labetalol. J Investig Allergol Clin Immunol. 2015;25(2):148–9 [A].

[16] Bebawi E, Jouni SS, Tessier AA, et al. A metoprolol-terbinafine combination induced bradycardia. Eur J Drug Metab Pharmacokinet. 2015;40(3):295–9 [A].

[17] Rietveld L, van der Hoek T, van Beek M, et al. Familial liability for metoprolol-induced psychosis. Gen Hosp Psychiatry. 2015;37:620. e5–6 [A].

[18] Carty O, Walsh E, Abdelsalem A, et al. Case report: drug-induced gingival overgrowth associated with the use of a calcium channel blocker (amlodipine). J Ir Dent Assoc. 2015;61(5):248–51 [A].

[19] Hammerstrong AE. Possible amlodipine-induced hepatotoxicity after stem cell transplant. Ann Pharmacother. 2015;49(1): 135–9 [A].

[20] Livada R, Shelton W, Bland PS, et al. Regression of calcium channel blocker—induced gingival enlargement in the absence of periodontal therapy. J Tenn Dent Assoc. 2015;95(2): 11–4 [A].

[21] Sarkar D, Kumar M. An interesting case of an antihypertensive causing post-prostatectomy incontinence. BMJ Case Rep. 2015;2015, http://dx.doi.org/10.1136/bcr-2015-211576, pii: bcr2015211576 [A].

[22] Vidal MA, Ferrando-Castagnetto F, Martínez F, et al. Myocardial infarction induced by oral terazosin in a patient with predisposing structural cardiomyopathy: case report. Med Chem Commun. 2016;16(5):e6480 [A].

[23] Shaw M, Matsa R. Clonidine withdrawal induced sympathetic surge. BMJ Case Rep. 2015;2015. http://dx.doi.org/10.1136/bcr-2015-210325, pii: bcr2015210325 [A].

[24] Adachi J, Mimura M, Minami I, et al. Thrombocytopenia induced by diazoxide in a patient with an insulinoma. Intern Med. 2014;53:759–62 [A].

[25] Kapelios CJ, Kaldara E, NtaliaNis A, et al. High furosemide dose has detrimental effects on survival of patients with stable heart failure. Hellenic J Cardiol. 2015;56:154–9 [c].

[26] Sardar GK, Eilbert WP. Severe hyponatremia associated with thiazide diuretic use. J Emerg Med. 2015;48(3):305–9 [A].

[27] Chen SH, Karanjia R, Chevrier RL, et al. Bilateral acute angle closure glaucoma associated with hydrochlorothiazide-induced hyponatraemia. BMJ Case Rep. 2014;2014. http://dx.doi.org/10.1136/bcr-2014-206690, pii: bcr2014206690.

[28] Warner C, Kwak Y, Blover MHB, et al. Bullous pemphigoid induced by hydrochlorothiazide therapy. J Drugs Dermatol. 2014;13(3):360–2 [A].

[29] Shafqet M, Brown T, Sharma R. Normal lipase drug-induced pancreatitis: a novel finding. Am J Emerg Med. 2015;33:476. e5–6 [A].

[30] Bertocchio JP, Barbe C, Lavaud S, et al. Safety of eplerenone for kidney-transplant recipients with impaired renal function and receiving cyclosporine A. PLoS One. 2016;11(4): e0153635 [C].

19

Diuretics

Yekaterina Opsha[1]

Ernest Mario School of Pharmacy, Rutgers, The State University of New Jersey, Piscataway, NJ, USA

Saint Barnabas Medical Center, Livingston, NJ, USA

[1]Corresponding author: kate.opsha@pharmacy.rutgers.edu

CARBONIC ANHYDRASE INHIBITORS [SEDA-35, 387; SEDA-36, 289; SEDA-37, 237]

Acetazolamide

Eyes

Patients suffering from glaucoma may require several therapies. Alaei and colleagues carried out an observational study in 50 glaucoma patients evaluating drug prescribing and adverse drug reactions associated with medications prescribed for this disease state. Acetazolamide was prescribed in 14 (28%) of patients, and other agents included timolol and dorzolamide. Over 50% of the patients reported adverse drug reactions (ADRs). Acetazolamide was associated with 14% of the total reported ADRs and ranged from mild to moderate severity and was topical in nature [1c].

Metabolic

Acetazolamide-related hypophosphatemia is very rare. The following is a case report of this type of hypophosphatemia which potentially led to a cardiac arrest in a 78-year-old female patient who was taking acetazolamide for glaucoma for a total of 1 day. The patient was successfully weaned from the ventilator after correction of hypophosphatemia and fully recovered. The risk of hypophosphatemia should be kept in mind by all physicians and an examination of serum metabolic panels may be indicated in patients at risk of hypophosphatemia [2A]. Other notable metabolic disturbances associated with the use of this agent are hyponatremia and hypokalemia [3M,4E]. As a general rule, when treating patients with diuretics, a basic metabolic panel should be obtained at baseline and monitored periodically.

LOOP DIURETICS [SEDA-35, 390; SEDA-36, 290; SEDA-37, 237]

Azosemide

Urinary System

A single-center study of 11 patients with type 2 diabetic kidney disease (DKD) and diuretic-resistant edema sought to evaluate the safety and efficacy of hydrochlorothiazide (HCTZ) in addition to other loop diuretics (azosemide or furosemide) and examine the clinical parameters of blood pressure (BP) control, proteinuria, and eGFR before and after addition of HCTZ. Each of the 11 patients had an estimated glomerular filtration rate (eGFR) $<30 \text{ mL/min}/1.73 \text{ m}^2$ and was suffering from severe edema despite being on adequate doses of loop diuretics. Patients were receiving either azosemide (60–120 mg/day) or furosemide (80–120 mg/day). In addition, patients were receiving a $13.6\pm3.8\text{-mg/day}$ dose of HCTZ. After the addition of HCTZ therapy, systolic blood pressure (SBP), diastolic blood pressures (DBP), as well as proteinuria significantly decreased (SBP: at 12 months, $p<0.01$, DBP: at 12 months, $p<0.05$, proteinuria: at 12 months, $p<0.01$). The annual change in eGFR was not significantly different before and after HCTZ therapy. These findings suggest that the combination of HCTZ and loop diuretics (specifically azosemide and furosemide) may improve SBP and DBP levels, and decreases proteinuria even in advanced stage type 2 DKD patients with severe edema in whom previously HCTZ was thought to be less beneficial [5A].

Bumetanide

A single-center retrospective study was conducted in 95 critically ill pediatric patients evaluating the use of bumetanide administered as a continuous infusion. Efficacy was defined as the ability to achieve negative fluid balance. Time to reach negative fluid balance was assessed at 12, 24, and 48 h. Safety was evaluated based on prevalence of adverse drug reactions. Adverse drug reactions were predefined as serum potassium concentration less than 3 mEq/L, serum chloride concentration less than 90 mEq/L, serum carbon dioxide concentration greater than 35 mEq/L, and serum creatinine increased greater than 1.5 times baseline and above patient-specific normal range. The mean dose of bumetanide was 5.7 ± 2.2 µg/kg/h (1–10 µg/kg/h) with median therapy duration of 3.3 days. The total percentage of patients achieving negative fluid balance by 48 h was 76% with more than half of patients reaching negative fluid balance within 12 h. Additionally, bumetanide appears to be a safe loop diuretic for use as a continuous infusion at the doses described in critically ill pediatric patients [6c].

Ethacrynic Acid

Ethacrynic acid has been used in clinical practice for several decades, particularly in patients who require loop diuretics but have a true sulfa allergy as all other loop diuretics contain a sulfa moiety. This is currently the only sulfonamide-free loop diuretic. However, this agent is not a very potent diuretic and should only be reserved for those patients who cannot tolerate or have failed other diuretic therapies. Ethacrynic acid is also rarely used because of its increased incidence of ototoxicity as compared to the other loop diuretics.

Oxidative Stress

It has been hypothesized that ethacrynic acid (EA) decreases the intracellular levels of glutathione. Whether the anticipated oxidative stress affects the structural integrity of DNA is not yet known. Therefore, DNA damage was assessed in EA-treated HCT116 cells, and the impact of several antioxidants was also determined. Ethacrynic acid caused both concentration-dependent and time-dependent DNA damage that eventually resulted in cell death. Unexpectedly, the DNA damage caused by EA was intensified by either ascorbic acid or trolox. In contrast, EA-induced DNA damage was reduced by N-acetylcysteine and by the iron chelator, deferoxamine. It was determined that EA increased the production of reactive oxygen species, which was inhibited by N-acetylcysteine and deferoxamine but not by ascorbic acid and trolox. Overall, it is concluded that EA has genotoxic properties that can be amplified by certain antioxidants, but if these effects are also seen in humans, it is not yet clear [7E].

Pediatrics

A prospective randomized double-blinded study was conducted in 74 infants undergoing surgery for congenital heart disease. The study evaluated the use and clinical effects of furosemide (F—administered to 38 patients) and ethacrynic acid (EA—administered to 36 patients) administered as a continuous infusion. The endpoints evaluated were: urine output (UO), fluid balance, renal, cardiac, respiratory, and metabolic functions. Patients received 0.2 mg/kg/h (up to 0.8 mg/kg/h) of either furosemide or ethacrynic acid. Serum creatinine and incidence of acute kidney injury did not show significant differences between groups. Metabolic alkalosis occurred frequently (about 70% of cases) in both groups, but mean bicarbonate level was higher in the ethacrynic acid group: 29.1 versus 27.8 in the furosemide group ($p=0.006$). No other adverse events were reported [8c].

Furosemide

High Dose Furosemide

A retrospective study was performed by Kapelios and colleagues in order to evaluate if furosemide exhibits the likelihood of major adverse clinical events when used in high doses in the long term on clinically stable patients during a first ambulatory HF department visit. A total of 173 prescribed doses of furosemide were evaluated. The low-dose group evaluated patients who received <80 mg of furosemide (103 patients). The high-dose group evaluated patients who received >80 mg of furosemide daily (70 patients). The baseline characteristics were similar between groups. According to the investigators "the 3-year survival free from the composite endpoint was significantly higher in the low-dose group than in the high-dose group (93.1% vs. 60.0%, $p<0.001$)". The study indicated that high dose furosemide was an independent predictor of an adverse outcome at 3 years (adjusted HR: 15.25; 95% CI: 1.06–219.39, $p=0.045$). The authors also concluded that the incidence of deterioration of renal function and episodes of hypokalemia during follow-up was also higher in the high furosemide dose (73.2% vs. 48.3, $p=0.003$, and 43.1% vs. 6.5%, $p<0.001$, respectively). One potential clinical reason for this is that in clinical practice it is more likely to prescribe high dose loop diuretics to sicker patients who have more frequent heart failure exacerbations [9C].

Pharmacokinetics/Pharmacodynamics

The coadministration of tolvaptan and furosemide, although done in practice, has not been extensively studied in a clinical setting. The use of tolvaptan has the potential to decrease the required doses of furosemide and hence decrease the side effect profile which frequently comes with the administration of loop diuretics such as electrolyte abnormalities and renal dysfunction. As a result of this clinical deficit, a study was conducted to investigate this drug interaction in 22 patients with CHF and advanced chronic kidney disease (CKD). Patients received tolvaptan 15 mg once daily for 7 days after single administration of furosemide. Patients' hemodynamic parameters, serum chemistry values, and body fluid status were assessed during the study. On day 8, serum sodium and potassium concentrations were significantly higher than baseline values. In addition, no significant changes in serum uric acid, blood pressure, or heart rate were observed in any patient in this study. Based on this short-term study, it appears that coadministration of these two agents appears to be safe in this patient population [10c].

Route of Furosemide Administration

In the following single-center, pilot, randomized trial involving patients with acute HF and renal dysfunction, the authors sought to investigate the difference in outcomes between continuous furosemide infusion (cIV) and bolus injections of furosemide (iIV). Primary end points were the evaluation of urine output volumes, renal function, and b-type natriuretic peptide (BNP) levels. A total of 57 patients were included in the study. The study observation was a significant increase in creatinine levels (1.78 ± 0.5 vs 1.41 ± 0.3 mg/dL, $p < 0.01$), and a reduction of the estimated glomerular filtration rate in cIV (44.8 ± 6.1 vs 46.7 ± 6.1 mL/min, $p < 0.05$). A significant increase of in-hospital additional treatment as well as length of hospitalization was observed in cIV. The authors also concluded that continuous furosemide administration revealed a higher rate of adverse events during the follow-up period ($p < 0.03$) [11c].

A Cochrane Review

A Cochrane review aimed to determine if the prophylactic administration of loop diuretics provides a therapeutic advantage in patients who are recipients of any blood product transfusion products versus placebo or general fluid restriction measures. It is well known that the use of furosemide (and other loop diuretics) can lead to hypovolemia which is the reason it may prove to be beneficial in patients who are receiving transfusions [12R]. The analysis evaluated four randomized controlled trials which involved 100 patients. Furosemide was the only diuretic investigated in all four studies and the primary focus of all the studies was on various markers of respiratory function. The results revealed an improvement in fraction of inspired oxygen (in favor of furosemide) in one study and an improvement in pulmonary capillary wedge pressure (in favor of furosemide) was noted in two studies. The reviewers concluded that "there was insufficient evidence to determine whether

premedicating people undergoing blood transfusion with loop diuretics prevents clinically important transfusion-related morbidity. Due to the continued use of prophylactic loop diuretics during transfusions, and because this review highlights the absence of evidence to justify this practice, well-conducted RCTs are urgently needed" [13R].

Torsemide

All-Cause Mortality

A study was performed at Duke University evaluating the potential risks and benefits of furosemide vs torsemide on all-cause mortality in the heart failure population. Patients receiving torsemide were more likely to be female and had more comorbidities compared with furosemide-treated patients. Survival was worse in torsemide-treated patients [5-year Kaplan–Meier estimated survival of 41.4% (95% CI: 36.7–46.0) vs. furosemide 51.5% (95% CI: 49.8–53.1)]. Further prospective studies are needed to evaluate the cardiac effects of these two loop diuretics in the heart failure patient population [14C].

THIAZIDE AND THIAZIDE-LIKE DIURETICS [SEDA-35, 388; SEDA-36, 292; SEDA-37, 239]

Chlorothiazide

Evaluation of the effectiveness of oral metolazone versus intravenous (IV) chlorothiazide as add-on therapy to loop diuretics in hospitalized patients with ADHF and renal dysfunction is the purpose of the following retrospective cohort study which enrolled 55 patients. The primary endpoint was net urine output (UOP) at 72 h after initiation of thiazide-like diuretics. Safety endpoints included worsening renal function, hypotension, and electrolyte abnormalities. The study reported no difference in median net UOP at 72 h in those receiving metolazone (4828 mL), compared to chlorothiazide (3779 mL, $p = 0.16$). There was no difference in hypotension, worsening renal function, hyponatremia, or hypokalemia ($p = NS$ for all comparisons). This study is important to consider when evaluating diuretic therapy in addition to loop diuretics considering the cost difference favoring oral metolazone [15c].

Chlorthalidone

Insulin Resistance

Chlorthalidone is commonly used for blood pressure control in hypertensive patients in Europe. However, there are reports to indicate that it can also lead to insulin resistance. Recent studies have demonstrated that some adverse effects of chlorthalidone can be avoided with spironolactone administration, but further prospective studies are necessary in this field [16H,17C].

Hydrochlorothiazide (HCTZ)

Metabolic Effects

The following article reviewed 9765 publications, and from these, it identified 14 randomized trials with 883 patients comparing HCTZ with indapamide (INDAP) and chlorthalidone on antihypertensive potency or metabolic effects. The authors concluded that there were no detectable differences between HCTZ and INDAP in metabolic adverse effects, including effects on serum potassium. These head-to-head comparisons demonstrated that, like chlorthalidone, INDAP is more potent than HCTZ at commonly prescribed doses without evidence for greater adverse metabolic effects. Greater efforts should be made to increase the use of these highly potent agents [18M].

Drug Toxicity

This study compared the clinical effectiveness and drug toxicity of chlorthalidone and hydrochlorothiazide. Mean systolic blood pressure/diastolic blood pressure values at least 30 days after initial prescription were lower with chlorthalidone 25 mg (132.2/74 mm Hg) compared with hydrochlorothiazide 25 mg (137/77.5 mm Hg) and hydrochlorothiazide 50 mg (138.6/78.5 mm Hg) ($p < 0.05$ for all comparisons). Goal systolic blood pressure/diastolic blood pressure values were achieved in a higher percentage of patients prescribed chlorthalidone without the compromise in renal function or significant difference in serum potassium [19C].

Hyponatraemia

The following study was seeking to evaluate the effect that HCTZ has on hyponatremia in 15 elderly hypertensive patients with a history of thiazide-induced hyponatraemia and 15 matched hypertensive controls using thiazide diuretics without previous hyponatraemia. After HCTZ administration, plasma sodium and osmolality significantly decreased and remained lower in patients compared with controls ($p < 0.001$). This study concluded that HCTZ is associated with impaired free water excretion and can cause thiazide-induced hyponatraemia. This effect is further exacerbated in patients previously exposed to HCTZ [20c]. Another case report reminds us of the importance for monitoring serum sodium in patients on thiazide diuretics since hyponatremia is associated with higher morbidity and mortality rates. A 69-year-old man with generalized weakness beginning

2 weeks after starting HCTZ presents to the emergency department with a serum sodium level of 120 mmol/L. The patient was admitted and successfully treated with free water restriction and discontinuation of the offending agent [21A].

A recent meta-analysis also revealed that thiazide-induced hyponatraemia occurs at approximately 19 days (95% CI 8, 30) after starting treatment, with mean trough serum sodium concentration of 116 mm (95% CI 113, 120) and serum potassium of 3.3 mm (95% CI 3.0, 3.5). The analysis concluded that patients who are prescribed thiazide diuretics should be aware of the symptoms of hyponatraemia and a physician follow-up within the first 14 days may not be sufficient in order to evaluate a patient for hyponatraemia secondary to thiazide therapy [22R].

HCTZ Potency

One study questioned if HCTZ is as potent as some of its competitors such as chlorthalidone (CTD) and bendroflumethiazide. The study found that HCTZ was less potent in lowering blood pressure in comparison to other agents in the same class. A recent meta-analysis also suggested that HCTZ (12.5–25 mg daily) to be less potent than antihypertensive agents from several other classes, including angiotensin-converting enzyme inhibitors, angiotensin-receptor blockers, and calcium antagonists. The risk of hyponatremia, hypokalemia, and hyperuricemia associated with HCTZ was lower than with CTD, while the risk of new onset or exacerbation of gouty arthritis was similar. Increasing evidence suggests inferiority of HCTZ in lowering BP and cardiovascular outcomes in hypertensive patients when compared with other drugs in the same class, particularly CTD and indapamide [23r,24R].

Indapamide (INDAP)

Systemic Review

Systemic review retrieved 9765 publications, and from these, it identified 14 randomized trials with 883 patients comparing HCTZ with INDAP and chlorthalidone on antihypertensive potency or metabolic effects. INDAP and chlorthalidone lowered systolic blood pressure more than HCTZ: −5.1 mm Hg (95% CI, −8.7 to −1.6); $p = 0.004$ and −3.6 mm Hg (95% CI, −7.3 to 0.0); $p = 0.052$, respectively. This review found no detectable differences between HCTZ and INDAP in metabolic adverse effects, including effects on serum potassium. In conclusion, these head-to-head comparisons demonstrate that, like chlorthalidone, INDAP is more potent than HCTZ at commonly prescribed doses without evidence for greater adverse metabolic effects [25R].

Case Report

On the contrary, a case report out of Denmark describes a 65-year-old male with type II diabetes and long-lasting treatment with indapamide for hypertension. In addition, he had a history of a high consumption of licorice. For 2 weeks, the patient suffered from myalgia, and upon admission to the hospital was found to have a reduced potassium concentration of 1.5 mmol/L (reference value: 3.6–5.1 mmol/L) and an elevated creatine kinase of 18 400 IU/L (reference value: 40–280 IU/L). It was believed that the patient developed rhabdomyolysis due to severe hypokalemia, possibly induced by a pharmacodynamic interaction between licorice and indapamide [26A].

Impaired Glucose Tolerance

An analysis of 26 randomized trials involving over 16 000 participants found a high probability between thiazide-type diuretics and an increase in fasting plasma glucose (FPG) compared with nonthiazide agents or placebo (mean difference [MD], 0.27 mmol/L [4.86 mg/dL]; 95% CI, 0.15–0.39). This effect seemed to be dose related [27R].

ALDOSTERONE RECEPTOR ANTAGONISTS [SEDA-35, 391; SEDA-36, 293; SEDA-37, 240]

Eplerenone

Hemodialysis

Eplerenone is a selective mineralocorticoid receptor antagonist and as such is generally well tolerated with most frequent adverse event being hyperkalemia, while the sexual adverse events (such as gynecomastia and vaginal bleeding such as in spironolactone) are limited with this agent [28r,29r].

It is well known that mineralocorticoid receptor antagonists reduce morbidity and mortality in patients with heart failure, but the safety of these drugs in patients receiving dialysis is unclear. The following randomized controlled Canadian trial evaluated whether hyperkalemia and/or hypotension should limit the use of eplerenone in hemodialysis patients. The evaluation was assessed in 146 patients for the primary outcome of discontinuation of the drug because of hyperkalemia or hypotension. Secondary outcomes included hyperkalemia, hypotension, and cardiovascular events. The primary outcome occurred in three patients (4.0%) in the eplerenone group and two (2.8%) in the placebo group, for an absolute risk difference of 1.2 (95% CI, −4.7 to 7.1). Eplerenone was interpreted as noninferior to placebo

with respect to the primary outcome but did have higher rates of hyperkalemia (9 patients, 11.7%) vs. 2 patients (2.6%) in the placebo arm. There was no significant effect on predialysis or postdialysis blood pressure. The study investigators concluded that eplerenone increased the risk of hyperkalemia but did not result in an excess need to permanently discontinue the drug [30c].

Arterial Hypertension

Scientific evidence accumulated so far supports the role of eplerenone as first-choice drug in heart failure, with lower prevalence rates of sex-related adverse effects associated with eplerenone as compared to spironolactone. A review of available scientific evidence, however, discloses that 11 randomized clinical trials assessing eplerenone in >3500 hypertensive patients have been reported so far. The results of these studies clearly show that eplerenone is an effective antihypertensive agent when used alone or in combination with other medications. Eplerenone monotherapy, in doses ranging from 25 to 100 mg daily, does show a promising result of a dose-dependent reduction in systolic blood pressure. Studies suggest that eplerenone administered at 100 mg daily has a blood pressure lowering that is 50–75% that of spironolactone, and comparison between eplerenone and amlodipine shows that both treatments decrease systolic blood pressure to a similar extent but eplerenone is better tolerated. The authors concluded that there is no evidence that eplerenone can play an important role in the treatment of mild to moderate arterial hypertension and therefore scientific experts and regulatory authorities should support its wider use in clinical practice worldwide [31r].

Spironolactone

Hyperkalemia

Hyperkalemia is a commonly known adverse effect of spironolactone. The following study wanted to evaluate the combined effect of spironolactone and ACE I/ARB therapy as frequently done in clinical practice for heart failure patients. Using a health insurance claims data, which covers over 30% of the German population ($n = 1491894$), the investigators evaluated the patient rates of hyperkalemia. Risk of hyperkalemia in heart failure patients was significantly associated with spironolactone use 95% [CI = 13.59 (11.63–15.88) in all and 11.05 (8.67–14.08)] in those with information on New York Heart Association (NYHA) stage of disease. This association was stronger in older (≥70 years of age) as compared with younger patients (<70 years of age). Careful potassium level monitoring in concomitant users of spironolactone and ACE/ARB is recommended in clinical practice [32MC].

Drug–Drug Interaction

Trimethoprim–sulfamethoxazole increases the risk of hyperkalemia when used with spironolactone. The investigators of the following study sought to evaluate if this therapy combination would be associated with an increased risk of sudden death (within 14 days after receiving the combination therapy), a consequence of severe hyperkalemia using a population-based nested case–control study involving patients aged 66 years or older who received spironolactone between 1994 and 2011 from Ontario. Of the 11968 patients who died of sudden death while receiving spironolactone, nearly 330 patients whose death occurred within 14 days after antibiotic exposure were identified. Compared with amoxicillin, trimethoprim–sulfamethoxazole was associated with a more than twofold increase in the risk of sudden death (adjusted OR 2.46, 95% CI 1.55–3.90). The evaluators concluded that when clinically appropriate, alternative antibiotics should be considered in these patients [33MC].

OSMOTIC DIURETICS

Mannitol [SEDA-35, 393; SEDA-36, 294; SEDA-37, 241]

Respiratory System

Evidence suggests that inhaled mannitol (available in Australia and some European counties) can be used to clear airway secretions in patients with cystic fibrosis for its increased mucociliary clearance ability. A Cochrane review was performed and found four studies which included a total of 667 participants for evaluation. Most studies compared inhaled mannitol to either placebo or standard of care. When compared to dornase alfa, the reported adverse effects were: haemoptysis, bronchospasm, pharyngolaryngeal pain and post-tussive vomiting which occurred at similar rates in both treatment arms. Cough was the most common side effect in the mannitol alone arm but there was no occurrence of cough in the dornase alfa alone arm and the most commonly reported reason of withdrawal from the mannitol plus dornase alfa arm was pulmonary exacerbations. There is evidence to show that treatment with mannitol over a 6-month period is associated with an improvement in some measures of lung function in people with cystic fibrosis compared to control. However, there is no evidence that quality of life is improved for participants taking mannitol compared to control [34R].

Kidney Injury

Mannitol has recently been linked to increasing the development of acute kidney injury (AKI). The following study investigated the incidence and risk factors of mannitol-related AKI in acute stroke patients. The study evaluated a total of 432 patients (ischemic stroke 62.3%) >20 years of age who were admitted to the neurocritical care center and were treated with mannitol therapy. The definition of AKI was defined as an absolute elevation in the serum creatinine (Scr) level of ≥ 0.3 mg/dL from the baseline or a $\geq 50\%$ increase in Scr. The results indicated that the incidence of mannitol-related AKI was similar among all stroke group patients: 6.5% in acute stroke patients, 6.3% in patients with ischemic stroke, and 6.7% in patients with intracerebral hemorrhage. Extra caution should be used in patients who are prescribed mannitol therapy especially in those with predisposing risk factors [35C].

References

Carbonic anhydrase inhibitors (CAIs)

[1] Alaei M, Najmi AK, Kausar H, et al. A prospective research study of anti-glaucoma drugs prescribing, utilization pattern and adverse drug reaction recording in a university hospital. Drug Res (Stuttg). 2015;65(3):164–8 [c].

[2] Hu CY, Lee BJ, Cheng HF, et al. Acetazolamide-related life-threatening hypophosphatemia in a glaucoma patient. J Glaucoma. 2016;24(4):e31–3 [A].

[3] Verbrugee FH, Steels P, Grieten L, et al. Hyponatremia in acute decompensated heart failure: depletion versus dilution. J Am Coll Cardiol. 2015;65:480–92 [M].

[4] Groot T, Sinke AP, Kortenoeven ML, et al. Acetazolamide attenuates lithium-induced nephrogenic diabetes insipidus. J Am Soc Nephrol. 2016;27(7):2082–91 [E].

Loops

[5] Hoshino T, Ookawara S, Miyazawa H. Renoprotective effects of thiazides combined with loop diuretics in patients with type 2 diabetic kidney disease. Clin Exp Nephrol. 2015;19(2):247–53 [A].

[6] McCallister KM, Chhim RF, Briceno-Medina M, et al. Bumetanide continuous infusions in critically ill pediatric patients. Pediatr Crit Care Med. 2015;16(2):e19–22 [c].

[7] Ward WM, Hoffman JD, Loo G. Genotoxic effect of ethacrynic acid and impact of antioxidants. Toxicol Appl Pharmacol. 2015;286(1):17–26 [E].

[8] Ricci Z, Haiberger R, Pezzella C, et al. Furosemide versus ethacrynic acid in pediatric patients undergoing cardiac surgery; a randomized controlled trial. Crit Care. 2015;19(1):1–9 [c].

[9] Kapelios C, Kaldara E, Ntalianis A, et al. High furosemide dose has detrimental effects on survival of patients with stable heart failure. Hellenic J Cardiol. 2015;56(2):154–9 [C].

[10] Tominaga N, Kida K, Matsumoto N, et al. Safety of add-on tolvaptan in patients with furosemide-resistant congestive heart failure complicated by advanced chronic kidney disease: a sub-analysis of a pharmacokinetics/pharmacodynamics study. Clin Nephrol. 2015;84(1):29–38 [c].

[11] Palazzuoli A, Pellegrini M, Franci B, et al. Short and long-term effects of continuous versus intermittent loop diuretics treatment in acute heart failure with renal dysfunction. Intern Emerg Med. 2015;10(1):41–9 [c].

[12] Oh SW, Han SY. Loop diuretics in clinical practice. Electrolyte Blood Press. 2015;13:17–21 [R].

[13] Sarai M, Tejani AM. Loop diuretics for patients receiving blood transfusions. Cochrane Database Syst Rev. 2015;(2):CD010138. http://dx.doi.org/10.1002/14651858.CD010138.pub2 [R].

[14] Mentz RJ, Buggey J, Fiuzat M, et al. Torsemide versus furosemide in heart failure: insights from Duke University hospital. J Cardiovasc Pharmacol. 2015;65(5):438–43 [C].

Thiazides

[15] Moranville MP, Choi S, Hogg J, et al. Comparison of metolazone versus chlorothiazide in acute decompensated heart failure with diuretic resistance. Cardiovasc Ther. 2015;33(2):42–9 [c].

[16] Castro-Torres Y, Fleites-Perez A, Carmona-Puerta R, et al. Negative effects of chlorthalidone on sympathetic nervous system and insulin resistance in hypertensive patients may be avoided with spironolactone: further studies are still needed. Ir J Med Sci. 2015;184(4):727–9 [H].

[17] Kipnes MS, Handley A, Lloyd E, et al. Safety, tolerability, and efficacy of azilsartan medoxomil with or without chlorthalidone during and after 8 months of treatment for hypertension. J Clin Hypertens. 2015;17(3):183–92 [C].

[18] Roush GC, Ernst ME, Kostis JB, et al. Head to head comparisons of hydrochlorothiazide with indapamide and chlorthalidone: antihypertensive and metabolic effects. Hypertension. 2015;65(5):1041–6 [M].

[19] Saseen JJ, Ghushchyan V, Nair KV. Comparing clinical effectiveness and drug toxicity with hydrochlorothiazide and chlorthalidone using two potency ratios in a managed care population. J Clin Hypertens. 2015;17(2):134–40 [C].

[20] Frenkel NJ, Vogt L, De Rooij SE, et al. Thiazide-induced hyponatraemia is associated with increased water intake and impaired urea-mediated water excretion at low plasma antidiuretic hormone and urine aquaporin-2. J Hypertens. 2015;33(3):627–33 [c].

[21] Sardar GK, Eilbert WP. Severe hyponatremia associated with thiazide diuretic use. J Emerg Med. 2015;48(3):305–9 [A].

[22] Barber J, McKeever TM, McDowell SE, et al. A systematic review and meta-analysis of thiazide-induced hyponatraemia: time to reconsider electrolyte monitoring regimens after thiazide initiation? Br J Clin Pharmacol. 2015;79(4):566–77 [R].

[23] Vongpatanasin W. Hydrochlorothiazide is not the most useful nor versatile thiazide diuretic. Curr Opin Cardiol. 2015;30(4):361–5 [r].

[24] Mohan JC, Jain R, Chamle V, et al. Short term safety and tolerability of a fixed dose combination of olmesartan, amlodipine and hydrochlorothiazide. J Clin Diagn Res. 2015;9(8):10–3 [R].

[25] Roush GF, Ernst ME, Kostis JB, et al. Head-to-head comparisons of hydrochlorothiazide with indapamide and chlorthalidone: antihypertensive and metabolic effects. Hypertension. 2015;65(5):1041–6 [R].

[26] Horwitz H, Woeien VA, Petersen LW, et al. Hypokalemia and rhabdomyolysis. J Pharmacol Pharmacother. 2015;6(2):98–9 [A].

[27] Zhang X, Xhao Q. Association of thiazide-type diuretics with glycemic changes in hypertensive patients: a systematic review and meta-analysis of randomized controlled clinical trials. J Clin Hypertens. 2016;18(4):342–51 [R].

Aldosterone antagonists

[28] Seferovic PM, Pelliccia F, Zivkovic I, et al. Mineralocorticoid receptor antagonists, a class beyond spironolactone—focus on the special pharmacologic properties of eplerenone. Int J Cardiol. 2015;200:3–7 [r].

[29] Lainscak M, Pelliccia F, Rosano G, et al. Safety profile of mineralocorticoid receptor antagonists: spironolactone and eplerenone. Int J Cardiol. 2015;200:25–9 [r].

[30] Walsh M, Manns B, Garg AX, et al. The safety of eplerenone in hemodialysis patients: a noninferiority randomized controlled trial. Clin J Am Soc Nephrol. 2015;10(9):1602–8 [c].

[31] Pelliccia F, Rosano G, Patti G, et al. Efficacy and safety of mineralocorticoid receptors in mild to moderate arterial hypertension. Int J Cardiol. 2015;200:8–11 [r].

[32] Abbas S, Ihle P, Harder S, et al. Risk of hyperkalemia and combined use of spironolactone and long-term ACE inhibitor/angiotensin receptor blocker therapy in heart failure using real-life data: a population- and insurance-based cohort. Pharmacoepidemiol Drug Saf. 2015;24(4):406–13 [MC].

[33] Antoniou T, Hallands S, Macdonald EM, et al. Trimethoprim-sulfamethoxazole and risk of sudden death among patients taking spironolactone. CMAJ. 2015;187(4):e138–43 [MC].

Osmotic diuretics

[34] Nolan SJ, Thornton J, Murray CS, et al. Inhaled mannitol for cystic fibrosis. Cochrane Database Syst Rev. 2015;9:10 [R].

[35] Lin SY, Tang SC, Tsai LK, et al. Incidence and risk factors for acute kidney injury following mannitol infusion in patients with acute stroke: a retrospective cohort study. Medicine. 2015;94(47):e2032 [C].

20

Metals

Lauren K. Roller[1], Laura J. Baumgartner

Department of Clinical Sciences, Touro University California College of Pharmacy, Vallejo, CA, USA

[1]Corresponding author: lauren.roller@tu.edu

ALUMINUM [SED-15, 97; SEDA-32, 413; SEDA-33, 447; SEDA-34, 349; SEDA-35, 397; SEDA-36, 297; SEDA-37, 243]

Multi-Organ Dysfunction

Increasing Rates of Death Following Aluminum Phosphide Ingestion

Aluminum phosphide is a well-known insecticide that has been banned in several countries due to its high fatality rate. However, it is still used in certain countries to help protect stored grains from pets and rodents. There is no effective antidote available, and the incidence of death secondary to exposure has been increasing Phosphine inhibits mitochondrial cytochrome oxidase. Effects of this inhibition ultimately lead to cellular damage by lipid peroxidation, cardiac myocyte and adrenal gland toxicity, and circulatory collapse [1c,2c].

An 8-year study conducted in Iran found an increasing rate of aluminum phosphide deaths (in 2006—5.22 cases per million and in 2013—37.02 cases per million), with the majority being suicide attempts. Although the substance is not legally available in Iran, it is imported illegally and sold in herbal drug stores [1c].

Respiratory

Smoking and Aluminum Exposure Impairs Lung Function

A cross-sectional comparative study was conducted to assess the effects of aluminum fumes on pulmonary function. Workers that were exposed to aluminum as a result of working in an aluminum foundry were compared to administrative workers with no exposure. The study found a potential combined negative effect of smoking and aluminum exposure on impairment of lung function, where as aluminum exposure alone had no impact on lung function [3c].

Gastrointestinal

Aluminum Phosphide Ingestion Leads to Gastrointestinal Hemorrhage

A case of gastrointestinal hemorrhage and ulcerations in the stomach, duodenum, jejunum, and ileum following consumption of five tablets of Celphos® (56% aluminum phosphide and 44% aluminum carbonate) has been reported. The patient eventually expired after 4 days of hospitalization from multi-organ failure and extensive gastrointestinal hemorrhage [2c].

Hematologic

Aluminum Linked to Oxidative Damage

The effect aluminum has on peripheral blood lymphocytes was studied. Aluminum was found to induce a mitochondrial membrane depolarization and a subsequent increase in production of reactive oxygen species and potential oxidative damage. This result was exacerbated when high aluminum concentrations were present [4c].

Drug Overdose

Gastrointestinal Hemorrhage Following Aluminum Phosphide Overdose

A 45-year-old male presented to the emergency department 7 hours after ingesting 5 tablets (3 g) of Celphos®. After ingestion, he had vomitus which was blood-tinged. On day two of hospitalization, the patient developed jaundice, oliguria, and electrolyte imbalances. He died on day four of hospitalization. Autopsy reports revealed multi-organ failure and gastrointestinal hemorrhage, including hemorrhages and ulcers on the gastric surface as well as extensively within the duodenum and jejunum and scant within the ileum [5A].

Lipid Emulsion Infusion for Aluminum Phosphide Overdose

Two separate case reports of intentional aluminum phosphide overdose have been reported. In both cases (Case 1: 40-year-old female; Case 2: 30-year-old male), each presented to the emergency department within 1–1.5 hours after ingesting 1 tablet (3 g) of Celphos®. Each patient immediately received fluids and gastric lavage on arrival. Within 12 hours of ingestion, they were started on an intralipid emulsion 20% at 10 mL/hour as well as magnesium sulfate 1 g over 20 minutes followed by 1 g/hour for 24 hours, then 1 g every 6 hours. Each patient improved by day 5 both infusions was discontinued. Both patients survived and were discharged within 10 days of admission [6A].

VA-ECMO as a Treatment for Aluminum Phosphine Poisoning

A case series using venoarterial extracorporeal membrane oxygenation (VA-ECMO) in 7 patients presenting with aluminum phosphine poisoning has been reported. In each case, patients presented 5–12 hours after ingestion with severe metabolic acidosis (pH ≤7) and refractory cardiogenic shock unresponsive to ionotropic agents, and left ventricular ejection fraction (LVEF) <35%. The mean time for each patient to receive VA-ECMO was 12.8 ± 2.9 hours (one patient was initiated at 28 hours). The patients began to show improvement in metabolic acidosis within 6–8 hours and improvement in cardiac function in 12–24 hours. All patients experienced local cannulation-site bleeding requiring blood transfusions. Ultimately, five of the seven patients survived to discharge. The two patients who expired experienced multiorgan failure before VA-ECMO was initiated. The average LVEF at discharge was $40.2 \pm 4.7\%$ [7c].

ARSENIC [SED-15, 339; SEDA-32, 414; SEDA-33, 448; SEDA-34, 351; SEDA-35, 399; SEDA-36, 298; SEDA-37, 244]

Respiratory

Respiratory Dysfunction Linked to Early Life Exposure to Arsenic

Several studies have reported a high prevalence of respiratory dysfunction in adult patients exposed to arsenic. It was recently found that *in utero* and early life exposure to arsenic may also have negative effects on respiratory function. These patients had a decrease in forced vital capacity with a restrictive spirometric pattern [8c].

Sweat Chloride Levels Elevated in Arsenic Exposed Patients

A cross-sectional study examined the effect arsenic exposure has on the results of a sweat chloride test, as the symptoms of arsenic toxicity often parallel the symptoms of cystic fibrosis. This study found that elevated sweat chloride levels were present among individuals who had been exposed to arsenic but had a negative genetic diagnosis of cystic fibrosis [9c].

Ear, Nose, Throat

Arsenic Exposure Is Associated with Nasal Polyposis

The association between blood arsenic levels and nasal polyposis, a chronic inflammatory disease of the nasal mucosa, was evaluated in a Tunisian population. Blood levels of arsenic were evaluated in patients with nasal polyposis and compared to patients without. Levels of arsenic were significantly higher in the nasal polyposis group, with smokers having higher levels than nonsmokers. On logistic regression, patients with a high arsenic level had 2.1-fold greater odds of having nasal polyposis than those with low arsenic levels [10C].

Psychiatric

Suicide Rates Increased Following Arsenic Exposure

The association of arsenic exposure and suicide mortality was evaluated over a 7-year period among 1639 Hungarian people. Levels of arsenic were split into three groups depending on level of arsenic found in drinking water between settlements (low: ≤10 μg/L vs. intermediate: 11–30 μg/L vs. high: 31–0 μg/L). The study found a positive association between age-standardized suicide rates and arsenic-contaminated drinking water [11C].

Endocrine

Cumulative Arsenic Exposure Predicts Hypothyroidism

The association of exposure to arsenic ground-water and hypothyroidism was evaluated in a 723 participants living in rural Texas. Logistic regression found groundwater containing arsenic ≥8 μg/L and cumulative arsenic exposure were significant predictors for hypothyroidism among Hispanics [12C].

Nutrition

Arsenic Exposure Is Associated with Increased Uric Acid Levels and Gout

A cross-sectional study examined the association between arsenic and serum uric acid levels or gout. A total of 5632 adults were included in the study. Results showed that arsenic exposure was associated with higher serum uric acid levels in men and an increased incidence of gout in women. After adjusting for confounders, increase in mean uric acid levels associated with arsenic exposure was 3% in men versus 1% in women. The odds ratio for gout based on arsenic exposure in women over 40 years of age was 5.46 (95% CI 1.7–17.6) [13C].

Urinary Tract

Arsenic Toxicity Linked to Nephrotoxicity

A review article examined the effects of arsenic-mediated nephrotoxicity. In cases of severe acute arsenic poisoning, acute tubular necrosis and acute interstitial nephritis have been reported with potential progression to chronic kidney disease. Causes may include direct toxicity on renal tubules, hypotensive shock, or hemoglobinuric tubular injury [14R].

Skin

Arsenic Contamined Drinking Water Increases Risk of Skin Lesions

The prevalence of skin lesions following arsenic exposure was evaluated in a field study in Kutahya. Villages were divided into two groups according to concentration of arsenic levels found in their drinking water (<20 µg/L vs >20 µg/L). The group with higher arsenic levels in their drinking water were found to have a higher cumulative arsenic index and more skin lesions [63c]. In addition, a review found a consistent dose–response relationship between arsenic contaminated water and development of skin lesions and skin cancers, with accumulating evidence suggesting risk may be prevalent at arsenic levels that were previously deemed harmless [15R].

Pregnancy

Arsenic Exposure Linked to Adverse Pregnancy Outcomes and Infant Mortality

Results from a systematic review and meta-analysis found an association between arsenic exposure and low birth weight. In addition, arsenic exposure was associated with an increased risk of spontaneous abortion (OR 1.98, 95% CI 1.27–3.1), stillbirth (OR = 1.77, 95% CI 1.32–2.36), and infant mortality (OR 1.35, 95% CI 1.12–1.62) [16R].

BARIUM [SEDA-31]

Electrolyte Imbalance

Profound Hyperkalemia Secondary to Barium Chloride Ingestion

A first case of massive overdose with barium chloride has been reported. A 23-year-old male ingested 100 g of pure analytical grade barium chloride as a suicidal agent. Three hours post-ingestion, the patient was experiencing nausea, vomiting, abdominal pain. The symptoms progressed to fatigue, abasia, and aconuresis. He received gastric lavage and magnesium sulfate catharsis. Six hours post ingestion, the patient was experiencing aphasia, hypersalivation, hyperhidrosis, respiratory insufficiency, limb weakness, and diminished neural reflexes. Laboratory work-up revealed severe hypokalemia (1.44 mmol/L) as well as acidosis (pH 7.23). The electrocardiogram showed flat ST segments and the presence of U waves. Gastric lavage and catharsis with sodium sulfate were repeated. Potassium replacement was initiated as an infusion of 16.8 mmol/hour. Sodium thiosulfate (8 g) was administered intravenously to reduce serum barium ions. Nine hours post-ingestion, hemoperfusion was initiated. Eleven hours post-ingestion, the patient was intubated secondary to respiratory failure. Electrocardiogram revealed premature ventricular beats and ventricular tachycardia. An amiodarone bolus of 150 mg was administered, and the potassium infusion was increased to 20 mmol/L. The patient transiently improved, but then decompensated shortly after. Twenty hours post-ingestion, potassium was 0.9 mmol/L, and the patient went into pulseless ventricular tachycardia. Cardiac resuscitation was initiated but ultimately unsuccessful. The basis of barium toxicity is rooted in the effects of profound persistent hypokalemia [17A].

CALCIUM SALTS [SED-15, 610; SEDA-33, 449; SEDA-34, 354; SEDA-35, 400; SEDA-36, 301; SEDA-37, 247]

Cardiovascular

Calcium Supplements May Affect Blood Pressure and Blood Coagulation

A randomized controlled trial examined the effect calcium supplementation had on blood pressure and blood coagulation in post-menopausal women. The reduction in systolic and diastolic blood pressure was smaller in the calcium supplementation group as compared to control. In addition, blood coagulability (assessed using thromboelastography) increased from baseline in both groups; however, at 4 hours, the calcium supplement group had a greater coagulation index [18C].

Sensory Systems

Age-Related Macular Degeneration Linked to Calcium Supplementation

A cross-sectional study was conducted to investigate the association between calcium supplementation and the prevalence of age-related macular degeneration

(AMD). Study participants who ingested more than 800 mg/day of supplemental calcium were found to have a higher chance of developing AMD (OR 1.85, 95% CI 1.25–2.75). This had a stronger association in patients who were older rather than younger (OR 2.63, 95% CI 1.52–4.54). Further, the results found that the development of AMD was more dependent on a dose threshold rather then a dose–response relationship [19C].

Systematic Reviews

Calcium Supplementation May Not Increase Coronary Heart Disease in Women

A meta-analysis of randomized controlled trials was conducted to determine if calcium supplementation, with or without vitamin D, increase coronary heart disease and all-cause mortality in elderly women. Results found a relative risk for calcium supplementation with or without vitamin D for all-cause mortality to be 0.96 (95% CI 0.91–1.02) and for MI to be 1.08 (95% CI 0.93–1.25). Based on this meta-analysis, the current evidence does not support the hypothesis that calcium supplementation increases all-cause mortality and coronary heart disease in elderly women; however, no conclusions can be made regarding men [20M,21r].

CHROMIUM [SED-15, 737; SEDA-32, 414; SEDA-33, 450; SEDA-34, 354; SEDA-35, 401; SEDA-36, 303; SEDA-37, 247]

Immunologic

Dermatitis Caused by Chromium-Containing Hip Implant

Metal-on-metal hip resurfacing is associated with corrosion, and this leads to release of metal ions into the blood. A case of a 60-year-old male with a 3-year history of unresponsive diffuse dermatitis secondary to a hypersensitivity reaction to cobalt–chrome–molybdenum alloy hip implant has been reported. The patient received a metal-on-metal (cobalt–chromium–molybdenum alloy) hip resurfacing procedure due to osteoarthritis. General pruritus and psoriatic-like dermatitis developed in 3 years after implantation which was unresponsive to antihistamines and corticosteroids. A patch test revealed chromium-sulfate hypersensitivity with a chromium blood level of 10.32 µg/L. Skin and right inguinal biopsies were completed, and the patient was diagnosed with Langerhans cell histiocytosis and type IV delayed-type hypersensitivity. Surgical removal of the implant was completed in and replaced with a cementless ceramic-on-ceramic implant. Three days after surgical removal, pruritus resolved. Spontaneous resolution of dermatitis

occurred by 3 months. The patient was symptom free 24 months after removal of the metal implant [22A].

Cancer

DNA Polymorphisms from Chromium Exposure and Lung Cancer

A case–control study in Slovakia was performed to assess the impact of DNA polymorphisms of DNA repair genes and the risk of lung cancer associated with chromium exposure. The DNA repair genes evaluated in the study included XPC (Lys939Gln), XPD (Lys751Gln), XRCC1(Arg399Gln), and hOGG1 (Ser326Ser). The study included 50 patients with chromium-exposed lung cancer subjects and 69 control subjects. Results indicated a significant increase in risk of lung cancer in XPD genotype Lys/Gln (OR = 1.94; 95% CI = 1.10–3.43; $p = 0.015$). Additionally, a significant increase in lung cancer was found in 2 different gene combinations which were XPD Lys/Gln + XPC Lys/Gln (OR = 6.5; 95% CI = 1.53–27.49; $p = 0.009$) and XPD Lys/Gln + XPC Gln/Gln (OR = 5.2; 95% CI = 1.07–25.32; $p = 0.04$). The study concluded that polymorphisms in DNA repair genes may contribute to an increased risk of lung cancer in those who have been exposed to chromium [23C].

Inhaled Chromium-VI Associated with Stomach Cancer

A meta-analysis of 56 case–control studies was conducted to evaluate the risk of stomach cancer from inhalation of chromium IV. The combined summary relative risk was 1.27 (95% CI 1.18–1.38; $p < 0.001$). Additionally, the relative risk for stomach cancer was higher in the studies that demonstrated an increased risk for lung cancer due to chromium IV inhalation (RR = 1.41, 95% CI 1.18–1.69: $p < 0.001$). The review concluded that an increased risk of stomach cancer exists following inhalation of chromium IV [24M].

Chromium Exposure Leading to Germinal Embryonal Carcinoma

The first two cases of germinal embryonal carcinoma secondary to chromium exposure have been reported.
Case 1

A 35-year-old male was hospitalized due to a pericardial effusion and subsequent pericardial drainage. He was diagnosed with extra gonadal mediastinal germinal cancer. In the 6 years leading up to his cancer diagnosis, the patient worked in a facility where he cleaned up chromium-containing dust and waste. Over an 8-year period, his disease continued to progress. He received multiple chemotherapy regimens and underwent surgical procedures, but ultimately died from complications.

Case 2

Another 35-year-old male who worked in the same facility as the patient in case 1 presented with poorly differentiated and extensively necrotic carcinoma. He was diagnosed with germinal embryonal carcinoma and began chemotherapy treatments. Over 14 months, the cancer continued to progress, and the patient eventually expired [25A].

COBALT [SED-15, 847; SEDA-32, 415; SEDA-33, 450; SEDA-34, 354; SEDA-35, 402; SEDA-36, 303; SEDA-37, 248]

Cardiovascular

Cobalt-Induced Cardiomyopathy

A case of cobalt-induced cardiomyopathy was reported in a 69-year-old woman with bilateral hip replacements. After obtaining further history, the patient noted that her hip prosthesis had been squeaking for the past 2 years and planned removal was in order due to recall status. A cobalt level was obtained and found to be 200–300 ng/mL (reference range: <1 ng/mL). The patient subsequently went into cardiogenic shock and received advanced heart failure treatment and removal of the hip prosthesis. Her postoperative course was complicated by stroke, and she eventually expired [26c].

Sensory Systems

High Concentrations of Cobalt Linked to Visual Loss

A systematic literature search was completed to evaluate the effects of cobalt on visual function. Eight case reports of cobalt were identified, five of which underwent metal hip arthroplasties, two of which had environmental exposure to cobalt, and one patient was treated medically with cobalt chloride. The results of these case reports showed that high serum concentrations of cobalt may be associated with both reversible and irreversible visual loss, optic atrophy, and optic neuropathy [27M].

Skin

Cobalt Allergy Linked to History of Dermatitis Following Leather Exposure

A questionnaire case–control study was conducted to examine the association between a history of dermatitis following exposure to leather and allergic cobalt dermatitis. A positive association was found between having a cobalt allergy and a history of dermatitis following leather exposure [28C].

Cobalt Spot Test Improves Diagnosis

Cobalt is a frequent cause of allergic contact dermatitis. A spot test specific for cobalt was recently developed and appears to be a useful tool in the diagnosis of allergic cobalt dermatitis.

A 28-year-old baker presents to clinic after suffering from persistent hand dermatitis over the past 6 months. He had contact with metal baking sheets 80–100× per work day for the past 12 years. A cobalt spot test was performed on the baking sheets, and the test resulted as positive [29c].

GADOLINIUM

Gadolinium is commonly found in magnetic resonance imaging contrast media, with each specific media containing different concentrations of gadolinium.

Respiratory

Acute Respiratory Distress Syndrome Following Gadolinium Contrast

A case of acute respiratory distress syndrome (ARDS) occurred in a 26-year-old female receiving gadolinium-based contrast media. She had no previous medical history or documented allergies. Soon after the gadolinium contrast media was administered, she developed respiratory distress and was treated with mechanical ventilation with eventual extubation [30c].

Electrolyte Balance

Gadolinium Linked to Hypophosphatemia

Triple dose gadolinium was administered to 877 patients undergoing a brain MRI, with 15.1% of those patients developing hypophosphatemia. The frequency of hypophosphatemia progressed with cumulative gadolinium administrations [31c].

Urinary Tract

Gadolinium-Based Contrast Media Associated with Nephrogenic Systemic Fibrosis

Administration of gadolinium-based contrast media is associated with nephrogenic systemic fibrosis (NSF), a rare fibrosing skin disorder that can develop in patients with kidney failure. NSF typically occurs weeks to months post-exposure, with the longest case being documented at 3.5 years. A recent case of NSF occurred in a patient 10 years after gadolinium exposure [32c].

IRON SALTS [SED-15, 1911; SEDA-32, 417; SEDA-33, 451; SEDA-34, 355; SEDA-35, 402; SEDA-36, 305, SEDA-37, 250]

Cardiovascular

Dietary-Heme Iron Intake Associated with Cardiovascular Risk

A meta-analysis was conduced to determine an association between intake of dietary iron and cardiovascular disease. Included in the meta-analysis were 13 prospective cohort studies that examined dietary iron intake and the risk of cardiovascular disease. Results of the meta-analysis showed that in the dietary intake of heme iron had an increased risk of cardiovascular disease. No association was found between dietary intake of non-heme iron and cardiovascular risk [33M].

Anaphylaxis

Anaphylaxis Risk Among Intravenous Iron Products

A retrospective new use cohort study was conducted to assess the risk of anaphylaxis with the various intravenous iron products on the market. Non-dialysis patients receiving first IV iron product dose and no more than one type of iron product were included. Patients were excluded if they received any blood transfusions within 30 days following the date of anaphylaxis. The primary outcome was to compare the risk between dextran and nondextran iron products. Risk of anaphylaxis between iron gluconate, iron sucrose, and ferumoxytol were analyzed as secondary outcomes. Results showed 274 cases of anaphylaxis with first IV dose and 170 additional cases with later administrations. The risk of anaphylaxis with dextran was higher than with nondextran products with an adjusted odds ratio of 2.6 (95% CI, 2.0–3.3; $p < 0.001$). The highest risk of anaphylaxis among the three iron products evaluated was iron sucrose with an odds ratio of 3.6 (95% CI, 2.4–5.4) [34C].

Pregnancy

Iron Supplementation in Non-Anemic Pregnant Females Associated with Low Birth Weight

A prospective observational study of non-anemic pregnant females was performed to evaluate the impact of receiving iron supplementation on birth outcomes. The study followed non-anemic females who received supplemental oral ferrous sulfate 150 mg (45 mg elemental iron) starting with the first day of the second trimester until delivery. Results showed that non-anemic females who received higher amounts of elemental iron per day had an increased risk of term low birth weight [35C].

LANTHANUM CARBONATE [SEDA-32, 417; SEDA-33, 451; SEDA-34, 356; SEDA-35, 404; SEDA-36, 306; SEDA-37, 250]

Gastrointestinal

Gastrointestinal Lesions Associated with Lanthanum Carbonate

Six cases of gastrointestinal histiocytic lesions associated with lanthanum carbonate (LC) ingestion have been reported. Three men and three women, all of which had end-stage renal disease and had been receiving LC for >21 months, were found to have a heavy burden of lanthanum in the gastroduodenal mucosa on gastrointestinal biopsy. Upon endoscopic examination, 3 patients were found to have gastric erosions, 2 were found to have gastric polyps, and 1 was found to have a gastric ulcer. A long-standing outcome for gastrointestinal side effects secondary to LC administration has not been established, and future research is needed [36c].

Systematic Reviews

Lanthanum Carbonate Improves Bone Outcomes

A systematic review consisting of randomized controlled trials comparing lanthanum carbonate (LC) with calcium-based phosphate binders was conducted to assess the safety and efficacy of LC. Eleven trials with 1501 patients were included. LC was found to be associated with a significant reduction in vascular calcification and incidence of hypercalcemia. In addition, LC had a beneficial effect on bone outcomes, such as a decreased number of patients developing low turnover bone disease [37M].

LEAD [SED-15, 2013; SEDA-28, 247; SEDA-35, 404; SEDA-36, 307; SEDA-37, 250]

Cardiovascular

Lead Exposures Contributes to Increased Blood Pressure

A cross-sectional study of 1447 participants in Zixing, China, an area with heavy metal exposure, were evaluated to investigate a connection between lead exposure, blood pressure, and kidney function. The patients were divided into two groups: low blood lead level (0–100 μg/L) and high blood lead level (≥100 μg/L). Statistically significant differences were detected between the low blood level and high blood lead level groups for systolic (121.92 mmHg vs 126.93 mmHg, $p < 0.001$) and diastolic (89.85 mmHg vs 95.09 mmHg, $p < 0.001$) blood pressures. No difference was observed serum creatinine and BUN [38C].

Hematologic

Lead Poisoning from Herbal Remedies Leading to Dysplastic Changes

A case report of a 61-year-old female receiving folk remedies in China for alleviation of a lumbar vertebral fracture and symptoms was found to have high lead blood levels causing dysplastic changes in erythroid precursors. Her symptoms included fatigue, pallor, chest tightness, shortness of breath with activity, poor appetite, and skin hyperalgesia. She was treated with CaNa$_2$-EDTA (calcium disodium versenate), her lead levels decreased, and blood counts normalized [39A].

MAGNESIUM SALTS [SED-15, 2196; SEDA-32, 417; SEDA-33, 452; SEDA-34, 356; SEDA-35, 406; SEDA-36, 309; SEDA-37, 251]

Neuromuscular Function

Recurarisation of Neuromuscular Blockade Caused by Magnesium Sulfate and Sugammadex Drug Interaction

Recurarisation of rocuronium-induced neuromuscular blockade was reported in a 61-year-old female with a history of atrial fibrillation during a surgical procedure under anesthesia. A dose of rocuronium 35 mg intravenously was administered for intubation. During the procedure, the patient developed tachycardia and atrial fibrillation for which metoprolol 5 mg IV was administered. When the procedure was finished, sugammadex 120 mg (2.1 mg/kg) was given to reverse neuromuscular blockade, and train of four was normalized within 120 seconds. Following reversal, magnesium sulfate 3600 mg (60 mg/kg) was given for conversion of atrial fibrillation to normal sinus rhythm. Recurarisation occurred after the initiation of the magnesium infusion, and the neuromuscular transmission nadir occurred 7 minutes post initiation. Train of four normalization reoccurred 50 minutes after the discontinuation of magnesium infusion [40A].

MANGANESE [SED-15, 2200; SEDA-32, 418; SEDA-33, 452; SEDA-34, 357; SEDA-35, 407; SEDA-36, 310]

Nervous System

Manganese Associated with Decreased Neurodevelopment

A study of 204 children from 6 months of age to 6 years of age were evaluated to determine if there is an association between infant neurodevelopment and manganese exposure. The study found that high manganese levels were associated with decreases of the mental developmental index at both 6 and 12 months of age. Higher levels of manganese were also associated with a decreased mental and physical development of girls within the first 12 months of age [41C].

Manganese Accumulation in Infants Receiving Parenteral Nutrition

A prospective observational study was conducted in 73 infants receiving parenteral nutrition to evaluate the effects of manganese on neuroimaging. Results showed a lower T1 relaxation time in those infants who received higher amounts of manganese. Additionally, an association between manganese levels, low T1 relaxation time, and elevated conjugated bilirubin was identified [42c].

Respiratory

Decreased Lung Function with Occupational Manganese Exposure

A retrospective review of 1658 ferromanganese workers in Guangxi, China was conducted to assess for the impact of manganese exposure on lung function as well as the effect of smoking on manganese exposure. The study found a decrease in lung function in male workers exposed to high levels of manganese (manganese-cumulative exposure index ≥ 1 mg/m^3 per year). When smokers were compared with non-smokers, there were statistically significant decreases in predicted forced vital capacity (FVC) and predicted maximal med-expiratory flow curve (MMEF) amongst those that were smokers [43C].

Immunologic

Contact Dermatitis from Manganese-Containing Implant

A case of a 60-year-old male with allergic contact dermatitis has been presented. The patient received a fixation of a malleolus fracture with a manganese-containing stainless steel plate. Patch testing confirmed 1+ positive (i.e., weak positive) for manganese chloride. The steel plate was removed and dermatitis symptoms resolved in 10 days [44A].

Genotoxicity

Manganese Exposure Associated with Gene Methylation and Parkinsonism

In previous accounts, manganese exposure has been linked to parkinsonism. A cohort study of 201 welders was conducted to evaluate whether manganese-induced DNA hypomethylation of the NOS2 exon 1 due to welding fumes was associated with Parkinsonism. Blood samples from each welder was collected and analyzed for

DNA methylation at 3 different CpG sites. Results concluded that hypomethylation occurred in the welders with parkinsonism [45C].

Pregnancy

Manganese Intake During Pregnancy Leads to Preterm Delivery

A cohort study of 1033 Iranian pregnant females was completed to evaluate the association between maternal nutritional status in the second trimester and preterm delivery. Using a questionnaire to assess dietary intake, the study found that intake was significantly higher in mothers who delivered preterm (<34 weeks gestation) than those that delivered at term [46C].

MERCURY AND MERCURIAL SALTS
[SED-15, 2259; SEDA-32, 419; SEDA-33, 453; SEDA-34, 358; SEDA-35, 407; SEDA-36, 311; SEDA-37, 251]

Respiratory

Respiratory Failure from Mercury Poisoning

A case of a 59-year-old male with mercury poisoning following gold and silver smelting has been reported. The patient was using mercury to smelt gold from computer chips on the stove. Within 5 minutes of beginning the process, he began to experience an itchy throat, shortness of breath, weakness, and tremors. He was admitted to the intensive care unit, intubated, and diagnosed with acute respiratory distress syndrome. After a month in the hospital, he was discharged to a long-term care facility for further treatment of pneumonitis [47S].

Nervous System

Mercury Exposure Associated with Developmental Differences in Female Newborns

A cross-sectional survey of preschool children under the age of 5 in a tin-ore mining town in Brazil was conducted to evaluate neurodevelopmental outcomes with exposure to organic mercury. Mercury concentrations were measured by hair samples for each infant. To account for ethylmercury exposure from thimerosal-containing vaccines (TCV), receipt of administration of TCVs for pregnant mothers and infants was collected. Mental developmental index (mean, SD) was significantly higher at 6 months in girls (95.37, 14.59) than in boys (90.19, 16.29). Psychomotor developmental index (median, min–max) was also significantly higher at 6 months in girls (99.11, 12.63) than in boys (96.01, 13.81). There was no difference in these indices at 24 months of age [48C].

Association of Prenatal Mercury Exposure and Autism

The CHARGE (Childhood Autism Risks from Genetics and the Environment) study was a case–control study evaluated the association of methylmercury exposure and autism and developmental delay. Children were included if they were between the ages of 24 months to 60 months. Infant blood mercury concentrations were obtained, and maternal fish consumption was assessed by a questionnaire. No association was found linking prenatal methylmercury exposure and risk of autism or developmental delay [49C].

Skin

Mercury Granuloma Development from a Mercury Thermometer

A case of a 28-year-old female nurse who developed a cutaneous mercury granuloma following an injury from a broken mercury thermometer has been reported. Twelve days following the injury, a lesion on the dorsum of her hand had increased. Upon excisional biopsy, histopathologic examination results showed a dense lympho-histiocytic infiltrate as well as a foreign body granulomatous reaction deep in the dermis. Once the mercury was excised, the swelling and itching resolved [50A].

Genotoxicity

Mercury Associated with Epigenetic Variability

Assessments of 138 mother–infant pairs were evaluated for an association between mercury exposure and DNA methylation as the composition of white blood cells in cord blood using toenail mercury levels and newborn cord blood. Increased toenail mercury levels that were associated with a decrease in monocytes by 2.5%. B-cells also increased by 3.5% with increased mercury concentrations. Additionally, enrichment of loci in the North shore regions of CpG islands, most of which were hypermethylated, was observed with toenail mercury levels. This study supports the theory that mercury may be involved in epigenetic variability as well as changes in immune cells [51C].

NICKEL [SED-15, 2502; SEDA-32, 419; SEDA-33, 453; SEDA-34, 358; SEDA-35, 409; SEDA-36, 313; SEDA-37, 252]

Immunologic

Allergic Nickel Dermatitis Caused by Nickel-Containing Screws

A case report of a 65-year-old male who developed allergic nickel dermatitis following internal fixation of a broken tibia with a screw and plating system made of stainless steel containing nickel has been reported. Approximately 6 months following fixation, the patient developed erythema and dermatitis around his surgical scar that was unresponsive to corticosteroids. Patch testing was performed and showed a 2+ positive (i.e., strong positive) reaction to nickel. The plate and screws were left in and the dermatitis symptoms resolved in 6 months [52A].

Nickel Allergy Leading to Hand Eczema Semi-Quantified with Dimethylglyoxime Testing

Dimethylglyoxime (DMG) testing is a semi-quantitative test that gives a positive result when $>0.5\ \mu g\ Ni/cm^2/week$ is released from a metallic surface. The test can also be used on skin after metal contact.

A case report of a 32-year-old female with a 5-year history of palmar hand eczema due to occupational nickel exposure has been reported. A patch test showed a 3+ reaction (i.e., extreme reaction) to nickel sulfate. The patient was tested using the DMG test for the presence of nickel. The DMG test performed on her hands 2 hours before work was negative for nickel and the DMG test performed 2 hours after work was positive for nickel. The DMG on the patient's skin showed stronger positive on her left-hand, which subsequently exhibited more severe dermatitis symptoms. This was associated with the patient handling more nickel-containing items with her left hand at work. When the patient wore nitrile rubber gloves, the DMG test was negative on the inside of the gloves. The patient began wearing nitrile rubber gloves at work and her eczema improved. This case report validates the usefulness of DMG testing on this skin [53A].

Cancer

Increased Cancer Mortality Associated with Nickel Exposure

An ecological study was completed evaluating the association of arsenic and nickel exposure with cancer mortality. The study was conducted in 83 towns of Suzhou, China using topsoil samples and death records. Results showed exposure to nickel-containing soil was related to liver (RR 1.022, CI 1.004–1.040; $p=0.022$) and nasopharyngeal cancer (RR 1.040, CI 1.014–1.067; $p=0.003$) mortality rates. Additionally, exposure to the combination of soil containing arsenic and nickel was associated with increased mortality in males from colon, gastric, kidney, and liver cancer [54C].

PALLADIUM [SEDA-22, 249; SEDA-33]

The main metal used in dental crowns and bridge work is palladium and accounts for the main source for palladium exposure. A more sensitive test allergen to palladium has been recently introduced, and the prevalence of contact allergy to palladium has risen.

Skin

Palladium Sensitization Linked to Dental Crowns

An observational study investigated whether sensitization to palladium was associated with clinical variables consisting of exposure to different dental allows and oral/skin complaints. Of the 906 patients included, 24.3% reacted to palladium. Factors associated with palladium sensitization were exposure to dental crowns, skin reactivity to metals, oral lichenoid lesions, xerostomia, and metal taste, but not eczema [55C].

SILVER SALTS AND DERIVATIVES [SED-15, 3140; SEDA-32, 420; SEDA-33, 454; SEDA-34, 359; SEDA-35, 409; SEDA-36, 314; SEDA-37, 253]

Respiratory

Safety Concerns Following Pleurodesis with Silver Nitrate

A double-blind, randomized, clinical trial evaluating the adverse events occurring from silver nitrate pleurodesis performed in patients with malignant plural effusion. A total of 60 patients were randomized to receive one of three doses of silver nitrate: 90 mg (0.3%, 30 mL), 180 mg (0.3%, 60 mL), 150 mg (0.5%, 30 mL). The solution was instilled into the pleural space via a catheter and held for 1 hour. Altogether, 199 adverse events occurred which included 23 serious adverse events. The number of adverse events was not statistically different amongst the three groups. Of the serious adverse events observed, hypoxia was most common (13/60 patients, 21.6%). Other common less serious adverse reactions included increase in serum creatinine (21/60 patients, 35%) and aspartate amino transferase (18/60, 30%) [56c].

Mouth and Teeth

Bisphosphonate-Related Osteonecrosis of the Jaw Induced by Silver Nitrate

A case of bisphosphonate-related osteonecrosis of the jaw due to silver nitrate application was reported in a 61-year-old male. The patient's past medical history included multiple myeloma, stage III IgG lambda for which he had been treated with a chemotherapy regimen that included zoledronic acid monthly as well as a bone marrow transplant (BMT). He continued his intravenous zoledronic acid after the chemotherapy regimen and BMT completion. He discovered a 'white patch' on his hard palate that was later diagnosed as a melanocytic macule. To confirmation this diagnosis, a biopsy was completed, and silver nitrate was used to achieve hemostasis on an exposed area of bone. Six weeks following the biopsy, a 4-mm diameter area of exposed bone was seen on examination. Further testing confirmed bisphosphonate-related osteonecrosis of the jaw [57A].

THALLIUM

Thallium is used for industrial use in optical lenses and light bulbs and for diagnostic purposes in the medical field for perfusion scintigraphy and tumor detection. Thallotoxicosis adverse effects include ascending peripheral neuropathy, gastrointestinal symptoms, and dermatological manifestations (including alopecia). The mechanism behind thallium toxicity is still unknown. Thallium found in any concentration in the body is abnormal.

Drug Abuse

Thallium Concentration Identified in Opioid Abusers

A case–control study of 150 subjects was conducted at a hospital in Iran. One hundred opioid abusers (i.e., raw opium, opium residue, crystal heroin, mixed abuse) admitted to the hospital for poisoning or rehabilitation were compared to 50 non-opioid abusers. Thallium concentrations were found in 19 subjects in the opioid-abuser group and 2 subjects in the control group. The mean (SE, min–max) urinary thallium concentration in the case group was 21 µg/L (5 µg/L, 0–346 µg/L) and 1 µg/L (0.14 µg/L, 0–26 µg/L) in the control group ($p = 0.001$). The results of this study suggest opioids may be adulterated with thallium [58c].

Intentional Thallium Intoxication

A case report of a 24-year-old male who ingested 100 mg of laboratory grade thallium monobromate and 0.1 dL of alcohol has been reported. He complained of painful paresthesia in the legs as well as worsening chronic depression. Within 8 hours of admission to the hospital, he was given Prussian blue (250 mg/kg), penicillamine, gastrointestinal decontamination with activated charcoal and lactulose, and forced diuresis. During his 30-day hospital stay, he developed acute cheilitis (week 2), diffuse alopecia (week 3), seborrheic dermatitis (week 3), and microbial eczema (week 4). Prussian blue and penicillamine were continued for the duration of his admission. He was transferred to a psychiatric facility after his hospital stay for management of anxious depression [59A].

Thallium Poisoning

A 46-year-old female and 50-year-old male married couple were poisoned with thallium (25 g of thallium mixed with table salt) on two separate occasions over 16 months. Immediately after ingestion, the first symptoms included sudden numbness and tingling of the hands and feet as well as alopecia within 1 week. Over the next several months, symptoms included numbness, allodynia, hyperesthesia, weakness, and muscular atrophy of the extremities. After the second poisoning with thallium, the subjects were hospitalized and treated with Prussian blue and hemoperfusion, but therapy was unsuccessful and both subjects eventually expired [60A].

URANIUM

Uranium is a natural occurring radioactive metal that is found in soil, water, plants, animals, food, and ambient air, with the most common source of exposure being food and water consumption.

Musculoskeletal

Uranium Exposure May Decrease Bone Development

Upon absorption, uranium may accumulate in renal and osseous tissues. It directly affects bone development and maintenance by inhibition of osteoblast differentiation. In addition, it may also inhibit the renal production of vitamin D, which will indirectly inhibit bone growth. Patient populations who may be at increased susceptibility to this adverse effect include both young and elderly patients [61M].

ZINC [SED-15, 3717; SEDA-32, 420; SEDA-33, 458; SEDA-34, 360; SEDA-35, 410; SEDA-36, 315; SEDA-37, 254]

Cardiovascular

Zinc Compound Air Releases Increases CVD Mortality

A retrospective ecological study was performed to determine if zinc exposure was associated with age adjusted cardiovascular disease mortality per 100 000 persons. The study was conducted across all of the counties in the United States. Toxic release inventory datasets compiled by the Environmental Protection Agency were used to collect air releases from over 53 000 facilities that manage toxic chemicals. In order to account for cardiovascular disease mortality, data were collected from the Center for Disease Control's Wonder website. Air releases containing zinc were associated with increased adjusted cardiovascular disease mortality [62C].

References

[1] Etemadi-Aleagha A, Akhgari M, Iravani FS, et al. Aluminum phosphide poisoning-related deaths in Tehran, Iran, 2006 to 2013. Medicine. 2015;94:e-1637 [c].

[2] Hugar BS, Praveen S, Hosahally JS, et al. Gastrointestinal hemorrhage in aluminum phosphide poisoning. J Forensic Sci. 2015;60:S261–3 [c].

[3] Elserougy S, Mahdy-Abdallah H, Hafez SF, et al. Impact of aluminum exposure on lung. Toxicol Ind Health. 2015;31:73–8 [c].

[4] Skarabahatava AS, Lukyanenko LM, Slobozhanina EI, et al. Plasma and mitochondrial membrane perturbation induced by aluminum in human peripheral blood lymphocytes. J Trace Elem Med Biol. 2015;31:37–44 [c].

[5] Hugar BS, Praveen S, Hosahally JS, et al. Gastrointestinal hemorrhage in aluminum phosphide poisoning. J Forensic Sci. 2015;60(Suppl 1):S261–3 [A].

[6] Baruah U, Sahni A, Sachdeva HC. Successful management of aluminium phosphide poisoning using intravenous lipid emulsion: report of two cases. Indian J Crit Care Med. 2015;19(12):735–8 [A].

[7] Mohan B, Gupta V, Ralhan S, et al. Role of extracorporeal membrane oxygenation in aluminum phosphide poisoning-induced reversible myocardial dysfunction: a novel therapeutic modality. J Emerg Med. 2015;49(5):651–6 [c].

[8] Recio-Vega R, Gonzalez-Cortes T, Olivas-Calderon E, et al. In utero and early childhood exposure to arsenic decreases lung function in children. J Appl Toxicol. 2015;35:358–66 [c].

[9] Christiani DC, Biswas SK, Ibne-Hasan OS. Elevated sweat chloride levels due to arsenic toxicity. N Engl J Med. 2015;372:582–3 [c].

[10] Khlifi R, Olmedo P, Gil F, et al. Association between blood arsenic levels and nasal polyposis disease risk in the Tunisian population. Environ Sci Pollut Res Int. 2015;22:14136–43 [C].

[11] Rihmer Z, Hal M, Kapitany B, et al. Preliminary investigation of the possible association between arsenic levels in drinking water and suicide mortality. J Affect Disord. 2015;182:23–5 [C].

[12] Gong G, Basom J, Mattevada S, et al. Association of hypothyroidism with low-level arsenic exposure in rural West Texas. Environ Res. 2015;138:154–60 [C].

[13] Kuo CC, Weaver V, Fadrowski JJ, et al. Arsenic exposure, hyperuricemia, and gout in US adults. Environ Int. 2015;76:32–40 [C].

[14] Robles-Osorio ML, Sabath-Silva E, Sabath E. Arsenic-mediated nephrotoxicity. Ren Fail. 2015;37:542–7 [R].

[15] Karagas MR, Gossai A, Pierce B, et al. Drinking water arsenic contamination, skin lesions, and malignancies: a systematic review of the global evidence. Curr Environ Health Rep. 2015;2:52–68 [R].

[16] Quansah R, Armah FA, Essumang DK, et al. Association of arsenic with adverse pregnancy outcomes/infant mortality: a systematic review and meta-analysis. Environ Health Perspect. 2015;123:412–21 [R].

[17] Yu D, Yi M, Jin L. Incorrigible hypokalemia caused by barium chloride ingestion. Am J Med Sci. 2015;349(3):279–81 [A].

[18] Bristow SM, Gamble GD, Stewart A, et al. Acute effects of calcium supplements on blood pressure and blood coagulation: secondary analysis of a randomized controlled trial in post-menopausal women. Br J Nutr. 2015;114:1868–74 [C].

[19] Kakigi CL, Singh K, Wang SY, et al. Self reported calcium supplementation and age-related macular degeneration. JAMA Ophthalmol. 2015;133:746–54 [C].

[20] Lewis JR, Radavelli-Bagatini S, Rejnmark L, et al. The effects of calcium supplementation on verified coronary heart disease hospitalization and death in postmenopausal women: a collaborative meta-analysis of randomized controlled trials. J Bone Miner Res. 2015;30:165–75 [M].

[21] Bolland MJ, Grey A, Avenell A, et al. Calcium supplements increase risk of myocardial infarction. J Bone Miner Res. 2015;30:389–90 [r].

[22] Bizzotto N, Sandri A, Trivellin G, et al. Chromium-induced diffuse dermatitis with lymph node involvement resulting from Langerhans cell histiocytosis after metal-on-metal hip resurfacing. Br J Dermatol. 2015;172(6):1633–6 [A].

[23] Sarlinova M, Majerova L, Matakova T, et al. Polymorphisms of DNA repair genes and lung cancer in chromium exposure. Adv Exp Med Biol. 2015;833:1–8 [C].

[24] Welling R, Beaumont JJ, Petersen SJ, et al. Chromium VI and stomach cancer: a meta-analysis of the current epidemiological evidence. Occup Environ Med. 2015;72(2):151–9 [M].

[25] Berardi R, Pellei C, Valeri G, et al. Chromium exposure and germinal embryonal carcinoma: first two cases and review of the literature. J Toxicol Environ Health A. 2015;78(1):1–6 [A].

[26] Khan AH, Verma R, Bajpai A, et al. Unusual case of congestive heart failure. Circ Cardiovasc Imaging. 2015;8:e003352 [c].

[27] Lim CA, Khan J, Chelva E, et al. The effect of cobalt on the human eye. Doc Ophthalmol. 2015;130:43–8 [M].

[28] Bregnbak D, Thyssen JP, Zachariae C, et al. Association between cobalt allergy and dermatitis caused by leather articles—a questionnaire study. Contact Dermatitis. 2015;72:106–14 [C].

[29] Bregnbak D, Zachariae C, Thyssen JP. Occupational exposure to metallic cobalt in a baker. Contact Dermatitis. 2015;72:115–26 [c].

[30] Park J, Byun IH, Park KH, et al. Acute respiratory distress syndrome after the use of gadolinium contrast media. Yonsei Med J. 2015;56:1155–7 [c].

[31] Wolansky LJ, Cadavid D, Punia V, et al. Hypophosphatemia is associated with the serial administration of triple-dose gadolinium to patients for brain MRI. J Neuroimaging. 2015;25:379–83 [c].

[32] Larson KN, Gagnon AL, Darling MD, et al. Nephrogenic systemic fibrosis manifesting a decade after exposure to gadolinium. JAMA Dermatol. 2015;151:1117–20 [c].

[33] Fang X, An P, Wang H, et al. Dietary intake of heme iron and risk of cardiovascular disease: a dose-response meta-analysis of prospective cohort studies. Nutr Metab Cardiovasc Dis. 2015;25(1):24–35 [M].

[34] Wang C, Graham DJ, Kane RC, et al. Comparative risk of anaphylactic reactions associated with intravenous iron products. JAMA. 2015;314(19):2062–8 [C].

[35] Shastri L, Mishra PE, Dwarkanath P, et al. Association of oral iron supplementation with birth outcomes in non-anaemic South Indian pregnant women. Eur J Clin Nutr. 2015;69(5):609–13 [C].

[36] Haratake J, Yasunaga C, Ootani A, et al. Peculiar histiocytic lesions with massive lanthanum deposition in dialysis patients treated with lanthanum carbonate. Am J Surg Pathol. 2015;39:767–71 [c].

[37] Zhai CJ, Yang XW, Sun J, et al. Efficacy and safety of lanthanum carbonate versus calcium-based phosphate binders in patients with chronic kidney disease: a systematic review and meta-analysis. Int Urol Nephrol. 2015;47:527–35 [M].

[38] Lu Y, Liu X, Deng Q, et al. Continuous lead exposure increases blood pressure but does not alter kidney function in adults 20-44 years of age in a lead-polluted region of China. Kidney Blood Press Res. 2015;40(3):207–14 [C].

[39] Lv C, Xu Y, Wang J, et al. Dysplastic changes in erythroid precursors as a manifestation of lead poisoning: report of a case and review of literature. Int J Clin Exp Pathol. 2015;8(1):818–23 [A].

[40] Unterbuchner C, Ziegleder R, Graf B, et al. Magnesium-induced recurarisation after reversal of rocuronium-induced neuromuscular block with sugammadex. Acta Anaesthesiol Scand. 2015;59(4):536–40 [A].

[41] Gunier RB, Arora M, Jerrett M, et al. Manganese in teeth and neurodevelopment in young Mexican-American children. Environ Res. 2015;142:688–95 [C].

[42] Aschner JL, Anderson A, Slaughter JC, et al. Neuroimaging identifies increased manganese deposition in infants receiving parenteral nutrition. Am J Clin Nutr. 2015;102(6):1482–9 [c].

[43] Wang F, Zou Y, Shen Y, et al. Synergistic impaired effect between smoking and manganese dust exposure on pulmonary ventilation function in Guangxi manganese-exposed workers healthy cohort (GXMEWHC). PLoS One. 2015;10(2):e0116558 [c].

[44] Watchmaker J, Collins R, Chaney K. Allergic contact dermatitis to manganese in metallic implant. Dermatitis. 2015;26(3):149–50 [A].

[45] Searles Nielsen S, Checkoway H, Criswell SR, et al. Inducible nitric oxide synthase gene methylation and parkinsonism in manganese-exposed welders. Parkinsonism Relat Disord. 2015;21(4):355–60 [C].

[46] Bakouei S, Reisian F, Lamyian M, et al. High intake of manganese during second trimester, increases the risk of preterm delivery: a large scale cohort study. Glob J Health Sci. 2015;7(5):226–32 [C].

[47] Koirala S, Leinenkugel K. Notes from the field: acute mercury poisoning after home gold and silver smelting—Iowa, 2014. MMWR Morb Mortal Wkly Rep. 2015;64(49):1365–6 [S].

[48] Marques RC, Bernardi JV, Abreu L, et al. Neurodevelopment outcomes in children exposed to organic mercury from multiple sources in a tin-ore mine environment in Brazil. Arch Environ Contam Toxicol. 2015;68(3):432–41 [c].

[49] McKean SJ, Bartell SM, Hansen RL, et al. Prenatal mercury exposure, autism, and developmental delay, using pharmacokinetic combination of newborn blood concentrations and questionnaire data: a case control study. Environ Health. 2015;14:62 [C].

[50] George A, Kwatra KS, Chandra S, et al. Cutaneous mercury granuloma following accidental occupational exposure. Indian J Dermatol Venereol Leprol. 2015;81(1):57–9 [A].

[51] Cardenas A, Koestler DC, Houseman EA, et al. Differential DNA methylation in umbilical cord blood of infants exposed to mercury and arsenic in utero. Epigenetics. 2015;10(6):508–15 [C].

[52] Bregnbak D, Menné T, Thyssen JP. Allergic nickel dermatitis following an occupational accident involving a mechanical rodeo bull. Contact Dermatitis. 2015;73(2):129–30 [A].

[53] Bangsgaard N, Thyssen JP, Hald M. Occupational hand eczema caused by nickel allergy and semi-quantified by dimethylglyoxime testing of the skin. Contact Dermatitis. 2015;73(1):65–7 [A].

[54] Chen K, Liao QL, Ma ZW, et al. Association of soil arsenic and nickel exposure with cancer mortality rates, a town-scale ecological study in Suzhou, China. Environ Sci Pollut Res Int. 2015;22(7):5395–404 [C].

[55] Muris J, Goossens A, Goncalo M, et al. Sensitization to palladium and nickel in Europe and the relationship with oral disease and dental alloys. Contact Dermatitis. 2015;72:286–96 [C].

[56] Terra RM, Bellato RT, Teixeira LR, et al. Safety and systemic consequences of pleurodesis with three different doses of silver nitrate in patients with malignant pleural effusion. Respiration. 2015;89(4):276–83 [c].

[57] de Souza MC, Stepavoi G. Case report: beware the silver nitrate stick—a risk factor for bisphosphonate-related osteonecrosis of the Jaw (BRONJ). Dent Update. 2015;42(8):735–6 738–40, 743 [A].

[58] Ghaderi A, Vahdati-Mashhadian N, Oghabian Z, et al. Thallium exists in opioid poisoned patients. Daru. 2015;23:39 [c].

[59] Sojáková M, Zigrai M, Karaman A, et al. Thallium intoxication. Case report. Neuro Endocrinol Lett. 2015;36(4):311–5 [A].

[60] Li S, Huang W, Duan Y, et al. Human fatality due to thallium poisoning: autopsy, microscopy, and mass spectrometry assays. J Forensic Sci. 2015;60(1):247–51 [A].

[61] Arzuaga X, Gehlhaus M, Strong J. Modes of action associated with uranium induced adverse effects in bone function and development. Toxicol Lett. 2015;236:123–30 [M].

[62] Chen B, Luo J, Hendryx M, et al. Zinc compound air releases from toxics release inventory facilities and cardiovascular disease mortality rates. Environ Res. 2015;142:96–103 [C].

[63] Arikan I, Namdar ND, Kahraman C, et al. Assessment of arsenic levels in body samples and chronic exposure in people using water with a high concentration of arsenic: a field study in Kutahya. Asian Pac J Cancer Prev. 2015;16(8):3183–8 [c].

Metal Antagonists

Joshua P. Gray*,1, *Sidhartha D. Ray*†

*Department of Science, United States Coast Guard Academy, New London, CT, USA
†Department of Pharmaceutical Sciences, Manchester University College of Pharmacy, Natural and Health Sciences,
Fort Wayne, IN, USA
1Corresponding author: joshua.p.gray@uscga.edu

COMBINATION THERAPIES

Combination therapies of metal antagonists are sometimes employed, such as combinations of deferoxamine and deferiprone or deferasirox and deferoxamine. Studies involving such combinations are described in this section.

A review discusses iron chelation therapy in transfusion-dependent thalassemia patients, reviews the mechanism of iron overload in the disease, and discusses the relative advantages and disadvantages of the chelators [1R]. An extensive review discusses the three iron chelating agents, deferoxamine, deferiprone, and deferasirox, highlighting methods to evaluate efficacy and risks and complications associated with the treatments [2R]. Another review discusses the use of chelators in metal intoxication, highlighting some of the adverse effects associated with treatment [3R]. Lead, copper, and mercury chelation are discussed in a review of metal chelators [4r].

Deferiprone and deferoxamine (group A) were compared with deferiprone and deferasirox (group B) in a prospective randomized clinical trial of 96 young beta thalassemia patients with severe iron overload [5C]. Initial gastrointestinal symptoms occurred in 11 (group A) and 8 (group B) patients. Neutropenia occurred in 3 (6.2%) and 5 (10.4%) patients, respectively, and was reversed by decreasing the deferiprone dose. Other adverse effects included arthralgia in 9 (18.7%) and 8 (16.6%) patients, ALT increase greater than threefold in 3 (6.25%) and 4 (8.33%), serum creatinine >33% above baseline in two occasions in 1 (2.08%) and 3 (6.2%), in groups A and B, respectively. Skin rash was reported in 2 (4.16%) of group B patients only. No adverse effects required the discontinuation of the study.

Deferiprone and deferasirox combination therapy for the treatment of iron overload in patients with beta thalassemia was evaluated for safety and efficacy in a trial of 36 patients (aged 13 ± 6.9 years). Adverse effects included transient gastrointestinal effects ($n=8$, 22%), persistent abdominal pain/diarrhea ($n=1$, who was discontinued for deferasirox), joint symptoms ($n=8$, 22%, of which 2 patients were discontinued for deferiprone), elevated AST/ALT enzymes ($n=4$, 11%, of which all were managed with temporary interruption of deferasirox treatment), and inconsistent elevation of creatine to >33% above baseline ($n=9$, 25%) [6c]. One patient experienced transient proteinuria.

HYPERION, an open-label single-arm prospective phase 2 study, evaluated combination deferasirox (average 30.5 mg/kg/day) and deferoxamine (average 36.3 mg/kg/day) high-dose treatment followed by deferasirox monotherapy upon clinical improvement in patients with severe transfusional myocardial siderosis [7c]. 90% ($n=54$ of 60 total) of the patients experienced an adverse effect. Adverse effects that led to discontinuation included abdominal pain ($n=2$), arthritis ($n=1$), drug rash with eosinophilia and systemic symptoms ($n=1$), and pruritus ($n=1$). Adverse effects that led to dose adjustment or interruption included urinary protein/creatinine ratio increase ($n=6$), abdominal pain ($n=5$), diarrhea ($n=5$), pyrexia ($n=4$), nausea ($n=3$), influenza ($n=3$), and blood creatinine increase ($n=3$).

A review discusses iron and oxidative stress in cardiomyopathy resulting from thalassemia [8R]. The authors stress the value of combination therapies such as deferasirox and deferiprone to prevent exposure of the heart to labile iron, reduce cardiac toxicity, and improve cardiac function.

An experimental paper discusses the mechanism of synergy between deferiprone and deferasirox, suggesting that one chelator has the physicochemical properties required to enter cells, chelate the intracellular iron, and subsequently donate the iron to the second "sink" chelator [9E]. These data suggest that the deferasirox dose required for a half-maximum effect can be reduced by 3.8-fold when only 1 μM deferiprone is added.

AMMONIUM TETRATHIOMOLYBDATE

Gastrointestinal

Emesis occurred after IV (2 dogs) and oral administration (3 dogs) in a pharmacologic evaluation of ammonium tetrathiomolybdate in 8 adult Beagles and Beagle crossbreds [10E]. The dogs received ammonium tetrathiomolybdate (1 mg/kg) IV and orally in a randomized crossover study. Serum copper concentrations increased significantly after IV and oral administration, suggesting the mobilization of tissue copper.

DEFERASIROX [SEDA-32, 426; SEDA-33, 466; SEDA-34, 368; SEDA-35, 420; SEDA-36, 323; SEDA-37, 259]

A review focuses on the use of deferasirox for the treatment of non-transfusional hemosiderosis in patients in the United States since its approval by the U.S. FDA in 2013 [11C]. The authors conclude that drug-related adverse effects were manageable, self-resolving, and typically did not require discontinuation of therapy.

Hematologic

Blood serum concentrations of deferasirox measured by HPLC were found to vary greatly in a trial of 80 patients with transfusion-dependent anemias [12c]. Deferasirox blood serum levels were inversely correlated with UGT1A1*28 polymorphism in patients with lean body mass below the media (p for interaction $= 0.05$).

Deferasirox, but not deferoxamine, stimulates reactive oxygen species signaling which leads to the differentiation of hematopoietic stem cells in vitro [13E]. These data suggest a mechanism of action unrelated to the iron chelation properties of deferasirox.

Gastrointestinal

A review article discusses the effect of gastrointestinal disturbances on patient compliance with deferasirox treatment and suggests strategies to increase compliance [14R]. Nausea, vomiting, diarrhea, and abdominal pain were common side effects observed in a retrospective study (February 2008–June 2012) of eight hemodialysis patients with end-stage renal disease prescribed deferasirox (15 mg/kg/day) for transfusion-induced iron overload [15c].

Five patients ($n = 74$) experienced adverse events in a 1-year nonrandomized extension to the CORDELIA study of patients with myocardial siderosis [16c]. Side effects included upper abdominal pain ($n = 5$) and diarrhea ($n = 4$). Mild, transient diarrhea ($n = 5$) and nausea ($n = 2$) were observed in an 12-month open-label, prospective, phase 2 study ($n = 10$) investigating deferasirox (10 ± 5 mg/kg/day) in patients with hereditary hemochromatosis and iron overload [17c].

Nausea (9.0%) and abdominal discomfort (8.3%) were observed in a multicenter DE02 trial ($n = 76$) investigating the safety, efficacy, and impact of deferasirox on iron homeostasis after allogenic hematopoietic stem cell transplant [18c]. Abdominal pain ($n = 23$, 38.3%) and diarrhea ($n = 16$, 26.7%) occurred in Taiwanese patients aged ≥ 2 years with transfusion-dependent beta-thalassemia whose serum ferritin levels were greater than 1000 ng/mL, who had started deferasirox since December 2005 [19c].

Liver

Reversible transaminitis occurred in 53% of patients ($n = 62$) in a retrospective study of children treated with deferasirox for sickle cell disease [20c]. Five patients ($n = 74$) experienced adverse events in a 1-year nonrandomized extension to the CORDELIA study of patients with myocardial siderosis [16c]. Side effects included upper abdominal pain ($n = 5$), increased ALT ($n = 8$), and increased aspartate aminotransferase ($n = 8$). Acute liver failure occurred in a 12-year-old girl with congenital dyserythropoietic anemia who had been treated with deferasirox [21A]. For 3 months prior, she had received deferasirox (26 mg/kg/day) due to iron overload (537.6 ng/mL). The patient was treated with N-acetyl cysteine on the second admission day and was followed by return of bilirubin, transaminases, and INR to baseline levels. NAC was halted after 5 days.

Urinary Tract

Five patients ($n = 74$) experienced adverse events in a 1-year nonrandomized extension to the CORDELIA study of patients with myocardial siderosis [16c]. Side effects increased blood creatinine ($n = 9$) and proteinuria ($n = 4$). Fanconi syndrome developed in 5 of 57 transfusion-dependent thalassemic patients receiving deferasirox after 6.9 ± 1.8 years of follow-up [22c]. Fanconi syndrome manifested with proximal renal tubular acidosis and hypophosphatemia, which required treatment and/or stoppage of treatment with deferasirox. Deferasirox had significant but reversible effects on renal hemodynamics for up to 2 years of treatment in a phase 1, open-label study in beta-thalassemia major patients with iron overload [23c]. Mean GFR and RPF declined from baseline to week 8 in a short-term study ($n = 11$), and a similar effect was found in a long-term study ($n = 5$), with mean GFR and RPF declining to week 52 (-17.7% and -26.1%, respectively).

Increased serum creatinine (23.5%) was observed in a 1-year, open-label, single-arm, phase 2 trial performed with deferasirox (10–40 mg/kg/day) ($n=102$; 42 with myelodysplastic syndromes, 29 with aplastic anemia, and 31 with other rare anemias) [24c]. Increased serum creatinine was primarily found in the myelodysplastic syndrome patients. Increased blood creatinine (26.5%) was observed in a multicenter DE02 trial ($n=76$) investigating the safety, efficacy, and impact of deferasirox on iron homeostasis after allogenic hematopoietic stem cell transplant [18c].

Skin

Skin rashes ($n=29$, 48.3%) occurred in Taiwanese patients aged ≥ 2 years with transfusion-dependent beta-thalassemia whose serum ferritin levels were greater than 1000 ng/mL, who had started deferasirox since December 2005 [19c]. Erythematous pruritic skin rashes developed 6 days after the initiation of treatment with deferasirox (750 mg/kg/day) in a 22-year-old female with thalassemia major [25A]. The rash started from the neck and spread over the whole body. On day 9, oral deferasirox was halted, and the patient was started on oral antihistaminics. The rashes subsided gradually, and the patient recovered by the ninth day after discontinuation of deferasirox.

Genotoxicity

Deferasirox significantly reduced the mitotic index value of bone marrow cells in human peripheral lymphocytes and the bone marrow of rats treated for 24 hour (500 mg/kg bw) [26E].

Age

Abdominal pain (41%), nausea (31%), vomiting (15%), jaundice (15%), and elevated serum creatinine (11.5%) were observed in a prospective study of pediatric thalassemia ($n=100$ children within 1 year of age 9) [27c].

DEFERIPRONE [SEDA-15, 1054; SEDA-32, 427; SEDA-33, 468; SEDA-34, 370; SEDA-35, 422; SEDA-36, 327; SEDA-37, 264]

Sensory Systems

Cerebellar ataxia, hypertonia, and bilateral cataract occurred in an 11-year-old boy with thalassemia major taking deferiprone [28A].

Age

Hemophagocytosis with cytopenia ($n=1$), neutropenia ($n=2$), thrombocytopenia ($n=2$), elevated alanine aminotransferase ($n=5$), elevated serum creatinine ($n=1$), proteinuria ($n=1$), and gastrointestinal discomfort ($n=4$) were identified adverse effects in a 3-year

study of children (9 with beta-thalassemia major and 33 with beta-thalassemia hemoglobin E; aged 3–18 years old) given daily oral deferiprone (50–100 mg/kg/day) combined with 40 mg/kg/dose subcutaneous desferrioxamine twice weekly [29c].

No adverse effects were detected in a safety profile study of nine children (four males) diagnosed with thalassemia ($n=8$) or hereditary spherocytosis ($n=1$) with serum ferritin >1000 microgram/L and treated with oral deferiprone [30c].

Hematologic

Neutropenia ($n=11$; incidence rate 6.5 per 100 patient-years) and severe neutropenia (agranulocytosis) ($n=5$; incidence rate 2.9 per 100 patient-years) occurred in a retrospective population-based cohort study of pediatric thalassemia patients from Hong Kong who had been treated with deferiprone [31c]. The patients also experienced severe arthropathy, elevated liver enzymes, and mild thrombocytopenia. The authors suggest that Chinese children might be more at risk for agranulocytosis and neutropenia in simultaneous combined therapy.

DEFEROXAMINE/DESFERRIOXAMINE [SEDA-15, 1058; SEDA-32, 429; SEDA-33, 471; SEDA-34, 371; SEDA-35, 423; SEDA-37, 265]

Nervous System

Deferoxamine-induced retinopathy was discussed in a review of the literature focused on multimodal technologies for retinal imaging [32r].

Hematologic

A model of deferoxamine dose optimization concluded that therapeutic intervention is not effective if >60% of doses are missed [33E]. The authors state that "poor quality of execution is preferable over drug holidays." An experimental study of HepG2 human liver cells demonstrated that deferoxamine stabilized low-density lipoprotein receptor mRNA and may be responsible for the hypocholesterolemic effect of iron reduction [34E].

DEFERITAZOLE (FORMERLY FBS0701)

Deferitazole is an orally active iron chelator which is a polyether derivative of desferrithiocin analogs. It has entered phase 1 and phase 2 clinical trials [35A]. Chelated iron (III)(deferitazole)$_2$ does not redox cycle.

HYDROXYUREA [SEDA-36, 330; SEDA-37, 266]

Hydroxyurea is used to treat sickle cell anemia patients and functions by inducing the expression of fetal hemoglobin. However, 25% of patients do not respond to hydroxyurea. A review discussed emerging drugs for sickle cell anemia treatments [36R]. A 1-year study of 48 patients with sickle cell disease with hydroxyurea (10 mg/kg/day) did not identify any significant side effects [37c].

Fever

A cross-sectional study of patients treated with hydroxyurea in an internal medicine department between 2006 and 2012 and a literature search identified 38 cases of hydroxyurea-induced fever [38A]. The fever appeared after a median duration of 21 days of treatment, with one-third of the patients presenting with either lung disease or hepatitis. Upon withdrawal of hydroxyurea, the fever disappeared in a median of 24 hours.

Myelotoxicity

Transient myelotoxicity was observed in 4.8% of 203 patients with HbSbeta(+)-thalassemia (IVS1-5(G → C) mutation) undergoing hydroxyurea treatment at 10 mg/kg/day [39c].

Dermal

Acral keratoses, psoriasiform plaques, and leucocytoclastic vasculitis were reported in a 69-year-old woman 4 years after commencing hydroxyurea [40A]. Upon increasing the dose of hydroxyurea, the lesions ulcerated, whereas upon cessation of treatment, rapid improvement occurred. Oral ulceration occurred in a patient 12 days after administration of the drug [41A].

D-PENICILLAMINE [SEDA-15, 2729; SEDA-32, 430; SEDA-33, 472; SEDA-34, 372; SEDA-35, 424; SEDA-36, 330; SEDA-37, 267]

Combination therapy of D-penicillamine plus zinc sulfate was associated with a significantly higher mortality rate compared to all other combination therapies (16.3% vs. 4.7%; RR: 3.51, 95% CI 1.54–8.00; $p < 0.001$) [42M]. The authors argue that any combination treatment involving zinc acetate should be avoided.

Dermal

Elastosis perforans serpiginosa and pseudopseudoxanthoma elasticum were diagnosed in a 57-year-old woman treated with D-penicillamine for 25 years [43A]. She reported a 5-month history of asymptomatic cutaneous lesions on her groin and a slow progressive thickening involving the neck and axillae which started 10 years prior. D-penicillamine deposits were detected in the affected skin.

Tense vesicubullous lesions filled with clear and hemorrhagic fluid over trauma-prone sites were detected in a 15-year-old girl treated for 2.5 years with 3 g/day D-penicillamine for Wilson's disease [44A]. These lesions ruptured in 7–10 days and healed with scarring within 1–2 months. Severe generalized dystonia was also detected involving the face, jaw, neck, trunk and limbs, with rigidity, and deep tendon jerks were difficult to elicit. Upon reduction of the dose of D-penicillamine to 1.5 g/day, her skin lesions improved over a period of 4–6 months.

Vesicubullous lesions over trauma-prone areas were detected in a 29-year-old man treated with D-penicillamine at 3 g/day for 4 years. The lesions healed with milia formation and scarring [44A]. Fragmented elastic fibers in the reticular dermis were detected in skin biopsies. Upon reduction of the dose of D-penicillamine to 1 g/day, the skin lesions significantly improved over 6 months.

GI

Elastosis perforans serpiginosa was diagnosed in a 32-year-old Chinese man treated with D-penicillamine for 2 years [45A]. The condition resolved upon treatment with 7.6% 5-aminolevulinic acid induced photodynamic therapy by a LED light of 633 nm at 130 J/cm^2, three sessions, 1-week interval.

Neurological

An experimental paper investigated the mechanism of neurological worsening in a mouse model of elevated copper [46E]. Free copper and hydroxyl radical were increased in the stratum of mice treated with D-penicillamine but not tetrathiomolybdate treatment, suggesting that D-penicillamine contributes to neurological deterioration, despite its chelation effects.

Silymarin

Silymarin is an extract from *Silybum marianum* (milk thistle) which contains various flavonolignans (including silybin). It is used as an herbal remedy for liver treatment. An extensive review discusses the potential mechanisms of action of silymarin, including direct scavenging of Fe and Cu in the gut, prevention of free radical formation by inhibition of ROS-producing enzymes, activation of nrf2 pathway genes, blocking NF-kappaB pathways, activating heat shock proteins, and affecting the microenvironment of the gut [47R]. A study of 80 beta thalassemic children (serum ferritin levels more than 1000 ng/mL) found that the group treated with both deferiprone (75 mg/kg/day, three times per day) and silymarin (oral silymarin in the form of Legalon tablets 140 mg, 1 hour before each meal (three times daily)) ($n=40$) had lower serum ferritin (989.5 ± 178.57 versus 1260 ± 212.26 ng/mL) and iron (156.55 ± 21.42 versus 172.40 ± 24.51) than the group treated with deferiprone alone ($n=40$) [48R].

A review article discusses some of the adverse effects of silymarin [48R]. Drug–drug interactions and liver toxicity by interference of metabolism of co-treated drugs due to induction or inhibition of cytochrome P450 is a concern. Studies suggest that the maximum recommended daily dose is 420 mg/day.

POLYSTYRENE SULPHONATES [SEDA-15, 2894; SEDA-32, 433; SEDA-33, 474; SEDA-34, 373; SEDA-35, 427; SEDA-36, 333; SEDA-37, 268]

Electrolyte disturbances and an increase in gastrointestinal side effects were noted in the test group of a double-blind randomized clinical trial of patients with mild hyperkalemia ($5.0–5.9$ mEq/L) ($n=33$) assigned either a placebo or sodium polystyrene sulfonate (30 g once daily for 7 days) [49c].

TRIENTINE [SEDA-15, 3508; SEDA-32, 431; SEDA-33, 474; SEDA-34, 373; SEDA-35, 427; SEDA-36, 333; SEDA-37, 267]

Serum ALT and AST levels fluctuated over the course of a 12-month study in two of eight patients participating in a clinical trial (22–71 years of age, 7 male) on a daily dose of trientine (15 mg/kg) for 12 months for the treatment of Wilson disease [50c].

Gastrointestinal

Active ileitis and moderate to severe pancolitis ceased upon withdrawal of trientine treatment and recurred upon rechallenge in a 40-year-old woman who had been on trientine therapy for 1 month for the treatment of Wilson disease [51A]. Upon switching to zinc therapy, the second incidence of colitis gradually resolved.

ZINC

Zinc salts function by blocking intestinal copper absorption [52c]. Zinc acetate induces the expression of enterocyte metallothionein, an endogenous chelator of metals that traps copper into enterocytes and causes the elimination of copper in the feces or with shedding of intestinal epithelial cells [53c].

1-(N-ACETYL-6-AMINOHEXYL)-3-HYDROXY-2-METHYLPYRIDIN-4-ONE (CM1)

A novel orally bioavailable chelator has been identified [54E]. The chelator forms a neutral iron (III) complex under physiological conditions. CM1 was tested and found to be orally active in a rat model.

References

[1] Saliba AN, Harb AR, Taher AT. Iron chelation therapy in transfusion-dependent thalassemia patients: current strategies and future directions. J Blood Med. 2015;6:197–209 [R].

[2] Saliba AN, El Rassi F, Taher AT. Clinical monitoring and management of complications related to chelation therapy in patients with beta-thalassemia. Expert Rev Hematol. 2016;9(2):151–68 [R].

[3] Aaseth J, Skaug MA, Cao Y, et al. Chelation in metal intoxication—principles and paradigms. J Trace Elem Med Biol. 2015;31:260–6 [R].

[4] Cao Y, Skaug MA, Andersen O, et al. Chelation therapy in intoxications with mercury, lead and copper. J Trace Elem Med Biol. 2015;31:188–92 [r].

[5] Elalfy MS, Adly AM, Wali Y, et al. Efficacy and safety of a novel combination of two oral chelators deferasirox/deferiprone over deferoxamine/deferiprone in severely iron overloaded young beta thalassemia major patients. Eur J Haematol. 2015;95(5):411–20 [C].

[6] Totadri S, Bansal D, Bhatia P, et al. The deferiprone and deferasirox combination is efficacious in iron overloaded patients with beta-thalassemia major: a prospective, single center, open-label study. Pediatr Blood Cancer. 2015;62(9):1592–6 [c].

[7] Aydinok Y, Kattamis A, Cappellini MD, et al. Effects of deferasirox-deferoxamine on myocardial and liver iron in patients with severe transfusional iron overload. Blood. 2015;125(25):3868–77 [c].

[8] Berdoukas V, Coates TD, Cabantchik ZI. Iron and oxidative stress in cardiomyopathy in thalassemia. Free Radic Biol Med. 2015;88 (Pt A):3–9 [R].

[9] Vlachodimitropoulou Koumoutsea E, Garbowski M, Porter J. Synergistic intracellular iron chelation combinations: mechanisms and conditions for optimizing iron mobilization. Br J Haematol. 2015;170(6):874–83 [E].

[10] Chan CM, Langlois DK, Buchweitz JP, et al. Pharmacologic evaluation of ammonium tetrathiomolybdate after intravenous and oral administration to healthy dogs. Am J Vet Res. 2015;76(5):445–53 [E].

[11] Ricchi P, Marsella M. Profile of deferasirox for the treatment of patients with non-transfusion-dependent thalassemia syndromes. Drug Des Devel Ther. 2015;9:6475–82 [C].

[12] Mattioli F, Puntoni M, Marini V, et al. Determination of deferasirox plasma concentrations: do gender, physical and genetic differences affect chelation efficacy? Eur J Haematol. 2015;94(4):310–7 [c].

[13] Tataranni T, Agriesti F, Mazzoccoli C, et al. The iron chelator deferasirox affects redox signalling in haematopoietic stem/progenitor cells. Br J Haematol. 2015;170(2):236–46 [E].

[14] Nolte F, Angelucci E, Breccia M, et al. Updated recommendations on the management of gastrointestinal disturbances during iron chelation therapy with Deferasirox in transfusion dependent patients with myelodysplastic syndrome—emphasis on optimized dosing schedules and new formulations. Leuk Res. 2015;39(10):1028–33 [R].

[15] Chen CH, Shu KH, Yang Y. Long-term effects of an oral iron chelator, deferasirox, in hemodialysis patients with iron overload. Hematology. 2015;20(5):304–10 [c].

[16] Pennell DJ, Porter JB, Piga A, et al. Sustained improvements in myocardial T2* over 2 years in severely iron-overloaded patients with beta thalassemia major treated with deferasirox or deferoxamine. Am J Hematol. 2015;90(2):91–6 [c].

[17] Cancado R, Melo MR, de Moraes Bastos R, et al. Deferasirox in patients with iron overload secondary to hereditary hemochromatosis: results of a 1-yr Phase 2 study. Eur J Haematol. 2015;95(6):545–50 [c].

[18] Jaekel N, Lieder K, Albrecht S, et al. Efficacy and safety of deferasirox in non-thalassemic patients with elevated ferritin levels after allogeneic hematopoietic stem cell transplantation. Bone Marrow Transplant. 2016;51(1):89–95 [c].

[19] Chang HH, Lu MY, Peng SS, et al. The long-term efficacy and tolerability of oral deferasirox for patients with transfusion-dependent beta-thalassemia in Taiwan. Ann Hematol. 2015;94(12):1945–52 [c].

[20] Tsouana E, Kaya B, Gadong N, et al. Deferasirox for iron chelation in multitransfused children with sickle cell disease; long-term experience in the East London clinical haemoglobinopathy network. Eur J Haematol. 2015;94(4):336–42 [c].

[21] Ling G, Pinsk V, Golan-Tripto I, et al. Acute liver failure in a pediatric patient with congenital dysery-thropoietic anemia type I treated with deferasirox. Hematol Rep. 2015;7(3):5987 [A].

[22] Capiello A. Elderly men should undergo an annual screening for prostate cancer. Infirm Aux. 1989;62(3):15 [c].

[23] Piga A, Fracchia S, Lai ME, et al. Deferasirox effect on renal haemodynamic parameters in patients with transfusion-dependent beta thalassaemia. Br J Haematol. 2015;168(6):882–90 [c].

[24] Kohgo Y, Urabe A, Kilinc Y, et al. Deferasirox decreases liver iron concentration in iron-overloaded patients with myelodysplastic syndromes, aplastic anemia and other rare anemias. Acta Haematol. 2015;134(4):233–42 [c].

[25] Sharma A, Arora E, Singh H. Hypersensitivity reaction with deferasirox. J Pharmacol Pharmacother. 2015;6(2):105–6 [A].

[26] Arslan M, Ila HB. Deferasirox-induced cytogenetic responses. Environ Toxicol Pharmacol. 2015;39(2):787–93 [E].

[27] Ejaz MS, Baloch S, Arif F. Efficacy and adverse effects of oral chelating therapy (deferasirox) in multi-transfused Pakistani children with beta-thalassemia major. Pak J Med Sci. 2015;31(3):621–5 [c].

[28] Parakh N, Sharma R, Prakash O, et al. Neurological complications and cataract in a child with thalassemia major treated with deferiprone. J Pediatr Hematol Oncol. 2015;37(7):e433–4 [A].

[29] Songdej D, Sirachainan N, Wongwerawattanakoon P, et al. Combined chelation therapy with daily oral deferiprone and twice-weekly subcutaneous infusion of desferrioxamine in children with beta-thalassemia: 3-year experience. Acta Haematol. 2015;133(2):226–36 [c].

[30] Chuansumrit A, Songdej D, Sirachainan N, et al. Safety profile of a liquid formulation of deferiprone in young children with transfusion-induced iron overload: a 1-year experience. Paediatr Int Child Health. 2016;36(3):209–13 2046905515Y0000000040. [c].

[31] Botzenhardt S, Sing CW, Wong IC, et al. Safety profile of oral iron chelator deferiprone in Chinese children with transfusion-dependent thalassaemia. Curr Drug Saf. 2016;11:137–44 [c].

[32] Di Nicola M, Barteselli G, Dell'Arti L, et al. Functional and structural abnormalities in deferoxamine retinopathy: a review of the literature. Biomed Res Int. 2015;2015:249617 [r].

[33] Bellanti F, Del Vecchio GC, Putti MC, et al. Model-based optimisation of deferoxamine chelation therapy. Pharm Res. 2016;33(2):498–509 [E].

[34] Guillemot J, Asselin MC, Susan-Resiga D, et al. Deferoxamine stimulates LDLR expression and LDL uptake in HepG2 cells. Mol Nutr Food Res. 2016;60(3):600–8 [E].

[35] Hider RC, Kong X, Abbate V, et al. Deferitazole, a new orally active iron chelator. Dalton Trans. 2015;44(11):5197–204 [A].

[36] Singh PC, Ballas SK. Emerging drugs for sickle cell anemia. Expert Opin Emerg Drugs. 2015;20(1):47–61 [R].

[37] Keikhaei B, Yousefi H, Bahadoram M. Hydroxyurea: clinical and hematological effects in patients with sickle cell anemia. Glob J Health Sci. 2016;8(3):47935 [c].

[38] Doutrelon C, Lazaro E, Ribeiro E, et al. Hydrocycarbamide induced fever: four cases and literature review. Rev Med Interne. 2015;36(2):73–7 [A].

[39] Dehury S, Purohit P, Patel S, et al. Low and fixed dose of hydroxyurea is effective and safe in patients with HbSbeta(+) thalassemia with IVS1-5(G→C) mutation. Pediatr Blood Cancer. 2015;62(6):1017–23 [c].

[40] Worley B, Glassman SJ. Acral keratoses and leucocytoclastic vasculitis occurring during treatment of essential thrombocythaemia with hydroxyurea. Clin Exp Dermatol. 2016;41(2):166–9 [A].

[41] Badawi M, Almazrooa S, Azher F, et al. Hydroxyurea-induced oral ulceration. Oral Surg Oral Med Oral Pathol Oral Radiol. 2015;120(6):e232–4 [A].

[42] Chen JC, Chuang CH, Wang JD, et al. Combination therapy using chelating agent and zinc for Wilson's disease. J Med Biol Eng. 2015;35(6):697–708 [M].

[43] Neri I, Gurioli C, Raggi MA, et al. Detection of D-penicillamine in skin lesions in a case of dermal elastosis after a previous long-term treatment for Wilson's disease. J Eur Acad Dermatol Venereol. 2015;29(2):383–6 [A].

[44] Khandpur S, Jain N, Singla S, et al. D-penicillamine induced degenerative dermopathy. Indian J Dermatol. 2015;60(4):406–9 [A].

[45] Wang D, Liang J, Xu J, et al. Effective treatment of d-penicillamine induced elastosis perforans serpiginosa with ALA-PDT. Photodiagnosis Photodyn Ther. 2015;12(1):140–2 [A].

[46] Zhang JW, Liu JX, Hou HM, et al. Effects of tetrathiomolybdate and penicillamine on brain hydroxyl radical and free copper levels: a microdialysis study in vivo. Biochem Biophys Res Commun. 2015;458(1):82–5 [E].

[47] Surai PF. Silymarin as a natural antioxidant: an overview of the current evidence and perspectives. Antioxidants (Basel). 2015;4(1):204–47 [R].

[48] Hagag AA, Elfaragy MS, Elrifaey SM, et al. Therapeutic value of combined therapy with deferiprone and silymarin as iron chelators in Egyptian children with beta thalassemia major. Infect Disord Drug Targets. 2015;15(3):189–95 [R].

[49] Lepage L, Dufour AC, Doiron J, et al. Randomized clinical trial of sodium polystyrene sulfonate for the treatment of mild hyperkalemia in CKD. Clin J Am Soc Nephrol. 2015;10(12):2136–42 [c].

[50] Ala A, Aliu E, Schilsky ML. Prospective pilot study of a single daily dosage of trientine for the treatment of Wilson disease. Dig Dis Sci. 2015;60(5):1433–9 [c].

[51] Boga S, Jain D, Schilsky ML. Trientine induced colitis during therapy for Wilson disease: a case report and review of the literature. BMC Pharmacol Toxicol. 2015;16:30 [A].

[52] Hoogenraad TU, Van den Hamer CJ. 3 Years of continuous oral zinc therapy in 4 patients with Wilson's disease. Acta Neurol Scand. 1983;67(6):356–64 [c].

[53] Sturniolo GC, Mestriner C, Irato P, et al. Zinc therapy increases duodenal concentrations of metallothionein and iron in Wilson's disease patients. Am J Gastroenterol. 1999;94(2):334–8 [c].

[54] Pangjit K, Banjerdpongchai R, Phisalaphong C, et al. Characterisation of a novel oral iron chelator: 1-(N-acetyl-6-aminohexyl)-3-hydroxy-2-methylpyridin-4-one. J Pharm Pharmacol. 2015;67(5):703–13 [E].

22

Antiseptic Drugs and Disinfectants

Dirk W. Lachenmeier[1]

Chemisches und Veterinäruntersuchungsamt (CVUA) Karlsruhe, Karlsruhe, Germany
[1]Corresponding author: lachenmeier@web.de

ALDEHYDES [SED-15, 1439, 1513; SEDA-31, 409; SEDA-32, 437; SEDA-33, 479; SEDA-34, 377; SEDA-36, 339; SEDA-37, 273]

Considering all disinfectants, aldehydes have a special status as they are able to pose occupational hazards even at very low concentrations in air (SEDA-36, 339; SEDA-37, 273). A novel observation during 2015 was the finding of potential formaldehyde intake due to use of electronic cigarettes [1E], which may contribute to cumulative human exposure. It has to be stressed that formaldehyde has not been directly contained in the liquids used for the electronic cigarettes (e.g. [2E]) but may only be formed when the electronic cigarette devices were set at extremely high voltages [1E].

Formaldehyde

Tumorigenicity

According to an updated assessment of the International Agency for Research on Cancer (IARC), formaldehyde was confirmed as carcinogenic to humans (Group 1). Formaldehyde causes cancer of the nasopharynx and leukemia [3S]. The IARC assessment and specifically the epidemiologic evidence on the association between formaldehyde exposure and risk of leukemia and other lymphohematopoietic malignancies have been previously discussed controversially [SEDA-36, 339; SEDA-37, 273]. A study in 43 formaldehyde-exposed workers compared to 51 unexposed workers in China found significantly lower circulating levels of two immune/inflammation markers, suggesting immunosuppression among the formaldehyde-exposed workers. The findings were judged as consistent with recently emerging understanding that immunosuppression might be associated with myeloid diseases [4c].

Teratogenicity

Using *ex vivo* and *in vitro* assays, it was demonstrated that formaldehyde (100 μM) may accumulate in the human placenta, cross to the fetal compartment, and affect human trophoblast differentiation and hormonal functions. These findings were suggested to corroborate the previous limited evidence in humans and animal models that formaldehyde may be associated with reproductive and developmental toxicity [5E].

Fertility

In a study of 114 male workers occupationally exposed to formaldehyde (0.22–2.91 mg/m^3 in air) compared to 76 controls, the semen quality assessed by several different parameters, especially sperm motion parameters, was significantly reduced. The results supported the hypothesis that formaldehyde exposure has negative effects on male reproduction [6c]. This association was also corroborated in an experiment in male rats that showed a dose-dependent (0.5, 5 and 10 mg/m^3 for 8 h/day) autopaghy in testicular tissue [7E].

Immunologic

In a retrospective analysis of patch test data (2003–2012) from a network of departments of dermatology in Germany, the results from 2248 nurses with occupational contact dermatitis (OCD) were compared to 2138 nurses without OCD. The results suggested that formaldehyde may have lost its particular importance in the health care sector, as an increased frequency of sensitization to formaldehyde among nurses with OCD was not observed. The age-standardized and sex-standardized reaction frequency for formaldehyde was 1.8% (95% CI: 1.3–2.3%) for nurses with OCD and 1.4% (95% CI: 0.7–2.1%) for nurses without OCD [8C]. In another retrospective analysis (1991–2011) of prick tests conducted in the context of the diagnosis of occupational contact urticarial and respiratory diseases in Finland, 21 patients out of 2703 (0.8%) had positive reactions to formaldehyde [9C]. A case of allergic contact dermatitis to formaldehyde contained in an alco-swab used for skin disinfecting was described. The formaldehyde content contained in the swabs was very low (76–96 ppm) and unlabeled [2A].

Glutaraldehyde (Glutaral)

Cardiovascular

Autologous pericardium may be treated with glutaraldehyde, but with treatment times over 60 min, excessive calcification of implants was observed. In a new case, pericardial calcification and progressive mitral stenosis were observed in a patient receiving an autologous pericardium treated with 0.625% glutaraldehyde for only 15 min and rinsed with saline for 6 min. The underlying mechanism of calcification is unclear [10A].

Gastrointestinal

A case of glutaraldehyde-induced colitis in a 56-year-old man was described following treatment of polyps by endoscopic mucosal resection. The patient developed mild abdominal pain, high fever, diarrhea, and progressed into some bloody stools 10 h after the procedure. The diagnosis of glutaraldehyde colitis was based on glutaraldehyde disinfectant (2%) retained in the endoscope channels because of inadequate flushing and rinsing the endoscope [11A].

Respiratory

A case of glutaraldehyde-induced occupational asthma was presented. The patient had frequent exposure to glutaraldehyde (2.5%) while working in an endoscopy lab and developed chronic upper and lower respiratory tract symptoms [12A].

Immunologic

In a retrospective analysis of patch test data (2003–2012) from a network of departments of dermatology in Germany, a reaction to glutaraldehyde was positive in 68 patients (3.8%) out of a sample of 1796 nurses with occupational contact dermatitis [8C]. In another retrospective analysis (1991–2011) of prick tests conducted in the context of the diagnosis of occupational contact urticarial and respiratory diseases in Finland, only 2 patients out of 1214 (0.16%) had positive reactions to glutaraldehyde [9C].

GUANIDINES

Chlorhexidine [SED-15, 714; SEDA-31, 410; SEDA-32, 439; SEDA-33, 480; SEDA-34, 378; SEDA-36, 340; SEDA-37, 273]

Drug Formulations

Chlorhexidine is used extensively in oral hygiene but can cause staining of the teeth and oral mucosa and adversely affect taste but rarely causes pain [SEDA-30, 278; SEDA-31, 416; SEDA-34, 378; SEDA-36, 340; SEDA-37, 273]. In Denmark, 42 chlorhexidine-containing medicinal products were available at hospital pharmacies, the major use being skin disinfectants (n=19) [13r]. In another market survey of cosmetic products in Denmark, chlorhexidine was identified in 80 of 2251 products (3.6%) with major occurrence in hair products (57/760) and in cosmetic products aimed at female consumers [14E].

A review of the literature published between 2007 and 2014 on the use of chlorhexidine in endodontics confirmed its efficacy but also the possibility of tooth staining and formation of brown precipitate when its use is associated with sodium hypochlorite [15R]. In a clinical trial of different mouthwashes, side effects such as short-term anesthesia were reported in 50% of subjects of the group using 0.2% chlorhexidine gluconate mouthwash (n=20) [16c]. Another review of in vitro data pointed out that the cytotoxic activity of chlorhexidine to human cells is not fully known and requires further study, especially because an absence of in vivo data was detected [17R].

Skin

A guideline regarding skin antisepsis for central neuraxial blockade (CNB) was published by several associations in the UK and Ireland. Chlorhexidine 0.5% in alcohol was suggested to be used for skin antisepsis before CNB. The potential neurotoxicity (of either the chlorhexidine or the alcohol ingredient) was determined to be outweighed by the superiority in reducing surgical site infection [18S].

Immunologic

A case of anaphylactic reaction to chlorhexidine 5 min following its application (concentration not provided) in a 72-year-old woman prior to surgical incision was reported [19A]. In a retrospective analysis (1991–2011) of prick tests conducted in the context of the diagnosis of occupational contact urticarial and respiratory diseases in Finland, only 1 patient out of 337 (0.3%) had a positive reaction to chlorhexidine [9C]. The utility of a new commercial assay for the measurement of allergen-specific IgE (sIgE) in serum was evaluated in a study of 130 patients; measurement of the chlorhexidine sIgE levels correlated well with skin test results [20c].

Polyhexamethylene Guanidine [SEDA-36, 341; SEDA-37, 273]

Polyhexamethylene guanidine (PHMG) has been used as an antiseptic, especially for the suppression of hospital infection in the Russian Federation and as a disinfectant for sterilization of household humidifiers in Korea [SEDA-36, 341; SEDA-37, 273].

Respiratory

Further evidence was gathered on the association of the disinfectants PHMG and oligo(2-(2-ethoxy)ethoxyethyl)-guanidinium-chloride (PGH) with lung disease (see SEDA-36, 341 and SEDA-37, 273 for description of cases). A comprehensive humidifier disinfectant exposure characterization was conducted for 374 patients with lung disease in Korea; the exposure intensities for those using guanidine disinfectants were higher than those for the non-guanidine disinfectants, and the association between guanidine disinfectant exposure and the development of lung disease continues to be investigated [21c]. In a 3-week in vivo experiment in rats, PHMG-phosphate aerosol particles in nanometer size (mean diameter 93.4 ± 1.7 nm with 56% of particles <100 nm) showed pulmonary inflammation and fibrosis including increased inflammatory cytokines and fibronectin mRNA [22E]. Furthermore, an in vitro model (a bronchial air–liquid interface co-culture model) showed that PHMG-phosphate triggered reactive oxygen species generation, airway barrier injuries and inflammatory responses [22E]. These in vivo and in vitro results provided plausible corroborating evidence for a causal association between PHMG exposure and pulmonary fibrosis reported in epidemiological studies [22E].

Polyhexamethylene Biguanidine [SEDA-36, 341; SEDA-37, 273]

Polyhexamethylene biguanidine (PHMB) has been applied as a substitute for chlorhexidine in local anti-infective treatments but is also used in different nonmedical fields (e.g. swimming pool sanitizer) [SEDA-36, 341; SEDA-37, 273]. The Scientific Committee on Consumer Safety (SCCS) of the European Commission recently published the second revision of its opinion on the safety of PHMB and concluded that PHMB is not safe for consumers when used as a preservative in all cosmetic products up to the maximum concentration of 0.3% [23S,24S].

Immunologic

A case of contact urticarial syndrome in a 39-year-old man following the use of wet wipes containing PHMB (concentration not reported) for intimate hygiene was reported [25A]. A second case of contact dermatitis due to use of PHMB was reported in a 59-year-old female patient. The symptoms included a worsening condition of her bilateral leg ulcers, perilesional eczema and mild hand dermatitis a few days following the application of PHMB-containing wound irrigation solution and application of PHMB-containing wound gel (both containing 0.1% PHMB). Patch tests to 2.5% and 5% PHMB were positive. Following avoidance of PHMB containing products, the symptoms disappeared [26A].

Skin

In a prospective and open-cohort clinical study ($n=31$), patients who underwent cardiac surgery received PHMB-containing wound antiseptics (0.5%). In 2 out of 15 patients in the PHMB group, adverse events occurred including pruritus, erythema, or both around the surgical wound [27c].

CETRIMIDE [SEDA-24, 225]

Cetrimide is a quaternary ammonium disinfectant, which is toxic to the endothelial and epithelial cells, and contact with the eyes should be avoided [SEDA-24, 225]. Cetrimide has been sometimes used as antiseptic in cosmetics [28c].

Immunologic

In a study of 1000 patients presenting with signs of allergic contact dermatitis in India in 1997–2006, 55 (5.5%) were patch test positive for cetrimide [29C]. In a smaller study in India, 4 out of 50 patients (8%) were tested positive for cetrimide [28c]. An interesting case was presented regarding severe swelling and redness of the scrotal and penile skin of a patient following a prostate cancer-related biopsy procedure. The antiseptic solution contained chlorhexidine and cetrimide 0.2%/0.1%. Patch tests showed no reaction to chlorhexidine (0.5%) but were positive to cetrimonium bromide (0.5%), an ingredient of cetrimide. The authors warned about the possibility of mislabeling of chlorhexidine allergy, because the combination of the two antiseptic agents is common, but chlorhexidine allergy is much more well known than cetrimide allergy [30A].

BENZALKONIUM COMPOUNDS [SED-15, 421; SEDA-32, 440; SEDA-33, 481; SEDA-34, 379; SEDA-36, 341; SEDA-37, 273]

Due to a large number of benzalkonium chloride intoxications of domestic cats ($n=245$, 1989–2014) mainly due to household antibacterial cleaners or disinfectants being reported [31E], the use of such products in households with animals as well as in veterinary environments was questioned and warnings for cat-owners were suggested [32E].

Sensory Systems

It is believed that eye drops containing benzalkonium chloride as preservative may contribute to ocular surface disease [see also SEDA-36, 341; SEDA-37, 273]. *In vitro* research using monolayer and stratified human corneal–limbal epithelial cells suggested that benzalkonium chloride (0.01–0.015%) in anti-allergic eye drop formulations contributes to cytotoxic effects (measured as reduced cell viability) as well as increased paracellular permeability and loss of transcellular barrier function [33E]. In *ex vivo* experiments, benzalkonium chloride (0.001%) induced a high level of DNA damage in human trabecular meshwork cells with the level of DNA fragmentation (Comet test) being 2.4-fold higher in subjects older than 50 years than in younger subjects [34E]. Another *ex vivo* study with 0.01% benzalkonium chloride in rabbit corneas detected an increase in corneal erosion size and lactate concentration, as well as severe alteration of the corneal structure, including breakdown of the corneal barrier function [35E]. *In vivo* research in eyes of rats topically treated with 0.01% benzalkonium chloride twice daily for 1 month reported a slight increase in fibroblast density and a more compact collagen deposition in the bulbar subepithelial connective tissues [36E]. In another 30-day *in vivo* study in mice, corneal damage, increased inflammation and apoptosis and low cell viability were observed in the group treated with 0.02% benzalkonium chloride eye drops once daily [37E]. In cats domestically exposed (e.g. from household disinfectants residues) by ingestion or dermally to benzalkonium chloride ($n = 245$), the most common adverse effects were hypersalivation/drooling (54%), tongue ulceration (40%), hyperthermia (40%) and oral ulceration (23%) [31E].

Immunologic

In a retrospective analysis of patch test data (2003–2012) from a network of departments of dermatology in Germany, a reaction to benzalkonium chloride was positive in 20 patients (1.1%) out of a sample of 1782 nurses with occupational contact dermatitis [8C].

ETHYLENE OXIDE [SED-15, 1296; SEDA-29, 242; SEDA-34, 379; SEDA-36, 341; SEDA-37, 273]

Ethylene oxide is used directly in the gaseous form to sterilize drugs, hospital equipment, disposable and reusable medical items, packaging materials, foods and other items [SEDA-36, 341; SEDA-37, 273].

Management of Adverse Drug Reactions

During an incident in an ethylene oxide producing plant, ethylene oxide vapor was released under high pressure (approximately 12 000 ppm at 1-m distance from the leak). The results of model estimates and actual biomonitoring data in the operators involved in the accident suggest that respiratory protection with independently supplied air is not sufficient because systemic exposure resulting from dermal absorption may reach levels of concern (two of three operators had exposure to ethylene oxide one to two orders of magnitude over the Dutch occupational exposure limit of 0.5 ppm based on hemoglobin adduct results). The authors suggested additional risk management measures such as wearing chemical impervious suits to control dermal uptake of ethylene oxide [38A].

HALOGENS

Sodium Hypochlorite [SED-15, 3157; SEDA-28, 262; SEDA-34, 380; SEDA-36, 342; SEDA-37, 273]

Teeth

Sodium hypochlorite is used to irrigate root canals in dentistry and can cause many adverse reactions [SEDA-34, 380; SEDA-36, 342; SEDA-37, 273]. Guidelines for management of sodium hypochlorite extrusion injuries were formulated [39R,40R]. A sodium hypochlorite accident resulting in life-threatening airway obstruction was reported in a 42-old female patient undergoing routine root canal therapy with 3% sodium hypochlorite (12 ml over 1 h); the patient was treated with 3 days on mechanical ventilation and fully recovered without any skin necrosis or nerve deficits within 3 weeks. Careful injection without pressure, the use of proper dam isolation, and the use of endodontic needles were suggested to avoid this type of complication [41A]. Another case of a hypochlorite (concentration not reported) accident during root canal treatment was described, in which significant right-sided facial swelling, bruising and pain were present 3 h following the dental appointment. A full recovery was made by the patient with no surgical intervention required, but significant bruising and swelling were present up to 4 weeks following the incident [42A].

Skin

Atypical ulcerations (epidermal necrosis) of the penis were described in a patient who had been using a diluted sodium hypochlorite (concentration not reported) lotion several times per day for cleaning his genitals; the lesions resolved within 8 weeks after the patient stopped to use sodium hypochlorite [43A,44A].

Cardiovascular

A case of stress cardiomyopathy induced by acute inhalation of hypochlorite fumes was reported in a 72-year-old woman, who had used sodium hypochlorite cleaners for cleaning a drain (concentration not reported). It was hypothesized that acute respiratory distress induced by toxic exhalation and possibly following adrenergic surge may have led to acute apical transient dysfunction, resembling stress cardiomyopathy [45A].

IODOPHORS [SED-15, 1896; SEDA-31, 411; SEDA-32, 440; SEDA-33, 485; SEDA-34, 380; SEDA-36, 342; SEDA-37, 273]

Polyvinylpyrrolidone (Povidone) and Povidone–Iodine

Skin

A 75-year-old male developed postoperative pain, which was found to be related to erythema consistent with the application area of 10% povidone–iodine below a tourniquet. To avoid such chemical burns associated with tourniquet use, a waterproof barrier was suggested to prevent pooling and impregnation of the padding [46A].

Immunologic

In a retrospective analysis of patch test data (2003–2012) from a network of departments of dermatology in Germany, a reaction to povidone–iodine was positive in 150 patients (8.7%) out of a sample of 1723 nurses with occupational contact dermatitis [8C].

References

[1] Jensen RP, Luo W, Pankow JF, et al. Hidden formaldehyde in e-cigarette aerosols. N Engl J Med. 2015;372(4):392–4 [E].

[2] Hahn J, Monakhova YB, Hengen J, et al. Electronic cigarettes: overview of chemical composition and exposure estimation. Tob Induc Dis. 2014;12(1):23 [E].

[3] IARC Working Group on the Evaluation of Carcinogenic Risks to Humans. Formaldehyde. IARC Monogr Eval Carcinog Risks Hum. 2012;100F:401–35 [S].

[4] Seow WJ, Zhang L, Vermeulen R, et al. Circulating immune/inflammation markers in Chinese workers occupationally exposed to formaldehyde. Carcinogenesis. 2015;36(8):852–7 [c].

[5] Pidoux G, Gerbaud P, Guibourdenche J, et al. Formaldehyde crosses the human placenta and affects human trophoblast differentiation and hormonal functions. PLoS One. 2015;10(7): e0133506 [E].

[6] Wang HX, Li HC, Lv MQ, et al. Associations between occupation exposure to formaldehyde and semen quality, a primary study. Sci Rep. 2015;5:15874 [c].

[7] Han SP, Zhou DX, Lin P, et al. Formaldehyde exposure induces autophagy in testicular tissues of adult male rats. Environ Toxicol. 2015;30(3):323–31 [E].

[8] Molin S, Bauer A, Schnuch A, et al. Occupational contact allergy in nurses: results from the Information Network of Departments of Dermatology 2003-2012. Contact Dermatitis. 2015;72(3):164–71 [C].

[9] Helaskoski E, Suojalehto H, Kuuliala O, et al. Prick testing with chemicals in the diagnosis of occupational contact urticaria and respiratory diseases. Contact Dermatitis. 2015;72(1):20–32 [C].

[10] Fukunaga N, Matsuo T, Saji Y, et al. Mitral valve stenosis progression due to severe calcification on glutaraldehyde-treated autologous pericardium: word of caution for an attractive repair technique. Ann Thorac Surg. 2015;99(6):2203–5 [A].

[11] Wang X, Han Z, Li Y, et al. A case of acute glutaraldehyde-induced colitis following polyps treated by EMR. Int J Colorectal Dis. 2015;30(2):277–8 [A].

[12] Copeland S, Nugent K. Persistent and unusual respiratory findings after prolonged glutaraldehyde exposure. Int J Occup Environ Med. 2015;6(3):177–83 [A].

[13] Opstrup MS, Johansen JD, Garvey LH. Chlorhexidine allergy: sources of exposure in the health-care setting. Br J Anaesth. 2015;114(4):704–5 [r].

[14] Opstrup MS, Johansen JD, Bossi R, et al. Chlorhexidine in cosmetic products—a market survey. Contact Dermatitis. 2015;72(1):55–8 [E].

[15] Bernardi A, Teixeira CS. The properties of chlorhexidine and undesired effects of its use in endodontics. Quintessence Int. 2015;46(7):575–82 [R].

[16] Sadat Sajadi F, Moradi M, Pardakhty A, et al. Effect of fluoride, chlorhexidine and fluoride-chlorhexidine mouthwashes on salivary Streptococcus mutans count and the prevalence of oral side effects. J Dent Res Dent Clin Dent Prospects. 2015;9(1):49–52 [c].

[17] Karpinski TM, Szkaradkiewicz AK. Chlorhexidine-pharmaco-biological activity and application. Eur Rev Med Pharmacol Sci. 2015;19(7):1321–6 [R].

[18] Association of Anaesthetists of Great Britain and Ireland, Obstetric Anaesthetists' Association, Regional Anaesthesia UK, et al. Safety guideline: skin antisepsis for central neuraxial blockade. Anaesthesia. 2014;69(11):1279–86 [S].

[19] Cuervo-Pardo L, Gonzalez-Estrada A, Fernandez J, et al. A rash during surgery: rounding up the usual suspects. BMJ Case Rep. 2015. http://dx.doi.org/10.1136/bcr-2015-209660 [A].

[20] Anderson J, Rose M, Green S, et al. The utility of specific IgE testing to chlorhexidine in the investigation of perioperative adverse reactions. Ann Allergy Asthma Immunol. 2015;114(5):425–6 [c].

[21] Park DU, Friesen MC, Roh HS, et al. Estimating retrospective exposure of household humidifier disinfectants. Indoor Air. 2015;25(6):631–40 [c].

[22] Kim HR, Lee K, Park CW, et al. Polyhexamethylene guanidine phosphate aerosol particles induce pulmonary inflammatory and fibrotic responses. Arch Toxicol. 2016;90(3):617–32 [E].

[23] Scientific Committee on Consumer Safety (SCCS), Bernauer U. Opinion of the scientific committee on consumer safety (SCCS)—2nd revision of the safety of the use of poly(hexamethylene) biguanide hydrochloride or polyaminopropyl biguanide (PHMB) in cosmetic products. Regul Toxicol Pharmacol. 2015;73(3):885–6 [S].

[24] The Scientific Committee on Consumer Safety of the European Commission. Opinion on the safety of poly(hexamethylene) biguanide hydrochloride (PHMB). Second revision of 13 July 2015, Luxembourg: European Commission; 2015 [S].

[25] Creytens K, Goossens A, Faber M, et al. Contact urticaria syndrome caused by polyaminopropyl biguanide in wipes for intimate hygiene. Contact Dermatitis. 2014;71(5):307–9 [A].

[26] Bervoets A, Aerts O. Polyhexamethylene biguanide in wound care products: a non-negligible cause of peri-ulcer dermatitis. Contact Dermatitis. 2016;74(1):53–5 [A].

[27] Ceviker K, Canikoglu M, Tatlioglu S, et al. Reducing the pathogen burden and promoting healing with polyhexanide in

non-healing wounds: a prospective study. J Wound Care. 2015;24(12):582–6 [c].

[28] Tomar J, Jain VK, Aggarwal K, et al. Contact allergies to cosmetics: testing with 52 cosmetic ingredients and personal products. J Dermatol. 2005;32(12):951–5 [c].

[29] Bajaj AK, Saraswat A, Mukhija G, et al. Patch testing experience with 1000 patients. Indian J Dermatol Venereol Leprol. 2007;73(5):313–8 [C].

[30] Engebretsen K, Hald M, Johansen JD, et al. Allergic contact dermatitis caused by an antiseptic containing cetrimide. Contact Dermatitis. 2015;72(1):60–1 [A].

[31] Bates N, Edwards N. Benzalkonium chloride exposure in cats: a retrospective analysis of 245 cases reported to the Veterinary Poisons Information Service (VPIS). Vet Rec. 2015;176(9):229 [E].

[32] Malik R, Page SW, Finlay-Jones G, et al. Benzalkonium chloride intoxication in cats. Vet Rec. 2015;176(9):226–8 [E].

[33] Guzman-Aranguez A, Calvo P, Ropero I, et al. In vitro effects of preserved and unpreserved anti-allergic drugs on human corneal epithelial cells. J Ocul Pharmacol Ther. 2014;30(9):790–8 [E].

[34] Izzotti A, La Maestra S, Micale RT, et al. Genomic and post-genomic effects of anti-glaucoma drugs preservatives in trabecular meshwork. Mutat Res. 2015;772:1–9 [E].

[35] Pinheiro R, Panfil C, Schrage N, et al. Comparison of the lubricant eyedrops Optive®, Vismed Multi®, and Cationorm® on the corneal healing process in an ex vivo model. Eur J Ophthalmol. 2015;25(5):379–84 [E].

[36] Huang C, Wang H, Pan J, et al. Benzalkonium chloride induces subconjunctival fibrosis through the COX-2-modulated activation of a TGF-1/Smad3 signaling pathway. Invest Ophthalmol Vis Sci. 2014;55(12):8111–22 [E].

[37] Kim JH, Kim EJ, Kim YH, et al. In vivo effects of preservative-free and preserved prostaglandin analogs: mouse ocular surface study. Korean J Ophthalmol. 2015;29(4):270 [E].

[38] Boogaard PJ, van Puijvelde MJP, Urbanus JH. Biological monitoring to assess dermal exposure to ethylene oxide vapours during an incidental release. Toxicol Lett. 2014;231(3):387–90 [A].

[39] Farook SA, Shah V, Lenouvel D, et al. Corrigendum. Practice article (BDJ 2014; 217: 679–684). Guidelines for management of sodium hypochlorite extrusion injuries. Br Dent J. 2015;218(4):230 [R].

[40] Farook SA, Shah V, Lenouvel D, et al. Guidelines for management of sodium hypochlorite extrusion injuries. Br Dent J. 2014;217(12):679–84 [R].

[41] Al-Sebaei M, Halabi O, El-Hakim I. Sodium hypochlorite accident resulting in life-threatening airway obstruction during root canal treatment: a case report. Clin Cosmet Investig Dent. 2015;7:41 [A].

[42] Hatton J, Walsh S, Wilson A. Management of the sodium hypochlorite accident: a rare but significant complication of root canal treatment. BMJ Case Rep. 2015. http://dx.doi.org/10.1136/bcr-2014-207480 [A].

[43] Gallais Sérézal I, Hillion B. Images in clinical medicine. Atypical ulcerations of the penis. N Engl J Med. 2015;372(6):555 [A].

[44] Füeßl HS. Mit der Genitalhygiene kann man es auch übertreiben [in German]. MMW Fortschr Med. 2015;157(7):35 [A].

[45] De Gennaro L, Brunetti ND, Buquicchio F, et al. Takotsubo cardiomyopathy induced by acute inhalation of hypochlorite drain gel exhalations. Int J Cardiol. 2015;180:216–7 [A].

[46] Ellanti P, Hurson C. Tourniquet-associated povidone-iodine-induced chemical burns. BMJ Case Rep. 2015. http://dx.doi.org/10.1136/bcr-2014-208967 [A].

23

Beta-Lactams and Tetracyclines

Lucia Rose*, Michelle M. Peahota†, Jason C. Gallagher‡,1

*Infectious Diseases, Cooper University Hospital, Camden, NJ, USA
†Infectious Diseases, Thomas Jefferson University Hospital, Philadelphia, PA, USA
‡Temple University, Philadelphia, PA, USA
1Corresponding author: jason.gallagher@temple.edu

CARBAPENEMS

Ertapenem

Organs and Systems

NERVOUS SYSTEM

Carbapenems, including ertapenem, have been associated with central nervous system (CNS) toxicity. Most ertapenem CNS toxicity studies have excluded patients receiving hemodialysis (HD). Lee and colleagues describe four cases of ertapenem-related CNS toxicity in HD patients that occurred in patients receiving the recommended ertapenem dose of 500 mg daily. A 72-year-old HD-dependent man was prescribed ertapenem for prophylaxis following a hernioplasty. He developed disorientation, incoherent speech, agitation, and visual hallucinations on the fifth day of ertapenem therapy. A 66-year-old HD-dependent man was prescribed ertapenem for pneumonia and developed generalized tonic–colonic seizures after the fourth dose of ertapenem. A 79-year-old woman, prescribed ertapenem for abdominal infection prophylaxis, developed confusion, agitation, and visual hallucinations on the third day of therapy during a HD session. A 73-year-old woman, prescribed ertapenem for an arteriovenous fistula wound, developed hallucinations and cognitive impairment during the fourth HD session. Ertapenem plasma levels were drawn and were noted to be 79.2 µg/mL 12 hours after the first ertapenem dose. Her plasma ertapenem level increased to 147.4 µg/mL prior to the second HD session and was recorded to be 150.7 µg/mL prior to the fourth HD session, both of which are much higher than would be predicted. Other than ertapenem therapy, there were no other described reasons for the CNS toxicity in the aforementioned cases. The authors highlight the risk of ertapenem-induced CNS toxicity in HD patients who are prescribed the recommended 500 mg daily dose. It should be noted that ertapenem concentrations are not widely available and have not been described to clinically monitor patients for risk of toxicity [1c].

BILIARY TRACT

A 56-year-old man developed jaundice 5 days after the initiation of ertapenem 500 mg daily for treatment of a urinary tract infection. During treatment, his total bilirubin and direct bilirubin became elevated, while his alanine aminotransferase, aspartate aminotransferase, and alkaline phosphatase remained within normal limits. Subsequent serologic tests for hepatitis and HIV were negative, and no significant findings were noted on abdominal imaging. His jaundice quickly resolved following ertapenem discontinuation. To their knowledge, the authors report the first case of ertapenem-induced hyperbilirubinemia [2c].

Meropenem

Organs and Systems

HEMATOLOGIC

Drug-induced immune hemolytic anemia (DIIHA) is a rare but potentially life-threatening condition associated with immune-mediated hemolysis. Various drugs, including antimicrobials, have been reported to induce DIIHA. However, there was no case report found related to meropenem use. A 76-year-old woman with no significant past medical history was prescribed 2 g of meropenem per day for the treatment of acute cholecystitis. Her baseline laboratory tests, including red blood cell count and hemoglobin, were within normal limits. On day

Side Effects of Drugs Annual, Volume 38
ISSN: 0378-6080
http://dx.doi.org/10.1016/bs.seda.2016.09.003

10 of meropenem therapy, she complained of lumbar pain, fever, and chills and subsequent laboratory testing revealed macroscopic hemolytic anemia. Given the concern for DIIHA, meropenem was discontinued and the woman was treated with prednisone, hydration, and blood transfusion. Meropenem serum antibodies were detected upon serologic testing, which confirmed a drug-induced reaction. The authors report, to their knowledge, the first case of meropenem-induced DIIHA. It is important to be aware of this rare but serious adverse effect in patients who receive meropenem and present with acute immune hemolysis [3c].

PENICILLINS

Amoxicillin

Organs and Systems

CARDIOVASCULAR

Kounis syndrome is the occurrence of an acute coronary syndrome secondary to mast cell degranulation during an allergic reaction. A-74-year-old male received amoxicillin/clavulanic acid IV for treatment of a urinary tract infection. Twenty minutes following administration, the man developed a generalized maculopapular rash on his trunk and limbs, substernal chest tightness, diaphoresis, and palpitations. He was treated for anaphylactic shock and an electrocardiogram revealed widespread ST elevation. Following diagnosis of an acute coronary syndrome, the man received aspirin 300 mg, clopidogrel 300 mg, and atorvastatin 40 mg. The patient was transferred to a coronary care unit and was managed for allergic myocardial infarction (Kounis Syndrome). The authors hope to increase awareness of Kounis Syndrome diagnosis in the setting of acute onset chest pain accompanied by an allergic reaction [4c].

URINARY TRACT

Crystalluria is a known adverse effect of amoxicillin and has been described with high-dose therapy. A 62-year-old woman was initiated on amoxicillin IV 200 mg/kg/day with gentamicin 240 mg IV once daily for *Streptococcus agalactiae* endocarditis. Her weight was not specified but her glomerular filtration rate (GFR) on admission was 82 mL/min per 1.73 m². Four days after antimicrobial therapy initiation, she developed cloudy urine with a granular appearance. Microscopic examination of her urine revealed large aggregated needle-shaped crystals, and she was diagnosed with amoxicillin-induced crystalluria. Her renal function progressively worsened as she developed oliguria and renal replacement therapy was initiated. Her renal function improved and she was discharged 1 month after admission without further renal replacement therapy. The case did not specify if changes were made to her antimicrobial regimen nor did it specify the time course in which her renal function improved. Nineteen months following her initial admission, her GFR was reported to be 45 mL/min per 1.73 m². The authors acknowledge that this woman's acute renal failure was likely multifactorial, but they speculate that amoxicillin crystalluria may have been involved in the process [5c].

SKIN

Acute generalized exanthematous pustulosis (AGEP), a skin reaction commonly elicited by antibiotics, is rarely associated with lymph node enlargement. A 37-year-old woman presented with a 12-hour history of fever and a rapidly progressing pruritic skin rash. Three days prior to presentation, she was initiated on oral amoxicillin/clavulanic acid for periodontitis. Her past medical history was significant for a similar reaction to amoxicillin when she was 16 years old. Multiple small (<5 mm in diameter), nonfollicular pustules with an erythematous base were noted on her trunk and limbs. Additionally, she had painful lymphadenopathy which involved the posterior cervical, postauricular, suboccipital, axillary, and inguinal regions. Serologic testing was negative for Epstein–Barr virus, human immunodeficiency virus, hepatitis B virus, and hepatitis C virus. Blood and pustule fluid bacterial cultures were also negative. Leukocytoclastic vasculitis was confirmed upon skin biopsy from a purpuric lesion. Subsequent allergic patch testing with beta-lactam antibiotics revealed a strong positivity for ampicillin, amoxicillin, and amoxicillin/clavulanic acid. Given the patient's history and presentation, she was definitively diagnosed with AGEP. This case describes lymphadenopathy associated with AGEP, a very rare manifestation of the reaction. Additionally, the authors suggest that patch testing may be beneficial in confirming the diagnosis of AGEP [6c].

Penicillin

Organs and Systems

SKIN

A 19-year-old woman presented with severe pain and edema in the right buttock and livedoid patches on her right lower limb. In addition, she was unable to move her right foot. The onset of her symptoms began minutes after the third injection of benzathine benzylpenicillin 2400000 IU IM for tonsillitis. A neurologic exam revealed hypoesthesia and decreased right lower limb muscle strength. Imaging and ultrasound did not reveal any signs of vascular occlusion. She was treated with IV pentoxifylline, prednisolone, meropenem, alprostadil, enoxaparin, and hyperbaric oxygen therapy (HBOT). Her symptoms progressively worsened. Upon further workup, she was diagnosed with compartment syndrome and underwent surgical debridement and fasciotomies. Biopsy showed muscle congestion, hemorrhage, necrosis, and inflammation, without vasculitis or bacteria. Given the appearance of a livedoid eruption shortly after IM injection and the exclusion of other causes (i.e. necrotizing fasciitis), she was diagnosed with Nicolau syndrome, a rare cutaneous drug reaction following IM administration. Subsequent management included 14 HBOT sessions, surgical debridement, and skin grafts. At her follow-up visit, the patient presented without any functional impairment. The authors suggest that HBOT, in addition to surgical intervention, should be considered early on in the management of Nicolau Syndrome [7c].

Piperacillin

Organs and Systems

NERVOUS SYSTEM

Antibiotic-induced neurotoxicity in hemodialysis patients has been described with ceftazidime and cefepime, but there only have been a few reports involving piperacillin/tazobactam use. A 67-year-old female with a history of ischemic stroke (10 years prior to admission), hypertension, and HD was hospitalized for pneumonia. She was initiated on cefepime 1 g after each HD session for treatment of pneumonia and developed a profound change in mental status, dysarthria, hemiparesia, and cranial nerve deficits after the second cefepime dose. Computed tomography (CT) imaging was negative for an acute process. Given the clinical findings, she was diagnosed as having cefepime-induced neurotoxicity, and cefepime was replaced with piperacillin/tazobactam 2.25 g every 6 hours. The patient's neurologic status recovered, but she developed new neurologic dysfunction 4 days after the initiation of piperacillin/tazobactam. A repeat brain CT showed no signs of acute stroke and an electroencephalogram showed disorganization of basal activity with no epileptiform paroxysms. Her neurologic status returned to baseline after discontinuation of piperacillin/tazobactam and two HD sessions. The authors suggest that HD patients with previous β-lactam-induced neurologic dysfunction may be more susceptible to neurotoxicity from other β-lactam agents [8c].

NEUROMUSCULAR FUNCTION

A 57-year-old man with a history of microscopic polyangiitis with renal dysfunction was admitted for bronchiectasis and hemoptysis and prescribed piperacillin/tazobactam 2.25 g every 8 hours. After the second dose, he developed myoclonic jerks of his limbs. His laboratory values, including serum potassium, calcium, and magnesium, were within normal limits. CT imaging of his brain and EEG was also normal. His myoclonus diminished following piperacillin/tazobactam discontinuation. This case describes drug-induced myoclonic jerks, a rare adverse effect associated with piperacillin/tazobactam [9c].

HEMATOLOGIC

The association of beta-lactam antibiotics and neutropenia has been documented, although the frequency at which it occurs appears to be rare. Lemieuz and colleagues performed a retrospective cohort study to evaluate the risk of developing neutropenia in a pediatricpopulation exposed to piperacillin/tazobactam vs those exposed to ticarcillin/clavulanate. Subjects were included if they were <18 years of age and had received at least 1 dose of either drug while hospitalized between January 2008 and June 2011. Exclusion criteria included active neoplasia, receipt of chemotherapy, neutropenia, receipt of immunosuppression, and human immunodeficiency virus (HIV) infection. Two hundred and ninety-nine cases were included in analysis: 65 (22%) in the piperacillin/tazobactam group and 234 (78%) in the ticarcillin/clavulanate group. Neutropenia was reported in 7/65 (10.8%) piperacillin/tazobactam patients and 6/235 (2.6%) ticarcillin/clavulanate patients. There was an increased risk of developing neutropenia in the piperacillin/tazobactam group vs ticarcillin/clavulanate group (unadjusted OR=4.59; 95% CI, 1.48–14.17). The study was unable to adjust for confounding variables given the low number of events. The authors acknowledge the value of piperacillin/tazobactam in clinical practice but recommend a risk/benefit assessment whenever using piperacillin/tazobactam [10C].

Thrombocytopenia, a known adverse effect of piperacillin/tazobactam, is often reported several days after use. A 47-year-old female with a history of chronic lung disease and HIV was treated with piperacillin/tazobactam 4.5 g IV every 6 hours for healthcare-associated pneumonia. Laboratory values on admission revealed hemoglobin of 11.2 g/dL, white blood cell count (WBC) of 17.76×10^3/mcL, and platelets of 198×10^3/mcL. Her platelet count decreased to 7×10^3/mcL after her second piperacillin/tazobactam dose. A 55-year-old female with rectal carcinoma status post resection was prescribed piperacillin/tazobactam 4.5 g IV every 6 hours for an abdominal fluid collection. Her baseline laboratory studies revealed hemoglobin of 8 g/dL, WBC of 5.74×10^3/mcL, and platelets of 325×10^3/mcL. Her platelet count decreased to 3×10^3/mcL after the third piperacillin/tazobactam dose. In both cases, there were no other etiologies that could explain the drop in platelets and thrombocytopenia quickly resolved following discontinuation of piperacillin/tazobactam. Although piperacillin/tazobactam-induced thrombocytopenia has been previously described with prolonged use, these cases show that near-immediate thrombocytopenia is possible. If drug-induced thrombocytopenia is suspected, prompt discontinuation of the inciting agent is critical [11c].

MONOBACTAMS

Aztreonam

Organs and Systems
HYPERSENSITIVITY

Aztreonam is considered a safe and effective alternative to other beta-lactams in patients with IgE-mediated hypersensitivity to penicillins. While cross-sensitivity is extremely rare between aztreonam and other beta-lactams, assessing this risk is important. Gaeta and colleagues conducted a study of 212 subjects between age 15 and 90 years who had a history of positive penicillin skin tests to at least one penicillin as well as IgE-mediated reactions to penicillins. Following positive penicillin skin testing, patients underwent skin testing to aztreonam and three carbapenems (imipenem, meropenem, ertapenem). None of the patients skin tested to aztreonam or carbapenems had positive skin tests. Since this study was purely for purposes of allergic research, patients were not initiated on any course of antibiotic therapy following skin testing. However, results can likely be extrapolated to clinical practice as skin testing is considered a reliable method for assessing allergy. In addition to supporting the use of aztreonam in patients who have IgE-mediated penicillin hypersensitivity, this data also support the safe use of carbapenems for the same population [12C].

CEPHALOSPORINS

All

Organs and Systems
IMMUNOLOGIC

A large Finnish pediatric case–control study was conducted to examine the risk of asthma with prenatal and postnatal exposure to various antimicrobials. The theory behind early antimicrobial exposure and asthma is likely linked to alteration of immunologically protective gut flora, as has been suggested previously. A total of 6690 case–control pairs were included in the analysis. Prenatal exposure to antimicrobials was significantly associated with an increased risk of asthma (OR=1.31) with the most commonly implicated antibiotic class

being cephalosporins (adjusted OR=1.46). In addition, pediatric use of antibiotics in the first year of life was found to be significantly associated with development of asthma (OR=1.60); cephalosporins were found to have the highest correlation of all antibiotic classes. The authors did not theorize why cephalosporins specifically were found to pose the highest risk for development of asthma. Unfortunately, the study did not specify which cephalosporins were administered to the patients evaluated. The student reinforces the importance of judicious prescribing of any antibiotics in pregnant women and in children, with particular attention to cephalosporins in this case [13MC].

Cefazolin

Organs and Systems
HYPERSENSITIVITY

Widely used for perioperative surgical prophylaxis, cefazolin is one of the most utilized antibiotics in hospitals. However, in patients with a history of penicillin allergy, alternative and possibly less preferred options are used due to the concern for cross-sensitivity. A large retrospective study among pediatric surgical patients at Nationwide Children's Hospital was conducted. The aim was to evaluate the incidence of adverse effects and allergic reactions in patients with a history of penicillin allergies that had received cephalosporins for surgical prophylaxis. Penicillin allergy history consisted of rash (40%), hives (27%), unknown (18%) and anaphylaxis (4%). A total of 513 penicillin-allergic patients were identified, representing 624 surgical cases. Of these, cephalosporins were administered in 153 cases (24.5%). Cefazolin was the most common cephalosporin administered (127 cases, 83%), followed by cefoxitin. Only one reaction (hives and erythema) was documented among the 153 (0.65%) patients that received a cephalosporin. Clindamycin was the most commonly substituted antibiotic, and the reaction rate was 1.5%. Therefore, the reaction rate to clindamycin was numerically higher than cephalosporins in penicillin-allergic patients, suggesting that a low cross-reactivity rate between these categories of beta-lactams and that it is likely safe to administer cephalosporins in patients with a history of non-anaphylactic penicillin allergies. If the penicillin reaction is severe such as anaphylaxis or Stevens–Johnson syndrome, cephalosporin test dosing should be performed or alternative options should be administered. These data are encouraging and correlate with other data suggesting a very low incidence of cross-sensitivity between penicillin and cephalosporin allergies, but it should be noted that limited duration of cephalosporin administration was given in this study [14C].

Cefepime

Organs and Systems

RENAL

Cefepime-induced nephrotoxicity has rarely been reported in the literature, although this toxicity is well known among other beta-lactams. A 62-year-old female was initiated on cefepime (6 g per day) for mastoiditis and temporal bone osteomyelitis for a planned duration of 6 weeks. At week 4, she developed acute kidney injury as evidenced by a rise in creatinine as well as proteinuria. Her dose of cefepime was reduced to 4 g per day, and by week 5, her creatinine continued to rise leading to a hospital admission. A renal biopsy was completed showing moderate interstitial fibrosis with patchy inflammatory infiltrates. Upon discontinuation of cefepime, her renal function rapidly improved within 1 week. She was diagnosed with acute interstitial nephritis secondary to cefepime. Using Naranjo criteria, this led to a score of six, showing cefepime to be a probable cause of nephrotoxicity. Of note, she was not initiated on any new medications other than cefepime, although her home medications were continued. It was also concluded that this toxicity may have been dose related [15A].

NERVOUS SYSTEM

Cefepime-induced neurotoxicity has been previously reported, particularly in patients with renal dysfunction who did not receive dose adjustment. An 88-year-old female with a creatinine clearance of 26 mL/min was initiated on cefepime 2 g IV q12h for left thigh cellulitis and an endovascular prosthetic infection due to *Enterobacter cloacae*. The patient was found to have rising serum creatinine. The day following initiation of cefepime, the patient developed sudden onset delirium and aphasia. At that point, she had received 6 g of total cefepime. A CT scan excluded other causes for this behavior. The following day, the patient experienced altered mental status associated with generalized myoclonic jerks. An electroencephalography (EEG) revealed diffuse slowing and triphasic elements. Cefepime-induced neurotoxicity was suspected, and the antibiotic was discontinued after a cumulative dose of 14 g. Two intermittent hemodialysis sessions were necessary to emergently clear drug. Serum cefepime concentrations were obtained, and levels were fourfold higher than the normal therapeutic range. After 48 hours, the patient had full neurologic recovery. The case was deemed highly probable based on a score of 9 on the Naranjo algorithm [16A].

Khasani reported two cases of jaw myoclonus within 48 hours of initiating cefepime. The myoclonus was described as repetitive bursts of 1-second duration, each with 3–5 clonic jaw jerks. Both patients had renal dysfunction and resolution of symptoms occurred within 24 hours of cefepime discontinuation [17A].

It appears that the risk of cefepime-induced neurotoxicity is highly correlated with renal dysfunction and likely related to supratherapeutic concentrations of cefepime.

GENERAL INFORMATION

A retrospective study aimed to evaluate differences in clinical and laboratory adverse events in infants who had received ceftazidime versus cefepime in the first 120 days of life between 1997 and 2012. A total of 2355 infants (1761 received ceftazidime, 594 received cefepime) and 17 921 days of therapy (13 293 days of ceftazidime, 4628 days of cefepime) were included in the analysis. The median gestational age of the ceftazidime recipients was 26 weeks versus 27 weeks in the cefepime group. Overall incidence of laboratory adverse events (373 versus 341/1000 infant days, $P < 0.001$) and severe adverse events (112 versus 87/1000 infant days, $P < 0.001$) were statistically higher in the ceftazidime group. Most of the differences were due to a higher incidence of leukocytosis, leukopenia and thrombocytopenia in the ceftazidime recipients. However, after adjustment for severity of illness, the difference was not significant. A potential explanation for this was that the ceftazidime group was generally sicker with higher numbers of positive blood cultures, mechanical ventilation and inotropic support. Hyperkalemia was also more common in the ceftazidime group (32 versus 21/1000 infant days, $P < 0.001$). Clinical adverse events were found to be similar in both groups. Seizure was the most commonly encountered clinical adverse event, albeit rare. Mortality rates were also not statistically different between both groups. The study suggested that there is no difference in toxicity between the two drugs in this page group [18MC].

Ceftaroline

Organs and Systems

HYPERSENSITIVITY

Ceftaroline desensitization was performed in a 32-year-old female with methicillin-resistant *Staphylococcus aureus* (MRSA) cellulitis and osteomyelitis for whom ceftaroline therapy was prescribed. The patient had never received ceftaroline previously, however, had a significant anaphylactic allergy history to various antibiotics including penicillin and ertapenem, two other beta-lactams that led to the concern of cross-reactivity with ceftaroline. The desensitization protocol used serial dilution to produce three solutions using a 20-mL vial of 600 mg of ceftaroline in 0.9% sodium chloride. A total of 14 infusion bags were made and administered to the patient totaling a cumulative dose of 574.94 mg. Ceftaroline 600 mg IV q12h was continued thereafter for 6 weeks. No acute hypersensitivity was reported during her 6 weeks of therapy. However, gastrointestinal (GI) symptoms including as nausea, vomiting and diarrhea were reported. These GI symptoms persisted after antibiotic discontinuation and were deemed to be secondary to her prior gastric bypass surgery [19A].

HEMATOLOGIC

Agranulocytosis and neutropenia are uncommon class effects of cephalosporins. Ceftaroline has been reported previously as a cause of hematologic toxicities. A retrospective cohort analysis evaluating the incidence of ceftaroline-induced neutropenia over a 1.5-year period was conducted. Patients were evaluated only if they received longer than 7 days of therapy. A total of 39 patients who received ceftaroline for a median duration of 27 days were included in the analysis. Seven of the 39 patients (18%) developed neutropenia while on therapy. Baseline characteristics between patients who developed neutropenia ($n=7$) and those who did not ($n=32$) were largely similar. The median time to development of neutropenia was 17 days. Of the seven patients who developed neutropenia, four of them had a nadir ANC of <500 cells/mm3. The authors recommend discontinuation of ceftaroline if the absolute neutrophil count (ANC) falls below 1500 cells/mm^3 [20c].

In a case series of patients receiving ceftaroline therapy at two institutions, four cases of agranulocytosis were reported. Twenty-nine patients were evaluated at site one; 11 received clindamycin in addition and the rest received ceftaroline monotherapy. In total, five patients developed a rash and two developed agranulocytosis. At site two, a total of 587 patients received ceftaroline; however, only 37 were on the antibiotic for more than 14 days at the higher dose of 600 mg IV q8h. Two of these 37 patients developed agranulocytosis. Three of the four cases reported necessitated treatment with G-CSF for restoration of neutrophil counts. The cases occurred more commonly in patients on 600 mg q8h, which is higher than the FDA approved dosing of 600 q12h. Generally this higher dose is used for off-label indications including severe infections due to MRSA such as bacteremia and endocarditis. At these higher doses, toxicities such as agranulocytosis may be more commonly noted. It is important to monitor these patients accordingly [21A].

Ceftolozane/Tazobactam

Organs and Systems
GENERAL INFORMATION

A randomized double-blind, phase 3 trial comparing levofloxacin to ceftolozane/tazobactam in adult patients with complicated urinary tract infections including pyelonephritis was performed. A total of 1068 patients were evaluated for safety. Incidence of adverse events was similar occurring in roughly 34% of patients in both treatment arms. Headache and gastrointestinal symptoms were the most common adverse events found in each group, which is consistent with other antimicrobials commonly prescribed. Two patients (<1%) on ceftolozane/tazobactam developed C. difficile diarrhea. Overall this antibiotic was well tolerated with similar toxicities as compared to other cephalosporins [22MC].

Ceftriaxone

Organs and Systems
HEMATOLOGIC

Acute hemolytic anemia is a rare but serious side effect of ceftriaxone. A 14-year-old boy developed pneumonia and was initiated on ceftriaxone for treatment. After 7 days of therapy, he continued to clinically decline and was transferred to the intensive care unit. Laboratory tests were performed revealing a hemoglobin of 2.6 g/dL (down from 9 g/dL 4 days prior). No overt source of acute bleeding was found, and workup for bleeding was negative. Acute hemolytic anemia was suspected, and a direct antibody test obtained was found to be positive. An agglutination test was performed on his plasma and in the presence of ceftriaxone, RBCs agglutinated. He subsequently developed acute tubular necrosis and acute liver insufficiency. Upon withdrawal of ceftriaxone, he was extubated within 24 hours and coagulopathy improved over the next few days. Treatment of this case mainly included supportive care including blood transfusions as well as immediate withdrawal of the offending agent. Due to the mortality associated with this rare side effect, early identification is imperative [23A].

A 49-year-old was initiated on a 6-week course of ceftriaxone 2 g IV q12h for vertebral osteomyelitis due to *Streptococcus intermedius*. Pretreatment laboratory markers were normal. On day 25 of therapy, a routine complete blood count revealed an ANC of 480/mm^3 (down from 4435/mm^3 12 days prior). Other laboratory parameters remained stable. On day 28, his ANC fell to zero. The patient developed a fever during the time his ANC had dropped and was subsequently broadened to cefepime and vancomycin for neutropenic fever. One week following discontinuation of ceftriaxone, his ANC normalized (2024/mm^3). Ceftriaxone was thought to be the sole cause of agranulocytosis in this case, due to the timing in relation to initiation and discontinuation of the drug. The authors concluded that the R2 side chain of ceftriaxone was the target for this immunologic reaction since the patient's ANC recovered on cefepime. This is a rare but serious toxicity of ceftriaxone, and early identification is crucial for optimal patient outcomes [24A].

BILIARY TRACT

A 79-year-old hemodialysis dependent patient was started on ceftriaxone for treatment of pneumonia. The dosing chosen was 1 g every other day. On the 13th day of therapy, the patient developed stomach pain in the right hypochondrium with a firm, round mass. CT scan revealed improved pneumonia; however, a 16 × 9-mm gallstone was found in the gallbladder with wall thickening. This abnormality was not detected in the original CT scan. Ceftriaxone-induced pseudolithiasis was suspected, and the antibiotic was discontinued. Improvement in the gallstone and gallbladder wall thickening began after a few weeks with complete resolution at day 48. Clinical and laboratory monitoring was required; however, intervention was not necessary. Although ceftriaxone-induced pseudolithiasis has been previously reported, this is the first case described in an adult hemodialysis-dependent patient [25A].

HYPERSENSITIVITY

A non-immediate T-cell-mediated reaction to both ceftriaxone and meropenem occurred in a 13-year-old male. The patient had been on high dose ceftriaxone for an extradural empyema, along with clindamycin and vancomycin. On day 7 of therapy, the patient developed a generalized maculopapular exanthema, fever and malaise. There was no eosinophilia, however. The regimen was then switched to meropenem and the cutaneous lesions worsened along with new lesions in the oral mucosa. The regimen was then switched to linezolid, amikacin and metronidazole and resolution of mucocutaneous lesions occurred promptly. Allergy testing via skin prick, intradermal and patch tests were performed for penicillin, ceftriaxone and meropenem and were all negative. Although lymphocyte transformation tests are not highly sensitive, it was performed for both agents and found to be positive for ceftriaxone but not meropenem. This case may have exhibited cross-sensitivity to ceftriaxone and meropenem, although it is difficult to definitively draw this conclusion [26A].

A skin test study of various cephalosporins was conducted among 102 patients aged 14–81 years with a history of cephalosporin allergy, documented by previous skin testing. The most commonly reported allergy was to ceftriaxone, followed by cefaclor and ceftazidime. The aim was to evaluate the presence of cross-sensitivity to alternative cephalosporins. Patients were divided into four groups based on the specific cephalosporin they were allergic to. Group A was the largest group, which included cephalosporins with a methoxyimino group in the R1 side chain plus ceftazidime. Group B were aminocephalosporins. Each group underwent skin test challenges to a variety of cephalosporins that were structurally different to the cephalosporin to which their allergy was reported. The 102 patients had 362 challenges with alternative cephalosporins (alternate side chains) and all were well tolerated indicating that cross-reactivity among cephalosporins is mainly connected to R1 side chains and not a class effect. Regardless, the authors still recommend pretreatment skin tests to alternative cephalosporins in patients with significant cephalosporin allergies [27C].

A 54-year-old male was prescribed ceftriaxone and clarithromycin for an upper respiratory infection. On the following day after initiation of these antibiotics, he complained of worsening dyspnea and a chest X-ray revealed worsening inflammation. He was then admitted to the hospital and started on cefepime and levofloxacin. His pneumonia continued to worsen, and on day 6 of admission, antibiotics were broadened to meropenem and ciprofloxacin with improvement. Antibiotics were then de-escalated to ceftazidime and levofloxacin, and he continued to improve. At some point during his treatment, the physician wrongly prescribed cefotaxime instead of ceftazidime and the patient began experiencing dyspnea, fever and gastrointestinal symptoms. On chest X-ray, opacities appeared worsened again and he underwent a bronchoalveolar lavage (BAL). The BAL showed lymphocytosis, increase in neutrophils and eosinophils, which the authors diagnosed as hypersensitivity pneumonitis in response to cefotaxime. The patient was given ceftriaxone 1 year later and again had rapid progression of pneumonitis as evidenced by symptomatic and radiologic worsening. The only cephalosporin that did not cause this patient to experience worsening pneumonitis was ceftazidime, which has a different R1 side chain than the others administered [28A].

Cefuroxime

Organs and Systems

SENSORY SYSTEMS

Intracameral cefuroxime is commonly used for prophylaxis in cataract surgery to prevent endopthalmitis. A retrospective case review evaluated the rate of postoperative endopthalmitis in patients who underwent cataract surgery and had received intracameral cefuroxime between 2007 and 2011 at an institution in Ireland. The institution had adopted usage of intracameral cefuroxime starting in 2007 for all cataract surgeries. A total of 8329 cataract surgeries were performed during the time period. There were only five cases of endopthalmitis (incidence of 0.06%). Of the five cases, three were culture positive (two coagulase-negative staphylococci and one *Pseudomonas aeruginosa*). Cefuroxime is not recommended to treat either of these two organisms, which is part of the debate as to whether this is the best agent for this indication. Regardless, the incidence was significantly lower compared to a previous study conducted at the same institution from 1997 to 2001, which was prior to usage of intracameral cefuroxime. In the earlier study, there were 43 of 8736 cases (incidence of 0.49%). Implementation of cefuroxime led to an eightfold reduction in the incidence of postoperative endopthalmitis for patients undergoing cataract surgery [29MC].

Although use of intracameral cefuroxime has lowered the incidence of endopthalmitis related to cataract surgery, reports of retinal toxicity have occurred. A 64-year-old male underwent cataract surgery in his left eye without complications. He received a standard dose (0.1 mL of 10 mg/mL) of intracameral cefuroxime at the end of surgery. Two days later, he complained of visual loss in the left eye. Retinal toxicity was observed as evidenced by diffuse retinal pallor with intraretinal cysts on fundoscopic examination. Global retinal dysfunction was noted on further testing as well as a large retinal serous detachment on the outer nuclear layer. One week after this occurred, visual acuity was completely recovered and abnormalities were no longer seen [30A].

HYPERSENSITIVITY

In Denmark as in other countries, cefuroxime is occasionally used for perioperative prophylaxis in various surgeries. A total of 413 adult patients developed perioperative drug-related hypersensitivity during a 9-year study period, of which 98 (23.7%) received cefuroxime for prophylaxis. Of the 98 patients who received cefuroxime, 89 (90.8%) of them had hypersensitivity reactions that were presumed to be due to cefuroxime. The intent of the study was to evaluate whether timing of cefuroxime administration in relation to onset of the reaction was a reliable method of concluding that the reaction was due to cefuroxime, since it is difficult to detect causes of hypersensitivity. Further investigation into cefuroxime hypersensitivity testing performed by skin tests, *in vitro* tests, and titrated provocations. After this testing, only 23 of the 89 patients (25.8%) were thought to have developed hypersensitivity due to cefuroxime. The other 66 patients tested negative to cefuroxime. All patients with confirmed cefuroxime hypersensitivity reacted within 15 minutes of antibiotic administration. However, a majority of cefuroxime-negative patients (65%) also reacted within 15 minutes of antibiotic administration. Therefore, timing of cefuroxime administration should not be considered a reliable predictor for identification of the etiology of hypersensitivity [31c].

A retrospective observational study was conducted with the aim to evaluate the cross-reactivity between penicillins and cephalosporins at one institution. Patients were included if they had an amoxicillin or penicillin allergy confirmed by skin test or oral challenge who had also received an oral challenge with a cephalosporin. Twenty-two patients were included in the study; 10 had skin reactions and 12 had respiratory or cardiovascular reactions. Patients with positive penicillin skin tests underwent skin tests most commonly with cefuroxime or cefixime. The culprit penicillins were amoxicillin (seven patients; 31.8%), amoxicillin/clavulanate (14 patients, 63%), and penicillin (one patient; 4.5%). Skin tests with oral cephalosporins were negative in all patients. In addition, 17 patients were challenged with both cefuroxime and cefixime, two with just cefuroxime and three with just cefixime. These penicillin-allergic patients tolerated cephalosporins as evidenced by skin tests and oral challenge. To note, the cephalosporins used were second or third generation with different side chains compared to amoxicillin or penicillin. It is likely that the side chain and not the beta-lactam ring plays a role in cross reactivity of these antibiotics [32c].

Cephalexin

Organs and Systems

HYPERSENSITIVITY

A large retrospective analysis was conducted to examine incidences of reported allergies and adverse drug reactions for intravenous versus oral cephalosporins. Over the 2-year study period, there were 901 908 courses of oral cephalosporins and 487 630 courses of intravenous cephalosporins prescribed. Women had higher rates of baseline and new penicillin or cephalosporin allergies as compared to men. In both men and women, cephalexin had a much higher rate of new allergies reported within 30 days (men—1187, women—2925); however, this was likely due to the fact that this was the most commonly prescribed cephalosporin, regardless of route. *Clostridium difficile* infection (CDI) within 90 days was most commonly reported with ceftriaxone (men—2048, women—3001), although this is not surprising given prior reports of third-generation cephalosporins and their link with causing CDI. Overall, anaphylaxis was extremely rare occurring in five oral and eight intravenous cephalosporin exposures. Overall, CDI appeared to pose a much greater risk as compared to serious allergic reactions. Patients should be educated about this risk prior to beginning any antibiotic, particularly cephalosporins [33MC].

TETRACYCLINES AND GLYCYLCYCLINES

Doxycycline

Organs and Systems

SKIN

An 87-year-old female was found to have developed a blue-gray discoloration on her face and extremities and darkening of subungal regions (melanonychia). Due to its slow progression, she was unaware of her skin findings. She had been taking oral doxycycline 200 mg daily, prescribed 11 years previously for bullous pemohigoid. Her medication list also consisted of losartan, metformin, atenolol-chlorthalidone, aspirin, levothyroxine, and atorvastatin. Utilizing the Naranjo algorithm, it was determined that her skin findings were a result of prolonged doxycycline use. The authors warn prescribers to be aware of possible skin and nail changes with chronic doxycyline use [34c].

Minocycline

Organs and Systems

EAR, NOSE, THROAT

A 40-year-old woman was referred to an otolaryngology clinic after incidental findings of speckled brownish pigmentation surrounding the umbo in both of her eardrums. The woman admitted to difficulty discerning speech in the setting of high background noise. She was prescribed daily minocycline for the treatment of acne vulgaris, which she used for the previous 14 years. She had no other significant past medical history and did not take any other medications. Upon examination, she was noted to have faint bluish color of the pinnae, sclera, and teeth, as well as brownish spots surrounding the umbo of both tympanic membranes. She underwent audiological evaluation which revealed normal hearing within speech range, but bilateral high-frequency hearing loss along with left ear low-frequency hearing loss. There were no findings of tinnitus, plugged sensation, or imbalance. It was advised that the woman discontinue minocycline, as it was thought that her findings were an adverse effect of minocycline. Nine months following minocycline discontinuation, a slight reduction in the blue color of her pinnae was noted. The authors cannot conclude if the woman's hearing loss was associated with the hyperpigmentation of her tympanic membrane, but suggest minocycline-induced hyperpigmentation should be considered when there is detection of blue brown spot on the ear drum [35c].

SKIN

Minocycline use is known to be associated with drug-induced skin pigmentation, which is characterized by a slate-grey coloring in affected areas. A 64-year-old woman presented with a 5-year history of upper-lip pigmentation. She had been prescribed minocycline 100 mg daily for cystic acne for 4 years. During the third year of minocycline treatment, she had non-fractionated carbon dioxide laser resurfacing of her upper lip to treat photodamage. Two months following laser treatment, she noticed discoloration of her upper lip area which was attributed to sun-induced damage. Further evaluation

with a cross-polarizing head lamp revealed slate-gray-sub-epidermal pigmentation, which is commonly observed with minocycline-induced pigmentation. Punch biopsy results of the affected area was also consistent with drug-induced pigmentation. The patient was treated with 4 sessions of Q-switched neodymium: yttrium, aluminum garnet laser treatment administered at 10-week intervals. A significant clearing of the gray pigment was noted 3 months following the fourth treatment. The authors recommend that patients taking minocycline, or other drugs associated with skin pigmentation, should discontinue therapy prior to ablative laser procedures [36c].

Persistent serpentine supravenous hyperpigmented eruption (PSSHE) is a cutaneous eruption characterized by hyperpigmented streaks over the venous network and is associated with patent vessels. A 40-year-old man with lepromatous leprosy (LL) and erythema nodosum leprosum (ENL) was prescribed clofazimine 50 mg daily, ofloxacin 400 mg daily, minocycline 100 mg daily, and prednisolone 40 mg daily. His ENL improved after 4 months of the drug regimen, and prednisone was subsequently discontinued. He began to develop asymptomatic erythematous hyperpigmented streaks over both thighs. Progressive pigmentation was also noted on his face. An examination noted that veins underlying the pigmentation were non-tender and patent. After 6 months of therapy, minocycline was discontinued and his hyperpigmentation became unnoticeable within 3 months. The authors hope to bring awareness of PSSHE in patients with LL who are receiving minocycline [37c].

Tetracycline

Organs and Systems

HEMATOLOGIC

The use of tetracyclines has been associated with pigmentation of various bodily areas, including skin, mucosa, nails, and bone. A revision tympanomastoidectomy was planned for a 52-year-old male with a history of chronic right ear infection and tympanic membrane perforation. During the procedure, the man's temporal bone was noted to be rusty green in color. His history was significant acne vulgaris, for which he received tetracycline from the ages of 14–19 years old. Notably, he underwent a tympanomastoidectomy when he was 14 years old (prior to tetracycline use), and no bone discoloration was documented at the time. A literature review, performed by the authors, found over 20 cases of intraoral bone and mucosal stating associated with tetracycline use. Although rare, it is important to be aware of potential diffuse tissue staining with prolonged tetracycline exposure [38c].

Tigecycline

Organs and Systems

HEMATOLOGIC

Tigecycline has been described to reduce fibrinogen levels, and this finding has been supported with more published reports [39c,40c]. Zhang and colleagues performed a retrospective analysis on the effects of tigecycline on coagulation and plasma fibrinogen levels in 20 patients with severe infection. Fibrinogen, activated partial thromboplastin time (APTT), thrombin time (TT), platelet count (PLT) were measured at baseline and throughout tigecycline treatment. Twenty-one patients treated with cefoperazone/sulbactam served as the control group. There were no differences in respect to age, gender, or acute physiology and chronic health evaluation (APACHE) II score. Three tigecycline patients received dosing higher than the package insert recommendation. Patients receiving tigecycline were noted to have decreased fibrinogen levels ($P < 0.001$). There was no significant fibrinogen level change in the control group. Additionally, tigecycline use was associated with prolonged PT, APTT, and TT ($P < 0.001$). Six tigecycline patients developed active bleeding which necessitated administration of plasma and/or fibrinogen. Following discontinuation of tigecycline therapy, fibrinogen levels improved. The authors conclude that tigecycline, used at both the recommended and higher than recommended dose, can result in a reduction of plasma fibrinogen levels. They suggest routine monitoring of coagulation parameters during tigecycline treatment [39c].

Long-Term Effects

DRUG RESISTANCE

Tigecycline, a broad spectrum antibiotic, lacks *in vitro* activity against *Pseudomonas aeruginosa*. Ulu-Klic and colleagues performed a single-center retrospective observational study to determine if tigecycline exposure is a risk factor for *P. aeruginosa* infection in ICU patients. Patients included in this study were hospitalized in an ICU and had documented infection with *P. aeruginosa* (case group) or had a documented nosocomial infection with an organism other than *P. aeruginosa* (control group). Patients with *P. aeruginosa* infection were evaluated for tigecycline exposure prior to infection. All patients with tigecycline exposure were included in the study.

A total of 1167 patients with nosocomial infection were included in the evaluation, of which, 278 (23.8%) patients had *P. aeruginosa* infection. Results were controlled for hospital length of stay. More patients in the case group received tigecycline before *P. aeruginosa* infection compared to the control group (21.2% vs 5.7%, $P < 0.01$). A multivariate analysis showed tigecycline use to be associated with an increased risk of *P. aeruginosa* infection

(3.992 OR [2.625–6.071] 95% CI, $P = 0.001$). Limitations include the retrospective design and lack of tigecycline treatment data, such as duration and initiation time prior to nosocomial infection. This study describes the risk of developing an infection with *P. aeruginosa* during tigecycline therapy in ICU patients and underscores the need for judicious tigecycline use [41C].

References

[1] Lee KH, Ueng YF, Wu CW, et al. The recommended dose of ertapenem poses a potential risk for central nervous system toxicity in haemodialysis patients—case reports and literature review. J Clin Pharm Ther. 2015;40:240–4 [c].

[2] Kaya B, Yilmaz B, Kiz F, et al. Ertapenem induced hyperbilirubinemia. Clin Res Hepatol Gastroenterol. 2015;39:e11 [c].

[3] Oka S, Shiragami H, Nohgaqa M. Intravascular hemolytic anemia in a patient with antibodies related to meropenem. Intern Med. 2015;54:1291–5 [c].

[4] Ralapanawa DM, Kularatne SA. Kounis syndrome secondary to amoxicillin/clavulanic acid administration: a case report and review of literature. BMC Res Notes. 2015;8:97. http://dx.doi.org/10.1186/s13104-015-1072-5 [c].

[5] Hentzien M, Lambert D, Limelette A, et al. Macroscopic amoxicillin crystalluria. Lancet. 2015;385:2296 [c].

[6] Syrigou E, Grapsa D, Charpidou A, et al. Acute generalized exanthematous pustulosis induced by amoxicillin/clavulanic acid: report of a case presenting with generalized lymphadenopathy. J Cutan Med Surg. 2016;19(6):592–4 [c].

[7] Lopes L, Alves A, Guerreiro F. Nicolau syndrome after benzathine penicillin treated with hyperbaric oxygen therapy. Int J Dermatol. 2015;54:103–5 [c].

[8] Diego P, Neves M, Freitas F, et al. Piperacillin/tazobactam-induced neurotoxicity in a hemodialysis patient: a case report. Hemodial Int. 2015;19:132–45 [c].

[9] Man L, Fu YP. Piperacillin/tazobactam-induced myoclonic jerks in a man with chronic renal failure. BMJ Case Rep. 2015; http://dx.doi.org/10.1136/bcr-2015-210184 [c].

[10] Lemieuz P, Gregoire JP, Thibeault R, et al. Higher risk of neutropenia associated with piperacillin-tazobactam compared with ticarcillin-clavulanate in children. Clin Infect Dis. 2015;60(2):203–7 [C].

[11] Shaik S, Kazi HA, Ender PT. Rapid-onset piperacillin-tazobactam induced thrombocytopenia. J Pharm Pract. 2015;28(2):2014–6 [c].

[12] Gaeta F, Valluzzi RL, Alonzi C, et al. Tolerability of aztreonam and carbapenems in patients with IGE-mediated hypersensitivity to penicillins. J Allergy Clin Immunol. 2015;135(4):972–6 [C].

[13] Metsala J, Lundqvist A, Virta LJ, et al. Prenatal and post-natal exposure to antibiotics and risk of asthma in childhood. Clin Exp Allergy. 2015;45:137–45 [MC].

[14] Beltran RJ, Kako H, Chovanec T, et al. Penicillin allergy and surgical prophylaxis: cephalosporin cross-reactivity risk in a pediatric tertiary care center. J Pediatr Surg. 2015;50:856–9 [C].

[15] Mac K, Chavada R, Paul S, et al. Cefepime induced acute interstitial nephritis—a case report. BMC Nephrol. 2015;16:15 [A].

[16] Mani LY, Kissling S, Viceic D, et al. Intermittent hemodialysis treatment in cefepime-induced neurotoxicity: case report, pharmacokinetic modeling, and review of the literature. Hemodial Int. 2015;19:330–51 [A].

[17] Khasani S. Cefepime-induced jaw myoclonus. Neurology. 2015;84:1183 [A].

[18] Arnold CJ, Ericson J, Cho N, et al. Cefepime and ceftazidime safety in hospitalized infants. Pediatr Infect Dis J. 2015;34:964–8 [MC].

[19] Jones JM, Richter LM, Alonto A, et al. Desensitization to ceftaroline in a patient with multiple medication hypersensitivity reactions. Am J Health Syst Pharm. 2015;72:198–202 [A].

[20] LaVie KW, Anderson SW, O'Neal HR, et al. Neutropenia associated with long-term ceftaroline use. Antimicrob Agents Chemother. 2015;60:264–9. http://dx.doi.org/10.1128/AAC.01471-15 [Epub ahead of print Oct 26, 2015]. [c].

[21] Varada NL, Sakoulas G, Lei LR, et al. Agranulocytosis with ceftaroline high-dose monotherapy or combination therapy with clindamycin. Pharmacother. 2015;35:608–12 [A].

[22] Wagenlehner FM, Umeh O, Steenbergen J, et al. Ceftolozane-tazobactam compared with levofloxacin in the treatment of complicated urinary-tract infections, including pyelonephritis: a randomised, double-blind, phase 3 trial (ASPECT-cUTI). Lancet. 2015;385:1949–56 [MC].

[23] Northrop MS, Agarwal HS. Ceftriaxone-induced hemolytic anemia: case report and review of literature. J Pediatr Hematol Oncol. 2015;37:e63–6 [A].

[24] Uy N, Thiagarajan P, Musher DM. Cephalosporin side chain idiosyncrasies: a case report of ceftriaxone-induced agranulocytosis and review of literature. Open Forum Infect Dis. 2015;2:1–4 [A].

[25] Shima A, Suehiro T, Takii M, et al. Reversible ceftriaxone-induced pseudolithiasis in an adult patient with maintenance hemodialysis. Case Rep Nephrol Dial. 2015;5:187–91 [A].

[26] Dias de Castro E, LeBlanc A, Sarmento A, et al. An unusual case of delayed-type hypersensitivity to ceftriaxone and meropenem. Eur Ann Allergy Clin Immunol. 2015;47:225–7 [A].

[27] Romano A, Gaeta F, Valuzzi RL, et al. IgE-mediated hypersensitivity to cephalosporins: cross reactivity and tolerability of alternative cephalosporins. J Allergy Clin Immunol. 2015;136:685–91 [C].

[28] Lee SH, Kim MH, Lee K, et al. Hypersensitivity pneumonitis caused by cephalosporins with identical R1 side chains. Allergy Asthma Immunol Res. 2015;7:518–22 [A].

[29] Rahman N, Murphy CC. Impact of intracameral cefuroxime on the incidence of postoperative endophthalmitis following cataract surgery in Ireland. Ir J Med Sci. 2015;184:395–8 [MC].

[30] Faure C, Perreira D, Audo I. Retinal toxicity after intracameral use of a standard dose of cefuroxime during cataract surgery. Doc Ophthalmol. 2015;130:57–63 [A].

[31] Christiansen IS, Kroigaard M, Mosbech H, et al. Clinical and diagnostic features of perioperative hypersensitivity to cefuroxime. Clin Exp Allergy. 2015;45:807–14 [c].

[32] Martinez Tadeo JA, Perez Rodriguez E, Almeida Sanchez Z, et al. No cross-reactivity with cephalosporins in patients with penicillin allergy. J Investig Allergol Clin Immunol. 2015;25:216–7 [c].

[33] Macy E, Contreras R. Adverse reactions associated with oral and parenteral use of cephalosporins: a retrospective population-based analysis. J Allergy Clin Immunol. 2015;135:745–52 [MC].

[34] Dowalit E, Dovico J, Unwin B. Skin hyperpigmentation and melanonychia from chronic doxycycline use. Ann Pharmacother. 2015;49(10):1175–6 [c].

[35] Reese S, Grundfast K. Minocycline-induced hyperpigmented of tympanic membrane, sclera, teeth, and pinna. Laryngoscope. 2015;125:2601–3 [c].

[36] Bernstein EF, Koblenzer C, Elenitsas R. Minocycline pigmentation following carbon dioxide laser resurfacing: treatment with the Q-switched Nd:YAG laser. J Drugs Dermatol. 2015;14(4):411–4 [c].

[37] Narang T, Dogra S, Sakia UN. Persistent serpentine supravenous hyperpigmented eruption in lepromatous leprosy after minocycline. Lepr Rev. 2015;86:191–4 [c].

[38] Farahnik B, Zaghi S, Hendizadeh L, et al. Rusty green stained temporal bone associated with exposure to tetracycline: an unusual presentation of black bone disease. J Laryngol Otol. 2015;129:276–8 [c].

[39] Zhang Q, Zhou S, Zhou J. Tigecycline treatment causes a decrease in fibrinogen levels. Antimicrob Agents Chemother. 2015;59(3):1650–5 [c].

[40] Routsi C, Kokkoris S, DOuka E, et al. High-dose tigecycline-associated alterations in coagulation parameters in critically ill patients with severe infections. Int J Antimicrob Agents. 2015;45:90–3 [c].

[41] Ulu-Klic A, Alp E, Altun D, et al. Increasing frequency of pseudomonas aeruginosa infections during tigecycline use. J Infect Dev Ctries. 2015;9(3):309–12 [C].

24

Miscellaneous Antibacterial Drugs

Saira B. Chaudhry[1]

Ernest Mario School of Pharmacy, Rutgers-The State University of New Jersey, Piscataway, NJ, USA
[1]Corresponding author: sairac@pharmacy.rutgers.edu

AMINOGLYCOSIDES [SED-15, 118; SEDA-32, 461; SEDA-33, 509; SEDA-34, 399; SEDA-35, 463; SEDA-36, 363; SEDA-37, 293]

Urinary Tract

A retrospective cohort study was conducted at two university hospitals to access when the risk of Acute Kidney Injury (AKI) increases after administration of an Aminoglycoside (AG), which were gentamicin and tobramycin for a minimum of 5 days. Patients had to have 2 AG levels >72 hours apart. AG-induced AKI was defined as ≥50% increase in serum creatinine (SCr) occurring after ≥5 days of AG initiation until a maximum of 7 days after cessation of the AG. AKI occurred 11 days (IQR 8–15) after AG administration. Independent risk factors associated with AKI were patients with heart failure, concomitant vancomycin, and high AG trough levels. A total of 56% of the patients had stage 1 AKI, 29% had stage 2, and 15% had stage 3. Only 51% of all AKI patients recovered their kidney function within 21 days from AG cessation. The median duration of AKI was 7 days (IQR 4–12). The authors did not express what doses of gentamicin and tobramycin the patients received [1c].

Amikacin [SED-15, 111; SEDA-32, 461; SEDA-33, 510; SEDA-34, 400; SEDA-35, 463; SEDA-36, 363; SEDA-37, 294]

Sensory Systems

Amikacin and kanamycin are mainly used for treating multi-drug resistant tuberculosis (MDR-TB) in developing countries where there is a high rate of MDR-TB. In a retrospective cohort study, Sagwa et al. compared the cumulative incidence of hearing loss in patients treated with amikacin or kanamycin for MDR-TB in Namibia. The study outcome was the occurrence of any hearing loss. A total of 353 patients were included in the study. Fifty-one (14%) of the patients were treated with amikacin-based regimen and 302 (86%) were treated with a kanamycin-based regimen. The cumulative hearing loss was greater among the amikacin-treated group than the kanamycin-based regimen group (75% vs. 56%, $p=0.01$). Also those treated with amikacin had more profound hearing loss than the kanamycin group (22% vs. 7%, $p=0.01$). Overall, this was a well-conducted study; however, one limitation is the authors did not discuss the doses of amikacin and kanamycin that were used [2c].

Urinary Tract

A retrospective study examined the outcomes of amikacin therapy for urinary tract infections (UTIs) caused by extended spectrum β-lactamase (ESBL) producing *E. coli*. One of the outcomes measured was AKI, which was defined as ≥50% increase in SCr levels <7 days or a urine output <0.5 ml/kg/hour for >6 hours according to the Risk, Injury, Failure, Loss, End-Stage classification (RIFLE). A total of 9 patients were evaluated. Only 1 patient had developed an increase in SCr from 3.64 to 4.76 mg/dl after amikacin treatment. There was no significant decrease in renal function according to the RIFLE classification. The authors did conclude that the increase in SCr in this patient could be contributed to the combined effects of treatment and other factors such as immunosuppressant therapy, graft kidney reflux, and rejection [3c].

Gentamicin [SED-15, 1500; SEDA-32, 461; SEDA-33, 510; SEDA-34, 400; SEDA-35, 463; SEDA-36, 364; SEDA-37, 294]

Pediatrics

A case controlled study was performed in a neonatal intensive care unit (NICU), between March 2012 to April

2013, to assess if extended interval dosing of gentamicin is associated with ototoxicity in neonates. Neonates received gentamicin 4 mg/kg/dose every 24 hours. Two staged Transient Evoked Otoacoustic Emissions (TEOAEs) screening tests were used. Initial TEOAEs were done after birth followed by a retest at discharge. Those who failed the TEOAE at discharge were then examined by auditory brain stem response (ABR) to confirm the hearing loss. There was no statistical difference in TEOAEs between the gentamicin group versus the non-gentamicin group. Those neonates treated with gentamicin for >5 days had a higher percentage of failure than those given gentamicin for <5 days (20% vs. 32%), no statistical significance was seen. This study suggests that extended interval dosing of gentamicin therapy in neonates does not increase the frequency of hearing loss [4c].

In an observational study, Cross et al. investigated if sepsis or systemic inflammatory response syndrome (SIRS) and gentamicin exposure would put neonates at risk of hearing loss in the NICU. The tests used to detect hearing loss were the distortion product otoacoustic emissions (DPOAE) and the automated auditory brainstem response (AABR), which was done at discharge. In order to pass the DPOAE screen, the neonates had to have responses in >6 of 10 frequencies in both ears. If patients did not pass, they would be considered a "referral" for potential hearing loss evaluation after discharge. Thirty-six (39.5%) of the 91 patients in the cohort were referred for follow-up evaluation for hearing loss. Seventy-four (81%) patients received gentamicin. Twenty patients (22%) had ≥4 days of gentamicin and 71 (78%) had <4 days. The risk ratio (RR) of referral with ≥4 days of gentamicin was 1.92 ($p=0.01$, 95% CI 1.22–3.03). Nine of the 18 patients with sepsis had ≥5 days of gentamicin and a DPOAE referral RR of 2.12 ($p=0.02$, 95% CI 1.35–3.34). Twenty subjects had gentamicin in combination with vancomycin or furosemide, with a RR of 1.77 ($p=0.05$, 95% CI 1.08–2.88). This study did demonstrate that exposure to gentamicin ≥4 days in neonates was associated with an increase risk of hearing loss [5c].

Musiime et al. conducted a systematic literature review and meta-analysis to assess the number of neonates at risk of gentamicin toxicity in low- and middle-income countries. The toxicities of interest were ototoxicity and nephrotoxicity. A total of 11 studies were included (9 were prospective randomized studies and 2 were prospective cohort studies). The studies were conducted between 1979 and 2004 in the United States, Thailand, India, and Germany. All the studies used intravenous gentamicin, except for one study that used intramuscular gentamicin. The dose of gentamicin ranged from 2.5 mg to 5 mg/kg/dose every 12–48 hours. Six trials assessed ototoxicity outcomes in neonates treated with gentamicin, and the meta-analysis estimate of hearing loss was 3% (95% CI 0–7%). Nephrotoxicity was not assessed due to variations in the definition among the studies [6M].

Urinary Tract

A retrospective, observational study compared the rate of nephrotoxicity with gentamicin perioperative prophylaxis versus no gentamicin use for selected orthopedic surgeries. The gentamicin was based on a weight-based protocol. The patients were calculated to receive a dose that approximated to 3–5 mg/kg of dosing body weight. The surgeries included were thoracolumbar spine fusions/refusions, total hip replacement and total knee replacements. The severity of nephrotoxicity was defined by RIFLE criteria. A total of 4177 surgeries were evaluated. Of those, 1590 received gentamicin. The rate of nephrotoxicity was 2.5% (39/1590) in the gentamicin group versus 1.8% (46/2587) in the group that did not receive gentamicin, $p=0.166$. Overall, the rate of nephrotoxicity was similar among the two groups [7c].

A retrospective observational study evaluated nephrotoxicity in patients exposed to extended interval dosing of gentamicin. The patients received doses ranging from 3 to 7 mg/kg every 24 or 36, or 48 hours, dependent on their renal function. Nephrotoxicity was defined as the incidence of receiving renal replacement therapy or an increase in SCr levels by at least 0.04 mmol/l from the mean during the 7 days before the gentamicin infusion to the maximum that occurred in 14 days after the first infusion. Nephrotoxicity was observed in 4% of the patients and was irreversible in 25% of these [8c].

Due to data lacking in the use of a single dose of an aminoglycoside in septic patients, Cobussen et al. retrospectively studied septic patients who received one dose of gentamicin (in combination with beta lactam antibiotics) versus those patients who were pneumoseptic only and did not receive gentamicin. RIFLE criteria were used to determine severity of AKI on admission and after admission. In a 12-month study period, a total of 179 patients were in the gentamicin group and 123 patients in the non-gentamicin group. After admission, AKI occurred in 12 patients (6.7%) in the gentamicin group and in four patients (3.3%) in the control group ($p=0.30$). This study demonstrated that there was no increased risk of developing nephrotoxicity after a single dose of gentamicin in septic patients [9c].

Tobramycin [SED-15, 3437; SEDA-32, 463; SEDA-33, 513; SEDA-35, 464; SEDA-36, 365; SEDA-37, 295]

Pediatrics

In an integrated analysis study, of the EDIT core trial and its extension studies, patients with Cystic Fibrosis

(CF) aged 6–21 years were given seven cycles of tobramycin powder for inhalation (TIP) over a period of 1 year. The total dose of tobramycin was 112 mg. Hearing loss of 20 dB at one frequency or 10–15 dB at two consecutive frequencies in either ear was reported in six patients. Two of the patients had a reported history of IV tobramycin and aminoglycoside use [10R].

In a randomized, multi-center, open-label, two period cross-over study, tobramycin inhalation solution (TIS) (300 mg/5 ml) was administered via PARI eFlow® rapid once daily or twice daily. There was no ototoxic or nephrotoxic effects found in patients [11c].

FLUOROQUINOLONES [SEDA-15, 1396; SEDA-32, 464; SEDA-33, 514; SEDA-34, 401; SEDA-36, 464; SEDA-36, 365; SEDA-37, 295]

Cardiovascular

In a meta-analysis, Mehrzad et al. reviewed clinical trials regarding QT prolongation, episodes of Tdp and adverse cardiac events with the use of fluoroquinolones (FQ). The analysis mainly focused on the 3 major FQ in the US market, ciprofloxacin, levofloxacin, and moxifloxacin. Moxifloxacin had a several fold higher risk of cardiac arrhythmias than levofloxacin or ciprofloxacin in randomized trials. Due to variations in the trials and also the relative rarity of cardiac events, the authors conclude that clinicians should not base their use solely on the concern for cardiac arrhythmias except in those who are at highest risk [12M].

Fluoroquinolones have been associated with collagen degradation leading to aortic aneurysms and dissections. A nested case–control study, using examined the relationship between FQ use and the risk of developing aortic aneurysm and dissection. Analysis of 1477 case patients and 147700 matched controls from the Taiwan National Health Insurance Research Database (NHIRD) from January 2000 to December 2011. Controls were matched based on age and sex. Use of FQ was assumed whenever there was any order for a reimbursement code of oral FQ with a prescription length of 3 days or longer. Current use of a FQ was defined as filling the prescription within 60 days of the index date. Past use was defined as filling the prescription 61–365 days prior to the index date. Current use of the FQ was associated with the highest risk of aortic aneurysm or dissection (RR 2.43 95% CI 1.83–3.22) as compared to past use (RR 1.48; 95% CI 1.18–1.86). Overall, there is an increased risk of developing an aortic aneurysm with FQ use [13A]. Another study used the same database to examine if there is an increased risk of ventricular arrhythmia and cardiovascular death with FQ use (ciprofloxacin, moxifloxacin, and levofloxacin) vs. amoxicillin–clavulanate and azithromycin. This study

found that moxifloxacin was associated with significant increases in ventricular arrhythmias and cardiovascular death. The adjusted OR for moxifloxacin was 3.30 (95% CI, 2.07–5.25) and 1.41 (95% CI 0.91–2.18) for levofloxacin. The adjusted OR for cardiovascular death was 2.31 (95% CI 1.39–3.48) and 1.77 (95% CI 1.22–2.59) for levofloxacin [14A].

Endocrine

A prospective, observational study found fluoroquinolones to cause dysglycemia in diabetic and non-diabetic patients. About 74.6% of the patients received the proper dose for indication. Dysglycemia occurred more frequently in those patients treated with ciprofloxacin (50%), followed by levofloxacin (42.4%), and moxifloxacin (7.6%). Hyperglycemia occurred more in the levofloxacin group (70%), followed by ciprofloxacin (39%), and moxifloxacin (33.3%) [15c].

Musculoskeletal

Arabyat et al. conducted an analysis of reports of tendon rupture contained in the FDA's Adverse Event Reporting System (FAERS) associated with Fluoroquinolone use. A total of 2495 reports of tendon rupture associated with FQ. Most of the reports were associated with levofloxacin (62%), followed by ciprofloxacin (24%) and moxifloxacin (9.2%). In conclusion, there is an association with FQ use and tendon rupture [16M].

A population-based longitudinal cohort study was conducted in Ontario, Canada, to determine collagen-associated adverse events (tendon rupture, retinal detachment, and aortic aneurysms) and their association with fluoroquinolone use. All three outcomes were more common in patients who received at least one FQ compared to patients who never received a FQ prescription. Those who received a FQ had a higher risk of tendon rupture (3.5% vs. 1.3%, $p < 0.01$), retinal detachment (0.26% vs. 0.14%, $p < 0.001$) and aortic aneurysm (1.7% vs. 0.7%, $p < 0.001$). This study demonstrated that FQ use is remarkably associated with tendon rupture, retinal detachment, and aortic aneurysms [17M].

Ciprofloxacin [SED-15, 783; SEDA-32, 465; SEDA-33, 514; SEDA-34, 402; SEDA-35, 465; SEDA-36, 365; SEDA-37, 295]

Drug–Drug Interaction

A 41-year-old African woman with a history of severe systemic lupus erythematosus (SLE) and severe glomerulonephritis presented to the Emergency room with severe myalgia and intense weakness for 3 days. The patient did require peritoneal dialysis (PD) and was on dialysis medications, as well as simvastatin 20 mg every other day. Nine days before she was admitted, the patient was diagnosed with PD-related peritonitis. She was given the following antimicrobial therapy to help treat it: vancomycin 2 g every 3 days, ciprofloxacin 500 mg twice a day, and single dose of gentamicin 80 mg. Four days later, the ciprofloxacin was stopped due the peritoneal fluid growing *Corynebacterium striatum*. The patient started to complain of severe muscle pain and intense weakness. She developed impressive rhabdomyolysis with a creatine kinase (CK) of 540 000 IU/l, lactate dehydrogenase of (LDH) of 19 200 IU/l, and aspartate aminotransferase of 1700 IU/l. She also developed severe electrolyte disturbances and a serum creatinine (SCr) of 12.4 mg/dl, of which she had to be admitted to the intensive care unit. The serum CK increased to 816 000 IU/l and progressively declined. The patient's electrolytes normalized and SCr returned to the patients baseline levels on day of 3 of ICU admission. It was believed that the patient developed rhabdomyolysis due to the drug interaction between simvastatin and ciprofloxacin [18A].

Hematologic

A case report of a 61-year-old female was given ciprofloxacin 500 mg twice daily for diarrhea, nausea, vomiting, and fever. After 5 days of treatment, the patient developed thrombocytopenia. The patient's thrombocyte count dropped to 16 000 per mm^3. Twelve units of thrombocyte suspension were given to the patient. The patient ended up receiving another 6 units of thrombocyte suspension, in turn, raising the thrombocyte count to 131 000 per mm^3 on the eighth day. The patient's thrombocyte count did normalize in the following days. The authors concluded that ciprofloxacin was the cause of thrombocytopenia in this patient [19A].

A 49-year-old African American woman was prescribed ciprofloxacin for a urinary tract infection (UTI). The patient presented with confusion, lethargy, and abdominal pain. Upon admission, the patient presented with anemia, thrombocytopenia, elevated lactate dehydrogenase, and SCr. The patient was diagnosed with thrombotic thrombocytopenic purpura (TTP). The patient received methylprednisolone 40 mg IV twice a day for 2 weeks and plasmapheresis. While on treatment, the patient's hematologic levels normalized. Ciprofloxacin was deemed to be the culprit in causing this patient to develop TTP [20A].

Musculoskeletal

A 72-year-old male presented with discitis and osteomyelitis, for which he received vancomycin and ciprofloxacin. Four days later, the patient complained of right hip pain. Magnetic resonance imaging (MRI) of the hip showed partial tearing of the right gluteus medius tendon insertion and at the origin of the right hamstring tendons. The patient was suspected to have FQ-induced tendinopathy and ciprofloxacin was discontinued. The

pain started to improve when the ciprofloxacin was discontinued [21A].

Nervous System

A 57-year-old Caucasian female was given ciprofloxacin 250 mg twice daily for 5 days for a UTI. Two months later, the patient presented with whole body burning and alopecia. She claimed the burning began 2 days after completing the ciprofloxacin. A neurological workup could not determine a unique cause of her symptoms. The patient still suffers from polyneuropathies chronologically related to ciprofloxacin use. The patient was placed on amitriptyline 20 mg daily to control her pain symptoms [22A].

Skin

Nair describes three case reports where the patients developed bullous fixed drug reactions caused by ciprofloxacin. All three developed lesions all over the body within 1 week after consuming ciprofloxacin. The lesions burned and itched. All the patients were treated with prednisolone 40 mg/day (then tapered), antihistamines, local soframycin, and topical steroids [23A].

A 92-old-year old female was prescribed ciprofloxacin for a UTI; after 8 days of treatment, she developed vesicular and bullous lesions on an erythematous base, distributed only on the trunk and upper extremities. A diagnosis of drug-induced bullous pemphigoid (DIBP) was made due to the ciprofloxacin. The ciprofloxacin was stopped and a topical corticosteroid was initiated for 20 days. The patient had complete resolution of their DIBP in 30 days [24A].

Levofloxacin [SED-15, 2047; SEDA-32, 467; SEDA-33, 516; SEDA-34, 403; SEDA-35, 465; SEDA-36, 366; SEDA-37, 296]

Cardiac

In a retrospective study, Stancampiano et al. investigated the incidence of ventricular tachycardia and ventricular fibrillation in patients with prolonged corrected QT interval (QTc) who received levofloxacin. Patients were excluded from the study if they received levofloxacin and azithromycin within 72 hours before the first ECG showing QTc prolongation or if the patients were using any concomitant antiarrhythmic medications at the time of admission. Patients received either oral or IV levofloxacin and the doses given ranged from 250 to 750 mg. A total of 1004 patients were selected (with QTc > 450 ms). Only 2 patients experienced sustained ventricular tachycardia after initiating levofloxacin (0.2%; 95% CI 0.0–0.7%). This study found that the short-term risk of sustained ventricular arrhythmia with prolonged QTc was rare [25c].

Drug–Drug Interactions

Five cases were reported to have a probable drug interaction between acenocoumarol and levofloxacin. All 5 patients were on long-term acenocoumarol with stable international normalized ratios (INR) for at least 6 months. All the patients received levofloxacin 500 mg daily for respiratory infections, and they all experienced elevated INRs requiring administration of vitamin K. In 2 patients, the acenocoumarol was switched to subcutaneous enoxaparin and the INR normalized. In two patients, the levofloxacin dose was reduced from 500 to 250 mg daily and the INR normalized. And in one patient, the acenocoumarol was held and the INR normalized the next day [26A].

Endocrine

Four days after starting levofloxacin (500 mg/day orally), a 56-year-old woman, with a history of diabetes mellitus (on metformin monotherapy) became unresponsive and severely hypoglycemic (blood glucose level of 15 mg/dl). She first received an ampule of 50% dextrose intravenously for this event. Over the next 2 days, the patient experienced episodes of hypoglycemia, which required dextrose infusion and glucagon; however, the patient's hypoglycemic events resolved by day 3. After ruling out all other causes, her hypoglycemia was thought be caused by the levofloxacin [27A].

Liver

A 53-year-old female was given levofloxacin 750 mg for one dose and developed toxic hepatitis and secondary multiple organ failure. The patient developed a rash after ingesting one dose of levofloxacin 750 mg for a pulmonary infection. The levofloxacin was discontinued; however, the patient within 3 days developed desquamation all over the body. After 5 days, the patient complained of abdominal pain and had yellowing of the skin. The patient was thought to be a candidate for liver transplant; however, she had a cardiopulmonary arrest and died [28A].

Musculoskeletal

A 53-year-old female received levofloxacin for a cat bite and developed an Achilles tendon rupture complicated by an abscess and hematoma. The patient underwent surgery for tendon repair and drainage of the abscess and hematoma. Five years post-op, the patient had full strength in her Achilles tendon and no restrictions in her daily activities [29A]. An 81-year-old male experienced bilateral Achilles tendon ruptures when he received levofloxacin 500 mg per day for 7 days for bronchitis. He required surgery to repair the ruptured Achilles tendons. He fully recovered and did not require any assistive device to walk [30A].

Neuromuscular Function

A 62-year-old Caucasian male developed craniocervical dystonia 3 days after initiating levofloxacin 500 mg orally twice daily for urinary symptoms. The levofloxacin was discontinued, and the patient's dystonic episodes completely resolved 7 days later [31A].

Two case reports describe patients developing CNS problems after initiating levofloxacin 750 mg daily. The first case is a 28-year-old female who became debilitated and bed ridden for a year after discontinuing the levofloxacin. She had could not bare weight on her feet and required assistance in feeding, bathing, and toileting because of the severe muscle pain and atrophy. The second case is a 46-year-old male also developed polyneuropathy of unknown origin and/or fibromyalgia due to levofloxacin. After discontinuing the levofloxacin, the patient was placed on citalopram 10 mg and Zinc to control the peripheral neuropathy [32].

Urinary Tract

Levofloxacin-induced crystal nephropathy was found to occur in a 64-year-old female after taking levofloxacin 500 mg daily for a possible respiratory infection. The patient was also started on amoxicillin sodium/sulbactam 4.5 g twice daily, as well. On the fifth day, the patients SCr increased from 80 to 368 μmol/l. Cotton-like crystals were also found in the urine sample. Levofloxacin was deemed the culprit to have caused this because the crystals matched the crystals in a healthy volunteer's urine sample. Both drugs were discontinued, and the patient was placed on hemodialysis. The patient's SCr levels normalized [33A].

Moxifloxacin [SED-15, 2392; SEDA-32, 468; SEDA-33, 518; SEDA-34, 404; SEDA-35, 466; SEDA-36, 367; SEDA-37, 297]

Cardiovascular

In a single-blinded, randomized, single-dose, placebo-controlled, two-period cross-over study, patients were placed in either of two groups: Group 1: moxifloxacin 400 mg tablet daily for 7 days then placebo for 7 days or Group 2: placebo for the first 7 days and then be switched moxifloxacin 400 mg orally daily. This studies primary outcome was to determine the QT/QTc effects of moxifloxacin. A total of 24 healthy patients were included in the study. It was found that moxifloxacin significantly prolonged the mean QTc at all times except 0.5 hours post-dose. The greatest time-matched difference in the QTc interval was 8.35 ms (90% CI: 5.43–11.27) at 4 h post-dose. In conclusion, moxifloxacin had a significant effect in prolonging the QTc interval [34c].

Nervous System

A 45-year-old female was prescribed moxifloxacin 400 mg orally once daily for sinus symptoms, which included ear pain, congestion, and low-grade fevers. Within 1 hour of taking the moxifloxacin, she felt nauseated, nervous, and agitate. Two hours after the first dose, she experienced a seizure that lasted for 10 min. The patient discontinued the moxifloxacin and fully recovered and did not have any recurring seizures [35].

Pediatric

A 10-year-old female was prescribed topical 0.5% preservative-free moxifloxacin four times daily for mucopurulent conjunctivitis. The patient returned 3 days later with redness, photophobia, watering and a drop in visual acuity in both eyes. She was also found to have circumcorneal congestion with corneal edema. The topical moxifloxacin was discontinued, and in a week, her cornea showed signs of clearing and her vision returned to normal [36].

Ofloxacin [SED-15, 2597; SEDA-34, 405; SEDA-35, 466; SEDA-36, 368; SEDA-37, 297]

Pediatric

Three case reports describe children developing ofloxacin induced cutaneous reactions. The first case describes a 5-year-old female given ofloxacin hydrochloride syrup 5 ml twice daily with paracetamol syrup 5 ml three times daily. The patient developed red colored papules all over the body with severe itching after 3 days. When the ofloxacin was withdrawn, the reactions subsided. The second case describes a 4-year-old boy who developed multiple itchy annular erythematous lesions all over the body 2 days after starting ofloxacin 7.5 ml twice daily and paracetamol 5 mg twice daily for enteric fever. After stopping the ofloxacin and substituting it with azithromycin, 48 hours later the patient's symptoms resolved. The third case is a 6-year-old female who developed erythema of eyelids with conjunctival congestion, buccal mucosal ulcerations, and painful red to black colored erythematous maculopapular blisters rapidly appeared all over the body 48 hours after taking ofloxacin. The ofloxacin was stopped, and the patient was given IV dexamethasone, chlorohexidine mouthwash, levocetrizine and calamine lotion. Ten days later, the patient's reaction resolved [37A].

GLYCOPEPTIDES [SEDA-32, 469; SEDA-33, 519; SEDA-34, 405; SEDA-35, 466; SEDA-36, 368; SEDA-37, 297]

Dalbavancin [SEDA-37, 297]

Cardiovascular

A randomized, partially double-blinded, single-center, parallel study was conducted to determine that dalbavancin had no effect on the 12-lead ECG QTc. A total of 200 patients were enrolled, and 50 patients were enrolled to each of the four treatment groups of dalbavancin 100 mg IV, dalbavancin 1500 mg IV, placebo IV, or moxifloxacin 400 mg oral. The study found that doses up to 1500 mg of dalbavancin had no effect on the QTc interval [38C].

Oritavancin [SEDA-37, 297]

Drug Studies

A major randomized, double-blinded trial studied patients who were given either oritavancin 1200 mg IV as a single dose or 7–10 days of intravenous vancomycin (1 g or 15 mg/kg of body weight) twice daily for acute bacterial skin and skin structure infections (SOLO II trial). The most frequently reported adverse events in the SOLO II were nausea, headache, vomiting, cellulitis, increased alanine aminotransferase and infusion site phlebitis [39].

Teicoplanin [SED-15, 3305; SEDA-32, 469; SEDA-33, 519; SEDA-34, 405; SEDA-35, 467; SEDA-36, 368; SEDA-37, 298]

Drug Studies

A retrospective, cohort study, observed if target trough concentrations of teicoplanin were achieved in hematologic malignant patients. The teicoplanin dose was 600 mg (800 mg if >80 kg) for 3 loading doses 12 hours apart, followed by a once daily maintenance dose. They also assessed if nephrotoxicity occurred based on the RIFLE criteria. The study found no evidence of renal impairment in 92.4% of teicoplanin treatments. Only 6.4% of treatments were classified to be in the 'Risk' category and 1.2% in the 'Injury' category. Overall, teicoplanin was renally tolerated in this patient population [40c].

Telavancin [SEDA-33, 520; SEDA-34, 405; SEDA-35, 467; SEDA-36, 369; SEDA-37, 298]

Drug Studies

In an open-label, single institution, pilot study, telavancin was given to cancer patients for uncomplicated bloodstream infections. The dose of telavancin used in the study was 10 mg/kg daily if CrCl >50 ml/min or 7.5 mg/kg daily if CrCl was 30–49 ml/min. The adverse events observed were nephrotoxicity, diarrhea, altered taste, nausea and vomiting, altered taste, skin rash, anorexia, palpitations, and confusion [41c].

Vancomycin [SED-15, 3593; SEDA-32, 470; SEDA-33, 520; SEDA-34, 406; SEDA-35, 467; SEDA-36, 369; SEDA-37, 298]

Hematologic

A 67-year-old male developed thrombocytopenia and hematuria 5 days after starting vancomycin 500 mg IV twice daily for pneumonia. The patient also became hemodynamically unstable. He required intravenous immunoglobulin, pulsed methylprednisolone, 13 units of packed red blood cells, 13 pools of platelets, and 4 units of fresh frozen plasma to reverse the thrombocytopenia. The patient's platelet count normalized after 3 days of treatment [42A].

A 62-year-old female was given heparin, vancomycin, and piperacillin/tazobactam for possible periprosthetic knee infection. She underwent extensive tissue debridement and explant of her prosthesis with placement of a vancomycin containing spacer. Eleven days after, her platelet count dropped, and the patient was switched from heparin to bivalirudin. However, the platelet count continued to drop by day 14. The vancomycin was substituted with daptomycin, and the piperacillin/tazobactam was continued. On day 17, the platelet count dramatically improved [43A].

Immunologic

Two case reports described the development of hypersensitivity syndrome/drug reaction with eosinophilia and systemic symptoms syndrome (HSS/DRESS), after initiating vancomycin 2 g IV per day and 4 g per day of vancomycin-containing bone cement spacers. Both patients had suffered from eosinophilia, rash, increased creatinine and abnormal liver function tests. In both cases, symptoms resolved after discontinuing vancomycin and initiating systemic corticosteroids [44A].

An unusual case of immune-mediated hypersensitivity reaction to intraperitoneal (IP) vancomycin was reported in a 49-year-old female. She was treated for 4 weeks of IP vancomycin once per week for peritonitis, after each dose she would experience general urticarial and prickling sensation, and the intensity increased gradually. The vancomycin was discontinued and the symptoms improved. AN intradermal skin test revealed a positive Immunoglobulin E-mediated hypersensitivity reaction to IP vancomycin [45A].

Pediatric

Moffett et al. conducted a case–control study to demonstrate if vancomycin may contribute to acute kidney injury (AKI) in pediatric patients admitted to the cardiac intensive care unit. Thirty patients out of 418 developed vancomycin-associated AKI (7.2%). This demonstrated that vancomycin-associated AKI in the pediatric cardiac intensive care unit is not very common [46c]. Another

propensity matched cohort study also demonstrated the infrequent occurrence of nephrotoxicity in neonates receiving vancomycin (16 neonates receiving vancomycin vs. 7 controls experienced AKI; OR 1.5; 95% CI 0.6–4.0) [47c].

A retrospective, cohort, single-center study was performed to determine the incidence of late-occurring AKI in children receiving ≥8days of vancomycin. This study enrolled 167 patients and found that late AKI occurred in 21 patients (12.6%). Majority of the patients also received concomitant therapy with IV acyclovir, amphotericin, or piperacillin–tazobactam [48c].

Pharmcogenomics

Van Driest et al. performed a genome wide association study of serum creatinine levels while on vancomycin. The study was conducted in 489 European American individuals. It was found that chromosome 6q22.31 locus was associated with increased SCr levels while on vancomycin therapy (most significant variant rs2789047, risk allele A, $\beta = -0.06$, $p = 1.1 \times 10^{-7}$) [49c].

Urinary Tract

Three case reports describe all the patients developing very high vancomycin trough levels (>40 µg/ml) and severe (stage 3) AKI. All 3 patients underwent kidney biopsies to reveal acute tubular necrosis. Vancomycin was discontinued. One patient required hemodialysis, but all 3 patient's kidney function returned to normal [50A].

KETOLIDES [SED-15, 1976; SEDA-32, 471; SEDA-33, 521; SEDA-34, 407; SEDA-35, 469; SEDA-36, 370; SEDA-37, 299]

Solithromycin [SEDA-35, 469; SEDA-36, 370; SEDA-37, 299]

Drug Study

A Phase 2 trial of 2 oral doses of solithromycin (1200 and 1000 mg) for treatment of uncomplicated gonorrhea. Twenty-eight patients received solithromycin 1200 mg and 31 received 1000 mg. The most common dose-related adverse effects seen were gastrointestinal, such as loose stools, nausea, and vomiting [51c].

Telithromycin [SEDA-35, 469; SEDA-36, 371; SEDA-37, 299]

Drug Study

In a literature search for randomized controlled trials to compare the efficacy and safety profile of commonly used antibiotics in the treatment of acute rhinosinusitis was conducted. This study found no major side effects noted with the use of telithromycin for this indication.

All the studies reviewed a dose of telithromycin 800 mg once daily [52M].

LINCOSAMIDES [SED-15, 2063; SEDA-32, 472; SEDA-33, 522; SEDA-34, 407; SEDA-35, 469; SEDA-36, 371; SEDA-37, 299]

Clindamycin

Immunologic

A 46-year-old female received IV clindamycin 900 mg for a periodontal abscess and developed severe anaphylaxis. The Clindamycin was immediately stopped and the patient was started on a bolus of normal saline, methylprednisolone 125 mg intravenous (IV), epinephrine 0.3 mg subcutaneously, diphenhydramine 25 mg IV and nebulized albuterol. After 10 min the patient stabilized. Her antibiotic was changed to amoxicillin/clavulanate 500 mg once daily [53A].

Liver

Clindamycin-induced acute symptomatic cholestatic hepatitis occurred in a 75-year-old female when she was prescribed oral clindamycin 450 mg every 6 hours for a UTI. Her symptoms started 3 days after initiating clindamycin. The clindamycin was discontinued, and she was started on N-acetyl cysteine (NAC) 10000 mg IV for 3 days and pentoxyphylline 400 mg three times a day. The patient was also started on solumedrol 125 mg IV twice a day for mild-to-moderate peri-portal chronic inflammation. The patient's symptoms began to improve, and she was discharged home with prednisone taper over 4 weeks [54A].

Skin

A 34-year-old female, 19 weeks pregnant, developed acute localized exanthematous pustulosis induced by clindamycin. She was given clindamycin oral 500 mg twice-daily prophylaxis for cervical cerclage. Three days later, she developed a pustular eruption on her right breast. The clindamycin was discontinued and the pustules resolved in 4 days [55A].

MACROLIDES [SED-15, 2183; SEDA-32, 472; SEDA-33, 522; SEDA-34, 408; SEDA-35, 469; SEDA-36, 371; SEDA-37, 299]

Azithromycin [SED-15, 389; SEDA-33, 522; SEDA-34, 408; SEDA-35, 469; SEDA-36, 371; SEDA-37, 299]

Cardiovascular

A Meta-analysis review was conducted to determine the all-cause mortality and cardiovascular death from azithromycin. This study found that azithromycin use was not associated with a higher risk of death from any cause (HR=0.99, CI 0.82–1.19) or cardiovascular cause (HR=1.15, CI 0.66–2) [56c]. Conversely, Goldstein et al. conducted a prospective study and found that azithromycin in a univariate analysis was not associated with QTc prolongation in patients with community acquired pneumonia [57c].

Drug–Drug Interactions

A 68-year-old male was being treated with ivabradine 7.5 mg twice a day for paroxysmal sinusal tachycardia. The patient was given azithromycin for acute sinusitis, and 5 days later, he experienced syncope. An ECG detected ventricular torsades de pointes (TdP). An infusion of magnesium was started and the TdP disappeared. There was a drug interaction between azithromycin and ivabradine, which blocks its metabolic breakdown, causing the TdP to occur. The patient was advised to avoid azithromycin [58A].

Liver

A 65-year-old male was prescribed azithromycin 1 g on day 1 and then 500 mg daily for the next 4 days. Fifteen days later, he developed an increase in liver enzymes and bilirubin. He underwent a liver biopsy, which revealed intracellular cholestasis in hepatocytes, bile duct epithelial injury, and bile duct loss. It was determined that the azithromycin caused cholestatic hepatitis in this patient. The patient was discharged with supportive care, and 4 months later, his bilirubin normalized and his symptoms resolved [59A].

Nervous System

A 45-year-old Chinese male was given azithromycin 500 mg to treat an upper airway infection. Within 2 hours, he developed a sensation that he could not sit still and had a sense of internal restlessness. The azithromycin was stopped and his symptoms resolved in 18 hours [60].

Pediatric

A retrospective chart review studied whether chronic azithromycin administration in pediatric cystic fibrosis patients led to increases in QTc intervals. This study found that no patients had clinically prolonged QTc intervals with azithromycin therapy. This study did find there to be more an inclination for adolescent males to have increase in QTc intervals [61c].

Clarithromycin [SED-15, 799; SEDA-32, 473; SEDA-33, 523; SEDA-34, 408; SEDA-35, 470; SEDA-36, 372; SEDA-37, 299]

Cardiovascular

In a self-controlled cases series and cross-over analysis study, Wong et al. were determining the cardiovascular outcomes in patients receiving clarithromycin or amoxicillin. In this study, they found that the propensity score adjusted rate ratio of myocardial infarction 14 days after starting the antibiotic treatment was 3.66 (95% CI 2.82–4.76) comparing clarithromycin use (132 events, rate 44.4 per 1000 person years) with amoxicillin use (149 events, 19.2 per 1000 person years). This study also found that clarithromycin was associated with an increased risk of arrhythmia and cardiac mortality [62c].

Drug–Drug Interactions

A 75-year-old female developed hypotension due to a drug interaction between her calcium channel blocker and clarithromycin. She was taking felodipine 10 mg, losartan 100 mg, and atenolol 100 mg daily for hypertension. She was started on clarithromycin for *H. pylori* gastritis. She developed hypotension, diaphoresis, and weakness, 3 days after beginning the clarithromycin. She was given intravenous glucagon, calcium gluconate, and normal saline. When her symptoms improved, she was discharged with metronidazole, amoxicillin, and omeprazole instead of clarithromycin. Significant hypotension can occur when clarithromycin is administered concomitantly with calcium channel blockers as seen in this case report [63A].

Erythromycin [SED-15, 1237; SEDA-32, 474; SEDA-33, 523; SEDA-34, 409; SEDA-35, 470; SEDA-36, 373; SEDA-37, 300]

Nervous System

A 28-year-old male, with a psychiatric history, maintained on olanzapine 10 mg daily and trihexyphenidyl 20 mg daily, developed akathisia after starting erythromycin for Pityriasis Rosea. He was started on erythromycin 250 mg four times a day with cetirizine 10 mg daily for 5 days. Four days later, he developed akathisia. Propranolol was given to help with the akathisia; however, the patient had no improvement. The propranolol was discontinued and when the erythromycin was stopped after 5 days the patient recovered [64A].

OXAZOLIDINONES [SED-15, 2645; SEDA-32, 474; SEDA-33, 525; SEDA-34, 409; SEDA-35, 471; SEDA-36, 373; SEDA-37, 300]

Linezolid [SEDA-35, 469; SEDA-36, 373; SEDA-37, 300]

Acid–Base Balance

Severe Lactic acidosis occurred in a 38-year-old cirrhotic female after taking linezolid. She was prescribed linezolid for a UTI and was advised to take it for 14 days. After 12 days of linezolid, she developed lactic acidosis. The linezolid was discontinued, and she was started on continuous dialysis and IV Thiamine. By day 7, her lab values returned to normal and dialysis was stopped [65A].

Tedizolid [SEDA-37, 301]

Drug Studies

In a *post hoc* analysis of the ESTABLISH-1 and 2 trials, Ortiz-Covarrubias et al. evaluated the safety and efficacy of tedizolid vs. Linezolid in Latino patients. Both studies compared tedizolid 200 mg daily with linezolid 600 mg twice daily. In this *post hoc* analysis, abnormal platelet counts were found to be threefold higher in the linezolid group (11.3%) than the tedizolid group (3.4%) at days 11–13 of therapy. Also a higher incidence of abnormal platelet counts was seen in the linezolid group (11.1%) than the tedizolid group (6.4%) after the last dose of therapy [66c].

POLYMYXINS [SED-15, 2891; SEDA-32, 476; SEDA-33, 527; SEDA-34, 412; SEDA-35, 473; SEDA-36, 374; SEDA-37, 301]

Colistin [SEDA-35, 473; SEDA-36, 374; SEDA-37, 301]

Urinary Tract

A retrospective cohort study investigated the development of nephrotoxicity associated with colistin dose, and whether it differs on renal function. The dosage of colistin in the study was 2.5–5 mg/kg/day divided in 2–4 doses. A total of 475 patients were included in this study. It was found that 43.5% of the patients experienced nephrotoxicity during treatment. Daily dosing of colistin (based on ideal body weight) was significantly associated with nephrotoxicity in patients with a glomerular filtration rate <60 ml/min/1.73 m^2 (OR, 2.34; 95% CI, 1.22–4.5) [67c]. A prospective, observational, cohort study in patients with severe sepsis or septic shock receiving colistin (at a median daily dose of 9 million IU) found that 44% of the patients developed acute kidney injury [68c].

STREPTOGRAMINS [SED-15, 3182; SEDA-32, 528; SEDA-34, 413; SEDA-35, 473; SEDA-36, 375; SEDA-37, 301]

Pristinamycin [SEDA-34, 413; SEDA-35, 469; SEDA-36, 375]

No adverse effects were reported during the time period of January 2015 to December 2015.

TRIMETHOPRIM, AND CO-TRIMOXAZOLE [SED-15, 3216, 3510; SEDA-32, 477; SEDA-33, 528; SEDA-34, 414; SEDA-35, 474; SEDA-36, 375; SEDA-37, 301]

Trimethoprim–sulfamethoxazole [SEDA-35, 474; SEDA-36, 375; SEDA-37, 301]

Drug–Drug Interaction

A population-based, nested, case–control study investigated whether trimethoprim–sulfamethoxazole when given with spironolactone caused a hyperkalemia and therefore an increased risk of death. It was found that when compared with amoxicillin, trimethoprim–sulfamethoxazole was associated with a more than twofold increase in the risk of sudden death (adjusted OR 2.46, 95% CI 1.55–3.90). Due to this interaction with spironolactone, it is recommended to choose an alternative antibiotic in place of trimethoprim–sulfamethoxazole [69c].

Electrolyte Balance

An 82-year-old woman was given trimethoprim–sulfamethoxazole (TMP–SMX) 160 mg/800 mg orally twice daily for a UTI for 7 days and experienced hyponatremia. Her Serum sodium level dropped from 132 to 121 mmol/l, the day after she finished her TMP–SMX. She was prescribed TMP–SMX several months later, and within several days, her serum sodium dropped from 138 to 129 mmol/l. The TMP–SMX was discontinued, and her serum sodium increased to 134 mmol/l [70].

Musculoskeletal

A 64-year-old male developed rhabdomyolysis after self-medicating himself with TMP–SMX 3 tablets daily for 2 weeks for a self-diagnosed UTI. During treatment, he started to have lower extremity pain, his aspartate aminotransferase was 66 U/l and creatinine kinase (CK) level was 1524 U/l. The patient was taking ketorolac 30 mg/ml, 2 vials per day, and meloxicam 15 mg, 2 vials per day, to help control his pain from a rheumatologist. Due to his pain not subsiding, he went to the hospital and was told to discontinue the TMP–SMX and NSAIDs. He was started on aggressive hydration with glucose 5% and 10% saline solution, 9% mannitol, and furosemide. After 16 days, the CK level normalized and the patient reported no more myalgias and was discharged [71A].

Pediatric

A 5-year-old girl Nigerian girl, infected with HIV, developed a hypersensitivity reaction to TMP–SMX. She was taking cotrimoxazole, 7 ml/day, three times/week (Septrim Pediatric oral suspension: 8 mg TMP/40 mg SMX/1 ml) for prevention of pneumonia. Two weeks after starting the cotrimoxazole, she developed pruritic erythematous maculopapular rash all over face, chest, and limbs. The patient was place a desensitization protocol of cotrimoxazole by gradually increasing doses by 0.5 ml every 3 days. After 28 days, the patient tolerated a daily dose of 5 ml [72A].

OTHER ANTIMICROBIAL DRUGS

Daptomycin [SED-15, 1053; SED-32, 478; SEDA-33, 529; SEDA-34, 416; SEDA-35, 474; SEDA-36, 375; SEDA-37, 302]

Musculoskeletal

A single case report describes a 46-year-old female developing rhabdomyolysis and eosinophilic pneumonia 2 days after initiating high dose daptomycin (10 mg/kg daily, 875 mg). The patient's CK level was 1754 IU/l; however, after immediately discontinuing the daptomycin, the patient's myalgias subsided. Seven days later, the patient developed a cough with mild hypoxemia and a CT scan of the chest demonstrated the patient had Eosinophilic pneumonia. His eosinophil count was 510/µl. His respiratory symptoms gradually resolved [73A].

Immunologic

A 76-year-old male developed eosinophilic pneumonia 2 weeks after starting daptomycin therapy for methicillin resistant *Staphylococcus aureus* (MRSA) septic knee and pacemaker lead vegetation. His eosinophilic count in the bronchoalveolar lavage (BAL) was 54% eosinophils. Daptomycin was immediately discontinued, and intravenous methylprednisolone was started. His respiratory symptoms subsided within 72 hours. He finished his therapy with vancomycin [74A].

Fosfomycin [SED-15, 1448; SEDA-34, 417; SEDA-35, 476; SEDA-36, 376; SEDA-37, 302]

Drug Studies

Iarikov et al. reviewed fosfomycin's Safety profile using the Food and Drug Administration Adverse Event (AE) Reporting System (FAERS) and published literature. The most common adverse events with parenteral fosfomycin were rash, peripheral phlebitis, hypokalemia, and gastrointestinal disorders, aplastic anemia, anaphylaxis, and liver toxicities. The most common adverse events reported with oral fosfomycin were gastrointestinal disorders [75c].

Fusidic Acid [SED-15, 1460; SEDA-32, 479; SEDA-33, 530; SEDA-34, 417; SEDA-35, 475; SEDA-36, 376; SEDA-37, 302]

No adverse effects were reported during the time period of January 2015 to December 2015.

References

[1] Paquette F, Bernier-Jean A, Brunette V, et al. Acute kidney injury and renal recovery with the use of aminoglycosides: a large retrospective study. Nephron. 2015;131(3):153–60 [c].

[2] Sagwa EL, Ruswa N, Mavhunga F, et al. Comparing amikacin and kanamycin-induced hearing loss in multidrug-resistant tuberculosis treatment under programmatic conditions in a Namibian retrospective cohort. BMC Pharmacol Toxicol. 2015;16(1):36 [c].

[3] Cho SY, Choi SM, Park SH, et al. Amikacin therapy for urinary tract infections caused by extended-spectrum beta-lactamase-producing Escherichia coli. Korean J Intern Med. 2016;31(1):156–61 [c].

[4] El-Barbary MN, Ismail RI, Ibrahim AA. Gentamicin extended interval regimen and ototoxicity in neonates. Int J Pediatr Otorhinolaryngol. 2015;79(8):1294–8 [c].

[5] Cross CP, Liao S, Urdang ZD, et al. Effect of sepsis and systemic inflammatory response syndrome on neonatal hearing screening outcomes following gentamicin exposure. Int J Pediatr Otorhinolaryngol. 2015;79(11):1915–9 [c].

[6] Musiime GM, Seale AC, Moxon SG, et al. Risk of gentamicin toxicity in neonates treated for possible severe bacterial infection in low- and middle-income countries: systematic review. Trop Med Int Health. 2015;20(12):1593–606 [M].

[7] Dubrovskaya Y, Tejada R, Bosco 3rd. J, et al. Single high dose gentamicin for perioperative prophylaxis in orthopedic surgery: evaluation of nephrotoxicity. SAGE Open Med. 2015;3:1–7 2050312115612803 [c].

[8] Plajer SM, Chin PK, Vella-Brincat JW, et al. Gentamicin and renal function: lessons from 15 years' experience of a pharmacokinetic service for extended interval dosing of gentamicin. Ther Drug Monit. 2015;37(1):98–103 [c].

[9] Cobussen M, de Kort JM, Dennert RM, et al. No increased risk of acute kidney injury after a single dose of gentamicin in patients with sepsis. Infect Dis (Lond). 2015;48(4):274–80 [c].

[10] Konstan MW, Flume PA, Galeva I, et al. One-year safety and efficacy of tobramycin powder for inhalation in patients with cystic fibrosis. Pediatr Pulmonol. 2016;51:372–8 [R].

[11] van Koningsbruggen-Rietschel S, Heuer HE, Merkel N, et al. Pharmacokinetics and safety of an 8 week continuous treatment with once-daily versus twice-daily inhalation of tobramycin in cystic fibrosis patients. J Antimicrob Chemother. 2016;71(3):711–7 [c].

[12] Mehrzad R, Barza M. Weighing the adverse cardiac effects of fluoroquinolones: a risk perspective. J Clin Pharmacol. 2015;55(11):1198–206 [M].

[13] Lee CC, Lee MT, Chen YS, et al. Risk of aortic dissection and aortic aneurysm in patients taking oral fluoroquinolone. JAMA Intern Med. 2015;175(11):1839–47 [A].

[14] Chou HW, Wang JL, Chang CH, et al. Risks of cardiac arrhythmia and mortality among patients using new-generation macrolides, fluoroquinolones, and beta-lactam/beta-lactamase inhibitors: a Taiwanese nationwide study. Clin Infect Dis. 2015;60(4):566–77 [A].

[15] Kabbara WK, Ramadan WH, Rahbany P, et al. Evaluation of the appropriate use of commonly prescribed fluoroquinolones and the risk of dysglycemia. Ther Clin Risk Manag. 2015;11:639–47 [c].

[16] Arabyat RM, Raisch DW, McKoy JM, et al. Fluoroquinolone-associated tendon-rupture: a summary of reports in the Food and Drug Administration's adverse event reporting system. Expert Opin Drug Saf. 2015;14(11):1653–60 [M].

[17] Daneman N, Lu H, Redelmeier DA. Fluoroquinolones and collagen associated severe adverse events: a longitudinal cohort study. BMJ Open. 2015;5(11):e010077 [M].

[18] De Schryver N, Wittebole X, Van den Bergh P, et al. Severe rhabdomyolysis associated with simvastatin and role of ciprofloxacin and amlodipine coadministration. Case Rep Nephrol. 2015;2015:761393 [A].

[19] Erdemli O, Timuroglu A, Oral I, et al. Ciprofloxacin-induced severe thrombocytopenia. Kaohsiung J Med Sci. 2015;31(2):110–1 [A].

[20] Hashmi HR, Diaz-Fuentes G, Jadhav P, et al. Ciprofloxacin-induced thrombotic thrombocytopenic purpura: a case of successful treatment and review of the literature. Case Rep Crit Care. 2015;2015:143832 [A].

[21] Goyal H, Dennehy J, Barker J, et al. Achilles is not alone!!! Ciprofloxacin induced tendinopathy of gluteal tendons. QJM. 2015;1–2 [A].

[22] Francis JK, Higgins E. Permanent peripheral neuropathy: a case report on a rare but serious debilitating side-effect of fluoroquinolone administration. J Investig Med High Impact Case Rep. 2014;2(3):1–4 2324709614545225 [A].

[23] Nair PA. Ciprofloxacin induced bullous fixed drug reaction: three case reports. J Family Med Prim Care. 2015;4(2):269–72 [A].

[24] Cozzani E, Chinazzo C, Burlando M, et al. Ciprofloxacin as a trigger for bullous pemphigoid: the second case in the literature. Am J Ther. 2015;1–3 [A].

[25] Stancampiano FF, Palmer WC, Getz TW, et al. Rare incidence of ventricular tachycardia and torsades de pointes in hospitalized patients with prolonged QT who later received levofloxacin: a retrospective study. Mayo Clin Proc. 2015;90(5):606–12 [c].

[26] Palacios-Zabalza I, Bustos-Martinez J, Peral-Aguirregoitia J, et al. Probable interaction between acenocoumarol and levofloxacin: a case series. J Clin Pharm Ther. 2015;40(6):693–5 [A].

[27] Bansal N, Manocha D, Madhira B. Life-threatening metabolic coma caused by levofloxacin. Am J Ther. 2015;22(2):e48–51 [A].

[28] Gulen M, Ay MO, Avci A, et al. Levofloxacin-induced hepatotoxicity and death. Am J Ther. 2015;22(3):e93–6 [A].

[29] Budny AM, Ley AN. Fluoroquinolone-mediated Achilles rupture: a case report and review of the literature. J Foot Ankle Surg. 2015;54(3):494–6 [A].

[30] Seidel J, Clarke T, Mathew B. To cipro or not to cipro: bilateral achilles ruptures with the use of quinolones. J Am Podiatr Med Assoc. 2015;105(2):185–8 [A].

[31] Lizarraga KJ, Lopez MR, Singer C. Reversible craniocervical dystonia associated with levofloxacin. J Clin Mov Disord. 2015;2:10 [A].

[32] Golomb BA, Koslik HJ, Redd AJ. Fluoroquinolone-induced serious, persistent, multisymptom adverse effects. BMJ Case Rep. 2015;2015:1–3.

[33] Liu Y, He Q, Wu M. Levofloxacin-induced crystal nephropathy. Nephrology (Carlton). 2015;20(6):437–8 [A].

[34] Chen Q, Liu YM, Liu Y, et al. Orally administered moxifloxacin prolongs QTc in healthy Chinese volunteers: a randomized, single-blind, crossover study. Acta Pharmacol Sin. 2015;36(4):448–53 [c].

[35] Cone C, Horowitz B. Convulsions associated with moxifloxacin. Am J Health Syst Pharm. 2015;72(11):910–2.

[36] Vignesh AP, Srinivasan R, Karanth S. A case report of severe corneal toxicity following 0.5% topical moxifloxacin use. Case Rep Ophthalmol. 2015;6(1):63–5.

[37] Ramani YR, Mishra SK, Rath B, et al. Ofloxacin induced cutaneous reactions in children. J Clin Diagn Res. 2015;9(6):FD01–2 [A].

[38] Dunne MW, Zhou M, Darpo B. A thorough QT study with dalbavancin: a novel lipoglycopeptide antibiotic for the treatment of acute bacterial skin and skin-structure infections. Int J Antimicrob Agents. 2015;45(4):393–8 [C].

[39] Corey GR, Good S, Jiang H, et al. Single-dose oritavancin versus 7-10 days of vancomycin in the treatment of gram-positive acute bacterial skin and skin structure infections: the SOLO II noninferiority study. Clin Infect Dis. 2015;60(2):254–62.

[40] Byrne CJ, Egan S, Fennell JP, et al. Teicoplanin use in adult patients with haematological malignancy: exploring relationships between dose, trough concentrations, efficacy and nephrotoxicity. Int J Antimicrob Agents. 2015;46(4):406–12 [c].

[41] Chaftari AM, Hachem R, Jordan M, et al. Case-control study of telavancin as an alternative treatment for gram-positive bloodstream infections in patients with cancer. Antimicrob Agents Chemother. 2015;60(1):239–44 [c].

[42] Lobo N, Ejiofor K, Thurairaja R, et al. Life-threatening haematuria caused by vancomycin-induced thrombocytopenia. BMJ Case Rep. 2015;2015:1–2 [A].

[43] Bose S, Wurm E, Popovich MJ, et al. Drug-induced immune-mediated thrombocytopenia in the intensive care unit. J Clin Anesth. 2015;27(7):602–5 [A].

[44] Guner MD, Tuncbilek S, Akan B, et al. Two cases with HSS/DRESS syndrome developing after prosthetic joint surgery: does vancomycin-laden bone cement play a role in this syndrome? BMJ Case Rep. 2015;2015:1–5 [A].

[45] Hwang MJ, Do JY, Choi EW, et al. Immunoglobulin E-mediated hypersensitivity reaction after intraperitoneal administration of vancomycin. Kidney Res Clin Pract. 2015;34(1):57–9 [A].

[46] Moffett BS, Hilvers PS, Dinh K, et al. Vancomycin-associated acute kidney injury in pediatric cardiac intensive care patients. Congenit Heart Dis. 2015;10(1):E6–E10 [c].

[47] Constance JE, Balch AH, Stockmann C, et al. A propensity-matched cohort study of vancomycin-associated nephrotoxicity in neonates. Arch Dis Child Fetal Neonatal Ed. 2016;101:F236–43 [c].

[48] Knoderer CA, Gritzman AL, Nichols KR, et al. Late-occurring vancomycin-associated acute kidney injury in children receiving prolonged therapy. Ann Pharmacother. 2015;49(10):1113–9 [c].

[49] Van Driest SL, McGregor TL, Velez Edwards DR, et al. Genome-wide association study of serum creatinine levels during vancomycin therapy. PLoS One. 2015;10(6):e0127791 [c].

[50] Katikaneni M, Lwin L, Villanueva H, et al. Acute kidney injury associated with vancomycin when laxity leads to injury and findings on kidney biopsy. Am J Ther. 2016;23:e1064–7 [A].

[51] Hook 3rd. EW, Golden M, Jamieson BD, et al. A phase 2 trial of oral solithromycin 1200 mg or 1000 mg as single-dose oral therapy for uncomplicated gonorrhea. Clin Infect Dis. 2015;61(7):1043–8 [c].

[52] Sng WJ, Wang DY. Efficacy and side effects of antibiotics in the treatment of acute rhinosinusitis: a systematic review. Rhinology. 2015;53(1):3–9 [M].

[53] Bulloch MN, Baccas JT, Arnold S. Clindamycin-induced hypersensitivity reaction. Infection. 2016;44:357–9 [A].

[54] Moole H, Ahmed Z, Saxena N, et al. Oral clindamycin causing acute cholestatic hepatitis without ductopenia: a brief review of idiosyncratic drug-induced liver injury and a case report. J Community Hosp Intern Med Perspect. 2015;5(5):28746 [A].

[55] De Cruz R, Ferguson J, Wee JS, et al. Acute localised exanthematous pustulosis (ALEP) induced by clindamycin in pregnancy. Australas J Dermatol. 2015;56(3):e55–8 [A].

[56] Bin Abdulhak AA, Khan AR, Garbati MA, et al. Azithromycin and risk of cardiovascular death: a meta-analytic review of observational studies. Am J Ther. 2015;22(5):e122–9 [c].

[57] Goldstein LH, Gabin A, Fawaz A, et al. Azithromycin is not associated with QT prolongation in hospitalized patients with community-acquired pneumonia. Pharmacoepidemiol Drug Saf. 2015;24(10):1042–8 [c].

[58] Cocco G, Jerie P. Torsades de pointes induced by the concomitant use of ivabradine and azithromycin: an unexpected dangerous interaction. Cardiovasc Toxicol. 2015;15(1):104–6 [A].

[59] Moy BT, Dojki FK, Scholes JV, et al. Azithromycin-induced cholestatic hepatitis. Conn Med. 2015;79(4):213–5 [A].

[60] Riesselman A, El-Mallakh RS. Akathisia with azithromycin. Ann Pharmacother. 2015;49(5):609.

[61] Lenehan PJ, Schramm CM, Collins MS. An evaluation strategy for potential QTc prolongation with chronic azithromycin therapy in cystic fibrosis. J Cyst Fibros. 2016;15:192–5 [c].

[62] Wong AY, Root A, Douglas IJ, et al. Cardiovascular outcomes associated with use of clarithromycin: population based study. BMJ. 2016;352:h6926 [c].

[63] Agrawal V, Chaudhari S, Sy A, et al. A case of hypotension and bradycardia precipitated by drug interaction of clarithromycin and calcium-channel blocker. J Am Geriatr Soc. 2015;63(9):1966–7 [A].

[64] Sachdeva A, Rathee R. Akathisia with erythromycin: induced or precipitated? Saudi Pharm J. 2015;23(5):541–3 [A].

[65] Hsu SN, Shih MF, Yang CW, et al. Severe linezolid-induced lactic acidosis in a cirrhosis patient. Nephrology (Carlton). 2015;20(1):47–8 [A].

[66] Ortiz-Covarrubias A, Fang E, Prokocimer PG, et al. Efficacy, safety, tolerability and population pharmacokinetics of tedizolid, a novel antibiotic, in Latino patients with acute bacterial skin and skin structure infections. Braz J Infect Dis. 2016;20(2):184–92 [c].

[67] Lee YJ, Wi YM, Kwon YJ, et al. Association between colistin dose and development of nephrotoxicity. Crit Care Med. 2015;43(6):1187–93 [c].

[68] Dalfino L, Puntillo F, Ondok MJ, et al. Colistin-associated acute kidney injury in severely Ill patients: a step toward a better renal care? A prospective cohort study. Clin Infect Dis. 2015;61(12):1771–7 [c].

[69] Antoniou T, Hollands S, Macdonald EM, et al. Trimethoprim-sulfamethoxazole and risk of sudden death among patients taking spironolactone. CMAJ. 2015;187(4):E138–43 [c].

[70] Huntsberry AM, Linnebur SA, Vejar M. Hyponatremia after initiation and rechallenge with trimethoprim-sulfamethoxazole in an older adult. Clin Interv Aging. 2015;10:1091–6.

[71] Petrov M, Yatsynovich Y, Lionte C. An unusual cause of rhabdomyolysis in emergency setting: challenges of diagnosis. Am J Emerg Med. 2015;33(1):123.e1–3 [A].

[72] Gomez-Traseira C, Boyano-Martinez T, Escosa-Garcia L, et al. Trimethoprim-sulfamethoxazole (cotrimoxazole) desensitization in an HIV-infected 5-yr-old girl. Pediatr Allergy Immunol. 2015;26(3):287–9 [A].

[73] Hagiya H, Hasegawa K, Asano K, et al. Myopathy and eosinophilic pneumonia coincidentally induced by treatment with daptomycin. Intern Med. 2015;54(5):525–9 [A].

[74] Wojtaszczyk A, Jankowich M. Dyspnea on daptomycin: eosinophilic pneumonia. R I Med J (2013). 2013; 98(6):41–3 [A].

[75] Iarikov D, Wassel R, Farley J, et al. Adverse events associated with fosfomycin use: review of the literature and analyses of the FDA adverse event reporting system database. Infect Dis Ther. 2015;4(4):433–58 [c].

25

Antifungal Drugs

Dayna S. McManus[1]

Department of Pharmacy Services, Yale-New Haven Hospital, Yale University, New Haven, CT, USA
[1]Corresponding author: dayna.mcmanus@ynhh.org

ALLYLAMINES [SEDA-34, 427; SEDA-35, 483; SEDA-36, 381; SEDA-37, 307]

Terbinafine [SEDA-34, 427; SEDA-35, 483; SEDA-36, 381; SEDA-37, 307]

Skin

A 25-year-old male with onychomycosis of the fingernail was prescribed terbinafine 250 mg by mouth daily. On day 18 of his terbinafine treatment he presented with an itchy rash that started on his chest and progressed to the rest of the body within 4 days. The rash consisted of scattered erythematous papules and plaques on the trunk, upper limbs, and gluteal region. Some plaques had peripheral collarettes of scaling. Erythematous tumid plaques were noted on the cheeks and a single erythematous papule on the penile shaft. The patient had no history of previous rash, fever, drug allergies and was not taking any other medications. Terbinafine was stopped and the patient was prescribed antihistamines and topical steroids which resulted in quick resolution of the rash. The patient was discharged from the hospital 4 days after initially presenting. The patients' presentation was similar to the erythematous papulosquamous eruptions that are usually seen with pityriasis rosea, which has been described with terbinafine before. The association between terbinafine and the rash was a 6 and therefore probably on the Naranjo causality assessment score. Patients starting terbinafine should be counseled on the possible skin reactions and recommended to discuss the reaction with their physician before using any more of the medicination [1A].

The clinical features of Roswell syndrome included lupus erythematosus, erythema multiforme-like lesions, a positive rheumatoid factor, and speckled pattern antinuclear antibodies (ANA). Case reports have implicated medications as a possible trigger for Roswell syndrome.

In the case report by Murad et al. an 81-year-old women presents with a generalised eruption that is mildly pruritic after starting terbinafine 5 weeks prior for an onychomycosis infection. The rash is present on the head, neck and back. Some areas are oedematous, some are crusted plaques and others are targetoid. A skin biopsy revealed vascular dermatitis with necrotic keratinocytes at the dermoepidermal junction and superficial dermal necrosis. Laboratory results were positive for speckled pattern antinuclear antibodies (ANA), extractable nuclear antigen (26.0; normal range <1.0), anti-RO antibody (237 U/mL; normal range <10.0) and C-reactive protein (36 mg/L; normal range <7). Terbinafine was discontinued and the patient was started on oral as well as topical steroids. After 10 days of topical treatment the patient's rash significantly improved and the patient had no additional episodes at 3-month follow-up. Based on the patient's presentation and laboratory finding it is likely that this was in fact a case of drug-induced Roswell syndrome. It is important to consider this overlapping syndrome when diagnosing patients with likely drug-related skin reactions [2A].

Bayata et al. present a case of a 14-year-old boy who presented with tiny, millimeter-sized pustules throughout his body and especially concentrated on the lower extremities. The rash started on the third day of treatment with oral terbinafine for treatment of tinea cruris. A skin biopsy revealed a normal granular layer, subcorneal pustules, dermal edema and a perivascular mixed inflammatory infiltrate with eosinophils. The patient's laboratory results revealed leukocytosis (18 600 cells/mm^3), neutrophilia (80.3%), eosinophilia (2.9%) and increased erythrocyte sedimentation rate (43 mm/hour). Based on these findings the patient was diagnosed with acute generalized exanthematous pustulosis. Since terbinafine was suspected to be the most likely cause it was discontinued and the patient received antipyretics and topical steroids.

Within 2 weeks the lesions resolved without reoccurrence. In addition to the other two cases this highlights the need to counsel patients to be aware of skin-related reactions while on terbinafine therapy [3A].

Drug–Drug Interactions

Tramadol

A randomized placebo-controlled crossover study was conducted with 12 healthy subjects to assess the interaction between terbinafine and tramadol. Because terbinafine inhibits CYP2D6 and tramadol is metabolized to its active metabolite, O-desmethyltramadol (M1), by CYP2D6 there may be a decrease in analgesic effect and possible increase in side effects with this combination. Of the patients included 8 were extensive and 4 were ultrarapid CYP2D6 metabolizers. Patients were given terbinafine 250 mg once daily by mouth in addition to tramadol 50 mg orally. The concentrations of tramadol and its primary active metabolite M1 were measured over 48 hours. Terbinafine was found to effect the area under the plasma concentration-time curve of tramadol by 115% and decrease M1 by 64% ($P < 0.001$). Terbinafine also increased the peak concentrations of tramadol by 53% and decrease M1 by 79% ($P < 0.001$). Finally terbinafine was found to increase the elimination half-life of tramadol by 48% and M1 by 50% ($P < 0.001$). Terbinafine also reduced the subjective drug effect of tramadol. Based on this study terbinafine may decrease the opioid effect of tramadol and lead to an increase in monoaminergic side effects given less metabolism of tramadol to M1. The effects may be less pronounced with poor metabolizers of CYP2D6 showing the benefit of possible pharmacogenomic testing to alter choice of medication and dose [4c].

Pharmacogenomics

The drug interactions in the cases presented above highlight the importance of pharmacogenomics in relation to terbinafine. Approximately 5–10% of Caucasians are categorized as "poor metabolisers" of drugs that are broken down by CYP2D6 due to a genetic polymorphism that results in a lack of functional CYP2D6 enzyme. Since terbinafine is an inhibitor of CYP2D6 it has the potential to cause significant drug–drug interactions especially when used in a patient who has a genetic polymorphism resulting in poor metabolism of drugs metabolized by CYP2D6. Consideration of pharmacogenetic testing for individuals who are on terbinafine in addition to other medications that undergo significant metabolized by CYP2D6 may be beneficial in preventing unwanted adverse effects [5A,6R].

AMPHOTERICIN [SEDA-33, 542; SEDA-34, 427; SEDA-35, 483; SEDA-36, 382; SEDA-37, 307]

Adverse Event Comparison of Available Amphotericin Formulations

A retrospective cohort study of 431 that received amphotericin B deoxycholate (d-AmB), liposomal AmB (L-AmB), or AmB lipid complex (ABLC) was conducted to compare nephrotoxicity risk with each formulation. Nephrotoxicity was determined according to modified RIFLE criteria. Of the 431 patients reviewed 236 received d-AmB, 105 received L-AmB, and 90 received ABLC. Severe nephrotoxicity (RIFLE 'Failure') was found to occur in 11.5%, 2.4% and 7.2% for d-AmB, L-AmB and ABLC, respectively ($P = 0.046$). L-AmB when compared with d-AmB, as a reference, was found to be an independent protective factor (OR: 0.18; 95% CI: 0.03–0.64; $P = 0.006$) for severe nephrotoxicity and also a protective factor for mortality (OR: 0.56; 95% CI: 0.32–0.99; $P = 0.046$). Overall 64.4% of patients experiences hypokalemia while 77.2% experienced hypomagnesaemia. Although there was no statistically significant difference in electrolyte abnormalities, there were more patients in the ABLC group that experienced hypokalemia than the L-AmB group at 72.4% versus 50%, respectively. This study showed that L-AmB was associated with a lower risk of severe nephrotoxicity as well as overall mortality. Limitations of the study included its retrospective design as this could be more susceptible to cofounding bias. There also was some missing values which could affect the nephrotoxicity data given the RIFLE score needs this information for its calculation. There was also data missing on the patient's race which could have affected the nephrotoxicity risk [7c].

A meta-analysis of randomized controlled trials that compared d-AmB with L-AmB to assess the effects of these medications on kidney function was conducted. A total of 12 studies, 2298 participants, were included in the analysis. Conventional amphotericin B, d-AmB, was found to increase serum creatinine significantly more so than L-AmB (RR 0.49, 95% CI 0.40–0.59). L-AmB was also found to have a significant decrease in all infusion-related reactions compared to d-AmB. These infusion-related reactions included: fever, chills and/or rigors, fever and/or rigors, nausea and vomiting. This study also was limited given it was retrospective and there was potentially bias as well as had multiple different study designs included. However, it does appear that liposomal amphotericin B is less nephrotoxic and has less infusion-related reactions than conventional amphotericin B [8M].

Liposomal Amphotericin (L-AmB)

Central Nervous System

A 39-year-old male was being treated with L-AmB in addition to oral fluconazole, due to acute renal dysfunction with flucytosine, for *Cryptococcus neoformans* meningitis. The patient was started on 150 mg daily of L-AmB which resulted in a decrease the cerebral spinal fluid (CSF) counts; however, the dose was eventually increased to 300 mg daily due to a lack of improvement in the patient's clinical symptoms. An MRI of the brain that was preformed 3 weeks after starting L-AmB showed white matter lesions in the bilateral frontal and occipital lobes. These lesions were characterized by hyperintensity of T2-weighted and FLAIR images. Although the CSF findings were improving, including the antigen titer for *Cryptococcus*, the patient's headache and right hemiparesis progressed. Therefore, the L-AmB was suspected as the cause of leukoencephalopathy and it was subsequently discontinued after 16 weeks of therapy. MRI of the brain 4 weeks after stopping L-AmB showed a dramatic improvement and near disappearance of almost all of the white matter lesions. Leukoencephalopathy related to amphotericin has been described in the past, but never with the liposomal formulation. The mechanism behind the neurotoxicity with amphotericin is thought to be caused by amphotericin's ability to bind to myelin and increase membrane permeability which results in leakage of the intracellular components from myelin. This case report demonstrates that although L-AmB may have less side effects than d-AmB neurotoxicity and leukoencephalopathy is still possible [9A].

Amphotericin B Deoxycholate (d-AmB)

Cardiovascular

A 45-year-old man without any past medical history was started on 0.6 mg/kg/day of d-AmB for treatment of visceral leishmaniasis. He received 18 days of d-AmB and 2 days prior to the completion of therapy he had an echocardiogram done that showed a left ventricular ejection fraction (LVEF) of 60% and was discharged without any symptoms. Five days after being discharged the patient was re-admitted with acute congestive heart failure (CHF). LVEF at this time was found to be reduced to 24%. Liver and kidney function were normal and all work-ups for acute CHF also came back unremarkable. An MRI of the heart revealed increased dimensions of ventricles, diffuse hypokinesia and severe systolic dysfunction. The patient's CHF was treated with captopril, furosemide, carvedilol and spironolactone. The patent's symptoms improved and a repeat echocardiogram 30 days after the original showed an LVEF of 58% with improvement in the size of the ventricles. Eventually the patient was weaned off all medications used to treat the CHF without any reoccurrence of symptoms. Unfortunately, the patient did not have a cardiac biopsy to definitively determine the cause of the acute CHF; however, the timing of the acute CHF seems to be related to d-AmB administration. Reversible cardiomyopathy has been reported with amphotericin use in the past; however, usually patients have a history of cardiovascular co-morbidities. A possible cause for this side effect is due to amphotericin's ability to cause direct cardiotoxicity via the interaction with cholesterol component of the plasma membrane. Because amphotericin can increase membrane permeability it results in loss for ions. When this occurs in the heart it can alter the sarcoplasmic reticular membrane ATPase system. In only one of the previously reported cases has a biopsy been performed. Results of the biopsy showed possible direct toxicity of the drug on cardiac cells. Neither the dose nor the duration appears to effect the development of this side effect. It is important to be aware of the possibility of cardiac toxicity with the use of amphotericin so that this can be appropriately considered on the differential [10A].

ANTIFUNGAL AZOLES [SEDA-33, 545; SEDA-34, 428; SEDA-35, 484; SEDA-36, 382; SEDA-37, 307]

For metronidazole see Chapter 27.

Fluconazole [SEDA-33, 551; SEDA-34, 430; SEDA-35, 485; SEDA-36, 382; SEDA-37, 307]

Skin

A 30-year-old women presented to the allergy department complaining of skin lesions that were papules with vesicles and crust on her lower lip with patchy areas of facial erythema. She had similar reactions over the last 3 months. A skin prick test was done with a wide range of food extracts and cosmetic products that she utilized and all were negative. Skin scrapings of the area were for a herpes viral infection despite the appearance being very similar to this type of infection. The patient reported taking oral fluconazole 150 mg monthly for recurrent vaginitis. Each episode of the rash over the last 3 months had occurred within 24 hours of taking the fluconazole. The patient had a skin test preformed with fluconazole, ketoconazole, itraconazole and voriconazole which were all negative. However, when an oral challenge test with fluconazole was done the patient broke out in the same rash on her face with blistering on her lips and elbows within 24 hours. An oral challenge was also done with itraconazole a month later which did not result in any reaction. There have been other cases of herpes like reactions to fluconazole presented in the literature before; however, there are very few. Although uncommon, it is important to consider fluconazole as a possible cause in someone that presents with a similar rash without a clear aetiology [11A].

Pregnancy

Frequently, pregnant women experience an episode of vulvovaginal candidiasis and receive treatment with fluconazole before they realize they are pregnant. Therefore, a retrospective study of published literature was conducted to determine the risk of congenital malformations in children born to mothers who were exposed to fluconazole in the first trimester of pregnancy. A total of 4 studies, one observational prospective study and 3 registry based, were included in the review. The rate for overall malformations was 1.10 (95% CI 0.98–1.25), for heart defect was 1.29 (95% CI 1.05–1.58), for craniofacial defects was 1.25 (95% CI 0.88–1.77), and for limb/musculoskeletal defects was 0.82 (95% CI 0.59–1.13). Compared to overall risk of malformations these odds ratios were not increased with fluconazole usage for vulvovaginal candidiasis. This study did not assess the risk of utilizing higher doses and longer durations of fluconazole for more serious infections and therefore this study cannot be used for treatment of these infections in pregnant patients [12M].

Itraconazole [SED-15, 1969; SEDA-33, 552; SEDA-34, 430; SEDA-35, 485; SEDA-36, 38; SEDA-37, 307]

Cardiovascular

A retrospective observational chart review study of pediatric patients with hemato-oncologic diseases who were treated with IV itraconazole from January 2012 to December 2013 was conducted to assess the risk of hypotension with itraconazole administration. There were a total of 180 patients that were reviewed who recieved itraconazole IV a total of 2627 times. Through chart review it was found that the systolic blood pressure (SBP) during the 4 hours following itraconazole administration was lower than during the 4 hours before administration (104 [53.0–160.33 mmHg] versus 105 [59.8–148.3 mmHg]; $P < 0.001$). The decrease in SBP was related to the use of continuous renal replacement therapy (CRRT) ($P = 0.012$) and the use of inotropic ($P = 0.005$) and hypotensive drugs ($P = 0.021$). Overall, a clinically meaningful SBP drop, defined as a $\geq 20\%$ drop in SBP, occurred in 5.37% of the administrations. Risk factors associated with clinically meaningful drops in SBP included the use of inotropes (OR 6.70, 95% CI 3.22–13.92; $P < 0.001$), reducing the dose of inotropes

(OR 8.08; 95% CI 1.39–46.94; $P = 0.02$), CRRT (OR 3.10, 95% CI 1.41–6.81; $P = 0.005$), and bacteremia (OR 2.70, 95% CI 1.32–5.51; $P = 0.007$), while age was a protective factor (OR 0.93, 95% CI 0.89–0.97; $P < 0.001$). Based on this study blood pressure should be very closely monitored when administering IV itraconazole especially in patients on CRRT, those taking hypotensive or inotropic medications and patients of younger age [13C].

Ketoconazole [SEDA-34, 430; SEDA-35, 486; SEDA-36, 383; SEDA-37, 307]

Skin

Sweet syndrome is an acute febrile neutrophilic dermatosis what results in erythematous papules and plaques usually in the upper extremities, face and/or neck. This syndrome has been shown to be caused by maliganancy and also medications. The most commonly associated medication has been granulocyte colony-stimulating factor (GM-CSF) but other medications have been reported as the cause as well. A 60-year-old Hispanic male presented with a history of pruritic burning and skin lesions on his upper extremities that looked very similar to the lesions described with sweet syndrome. Two days before the onset of the lesions the patient started ketoconazole 200 mg daily for treatment of Pityrosporum folliculitis. Microscopic examination of the lesions showed a dense neutrophilic infiltrate in superficial and mid-dermis, associated with marked papillary dermal edema. All other work-ups including infectious etiology were negative. The patient was diagnosed with sweet syndrome, given that he met all 4 of 5 diagnostic criteria with fever being the only absent symptom. However, fever is not always reported with sweet syndrome. Ketoconazole was discontinued. Two weeks later the lesions resolved on their own. Ketoconazole has been shown to stimulate chemotaxis which could be the mechanism behind the cause of sweet syndrome. Although there have not been a significant number of reports of sweet syndrome with ketoconazole, it is important to keep this on the differential in a patient that presents with these lesions who is on ketoconazole [14A].

A review of published literature on oral ketoconazole and reported adverse events was recently published. This review found that oral ketoconazole, in comparison to other antifungal agents, is very commonly associated with serious drug-related adverse events. There have been cases of hepatotoxicity that have resulted in liver transplantation and death worldwide. These cases have caused countries to no longer recommend utilizing this agent for fungal infections or change the product's labeling to include this strict safety warning. The study also found a large number of reports of endocrine dysregulation as well. Gynecomastia is the most commonly reported endocrine dysregulation related to the medication. Ketoconazole inhibits testosterone synthesis via CYP17A1 and selectively displaces dihydrotestosterone and estradiol from serum-binding globulins. This mechanism is likely how ketoconazole also can cause gynecomastia. Based on the significant reports of common and severe adverse events related to ketoconazole use it is recommended that newer antifungal agents with better safety profiles are utilized in ketoconazole's place [15M].

Posaconazole [SEDA-33, 553; SEDA-34, 430; SEDA-35, 486; SEDA-36, 383; SEDA-37, 307]

A 13-year-old female with an osteosarcoma-like tumor involving the maxillary sinus was started on posaconazole as step down therapy for treatment of a *Coniothyrium fuckelii* sinus infection. While inpatient the patient was receiving posaconazole suspension at 400 mg twice daily and at discharge it was accidentally changed to posaconazole delayed release tablets 400 mg twice daily instead of the correct dose of daily. Two weeks after discharge the patient developed fatigue, decreased appetite, and musculoskeletal pain. In addition she was found to have a potassium of 2.7 mEq/L and oral potassium supplements were therefore prescribed. Over the next few weeks her nausea, fatigue, and bone pain worsened and she began to have decreased enteral intake. In addition her hypokalemia (3.1 mEq/L) continued and she developed progressive anemia with hemoglobin that dropped from 9.1 to 8.3 g/dL. At this time she was admitted to the hospital where the mistake in the prescribing was discovered. The posaconazole dose was held and a level was checked that came back at 9.5 mcg/mL. One week after stopping the posaconazole the patient's symptoms resolved. It is important to be aware of the differences in dosing between the suspension and delayed release tablets of posaconazole. Because the dosing of these two different dosage forms is not interchangeable it is possible that it can lead to overdosing of the tablet formulation that can result in the adverse effects described here [16A].

Voriconazole [SEDA-33, 554; SEDA-34, 431; SEDA-35, 486; SEDA-36, 384; SEDA-37, 307]

Sensory System

A 16-year-old girl with a past medical history of T-cell leukemia was started on voriconazole IV 400 mg/day for treatment of invasive pulmonary aspergillosis given a positive galactomannan as well as imaging. On the fourth day of treatment the patient developed visual and auditory hallucinations and disturbances. She reported seeing discolorations of yellow and green as well as strangers walking around her room and talking with her. She was completely conscious during these hallucinations and there was no concern for psychiatric illness. All her exams were normal and no other causes other than voriconazole could be identified. On the Naranjo Adverse Drug Reaction Probability Scale it scored a 5 which was a probably relationship. Voriconazole was continued because it was considered the best agent for her infection. She took the voriconazole for 70 days total and the hallucinations only persisted for the first 4 days and then resolved completely. This case highlights that the visual disturbances and hallucinations may resolve on their own [17A].

Skin

A 69-year-old male with a history of chronic lymphocytic leukemia (CLL) presented with a recurrent biopsy-proven squamous cell carcinoma (SCC) of the scalp. The patient had multiple surgeries for SCC on his scalp, nose, shoulders and forearms in the past. Despite the resection of the SCC with clear margins as well as cetuximab treatment the patient continued to develop new SCC lesions and re-growth of the lesion on his cheek and scalp. At a follow-up appointment the patient mentioned that he had been taking voriconazole on and off for prophylaxis whenever he had worsening sinus symptoms. The patient stated that he had taken the voriconazole about every 2–3 months over the last 5 years. The patient was advised to stop his voriconazole. After stopping the voriconazole he had improvement in his current lesions and a decrease in the number of new lesions. However, one of the lesions on his scalp continued to progress and eventually the patient passed away from the disease [18A].

A retrospective review of 381 allogenic hematopoietic stem cell transplant patients (all-HSCT) was conducted to evaluate the risk of voriconazole-induced squamous cell carcinoma (SCC). Patients that received voriconazole as well as other forms of antifungals were included to compare the risk of SCC with patients on voriconazole versus other antifungals. SCC developed in 26 of 312 patients who were exposed to voriconazole and only 1 of 69 patients on antifungals other than voriconazole. Therefore, the risk of SCC was found to be 19% at 5 years post allo-transplant. Cumulative days of voriconazole use were found to be a risk factor for SCC with a hazard ratio of 1.859 for each 180 days of use ($P < 0.001$). This study helps understand the SCC risk when using voriconazole prophylaxis in allogenic HSCT patients [19C].

A retrospective chart review of 430 pediatric patients who received voriconazole from 2003 to 2013 was done to assess the risk of voriconazole-induced phototoxicity. The overall incidence of phototoxicity was 20% in children treated with voriconazole. The incidence increased to 47% when patients were treated for 6 months or longer. Additional risk factors for the development of phototoxicity in addition to voriconazole use were found to be white race, cystic fibrosis, cumulative treatment time, and cumulative dose. Four patients (1%) had nonmelanoma skin cancer and all of them experienced a phototoxic reaction during voriconazole treatment. Of those with phototoxicity, 5% were discontinued on voriconazole, 6% were referred to dermatology, and 26% received counseling about sun protection from their primary physician. This study shows the overall risk of voriconazole-associated phototoxicty in pediatric patients [20C].

Periostitis

Cases of voriconazole-induced periostitis continue to be reported. Voriconazole preparations contain fluoride and the mechanism of this adverse effect has been linked to the accumulation of fluoride which usually results in elevated levels in patients on therapy for at least 6 months. In most cases, the periostitis and fluoride accumulation ceases once voriconazole is stopped. The EIDOS and DoTS descriptions of this reaction are shown in Figure 27.2 (SEDA-37).

Fluoride integrates as fluorapatite into the bone crystal structure and promotes bone formation by stimulating osteoblasts. The integration of fluorapatite into bone causes alterations in bone crystal size and structure, making these more resistant to resorption. Ultimately this increases bone density and leads to osteosclerosis associated with brittleness, exostoses, pain, decreased mechanical competence of bone and increased susceptibility to fractures [21C].

Fluoride intoxication resembles hypertrophic osteoarthropathy and periostitis deformans, and several common features have been observed in skeletal imaging. Symmetric diffuse periosteal reactions including osteosclerosis and hyperostotic periostitis have been described together with osteoporosis, ligamentous calcification and periarticular changes; these have been located in various parts of the skeleton. Contrary to hypertrophic osteoarthropathy, voriconazole-induced periostitis is strongly associated with an elevated alkaline phosphatase and shows characteristically no digital clubbing [21C,22H].

Several etiological explanations may be considered for voriconazole-associated fluorosis. Fluorine is organically bound in voriconazole and hepatic oxidative metabolism may increase unbound fluoride levels after extensive voriconazole administration. Pharmacogenomic variations, especially polymorphisms in CYP2C19 enzyme may further alleviate this phenomena. Secondly, renal insufficiency or failure may increase the risk for toxicity during fluorine exposure, since its renal clearance is dependent on the patients renal function [22H].

Periostitis Cases

A 66-year-old woman was admitted with severe and disabling left shoulder pain that had worsened over the course of about 10 months. The patient had a past medical history significant for T-cell prolymphocytic leukemia and was on voriconazole 300 mg twice daily by mouth for treatment of an invasive neurohistoplasmosis infection. Radiographic finders were significant for smooth periosteal thickening of the left clavicle and bone scan showed multiple areas of increased tracer activity. After ruling out many potential causes for these findings the patient was diagnosed with voriconazole-induced periostitis given the patient started taking the voriconazole around the same time the shoulder pain started. The voriconazole was discontinued and the pain resolved within 48 hours of discontinuing. At 3-month follow-up a repeat bone scan was normal [23A].

A 74-year-old woman was started on voriconazole for an Aspergillus infection of the lung after her lung transplant. Over a 7-year period the patient was on and off the voriconazole treatment. Most recently the patient was on voriconazole for about 8 months when she presented to the orthopedic clinic with diffuse bone pain. A bone scan was preformed and it revealed a linear area of increased uptake in the sixth, seventh, eighth rib, as well as the clavicle and the acetabulum. Further workup did not revile any underlying malignancy. Therefore, the patient was diagnosed with voriconazole-induced periostitis. Voriconazole was discontinued and at 6-week follow-up the patient's pain resolved. Although voriconazole-induced periostitis is rare, cases continue to be reported in the literature [24A].

A 64-year-old man presented with diffuse migratory arthralgias and myalgias. The patient had a history of renal cell carcinoma and acute myelogenous leukemia and a matched sibling allogenic stem cell transplant 3 months prior to the onset of the pain. Bone scan revealed multiple osteoblastic lesions consistent with periostitis. The patient had been on voriconazole 400 mg daily for about 4 months prior to the onset of pain for treatment of a fungal pneumonia. Voriconazole was changed to caspofungin and the pain resolved within 4 days of stopping the voriconazole. Voriconazole-induced periostitis should be on the differential for patients on voriconazole who present with bone pain [25A].

Although complications of voriconazole treatment in relation to elevated fluoride levels have been well documented in adult patients, it is not as well described in pediatric patients. Therefore, a retrospective review of 5 pediatric hematopoietic stem cell transplant (HSCT) patients on voriconazole therapy was conducted to assess their fluoride levels as well as clinical and other laboratory data. The patients in the case series ranged from 3 months of age to 19 years of age. The duration of voriconazole therapy ranged from 3 months to greater than 12 months. All 5 patients in the study had elevated fluoride levels ranging from 6.2 to 23.8 μmol/L. The child with the fluoride level of 23.8 μmol/L started to have irritability that seemed to be triggered by any movement.

Imaging studies were done on the child and it appeared that she had a bilateral diffuse periosteal reaction with widening in the femur, tibia and fibula. The child also had an elevated alkaline phosphatase (ALP) level of 2416 IU/L. Elevated ALP levels have also been found to be associated with voriconazole-induced periostitis. The patient was changed from voriconazole to posaconazole and within 48 hours she was less irritable and was able to tolerate movements better. Within 3 weeks her ALP and fluoride levels were normal and she had improved movement. Pediatric patients are possibly even more at risk for fluoride accumulation and periostitis and therefore they should be closely monitored for signs and symptoms of voriconazole periostitis while on long-term voriconazole therapy [26c].

Isavuconazole

Isavuconazole or Cresemba™ is the newest azole antifungal approved that comes as the salt formulation isavuconazonium. The United States Food and Drug Administration approved isavuconazole in March of 2015 for the treatment of invasive aspergillosis and invasive mucormycosis. Isavuconazole is available as an oral and intravenous formulation. The intravenous formulation is available without a cyclodextrin-solvent ingredient, which may be more favorable compared to voriconazole and posaconazole intravenous, which do contain this ingredient. Not having this solvent is an advantage because although the clinical data do not suggest accumulation of cyclodextrin-solvent results in acute kidney injury caution is advised in patients with decreased renal function. Isavuconazole has a broad spectrum of activity including most yeast species, *Aspergillus* species, and mucormycosis. Oral bioavailability is good at approximately 98%. The drug is mostly metabolized via the liver and is a substrate of and mild to moderate inhibitor of CYP3A4 which does result in some drug–drug interactions, similar to the other azole antifungals.

When combining the three trials that isavuconazole was studied in there were about 1700 patients in total who were treated with this medication. In the SECURE trial the safety and efficacy of isavuconazole were compared to voriconazole and were found to be better tolerated with 42.4% of patients experiencing an adverse event in the isavuconazole group versus 59.8% in the voriconazole group. The most common side effects seen with isavuconazole use from the trials included mild gastrointestinal disorders, pyrexia, hypokalemia, headache, constipation, and cough. Compared to voriconazole, isavuconazole had statistically significantly less eye disorders (26.6% versus 15.2%), skin and subcutaneous tissue disorders (42.5% versus 33.5%), and hepatobiliary disorders (16.2% versus 8.9%). Isavuconazole also appears to shorten the QT interval instead of prolonging it like the other azole antifungals and therefore may

provide a benefit in patients needing antifungal therapy with a prolonged QT interval.

It will be important to monitor the post-marketing data and literature surrounding this drug to further understand the side effects associated with the medication and its place in therapy [27R].

Rx
Special Review

Drug–Drug Interactions and Pharmacogenomics of the Azoles Antifungal

Since many of the azole antifungals affect the hepatic cytochrome P450 system there are a large number of drug–drug interactions with many of these agents. Because of the large number of drug–drug interactions associated with the azole antifungals it is important to always review all medications, both prescription and over-the-counter, whenever starting a patient on an azole antifungal. The chart below shows the extent of the interactions with cytochrome P450 system that are commonly associated with drug interactions and the different azole antifungals affect on those cytochromes.

The other important factor that affects the potential severity with these drug–drug interactions involved pharmacogenomics. As discussed briefly in Section "Terbinafine", some individuals are classified as poor metabolizers or rapid metabolizers of certain cytochrome P450 enzyme systems. Depending on the patient's pharmacogenomics and therefore ability to metabolize certain medications through the CYP 450 system they may be at risk of being undertreated by a certain medication or potentially being over treated and therefore at risk for developing more side effects [28H,29R].

Voriconazole, in particular, has been one of the most difficult azoles to utilize effective dosing strategies because of the significant intra-patient variability in plasma concentrations due to nonlinear pharmacokinetics and patient characteristics such as age, sex, weight, liver disease, and genetic polymorphisms in the cytochrome P450 2C19 gene (CYP2C19) encoding for the CYP2C19 enzyme. The largest portion in variability in voriconazole dosing is the CYP2C19 polymorphisms and therefore it may be important, especially from an efficacy standpoint, to test CYP2C19 genotypes to help optimize the efficacy of voriconazole while decreasing the toxicity [29R].

A study done in pediatric patients in Japan highlight that there is a value to identifying these polymorphisms because they found there is an association between voriconazole plasma concentrations and the CYP2C19 phenotype. In this study 37 pediatric patients who had voriconazole plasma concentrations measured and were categorized as normal metabolizers, intermediate metabolizers, poor metabolizers, or hypermetabolizers based on genotype testing were retrospectively reviewed. Trough plasma concentrations of voriconazole were statistically significantly higher in the poor metabolizer and intermediate metabolizer groups compared with the normal metabolizer

	CYP3A4		CYP2C9		CYP2C19	
	Substrate	Inhibitor	Substrate	Inhibitor	Substrate	Inhibitor
Fluconazole		Moderate		Moderate		Strong
Itraconazole	Major	Strong				
Voriconazole	Minor	Strong	Major	Moderate	Major	Moderate
Posaconazole		Strong				
Ketoconazole	Major	Strong		Moderate		Moderate
Miconazole						
Isavuconazole	Major	Moderate				Weak

This figure highlights some of the most common cytochrome P450 enzymes that are affected by antifungals and therefore are important to be aware of for pharmacogenomics differences as well as drug–drug interactions [28H,29R].

and hypermetabolizer groups (P = 0.004). Syndromes of inappropriate antidiuretic hormone secretion and cardiac toxicities were experienced by two patients in the high voriconazole concentration group. Dose adjustment based on CYP2C19 phenotype therefore may be useful during voriconazole therapy to improve efficacy and avoid toxicity. Japanese children, in particular, may benefit from this since they have a higher incidence of the poor metabolizer and intermediate metabolizer phenotypes as a group [30c].

Clozapine

A case of a 29-year-old Caucasian female was admitted to the hospital due to acute psychosis and was diagnosed with schizoaffective disorder. The patient was on long-term oral contraceptive therapy as well as fluconazole oral therapy for oral candidiasis and miconazole gel. The patient was on this combination for 29 days during her admission. On the last day of antifungal therapy she was ordered for clozapine. Clozapine was started at 25 mg daily and then eventually increased to 225 mg daily. After 3 weeks of clozapine therapy her level came back supratherapeutic at 542 ng/mL (therapeutic range is 350–450 ng/mL). In addition the patient was found to have an elevated eosinophilia and C-reactive protein. The patient was also complaining of nausea, vomiting, and palpitations. On physical exam she was found to have tachycardia and gallop rhythm and an echocardiogram showed small pericardial effusion suggestive of iatrogenic pericarditis. Both the oral contraceptive and clozapine were held and within 4 days she had resolution of her symptoms and recovery of her pericardial effusion. On the drug interaction probability scare (DIPS) the combination of clozapine with the antifungal and the oral contraceptive scored a 5 which is a probable cause. Fluconazole and miconazole do inhibit CYP3A4 which is how clozapine is metabolized. Given with the oral contraceptives the antifungals effect on the CYP enzymes were likely prolonged even after therapy was stopped.

It is important to closely monitor the level and for side effects with clozapine in combination with these other agents [31A].

Everolimus

A 66-year-old man who had a past medical history of renal transplant was on everolimus 1.5 mg twice for immunosuppression post-transplant. One month after initiating the everolimus the patient was started on voriconazole orally at 400 mg twice daily one day one followed by 200 mg twice daily for treatment of an *Aspergillus fumigatus* pulmonary infection. The everolimus dose was empirically reduced to 1.5 mg in the morning and 1 mg in the evening on the day of starting voriconazole and then reduced further to 1 mg twice daily starting on the second day of voriconazole therapy. On the third day of voriconazole therapy the everolimus level was 24.7 ng/mL, which was about 5 times higher than before voriconazole therapy. Everolimus was held due to the high level and 3 days later it was back in the therapeutic range of 8 ng/mL. Despite the patient's supratherapeutic voriconazole level of 10.7 mg/L the patient was transferred to the ICU due to worsening respiratory status requiring mechanical ventilation. Chest X-ray and lung computed tomography scans showed images consistent with everolimus-associated pneumonia. This interaction is likely due to voriconazole's inhibition of CYP3A4 which is how everolimus is mainly metabolized. Previous studies have suggested a 65% decrease in the everolimus dose should be applied when starting patients on voriconazole; however, this case highlights that an 80% reduction may be more appropriate to prevent this drug interaction-related side effect [32A].

Sirolimus

In order to determine the empiric dose adjustment necessary for sirolimus therapy when patients are started on posaconazole oral suspension a retrospective cohort study was conducted. Hematopoietic stem cell transplant (HSCT) patients who received posaconazole oral suspension and oral sirolimus between 2009 and 2011 were included. Sirolimus concentrations were measured at baseline and then up to 28 days after starting posaconazole. The sirolimus concentration/dose (C/D) ratio was determined for each sirolimus concentration obtained for all of the 75 patients included in the study. The C/D ratio for sirolimus was 2.29 ng/mL/mg prior to posaconazole initiation which increased to 6.24 ng/mL/mg approximately 17–20 days after initiation of posaconazole. Therefore, the C/D ratio increased approximately 2.7-fold in HSCT patients who were started on posaconazole. Therefore, a sirolimus dose reduction of 50–65% may be necessary in patients who are started on posaconazole therapy due to the CYP3A4 inhibition posaconazole causes [33c].

A retrospective review of 67 HSCT patients who received sirolimus, tacrolimus and low-dose methotrexate in addition to voriconazole was reviewed. The review was to assess the effect of voriconazole on sirolimus concentrations due to the CYP3A4 inhibition voriconazole causes which results in a decreased metabolism of sirolimus. When voriconazole was started the dose of sirolimus was reduced by 90% in all 67 patients. The median serum sirolimus levels before and after the start of voriconazole therapy were 5.8 ng/mL (range: 0–47.6) and 6.1 ng/mL (range: 1–14.2) ($P=0.45$). Only one patient developed an adverse effect of sirolimus-related thrombotic microangiopathy that resolved after sirolimus discontinuation and their average level was 6 ng/mL. Therefore, a sirolimus dose reduction of about 90% when starting voriconazole therapy results in similar levels prior to the initiation of voriconazole therapy [34c].

Vincristine

Vincristine, a chemotherapeutic agent, in combination with azole antifungals, has shown to increase adverse drug reactions. The most common adverse reactions that have been reported include gastrointestinal toxicity, peripheral neuropathy, electrolyte abnormalities, cranial neuropathy and seizures. These increased adverse events are thought to be related to the azole antifungal's inhibition of the cytochrome P450 (CYP) which results in inhibition of the metabolism of vincristine and therefore an increase in adverse effects. A retrospective study of 68 children with acute lymphoblastic leukemia (ALL) who received vincristine and azole antifungals was conducted. Patients were divided into different groups depending on the antifungal agent they received. The control group who just received vincristine had 44 patients, the itraconazole group at 44 patients, the fluconazole group had 42 patients and the voriconazole group had 6 patients. Overall there were significantly more adverse drug events in the itraconazole group and the voriconazole group compared to the fluconazole and control group ($P < 0.05$). There was no major difference between fluconazole and the control group. This is likely because fluconazole does not inhibit CYP3A4 as significantly the other azole antifungal agents. The side effects seen were similar to what has been reported before with gastrointestinal toxicity and peripheral neuropathy being the most common side effects. Therefore, when utilizing vincristine in this patient population fluconazole appears to be the safest azole antifungal to utilize for treatment and or prophylaxis of fungal infections [35c].

PYRIMADINE ANALOGUES [SEDA-36, 383; SEDA-37, 307]

Flucytosine

There are no new studies or reports of side effects related to flucytosine at this time.

ECHINOCANDINS [SEDA-33, 556; SEDA-34, 434; SEDA-35, 489; SEDA-36, 388; SEDA-37, 307]

Hemodynamic Effects of the Echinocandins

Administration of the echinocandins has been associated with temporary hemodynamic deterioration. Therefore, a prospective study in patients in the medical intensive care unit (ICU) who received echinocandins was conducted to assess this association. A transpulmonary thermodilution (TPTD) was used with measurements being taken immediately before, after and 4 hours after echinocandin administration for 2 days. All 15 patients in the study received either caspofungin or anidulafungin at the standard doses of 70 mg on the first day followed by 50 mg on the second day for caspofungin and 200 mg on the first day followed by 100 mg on the second day for anidulafungin. There was a significant change found in mean arterial pressure as well as diastolic blood pressure immediately after echinocandin administration ($P < 0.042$ and $P < 0.007$, respectively). In patients on norepinephrine there were no significant changes in the vasopressor dose. There was also no change found at the 4-hour after administration time period. Therefore, it may be important to closely monitor ICU patient's hemodynamics for any significant changes immediately after administration of echinocandin therapy [36c].

Anidulafungin [SEDA-35, 489; SEDA-36, 388; SEDA-37, 307]

There are no new studies or reports of side effects realted to anidulafungin at this time.

Caspofungin [SEDA-33, 556; SEDA-34, 434; SEDA-35, 490; SEDA-36, 389; SEDA-37, 307]

Hepatic

A retrospective review of 61 cancer patients who received anidulafungin treatment after caspofungin at M.D. Anderson Cancer Center was conducted to access the effect of the switch on hepatotoxicity. Since anidulafungin does not undergo hepatic metabolism, like the other echinocandins, it is suspected that there will be less hepatotoxicity associated with the use of this medication. Many patients in the study received medications and chemotherapy that can be considered hepatotoxic (77% and 62%, respectively). Alanine aminotransferase (ALT) and Aspartate transaminase (AST) were found to have decreased significantly when anidulafungin was changed to caspofungin and when anidulafungin was stopped ($P < 0.029$ and $P < 0.0017$, respectively). The median changes in AST, ALT and total bilirubin (TB) during anidulafungin therapy were found to be −43, −25 and −0.15 mg/dL, respectively. Over 70% of patients had a decrease in their hepatic enzymes that resulted in stable and decreased levels by the end of anidulafungin therapy. The common terminology criteria for adverse events (CTCAE) were utilized to define the liver injury/hepatotoxicity. Among 54 patients who had ALT with CTCAE grade ≥2 at the time of switching to anidulafungin therapy, 34 (63%) had decreased values and 12 (22%) had stable values at the end of anidulafungin therapy. Among 33 patients who had AST with CTCAE grade ≥2 at the time of switching, 18 (55%) who had decreased values and 8 (24%) had stable values at the end of anidulafungin therapy. Among 54 patients who had TB of CTCAE grade ≥2 at the time of switching, 28 (52%) had decreased values at the end of anidulafungin therapy. This study suggests anidulafungin does have less of an effect on hepatic enzymes and hepatotoxicity and therefore may be a favorable alternative to caspofungin for patients that develop hepatotoxicity while on therapy with this medication [37c].

References

[1] George A, Bhatia A, Kanish B, et al. Terbinafine induced pityriasis rosea-like eruption. Indian J Pharmacol. 2015;47(6):680–1 [A].

[2] Murad A, Shudell E, Mulligan N. Rowell's syndrome induced by terbinafine. BMJ Case Rep. 2015;28:1–2 [A].

[3] Bayata S, Ermertcan AT, Ates M, et al. Acute generalized exanthematous pustulosis in a child probably induced by terbinafine. Indian J Dermatol Venereol Leprol. 2015;81(1):95 [A].

[4] Saarikoski T, Saari TI, et al. Effects of terbinafine and itraconazole on the pharmacokinetics of orally administered tramadol. Eur J Clin Pharmacol. 2015;71(3):321–7 [c].

[5] Sheikh AR, Westley I, Sallustio B, et al. Interaction of terbinafine (an anti-fungal agent) with perhexiline: a case report. Heart Lung Circ. 2014;23(6):e149–51 [A].

[6] Meletiadis J, Chanock S, Walsh TJ. Defining targets for investigating the pharmacogenomics of adverse drug reactions to antifungal agents. Pharmacogenomics. 2008;9(5):561–84 [R].

[7] Falci DR, da Rosa FB, Pasqualotto AC. Comparison of nephrotoxicity associated to different lipid formulations of amphotericin B: a real-life study. Mycoses. 2015;58(2):104–12 [c].

[8] Botero Aguirre JP, Restrepo Hamid AM. Amphotericin B deoxycholate versus liposomal amphotericin B: effects on kidney function. Cochrane Database Syst Rev. 2015;11:CD01048 [M].

[9] Sato M, Hirayanagi K, Makioka K, et al. Reversal of leukoencephalopathy induced by liposomal amphotericin B in a patient with cryptococcal meningitis. J Neurol Sci. 2015;350(1–2):118–9 [A].

[10] Soares JR, Nunes MC, Leite AF, et al. Reversible dilated cardiomyopathy associated with amphotericin B therapy. J Clin Pharm Ther. 2015;40(3):333–5 [A].

[11] González-Fernández T, López-Freire S, et al. Herpes-like eruption due to fluconazole. J Investig Allergol Clin Immunol. 2015;25(2):135–6 [A].

[12] Alsaad AM, Kaplan YC, Koren G. Exposure to fluconazole and risk of congenital malformations in the offspring: a systematic review and meta-analysis. Reprod Toxicol. 2015;52:78–82 [M].

[13] Lee HJ, Lee B. Association of systolic blood pressure drop with intravenous administration of itraconazole in children with hemato-oncologic disease. Drug Des Devel Ther. 2015;9:6489–95 [C].

[14] Baquerizo Nole KL, Lee E, Villada G, et al. Ketoconazole-induced Sweet syndrome: a new association. Am J Dermatopathol. 2015;37(5):419–22 [A].

[15] Gupta AK, Daigle D, Foley KA. Drug safety assessment of oral formulations of ketoconazole. Expert Opin Drug Saf. 2015;14(2):325–34 [M].

[16] Martino J, Fisher BT, Bosse KR, et al. Suspected posaconazole toxicity in a pediatric oncology patient. Pediatr Blood Cancer. 2015;62(9):1682 [A].

[17] Bayhan GI, Garipardic M, Karaman K, et al. Voriconazole-associated visual disturbances and hallucinations. Cutan Ocul Toxicol. 2016;35(1):80–2 [A].

[18] Patel VA, Parikh SA, Nayyar PM, et al. Voriconazole-induced multiple squamous cell carcinomas in a patient with chronic lymphocytic leukemia. Dermatol Surg. 2015;41(6):747–9 [A].

[19] Wojenski DJ, Bartoo GT, et al. Voriconazole exposure and the risk of cutaneous squamous cell carcinoma in allogeneic hematopoietic stem cell transplant patients. Transpl Infect Dis. 2015;17(2):250–8 [C].

[20] Sheu J, Hawryluk EB, et al. Voriconazole phototoxicity in children: a retrospective review. J Am Acad Dermatol. 2015;72(2):314–20 [C].

[21] Lindsay R. Fluoride and bone—quantity versus quality. N Engl J Med. 1990;322(12):845–6 [C].

[22] Whitford GM. Intake and metabolism of fluoride. Adv Dent Res. 1994;8(1):5–14 [H].

[23] Glushko T, Colmegna I. Voriconazole-induced periostitis. CMAJ. 2015;187(14):1075 [A].

[24] Tailor TD, Richardson ML. Case 215: voriconazole-induced periostitis. Radiology. 2015;274(3):930–5 [A].

[25] Baird JH, Birnbaum BK, Porter DL, et al. Voriconazole-induced periostitis after allogeneic stem cell transplantation. Am J Hematol. 2015;90(6):574–5 [A].

[26] Tarlock K, Johnson D, et al. Elevated fluoride levels and periostitis in pediatric hematopoietic stem cell transplant recipients receiving long-term voriconazole. Pediatr Blood Cancer. 2015;62(5):918–20 [c].

[27] Rybak JM, Marx KR, et al. Isavuconazole: pharmacology, pharmacodynamics, and current clinical experience with a new triazole antifungal agent. Pharmacotherapy. 2015;35(11):1037–51 [R].

[28] Ashbee HR, Gilleece MH. Has the era of individualized medicine arrived for antifungals? A review of antifungal pharmacogenomics. Bone Marrow Transplan. 2012;47(7):881–94 [H].

[29] Owusu Obeng A, Egelund EF, Alsultan A, et al. CYP2C19 polymorphisms and therapeutic drug monitoring of voriconazole: are we ready for the clinical implication of pharmacogenomics? Pharmacotherapy. 2014;34(7):703–18 [R].

[30] Narita A, Muramatsu H, Sakaguchi H. Correlation of CYP2C19 phenotype with voriconazole plasma concentration in children. J Pediatr Hematol Oncol. 2013;35(5):e219–23 [c].

[31] Cadeddu G, Deidda A, et al. Clozapine toxicity due to a multiple drug interaction: a case report. J Med Case Rep. 2015;9:77 [A].

[32] Lecefel C, Eloy P, et al. Worsening pneumonitis due to a pharmacokinetic drug-drug interaction between everolimus and voriconazole in a renal transplant patient. J Clin Pharm Ther. 2015;40(1):119–20 [A].

[33] Cho E, Chan H, et al. Management of drug interaction between posaconazole and sirolimus in patients who undergo hematopoietic stem cell transplant. Pharmacotherapy. 2015;35(6):578–85 [c].

[34] Ceberio I, Dai K, et al. Safety of voriconazole and sirolimus coadministration after allogeneic hematopoietic SCT. Bone Marrow Transplant. 2015;50(3):438–43 [c].

[35] Yang L, Yu L, et al. Clinical analysis of adverse drug reactions between vincristine and triazoles in children with acute lymphoblastic leukemia. Med Sci Monit. 2015;21:1656–61 [c].

[36] Lahmer T, Schnappauf C. Influence of echinocandin administration on hemodynamic parameters in medical intensive care unit patients: a single center prospective study. Infection. 2015;43(6):723–7 [c].

[37] Jung DS, Tverdek FP, et al. Switching to anidulafungin from caspofungin in cancer patients in the setting of liver dysfunction is associated with improvement of liver function tests. J Antimicrob Chemother. 2015;70(11):3100–6 [c].

26

Antiprotozoal Drugs

Dayna S. McManus*, *Kristopher G. Hall*[†], *Sidhartha D. Ray*[†,1]

*Department of Pharmacy Services, Yale-New Haven Hospital, Yale University, New Haven, CT, USA
[†]Department of Pharmaceutical Sciences, Manchester University College of Pharmacy, Natural and Health Sciences, Fort Wayne, IN, USA
[1]Corresponding author: sdray@manchester.edu

ALBENDAZOLE

Liver

A 6-year-old girl was started on albendazole 15 mg/kg/day for treatment of a liver hydatid cyst. Two months later she was admitted with abdominal pain and elevated Aspartate aminotransferase (AST) and alanine aminotransferase (ALT) levels of 663 and 800 IU/L, respectively. Albendazole was stopped and the patient underwent work-up for possible causes of the elevated liver enzymes. After stopping the albendazole her transaminitis resolved. About 7 months later the patient's showed significant increase in her cyst and therefore albendazole was re-started at 15 mg/kg/day. Three weeks after starting albendazole the patient's AST and ALT were elevated again at 496 and 468 IU/L, respectively. The patient's ANA titer was also positive (1:100). To try to diagnose the cause of the hepatic injury a liver biopsy was performed which showed portal lymphoplasmacytic inflammation with extensive necrosis. Albendazole was again stopped and the patient was started on prednisolone and azathioprine. After these medication changes the patient's liver enzyme levels began to return to normal over the course of 2 weeks. Over the next few months the patient's physical exam as well as laboratory findings remained normal and the steroid and azathioprine were tapered off. There were a few factors that made it likely that the patient's autoimmune hepatitis was caused by albendazole. First, the patient's transaminitis was apparent each time the patient started albendazole and it resolved every time albendazole was stopped as well as when steroids and azathioprine were started. In addition, the patient's biopsy was consistent with drug-induced hepatitis and work-up for all other causes of hepatitis was negative. This is the first reported case of likely albendazole-induced autoimmune hepatitis [1A].

Drug–Drug Interactions

A systematic review of the literature on the pharmacokinetics and drug interactions of albendazole or mebendazole was published. A total of 17 articles were included in the final review. Overall it was found that strong inhibitors of CYP3A4 such as cimetidine increase the elimination half-life and can result in side effects due to higher than expected levels of cimetidine. Cases of this interaction were reported in the literature as well as pharmacokinetic reviews of healthy volunteers taking both medications to find out their effect on one another. Another interesting drug–drug interaction that noted was that dexamethasone appears to increase levels of albendazole by inhibiting its elimination. The exact mechanism of this drug–drug interaction is largely unknown; however, the interaction was published in the literature. On the other hand, strong inducers of CYP3A4 such as phenytoin, phenobarbital and carbamazepine decrease the area under the curve (AUC) of albendazole, which may lead to decreased efficacy of these agents. Significant number of publications demonstrates this drug interaction. Reviews of ritonavir use with albendazole show that with short-term use there is no effect on albendazole levels; however, with long-term use the levels of albendazole begin to decrease. Based on this review it is imperative that providers review patient's medication lists to identify any medications that may alter the effect of the patient's albendazole therapy [2M].

ISSN: 0378-6080
http://dx.doi.org/10.1016/bs.seda.2016.08.018

ARTEMETHER–LUMEFANTRINE

An observational cohort study of pregnant women who were inadvertently exposed to artemether–lumefantrine in their first trimester was conducted since the effect of exposure during pregnancy is unknown. Women were followed up until 6 weeks post-delivery and children for 12 months after birth. Women were also included if they received sulphadoxine–pyrimethamine (SP) and/or quinine. There was a total of 294 exposure in the cohort 150 were to artemether–lumefantrine (AL), 9 for sulphadoxine–pyrimethamine with artemether–lumefantrine and 135 with sulphadoxine–pyrimethamine and/or quinine. Perinatal mortality, including stillbirths and neonatal deaths, was similar in each of the treatment arms (AL 4.4%, SP and/or quinine 3.9%). Low birth weights were reported in 10.2% (95% CI 6.0, 16.6) and 6.7% (95% CI 3.4, 12.6) of newborns in the AL and SP and/or quinine arms, respectively. Overall development was similar between the two arms, both at 14 weeks and 12 months of age. Based on this observational study it appears that AL and SP are not associated with any safety risks when utilized in the first trimester of pregnancy [3c].

A 5-year surveillance of all adults and pediatric patients who were treated with artemether–lumefantrine for malaria in the US was conducted. The goal was to identify the safety and efficacy of this medication were was any different for patients in the USA versus endemic settings. A total of 108 patients were evaluated for safety. A total of 4 patients (3.7%) were found to have adverse events in the study. The side effects included anemia in two patients and nausea in another. These side effects were no different than those seen when the drug was used in patients outside the US [4M].

DIHYDROARTEMISININ–PIPERAQUINE

A randomized controlled non-inferiority trial was conducted to compare the safety and efficacy of dihydroartemisinin–piperaquine and artesunate–amodiaquine versus artemether–lumefantrine in children less than 10 years of age for acute uncomplicated *Plasmodium falciparum* infection. The primary outcome was PCR-corrected day-42 cure rates. PCR-corrected PP cure rates of 96.7, 98.1 and 96.3, respectively, for artemether–lumefantrine, artesunate–amodiaquine and dihydroartemisinin–piperaquine was observed. In terms of side effects there were not major differences in terms of type of side effect (all P values < 0.05). Although there was no significant statistical differences ($P = 0.09$) there was slight more side effects with artesunate–amodiaquine (35.5%) and dihydroartemisinin–piperaquine (37.9%) compared with artemether–lumefantrine (27.5%). The most common side effects for all of the agents were vomiting, cough, rashes, and anorexia. One serious AE occurred involving a child who experienced severe fatigue after artemether–lumefantrine ingestion. After 3 days of hospitalization the patient was discharged without complications. There was a slight decrease in mean hemoglobin levels in all treatment groups on days 0 through 7. Although there were changes in all groups the change was statically significant for dihydroartemisinin–piperaquine ($P = 0.0001$) and artemether–lumefantrine ($P = 0.003$). Similar to hemoglobin changes there was also slight increases in alanine transferase activity and creatinine levels in all treatment groups; however, the differences were not statistically significant between groups [5C].

OXANTEL PAMOATE–ALBENDAZOLE

A randomized controlled trial was conducted to determine the safety and efficacy of combination versus standard therapy for *T. trichiura* and concomitant intestinal nematodes in children aged 6–14 in Tanzania. Children were randomized to receive either albendazole (400 mg) plus ivermectin (200 µg/kg), albendazole (400 mg) plus mebendazole (500 mg), albendazole (400 mg) plus oxantel pamoate (20 mg/kg), or mebendazole (500 mg) alone. The primary outcome of the study was the number of children who were cured of *T. trichiura* infection. Additionally the study set out to determine the reduction of *T. trichiura* eggs in stool with the different therapy regimens based on geometric means when available. A total of 440 children were included in the study and 431 were included in the final analysis. Out of 108 children 74 were cured in the albendazole plus oxantel pamoate group [(68.5%, 95% CI 59.6–77.4); egg reduction 99.2%, 98.7–99.6], 30 of 109 in the albendazole plus ivermectin group [(27.5%, 19.0–36.0); egg reduction 94.5%, 91.7–96.3]. The mebendazole alone group cured 9 of 107 ([8.4%, 3.1–13.8]; egg reduction 58.5%, 45.2–70.9) and albendazole plus mebendazole had the same 9 of 107 patients cured [(8.4%, 3.1–13.8); egg reduction 51.6%, 35.0–65.3]. About a fifth of the children reported adverse events, which majority were described as mild. The most commonly reported adverse effects were abdominal cramps and headache. Albendazole plus oxantel pamoate had the highest number of reports of abdominal cramps at 20 patients (18.2%), 13 patients (12%) for albendazole plus ivermectin, 10 (9.3%) for albendazole plus mebendazole, and 16 (14.5%) for mebendazole. Headaches were reported by 5 (4.6%) children for albendazole plus ivermectin, 6 (5.6%) for albendazole plus mebendazole, 12 (10.9%) for albendazole plus oxantel pamoate, and 7 (6.4%) for mebendazole. Overall albendazole plus oxantel pamoate was the most efficacious for the treatment of infection with *T. trichiura* but did have the most headaches and abdominal cramps associated with it [6C].

PRIMAQUINE

A review of 50 patients with *vivax* malaria in Mâncio Lima, Acre, who were treated with chloroquine and primaquine, was reviewed to assess for side effects associated with these medications. Patients were assessed for 21 different symptoms before and after treatment and for reported side effects of these drugs after treatment were started. Prior to starting medication the most frequent symptoms were headache, fever, chills, sweating, arthralgia, back pain, and weakness. These side effects were present 40–76% of respondents. Once medication was started there was a reduction the occurrence of most of these symptoms. Appetite also improved after starting medication, but gastrointestinal symptoms and choluria increased in frequency after starting. There were no reports of pale stools before medication, but 12% reported the occurrence of this symptom after treatment started. Other symptoms such as blurred vision (54%), pruritus (22%), paresthesia (6%), insomnia (46%), and "stings" into the skin (22%) were reported after chloroquine was taken. Overall, chloroquine and primaquine reduced many of the systemic symptoms caused by *P. vivax* malaria; however, gastrointestinal side effects were the main side effect that persisted. It is important to discuss this with patients to encourage them to continue their medication because if not it may lead to lack of adherence to drug treatment [7c].

Currently, in Cambodia primaquine is often not utilized because of the concern for patients who are G6PD deficient and the lack of ability to test for thus. Therefore, a safety and efficacy study was conducted to assess the possibility of utilizing a weekly primaquine regimen in patients who were not tested for G6PD. A total of 75 Cambodian patients who were treated for malaria with dihydroartemisinin/piperaquine on days (D) 0, 1 and 2 were included. Then the included patients received weekly doses of primaquine 0.75 mg/kg for 8 weeks (starting on D0, last dose on D49), and followed until D56 were enrolled. Participants' G6PD status was confirmed by G6PD genotype and measured G6PD activity. The primary outcome of the study was treatment completion without primaquine toxicity. Primaquine toxicity was defined as any one of: severe anemia (haemoglobin [Hb] <7 g/dL), a >25% fractional fall in Hb from D0, the need for a blood transfusion, haemoglobinuria, acute kidney injury (an increase in baseline serum creatinine >50%) or methaemoglobinaemia >20%. Of the enrolled patients 18 were G6PD positive and had D0 G6PD activity ranging from 0.1 to 1.5 U/g Hb (median 0.85 U/g Hb).

In the 57 patients with normal G6PD, D0 G6PD activity ranged from 6.9 to 18.5 U/g Hb (median 12 U/g Hb). Median D0 Hb concentrations were similar ($P=0.46$) between G6PD positive (13 g/dL, range 9.6–16) and G6PD negative (13.5 g/dL, range 9–16.3). Both groups reached a nadir in terms of Hb concentrations on D2. (10.8 g/dL (8.2–15.3) in the G6PD positive versus 12.4 g/dL (8.8–15.2) in the G6PD negative ($P=0.006$)). By D7, five G6PD positive patients (27.7%) had a >25% fall in Hb, compared to 0 G6PD negative patients ($P=0.00049$). One of these G6PDd patients required a blood transfusion. No patients in any group developed severe anaemia, haemoglobinuria, a methaemoglobin concentration >4.9%, or acute kidney injury. Overall patient with G6PD positivity demonstrated significant, mostly transient, falls in Hb and one received a blood transfusion. Weekly primaquine in patients mandates medical supervision and pre-treatment screening for G6PD status, but may be a helpful future option pending additional studies [8c].

QUINACRINE

A case of a 45-year-old African American woman with possible quinacrine-induced cholestatic hepatitis was presented. The patient presented to the rheumatology clinic with a history of undifferentiated connective tissue disease (UCTD). The disease had manifested as biopsy-proven urticarial dermatitis, inflammatory arthritis, fatigue, and weight loss in the setting of positive immunofluorescence antinuclear antibodies (1:160, speckled pattern), anti-RNP, anti-Sm/RNP, and antichromatin antibodies. For treatment the patient was started on quinacrine 100 mg per day. The patient initially was started on hydroxychloroquine, but 2 months after starting she developed a pruritic rash and so it was changed to quinacrine. At the time she started treatment with quinacrine, she was also receiving 5 mg of prednisone, diphenhydramine as needed, ergocalciferol, and norgestimate–ethinyl estradiol. All of these were long-term medications, which were not new to her. Four weeks after starting quinacrine, she presented to the emergency department with generalized fatigue, loss of appetite, nausea, diffuse abdominal pain, scleral icterus, and dark tea-colored urine. The medications she was taking remained the same with no history of new medications, supplements, or alcohol intake.

Analysis of serum chemistry (blood work) demonstrated aspartate aminotransferase (AST) 629 (8–30 IU/L), alanine aminotransferase (ALT) 913 (≤35 IU/L), alkaline phosphatase 914 (30–130 IU/L), total bilirubin 11.0 (0.2–1.2 mg/dL), direct bilirubin 9.0, and indirect bilirubin 2.0. Abdominal ultrasound was performed and was found to be unremarkable. She was initially diagnosed with acute cholestatic hepatitis. Work-up for both infectious and autoimmune hepatitis causes was all-negative and therefore the hepatologists felt the liver injury could be secondary to the quinacrine. After negative work-ups the patient was discharged from the hospital. A week later, her liver function tests worsened with an AST level of 540, ALT 856, alkaline phosphatase 1300, and total bilirubin 22.9. Due to worsening live function tests it was decided she would undergo a liver biopsy. Results from the biopsy showed canalicular cholestasis without comparable periportal cholestatic ductular reaction, strongly suggesting a metabolic cause such as drug therapy. The Roussel Uclaf Causality Assessment Method scale was calculated to determine how likely the hepatic injury could be from the quinacrine. The score calculated to be 6, which indicates probable causal relationship between the offending drug and liver damage. In the context of the clinical history, laboratory investigations, and liver biopsy findings, the diagnosis of quinacrine-induced cholestatic hepatitis was made. Despite holding all of her medications, except the 5 mg of prednisone, her bilirubin and transaminases did not peak until 3 weeks after she initially developed the cholestatic jaundice. Liver enzymes normalized over a period of about 5 months after stopping the quinacrine. Long-term, high-dose quinacrine for treatment of malaria was occasionally reported to be associated with reversible hepatitis, presumably because of its tendency to concentrate in the liver. Transient acute quinacrine hepatitis has been reported on 1 occasion in 1985 in a patient with UCTD; however, this patient was prescribed 3 times the normal recommended dose. This is the first reported case of quinacrine-induced cholestatic hepatitis in UCTD when the medication was utilized at the appropriate dose. Because this is a new and serious complication of quinacrine use physicians should be aware and suspect this in patients presenting with a similar presentation [9A].

ARTESUNATE

A case of fevers and delayed hemolysis in a patient receiving artesunate was reported. The patient was a 68-year-old African American woman who presented with a 3-day history of fever to 102.8°F. The patient also reported periods of intermittent confusion, fatigue, anorexia, and myalgia. Prior to presenting with these symptoms the patient had been receiving artesunate in Nigeria for 3 weeks for the treatment of malaria. She returned to the USA 1 week before presentation. The patient's temperature was 101.6°8 F, with a pulse of 106 beats/min, blood pressure of 125/80 and oxygen saturation of 99% on room air. Laboratory examination revealed a leukocyte count of 21 000/mL with 70% neutrophils, 23% lymphocytes, 4% monocytes and 3% eosinophils, hemoglobin of 8.4 g/dL which dropped to 7.0 on

the fifth day of hospitalization, and a platelet count of 306 000. The serum in the chemistry tube was grossly hemolyzed, with potassium of 15 mEq/L and normal renal function. These findings were noted on multiple specimens. Wright–Giemsa stain from multiple blood samples did not reveal intraerythrocytic parasites. However, the peripheral smear was remarkable for rouleaux formation and erythrocytes with atypical diamond-shaped central blanched pitting. Further laboratory testing on hospital day 2 revealed an indirect bilirubin of 3.2 mg/dL, total bilirubin 4.4 mg/dL, LDH 965 IU/dL and haptoglobin 326 mg/dL (normal 43–212). The anemia and hemolytic picture continued to worsen over the next few days, before eventually improving. From 2010 to 2012 there have been 19 reported cases of delayed hemolytic anemia after treatment of severe malaria with artesunate.

Worldwide, there have been 37 reported cases of hemolysis associated with the use of artemisinin derivatives in the treatment of severe malaria. There are two distinct patterns of hemolysis after artesunate therapies that have been described. The first pattern involves a delayed onset and the second is a persistent pattern of hemolysis, which continues from about day 7 to 14. Delayed hemolysis typically occurs 2–3 weeks after completion of artesunate therapy, which was the exact presentation of this patient. A delayed hemolytic pattern is defined by a decrease in hemoglobin associated with a low haptoglobin or increase in LDH occurring at least 7 days following artesunate treatment, which was the presentation of this patient. The mechanism behind the hemolysis from artesunate is still unclear. A potential explanation is a process performed by the spleen called pitting. Pitting occurs when artesunate exposed parasites are expelled from infected erythrocytes in the spleen. The erythrocytes then reseal and reenter circulation as pitted erythrocytes that have a shortened lifespan. The delayed clearance of these pitted erythrocytes by the spleen may explain the features of post artesunate delayed hemolysis. The degree of initial parasitemia has been shown to increase the risk of this occurrence. It is imperative that providers should be aware of this delayed side effect in order to prevent unnecessary further treatment of presumed malaria [10A].

A prospective cohort study of 123 patients in France who had severe malaria that was treated with artesunate was conducted to evaluate the risk of delayed-onset hemolysis. The evaluation reviewed the outcomes, adverse events, and postartesunate delayed-onset hemolysis (PADH). Of the 123 patients who were reviewed there were a total of 97 adverse events that occurred. Among the 78 patients who received follow-up for >8 days after treatment initiation, 76 (97%) had anemia. 21 (27%) of the 78 cases on anemia that were reported were noted to be PADH. The median drop in hemoglobin levels was 1.3 g/dL and 15% of patients with PADH had hemoglobin levels of <7 g/dL. Only one of these patients required a transfusion. Despite the high incidence of PADH, the resulting anemia remained mild in 85% of cases. It is helpful to note that majority of cases were mild; however, providers should still be aware of this adverse effect when treating patients [11c].

MEFLOQUINE

A database analysis was conducted to review the reports of eye disorder adverse events related to mefloquine (as Lariam®) use. The F. Hoffmann-La Roche global drug safety database was utilized for the review. Any reports of adverse event were also reviewed and verified by a trained ophthalmologist. The analysis focused on 3 categories of eye disorders including visual acuity, anatomical parts of the eye and neuro-ophthalmic events. To put our analysis in context, an extensive literature search on "mefloquine" and "eye disorders" was conducted. A total of 591 cases with 695 events associated with "Eye disorder" in individuals exposed to mefloquine were reported. The majority of the events ($n = 493$, 70.9%) were related to visual acuity (mainly visual impairment and blurred vision), followed by neuro-ophthalmic events ($n = 124$, 17.8%). The majority of visual adverse events were non-serious but 37.7% ($n = 223$) of cases were classified as serious. Nine events of maculopathy were reported and 48 cases with 53 events described symptoms of optic neuropathy. Based on this review it does appear that mefloquineis likely to be associated with eye disorders. Therefore, providers should be aware of these risks and discuss the risk with travelers [12M].

A national Danish registry was utilitized to review the acute psychiatric side effects associated with mefloquine usage. A total of 73 patients treated with mefloquine reported to the national register during 5 consecutive years. Acute psychiatric side effects were retrospectively assessed using the Symptom Check List (SCL-90-R) and questions based on Present State Examination (PSE). Subjects reporting suspected psychotic states were contacted for a personal PSE interview. Long-term effects were evaluated with short form (SF-36). In the SCL-90-R, clinically significant scores for anxiety, phobic anxiety and depression were found in 55%, 51%, and 44% of patients treated with mefloquine. Substantial acute phase psychotic symptoms were found in 15% and were time-limited. Cases of hypomania/mania in the acute phase were 5.5% in patients treated with mefloquine. Significant long-term mental health effects were demonstrated for the SF-36 subscales mental health (MH), role

emotional (RE), and vitality (VT) in the mefloquine group compared to matched controls. The most frequent acute psychiatric problems were anxiety, depression, and psychotic symptoms. Providers should be aware of these side effects when prescribing mefloquine specifically in patients that already have a history of psychiatric disease [13M].

References

[1] Koca T, Akcam M. Albendazole-induced autoimmune hepatitis. Indian Pediatr. 2015;52(1):78–9 [A].

[2] Pawluk SA, Roels CA, et al. A review of pharmacokinetic drug-drug interactions with the anthelmintic medications albendazole and mebendazole. Clin Pharmacokinet. 2015;4: 371–383 [M].

[3] Manyando C, Njunju EM, Virtanen M, et al. Exposure to artemether-lumefantrine (Coartem) in first trimester pregnancy in an observational study in Zambia. Malar J. 2015;14:77 [c].

[4] Gray AM, Arguin PM, Hamed K. Surveillance for the safety and effectiveness of artemether-lumefantrine in patients with uncomplicated Plasmodium falciparum malaria in the USA: a descriptive analysis. Malar J. 2015;14:349 [M].

[5] Nji AM, Ali IM, Moyeh MN, et al. Randomized non-inferiority and safety trial of dihydroartemisin-piperaquine and artesunate-amodiaquine versus artemether-lumefantrine in the treatment of uncomplicated Plasmodium falciparum malaria in Cameroonian children. Malar J. 2015;14:27 [C].

[6] Speich B, Ali SM, Ame SM, et al. Efficacy and safety of albendazole plus ivermectin, albendazole plus mebendazole, albendazole plus oxantel pamoate, and mebendazole alone against Trichuris trichiura and concomitant soil-transmitted helminth infections: a four-arm, randomised controlled trial. Lancet Infect Dis. 2015;15(3):277–84 [C].

[7] Braga CB, Martins AC, Cayotopa AD, et al. Side effects of chloroquine and primaquine and symptom reduction in malaria endemic area (Mâncio Lima, Acre, Brazil). Interdiscip Perspect Infect Dis. 2015;2015:346853 [c].

[8] Kheng S, Muth S, Taylor WR, et al. Tolerability and safety of weekly primaquine against relapse of Plasmodium vivax in Cambodians with glucose-6-phosphate dehydrogenase deficiency. BMC Med. 2015;13:203 [c].

[9] Namas R, Marquardt A. Case report and literature review: quinacrine-induced cholestatic hepatitis in undifferentiated connective tissue disease. J Rheumatol. 2015;42(7): 1354–1355 [A].

[10] Lahoud JS, Lahoud OB, Lin YS, et al. Artesunate-related fever and delayed hemolysis in a returning traveler. IDCases. 2015;2(2):63–5 [A].

[11] Jauréguiberry S, Thellier M, Ndour PA, et al. Delayed-onset hemolytic anemia in patients with travel-associated severe malaria treated with artesunate, France, 2011–2013. Emerg Infect Dis. 2015;21(5):804–12 [c].

[12] Adamcova M, Schaerer MT, Bercaru I, et al. Eye disorders reported with the use of mefloquine (Lariam(®)) chemoprophylaxis—a drug safety database analysis. Travel Med Infect Dis. 2015;13(5):400–8 [M].

[13] Ringqvist Å, Bech P, Glenthøj B, et al. Acute and long-term psychiatric side effects of mefloquine: a follow-up on Danish adverse event reports. Travel Med Infect Dis. 2015;13(1): 80–88 [M].

27

Antiviral Drugs

Sreekumar Othumpangat*,¹, Sidhartha D. Ray†, John D. Noti*

*Allergy and Clinical Immunology Branch, Health Effects Laboratory Division, National Institute for Occupational Safety and Health, Centers for Disease Control and Prevention, Morgantown, WV, USA

†Department of Pharmaceutical Sciences, Manchester University College of Pharmacy, Natural and Health Sciences, Fort Wayne, IN, USA

¹Corresponding author: seo8@cdc.gov

Key to abbreviations and alternative names of some antiviral drugs

3TC	lamivudine (dideoxythiacytidine)
AZT	zidovudine (azidothymidine)
D4T	stavudine (didehydrodideoxythymidine)
DDI	didanosine (dideoxyinosine)
FTC	emtricitabine
SOF	sofosbuvir
TMC 278	rilpivirine
TMC125	etravirine

DRUGS ACTIVE AGAINST CYTOMEGALOVIRUS

Cidofovir [SED-15, 771; SEDA-32, 529; SEDA-33, 577; SEDA-34, 447; SEDA-35, 503; SEDA-36, 401; SEDA-37, 329]

Observational Studies

An open-label, non-randomized, single-dose pilot study reported on the safety and pharmacokinetics of cidofovir in pediatric hematopoietic stem cell transplant (HSCT) recipients with symptomatic adenovirus, nucleoside-resistant cytomegalovirus (CMV) or herpes simplex virus (HSV), and/or human papovavirus infections. Twelve patients were enrolled in the study (median age, 9 years; 33.5 days post-transplantation). Four out of seven patients with adenovirus infection were treated with cidofovir and eventually cleared their infections. Four out of 12 patients died of disseminated viral disease and multi-organ failure. Two out of 12 patients had evidence of acute kidney injury after the first dose, and one of these patients developed chronic kidney disease; two other patients developed late nephrotoxicity. The mean drug half-life was 9.5 h. Pharmacokinetics were similar to those reported for adults, although the drug half-life was significantly longer than that for adults. Cidofovir was well tolerated in the majority of patients [1c].

In another study, the structural, topological and vibrational properties of cidofovir and brincidofovir were studied to understand the structural and functional properties by using density functional theory, natural bond orbital theory, atoms in molecules theory, frontier orbitals and molecular electrostatic potential calculations and the hybrid B3LYP/6-31G method [2c].

Letermovir

Infection with CMV is prevalent in immunosuppressed patients. In solid organ transplant and HSCT recipients, CMV infection is associated with high morbidity and preventable mortality. Prevention and treatment of cytomegalovirus with currently approved antiviral drugs is often associated with side effects that sometimes preclude their use. Moreover, CMV has developed mutations that confer resistance to standard antiviral drugs. During the last decade, there have been calls to develop novel antiviral drugs that could provide better options for prevention and treatment of CMV. Letermovir is a highly specific antiviral drug that is currently undergoing clinical development for the management of CMV infection. It acts by inhibiting the viral terminase complex. Letermovir is highly potent in vitro and in vivo against CMV. Due to a distinct mechanism of action, letermovir does not exhibit cross-resistance with other antiviral drugs. It is predicted to be active against strains that are resistant to ganciclovir, foscarnet, and cidofovir. To date, early-phase clinical trials suggest a very low incidence of adverse effects [3r].

Foscarnet [SED-15, 1447; SEDA-34, 448; SEDA-35, 504; SEDA-36, 403; SEDA-37, 329]

Observational Study

The safety and efficacy of foscarnet was evaluated in people diagnosed with CMV antigenemia following bone marrow transplantation between unrelated people and the administration of foscarnet. The study examined 59 patients at the National Cancer Center Hospital between June 2004 and November 2011. Renal dysfunction was observed in 11 cases (Grade 1 in 3 cases, Grade 2 in 7 cases, and Grade 3 in one case). The drug was discontinued or the dose was adjusted in 4 cases. Hypocalcemia was observed in 27 cases, hypokalemia in 17 cases, and hypomagnesemia in 17 cases. In the following cases, the severity of bone marrow suppression turned to Grade 4 following the start of treatment: 2 cases of leucopenia, 5 cases of decreased platelet count, 2 cases of decreased hemoglobin level in the blood, and 4 cases of a decreased neutrophil counts were observed. The authors' conclusion was that foscarnet may be safely and effectively used as a remedy for CMV antigenemia following bone marrow transplantation between unrelated people [4c].

Foscarnet-induced adverse drug reaction (ADR) in the Beijing, China from March 2008 to December 2014 in CMV patients has been reported. The study evaluated 152 case reports received from Beijing drug Adverse Reaction Monitoring Center. The type and time of ADR, the age of patient, the gender and nationality of patient, serious adverse reactions, allergy history, administration, dosage, preparation, the indication, ADR history, ADR involved organ and system, the causal relationship, treatments and prognosis were retrospectively analyzed. The ADR induced by foscarnet more often occurred in patients aged from 31 to 60, appearing within 24 h (55.3%) after drug administration. ADR involved different systems and organs, predominantly the renal function and epileptic seizures [5C].

A case report demonstrated the difficulties in managing CMV retinitis in severely immunocompromised patients. A 40-year-old man diagnosed with HIV in 2011, had a CD4 count of 50 cells/μL and a HIV viral load 10000000 copies/mL. At the time, he was also diagnosed with diffuse large B cell lymphoma with liver metastasis. He received chemotherapy, achieved virological suppression on antiretroviral therapy and his CD4 count rose to 120 cells/μL. Six months later, he was diagnosed with CMV retinitis. CMV load in the plasma was 400000 and 600000 copies/mL in the cerebrospinal fluid (CSF). Intravitreal ganciclovir and foscarnet were administered with IV ganciclovir for 3 weeks, after which the patient was discharged home on maintenance treatment of oral 900 mg valganciclovir daily. His CD4 count was 140 cells/μL, HIV viral load was undetectable and plasma CMV load was 16000 copies/mL. Ten weeks later, he had a drop in visual acuity from 6/38 to hand movements in the right eye. Detachment of the right retina and active retinal inflammation in the left eye, along with ataxia and nystagmus were observed. The CMV load in the plasma was 550000 and 198554 copies/mL in the CSF. UL 97 mutations C592G and C607Y, associated with ganciclovir resistance were detected in peripheral blood but not in CSF. Intravitreal ganciclovir and foscarnet were administered to the left eye in conjunction with systemic antiviral therapy with IV foscarnet and ganciclovir. Subsequently, there was significant improvement in left retina with no evidence of active inflammation and 4 weeks later his CMV load in both plasma and CSF was undetectable. IV foscarnet monotherapy was continued for additional 4 weeks until CD4 count rose above 100 cells/μL. There was significant reduction in CMV load and retinal improvement when IV foscarnet combined with ganciclovir was given [6A].

Ganciclovir and Valganciclovir [SED-15, 1480; SEDA-34, 449, SEDA-35, 504, SEDA-36, 404, SEDA-37, 330]

Observational Study

A multicenter, double-blind, placebo-controlled, randomized clinical trial reported on valganciclovir for the prevention of complications of late CMV infection after HSCT at the Fred Hutchinson Cancer Research Center. Patients were randomly assigned to receive valganciclovir (900 mg once per day) or matching placebo between 1999 and 2008. The study drug was withdrawn when CMV viral load was greater than 1000 copies/mL or greater than five times than the baseline, and preemptive therapy was started with IV ganciclovir (5 mg/kg twice daily) or valganciclovir (900 mg twice daily); if neutropenia was detected, foscarnet (90 mg/kg twice daily) was used. The number of patients with adverse events (AEs) and serious AEs did not differ. More patients with drug-related Grade 2 AEs were reported in the valganciclovir group, which was driven by neutropenia (40% in the placebo group vs. 55% in the valganciclovir group), but there were no differences between the groups at Grade 3 or greater levels. The proportion of patients with gastrointestinal or renal AEs did not differ between groups [7C].

Five cases of renal transplant recipients at the University of Chicago Medical Center with resistant CMV infection were successfully treated with leflunomide. Five renal transplant recipients (2 simultaneous pancreas/kidney transplants, 3 deceased donor kidney transplants) were diagnosed with ganciclovir-resistant CMV infection from 2003 to 2011. Of the 4 patients who had resistance genotype testing, 3 showed a UL97 mutation and 1 patient had a clinically resistant CMV infection. All patients received CMV prophylaxis with valganciclovir for 3 months. All 5 patients received other antiviral agents (e.g. ganciclovir, foscarnet), and in 4 patients, viremia was cleared before leflunomide was initiated as maintenance therapy. The beneficial effect of leflunomide in this setting warrants further investigation. The only known AEs is abnormal liver function tests. In light of the long half-life of teriflunomide ($\sim$15 days), it may take several weeks for liver function tests to return to normal after discontinuation of the drug. In the authors' opinion leflunomide is effective in preventing viral recurrence, when used with short-term foscarnet in treating ganciclovir-resistant CMV infection [8c].

A retrospective study reported on 71 HIV-infected patients who had detectable CMV viremia between 1 January 2007 and 31 December 2007. The study evaluated the efficacy and safety of pre-emptive anti-CMV therapy (PACT). Sixteen patients who had lower CD4 cell counts and higher blood CMV DNA levels received PACT (valganciclovir). The cumulative incidence of CMV end-organ disease (EOD) and death at 1 year was 44% and 21% in patients with and without PACT, respectively ($p = 0.013$). Both PACT and high blood CMV DNA levels were significantly associated with CMV EOD and death in an unadjusted analysis. Five patients with PACT experienced severe drug-related AEs. Safety data were available for 14 of the 16 patients who received PACT, and severe drug-related AEs occurred in 5 (36%). Three patients treated with valganciclovir experienced Grade 3 or 4 neutropenia ($n=2$), or Grade 3 anemia ($n=1$), all received hematopoietic growth factors and one received a blood transfusion. Of note, only one patient in the PACT group received zidovudine (AZT), but no safety data were available for this patient. Two patients treated with foscarnet experienced Grade 3 and 4 metabolic AEs (hypocalcaemia ($n=2$), hypophosphatemia [$n=1$]) [9C].

Combination Study

Although no licensed drugs are available for therapy of congenital CMV infection, ganciclovir and its oral pro-drug, valganciclovir, were administered to symptomatic infants to improve neuro-developmental and auditory outcome. Other potentially efficacious drug therapies for congenital CMV disease are foscarnet and cidofovir, which are administered in a few cases. A literature search was reported looking for evidence on pharmacokinetics, efficacy, and side effects of ganciclovir/valganciclovir and the other two antiviral drugs [10R].

DRUGS ACTIVE AGAINST HERPES VIRUSES [SEDA-32, 530; SEDA-33, 577; SEDA-34, 450; SEDA-35, 507; SEDA-36, 407; SEDA-37, 332]

Acyclovir

Observational Studies

A retrospective case–control study of patients admitted to Children's Hospital Colorado from October 2006 to January 2009 who received treatment doses of IV acyclovir has been reported. Renal dysfunction occurred in 131 of 373 (35%) of the patients studied. Median times to risk, injury, and failure were 0.8, 0.7, and 1.4 days, respectively. In aggregate analyses, failure cases were older, had greater BMI and weight, and received fewer doses of acyclovir compared with failure controls. Urinalysis abnormalities were seen in 18 of 42 (43%), 14 of 23 (61%), and 4 of 9 (44%) cases with results available in the risk, injury, and failure groups, respectively, compared with 45 of 113 (40%) of controls. Hematuria, proteinuria, white blood cells, and granular casts were the most common findings in patients with renal dysfunction, but without significant differences between cases and controls. No patients required dialysis. Authors found that the concomitant ceftriaxone administration with acyclovir is a risk factor [11C].

Neurological

A retrospective observational study evaluated the role of antiviral therapy in immunocompromised patients with HSV meningitis. Authors reviewed the charts of 53 patients with CSF specimens positive for HSV-1 or HSV-2 by polymerase chain reaction (PCR) between July 2000 and November 2012 in Minneapolis, Minnesota. Six patients with meningitis did not receive antivirals, whereas the remaining patients were treated with an oral antiviral ($n=11$ [26.2%]), combination IV and oral therapy ($n=22$ [52.4%]), or IV acyclovir alone ($n=3$ [7.1%]). Authors recommend treating immunocompromised patients with HSV meningitis with a 7–10-day course of specific antiviral therapy to improve neurologic outcomes [12c].

A 58-year-old Japanese man, who underwent surgery to remove a thymoma at the age of 54, acutely developed speech difficulties and was admitted on suspicion of stroke. Vital signs were normal except for a mild fever (37.8 °C). His general condition was normal (height: 160 cm, weight: 60 kg). Brain MRI demonstrated multiple lesions in the frontal lobes. Although the CSF findings were normal, acyclovir (10 mg/kg, three times a day) was administered, and his fever and neurological symptoms fully recovered. Later neurological examination revealed the reappearance of motor aphasia and mild right hemiparesis. The MRI demonstrated an increase in size of the lesion in the left cingulate gyrus, an abnormal signal intensity lesion in the left corona radiata, and edematous swelling of the bilateral medial temporal regions. The patient's serum had increased levels of CMV pp65 antigen-positive leukocytes and the patient was diagnosed as having Good's syndrome, resulting in opportunistic infections in the brain. Since the patient was positive for CMV antigen, antiviral therapy was performed using ganciclovir, 5 mg/kg, twice a day for 2 weeks, along with immunoglobulin replacement therapy (5 g/day, for 3 days). The patient became free from any neurological symptoms for 1 year, and the brain lesions were improved without any AEs [13A].

A 65-year-old woman who was diagnosed with a multidermatomal herpes zoster infection and taking valacyclovir, 1 g every 8 h along with prednisone, developed neurological abnormalities. Antiviral drugs were discontinued in the patient and dialysis started. Serum acyclovir levels significantly dropped after the first two sessions of hemodialysis and the patient returned to baseline from neurological disorders. The authors suggests that patients with a history of herpes zoster infection and CDK are the population most vulnerable to develop acyclovir-induced neurotoxicity[14A].

Immune Response

Fifty-one patients were recruited from Birmingham Heartlands Hospital to evaluate the immune response to acyclovir, of which 24 were CMV-seropositive (median age 41 years; range 21–74 years). Patients were receiving long-term treatment with acyclovir at a dose of 400 mg twice a day for suppression of recurrent herpesvirus (HSV-1 and HSV-2) infection. The treatment duration ranged between 1 and 108 months with a median of 28 months. Acyclovir treatment was able to reduce the functional immune response against the late CMV protein, and the absolute frequency of CD8+ T cells specific for IE-1 and pp65 using a panel of HLA-peptide tetramers. The study revealed that acyclovir therapy has the potential to reduce some components of the CMV-specific T cell response [15c].

Famciclovir

Renal Function

Abnormal penciclovir blood concentration increased by famciclovir has been reported in a 91-year-old woman admitted for anorexia and general fatigue. The patient was diagnosed as having dehydration based on the blood test. The patient, receiving 1500 mg of famciclovir per day developed acute renal failure. Famciclovir was discontinued immediately, and the patient was advised to drink more water, which improved the renal condition [16A].

Famciclovir combined with oxymatrine improved clinical efficacy, prevented the development of liver fibrosis, and improved the T lymphocyte subsets in peripheral blood in patients with chronic severe viral hepatitis B [17c].

Valacyclovir

Skin Lesions

Acyclovir and valacyclovir allergies were rarely reported in the literature. A 60-year-old woman was admitted with a stage III non-secretory multiple myeloma and a history of hypothyroidism secondary to Hashimoto's thyroiditis. She underwent induction chemotherapy and eventual auto-HSCT. Her home medications included a compounded thyroid supplement and occasional ibuprofen with no known drug allergies. Her induction chemotherapy consisted of bortezomib, lenalidomide, liposomal doxorubicin, and dexamethasone. She was started on aspirin 81 mg daily, zolpidem 5 mg at bedtime and valacyclovir 500 mg daily on day 1 of chemotherapy. On day 15 of induction chemotherapy, she developed an urticarial-type rash bilaterally on her torso and, back thighs, which was treated with a 10-day methylprednisolone administration. Two weeks later, her rash had subsided. She was re-challenged with valacyclovir and similar symptoms reappeared, without any other systemic manifestations. These sequences of reactions were due to oral valacyclovir. Two months later, she returned for stem cell mobilization with filgrastim followed by high dose melphalan (200 mg) and auto-HSCT. The day prior to her auto-HSCT she was started on levofloxacin 500 mg daily, fluconazole 400 mg daily and famciclovir 500 mg daily for prophylaxis. By day 11 post-HSCT, she stopped anti-fungal and bacterial prophylaxis and continued antiviral prophylaxis without any reported issues. After 6 months, post-HSCT famciclovir and sulfamethoxazole/trimethoprim were discontinued. She continues to be in remission without any transplant or infection-related complications [18A].

DRUGS ACTIVE AGAINST HEPATITIS VIRUSES

Adefovir [SED-15, 35; SEDA-32, 530; SEDA-33, 578; SEDA-34, 452; SEDA-35, 507; SEDA-36, 409; SEDA-37, 333]

Urinary Tract

Adefovir (ADV), a nucleotide analog, has moderate potency and potential nephrotoxicity. ADV was recommended by certain scholars because it has less drug resistance ratio than lamivudine (LMV). In a prospective double-blind study, 252 patients diagnosed with chronic hepatitis B virus (HBV) infection between January 2006 and August 2014 were recruited and screened for resistance to ADV. The patients were randomly divided into three groups: LMV+ADV ($n=88$), telbivudine (LdT)+ADV ($n=84$), entecavir (ETV) + ADV ($n=80$). The patients were administered with LMV 100 mg a day; LdT 600 mg once a day; ADV 10 mg once a day; ETV 0.5 mg once a day. All the patients tolerated treatment well, and no patient discontinued the therapy. At week 36 of treatment, the rate of side effects in the LMV+ADV group was 1.1%, with one patient demonstrating blood urea nitrogen (BUN) elevation (14.2 mmol/L). In the LdT + ADV group, the rate was 1.2%, with one patient demonstrating BUN elevation (14.7 mmol/L) and one patient with creatine kinase elevation (138.6 μmol/L), the rate of side effects happening in the ETV + ADV group was 1.3%, with one patient demonstrating BUN elevation (14.6 mmol/L). At week 96 of treatment, the rate of side effects happening in the LMV + ADV 4.5%, with two patients having blood urea BUN elevation (mean 13.9 mmol/L), one patient having diarrhea, and one patient having nausea; the ratio of side effects in the LdT + ADV group was 7.1%, with two patients having BUN elevation (mean 14.5 mmol/L), one patient having creatine kinase elevation (142.3 μmol/L). The rate of side effects in the ETV + ADV group was 5.0%, with two patients having BUN, one patient having headache, and one patient having dizziness. None of the patients developed acute renal failure or myopathy during the rescue therapy. The patients suffering side effects recovered after undergoing symptomatic treatments [19c].

Comparative Study

The efficacy of tenofovir (TDF) in 3TC-resistant patients with a suboptimal response to 3TC plus ADV was reported. HBV serological markers and biochemistry were assessed at baseline at weeks 12, 24, and 48. Resistance surveillance and side effects were monitored during therapy. Fifty-nine patients were randomized to switch to TDF ($n=28$) or continuation with 3TC plus ADV ($n=31$). No significant differences were found between the groups at baseline [20c].

The clinical effects of ADV combined with ETV in the treatment of chronic HBV in 68 patients with decompensated cirrhosis has been reported. In these patients, ADV combined with ETV treatment effectively delayed the progression of liver cirrhosis, improved the liver function and sleep quality, and reduced the risk of hepatocellular carcinoma [21c].

A retrospective study conducted in Korean population evaluated the efficacy of TDF treatment for more than 6 months in 151 nucleos(t)ide-naïve HBV patients. The study found that the cumulative rates of virologic response at 6, 9, 12, and 18 months were 47.0%, 59.4%, 67.9%, and 69.3%, respectively. Most of the AEs were mild. No significant changes were observed in serum creatinine and phosphorus levels [22C].

Combination

Sixty-eight patients were enrolled in a study to understand the effect of Peg-IFN α-2 α combined with ADV in HBV postpartum women with normal levels of ALT and high levels of HBV DNA. Thirty (30/68) patients were switched to CPIA treatment after childbirth, 93.3% (28/30) achieved virological response, 56.7% (17/30) achieved Hepatitis B virus e antigen (HBVeAg)

seroclearance and 26.7% (8/30) cleared HBsAg after the treatment period. The HBV DNA and HBVeAg levels before CPIA treatment were negatively associated with HBeAg seroclearance. HBVsAg and HBVeAg levels in week 12 and week 24 after CPIA treatment were negatively associated with HBsAg seroclearance. Thirty-eight (38/68) patients did not receive antiviral treatment after childbirth, and none of them had HBVeAg or HBVsAg clearance. Authors suggests that it is safe to treat postpartum women who have HBV with a combination of drugs [23c].

DIRECT-ACTING ANTIVIRAL PROTEASE INHIBITORS [SEDA-35, 508; SEDA-36, 409; SEDA-37, 334]

Boceprevir

Intraocular pressure increased in patients with hepatitis C virus (HCV) treated with Peg-IFN-a-2a, RBV, and boceprevir [24c].

Hematological Toxicity

A cohort study involving 81 liver transplant patients (Male: 76%, mean age: 55.8 ± 9.7 years) with severe HCV recurrence (F3 or F4: $n=34$ (42%)) has been reported. The patients were treated with boceprevir ($n=36$) or telaprevir ($n=45$). A premature discontinuation of anti-HCV therapy due to a serious AE reported in 22 patients (27%) due to boceprevir. Hematological toxicity was reported as a side effect of boceprevir in 95% of patients, infections in 28% and death in 7% [25c].

Telaprevir

Observational Study

An observational study was reported to evaluate the safety and efficacy of telaprevir (TVR), in combination with Peg-IFNa-2b and RBV in 3563 chronic HCV patients. Patients were treated with TVR, Peg-IFN and RBV for 12 weeks followed by Peg-IFN and RBV for 12 weeks (triple therapy). Serious ADR were observed in 96.5% patients. ADR related to skin disorders and anemia were frequently observed in addition to serious renal dysfunction [26C].

The safety and efficacy of a triple therapy in HCV and HIV co-infected patients was reported. Five hundred eighty-four patients from 24 health care settings in Austria, Germany, Spain, Switzerland and the United Kingdom were included in the observational study. The patients, who were over 18 years old and were co-infected with HIV, were given triple therapy against HCV including BOC or TVR in combination with Peg-IFN plus RBV with HCV genotype 1 at the time of starting therapy. Patients received a three-drug combination based on Peg-IFN alfa-2a or Peg-IFN alfa-2b at a dose of 180 μg or 1.5 μg/kg once per week, respectively, and oral RBV at daily doses of 800–1200 mg. BOC was administered orally at doses of 800 mg every 8 h for 44 weeks. Oral TVR was given at doses of 750 mg every 8 h or 1125 mg twice a day during the first 12 weeks of therapy. Of these, 159 patients reached the 60-week follow-up analysis. Treatment was discontinued due to AEs in 13/159 (8.2%; 95% CI: 4.4–13.6%) subjects. Any AE were reported in 38/46 (82.6%) of the patients treated with BOC and 92/113 (81.4%) of those treated with TVR. Grade 3 or 4 anemia was reported in 9 (7%) patients, Grade 3 or 4 thrombocytopenia was observed in 22 (17.2%) patients and 21 (16.4%) individuals presented Grade 3 or 4 neutropenia. Erythropoietin was administered to 36 (22.6%) individuals and nine (5.7%) received blood transfusion. General dose reductions of Peg-IFN and RBV were reported in 16 (17.4%) and 40 (43.5%) patients of the 92 subjects, respectively [27C].

Triple therapy involving TVR, Peg-IFN and RBV were reported to improve antiviral efficacy but had potentially severe AEs in patients with chronic HCV [28c].

TVR treatment has caused elevated levels of serum creatinine and anemia in chronic HCV patients [29c]. Another study involving 112 patients infected with hepatitis C genotype 1 treated with Peg-IFN/RBV/TVR triple therapy developed significant renal impairment and anemia [30].

Bacterial infection as an AE of TVR-based triple therapy in HCV patients has been reported. Bacterial infections occurred in 21 of the 430 (4.9%) patients during TVR-based triple therapy. Among these subjects, 71.4% (15 of 21) experienced bacterial infections during the initial 8 weeks of treatment. Urinary tract infections were observed in 2.8% of cases (12 of 430) and were more prevalent in women (11 of 215, 5.1%) than in men (1 of 215) [31c].

A multicenter center study in patients with recurrent advanced HCV, who had undergone liver transplants showed serious AEs on TVR-based triple therapy [32c].

Skin Toxicity

Skin eruption has been reported as a side effect caused by TVR in a case study. A 53-year-old male patient with genotype 1 HCV cirrhosis, who was not previously treated for the disease, was treated with Peg-IFN-a in a single 180-μg subcutaneous injection, weekly with 1250 mg oral RBV per day and 750 mg oral TVR three times daily. After 4 weeks of treatment, a non-pruriginous erythematous macule was observed in the right inframammary region, which was treated with dexamethasone cream. On ninth week, the patient showed nausea, confluent pruriginous maculopapular eruption, lesions on more than 50% of the body surface, enanthem and ulcers on the oral mucosa, as well as purpuric lesions on the legs. TVR was removed from the treatment course with maintenance of Peg-IFN and RBV until the end of the 48 weeks. Orobase triamcinolone was applied to the lesions of the oral mucosa and clobetasol cream to the cutaneous lesions, which cured the eruption within 15 days of treatment. Twelve to 24 weeks of the treatment, the PCR-HCV remained negative and the patient did not present recurrence of the cutaneous lesions [33A].

A 50-year-old woman having HCV genotype 1b experienced TVR-related severe cutaneous eruptions 8 weeks after starting a triple antiviral therapy. Adverse cutaneous reactions were caused by a TVR-induced T-cell dependent immune mechanism in this patient [34c].

Efficacy and safety of TVR, Peg-IFNα-2b and RBV triple therapy in 106 Japanese patients infected with hepatitis C virus genotype 1b has been reported [35C].

Entecavir [SEDA-33, 578; SEDA-34, 452; SEDA-35, 512; SEDA-36, 411; SEDA-37, 335]

Observational Study

A prospective study was conducted in 34 antiviral treatment-naïve patients with chronic HBV who received ETV monotherapy and were followed up for 4 years, the mtDNA contents initially decreased and then increased, while the mtDNA4977 depletion rates first increased and then decreased. A long-term ETV monotherapy induced mitochondrial toxicity in patients with chronic HBV [36E].

A comparative study showed the effectiveness of TDF and ETV in treating chronic HBV. From 2008 to 2013, 189 consecutive treatment-naive chronic HBV patients receiving TDF ($n = 41$) or ETV ($n = 148$) for severe acute exacerbation participated in this study. Among the patients who survived by week 24, showed no difference between the two groups in the percentage of patients who had a serum creatinine increase of ≥ 0.5 mg/dL from baseline (6.7%) vs. 2.0% in the TDF and ETV groups, respectively. However, a significant reduction in the estimated glomerular filtration rate (eGFR) was found in both groups [37C].

A similar comparative study of the efficacy of TDF and ETV for initial treatment of 90 patients with chronic HBV in China has also been reported [38c].

A retrospective study reported the efficacy and safety of ETV in white patients with chronic HBV. The study was conducted at 23 Spanish centers in 237 chronic HBV patients treated with ETV (0.5 mg/day). The mean age of the cohort was 43 years (range: 19–82 years); 73% were male, 83% were white, and 33% were HBeAg positive. There were no treatment discontinuations due to AEs. Three patients were diagnosed with hepatocellular carcinoma at months 12, 30 and 54, and six experienced hepatic decompensation during follow-up [39C].

Ribavirin [SEDA-33, 578; SEDA-34, 452; SEDA-35, 512; SEDA-36, 412; SEDA-37, 335]

Neurological

A study was conducted to evaluate neuropsychiatric AEs of interferon-based treatment for HCV in standard multidisciplinary clinical practice. Patients with chronic HCV who completed treatment with Peg-IFN and RBV between 2005 and 2013 were included in the study. All patients underwent a multidisciplinary follow-up during treatment. During treatment, 1679 neuropsychiatric AEs in 618 patients (86.2%) generated 1737 clinical interventions. Fifty-seven (3.3%) neuropsychiatric AEs were severe and 2 (0.1%) life-threatening (suicidal attempts). Most neuropsychiatric AEs (1555 events, 92.6%) resolved without sequelae. Psychiatric medication was required in 289 patients (40.3%) [40C].

A prospective cohort study in 30 patients (median age 59 years and 57% of women) with HCV associated–mixed cryoglobulinemia vasculitis has been reported. All patients received antiviral therapy with Peg-IFNα-2a (180 μg/week, $n=20$) or 2b (1.5 μg/kg/week, $n=10$), subcutaneously plus RBV (600–1200 mg/day orally) for 48 weeks. Treatment with the protease inhibitor consisted of oral administration of TVR at a dose of 750 mg three times daily for 12 weeks or boceprevir at a dose of 800 mg three times daily for 44 weeks ($n=13$). The main side effects of antiviral therapy included fatigue (87%), neutropenia (78.3%), anemia (73.9%), thrombocytopenia (65.2%), infection (47.8%), pruritus (39.1%), depression (21.7%), and nausea (21.7%). A high incidence of serious AEs (14 patients) was observed during the 72 weeks of follow-up [41c].

Telbivudine [SEDA-33, 582; SEDA-34, 455; SEDA-35, 515; SEDA-36, 412; SEDA-37, 335]

One study examined 153 chronic hepatitis B patients infected with HBV variants resistant to 3TC. Patients were divided into two groups: the TDF monotherapy group included 33 patients and the combination therapy group (TDF plus 3TC or LdT) had 120 patients. No patient experienced any significant renal dysfunction during the treatment period. Authors conclude that TDF monotherapy has antiviral efficacy comparable to that of TDF plus 3TC or LdT combination therapy [42C].

Vertical Transmission

A prospective long-term study evaluated the efficacy of LdT in preventing vertical transmission of HBV from mothers to their infants. Four hundred and fifty hepatitis B e antigen-positive pregnant women with HBV DNA levels greater than 106 IU/mL were studied. Two hundred seventy-nine women received LdT (600 mg/day) during weeks 24–32 of gestation, and 171 women who were unwilling to take antiviral drugs participated as controls. Mother-to-child transmission of HBV was determined by detection of hepatitis B surface antigen and HBV DNA in the infant 6 months after birth. None of the infants whose mothers were given LdT tested positive for of hepatitis B surface antigen at 6 months, compared with 14.7% of infants in the control group ($p=5.317 \times 10^{-8}$). Levels of HBV DNA also decreased among women given LdT. No severe AEs or complications were observed in women or infants treated with LdT [43C].

Neurological

A randomized, open-label, international, multicenter study compared the combination of LdT plus Peg-IFN vs. monotherapy in 159 adults HBV patients. Patients were divided into three groups. All received LdT 600 mg once daily for 104 weeks. In addition, 50 patients received Peg-IFN 180 μg subcutaneously once per week for the first 52 weeks, 55 patients received LdT 600 mg once daily for 104 weeks, and 54 patients received Peg-IFN 180 μg subcutaneously once per week for 52 weeks. Despite the different drug exposure times, the percentage of patients who experienced AEs was higher in the Peg-IFN monotherapy group (90.7%) and in the combination-therapy group (88.0%) than in the LdT monotherapy group (70.4%). No patient died during the study and the rates of SAEs in the combination therapy were higher when compared to other groups. Peripheral neuropathy occurred in 8 patients and was judged as being a drug-related serious AE; of these, 7 cases occurred in the combination-therapy group and, at the last follow-up, 3 patients had improved and 4 completely recovered. One case of peripheral neuropathy occurred in the LdT monotherapy group and, at the last follow-up, the patient showed improvement. The most frequent AEs in the Peg-IFN monotherapy group were headache (17 [32%]), pyrexia (14 [26%]) and alopecia (15 [28%]), while discontinuation due to AEs occurred in 3 patients (feeling abnormal, neutropenia and impotence). In the LdT monotherapy group, the most frequent AEs were upper respiratory tract infections ($n=11$, 20%) and headache ($n=9$, 17%). On-treatment ALT flares were 6% (3/47) in the LdT plus Peg-IFN combination group and 4% (2/53) in each monotherapy group [44C].

Faldaprevir

The safety of faldaprevir, deleobuvir, and ribavirin in patients with chronic HCV infection was reported in a recent study. The most frequent AEs with faldaprevir, deleobuvir, and RBV in patients with or without cirrhosis were mild or moderate gastrointestinal and skin AEs [45c].

Sofosbuvir [SEDA-37, 335]

Sofosbuvir (SOF)-based regimens appear to be well tolerated with headache and fatigue being the most common side effects [46R].

A recent analysis showed that the combination of SOF and simprevir was more effective than RBV. A prospective open-label study looked at 82 patients with chronic HCV genotype 1 A infection and Child's Grade A cirrhosis. Patients were enrolled from 2 clinics in Atlanta, Georgia, from December 2013 through January 2014. Subjects were assigned randomly to groups given simeprevir (150 mg/day) and SOF (400 mg/day) ($n=58$ in the final analysis) or Peg-IFN-a-2b (1.5 mcg/kg/week), ribavirin (1000–1200 mg/day), and SOF (400 mg/day) ($n=24$ in the final analysis) [47C].

An open-label, non-randomized study reported on direct-acting antiviral regimens in non-cirrhotic patients with HCV was conducted at National Institutes of Health (NIH) Clinical Center in Bethesda, Maryland. Treatment-naive and predominantly African American patients with HCV genotype 1 infection and early-stage liver fibrosis were enrolled from January 2014 to May 2015. Forty-nine of 50 patients completed 4 weeks of treatment with study medications, and primary endpoint results were obtained for them. Twenty-five patients received a 3-drug regimen consisting of ledipasvir and SOF plus GS-9451 for 4 weeks, and 25 received a 4-drug regimen consisting of ledipasvir, SOF, GS-9451, and GS-9669 for 4 weeks. Forty-eight percent (12 of 25) of patients receiving the 3-drug regimen and 72% (18 of 25) of those receiving the 4-drug regimen had mild AEs reported. The most common AEs were fatigue, diarrhea, and headache. Two serious AEs occurred: vertigo for 3 days in a patient with a heart rate of 57 beats/min who was not receiving antiarrhythmic agents, and angioedema. Both events occurred in patients receiving the 4-drug regimen but were deemed to be unrelated to the study drugs [48C].

A randomized, phase 2, open-label study was conducted at 48 U.S. sites with 377 treatment-naive non-cirrhotic patients. The patients having HCV genotypes 1–6 were randomly assigned to SOF, 400 mg, with velpatasvir, 25 or 100 mg, for 12 weeks. Another group of patients with genotype 1 or 2 HCV infection was randomly assigned to SOF, 400 mg, and velpatasvir, 25 or 100 mg, with or without ribavirin for 8 weeks. The AEs were reported in 262 (69%) patients. AEs experienced by more than 10% of patients were fatigue (21%), headache (20%), and nausea (12%). One patient committed suicide. Incidence of fatigue, insomnia, and rash were higher in patients treated with ribavirin-containing regimens. One patient, a 19-year-old white woman with genotype 1 HCV infection who was receiving 8 weeks of SOF plus velpatasvir, 25 mg (group 1), developed mild

abdominal pain, mild palpitations, and moderate dizziness on treatment day 6 [49C].

A prospective cohort study reported on fibrosing cholestatic hepatitis (FCH) patients in France and Belgium from October 2013 through April 2014. Twenty-three FCH patients were included in the study on the effects of antiviral agents with recurrence of HCV infection after liver transplantation. Most of the patients had genotype 1 infections that had not responded to previous treatment; 4 patients were co-infected with HIV. Treatment regimens were divided into 2 groups: SOF+RBV+Peg-IFNα (SOF+RBV group; $n=8$) SOF+daclatasvir+RBV (SOF+daclatasvir group; $n=15$). Dosages were 400 mg/day for SOF and 60 mg/day for daclatasvir, whereas the RBV was given at different concentrations, 400 mg ($n=5$), 600 mg ($n=2$), 800 mg ($n=8$), and 1000 mg ($n=6$). The planned duration of treatment was 24 weeks for all regimens. All patients survived, without re-transplantation, until week 36. There was no Grade 3 or 4 AEs related to SOF or daclatasvir and no significant interactions among drugs. Fifteen patients (65%) experienced at least 1 serious AEs, which were considered unrelated to drugs. Infection was the most common AE, including urinary tract infection ($n=4$), spontaneous bacterial peritonitis ($n=3$), undetermined sepsis ($n=3$), fungal infection ($n=1$), and cytomegalovirus reactivation ($n=1$). Most infections (93%) were observed within the first 8 weeks of treatment, before achievement of complete clinical response. Other clinical AEs included ascites, severe denutrition, and hepatic encephalopathy, all directly related to FCH. Anemia was observed in almost two thirds of patients and led to a RBV dose reduction (up to 200 mg/day) in 61% and discontinuation in 22% of cases. Mild to moderate renal failure was observed in 43% of cases, but creatinine values remained stable over time during treatment and follow-up periods. Severe renal failure (eGFR, <30 mL/min) was observed in 1 patient during a septic episode, but values returned to normal after infection resolution. One patient on SOF+daclatasvir displayed worsening of cholestasis with bilirubin level greater than 100 µmol/L at week 12. Cholestasis persisted after discontinuing daclatasvir at week 16, and improved the condition after SOF stopped at week 24 [50c].

An open-label study was conducted in 151 patients who were naïve to HCV treatment and 52 patients who were previously treated; all of them were co-infected with HIV-1. Previously untreated patients were randomly assigned in a 2:1 ratio to receive either 12 or 8 weeks of daclatasvir at a standard dose of 60 mg plus 400 mg of SOF daily. Previously treated patients underwent 12 weeks of therapy at the same doses. Patients had HCV genotypes 1 through 4 (83% with genotype 1), and 14% had compensated cirrhosis; 98% were receiving antiretroviral therapy. Among patients with genotype 1, a sustained virologic response was reported in 96.4% who were treated for 12 weeks and in 75.6% who were treated for 8 weeks among previously untreated patients. The most common AEs were fatigue, nausea, and headache. There were no study drug discontinuations because of AEs [51C].

A double-blind trial from October 2013 to October 2014 was conducted in 155 HCV genotype 1 patients having compensated cirrhosis who had not achieved sustained virological response (SVR) after successive treatments with Peg-IFN and protease-inhibitor regimens. The patients were assigned in a 1:1 ratio to receive placebo matched in appearance to study drugs for 12 weeks followed by once daily combination fixed-dose tablets of 90 mg ledipasvir and 400 mg SOF plus weight-based RBV for 12 weeks, or ledipasvir-SOF plus placebo once daily for 24 weeks. One patient discontinued treatment because of AEs while receiving only placebo drug. The most common event in the two groups was asthenia, followed by pruritus and headache in the ledipasvir-SOF plus RBV group and headache and fatigue in the ledipasvir-SOF group [52C].

A phase 2, open-label study reported the efficacy and safety of ledipasvir and SOF, with or without RBV, in patients infected with HCV genotype 3 or 6. The study was conducted in 126 patients with HCV infections at 2 centers in New Zealand from April 2013 through October 2014. Previously untreated patients with HCV genotype 3 were given fixed-dose combination tablet of ledipasvir and SOF ($n=25$) or ledipasvir and SOF along with RBV ($n=26$). Treatment-experienced patients with HCV genotype 3 ($n=50$) received ledipasvir and SOF and RBV. The most common AEs were headache, upper respiratory infection, and fatigue and nausea. Six patients experienced serious AEs. Two of the events, upper abdominal pain and abdominal pain, were treatment related. Only 1 patient, with HCV genotype 3 receiving ledipasvir and SOF alone, discontinued treatment because of an AE. A 49-year-old patient discontinued RBV after acute agitation. Seven patients taking RBV experienced anemia. Six patients had their dose of RBV reduced and one patient discontinued RBV [53C].

SOF plus RBV for the treatment of chronic genotype 4 HCV infection in 60 patients of Egyptian ancestry has been reported. The most common AEs were headache, insomnia, and fatigue. No patients had AEs leading to dose modification, interruption, or discontinuation of SOF [54c].

The challenges for direct-acting antiviral therapy have been reviewed [55R]. The safety of direct-acting antiviral agents in HCV patients co-infected with hepatitis B virus (HBV) or HIV has been evaluated in a recent review [56R].

Simeprevir

A review published the use of simeprevir in HCV treatment and evaluated the efficacy. Grade 3–4 AE, serious AE and treatment withdrawal rates with simeprevir plus Peg-IFN-α/RBV were similar to those with placebo plus Peg-IFN-α/RBV. Skin rashes with simeprevir were mostly mild or moderate; serious photosensitivity reactions rarely reported. Simeprevir is efficacious and generally well tolerated in patients with chronic HCV genotypes 1 and 4 infection [57R].

DRUGS ACTIVE AGAINST HUMAN IMMUNODEFICIENCY VIRUS: COMBINATIONS

Abacavir/Lamivudine

Observational Study

Between 1998 and 2011, 1309 HIV-infected patients from different countries in Europe who had a chronic HCV infection were treated with a combination of Peg-IFN and RBV. Patients using an ABC-containing regimen showed no difference in response to HCV treatment compared to those using an FTC + TDF-containing backbone [58C].

Abacavir/Lamivudine/DTG

A randomized, double-blind, non-inferiority study in 833 ART-naive HIV-1 patients evaluated the safety and efficacy of 50 mg DTG + ABC/3TC vs. efavirenz (EFV)/ TDF/FTC. Of the 833 participants, 342 in the DTG + ABC/3TC arm and 310 in the efavirenz/TDF/FTC arm were treated for 96 weeks. Nine drug-related serious AEs occurred in the efavirenz/TDF/FTC arm compared with 2 (<1%) in the DTG + ABC/3TC arm through week 144. During the double-blind phase, ABC hypersensitivity was reported in 5 participants (1%) in the EFV/TDF/ FTC arm and in 2 participants (0.5%) in the DTG + ABC/ 3TC arm. Two fatalities were previously reported in the week 48 analysis; no additional fatalities occurred through week 144. Two new drug-related SAEs occurred, 1 in the EFV/TDF/FTC arm (renal failure between week 48 and week 96) and 1 in the DTG + ABC/3TC arm (osteonecrosis between week 96 and week 144). A greater increase in high-density lipoprotein cholesterol for the EFV/TDF/FTC arm compared with the DTG + ABV/ 3TC arm was seen through week 144. Five participants presented with Grade 2 elevations in creatinine levels in the DTG + ABC/3TC arm. Six participants had Grade 3/4 alanine aminotransferase (ALT) elevations in the DTG + ABC/3TC arm [59r].

Elvitegravir

Observational Studies

A 96-week, phase 3, open-label, multicenter cohort study evaluated the safety and efficacy of Cobistat-containing regimens in HIV-1-infected adult patients who are either treatment-naive (STB cohort) or treatment-experienced (COBI cohort: switch ritonavir to COBI) with stable, mild-to-moderate renal impairment. Thirty-three patients were enrolled and received at least one dose of STB elvitegravir/COBI/FTC/TDF (STB, $n=33$). Serious AEs were reported for 12% of patients ($n=4$), increased blood creatine phosphokinase ($n=1$), infected cyst ($n=1$), right ventricular failure and lymphoma (both in the same patient; $n=1$), and hepatitis C and Hodgkin's disease (both in the same patient; $n=1$). None of the AEs was considered related to study drug except for the serious AE of increased blood creatinine phosphokinase. The most frequent AEs were diarrhea (30%), insomnia (21%), and nausea and headache (each 18%). AEs considered related to study drug by the investigator were reported for 45% of patients (15/33 patients). The most frequently reported AEs considered related to study drug by the investigator were nausea (3 patients) and blurred vision, upper abdominal pain, vomiting, decreased eGFR, hyperglycemia, headache, and insomnia (each reported for 2 patients). Four patients (12%) discontinued study drug due to an AE. One patient discontinued due to HCV and Hodgkin's disease. The other 3 patients discontinued due to renal AEs, 2 of whom met the protocol-defined criterion for potential discontinuation. All 3 patients had baseline CrCl between 50 and 55 mL/min and developed CrCl <50 mL/min without evidence of PRT. Only 1 patient had cystatin C-based eGFR <50 mL/min·1.73 m^{-2} at the time of discontinuation, which was preexisting at baseline. CrCl returned to baseline after STB discontinuation in 2 patients. One patient had confirmed increase in serum creatinine >0.4 mg/dL and the study drug discontinued [60c].

Cobicistat

Observational Studies

The pharmacokinetics, pharmacodynamics, and safety of both pharmacoenhancers and the clinical utility of COBI in future HIV therapy is reviewed [61R].

Elvitegravir/Cobicistat/FTC/Tenofovir

A cross-sectional study was carried out between April and July 2014 at the Buea, Limbe and Kumba government Hospitals in South-Western Region of Cameroon on the efficacy of combination ARV therapy. Two hundred participants on HAART, DOTS were enrolled into the study. The ages ranged from 21–65 years with the mean age being 38.04 ($\pm$10.52) years. The 200 participants were divided into three treatment groups. Sixty (30%) participants were on HAART and DOTS combined treatment, 70 (35%) were on HAART and 70 (35%) were on DOTS.

Out of 130 participants on HAART and HAART/DOTS, 80 (61.54%) were treated with the combination of AZT, 3TC, and NVP; 6 patients were on AZT, 3TC, and EFV while 44 patients were on TDF, 3TC, and EFV. Regarding the 130 participants on DOTS and HAART/DOTS, 63 (48.5%) were on the drug regimen rifamycin, isoniazid, ethambutol, pyrazinamide (intensive phase) and 67 (51.5%) were on rifamycin, isoniazid (continuation phase). The mean eGFR was significantly higher in patients on HAART than in the patients on HAART/DOTS with respect to AZT, 3TC, NVP combination [126.0 ($\pm$83.44) and 95.38 ($\pm$26.51), $p=0.039$]. In addition, the mean serum albumin was significantly higher in patients on HAART alone than those on HAART/DOTS with respect to AZT, 3TC, NVP combination [49.26 ($\pm$5.76) and 38.07 ($\pm$8.95), $p=0.001$]. No significant difference was found in mean serum creatinine between patients on HAART and those on HAART/DOTS with respect to TDF, 3TC, EFV combination. However, patients on HAART had abnormal higher value of mean serum creatinine compared to those on HAART/DOTS [2.06 ($\pm$4.16) and 0.97 ($\pm$0.28), $p=0.217$]. Authors concluded that the use of the HAART regimen (TNF, 3TC and EFV combination) among the HAART-treated adults was nephrotoxic. The other combined HAART and DOTS regimens had no nephrotoxic effect. Abnormal kidney function could be associated with HAART use [62C].

DRUGS ACTIVE AGAINST HUMAN IMMUNODEFICIENCY VIRUS: NUCLEOSIDE ANALOGUE REVERSE TRANSCRIPTASE INHIBITORS (NRTI) [SEDA-15, 2586; SEDA-32, 534; SEDA-33, 585; SEDA-34, 456; SEDA-35, 516; SEDA-36, 415; SEDA-37, 337]

Abacavir [SEDA-15, 3; SEDA-32, 534; SEDA-33, 585; SEDA-34, 456; SEDA-35, 516; SEDA-36, 415; SEDA-37, 337]

Observational Studies

A descriptive study of HIV-infected patients in Bangkok, Thailand was conducted in 103 patients with a median age of 46 (range 20–85) years during January 2011 to November 2014. Most of the participants (97%) were on ARV, and more than half of the patients had undetectable HIV RNA at the end of the study. The most common ARV regimen was TDF, 3TC, and EFV (25%). Two out of four patients who had positive HLA-B*5701 developed hypersensitivity after receiving ABC. One out of five patients who undergone HLA-B*4001 genotyping developed lipodystrophy after receiving d4T. One out of two patients who had positive HLA-B*3505 developed skin rash after receiving NVP. There were

45 ADRs reported that includes skin rashes, of which 18 were from TDF, 17 from EFV, four from AZT, two from ABC, and one each from NVP, raltegravir, ritonavir, and DDI. The most common ADRs of other types from each drug were AKI from TDF, dizziness from EFV, anemia from AZT, hypersensitivity reaction from ABC, and drug rash from NVP. ADRs, such as dizziness, insomnia, or depression from EFV or skin rash from ABC, EFV, or NVP, were improved in 96.4% of patients [63c].

SINGLE is an ongoing, phase 3, multicenter, randomized, double-blind, non-inferiority study involving treatment-naive HIV-infected participants. The safety profile of DTG + ABC/3TC through week 96 and week 144 was similar to week 48 and was generally favorable compared with the efavirenz/T DF/FTC arm throughout. The most common drug-related AEs in the EFV/TDF/FTC arm, which differed by more than 2% from the DTG + ABC/3TC arm, were dizziness [140 (33%) vs. 29 (7%)], abnormal dreams [67 (16%) vs. 27 (7%)], and rash [34 (8%) vs. 4 (<1%)]. The drug-related AE of insomnia was more commonly reported in the DTG + ABC/3TC arm (n = 41, 10%) than in the EFV/TDF/FTC arm (n = 28, 7%). The overall incidence of serious AEs was low and comparable across the DTG + ABC/3TC and efavirenz/TDF/FTC arms through week 96 [44 (11%) vs. 51 (12%), respectively] and week 144 [65 (16%) vs. 60 (14%), respectively]. Nine drug-related serious AEs occurred in the EFV/TDF/FTC arm compared with two in the DTG + ABC/3TC arm through week 144. During the double-blind phase, ABC hypersensitivity was reported in five participants in the EFV/TDF/FTC arm and in two (0.5%) participants in the DTG + ABC/3TC arm. Two fatalities were previously reported in the week 48 analysis 1; no additional fatalities occurred through week 144. Two new drug-related SAEs occurred, 1 in the EFV/TDF/FTC arm (renal failure between week 48 and week 96) and 1 in the DTG + ABC/3TC arm (osteonecrosis between week 96 and week 144). No clinically significant differences in laboratory parameters between the arms emerged from week 48. A greater increase in high-density lipoprotein cholesterol for the EFV/TDF/FTC arm compared with the DTG + ABC/3TC arm was seen through week 144; overall, both groups showed a small increase in the ratio of total cholesterol to high-density lipoprotein cholesterol. A comparable and modest rise in mean total triglycerides was seen through week 96 in both groups; however, the increase in triglycerides in the EFV/TDF/FTC arm was greater than in the DTG + ABC/3TC arm at week 144. Mean serum creatinine level in patients receiving DTG + ABC/3TC remained stable through week 144. Five participants presented with Grade 2 elevations in creatinine levels in the DTG + ABC/3TC arm on a single occasion through week 144. Overall, there was a low rate of elevated liver enzymes in both treatment groups across the study period. Six

participants had Grade 3/4 ALT elevations in the DTG + ABC/3TC arm. Three were due to acute HCV infections, and 3 due to concurrent use of hepatotoxic drugs (anabolic steroids, naltrexone, and duloxetine). Three Grade 3/4 ALT elevations were observed in the EFV/TDF/FTC arm; two of these were due to acute HCV infections and one due to the use of anabolic steroids. Two participants (one in each study arm) with acute HCV infections were withdrawn from the study [64c].

An overview compared the efficacy and safety of the combined DTG/ABC/3TC co-formulation to single tablet regimen (STR). The DTG/ABC/3TC regimen is highly effective in achieving sustained suppression of HIV-1 RNA in plasma. The STR has a favorable safety profile and a low potential for drug interactions, which will contribute to a prominent role in therapy with ABC as backbone component [65R].

Lamivudine [SED-15, 1989; SEDA-32, 531; SEDA-33, 587; SEDA-34, 456; SEDA-35, 517; SEDA-36, 416; SEDA-37, 338]

Observational Studies

A 48-week randomized, parallel, open-label, multicenter, non-inferiority trial to compare the efficacy and safety of three PI-based second-line antiretroviral combinations in three African countries has been reported. The patients (454) were randomized to three groups to receive LPV/r (co-formulated LPV 200 mg/ritonavir 50 mg two tablets twice daily) with TDF 300 mg/FTC 200 mg (one tablet daily with food) (control group); ABC (600 mg tablet) with ddI (enteric-coated capsule of 250 or 400 mg based on body weight) once daily fasting, and LPV/r twice daily (ABC/ddI group); or DRV 800 mg (two 400 mg tablets) boosted with ritonavir (100 mg tablet) and TDF/FTC, all taken with food once daily (DRV group). Participants in the ABC/ddI group with chronic HBV continued on 3TC 150 mg/day. Gastrointestinal complaints were common and significantly different between the DRV/r and the LPV/r groups [26 (17%) vs. 48 and 50 (33%)]. Twenty-four (5%) participants reported symptoms of neuropathy, mainly from baseline: 11 were in ABC/ddI group. No statistically significant differences were recorded across groups for liver and kidney toxicity: only one patient had increased alanine aminotransferase (>5 × upper limit of normal). Sixty-one (14%) participants experienced a 25% decrease in estimated eGFR between baseline and week 48, with a higher frequency in those taking TDF. Grade 3 or 4 AEs occurred in 58 (13%) patients, with no difference between groups. Only five patients stopped assigned treatment because of AEs: one for suspected ABC reaction, one in DRV group for severe kidney failure that was not related to the study drug, two for progressive neuropathy in ddI in patients with pre-existent d4T-related neuropathic pain, and one patient requesting to reduce the pill burden (ABC/ddI group on TB treatment). The authors suggests that patients with high viral load at first-line failure may need special management to avoid early second-line failure [66C].

Stavudine [SED-15, 3180; SEDA-32, 535; SEDA-33, 587; SEDA-34, 456; SEDA-35, 517; SEDA-36, 417; SEDA-37, 338]

See also Section Zidovudine.

Observational Studies

The long-term side effects of d4T led to recommendations in 2009 to phase out the use of this drug. A prospective observational cohort study was conducted with 18 786 HIV-1-infected patients from 107 clinics in 37 countries. Overall, 963 of 13 246 (7.3%) EuroSIDA patients under follow-up during the study period received a d4T-based cART regimen. There were 392 patients taking d4T in 1 January 2006, of whom 381 (97.2%) discontinued before 1 January 2013. The majority of patients, 288 (75.6%), discontinued d4T together with at least one other ARV drug. The most frequent reason for discontinuation was indicated as physician's choice (26.5%), followed by unknown reasons (17.6%), abnormal fat distribution (15.8%), treatment failure (virological, immunological and/or clinical) (15.0%), other reasons (9.2%), patient's wish (6.0%) and toxicity (5.5%). Among those who discontinued d4T alone ($n = 93$; 24.4%), d4T-related toxicities such as abnormal fat distribution, dyslipidaemia and nervous system toxicity were frequently indicated (24.7%, 4.3% and 3.2%, respectively) However, the proportions of d4T discontinuations were very high because of physician's decision, unknown and treatment failure (23.7%, 19.4% and 7.5% respectively). In authors opinion, all HIV clinicians should be aware of the potential harmful effects associated with d4T treatment and avoid the drug as much as possible [67M].

Zidovudine [SED-15, 3713; SEDA-32, 536; SEDA-33, 588; SEDA-34, 458; SEDA-35, 517; SEDA-36, 417, SEDA-37, 338]

Eight hundred and fifty-two patients received three different backbones of nucleoside reverse transcriptase inhibitor in a non-randomized manner. Of these 161 patients were on AZT, 628 on d4T, and 63 on TDF; all received lamvudine. Grade 4 anemia was higher for those receiving ZDV than the d4T group. The patients taking d4T had a higher increase in hemoglobin than those were on ZDV [68C].

A prospective cohort study was conducted in 211 adult patients (≥18 years of age) with HIV/AIDS who commenced ART. All ADRs in the first 12 months of therapy were recorded, and the severity, causality, and preventability were assessed. Of these, 181 (85.7%) experienced at least one ADR and 66 (31.3%) experienced at least one severe ADR within 12 months of commencing ART. The patients taking AZT-containing regimens experienced severe ADRs [69C].

DRUGS ACTIVE AGAINST HUMAN IMMUNODEFICIENCY VIRUS: NUCLEOTIDE ANALOGUE REVERSE TRANSCRIPTASE INHIBITORS

Tenofovir [SED-15, 3314; SEDA-32, 537; SEDA-33, 588; SEDA-34, 458; SEDA-35, 518; SEDA-36, 418; SEDA-37, 338]

The safety and efficacy of TDF in HIV-1-infected children has been evaluated in a randomized-controlled trial. Ninety-seven children were in the age group of 2 to <16 years were on a d4T (d4T) or AZT-containing regimen. They had HIV-1 RNA <400 copies/mL and were randomized to either switch d4T or ZDV to TDF or continue d4T or ZDV. No subjects discontinued the study drug because of an AE in the 48 weeks of treatment. Only four subjects discontinued TDF because of proximal renal tubulopathy in the extension phase [70c].

Renal Toxicity

A retrospective, longitudinal observational study was conducted in 451 adult HIV-1-infected patients treated with TDF to assess the incidence of renal damage and to identify the associated potential risk factors. Patients treated with TDF from January 2010 to December 2012 were included in the study. Patient follow-up started when initiating treatment with TDF until the end of the study period (July 31, 2013). Renal toxicity was classified as moderate eGFR < 60 mL/min or severe eGFR < 30 mL/min. The incidence rate for moderate and severe renal insufficiency was calculated as number of cases per 1000 patient-year. The incidence rate of moderate severe renal insufficiency (RI) was 29.2 cases per 1000 person-year (95%), whereas the incidence of severe RI was 2.2 cases per 1000 person-year (95%). Multivariate analysis confirmed an independent association with the risk of kidney damage for age (OR 1.08 95%), time on treatment with TDF (OR 1.16 95%), baseline creatinine (OR 49.80 95%) and treatment with NNRTIs (OR 0.45 95%). Mild to moderate renal failure is a frequent complication during treatment with TDF although severe renal impairment is rare. Risk factors included age, duration of treatment with TDF, elevated baseline creatinine levels, and treatment with protease inhibitor boosted with ritonavir combinations [71C].

Renal overload of TDF in patients with a pre-existing kidney impairment resulting in worsening renal function has been reviewed [72R].

DRUGS ACTIVE AGAINST HUMAN IMMUNODEFICIENCY VIRUS: NON-NUCLEOSIDE REVERSE TRANSCRIPTASE INHIBITORS (NNRTI) [SEDA-15, 2553; SEDA-31, 486; SEDA-32, 537; SEDA-33, 590; SED-34, 459; SEDA-35, 519; SEDA-36, 420; SEDA-37, 339]

Efavirenz [SEDA-15, 1204; SEDA-32, 537; SEDA-33, 590; SEDA-34, 459; SEDA-35, 519; SEDA-36, 420; SEDA-37, 339]

A systematic review and meta-analysis of randomized-controlled trials on EFV-based regimens in antiretroviral-naive HIV-infected patients was conducted [73R]. The authors are of the opinion that there is good efficacy and beneficial safety profile of drugs from new classes of antiretroviral agents (integrase inhibitors, CCR5 antagonists) compared with other initial regimens used in clinical practice for the treatment of HIV-infected patients.

Observational Studies

A retrospective cohort study was reported using clinical data from HIV-1 infected adults (aged ≥15 years), who received EFV as part of their initial antiretroviral therapy between January 2004 and December 2011. HIV-positive patients (2920) were on non-nucleoside reverse-transcriptase inhibitors, NVP or EFV plus two nucleoside reverse-transcriptase inhibitors (NRTIs), often d4T, DDI, AZT, TDF, or ABC plus 3TC. Three hundred fifty-eight ADRs were reported during 8834 person-years of follow-up, with an incidence rate (IR) of 40.5 ADRs per 1000 person-years on EFV-based regimens. ADRs were reported in 195 patients (55%) within 12 months of treatment initiation, 50 patients (14%) within 13–24 months, 36 (10.1%) within 25–36 months, and 77 (21.5%) more than 36 months after commencement of treatment. The majority (55%) of the ADRs were Grade 3 in terms of severity while Grade 2 and Grade 1 ADRs accounted for 31.3% and 12.3%, respectively. The proportion of life-threatening (Grade 4) ADRs was 1.4%. The incidence of ADRs varied across the NRTIs, and was 151 per 1000 person-year (31 events) for d4T-containing regimens, 51.7 (6 events) for ABC, 40.2 (176 events) for TDF, 34.7 (128 events) for AZT and 33.8 (15 events) for DDI. Of

those that experienced an ADR, 48.9% (n=175) had EFV substituted with NVP. The most common ADR was lipodystrophy, with an incidence of 63.1 per 1000 person-year (184 events) followed by neuropsychiatric symptoms with an incidence of 29.9 per 1000 person (88 events). More than one-third (33 out of 88) of the neuropsychiatric AEs occurred within 12 months of starting ART, while 12 (13.6%), 13 (14.8%) and 30 (34.1%) were within 13–24, 25 to 36 and more than 36 months of treatment. Lipo-accumulation was the most common lipodystrophy syndrome reported, while nightmares were the most frequently reported neuropsychiatric symptom (incidence of 6.8 per 1000). Twenty-four incidents of gynecomastia were recorded, mainly in patients who received regimens containing d4T (incidence 107 per 1000 person-year), while seizures were rare, with only two incidents reported among patients on AZT-based NRTI. Neuropsychiatric ADRs associated with EFV-based ART had both early and late onset patients on chronic EFV therapy [74C].

Twelve patients with R5-tropic virus and suppressed viral load on two NRTIs plus EFV switched to MVC 600 mg twice daily for 14 days, and then to MVC 300 mg twice daily. MVC was well-tolerated with no Grade 3/4 adverse events; all subjects maintained viral suppression to the end of the study. One subject experienced a transient Grade 1 aspartate transaminase (AST) elevation during the 600 mg twice daily in MVC treatment. The authors suggests that when switching from EFV to MVC, increasing the dose of MVC from 300 mg twice daily to 600 mg twice daily for 1 week would be sufficient to compensate for the prolonged induction effect of EFV [75c].

A study compared semen characteristics across 378 HIV-1-infected patients receiving different antiretroviral regimens or never treated by antiretroviral drugs. This study was done between 2001 and 2007. Sperm motility was the only semen parameter that significantly varied. The median percentage of rapid spermatozoa was 5% in the group of patients receiving a regimen including EFV vs. 20% in the other groups and the sperm velocity was reduced by about 30% in this group [76C].

A review describes the epidemiology, severity and management of neuropsychiatric side effects of EFV [77R].

Etravirine [SEDA-33, 592; SEDA-34, 459; SEDA-35, 520; SEDA-36, 421; SEDA-37, 339]

Observational Studies

The successful use of a TMC125-based regimen in a patient treated with chemotherapy for advanced Hodgkin's lymphoma has been reported. TMC125 constitutes a valuable option for concomitant use with chemotherapy due to its moderate inducing effect on drug-metabolizing enzymes [78c].

Data from cohorts of the EuroSIDA and EUResist Network in France, Italy, Spain, Switzerland and UK collected in 2007 to 2012 from HIV-1-infected patients undergone antiretroviral treatment showed the efficacy of TMC125 plus darunavir/ritonavir (DRV group; n=999) vs. TMC125 plus an alternative boosted protease inhibitor (other PI group; n=116) were evaluated. The drug responses measured for 24 weeks and the DRV group and PI group showed no significant difference in antiretroviral treatment efficiency. These data do not indicate a difference in response between the DRV and other PI groups [79C].

A prospective study evaluated 25 virologically suppressed patients, largely pretreated (15.6 years on therapy) with antiretroviral drug toxicity (n=19) or interactions (n=9, mainly with chemotherapy against non-Hodgkin lymphoma or anti-HCV therapy), who switched to a dual therapy with TMC125 plus RAL. Patients were not required have prior virological failure or resistance to both drugs. After a median follow-up of 722 days (473–1088: 53.3 patients-year), there were no cases of transient virological replication or failure. Only 1 patient left therapy at day 10 due to a Grade 2 rash. There were no cases of Grade 3-4 liver toxicity and total cholesterol and triglycerides levels decrease significantly after initiation [80c].

Nevirapine [SEDA-33, 593; SEDA-34, 460; SEDA-35, 521; SEDA-36, 421; SEDA-37, 339]

Observational Study

A prospective, observational study was conducted in the outpatient department of skin and venereal disease reported with cutaneous adverse drug reactions (CADRs). Ninety patients were enrolled in the study. Male to female ratio for CADRs was 1:2. The most commonly encountered CADR was maculopapular rash in 76.67% cases followed by urticaria (8.89%), Stevens-Johnson syndrome (4.4%) and fixed dose eruptions (3.33%). NVP was suspected in 52 out of 90 (57.77%) cases of CADRs which included 39 cases of maculopapular rash, five cases of urticaria, four cases of Stevens-Johnson syndrome, and two cases each of pustular rash and angioedema, respectively [81c].

Tuberculosis and HIV co-infected patients having the NVP concentrations <3000 ng/mL were found to be a risk factor for virological failure [82C].

A retrospective study showed the incidence of NVP toxicity in children who were switched from EFV to NVP compared with that of children who had started NVP-based antiretroviral therapy directly. Children in the switched group who developed NVP toxicity had higher mean CD4 cell counts than children in treatment naïve group with NVP [83c].

Rilpivirine [SEDA-35, 521; SEDA-36, 423; SEDA-37, 340]

A phase 3, 96-week, randomized, open-label, international, non-inferiority study was conducted in 799 patients who received RPV/FTC/TDF or EFV/FTC/TDF. At week 96, trial completion RPV/FTC/TDF was non-inferior to EFV/FTC/TDF [HIV-1 RNA <50 copies/mL: 77.9% vs. 72.4%, respectively]. Compared with EFV/FTC/TDF, RPV/FTC/TDF group had fewer AE-related discontinuations (3.0% vs. 11.0%), significantly fewer AEs. Overall, the 96-week RPV/FTC/TDF treatment demonstrated non-inferior in efficacy and tolerability than EFV/FTC/TDF [84C].

An open-label, single-arm study at two public sexual health clinics and two hospital emergency departments in urban Australia reported the safety of co-formulated FTC, RPV, and TDF as a 3-drug, single-tablet regimen for post-exposure prophylaxis (PEP) in men who have sex with men (MSM). Single-tablet FTC-RPV-TDF once daily for 28 days were given to 100 HIV-uninfected PEP in MSM. PEP completion was 92%; premature cessation resulted from loss to follow-up (6%), AEs (1%), or study burden (1%). No participant was found to acquire HIV through week 12. Eighty-eight participants experienced at least one clinical AE; 4 patients had Grade 3 AEs or higher, possibly attributable to study drug. Fifty-six participants experienced at least one laboratory AE; 4 had AEs of Grade 3 or higher, due to the single tablet [85c].

DRUGS ACTIVE AGAINST HUMAN IMMUNODEFICIENCY VIRUS: PROTEASE INHIBITORS [SED-15, 2586; SEDA-32, 541; SEDA-33, 593; SEDA-34, 461, SEDA-35, 522; SEDA-36, 423; SEDA-37, 340]

Atazanavir

Observational Study

Ritonavir-boosted atazanavir (ATV/r) is a relatively well-tolerated antiretroviral drug. A retrospective analysis of routine TDM of ATV carried out as day-by-day clinical practice for the optimization of drug dosing in HIV-infected 240 adult patients between January 2010 and May 2013 participated in the study. HIV-infected patients treated with ATV for at least 3 months and with one assessment of ATV plasma were included in the study. Patients were at 901±870 days of therapy with ATV, mainly treated at the conventional ATV/r dosage 300/100 mg q.d. (68%), given concomitantly with tenofovir-based antiretroviral regimens. One hundred forty-seven (61%) out of the 240 HIV-positive patients enrolled in the present study experienced hyperbilirubinemia of Grade ≥1. Overall,

55 out of the 240 HIV-positive patients developed dyslipidemia, namely hypercholesterolemia ($n=26$) or hypertriglyceridemia ($n=45$). Patients with dyslipidemia had ATV concentrations significantly higher as compared with patients with no ATV-related complications [86C].

An international phase 3 double-blind and double-dummy study was conducted in 692 HIV-1-infected adults. Patients had estimated eGFR of at least 70 mL/min and genotypic sensitivity to ATV, FTC, and TDF. Eligible patients were randomized 1:1 to receive either COBI ($n=344$) or RTV ($n=348$) and matching placebo, each administered once daily with ATV plus FTC/TDF. After week 48, study visits occurred every 12 weeks until week 144. At week 144, a small increase in serum creatinine (median change from baseline +0.13 vs. +0.07 mg/dL) and a corresponding decrease in eGFR (median change −15.1 vs. −7.5 mL/min) were observed in both groups. Seven patients (2.0%) in each group developed proximal renal tubulopathy (PRT). In 5 of the 7 patients in the COBI group and 6 of the 7 patients in the RTV group, PRT occurred after week 48. In the COBI-containing regimen, reversibility of renal laboratory abnormalities was seen in 6 of the 7 patients after discontinuation of the study drug [87C].

An open-label, single-center, single-dose, crossover study, randomized study reported in 64 healthy subjects to one of eight treatment sequences, in a single center in the United States between 25 April 2013 and 20 June 2013. Subjects were randomized equally to one of eight treatment sequences in which treatments were administered over four or five study periods. Subjects received a 300 mg ATV capsule co-administered with a 150 mg COBI tablet or an FDC tablet of ATV/COBI (300/150 mg) following a light meal (treatment A or B, respectively), according to the assigned treatment sequences on day 1 (period 1) and day 8 (period 2). On day 15 (period 3) and day 22 (period 4), subjects received a 300 mg ATV capsule co-administered with a 150 mg COBI tablet or an FDC tablet of ATV/COBI (300/150 mg) under fasted conditions (treatment C or D, respectively). Thirty-two subjects were assigned to receive the ATV/COBI (300/150 mg) FDC tablet following a high-fat meal (treatment E) on day 29 (period 5). Study drugs were administered in the morning within approximately 5 min after a meal in periods 1, 2 and 5, or after fasting for approximately 10 h in periods 3 and 4. Overall, the most common AEs were dizziness (6.3%), abdominal discomfort (4.7%), musculoskeletal chest pain (4.7%) and nasopharyngitis (4.7%); all were mild to moderate in severity and had resolved by study completion. For laboratory abnormalities, 6 subjects (9.4%) experienced elevations in total bilirubin, with the highest observed in the subject who received duplicate doses of study drugs on study day 1. Other laboratory abnormalities that occurred in two or more subjects included: creatine kinase ($n=2$, 3.1%), low leukocytes ($n=4$, 6.3%), low neutrophils ($n=5$, 7.8%), urinary red blood cells ($n=2$, 3.1%) and urinary white blood cells ($n=7$, 10.9%) [88c].

Norethindrone-based progestin-only contraceptives exhibited greater drug exposure, when co-administered with RTV-boosted ATV regimen in women infected with HIV [89c].

Ritonavir (r)

In Nigeria, atazanavir/ritonavir (ATV/r) is the preferred protease inhibitor (PI) as it cause fewer side effects than lopinavir/ritonavir (LPV/r). A recent study evaluated the immunologic and virologic effects of switching 400 patients to an ATV/r-containing regimen from LPV/r at the Lagos University Teaching Hospital in Nigeria. Two hundred and fifty-five patients were virologically suppressed on LPV/r prior to switch, 107 patients were switched due to failure on a first-line line of treatment, 28 were on saquinavir/ritonavir (SQV/r)-based regimen, and 10 were unintentionally switched. Ninety-nine patients evaluated for 12 months after ATV/r switch and only two showed detectable viral load. Twenty-six patients from this group did not show any viral load after 24 months of treatment. In a comparison group of 576 patients who were maintained on LPV/r-based regimens, 359 patients had undetectable viral loads after 24 months of treatment. The study concluded that there was no significant difference between LPV/r and ATV/r in virologic failure [90C].

DRUGS ACTIVE AGAINST HUMAN IMMUNODEFICIENCY VIRUS: INHIBITORS OF HIV FUSION [SEDA-33, 598; SEDA-34, 464; SEDA-35, 525; SEDA-36, 428; SEDA-37, 341]

Enfuvirtide

Participants were enrolled between March 2008 and May 2011 at 62 centers in the United States, with follow-up through 48 weeks. Of 720 potential participants screened for resistance testing, 360 patients were randomly assigned and 337 participants completed the study. Patients received 600 mg of darunavir with 100 mg of RTV, 90 mg of enfuvirtide (ENF) by subcutaneous injection, 200 mg of TMC125 (ETR), 400 mg of RAL, and 500 mg of tipranavir with 200 mg of RTV. The most common antiretroviral regimen was RAL plus RTV-boosted darunavir with ENF, ETR (56%); in the add-NRTIs group, 81% of participants used TDF plus FTC (or 3TC), Thirty-seven (21%) and 44 (24%) participants in the omit- and add-NRTIs groups, respectively, had a serious AE. Three serious AEs in the omit-NRTIs group and 13 in the add-NRTIs group were related to antiretroviral therapy. After treatment initiation, there were no deaths in the omit-NRTIs group and 6 deaths in the add-NRTIs group. The causes of death were as follows: heart failure in a participant with lymphoma (9 weeks on study treatment), Listeria meningitis (17 weeks), renal failure (21 weeks), sepsis with liver failure (25 weeks), progressive multifocal leukoencephalopathy (30 weeks), and abdominal bleeding in a participant with HCV and cirrhosis (52 weeks). Three deaths occurred during the pre-randomization screening period [91C].

DRUGS ACTIVE AGAINST HUMAN IMMUNODEFICIENCY VIRUS: INTEGRASE INHIBITORS [SEDA-33, 599; SEDA-34, 465; SEDA-35, 525; SEDA-36, 428; SEDA-37, 342]

Dolutegravir

The side effect profiles of DTG are similar to RTV and have been found to be well tolerated. DTG has a long plasma half-life and is suitable for once daily use without the need for a boosting agent. The clinical effectiveness of DTG is reviewed here [92R]. Clinical effectiveness of DTG in the treatment of HIV was also reviewed [92R]. Clinical effectiveness of DTG in the treatment of HIV/AIDS has been reviewed and the side effect profiles of DTG are similar to RTG [93R].

Observational Studies

An open-label, non-randomized, multicenter phase I/II study of HIV-infected, treatment-experienced children between 4 weeks and <18 years in age was conducted. DTG dose was prescribed using the weight of the patients: 50 mg for children >=40 kg, 35 mg for children between 30 and 40 kg, and DTG was available as 50, 25 and 10 mg tablets. Most frequent reported events were as follows: gastrointestinal diarrhea in 8 (35%), decrease appetite in 7 (30%), abdominal pain in 5 (21%) and nausea in 3 (13%); respiratory cough in 13 (56%), pharyngeal pain in 8 (35%), nasal congestion in 7 (30%) and sinus congestion in 4 (17%); musculoskeletal extremity pain in 6 (26%), arthralgia in 3 (13%) and back pain in 3 (13%) and general fever in 7 (30%), lymphadenopathy in 6 (26%), headache in 6 (26%) and dizziness in 4 (17%). None of these were considered related to DTG and are common events among adolescents with other illnesses. There were two Grade 3 clinical events: gastritis and deep vein thrombosis, not considered related to DTG that resolved without DTG discontinuation. Two subjects experienced Grade 3 laboratory abnormalities; one patient developed unconjugated bilirubin elevation while on ATV [94c].

Raltegravir (RTG)

Observational Study

This review provide an overview of RTG role in the management of HIV-1 infection, highlighting its key pharmacokinetic and pharmacodynamic properties. Due to RTGs' tolerability, efficacy, few drug-to-drug interactions and its weak genetic barrier to resistance, the authors' are of the opinion that RTG should be administered twice daily and with fully active companion antiretrovirals [95R].

RTG is the first human immunodeficiency virus (HIV) integrase strand transfer inhibitor approved by the US FDA and the European Medicines Agency (EMA) for treatment of HIV infection in children. A new pediatric formulation of RTG has been introduced with 25-mg and 100-mg tablets that can be chewed or swallowed whole [96L].

A 23-year-old man was admitted with severe thrombocytopaenia. He was diagnosed with acute HIV infection and HIV-associated thrombocytopaenia. Although his thrombocytopaenia improved immediately with short-term dexamethasone therapy, this effect was not sustained after cessation of therapy. Antiretroviral therapy including RTG was initiated, and the patient recovered from severe thrombocytopaenia within several days. No significant AES reported [97c].

The data on efficacy and safety of integrase strand transfer inhibitors in antiretroviral-naive HIV patients and the strengths and weaknesses of drugs within this class are reviewed here. Integrase strand transfer inhibitors cause a rapid drop in viral load, exhibit very low drug interactions (except elvitegravir/ COBI), and have low pill burden and convenient dosing frequency. RTG was also superior to atazanavir/ritonavir and darunavir/ritonavir in the ACTG 5257 study for the combined virologic/tolerability endpoint. Elvitegravir/ COBI/FTC/TDF was non-inferior to efavirenz/FTC/ TDF and to atazanavir/ritonavir plus FTC/TDF in terms of confirmed virologic response in the GS-US-236-0102 and GS-US-236-0103 studies, respectively. DTG showed non-inferiority compared to RTG in the SPRING-2 study and was superior to efavirenz and darunavir/ritonavir in the SINGLE and FLAMINGO trials, respectively [98R].

DRUGS ACTIVE AGAINST HUMAN IMMUNODEFICIENCY VIRUS: CHEMOKINE RECEPTOR CCR5 ANTAGONISTS [SEDA-33, 600; SEDA-34, 465; SEDA-35, 528; SEDA-36, 430; SEDA-37, 343]

Maraviroc

Observational Study

An open-label safety study of MVC was conducted at 262 sites worldwide in 1032 R5 HIV-positive treatment-experienced patients. Safety data were analyzed overall and by subgroup based on ARV combination [MVC+ optimized background therapy (OBT), MVC±OBT + DRV/r, MVC±OBT+RAL, MVC±OBT+RAL+DRV/r, MVC±OBT+RAL+ETV±DRV/r]. Most (90.3%) AEs (AEs) were of mild or moderate severity with few Grade 3/4 events, discontinuations, or temporary discontinuations/dose reductions due to AEs or serious AEs [99C].

The role of CCR5 in HIV-1 infection, the development of the CCR5 antagonist MVC, its pharmacokinetics, pharmacodynamics, drug–drug interactions, and the implications of these interactions on treatment outcomes, including viral mutations and drug resistance, and the mechanisms associated with the development of resistance to MVC are reviewed [100R].

DRUGS ACTIVE AGAINST INFLUENZA VIRUSES: ION CHANNEL INHIBITORS [SED-15, 105, 3051; SEDA-32, 544; SEDA-33, 269, 602; SEDA-34, 467; SEDA-35, 529; SEDA-36, 430; SEDA-37, 344]

Amantadine

A meta-analysis was performed in palliative care patients with fatigue that is common in patients with an incurable disease (terminal illness) such as advanced cancer, HIV/AIDS, multiple sclerosis, amyotrophic lateral sclerosis, or cardiac, lung or kidney failure. Data from 18 drugs and 4696 participants were included in the study. Treatment results pointed to weak and inconclusive evidence for the efficacy of amantadine, pemoline and modafinil in multiple sclerosis and for carnitine and donepezil in cancer-related fatigue. Adverse reactions were mild and had little or no impact [101M].

Study reported the effect of amantadine on irritability in persons in the post-acute period after traumatic brain injury (TBI) [102c].

DRUGS ACTIVE AGAINST INFLUENZA VIRUSES: NEURAMINIDASE INHIBITORS [SED-15, 2436; SEDA-32, 544; SEDA-33, 601; SEDA-34, 466; SEDA-35, 528; SEDA-36, 431; SEDA-37, 344]

Oseltamivir (Tamiflu)

Influenza is a seasonal disease affecting both adults and children. Influenza, if untreated could lead to severe lower respiratory tract infections, acute otitis media, rhinosinusitis, febrile seizures, dehydration or encephalopathy. Oseltamivir is a well-studied drug for the treatment of the influenza virus for both the treatment and prevention of infection. Oseltamivir treatment should only be recommended in severe influenza cases where it is confirmed by reliable laboratory tests [103c].

A 15-year-old Japanese female with influenza infection developed abnormal psychiatric symptoms after administration of standard doses of oseltamivir. She had no history of neurological illness, had never previously taken oseltamivir, and had not developed psychiatric reactions during previous influenza infection. Her delirium-like symptoms, including insomnia, visual hallucinations, and a long-term memory deficit, disappeared after cessation of oseltamivir and administration of benzodiazepine. A detailed assessment was performed, including neurological examination (electroencephalogram, brain magnetic resonance imaging, single photon emission computed tomography with 99mTc-ethyl cysteinate dimer and with 123I-iomazenil, cerebrospinal fluid analysis and glutamate receptor autoantibodies), drug level determination and simulation, and genetic assessment (OAT1, OAT3, CES1, Neu2). Abnormal slowing in the electroencephalogram, which is characteristic of influenza-associated encephalopathy, was not observed in repeated recordings. The serum level determination of active metabolite Ro 64-0802 determined at 154 h after final dosing of oseltamivir was higher than the expected value, suggesting delayed elimination of Ro 64-0802. Thus, abnormal exposure to Ro 64-0802 might have contributed, at least in part, to the development of neuropsychiatric symptoms in this patient. The score on Naranjo's ADR probability scale was 6. Mutation of c.122G>A (R41Q) in the sialidase Neu2 gene, increased CSF glutamate receptor autoantibodies, and limbic GABAergic dysfunction indicated by SPECT with 123I-iomazenil were found as possible contributory factors to the CNS side effects [104S].

In an in vivo animal study, mice were infected with influenza A virus. The infected mice were then orally administered with polyphylla saponin I and oseltamivir twice a day for 5 days. In vitro studies in MDCK cells have shown that polyphylla saponin I (6.25, 12.5, 25 and 50 μg/mL) and oseltamivir (40 μg/mL) could inactivate the influenza virus. Studies in mice showed that polyphylla saponin I (5 and 10 mg/kg), and oseltamivir (3 mg/kg) reduced viral hemagglutination titer, improved the pathology of lung, and increased the survival time from 8.5 ± 0.3 to 13.2 ± 0.5 days. The experimental data suggests that the polyphylla saponin I may have antiviral activity on influenza A virus [105E].

OTHER DRUGS

Imiquimod [SED-15, 1718; SEDA-35, 530; SEDA-36, 431; SEDA-37, 344]

Dermatological Studies

A 38-year-old HIV-1-positive African woman established on cART presented with a 3-week history of a large, tender hypertrophic ulcer on the left labium majus. She was commenced on acyclovir (400 mg TDS for 2 weeks), and a PCR swab of the ulcer was positive for HSV-2. The treatment was switched to valaciclovir 500 mg BD (for 3 weeks) and then 1 g BD (for 4 weeks). The ulcer persisted (still PCR positive for HSV-2) and a biopsy showed extensive ulceration with non-specific inflammatory changes. Further treatment with valganciclovir and topical foscarnet led to minimal improvement for 12 months. Topical imiquimod (three times a week) was commenced and within 2 months the ulcer had completely resolved without any noticeable side effects.

A 44-year-old man of West African origin presented with genital ulceration. The ulcers resolved after empirical acyclovir treatment. He was also diagnosed with HIV-2 and hepatitis B co-infection (CD4 60 cells/mm^3) but then defaulted care prior to starting cART. Three years later, he re-presented with a 6-month history of intermittently recurring genital ulceration of HSV. He had three painless hypertrophic ulcers on his scrotum and one on his penile shaft. Acyclovir 800 mg TDS, PCP and MAI prophylaxis and cART (Truvada, darunavir and ritonavir) were commenced. The ulcers were positive on PCR testing. After 4 weeks, the ulcers had fully healed and the acyclovir dose was reduced to 400 mg BD. Seven months later the genital ulceration recurred and acyclovir was increased (400 mg TDS). He was on cART with good adherence, CD4 200 cells/mm^3 and HIV-VL <50 copies/mL. The ulcers were again HSV-2 positive on PCR testing and showed no improvement after 4 weeks of acyclovir. Tests for other STIs including syphilis were negative. The drugs were switched to valaciclovir for 2 weeks, followed by topical foscarnet cream for 3 months. However, there was no improvement and the ulcer remained positive for HSV-2. A biopsy showed a nonspecific inflammatory infiltrate with no viral inclusions seen and no pathogens identified on staining. Administration of valganciclovir and topical foscarnet cream did not show any improvement in ulceration. Three times weekly topical imiquimod therapy healed the ulcers completely within 8 weeks of treatment. He suffered a recurrence several months later which also fully responded to a 2-week course of imiquimod [106c].

Acknowledgements

Disclaimer: The findings and the conclusions in this report are those of the authors and do not necessarily represent the views of the National Institute for Occupational Safety and Health.

References

[1] Caruso Brown AE, et al. Pharmacokinetics and safety of intravenous cidofovir for life-threatening viral infections in pediatric hematopoietic stem cell transplant recipients. Antimicrob Agents Chemother. 2015;59(7):3718–25 [c].

[2] Romani D, Brandán SA. Effect of the side chain on the properties from cidofovir to brincidofovir, an experimental antiviral drug against to Ebola virus disease. Arab J Chem. 2015; http://dx.doi.org/10.1016/j.arabjc.2015.06.030, in press [c].

[3] Melendez DP, Razonable RR. Letermovir and inhibitors of the terminase complex: a promising new class of investigational antiviral drugs against human cytomegalovirus. Infect Drug Resist. 2015;8:269–77 [r].

[4] Sano T. Safety and efficacy of foscarnet for preemptive therapy against cytomegalovirus reactivation following unrelated bone marrow transplantation. Jpn J Chemother. 2015;63(6):568–75 [c].

[5] Hu Y, Liu Y, Liu S, et al. Analysis of foscarnet-induced adverse drug reaction in Beijing area from 2008 to 2014. Chin Pharm J. 2015;50(18):1634–8 [C].

[6] Timperley A, Taha H, Das S. Management of cytomegalovirus retinitis in HIV infection in the era of highly active antiretroviral therapy. Int J STD AIDS. 2015;26(10):757–8 [A].

[7] Boeckh M, et al. Valganciclovir for the prevention of complications of late cytomegalovirus infection after allogeneic hematopoietic cell transplantation: a randomized trial. Ann Intern Med. 2015;162(1):1–10 [C].

[8] Chon WJ, et al. Use of leflunomide in renal transplant recipients with ganciclovir-resistant/refractory cytomegalovirus infection: a case series from the University of Chicago. Case Rep Nephrol Dial. 2015;5(1):96–105 [c].

[9] Mattioni S, et al. Assessment of the efficacy and safety of pre-emptive anti-cytomegalovirus (CMV) therapy in HIV-infected patients with CMV viraemia. Int J STD AIDS. 2015;26(5):306–12 [C].

[10] Mareri A, et al. Anti-viral therapy for congenital cytomegalovirus infection: pharmacokinetics, efficacy and side effects. Journal Matern Fetal Neonatal Med. 2016;29(10):1657–64 [R].

[11] Rao S, et al. Intravenous acyclovir and renal dysfunction in children: a matched case control study. J Pediatr. 2015;166(6).1462–1468.e4, [C].

[12] Noska A, et al. The role of antiviral therapy in immunocompromised patients with herpes simplex virus meningitis. Clin Infect Dis. 2015;60(2):237–42 [c].

[13] Ueno S, et al. Good's syndrome with opportunistic infection of the central nervous system: a case report. BMC Neurol. 2015;15(1):1–4 [A].

[14] Gentry Iii JL, Peterson C. Death delusions and myoclonus: acyclovir toxicity. Am J Med. 2015;128(7):692–4 [A].

[15] Pachnio A, et al. Acyclovir therapy reduces the CD4+ T cell response against the immunodominant pp65 protein from cytomegalovirus in immune competent individuals. PLoS One. 2015;10(4):e0125287 [c].

[16] Ide N. An elderly patient presenting with abnormal penciclovir blood concentration increased by famciclovir at the usual dose: a case report. Jpn J Chemother. 2015;63(5):469–72 [A].

[17] Shen XJ. Effect of famciclovir combined with oxymatrine on T lymphocyte subsets in patients with chronic severe viral hepatitis B. World Chin J Digestol. 2015;23(18):2961–5 [c].

[18] Shah SA, Gulbis A, Wilhelm K. A case series using famciclovir in stem cell transplant recipients with valacyclovir hypersensitivity reactions. J Oncol Pharm Pract. 2015;21(4):305–9 [A].

[19] Wang G, et al. Cost-effectiveness analysis of lamivudine, telbivudine, and entecavir in treatment of chronic hepatitis B with adefovir dipivoxil resistance. Drug Des Devel Ther. 2015;9:2839–46 [c].

[20] Yang DH, et al. Tenofovir disoproxil fumarate is superior to lamivudine plus adefovir in lamivudine-resistant chronic hepatitis B patients. World J Gastroenterol. 2015;21(9):2746–53 [c].

[21] Li BX, et al. Clinical effects of entecavir and adefovir dipivoxil in treatment of hepatitis B associated decompensated cirrhosis. World Chin J Digestol. 2015;23(21):3460–3 [c].

[22] Kim J, et al. Efficacy and safety of tenofovir in nucleos(t)ide-naïve patients with genotype C chronic hepatitis B in real-life practice. Int J Clin Pharm. 2015;37(6):1228–34 [C].

[23] Lu J, et al. Effect of Peg-interferon α-2a combined with adefovir in HBV postpartum women with normal levels of ALT and high levels of HBV DNA. Liver Int. 2015;35(6):1692–9 [c].

[24] Ilyas F, et al. Intraocular pressure rise in the course of peginterferon alpha-2a, ribavirin, and boceprevir therapy for hepatitis C. Can J Ophthalmol. 2015;50(6):e112–4 [c].

[25] Coilly A, et al. Multicenter experience with boceprevir or telaprevir to treat hepatitis C recurrence after liver transplantation: when present becomes past, what lessons for future? PLoS One. 2015;10(9):e0138091 [c].

[26] Shiraishi M, et al. Postmarketing surveillance of telaprevir-based triple therapy for chronic hepatitis C in Japan. Hepatol Res. 2015;45(13):1267–75 [c].

[27] Neukam K, Munteanu DI, Rivero-Juarez A, et al. Boceprevir or telaprevir based triple therapy against chronic hepatitis C in HIV coinfection: real-life safety and efficacy. PLoS One. 2015;10(4): e0125080 [C].

[28] Oze T, et al. The real impact of telaprevir dosage on the antiviral and side effects of telaprevir, pegylated interferon and ribavirin therapy for chronic hepatitis C patients with HCV genotype 1. J Viral Hepat. 2015;22(3):254–62 [c].

[29] Matsui K, et al. Does elevation of serum creatinine in patients with chronic hepatitis C under therapy of telaprevir mean renal impairment? Nephrology. 2015;20(11):843–8 [c].

[30] Morihara D, et al. Adjusting the starting dose of telaprevir according to renal function decreases adverse effects and affects the sustained virological response rate. Eur J Gastroenterol Hepatol. 2015;27(1):55–64.

[31] Kawano A, et al. Bacterial infection as an adverse effect of telaprevir-based triple therapy for chronic hepatitis C infection. Intern Med. 2015;54(6):567–72 [c].

[32] Verna EC, et al. Telaprevir- and boceprevir-based triple therapy for hepatitis C in liver transplant recipients with advanced recurrent disease: a multicenter study. Transplantation. 2015;99(8):1644–51 [c].

[33] Falcaõ EMM, et al. Cutaneous eruption due to telaprevir. Case Rep Dermatol. 2015;7(3):253–62 [A].

[34] Federico A, et al. Telaprevir may induce adverse cutaneous reactions by a T cell immune-mediated mechanism. Ann Hepatol. 2015;14(3):420–4 [c].

[35] Kawaguchi Y, et al. Efficacy and safety of telaprevir, pegylated interferon α-2b and ribavirin triple therapy in Japanese patients infected with hepatitis C virus genotype 1b. Intern Med. 2015;54(20):2551–60 [C].

[36] Zhou L, et al. Changes in mitochondrial toxicity in peripheral blood mononuclear cells during four-year administration of entecavir monotherapy in Chinese patients with chronic hepatitis B. Med Sci Monit. 2015;21:2058–63 [E].

[37] Hung CH, et al. Tenofovir versus entecavir in treatment of chronic hepatitis B virus with severe acute exacerbation. Antimicrob Agents Chemother. 2015;59(6):3168–73 [C].

[38] Huang M, et al. Comparison of the efficacy of tenofovir disoproxil fumarate and entecavir for initial treatment of patient with chronic hepatitis B in China. Int J Clin Exp Med. 2015;8(1):666–73 [c].

[39] Buti M, et al. Entecavir has high efficacy and safety in white patients with chronic hepatitis B and comorbidities. Eur J Gastroenterol Hepatol. 2015;27(1):46–54 [C].

[40] Masip M, et al. Prevalence and detection of neuropsychiatric adverse effects during hepatitis C treatment. Int J Clin Pharm. 2015;37(6):1143–51 [C].

[41] Saadoun D, et al. PegIFNα/ribavirin/protease inhibitor combination in severe hepatitis C virus-associated mixed cryoglobulinemia vasculitis. J Hepatol. 2015;62(1):24–30 [c].

[42] Jung E, et al. Tenofovir monotherapy versus tenofovir plus lamivudine or telbivudine combination therapy in treatment of lamivudine-resistant chronic hepatitis B. Antimicrob Agents Chemother. 2015;59(2):972–8 [C].

[43] Wu Q, et al. Telbivudine prevents vertical transmission of hepatitis B virus from women with high viral loads: a prospective long-term study. Clin Gastroenterol Hepatol. 2015;13(6):1170–6 [C].

[44] Marcellin P, et al. Telbivudine plus pegylated interferon alfa-2a in a randomized study in chronic hepatitis B is associated with an unexpected high rate of peripheral neuropathy. J Hepatol. 2015;62(1):41–7 [C].

[45] Zeuzem S. Efficacy and safety of faldaprevir, deleobuvir, and ribavirin in treatment-naive patients with chronic hepatitis C virus infection and advanced liver fibrosis or cirrhosis. Antimicrob Agents Chemother. 2015;59(2): 1282–91 [c].

[46] Noell BC, Besur SV, deLemos AS. Changing the face of hepatitis C management—the design and development of sofosbuvir. Drug Des Devel Ther. 2015;9:2367–74 [R].

[47] Pearlman BL, Ehleben C, Perrys M. The combination of simeprevir and sofosbuvir is more effective than that of peginterferon, ribavirin, and sofosbuvir for patients with hepatitis C-related Child's Class A cirrhosis. Gastroenterology. 2015;148(4). 762–770. e2, [C].

[48] Kohli A, Kattakuzhy S, Sidharthan S, et al. Four-week direct-acting antiviral regimens in noncirrhotic patients with hepatitis C virus genotype 1 infection: an open-label, nonrandomized trial. Ann Intern Med. 2015;163(12):899–907 [C].

[49] Everson GT, Towner WJ, Davis MN, et al. Sofosbuvir with velpatasvir in treatment-naive noncirrhotic patients with genotype 1 to 6 hepatitis C virus infection: a randomized trial. Ann Intern Med. 2015;163(11):818–26 [C].

[50] Leroy V, et al. Efficacy of sofosbuvir and daclatasvir in patients with fibrosing cholestatic hepatitis C after liver transplantation. Clin Gastroenterol Hepatol. 2015;13(11). 1993-2001.e2, [C].

[51] Wyles DL, et al. Daclatasvir plus sofosbuvir for HCV in patients coinfected with HIV-1. N Engl J Med. 2015;373(8):714–25 [C].

[52] Bourlière M, et al. Ledipasvir-sofosbuvir with or without ribavirin to treat patients with HCV genotype 1 infection and cirrhosis non-responsive to previous protease-inhibitor therapy: a randomised, double-blind, phase 2 trial (SIRIUS). Lancet Infect Dis. 2015;15(4):397–404 [C].

[53] Gane EJ, et al. Efficacy of ledipasvir and sofosbuvir, with or without ribavirin, for 12 weeks in patients with HCV genotype 3 or 6 infection. Gastroenterology. 2015;149(6). 1454–1461.e1, [C].

[54] Ruane PJ, et al. Sofosbuvir plus ribavirin for the treatment of chronic genotype 4 hepatitis C virus infection in patients of Egyptian ancestry. J Hepatol. 2015;62(5):1040–6 [c].

[55] Majumdar A, Kitson MT, Roberts SK. Treatment of hepatitis C in patients with cirrhosis: remaining challenges for direct-acting antiviral therapy. Drugs. 2015;75(8):823–34 [R].

[56] Jafari A, et al. Safely treating hepatitis C in patients with HIV or hepatitis B virus coinfection. Expert Opin Drug Saf. 2015;14(5):713–31 [R].

[57] Sanford M. Simeprevir: a review of its use in patients with chronic hepatitis C virus infection. Drugs. 2015;75(2):183–96 [R].

[58] Smit C, et al. Effect of abacavir on sustained virologic response to HCV treatment in HIV/HCV co-infected patients, Cohere in Eurocoord. BMC Infect Dis. 2015;15(1):1–10 [C].

[59] Walmsley S, Baumgarten A, Berenguer J, et al. Brief report: dolutegravir plus abacavir/lamivudine for the treatment of HIV-1 infection in antiretroviral therapy-naive patients: week 96 and week 144 results from the SINGLE randomized clinical trial. J Acquir Immune Defic Syndr. 2015;70(5):515–9 [R].

[60] Post FA, et al. Elvitegravir/cobicistat/emtricitabine/tenofovir DF in HIV-infected patients with mild-to-moderate renal impairment. J Acquir Immune Defic Syndr. 2015;68(3):310–3 [c].

[61] von Hentig N. Clinical use of cobicistat as a pharmacoenhancer of human immunodeficiency virus therapy. HIV/AIDS. 2015;8:1–16 [R].

[62] Nsagha DS, Pokam BT, Assob JC. HAART, DOTS and renal disease of patients co-infected with HIV/AIDS and TB in the South West Region of Cameroon. BMC Public Health. 2015;15(1):1040 [C].

[63] Kiertiburanakul S, et al. The use of pharmacogenetics in clinical practice for the treatment of individuals with HIV infection in Thailand. Pharm Pers Med. 2015;8:163–70 [c].

[64] Walmsley S, et al. Dolutegravir plus abacavir/lamivudine for the treatment of HIV-1 infection in antiretroviral therapy-naive patients: week 96 and week 144 results from the SINGLE randomized clinical trial. J Acquir Immune Defic Syndr. 2015;70(5):515–9 [c].

[65] Bollen P, et al. Clinical pharmacokinetics and pharmacodynamics of dolutegravir used as a single tablet regimen for the treatment of HIV-1 infection. Expert Opin Drug Saf. 2015;14(9):1457–72 [R].

[66] Ciaffi L, et al. Efficacy and safety of three second-line antiretroviral regimens in HIV-infected patients in Africa. AIDS. 2015;29(12):1473–81 [C].

[67] Podlekareva D, et al. Changing utilization of stavudine (d4T) in HIV-positive people in 2006–2013 in the EuroSIDA study. HIV Med. 2015;16(9):533–43 [M].

[68] Parkes Ratanshi R, et al. Development of severe anemia and changes in hemoglobin in a cohort of HIV-infected Ugandan adults receiving zidovudine-, stavudine-, and tenofovir-containing antiretroviral regimens. J Int Assoc Provid AIDS Care (JIAPAC). 2015;14(5):455–62 [C].

[69] Bezabhe WM, et al. Adverse drug reactions and clinical outcomes in patients initiated on antiretroviral therapy: a prospective cohort study from Ethiopia. Drug Saf. 2015;38(7):629–39 [C].

[70] Saez-Llorens X, et al. A randomized, open-label study of the safety and efficacy of switching stavudine or zidovudine to tenofovir disoproxil fumarate in HIV-1-infected children with virologic suppression. Pediatr Infect Dis J. 2015;34(4):376–82 [c].

[71] Quesada PR, et al. Incidence and risk factors for tenofovir-associated renal toxicity in HIV-infected patients. Int J Clin Pharm. 2015;37(5):865–72 [C].

[72] Coppolino G, et al. The case of chronic hepatitis B treatment with tenofovir: an update for nephrologists. J Nephrol. 2015;28(4):393–402 [R].

[73] Kryst J, et al. Efavirenz-based regimens in antiretroviral-naive HIV-infected patients: a systematic review and meta-analysis of randomized controlled trials. PLoS One. 2015;10(5):e0124279 [R].

[74] Abah IO, et al. Incidence and predictors of adverse drug events in an African cohort of HIV-infected adults treated with efavirenz. Germs. 2015;5(3):83–91 [C].

[75] Waters L, et al. Switching safely: pharmacokinetics, efficacy and safety of switching efavirenz to maraviroc twice-daily in patients on suppressive antiretroviral therapy. Antivir Ther. 2014;20(2):157–63 [c].

[76] Frapsauce C, et al. Impaired sperm motility in HIV-infected men: an unexpected adverse effect of efavirenz? Hum Reprod. 2015;30(8):1797–806 [C].

[77] Gaida R, Truter I, Grobler C. Efavirenz: a review of the epidemiology, severity and management of neuropsychiatric side-effects. S Afr J Psychiatr. 2015;21(3):94–7 [R].

[78] Kurz M, et al. Etravirine: a good option for concomitant use with chemotherapy for Hodgkin's lymphoma. Int J STD AIDS. 2015;26(3):212–4 [c].

[79] Vingerhoets J, et al. Efficacy of etravirine combined with darunavir or other ritonavir-boosted protease inhibitors in HIV-1-infected patients: an observational study using pooled European cohort data. HIV Med. 2015;16(5):297–306 [C].

[80] Casado JL, et al. Efficacy and pharmacokinetics of the combination of etravirine plus raltegravir as novel dual antiretroviral maintenance regimen in HIV-infected patients. Antiviral Res. 2015;113:103–6 [c].

[81] Pawar MP, et al. Nevirapine: most common cause of cutaneous adverse drug reactions in an outpatient department of a tertiary care hospital. J Clin Diagn Res. 2015;9(11):FC17–20 [c].

[82] Bhatt NB, et al. Nevirapine or efavirenz for tuberculosis and HIV coinfected patients: exposure and virological failure relationship. J Antimicrob Chemother. 2015;70(1):225–32 [C].

[83] Sanjeeva GN, et al. Nevirapine-related adverse events among children switched from efavirenz to nevirapine as compared to children who were started on nevirapine-based antiretroviral therapy directly. AIDS Care. 2015;27(5):655–9 [c].

[84] van Lunzen J, et al. Rilpivirine vs. efavirenz-based single-tablet regimens in treatment-naive adults: week 96 efficacy and safety from a randomized phase 3b study. AIDS. 2016;30(2):251–9 [C].

[85] Foster R, et al. Single-tablet emtricitabine-rilpivirine-tenofovir as HIV postexposure prophylaxis in men who have sex with men. Clin Infect Dis. 2015;61(8):1336–41 [c].

[86] Gervasoni C, Meraviglia P, Minisci D, et al. Metabolic and kidney disorders correlate with high atazanavir concentrations in HIV-infected patients: is it time to revise atazanavir dosages? PLoS One. 2015;10(4):e0123670 [C].

[87] Gallant JE, et al. Cobicistat compared with ritonavir as a pharmacoenhancer for atazanavir in combination with emtricitabine/tenofovir disoproxil fumarate: week 144 results. J Acquir Immune Defic Syndr. 2015;69(3):338–40 [C].

[88] Sevinsky H, et al. A randomized trial in healthy subjects to assess the bioequivalence of an atazanavir/cobicistat fixed-dose combination tablet versus administration as separate agents. Antivir Ther. 2015;20(5):493–500 [c].

[89] DuBois BN, et al. Increased exposure of norethindrone in HIV+ women treated with ritonavir-boosted atazanavir therapy. Contraception. 2015;91(1):71–5 [c].

[90] Akanmu AS, et al. Immunological and virological outcomes of patients switched from LPV/r to ATV/r-containing second-line regimens. Curr HIV Res. 2015;13(3):176–83 [C].

[91] Tashima KT, et al. HIV salvage therapy does not require nucleoside reverse transcriptase inhibitors a randomized, controlled trial. Ann Intern Med. 2015;163(12):908–17 [C].

[92] Das S, Taha H, Das A. Clinical effectiveness of dolutegravir in the treatment of HIV/AIDS. Infect Drug Resist. 2015;8:339–52 [R].

[93] Taha H, Das A, Das S. Clinical effectiveness of dolutegravir in the treatment of HIV/AIDS. Infect Drug Resist. 2015;8:339–52 [R].

[94] Viani R, et al. Safety, pharmacokinetics and efficacy of dolutegravir in treatment-experienced HIV-1 infected adolescents. Pediatr Infect Dis J. 2015;34(11):1207–13 [c].

[95] Calcagno A, D'Avolio A, Bonora S. Pharmacokinetic and pharmacodynamic evaluation of raltegravir and experience from clinical trials in HIV-positive patients. Expert Opin Drug Metab Toxicol. 2015;11(7):1167–76 [R].

[96] Blonk MI, et al. Dose optimization of raltegravir chewable tablets in a 4-year-old HIV-infected child. Clin Infect Dis. 2015;61(2):294–5 [L].

[97] Aoki A, et al. A case of severe thrombocytopaenia associated with acute HIV-1 infection. Int J STD AIDS. 2015;26(3):209–11 [c].

[98] D'Abbraccio M, et al. Efficacy and tolerability of integrase inhibitors in antiretroviral-naive patients. AIDS Rev. 2015;17(3):171–85 [R].

[99] Lazzarin A, et al. The maraviroc expanded access program—safety and efficacy data from an open-label study. HIV Clin Trials. 2015;16(1):10–21 [C].

[100] Kanmogne G, Woollard S. Maraviroc: a review of its use in HIV infection and beyond. Drug Des Devel Ther. 2015;9:5447–68 [R].

[101] Mücke M, et al. Pharmacological treatments for fatigue associated with palliative care cochrane database of systematic reviews. Cochrane Database Syst Rev. 1996;5: CD006788 [M].

[102] Hammond FM, et al. Amantadine effect on perceptions of irritability after traumatic brain injury: results of the amantadine irritability multisite study. J Neurotrauma. 2015;32(16):1230–8 [c].

[103] Esposito S, Principi N. Oseltamivir for influenza infection in children: risks and benefits. Expert Rev Respir Med. 2016;10:79–87 [c].

[104] Morimoto K, et al. Analysis of a child who developed abnormal neuropsychiatric symptoms after administration of oseltamivir: a case report. BMC Neurol. 2015;15(1):1–5 [S].

[105] Pu X, et al. Polyphylla saponin I has antiviral activity against influenza A virus. Int J Clin Exp Med. 2015;8(10):18963–71 [E].

[106] McKendry A, Narayana S, Browne R. Atypical presentations of genital herpes simplex virus in HIV-1 and HIV-2 effectively treated by imiquimod. Int J STD AIDS. 2015;26(6):441–3 [c].

28

Drugs Used in Tuberculosis and Leprosy

M. Smith[1], A. Accinelli[1], F.R. Tejada[2], M.K. Kharel[2]

School of Pharmacy and Health Professions, University of Maryland at Eastern Shore, Princess Anne, MD, USA
[2]Corresponding authors: frtejada@umes.edu; mkkharel@umes.edu

BEDAQUILINE

Bedaquiline (BDQ) is a recently approved fast-tracked antibiotic for the treatment of multidrug-resistant tuberculosis (MDR-TB). Many common adverse events have been reported in patients receiving BDQ therapy in clinical trials such as nausea, unilateral deafness, arthralgias, hemoptysis, hyperuricemia, rash, extremity, chest pain, and QTC prolongation [1r]. A recent phase 2, multicenter, open-label, single-arm trial, indicated that addition of BDQ to a background regimen was well tolerated and led to good outcomes in patients with MDR-TB [2MC]. A separate study reported nausea, arthralgia, and anorexia and subjective fever in 60%, 40% and 30% of patients with *Mycobacterium avium* and *Mycobacterium abscessus* infections, respectively [3c]. Less common adverse effects included neuropathy, fever, diarrhea, vomiting, headache, weight loss, insomnia, fatigue, dizziness, tinnitus, ataxia, and blurred vision. The continuing education provider Prescrire labeled BDQ as a dangerous drug based on adverse effects observed in a double-blind, randomized, placebo-controlled trial which included 160 patients with multidrug-resistant pulmonary TB [4C]. Notably, there were 10 deaths in BDQ group compared to 2 deaths in placebo group. The adverse effects of BDQ included prolongation of QT segment in addition to hepatic and pancreatic disorders. A separate cohort study also indicated the association of BDQ with prolongation of QTcB [5c]. While there is limited information on the use of BDQ in HIV co-infected patients including those on antiretroviral treatment (ART), an interim study concluded BDQ therapy may be both efficacious and safe [6c]. Further studies are needed to validate these initial findings.

CLOFAZIMINE

Clofazimine (CFZ) is used in combination with rifampicin and dapsone as multidrug therapy for the treatment of multibacillary (MB) leprosy. CFZ is also used as a second-line treatment agent in multi-drug resistant (MDR) TB and infections caused by several mycobacterial strains. Due to its high lipophilicity, CFZ accumulates in the skin, subcutaneous fat, liver, lungs, adrenals, kidneys, lymph nodes, and gastrointestinal tract. Accumulation in the tissues results in a red discoloration of the organs and the skin. It is more marked on sun-exposed areas including the face and results in low acceptability amongst fairer skinned individuals. Persistent serpentine supravenous hyperpigmented eruption, xerosis and icthyosis of the skin were also noted as adverse effects of CFZ therapy [7c,8C,9C]. Depression and hallucinations as a result of CFZ intake were also reported in 2015 in addition to gastrointestinal disturbances such as abdominal pain, malabsorption and combined-degeneration in patients who were deficient in iron and vitamin B12 [9C].

CYCLOSERINE

Cycloserine (CS) (4-amino-3-isoxazolidinone) is a broad-spectrum antibiotic that is used to treat TB. CS's propensity to cause numerous CNS side effects has relegated its use to second-line treatment. However, with the emergence of MDR-TB and XDR-TB, second-line drugs like CS are being further utilized. Case reports have noted CS's potential to cause psychosis, dizziness, vertigo, headache, sleep disturbances, peripheral neuropathy and depression [10c,11c]. Gastrointestinal trouble, rash, allergy, fever, and cardiovascular problems (including cardiac arrhythmia) are also described on rare occasions [12R]. A meta-analysis that analyzed approximately 1100

---

[1] Authors contributed equally to the work.

patients reiterated the occurrence of these adverse effects on patients who were treated with 500–1000 mg of CS daily for 6–24 months [13c]. In addition, the report indicated CS was associated with tinnitus, visual disturbances, seizures, and psychosis in 3–5% of patients. CS-induced neuroleptic malignant syndrome (NMS) and hepatotoxicity were also reported in separate case reports [10c,11c,14c].

DELAMANID

Delamanid is a relatively new experimental drug that has exhibited potency against both drug-susceptible and drug-resistant strains of *Mycobacterium tuberculosis*. It has been approved for treating TB both in European Union countries (under the trade name Deltyba) and in Japan as a part of combination therapy to treat MDR-TB [15R]. During clinical trials, delamanid was subjected to small-cohort studies aimed at determining safety and efficacy. Common adverse effects of delamanid were observed in healthy subjects during clinical studies. These adverse effects included headache, nausea and dizziness. In a recent clinical trial, 481 MDR-TB patients receiving a background drug regimen for MDR TB were randomized to receive delamanid 100 mg twice daily, delamanid 200 mg twice daily, or placebo. Delamanid exhibited asymptomatic QT segment prolongation in both treatment groups (13.1% and 9.9%) compared to placebo group (3.8%) [16s]. Such QT prolongation could be of clinical concern if delamanid is ever administered with flouroquinolones [17r]. Limited information is available concerning the interaction of delamanid with other drugs/foods. Although clinical efficacy and safety of delamanid looks promising, further clinical studies in bigger subject populations are necessary to validate these initial findings.

DAPSONE

Dapsone (4,4′-diaminodiphenylsulfone) has been widely used in the treatment of leprosy since its discovery in the 1940s. Previous studies have described the genetic susceptibility associated with dapsone-related adverse effects. A handful of adverse effects of dapsone therapy were reported in 2015. They include drug-induced hypersensitivity syndrome (DIH), hepatitis, hematological disorders and photosensitive dermatitis [18c,19c,20c,21c].

Hematologic Disorders

Methemoglobinemia and hemolysis were two major adverse effects of dapsone reported in 2015 [22c,23c,24r].

Severe ischemic retinal injury as a result dapsone-induced methemoglobinemia was also reported in a separate case study [25c]. Hemolysis is thought to be a result of oxidative stress on red blood cells induced by dapsone metabolites which produce reactive oxygen species that disrupt the red blood cell membrane and promote splenic sequestration. Such effects of dapsone in children have been underreported. A recent case study described a dapsone-induced hematologic disorder in a 3-year-old child [26c].

- A 3-year-old boy was brought to the hospital after accidentally ingesting an unknown amount of dapsone. At the onset of admission, the boy was lethargic, with vomiting and unsteadiness. An initial methemoglobin (MHbA) level of 19.4% confirmed acute dapsone-induced methemoglobinemia. Oxygen inhalation and ascorbic acid was administered via nasogastric tube along with ranitidine and ondansetron. Methylene blue 0.1% (2 mg/kg) was administered via IV route. Follow-up packed red cell transfusion (on days 2 and 3) and a second dose of methylene blue (on day 7) helped the child recover fully [26c].

Drug–Drug Interaction

A new drug–drug interaction between dapsone and vorinostat (when used for anti-bacterial prophylaxis in the treatment of glioblastoma multiforme) has been recently described. The potential interactions between dapsone and vorinostat may have important clinical implications as more than 10 clinical trials evaluating drug combinations with vorinostat in patients with malignant glioma are either ongoing or planned in North America [27c]. Patients undergoing treatment for glioblastoma multiforme are routinely placed on Dapsone prophylactic treatment for *Pneumocystis jirovecii* pneumonia. Two patients with glioblastoma multiforme developed severe hemolytic anemia shortly after initiating therapy with vorinostat, a pan-active histone deacetylase inhibitor, while they were on prophylactic dapsone. There are several proposed mechanisms by which histone deacetylase inhibition may alter dapsone metabolism including changes in hepatic acetylation or N-glucuronidation leading to an increase in the bioavailability of dapsone's hematotoxic metabolites [27c].

ETHAMBUTOL

Ethambutol (EMB) is a first-line anti-TB therapeutic agent used only in conjunction with other agents such as isoniazid (INH) and rifampin (RMP). With the widespread use of this drug, numerous adverse effects have been reported. During 2015, many reports reiterated previously observed adverse effects of EMB such as ocular toxicity, peripheral neuropathy, and hyperuricemia [28c,29C,30c,31c,32c]. A retrospective study involving 1004 patients reported EMB-related optic neuropathy in 1.29% of patients where visual improvement occurred in only half of the patients after discontinuation of EMB therapy [29C]. A separate study indicated the beneficial effects of Vitamins E and B1 in preventing EMB-mediated optic neuropathy [33c].

Psychiatric

Depression disorder and TB both are known to share a number of risk factors such as poor economy and homelessness. Notably, anti-TB medications have been identified to be contributing to exacerbate depression [34R]. A nation-wide cohort study in Taiwan that involved 23 145 patients revealed the incidence of depression in 1.71% patients who are on at least two anti-TB medications (out of INH, EMB, RMP and pyrazinamide (PZA)) compared to 1.2% subjects (without TB) in the control group during the mean follow-up period of 6.53 years [35E]. Notably, the risk of incident depressive disorder was significantly higher (adjusted HR 2.54, 95% CI, 1.19–5.45) in patients with TB who received more than 60 defined daily doses of EMB. This effect was shown to be dose dependent as the risk of depression increased with the increase in defined daily doses (DDDs) of EMB. The report highlights a need for further assessment of depression for patients who are on EMB [35E].

Dermatologic

Fixed drug eruption (FDE) is a cutaneous reaction that occurs most commonly with RMP, and rarely with INH and PZA. The following case study reports an incidence of FDE in a patient after taking EMB [36c].

- A 32-year-old patient treated for pulmonary TB presented with pruritus and burning localized to the internal surface of the lips and interdigital folds during the fourth month of treatment with RMP, INH, and EMB. Erythema was found on the inner and outer faces of the lips with inflammation and cracking at the corners. The lesions appearance was consistent with FDE and reoccurred when the same triple therapy regimen was accidentally reintroduced. EMB was discontinued, and the FDE was completely resolved during the course of rifamycin and INH treatment. The patient was eventually declared cured of FDE. A year after the end of TB treatment, dermatological examination revealed a residual depigmentation of the two lips and the complete cleaning of interdigital fold lesions [36c].

FLUOROQUINOLONES

Fluoroquinolone (FQ) antibiotics used in the treatment of TB include levofloxacin, moxifloxacin, ofloxacin, and ciprofloxacin. FQs have a wide variety of common adverse effects that impact the GI (e.g. nausea, vomiting, and diarrhea), CNS (insomnia, dizziness, headache, psychosis) and the CV system (QT prolongation). These effects are usually mild and are generally well tolerated with short-term use of FQs. However, serious and rare side effects of FQs also exist. These include Stevens–Johnson syndrome, toxic epidermal necrolysis, and dysglycaemia [37R,38c]. Levofloxacin was reported to induce drug rash with eosinophilia and systemic symptoms (DRESS syndrome) [39c]. Fluoroquinolone-induced disabling symptoms are also of particular concern [40c]. These symptoms include tendinopathy, muscle weakness, peripheral neuropathy, sleep disorders, autonomic dysfunction and cognitive dysfunction. A multicenter randomized trial reported tenosynovitis in 18.2% of patients taking levofloxacin [41MC]. Other studies reported that FQs increase the risk of aortic dissection and aortic aneurysm [41MC,42MC]. However, a meta-analysis that analyzed 2056 patients revealed no difference in the rate of serious adverse effects between moxifloxacin and other first-line medications [43M]. Similarly, a meta-analysis of observational studies disputed literature reports that suggested a higher risk of retinal detachment associated with FQ therapy [44M]. Ciprofloxacin-induced thrombocytopenia represents a rare adverse effect [45c].

Reproductive

FQs have also been shown to negatively impact the male reproductive system, causing decreased testicle and seminal vesicle weight, and decreased the motility of sperm (after thawing) [46R]. The impact of FQs on the female reproductive system has not yet been fully established.

Dermatologic

An analysis of 18 cohort studies on Indian patients with cutaneous adverse drug reactions indicated that FQs accounted for 5.12% of the suspected causative drugs. FQs also had a high severe to non-severe ratio of cutaneous adverse drug reactions (1:9.07) [47R]. These findings were consistent with the case reports of FQ-induced cutaneous adverse reactions in children [38c]. The reactions included severe itching, formation of rash and red papules and ulceration in the buccal cavity.

ISONIAZID

Isoniazid (INH, pyridine-4-carboxy hydrazide) is considered one of the most reliable and cost-effective therapeutic options to treat TB [48E]. This drug is routinely included in regimens to treat various stages of Mycobacterial infections ranging from preventive therapy for patients with latent TB to multi-drug therapy for patients with drug-resistant active TB [49C]. Studies suggested that monotherapy of INH is as effective as the combination therapy involving INH and RPT in treating TB in adolescents and children [50MC]. Although isoniazid preventive therapy (IPT) is recommended for 6–12 months among patients with positive tuberculin skin test [51r,52M], the protective effect of INH therapy wanes over time providing justification for a lifetime treatment [53R,54C,55c]. In this context, the World Health Organization (WHO) recently recommended 36 weeks of IPT for HIV infected persons in those regions where there is a high rate of transmission of TB [56s]. With the growing trend of INH treatment for an extended period, concerns over the drug-related adverse effects are increasing. Isoniazid is known to cause numerous side effects including hepatotoxicity, gastrointestinal and dermatological disorders, neurotoxicity, autoimmune and psychiatric disorders in addition to contributing to patients' noncompliance [57R,58C]. This section covers the highlights of the adverse effects of INH treatment reported during the year of 2015.

Neurological and Psychiatric Disorders

A handful of reports concerning INH-induced neurological adverse effects were published in 2015. Mafukidze et al. reported a case report of polyneuropathy in a patient receiving anti-TB medication including INH. This is an addition to existing literature reports on INH-induced neuropathy [59c]. A therapeutic dose of INH was reported to be associated with inducing convulsions in an alcoholic patient [60c]. This raised additional concerns of INH-related adverse neurological effects among alcoholic patients. Induction of numerous psychiatric disorders such as psychosis, obsessive–compulsive disorders, mania, and suicidal tendencies as a result of INH therapy has been reported in literatures [61c,62r,63R]. Case reports of INH-induced psychosis and obsessive–compulsive disorders available in 2015 were new additions to pre-existing literatures [64c,65c]. While the detailed mechanisms of these adverse effects are not well understood, the reports highlight a need for a close monitoring for side effects of INH among patients.

Hematologic Disorders and Hypersensitivity Reactions

INH-induced DRESS syndrome is a rare but severe reaction characterized by rashes, fever and multi-organ failure. Eosinophil count elevates significantly in hypereosinophilic syndrome (HES) a form of DRESS which follows organ damage. Zhang et al. have reported a case of INH-induced DRESS syndrome [66c].

- A 43-year-old man was presented with the complaints of chest pain, tightness and fever. Multi-drug treatment regimen including RMP, INH, EMB and PZA was initiated following the diagnosis of tuberculous meningitis. The patient developed hepatic dysfunction shortly after the initiation of anti-TB therapy. RMP was suspected for this adverse effect, and this drug was omitted from the regimen. Although CT analysis indicated pericardial effusion, no abnormality was detected on coronary angiography. Hematologic analysis revealed a significant drop in platelet count (to $34 \times 10^9/L$) and $\sim44.5\%$ elevation of eosinophil from the normal range. The patient shortly experienced cardiac arrest requiring CPR and mechanical ventilation and drug therapy including noradrenaline and methylprednisolone. Based on biopsy analysis, the patient was diagnosed with eosinophilic myocarditis. EMB was replaced with ofloxacin and RMP was reintroduced in the anti-TB drug regimen. After the removal of steroid from the regimen, eosinophil level elevated again. Notably, eosinophil count returned to normal level following the withdrawal of INH, while other drugs were kept intact in the regimen concluding the association of INH with eosinophilic myocarditis.

Although INH rarely produces cutaneous adverse reactions, Bondalpati et al. have reported leukocytoclastic vasculitis in a 64-year-old patient with extra pulmonary TB (Pott's Spine) following the 4-days of treatment with a multi-drug regimen containing INH, RMP, PZA and EMB [67c]. Through a low-dose challenge study, authors confirmed this adverse effect was associated with INH. The report highlights the need of vigilance and awareness while prescribing INH to patients.

Hepatotoxicity and Pancreatitis

Hepatotoxicity represents one of the classic adverse effects of INH therapy. Given that INH is often administered in conjunction with other drugs, there is an increased concern over the exacerbation of adverse effects particularly, among patients taking multi-drug antiretroviral therapy (ART) and IPT. Tedla et al. addressed this question by conducting a randomized trial study among 1006 HIV patients who received IPT for 36 months and ART in conjunction with or after IPT therapy [68C]. The study revealed mild, moderate and severe levels hepatitis among 12.8%, 3.4%, 1.6% patients, respectively. Notably, 40% of the moderate to severe cases were reported during first 2 months of IPT initiation, whereas

84% of severe cases were reported within first 9 months of IPT treatment. Jaundice and hepatic encephalopathy were most common among patients with severe hepatotoxicity. As acetylation represents the major route for metabolism of INH, fast acetylators are less likely to experience INH-related adverse effects compared to slow acetylators. This was further corroborated by a retrospective study, which revealed a positive correlation of plasma INH level with hepatotoxicity. In a study of 195 TB patients, Jeong et al. noted a lower ratio of acetylated-INH to INH among patients with hepatotoxicity compared to patients without hepatotoxicity [69C]. While a mild to moderate level of INH-induced liver injuries has been well known for years, acute pancreatitis leading to liver failure is quite rare. Saleem et al. reported such case where an 11-year-old girl developed acute pancreatitis after 2 weeks of INH therapy. Discontinuation of INH therapy reverted this adverse effect in its own [70c]. Notably, Miyazawa et al. reported a fatal liver injury caused by INH in otherwise a healthy patient [71c]. The details of this case are summarized below.

- A 53-year-old Japanese man with l LTBI was given with INH (daily dose of 300 mg) as a preventive therapy following his exposure to a person with active TB despite the negative diagnostic tests for active TB such as chest X-ray and QuantiFERON-TB2 G blood test (QFTs). After 70 days of treatment, the patient developed jaundice and general malaise. The treatment was continued for additional 10 days, and the patient was referred to the hospital for possible hepatic disorder. He was presented with severe jaundice as indicated by scleral icterus. Further lab analysis revealed an extremely elevated level of liver enzymes such as aspartate aminotransferase (AST, 1581 IU/L) alanine aminotransferase (ALT, 2540 IU/L) and γ-glutamyl transpeptidase (γ-GTP, 553 IU/L). However, common markers for viral hepatitis were all negative. Treatment with ursodeoxycholic acid temporarily improve the level of liver enzymes, he was diagnosed with liver atrophy within 12 days of admission. The patient was then suffered from infection of *Enterobacter aerogenes* which followed the diagnosis of Grade II hepatic encephalopathy. Although the patient's hepatic encephalopathy improved to grade I level following hemodiafiltration (HDF) for 3 days, further liver atrophy was detected on a computed tomography (CT) scan on the 18th day indicating an irreversible nature of liver damage. The patient died of liver failure after 4 months.

Erythroderma

Although erythroderma is known to be a rare, yet potentially a fatal adverse effect of anti-TB treatment, Garg

et al. have presented this adverse effect associated with INH therapy in a case report [72c]. Authors reported the development of generalized redness, scaling and itching after 8 weeks of anti-TB drugs therapy. Sequential challenge study confirmed the association of these adverse effects with the INH. A similar incidence was also reported in a patient with tubercular lymphadenitis [73c].

Pulmonary Fibrosis

Although there are handful of reports on INH-induced pneumonitis [74c,75c], pulmonary fibrosis represents a rare side effect of anti-TB medications. Chung et al. recently reported such case [76c].

- A 42-year-old man was presented with symptoms typical of TB such as night sweating, uninterrupted fever, weight loss and dyspnea on exercise. CT scan indicated pleural effusion on the right side, and further analysis of biopsy suggested that pleurisy was associated with TB. The treatment of the patient with INH, RPT, EMB and PZA diminished the symptoms gradually. However, the patient complained of worsened dyspnea and cough again. The chest images revealed bilateral lung infiltrations, glass ground opacity and reticular opacity. Biopsy data indicated interstitial inflammation with fibrosis. Although authors could not confirm the exact cause of this condition, INH was suspected to cause pneumonitis at early stage which might have then progressed to lung fibrosis within couple of weeks of treatment. Further studies are needed to identify the definitive cause.

Metabolic Disorders

Literatures concerning drug-induced metabolic disorders are rapidly growing. This is particularly the case for polypharmacy. Among them, drug-induced hyperglycemia has recently received significant attention [77H]. Such metabolic conditions as a result of adverse effects of anti-TB drugs are quite rare. Notably, Manish and co-workers have reported an INH-induced diabetes in a 6-year-old female alerting practitioners for a need to a close monitoring of blood sugar level patients while they are on INH therapy [78c]. Metabolic acidosis is another common side effect of INH therapy. However, it is quite rare with commonly used doses. There were a handful of case reports of INH-indicated metabolic acidosis and renal damage induced by INH therapy [79c,80c].

LINEZOLID

A systematic review and meta-analysis in the period January 2000 to May 2014, suggested that linezolid

(LNZ) is a promising and viable option for treating DR-TB patients. The pooled analysis showed that LNZ was associated with a promising favorable outcome in 83% of treated patients with sputum conversion in 89% of them [81M]. In Madrid Spain, a retrospective study of a series of MDR-TB diagnosed patients suggested that a 600 mg daily LNZ dosage as safe, with rare adverse effects [82R]. In the period 1998–2014, only 4 of 21 patients with MDR-TB that received LNZ treatment developed toxicity attributed to LNZ. The most serious adverse events in these patients were anemia in the 2 patients treated with 1200 mg per day and moderate paresthesia in 1 patient. In both cases, anemia and paresthesia improved when the dosage was reduced to 600 mg per day. Similarly, a retrospective study conducted in Chinese adults indicated that LNZ was a well-tolerated and efficient treatment for extensively drug-resistant (XDR) pulmonary TB [83c]. Of the 16 patients who received LNZ (600 mg daily) as part of their individualized treatment regimens, 11 had successfully completed therapy with documented negative quantitative PCR (qPCR) data and cultures at follow-up (mean = 12 months). LNZ was discontinued for 2 patients because of intractable diarrhea and nausea shortly after beginning treatment.

Several prospective studies of LNZ for the treatment of extensively drug-resistant tuberculosis (XDR-TB) have been conducted [84r,85c,86c]. However, these studies were limited by the small number of patients enrolled. A prospective controlled trial monitored the translational competence of mitochondria isolated from peripheral blood of the 38 participants. Those on 600 mg once a day of LNZ had a significantly higher risk of mitochondrial toxicity-associated adverse events than those on 300 mg [85c]. The second study monitored 38 patients with chronic XDR-TB who were receiving LNZ treatment. Of the 38 patients, 27 had negative results on sputum culture 1 year after the end of treatment. Of the 27, eventually 14 had dose reductions from 600 to 300 mg due to adverse events. Additional serious adverse events were resolved after the discontinuation of LNZ. Twenty-seven of 38 patients were cured of the infection at 1 year after the termination of the study. Notably, there were no relapses in the patients in the first year [84r]. The third prospective study involved a randomized, controlled clinical trial, recruiting 65 XDR-TB patients who started individualized anti-TB regimens containing LNZ (600 mg twice a day) for ~1 month and were then shifted to 600 or 300 mg once a day. LNZ was prescribed to 33 patients. After 2 years, the proportion of sputum-culture conversion was outstanding in those exposed to LNZ-containing regimens when compared with those in the control arm (78.8% versus 37.6%) [86c].

Visual Disturbance

A case illustrated that even moderate doses of LNZ taken over a short period of time can be associated with reversible optic neuropathy [87c]. The results supported the hypothesis that the optic nerve changes were most likely secondary to LNZ therapy.

- A 22-year-Indian male with multidrug resistant spinal TB and TB meningitis was started on second-line anti-TB drugs. The patient had been on 600 mg daily dose of LNZ for only 4 weeks along with PZA 2 g once daily, moxifloxacin 400 mg once daily and CS 250 mg twice daily. Following the treatment, the patient developed progressive asymmetrical optic neuropathy with a peripapillary nerve fiber layer hemorrhage and a relative afferent papillary defect (RAPD). Visual fields showed defects typical of optic neuropathy. Electrodiagnostics revealed low-amplitude waves on pattern visual evoked potentials (VEP), which indicated that optic nerve function was suboptimal. Besides the fact that the visual acuity and color vision of the patient improved dramatically on stopping LNZ, the RAPD also resolved, as did the visual field changes.

Optic neuropathy is a well-known cause of visual disturbances in LNZ-treated patients. However, the possibility of LNZ-related retinopathy has not been investigated. A case of retinopathy demonstrated by multifocal electroretinogram (mfERG) has been reported in a LNZ-treated patient [88c]. The mfERG findings suggest the possibility of a retinopathy through cone dysfunction.

- A 61-year-old man with extensively drug-resistant pulmonary TB treated with LNZ for 5 months presented with painless loss of vision in both eyes. The patient's best corrected visual acuity was 20/50 in the right eye and 20/100 in the left eye. Fundus examination revealed mild disc edema, and color vision was defective in both eyes. Humphrey visual field tests showed a superotemporal field defect in the right eye, and central and pericentral field defect in the left eye. Optical coherence tomography (OCT) revealed only mild optic disc swelling. In mfERG, central amplitudes were depressed in both eyes. Four months after the cessation of LNZ, visual acuity was restored to 20/20 right eye and 20/25 left eye. The color vision and visual field had improved. The OCT and mfERG findings improved as well.

The long-term use of LNZ has shown to be toxic in patients. A preclinical study reported exposure-dependent killing of M. tuberculosis by LNZ. Notably, 300 mg LNZ given every 12 hours generated more bacterial kill but caused more toxicity than 600 mg LNZ given once daily. Although the latter regimen was safer from the toxicity standpoint, none of the regimens prevented LNZ resistance [89E].

PYRAZINAMIDE

Pyrazinamide (PZA) is a first-line agent used for the treatment of TB. PZA's ability to reduce treatment time makes it one of the few anti-TB drugs that is usually maintained in all new regimens for multi-drug resistant (MDR) and extensively drug-resistant (XDR) TB. PZA is known to cause numerous adverse effects including joint pain, hepatotoxicity (hepatitis), nausea, vomiting, anorexia, anemia, urticaria, hyperuricemia, interstitial nephritis, hypersensitivity, olfactory disturbance and fever. A case report concerning PZA-induced hepatotoxicity and gastritis is presented in the following paragraph [90c].

• A 51-year-old woman with tubercular pericardial effusion received an anti-TB treatment (ATT) regimen comprised of INH 300 mg, RMP 450 mg and PZA 1500 mg, daily. Soon after starting the regimen, she developed persistent vomiting and GI irritation due to multiple hemorrhagic erosions (grade III gastritis) observed via GI scopy. Her elevated level of liver enzymes was indicative of hepatotoxicity. PZA was suspected to cause these adverse effects. As a result, PZA was replaced with EMB (1 g), and the patient was treated symptomatically with pantoprazole (40 mg, IV) BD for Gastritis, domperidone (10 mg, twice daily) for vomiting, and livogen (500 mg) for anemia. Adverse effects eventually diminished after removing PZA; GI scopy report was normal on day 15, and the patient was discharged in stable condition.

Although the mechanism of PZA-induced hepatotoxicity is not well understood, recent biochemical analysis revealed that the hydroxylated metabolite of PZA (5-OH-PZA), produced through the activity of xanthine oxidase, is responsible for the hepatotoxic effects [91E]. Notably, a retrospective analysis revealed PZA-related hepatotoxicity occurred in 10 out of 17 patients who were on anti-TB regimens containing PZA [69C].

Rare side effects of PZA that were recently observed include olfactory disturbance [92c] and myopathy [93c].

• A 63-year-old man with TB was treated with a multi-drug regimen including INH (400 mg), RMP (600 mg), PZA (1250 mg), EMB (800 mg) and streptomycin (STR, 750 mg). On the fourth day of treatment, the patient complained of poor appetite, itchy skin, and nausea. In addition, the patient also notated a major change in the original smell of food, which severely impacted his appetite. Discontinuation of the regimen relieved the symptoms gradually. After being re-challenged with PZA (1500 mg), the patient noted similar side effects as before. Discontinuation of PZA again resolved the symptoms gradually [92c].

Although the exact mechanism of PZA-mediated dysomia has not been well established, it is proposed that pyrazinoic acid—the active metabolite of PZA—accumulates within native bacilli, killing the bacteria and contributing to olfactory disturbances [92c,94E].

• A 26-year-old man with pulmonary TB developed polyarthralgia, myalgia, weakness, elevated levels of creatine kinase (CK) and uric after receiving PZA therapy. Upon cessation of PZA, the patient experienced immediate improvements in polyarthralgia. Discontinuation also resulted in improvements in myalgia and CK, but these improvements were delayed [93c].

RIFAMYCIN

Rifamycin antibiotics—also known as rifamycins—are first-line tuberculosis (TB) treatments with rifamycin SV, rifampicin (or rifampin, RMP), rifaximin, rifabutin (RBT), and rifapentine (RPT) approved by the U.S. Food and Drug Administration (FDA). Of these, RMP is most commonly used as first-line therapy alone or in combination with other agents for treatment of mycobacterial diseases including TB. Many of the previously known adverse effects of rifamycins were reiterated in literature during 2015. The notable ones include RMP-induced renal toxicity, immunologic reactions and hepatotoxicity. Although RMP-induced acute kidney injuries including interstitial nephritis commonly occur at higher doses [95R], reports of minimal change disease (MCD) caused by this drug are quite rare. Park and co-workers have reported an incident in a 68-year-old female patient with pleural TB [96c]. A separate case study noted the induction of leukocytoclastic vasculitis (LCV) by RMP therapy in a 12-year-old female pulmonary TB patient [97c]. LCV is characterized by inflammation of the small vessels causing palpable purpura and other symptoms including petechial, exhaustion, myalgia, arthralgia, and pyrexia. Although LCV caused by anti-TB drugs is rarely observed, it can occur during multi-drug therapy prompting for alternative therapies.

Variations exist among members of rifamycins resulting in differing inclusion in multi-drug regimens and dosing. The differences in therapeutic outcomes and adverse effects among members of rifamycins when used in conjunction with other drugs are not fully established yet. In this context, a study investigated TB patients receiving either RPT 450, RPT 600, or RMP 600 daily for 8 weeks with INH, PZA, and EMB. Notably, adverse effects were similar among the groups. The most common side effects included pruritus/rash, nausea and/or vomiting, diarrhea, musculoskeletal and haemoptysis [98c].

Teratogenic

Although the risk of teratogenic effects of first-line anti-TB drugs during pregnancy is considered minimal, a case of limb deformity has been reported in the following case study [99c].

- A male newborn was born with a hypoplastic right forearm to a mother with TB who was on isoniazid and RMP during the first 2 months of her pregnancy. In the absence of other risk factors such as exposure to medications other than anti-TB drugs, chronic disease, diabetes mellitus, smoking history and viral infections during and after conceptions, the anomaly could be attributed to RMP/INH usage during the first trimester of pregnancy. However, more studies are needed to validate/refute this hypothesis.

Hepatotoxicity

Hepatotoxicity is one of the most common side effects of RMP and INH. A study was conducted to determine risk factors for drug-induced hepatotoxicity from anti-TB therapy. Patients received the following anti-TB regimen: streptomycin (STR) 0.75 gm IM (<50 years) and 0.50 gm (>50 years), RMP: <450 mg/day (for patients with body weight <50 kg); 600 mg (patients with body weight >50 kg); INH: 600 mg (10–15 mg/kg), EMB: 1200 mg (30 mg/kg), and PZA: 1500 mg (30–35 mg/kg). Notably, drug-induced liver injury (DILI) occurred in 3.8% of the patients in the study (150 patients out of total cohort of 3900 patients). DILI developed after starting anti-TB therapy in 20 days and lasted 14 days on average. The study showed several risk factors for developing DILI including: prior history of hepatitis, age >60 years, female sex, alcohol consumption, previous anti-TB therapy, hypoalbuminemia, extensive nature of disease, and diabetes mellitus [100C]. Liver toxicity was observed in 33% (23 of 69 patients) of patients with solid organ transplants [101c]. The authors concluded the daily doses (≥600 mg) of RMP to be an independent risk factor ($p=0.016$; OR 2.47; 95% CI: 1.18–5.15). Mortality in patients with hepatotoxicity (43.5%) was more than twofold that of patients with normal liver function (19.6%). Jeong et al. also reported hepatotoxicity in 17 (8.7%) of the 195 TB patients who were on multi-drug (INH, RMP, PZA, and EMB) therapy [69C]. The report fell short in identifying/quantifying the extent of liver injury caused by individual drug, and intergroup differences of serum concentration of individual drug were not statistically significant.

Drug–Drug Interaction

RMP is a well known inducer of cytochrome P450 3A4 isoform (CYP3A4). Many studies reported interactions of RMP with other drugs in 2015. A case report indicated a need of increasing the dose of clozapine from the regular dose (300 mg/day) to the maximum dose 1000 mg/day to control schizophrenia in a patient, while he was treated for TB with a four-drug (RMP, INH, PZA and moxifloxacin) regimen. RMP-induced metabolism of clozapine can be hypothesized for faster clearance of clozapine thereby producing inadequate pharmacological outcome [102R]. Similarly, a Phase I study involving 32 patients showed that RMP and RBT can contribute to decrease plasma levels of BDQ. Pharmacokinetic analysis revealed 4.78- and 3.96-fold increase in clearance of BDQ with RMP and RBT, respectively [103c]. These reports align well with the literature precedent concerning interactions of rifamycins with other drugs, particularly those which are metabolized by CYP3A4.

Latent Tuberculosis Infection

Latent tuberculosis infection (LTBI) and human immunodeficiency virus (HIV)-coinfection are challenges in the control of TB transmission. In December 2, 2014, the U.S. FDA approved RPT in combination with INH for a new indication for the treatment of LTBI in patients 2 years of age and older at high risk of progression to TB disease [104r]. Evidence summarized from systematic literature search and data extraction of effectiveness and safety of RPT–INH combination therapy compared to LTBI INH monotherapy in the general and HIV-positive population, suggested no differences between RPT–INH short-course treatment and the standard INH therapy in reducing active TB incidence or death [105R]. However, there is limited data for a 3-month once-weekly combination of RPT and INH for treatment of LTBI in children. A recent clinical trial results showed treatment with the combination-therapy group was as effective as INH-only treatment for the prevention of TB in children aged 2–17 years [106MC]. The combination-therapy group reportedly had a higher treatment completion rate than did the INH-only group and was safe. In the safety population, 3 of 539 participants (0.6%) in the combination-therapy group had a grade 3 adverse events (AE) vs 1 of 493 (0.2%) who received INH only. Neither arm had any hepatotoxicity, grade 4 AEs, or treatment-attributed death [106MC].

Pediatrics

For young children (≤5 years of age) undergoing co-treatment of HIV and TB, it remains unclear whether a safe and effective RBT dose exists. In an open-label study with 6 children, when RBT dosed at 5 mg/kg three times a week was given to children receiving lopinavir/ritonavir, a decline in neutrophil count was observed in all children while two children experienced grade 4 neutropenia which resolved rapidly without complications [107c]. Although these observations caution practitioners, further studies involving larger sample sizes are needed to confirm these adverse effects.

STREPTOMYCIN

The increased prevalence of MDR-TB has caused an increase in the use of second-line treatment agents. Streptomycin (STR) use in MDR-TB has decreased in recent years because of the development of bacterial resistance and adverse effects. Published adverse effects of STR include fever, rash, tinnitus, ataxia and nephrotoxicity. A study by Tag El Din et al. assessed the adverse reactions of second-line TB drugs, including STR, in patients being treated for MDR-TB. The study included 107 patients during the period of January 2009 to January 2012. To be included, patients had to be resistant to at least RMP and INH. Of the patients that received STR ($n = 7$), 5.3% developed ototoxicity ($p = 0.084\%$), 7.1% developed hypokalemia ($p = 0.881$), 10% developed hepatotoxicity ($p = 0.642$), 0% developed hypothyroidism ($p = 0.629$), 8.2% developed GIT manifestations ($p = 0.927$), and 28.6% developed PN ($p = 0.175$) [108C]. A literature review also revealed alterations in male reproductive organs as a result of STR therapy in addition to low sperm count and poor sperm motility [46R].

References

[1] Field SK. Bedaquiline for the treatment of multidrug-resistant tuberculosis: great promise or disappointment? Ther Adv Chronic Dis. 2015;6:170–84 [r].

[2] Pym AS, Diacon AH, Tang SJ, et al. Bedaquiline in the treatment of multidrug- and extensively drug-resistant tuberculosis. Eur Respir J. 2016;47:564–74 [MC].

[3] Philley JV, Wallace Jr. RJ, Benwill JL, et al. Preliminary results of bedaquiline as salvage therapy for patients with nontuberculous mycobacterial lung disease. Chest. 2015;148:499–506 [c].

[4] Bedaquiline. More data needed on this dangerous antitubercular drug. Prescrire Int. 2014;23:232–4 [C].

[5] Guglielmetti L, Le Du D, Jachym M, et al. Compassionate use of bedaquiline for the treatment of multidrug-resistant and extensively drug-resistant tuberculosis: interim analysis of a French cohort. Clin Infect Dis. 2015;60:188–94 [c].

[6] Ndjeka N, Conradie F, Schnippel K, et al. Treatment of drug-resistant tuberculosis with bedaquiline in a high HIV prevalence setting: an interim cohort analysis. Int J Tuberc Lung Dis. 2015;19:979–85 [c].

[7] Narang T, Dogra S, Sakia UN. Persistent serpentine supravenous hyperpigmented eruption in lepromatous leprosy after minocycline. Lepr Rev. 2015;86:191–4 [c].

[8] Tang S, Yao L, Hao X, et al. Clofazimine for the treatment of multidrug-resistant tuberculosis: prospective, multicenter, randomized controlled study in China. Clin Infect Dis. 2015;60:1361–7 [C].

[9] Jarand J, Davis JP, Cowie RL, et al. Long term follow up of Mycobacterium avium complex lung disease in patients treated with regimens including clofazimine and/or rifampin. Chest. 2016;149:1285–93 [C].

[10] Saraf G, Akshata JS, Kuruthukulangara S, et al. Cycloserine induced delirium during treatment of multi-drug resistant tuberculosis (MDR-TB). Egypt J Chest Dis Tuberc. 2015;64:449–51 [c].

[11] Tandon VR, Rani N, Roshi, et al. Cycloserine induced psychosis with hepatic dysfunction. Indian J Pharmacol. 2015;47:230–1 [c].

[12] Schade S, Paulus W. D-cycloserine in neuropsychiatric diseases: a systematic. Int J Neuropsychopharmacol. 2016;19:1–7 [R].

[13] Kantrowitz JT, Halberstam B, Gangwisch J. Single-dose ketamine followed by daily D-cycloserine in treatment-resistant bipolar depression. J Clin Psychiatry. 2015;76:737–8 [c].

[14] Sawant NS, Kate NS, Bhatankar SS, et al. Neuroleptic malignant syndrome in cycloserine-induced psychosis. Indian J Pharmacol. 2015;47:328–9 [c].

[15] Blair HA, Scott LJ. Delamanid: a review of its use in patients with multidrug-resistant tuberculosis. Drugs. 2015;75:91–100 [R].

[16] World Health Organization Interim Policy Guidance. The use of delamanid in the treatment of multidrug-resistant tuberculosis. Geneva, Switzerland: WHO Press; 2014 [s].

[17] Szumowski JD, Lynch JB. Profile of delamanid for the treatment of multidrug-resistant tuberculosis. Drug Des Devel Ther. 2015;9:677–82 [r].

[18] Karjigi S, Murthy SC, Kallappa H, et al. Early onset dapsone-induced photosensitive dermatitis: a rare side effect of a common drug. Indian J Lepr. 2015;87:161–4 [c].

[19] Gavilanes MC, Palacio AL, Chellini PR, et al. Dapsone hypersensitivity syndrome in a lepromatous leprosy patient—a case report. Lepr Rev. 2015;86:186–90 [c].

[20] Quaresma MV, Bernardes Filho F, Hezel J, et al. Dapsone in the treatment of pemphigus vulgaris: adverse effects and its importance as a corticosteroid sparing agent. An Bras Dermatol. 2015;90:51–4 [c].

[21] Sauvetre G, MahEvas M, Limal N, et al. Cutaneous rash and dapsone-induced hypersensitivity syndrome a common manifestation in adult immune thrombocytopenia. Presentation and outcome in 16 cases. Am J Hematol. 2015;90:E201–2 [c].

[22] Furuta K, Ikeo S, Takaiwa T, et al. Identifying the cause of the "Saturation Gap": two cases of dapsone-induced methemoglobinemia. Intern Med. 2015;54:1639–41 [c].

[23] Swartzentruber GS, Yanta JH, Pizon AF. Methemoglobinemia as a complication of topical dapsone. N Engl J Med. 2015;372:491–2 [c].

[24] Watton C, Smith K, Carter E. Methemoglobinemia as a complication of topical dapsone. N Engl J Med. 2015;372:492 [r].

[25] Hanuschk D, Kozyreff A, Tafzi N, et al. Acute visual loss following dapsone-induced methemoglobinemia and hemolysis. Clin Toxicol (Phila). 2015;53:489–92 [c].

[26] Sunilkumar MN, Ajith TA, Parvathy VK. Acute dapsone poisoning in a 3-year-old child: case report with review of literature. World J Clin Cases. 2015;3:911–4 [c].

[27] Lewis JA, Petty WJ, Harmon M, et al. Hemolytic anemia in two patients with glioblastoma multiforme: a possible interaction between vorinostat and dapsone. J Oncol Pharm Pract. 2015;21:220–3 [c].

[28] Kim KL, Park SP. Visual function test for early detection of ethambutol induced ocular toxicity at the subclinical level. Cutan Ocul Toxicol. 2016;35:228–32 [c].

[29] Chen SC, Lin MC, Sheu SJ. Incidence and prognostic factor of ethambutol-related optic neuropathy: 10-year experience in southern Taiwan. Kaohsiung J Med Sci. 2015;31:358–62 [C].

[30] Louthrenoo W, Hongsongkiat S, Kasitanon N, et al. Effect of antituberculous drugs on serum uric acid and urine uric acid excretion. J Clin Rheumatol. 2015;21:346–8 [c].

[31] Holla S, Amberkar MB, Bhandarypanambur R, et al. Cycloserine induced late onset psychosis and ethambutol induced peripheral neuropathy associated with MDR-TB treatment in an Indian patient—a rare case report. J Clin Diagn Res. 2015;9:FD01–3 [c].

[32] Han J, Byun MK, Lee J, et al. Longitudinal analysis of retinal nerve fiber layer and ganglion cell-inner plexiform layer thickness in ethambutol-induced optic neuropathy. Graefes Arch Clin Exp Ophthalmol. 2015;253:2293–9 [c].

[33] Rasool M, Malik A, Manan A, et al. Determination of potential role of antioxidative status and circulating biochemical markers in the pathogenesis of ethambutol induced toxic optic neuropathy among diabetic and non-diabetic patients. Saudi J Biol Sci. 2015;22:739–43 [c].

[34] Doherty AM, Kelly J, McDonald C, et al. A review of the interplay between tuberculosis and mental health. Gen Hosp Psychiatry. 2013;35:398–406 [R].

[35] Yen YF, Chung MS, Hu HY, et al. Association of pulmonary tuberculosis and ethambutol with incident depressive disorder: a nationwide, population-based cohort study. J Clin Psychiatry. 2015;76:e505–11 [E].

[36] Bakayoko AS, Kaloga M, Kamagate M, et al. Fixed drug eruption after taking ethambutol. Rev Mal Respir. 2015;32:48–51 [c].

[37] Ramachandran G, Swaminathan S. Safety and tolerability profile of second-line anti-tuberculosis medications. Drug Saf. 2015;38:253–69 [R].

[38] Ramani YR, Mishra SK, Rath B, et al. Ofloxacin induced cutaneous reactions in children. J Clin Diagn Res. 2015;9:Fd01–2 [c].

[39] Charfi O, Lakhoua G, Sahnoun R, et al. DRESS syndrome following levofloxacin exposure with positive patch-test. Therapie. 2015;70:547–9 [c].

[40] Golomb BA, Koslik HJ, Redd AJ. Fluoroquinolone-induced serious, persistent, multisymptom adverse effects. BMJ Case Rep. 2015;2015:1–10 [c].

[41] Torre-Cisneros J, San-Juan R, Rosso-Fernandez CM, et al. Tuberculosis prophylaxis with levofloxacin in liver transplant patients is associated with a high incidence of tenosynovitis: safety analysis of a multicenter randomized trial. Clin Infect Dis. 2015;60:1642–9 [MC].

[42] Lee CC, Lee MT, Chen YS, et al. Risk of aortic dissection and aortic aneurysm in patients taking oral fluoroquinolone. JAMA Intern Med. 2015;175:1839–47 [MC].

[43] Chen Z, Liang JQ, Wang JH, et al. Moxifloxacin plus standard first-line therapy in the treatment of pulmonary tuberculosis: a meta-analysis. Tuberculosis (Edinb). 2015;95:490–6 [M].

[44] Chui CS, Wong IC, Wong LY, et al. Association between oral fluoroquinolone use and the development of retinal detachment: a systematic review and meta-analysis of observational studies. J Antimicrob Chemother. 2015;70:971–8 [M].

[45] Erdemli O, Timuroglu A, Oral I, et al. Ciprofloxacin-induced severe thrombocytopenia. Kaohsiung J Med Sci. 2015;31:110–1 [c].

[46] Khaki A. Assessment on the adverse effects of aminoglycosides and flouroquinolone on sperm parameters and male reproductive tissue: a systematic review. Iran J Reprod Med. 2015;13:125–34 [R].

[47] Patel TK, Thakkar SH, Sharma D. Cutaneous adverse drug reactions in Indian population: a systematic review. Indian Dermatol Online J. 2014;5:S76–86 [R].

[48] Shayakhmetova GM, Bondarenko LB, Voronina AK, et al. Induction of CYP2E1 in testes of isoniazid-treated rats as possible cause of testicular disorders. Toxicol Lett. 2015;234:59–66 [E].

[49] Group TAS, Danel C, Moh R, et al. A trial of early antiretrovirals and isoniazid preventive therapy in Africa. N Engl J Med. 2015;373:808–22 [C].

[50] Villarino ME, Scott NA, Weis SE, et al. Treatment for preventing tuberculosis in children and adolescents: a randomized clinical trial of a 3-month, 12-dose regimen of a combination of rifapentine and isoniazid. JAMA Pediatr. 2015;169:247–55 [MC].

[51] Horsburgh Jr. CR, Rubin EJ. Clinical practice. Latent tuberculosis infection in the United States. N Engl J Med. 2011;364:1441–8 [r].

[52] Akolo C, Adetifa I, Shepperd S, et al. Treatment of latent tuberculosis infection in HIV infected persons. Cochrane Database Syst Rev. 2010;20:CD000171 [M].

[53] Getahun H, Matteelli A, Chaisson RE, et al. Latent Mycobacterium tuberculosis infection. N Engl J Med. 2015;372:2127–35 [R].

[54] Churchyard GJ, Fielding KL, Grant AD. A trial of mass isoniazid preventive therapy for tuberculosis control. N Engl J Med. 2014;370:1662–3 [C].

[55] Samandari T, Agizew TB, Nyirenda S, et al. Tuberculosis incidence after 36 months' isoniazid prophylaxis in HIV-infected adults in Botswana: a posttrial observational analysis. AIDS. 2015;29:351–9 [c].

[56] World Health Organization (WHO). Guidelines for intensified tuberculosis case-finding and isoniazid preventive therapy for people living with HIV in resource constrained setting. Geneva, Switzerland: WHO Press; 2011 [s].

[57] Tejada F, Walk A, Kharel M. Drugs used in tuberculosis and leprosy. Side Effects Drugs Annual. 2015;37:349–65 [R].

[58] Stennis NL, Burzynski JN, Herbert C, et al. Treatment for tuberculosis infection with 3 months of isoniazid and rifapentine in New York City Health Department Clinics. Clin Infect Dis. 2016;62:53–9 [C].

[59] Mafukidze AT, Calnan M, Furin J. Peripheral neuropathy in persons with tuberculosis. J Clin Tuberc Other Mycobact Dis. 2016;2:5–11 [c].

[60] Aiwale AS, Patel UA, Barvaliya MJ, et al. Isoniazid induced convulsions at therapeutic dose in an alcoholic and smoker patient. Curr Drug Saf. 2015;10:94–5 [c].

[61] Iannaccone R, Sue YJ, Avner JR. Suicidal psychosis secondary to isoniazid. Pediatr Emerg Care. 2002;18:25–7 [c].

[62] Schrestha S, Alao A. Isoniazid-induced psychosis. Psychosomatics. 2009;50:640–1 [r].

[63] Alao AO, Yolles JC. Isoniazid-induced psychosis. Ann Pharmacother. 1998;32:889–91 [R].

[64] Baytunca MB, Erermis S, Bildik T, et al. Isoniazid-induced psychosis with obsessive-compulsive symptoms (schizo-obsessive disorder) in a female child. J Child Adolesc Psychopharmacol. 2015;25:819–20 [c].

[65] Onila SO, Oyedeji GA, Oninla OA, et al. Isoniazid-induced psychosis in 2 children treated for tuberculosis: case reports and literature review. Int J Med Pharm Case Reports. 2016;6:1–6 [c].

[66] Zhang SN, He QX, Yang NB, et al. Isoniazid-induced drug rash with eosinophilia and systemic symptoms (DRESS) syndrome presenting as acute eosinophilic myocarditis. Intern Med. 2015;54:1227–30 [c].

[67] Bondalapati S, DR V, Rampure D, et al. Isoniazid induced cutaneous leukocytoclastic vasculitis in extra pulmonary tuberculosis (Pott's spine): a case report. J Clin Diagn Res. 2014;8:MD03–5 [c].

[68] Tedla Z, Nguyen ML, Sibanda T, et al. Isoniazid-associated hepatitis in adults infected with HIV receiving 36 months of isoniazid prophylaxis in Botswana. Chest. 2015;147:1376–84 [C].

[69] Jeong I, Park JS, Cho YJ, et al. Drug-induced hepatotoxicity of anti-tuberculosis drugs and their serum levels. J Korean Med Sci. 2015;30:167–72 [C].

[70] Saleem AF, Arbab S, Naz FQ. Isoniazid induced acute pancreatitis in a young girl. J Coll Physicians Surg Pak. 2015;25:299–300 [c].

[71] Miyazawa S, Matsuoka S, Hamana S, et al. Isoniazid-induced acute liver failure during preventive therapy for latent tuberculosis infection. Intern Med. 2015;54:591–5 [c].

[72] Garg Y, Gore R, Jain S, et al. A rare case of isoniazid-induced erythroderma. Indian J Pharmacol. 2015;47:682–4 [c].

[73] Uppu B, Muppur A, Devi V. A case report—INH induced erythroderma in a patient with tubercular lymphadenitis. IOSR J Dent Med Sci. 2015;14:17–9 [c].

[74] Endo T, Saito T, Nakayama M, et al. A case of isoniazid-induced pneumonitis. Nihon Kokyuki Gakkai Zasshi. 1998;36:100–5 [c].

[75] Suzuki N, Ohno S, Takeuchi Y, et al. A case of isoniazid (INH)-induced pneumonitis. Nihon Kyobu Shikkan Gakkai Zasshi. 1992;30:1563–8 [c].

[76] Chung CU, Park DI, Lee CS, et al. Isoniazid and pulmonary fibrosis. Chin Med J (Engl). 2015;128:702–3 [c].

[77] American Diabetes Association. Diagnosis and classification of diabetes mellitus. Diabetes Care. 2013;36:S67–74 [H].

[78] Manish G, Keshav GK, Syed RM, et al. Isoniazid induced childhood diabetes: a rare phenomenon. J Basic Clin Pharm. 2015;6:74–6 [c].

[79] Kaur U, Chakrabarti SS, Gambhir IS. Isoniazid induced metabolic acidosis and renal dysfunction in an elderly patient with chronic renal disease. Curr Drug Saf. 2015;11:181–3 [c].

[80] Stettner M, Steinberger D, Hartmann CJ, et al. Isoniazid-induced polyneuropathy in a tuberculosis patient—implication for individual risk stratification with genotyping? Brain Behav. 2015;5:e00326 [c].

[81] Zhang X, Falagas ME, Vardakas KZ, et al. Systematic review and meta-analysis of the efficacy and safety of therapy with linezolid containing regimens in the treatment of multidrug-resistant and extensively drug-resistant tuberculosis. J Thorac Dis. 2015;7:603–15 [M].

[82] Ramirez-Lapausa M, Pascual Pareja JF, Carrillo Gomez R, et al. Retrospective study of tolerability and efficacy of linezolid in patients with multidrug-resistant tuberculosis (1998–2014). Enferm Infecc Microbiol Clin. 2016;34:85–90 [R].

[83] Liu Y, Bao P, Wang D, et al. Clinical outcomes of linezolid treatment for extensively drug-resistant tuberculosis in Beijing, China: a hospital-based retrospective study. Jpn J Infect Dis. 2015;68:244–7 [c].

[84] Lee M, Cho SN, Barry 3rd CE, et al. Linezolid for XDR-TB—final study outcomes. N Engl J Med. 2015;373:290–1 [r].

[85] Song T, Lee M, Jeon HS, et al. Linezolid trough concentrations correlate with mitochondrial toxicity-related adverse events in the treatment of chronic extensively drug-resistant tuberculosis. EBioMedicine. 2015;2:1627–33 [c].

[86] Tang S, Yao L, Hao X, et al. Efficacy, safety and tolerability of linezolid for the treatment of XDR-TB: a study in China. Eur Respir J. 2015;45:161–70 [c].

[87] Agrawal R, Addison P, Saihan Z, et al. Optic neuropathy secondary to linezolid for multidrug-resistant mycobacterial spinal tuberculosis. Ocul Immunol Inflamm. 2015;23:90–2 [c].

[88] Park DH, Park TK, Ohn YH, et al. Linezolid induced retinopathy. Doc Ophthalmol. 2015;131:237–44 [c].

[89] Brown AN, Drusano GL, Adams JR, et al. Preclinical evaluations to identify optimal linezolid regimens for tuberculosis therapy. MBio. 2015;6:1–8 [E].

[90] Yasaswini B, James A, Sudhakar R, et al. Pyrazinamide induced multiple adverse drug reactions: a case report. World J Pharmacy Pharm Sci. 2015;4:1317–20 [c].

[91] Shih TY, Pai CY, Yang P, et al. A novel mechanism underlies the hepatotoxicity of pyrazinamide. Antimicrob Agents Chemother. 2013;57:1685–90 [E].

[92] Tsou CC, Chien JY. Olfactory disturbance related to pyrazinamide. QJM. 2014;107:217–8 [c].

[93] Shah R, Venkatesan P. Drug-induced myopathy in a patient with pulmonary tuberculosis. BMJ Case Rep. 2015;2015. http://dx.doi.org/10.1136/bcr-2014-206906 PMID:26177994, [c].

[94] Shi W, Zhang X, Jiang X, et al. Pyrazinamide inhibits trans-translation in Mycobacterium tuberculosis. Science. 2011;333:1630–2 [E].

[95] Silva Junior GB, Daher Ede F, Pires Neto Rda J, et al. Leprosy nephropathy: a review of clinical and histopathological features. Rev Inst Med Trop Sao Paulo. 2015;57:15–20 [R].

[96] Park DH, Lee SA, Jeong HJ, et al. Rifampicin-induced minimal change disease is improved after cessation of rifampicin without steroid therapy. Yonsei Med J. 2015;56:582–5 [c].

[97] Avcu G, Sensoy G, Celiksoy MH, et al. Cutaneous leukocytoclastic vasculitis associated with anti-tuberculosis drugs. Pediatr Int. 2015;57:155–7 [c].

[98] Dawson R, Narunsky K, Carman D, et al. Two-stage activity-safety study of daily rifapentine during intensive phase treatment of pulmonary tuberculosis. Int J Tuberc Lung Dis. 2015;19:780–6 [c].

[99] Kalayci T, Erener-Ercan T, Buyukkale G, et al. Limb deformity in a newborn. Is rifampicin just an innocent bystander? Eur Rev Med Pharmacol Sci. 2015;19:517–9 [c].

[100] Gaude GS, Chaudhury A, Hattiholi J. Drug-induced hepatitis and the risk factors for liver injury in pulmonary tuberculosis patients. J Family Med Prim Care. 2015;4:238–43 [C].

[101] Schultz V, Marroni CA, Amorim CS, et al. Risk factors for hepatotoxicity in solid organ transplants recipients being treated for tuberculosis. Transplant Proc. 2014;46:3606–10 [c].

[102] Gee S, Dixon T, Docherty M, et al. Optimising plasma levels of clozapine during metabolic interactions: a review and case report with adjunct rifampicin treatment. BMC Psychiatry. 2015;15:195 [R].

[103] Svensson EM, Murray S, Karlsson MO, et al. Rifampicin and rifapentine significantly reduce concentrations of bedaquiline, a new anti-TB drug. J Antimicrob Chemother. 2015;70:1106–14 [c].

[104] Sanofi. Sanofi receives fda approval of priftin® (rifapentine) tablets for the treatment of latent tuberculosis infection. http://www.news.sanofi.us/press-releases?item=136875. Accessed April 27, 2015. [r].

[105] Vidal JS, Silva MT, Sanchez MN. Rifapentine for latent tuberculosis infection treatment in the general population and human immunodeficiency virus-positive patients: summary of evidence. Rev Soc Bras Med Trop. 2015;48:507–13 [R].

[106] Villarino ME, Scott NA, Weis SE, et al. Treatment for preventing tuberculosis in children and adolescents: a randomized clinical trial of a 3-month, 12-dose regimen of a combination of rifapentine and isoniazid. JAMA Pediatr. 2015;169:247–55 [MC].

[107] Moultrie H, McIlleron H, Sawry S, et al. Pharmacokinetics and safety of rifabutin in young HIV-infected children receiving rifabutin and lopinavir/ritonavir. J Antimicrob Chemother. 2015;70:543–9 [c].

[108] Tag El Din M, El Maraghy A, Abdel Hay A. Adverse reactions among patients being treated for multi-drug resistant tuberculosis at Abbassia Chest Hospital. Egypt J Chest Dis Tuberc. 2015;64:939–52 [C].

29

Antihelminthic Drugs

Igho J. Onakpoya[1]

Nuffield Department of Primary Care Health Sciences, Oxford, United Kingdom
[1]Corresponding author: igho.onakpoya@phc.ox.ac.uk

ALBENDAZOLE [SEDA-35, 565; SEDA-36, 457; SEDA-37, 367]

Drug Combination Studies

The safety of albendazole in combination with ivermectin, mebendazole, or oxantel pamoate in the treatment of *Trichuris trichiura* infection has been evaluated in a randomized comparative clinical trial including 440 children [1C]. Abdominal cramps and headaches were the most common adverse events observed. No serious adverse events were observed.

The safety and pharmacokinetics of albendazole coadministered with diethylcarbamazine and ivermectin in the treatment of *Wuchereria bancrofti* infestation has been examined in a randomized clinical trial of 24 adults [2c]. Adverse events most frequently reported were headache, fever and joint pain. None of these were considered serious.

Dose Comparison Studies

In a randomized, open-label study including 70 adults participants, three modified dosage combinations were compared with standard dosage of albendazole and ivermectin for treatment of *Wuchereria bancrofti* infestation [3c]. Adverse events most commonly reported were fever, headache, joint and abdominal pains; none of these events were considered serious. There was no significant difference in adverse event rates across groups.

In a randomized four-arm trial of 104 adults with *Wuchereria bancrofti* infestation, increased dosages and frequency of administration (800 mg 6 monthly or annually) with albendazole was compared with the standard dose (300 mg annually) [4c]. The most frequent adverse events reported were light headedness, fever, body ache and

unsteadiness; none of these events was severe. At 12 months, the biannual arms had a lower frequency of adverse events compared with annual arms (3.8% vs. 28%).

Liver

Albendazole-included cirrhosis has been reported [5A].

• A 65-year-old woman followed up for Child-Pugh class A cirrhosis secondary to autoimmune hepatitis, who was treated with prednisolone and azathioprine for 5 years, was evaluated for hemoptysis. Thoracic CT showed an area of consolidation. Fine-needle aspiration biopsy was compatible with a hydatid cyst. Albendazole treatment was started. On the sixth day of therapy, she was hospitalized with abdominal distention and pruritus. Physical examination was normal except for abdominal distention. Hemoglobin was 6.6 g/dL, leucocytes $0.6 \times 10^3/\mu L$, platelets $86 \times 10^3/\mu L$, alanine aminotransferase 56 U/L, aspartate aminotransferase 57 U/L, alkaline phosphatase 184 U/L, gamma glutamyl transferase 172 U/L, total bilirubin 1.9 g/dL, albumin 2.9 g/dL, and international normalized ratio 1.4. All these parameters were normal before using albendazole. Hepatitis B virus surface antigen, hepatitis C virus antibody, and hepatitis A IgA antibody were negative. Serum ceruloplasmin level was 38 mg/dL (normal = 20–50 mg/dL). The patient had no alcohol or herbal medicine exposure. She showed no confusion. Abdominal USS revealed hepatosplenomegaly with diffuse abdominal fluid. Albendazole was stopped on admission, and clinical symptoms resolved within 1 week. Laboratory findings improved within 30 days.

The first case of autoimmune hepatitis induced by albendazole has been reported [6A].

- A 6-year-old girl was referred to an outpatient clinic with the diagnosis of liver hydatid cyst. Her physical examination and routine laboratory analyses were unremarkable. Albendazole treatment (15 mg/kg/day) was given for 2 weeks prior to performing puncture, aspiration, injection and re-aspiration (PAIR). But she was lost to follow-up and was readmitted 2 months later with abdominal pain. AST, ALT, and GGT were 663, 800, and 92 IU/L, respectively. Laboratory investigations to exclude infectious, autoimmune, and metabolic liver disease were normal. The elevated transaminase levels returned to the normal range after cessation of albendazole. At ninth month, abdominal USS revealed a progressive increase in the size of the cyst. Treatment with PAIR technique was considered. Albendazole treatment (15 mg/kg/day) was initiated again 2 weeks before the PAIR procedure. She had mild elevation of transaminase levels at time of the procedure, but albendazole was continued for a week. Three weeks later, AST and ALT were 496 and 468 IU/L. ANA titers became positive (1:100; granular pattern). Liver biopsy showed widespread portal lymphoplasmacytic inflammation with extensive interface (piecemeal) necrosis. Prednisolone and azathioprine were started. Transaminase levels rapidly decreased to normal ranges in 2 weeks. One month later, she had no complaints; physical examination and laboratory parameters were all normal. The steroid dose was tapered. Four months later, laboratory findings and clinical features were also normal. Afterwards, the dose of azathioprine was also tapered.

Hematologic

Medullary aplasia in a patient has been described [7A].

- A 57-year-old male patient with a previous diagnosis of peritoneal hydatid cyst presented with features suggestive renal insufficiency secondary to post renal compression by a hydatid cyst. Clinical investigation revealed coinfection HIV, HBV and HCV, with signs of chronic liver disease with macrocytic anemia and chronic thrombocytopenia. Four years earlier, he underwent total cystopericystectomy due to a hepatic hydatid cyst. Treatment was initiated with oral albendazole 400 mg 12 hourly prior to surgery and a progressive decrease in hematological values was observed. Due to suspected toxicity, albendazole treatment was stopped. Despite the discontinuation of albendazole, a decreased blood count in the three cell lines below normal was observed. Through blood transfusions and administration of colony-stimulating factors granulocyte, hematological parameters of the three cell lines returned to baseline 10 days later.

Route of Administration

A 21-month-old girl, 12 kg in weight, was hospitalized because of ascariasis infection complicated by intestinal perforation. After surgical management, treatment with oral albendazole (Zentel 0.4 g/10 mL containing Glycerol 0.5 g/10 mL, sorbic acid, potassium sorbate and benzoic acid) was started. On day 4, she mistakenly received an intravenous injection of the daily oral dose of albendazole (200 mg). Within 12 h, she developed hemolytic anemia with liver cytolysis and anuric acute renal failure requiring dialysis (Sodium 122 mmol/L, potassium 6.8 mmol/L, BUN 24.9 mmol/L, creatinine 316 μmol/L, and uric acid 660 μmol/L). Upon admission, she had spontaneous breathing with 2 L/min oxygen, her hemodynamic status was normal. Glasgow Coma Score was 12/15 without any focal neurological signs. Kidney ultrasound and Magnetic Resonance Imaging (MRI) showed bilateral kidney cortical necrosis. A cerebral MRI performed 5 weeks after poisoning because of intermittent action-related shaking and strabismus showed diffuse brain lesions. Ophthalmologic examination revealed an ischemic lesion of the left retina with papillary and retinal pallor. Diuresis resumed within 10 days under high dose of furosemide (8 mg/kg/day) and dialysis was discontinued after 15 days, but she developed a chronic kidney disease, with an eGFR of 17 mL/min/1.73 m2. Her neurological status totally recovered [8A].

Drug–Drug Interaction

In a systematic review of pharmacokinetic studies, the elimination half-life of albendazole was increased by cimetidine, while dexamethasone and praziquantel increased the area under the plasma concentration–time curve (AUC) [9M]. Levamisole and ritonavir decreased the AUC of albendazole.

IVERMECTIN

See SEDA-35, 565; SEDA-36, 457; SEDA-37, 367.

LEVAMISOLE

Hematologic

- A 22-year-old female was admitted with fever and diarrhea. Clinical evaluation was unremarkable except for fever and mild dehydration. Her initial evaluation revealed the presence of marked agranulocytosis (total leukocyte count: 460/mm^3; differential leukocyte count: N 0%, L 24%, M 1%—out of 25 cells). The rest of the counts were normal. Stool culture yielded *Salmonella* species. The exact species could not be ascertained as the isolate was non-reacting to the available antisera, including typhi and para typhi. Other cultures were negative. She was started on broad spectrum antibiotics. Antifungals were also initiated empirically in view of the severe neutropenia. Simultaneously, granulocyte-colony stimulating factor (G-CSF) was also started. There was a steady improvement in her counts, which normalized by the fifth day of initiating G-CSF, and the patient was soon discharged thereafter. Among her other investigations, peripheral smear showed "marked leukopenia and neutropenia," other cell lines being normal. Bone marrow study was also done prior to the administration of G-CSF, which was reported as "hypoplastic." Subsequent peripheral smear after the normalization of white blood cell count was normal. The patient had denied intake of any drugs from outside. Other investigations, including B$_{12}$ assay, serum uric acid, lactate dehydrogenase levels, HIV, hepatitis B surface antigen, hepatitis C virus, and rheumatoid arthritis (RA) factor, were essentially normal. Only anti-nuclear antibody (ANA) was reported as positive. Anti-double-stranded DNA test was insignificant. The patient was followed up as an outpatient for one more month without any incident. Two months after discharge, the patient again presented with fever. This time she had tonsillitis. Clinical examination did not reveal anything else. Again, she was found to have marked agranulocytosis (total leukocyte count: 800/mm^3; differential leukocyte count: N 1%, L 22%, E 1%, M 1%—out of 25 cells). The rest of the counts were normal. Cultures including throat swab cultures were negative. Again, the intake of any drugs from outside was denied. The patient was started on broad spectrum antibiotics and G-CSF. Antifungals were added empirically as before. Clinical response and counts mirrored the earlier admission; by the fifth day of initiating G-CSF, her counts normalized. Six days into the treatment, the patient's father brought a tablet strip which was prescribed to her by a local GP for some "illness" causing hair fall; the details of which were unclear. The drug was identified as levamisole. She had taken one tablet (50 mg) 15 days prior to her first admission and again 15 days prior to her second admission. This information was not revealed by the family since they considered the drug to be "insignificant." The patient was followed up as an outpatient for another 3 months and continued to be normal [10A].

Immunologic

Vasculitis with extensive skin involvement has been reported [11A].

- A 38-year-old African-American woman patient presented with a 2-week history of dark and painful discoloration of her right second and third finger tips. She also had a 1-day history of generalized body aches, pruritic and painful rashes on all extremities, right ankle pain, erythema, and edema affecting her ambulation. She also complained of a whitish vaginal discharge. Past medical history was significant for prior episodes of gonorrhea, poly-substance abuse (alcohol, opioid, and inhaled cocaine), depression, and anemia. She denied fever, chills, dyspnea, nausea, vomiting, or diarrhea. She stated that her last cocaine use was 2 weeks prior to her symptom onset. On physical examination, vital signs were normal. Multiple coin-like, erythematous tender indurated swellings with a central pustule or vesicle were noted, particularly on the lower extremities. The right ankle was red, tender, and swollen, and a joint effusion could be palpated. She had right ankle arthritis with decreased range of motion. The distal right hand second and third fingertips were necrotic and draining frank pus, which suggested super-added infection. Chest, abdominal, and neurological examinations were unremarkable. Pelvic examination showed whitish discharge without cervicitis. Metabolic panel and complete blood count with differential were unremarkable except for mild iron-deficiency anemia. Total WBC count was normal (8.7×10^3/μL). Differential count revealed mild eosinophilia 7.1%. ESR was 59 mm/h and C-reactive protein was elevated to 19.4 mg/L (normal 0–5 mg/L). Urine drug screening was negative for cocaine, cannabis, amphetamines, barbiturates, and benzodiazepine. She was initially treated with daily ceftriaxone because of suspected disseminated gonococcal infection (DGI). However, multiple sets of blood cultures, and urine, throat and vaginal cultures were negative. Urine gonococcal and chlamydia DNA nucleic acid amplification tests were negative. Further laboratory testing showed negative hepatitis screen, HIV screen, and negative RPR. Lyme disease panel was negative. Right ankle joint fluid analysis did not show any evidence of bacterial infection or crystal-induced arthropathy. Serological testing showed negative antinuclear antibody, a positive perinuclear anti-neutrophil cytoplasmic antibody (p-ANCA), and elevated antiproteinase-3 (18.8 U/mL), thereby supporting the diagnosis of LIV. Cytoplasmic ANCA (c-ANCA) and anti-myeloperoxidase antibodies (MPO) were negative. C3 complement was normal, and C4 complement was mildly low 13.6 (normal 15–53). Rheumatoid factor was negative. Appropriate antibiotics for the fingertip infection and supportive therapy were instituted. On further questioning, she endorsed having had a similar but milder rash on her lower extremities in the past, for which she had never sought any medical attention. The patient fully recovered over the next few weeks.

Levamisole-Contaminated Cocaine

Abuse of cocaine-tainted with levamisole is becoming a public health challenge [12A], and adverse reactions related to the use of levamisole almost invariably involved abuse of levamisole-contaminated cocaine. In this section, descriptions of varied case presentations attributed to consumption of levamisole-contaminated cocaine are described.

Nervous System

Two cases of progressive multifocal leukoencephalopathy have been reported [13A].

- *A 25-year-old man with history of cocaine use presented to the emergency room with left-sided upper and lower limb weakness as well as sensory impairment involving the face. The symptoms evolved such that he was bed-ridden after 48 h. He had no history of previous neurological or systemic symptoms. Computed tomography (CT) of the brain showed bilateral periventricular hypo-densities. CT angiography of cervical and intracranial vessels was unremarkable. An MRI study of the brain demonstrated increased FLAIR signal deep in the right and left hemispheres, which also displayed patchy gadolinium enhancement and restricted diffusion. Five days after admission, he developed dysphagia, dysarthria, and confusion. In addition to the previously noted MRI abnormalities, repeat imaging showed new lesions in the left internal and external capsules, putamen and corona radiata, right medial pons and left cerebellar peduncle, with heterogenous gadolinium enhancement. The neuroradiological impression was that the lesions were most compatible with demyelinating disease. A urine screen was positive for cocaine, cannabinoids, and oxycodone, and negative for amphetamine, methadone, benzodiazepines, and barbiturates. Complete blood count, ESR, serum electrolytes, urea, creatinine, and glucose were normal. Antinuclear antibodies, rheumatoid factor, perinuclear and cytoplasmic anti-neutrophil cytoplasmic antibodies (pANCA and cANCA, respectively), urinalysis, viral serology for HIV, CMV, Hepatitis A, B, and C, Lyme serology, syphilis were all negative. Liver enzymes (AST, ALT and GGT) were mild to moderately elevated and subsequently normalized over a period of 6 months. Cerebrospinal fluid (CSF) results included: slightly elevated protein at 0.50 g/L (normal 0.20–0.40 g/L), normal glucose and chloride, normal total cell count (3×10^6/L), negative oligoclonal bands, normal IgG index, elevated albumin index at 9.0 (2.7–4.7), negative cryptoccocal antigen, negative cultures for bacteria and fungi, negative polymerase chain reaction (PCR) studies for CMV and HSV 1–2, and normal cytology. He was treated with intravenous methylprednisolone, 1000 mg daily for five consecutive days, and subsequently underwent plasma exchange. During plasma exchange, his neurological condition stabilized and he subsequently achieved good, albeit partial, recovery. At 3 months follow-up, he had mild residual left-sided hemiplegia but was otherwise independent in activities of daily living and starting to return to work. Follow-up MRI 5 months after presentation showed reduction in the size of lesions, no enhancement, and no new lesions. MRI 21 months after the initial presentation also showed no new lesions.*

- *A 41-year-old woman presented to the emergency room with a history of recent confusion and impaired balance. She had been using cocaine daily for 7 months. MRI FLAIR images showed multiple white matter signal changes in both cerebral hemispheres in a predominantly periventricular distribution sparing the corpus callosum, cerebellum and brainstem. Subtle gadolinium enhancement was present in a few lesions. She was treated with supportive care for 1 week and then discharged with partial recovery. She resumed cocaine use and was readmitted 6 weeks after the previous hospital discharge because of worsening neurological symptoms. She was completely bedridden with inability to walk, incontinence, severely impaired communication skills, behavioural problems, cognitive impairment, and multifocal neurological deficits. MRI FLAIR images showed marked progression compared to the previous results. Confluent white matter abnormalities involved both cerebral hemispheres. There was subtle scattered restricted diffusion and no gadolinium enhancement. Urine testing was positive for cocaine, oxycodone, opiates, benzodiazepines, tramadol and citalopram, and negative for cannabinoids, amphetamine and methadone. Complete blood count, electrolytes, glucose, liver enzymes and creatinine kinase, were within normal limits. Serologic tests for HIV, Hepatitis A, B, and C, Lyme disease and syphilis were negative. The serum creatinine was elevated (137 μmol/L) as was the urea (7.6 mmol/L). Serum albumin was low (29 g/L). The ESR ranged from 22 to 64 on multiple samplings, C-reactive protein was elevated at 11 mg/L, while antinuclear antibodies, pANCA, cANCA, C3, C4, NMDA receptor and anti-thyroid peroxidase antibodies were normal. The vitamin B_{12} level was low at 166 pmol/L (normal >180). Copper, zinc and ceruloplasmin levels were normal. CSF protein was slightly elevated at 0.48 g/L. The glucose, chloride and cell count (4×10^6/L) were normal. No CSF acid fast bacilli were seen, and cultures for bacteria and fungi were negative. CSF PCR for CMV and HSV1–2 were negative. She was treated with intravenous* methylprednisolone, 1000 mg/day for 5 days, and plasma exchange. She showed substantial, albeit partial, recovery soon thereafter which continued over the course of several months. At 4 months follow-up, multiple domains of cognitive function were improved, but she had some residual deficits in attention, calculation, and visuospatial function. She was independent with respect to walking and most activities of daily living. Follow-up MRI at that time showed improvement of the subcortical and periventricular signal abnormalities and no new lesions. Similarly, no new lesions were seen on MRI 13 months after presentation.

Sensory Systems

Necrosis of the eyelids with secondary ectropion has been reported [14A].

* A 56-year-old female presented with eyelid necrosis secondary to systemic levamisole-induced vasculitis. Skin biopsy revealed necrotic epidermis with small-vessel thrombosis, fibrinoid reaction, and neutrophilic infiltration of vessel walls in the dermis with positive pANCA. She was treated with plasmapheresis and steroids. Six months later, she developed severe, symptomatic cicatricial ectropion with marked anterior lamellar shortage and middle lamellar contracture. Scar release in the middle lamellar plane with lateral tarsal strip procedures was performed, with full-thickness skin grafts from the upper eyelids. She remained fully epithelialized postoperatively with improvement in symptoms, although she had incomplete graft intake due to her eyelid necrosis and compromised dermal blood supply.

Pancreas

Acute pancreatitis with subsequent renal failure has been reported [15A].

* A 22-year-old male presented with shortness of breath and mid-abdominal pain radiating to the chest. He was sent for emergency chest CT scan after a routine laboratory test showed elevated D-dimer levels. The patient denied any fever, chills, recent travel or prior history of thromboembolic disease. He admitted to drinking some whiskey daily. His blood pressure was 139/74 mmHg, heart rate 67 beats/min; respiratory rate 18 cycles/min, oxygen saturation was 98% on room air. Clinical examination revealed mild epigastric tenderness, otherwise unremarkable. His chest CT scan was negative for pulmonary embolism but showed some stranding at the tail of the pancreas suspicious for acute pancreatitis. Routine laboratory tests showed white blood cell count of 14.4/μL, elevated lipase (754 U/L), creatinine (0.79 mg/dL), ESR (1 mm/h), C-reactive protein (0.08 mg/dL), alanine aminotransferase (23 U/L), aspartate aminotransferase (71 U/L), alkaline phosphatase (139 U/L), gamma-glutamyltransferase (209 U/L). He was kept nil per oral, intravenous normal saline and pain medications were commenced. A right upper quadrant ultrasound did not show any evidence of gallstones but revealed a fatty liver.

His lipid panel and triglycerides were normal. A urine toxicology screen was positive for cocaine and marijuana. His ethanol blood level was normal. On day 2–3 of admission, the patient was noticed to have elevated creatinine (3.71 mg/dL) with an initial normal baseline creatinine and thrombocytopenia (59/μL). Subcutaneous heparin used for deep vein thrombosis prophylaxis was stopped due to suspected heparin-induced thrombocytopenia, and a platelet factor-4 antibody test was requested. The patient subsequently became oliguric with a urine output of (200 mL in 24 h) despite adequate fluid hydration (8 L/12 h). A renal ultrasound did not show any hydronephrosis or stones. A follow-up magnetic resonance cholangiopancreatography (MRCP) showed heterogeneous pancreas suggesting inflammation. The patient was thought to have an atypical form of pancreatitis since his clinical condition was fairly stable but his laboratory indices were worsening. An immunoglobulin g4 test to rule out auto-immune pancreatitis was negative. Laboratory results showed thrombocytopenia, anemia, negative platelet factor-4, elevated direct bilirubin, low haptoglobin, high lactate dehydrogenase, elevated D-dimer and positive fibrin degradation products. Schistocytes were seen on blood microscopy. An ADAMS-13 level to rule out TTP was negative. The patient eventually became anuric and developed azotemia. A diagnosis of acute renal failure with a likely vasculitic process was made. Urinalysis showed muddy brown casts, proteinuria and white blood cells. Fractional excretion of sodium was 3.57. Work-up for glomerulonephritis which included tests for human immunodeficiency virus (HIV), hepatitis, anti-neutrophil cytoplasmic antibody (ANCA), anti-nuclear antibody (ANA), anti-glomerular basement membrane antibody, anti-cardiolipin antibody, scleroderma antibody, complement C3/C4 were all negative. Hemodialysis was subsequently initiated and a kidney biopsy revealed pauci-immune necrotizing glomerulonephritis with features of glomerular thrombotic microangiopathy consistent with the patient's ingestion of levamisole. The patient was commenced on high dose intravenous solumedrol and rituximab. He was transfused with nine units of packed red blood cells and he also had nine sessions of plasmapheresis. His renal function and hematological indices improved over 2 months of treatment, and he was discharged in stable clinical condition with no abdominal pain.

Hematologic

Neutropenia and thrombocytopenia induced by levamisole has again been reported [16A].

* A 36-year-old man was admitted to the intensive care unit with fever, right gluteal pain and swelling of 3-day duration. He denied trauma, rash, flu-like symptoms, or sick contacts. Medical history included continuous cocaine abuse (sniffing), paroxysmal atrial fibrillation, and two

episodes of febrile neutropenia in the past. On examination, the patient was awake, alert, comfortable, febrile 103.1 F and tachycardic (120 bpm). An abscess was found on the gluteal area. The rest of the skin was intact, and the rest of the exam was unremarkable. Laboratory findings showed severe leukopenia with neutropenia and thrombocytopenia. Urine toxicology was positive for cocaine and cannabinoids. He was managed for severe sepsis and febrile neutropenia with drainage of his gluteal abscess, fluids, broad spectrum antibiotics, including caspofungin, and granulocyte colony-stimulating factor (G-CSF). Serum and urine levamisole levels performed by high-performance liquid chromatography/tandem mass spectrometry (LC–MS/MS) 5 days after admission were negative. Flow cytometry, cultures, serology, HIV, and vasculitis work-up were done and ruled out other common causes of neutropenia and thrombocytopenia. Despite high fevers, the patient remained stable, and asymptomatic. Clinical course was complicated by acute kidney injury on day 5 of admission. Urine analysis revealed no eosinophils and benign sediment. On review of medical records, the patient had been admitted to our institution twice during the last 12 months for febrile neutropenia. He became afebrile on day 7 of admission with resolution of thrombocytopenia and some improvement of WBC. He was discharged home in stable condition, and he was lost to follow-up.

Skin

Necrosis of the skin with neutropenia has been reported in a middle-aged male [17A].

- *A 53-year-old man presented to the emergency department with symptoms of bilateral ear pain that developed over the past 8 h. The patient was a chronic cocaine user for the past 35 years and had last inhaled 'crack cocaine' on the day of presentation. On examination, both auricles were erythematous and painful to the touch. Palpable, non-blanching retiform purpura was evident with a similar non-blanching erythematous patch on both cheeks. The anterior portions of both lower extremities had developing purpura. Skin necrosis was also found on the right hand. Initial laboratory findings showed leukopenia with isolated neutropenia, normal platelet count and normal complete metabolic panel. Urine toxicology was positive for cocaine. Coagulation panel was within normal limits. Further autoimmune work-up revealed perinuclear antineutrophil cytoplasmic antibodies (p-ANCA) positive and elevated IgM anticardiolipin antibodies with negative antinuclear antibodies. Hepatitis viral panel, cryoglobulins and HIV tests were negative. Based on his clinical picture, laboratory findings and a detected serum levamisole level, the diagnosis of drug-induced ANCA-associated vasculitis secondary to levamisole-adulterated cocaine was made. Rheumatology follow-up within 10 days showed complete resolution of the purpuric lesions on the ears and healing of the skin*

necrosis on the hand within 10 days of abstinence from cocaine.

- *A 52-year-old man presented to the emergency department with skin pain. Although he felt well, he reported that he had developed skin sores 3 weeks prior to presentation that were progressively causing skin pain and sleeplessness. He acknowledged smoking cigarettes and snorting cocaine but denied intravenous use of cocaine or using any other drugs. His usual medications were lisinopril and tramadol, and he had no known drug allergies. His history was remarkable for methicillin-resistant Staphylococcus aureus (MRSA) septic arthritis of the shoulder and MRSA prepatellar bursitis within the last 2 years. During examination in the emergency department, he was alert, afebrile, nontoxic, generally healthy, and in no acute distress. Extensive necrotic skin lesions were present on the trunk, extremities, and both ears. The lesions were large necrotic patches with irregular, sharply angulated borders with thin or ulcerated epidermis surrounded by a bright halo of erythema. Ulcers were noted on the tongue. The clinical diagnosis was probable thrombosis of skin vessels with skin necrosis due to cocaine that was likely contaminated with levamisole. Blood cell counts showed mild anemia and mild leukopenia. Liver function tests, serum protein electrophoresis, hepatitis profile, human immunodeficiency virus 1 and 2, rapid plasma reagin, antinuclear antibody, normal antithrombin III, protein C, protein S, factor V Leiden, prothrombin mutation G20210A, anticardiolipin IgG, IgM, and IgA were all within normal ranges. ESR was elevated (26 mm/h); perinuclear antineutrophil cytoplasmic antibody greater than 1:320 (reference range, <1:20) with normal proteinase 3 and myeloperoxidase antibodies; urine toxicology was positive for cocaine. The patient was stable with good family support and was discharged from the emergency department to be followed in our dermatology office. The following day, his skin biopsies were interpreted as neutrophilic vasculitis with extensive intravascular early and organizing thrombi involving all small- and medium-sized blood vessels consistent with levamisole-induced necrosis or septic vasculitis. Based on his history of MRSA septic arthritis and bursitis, he was hospitalized for treatment with intravenous vancomycin pending further studies. Skin biopsy for direct immunofluorescence revealed granular deposits of IgM and linear deposits of C3 at the dermoepidermal junction and in blood vessel walls. Two tissue cultures for bacteria and fungi were negative and 2 blood cultures were negative. An echocardiogram was normal and without evidence of emboli. The patient remained stable, and antibiotics were discontinued. He was released from the hospital, and his skin lesions healed satisfactorily with showering and mupirocin ointment [18A].*

Immunologic

Delayed recurrent vasculitis in a middle-aged female has been reported [19A].

• *A 51-year-old woman complained of painful erythematous rash that started a few hours after smoking cocaine and progressed to blistering dark lesions involving her lower extremities and hands. She had similar episodes of skin eruptions in the past that always occurred after cocaine use, but she was not on any long-term treatment. Although she has been smoking cocaine for more than 35 years, these skin eruptions started 4 years ago. Two years ago, she had a severe skin eruption with necrosis which required skin grafting. Her other medical problems were hepatitis C, for which she never received treatment, and she had an excision of melanoma 10 years ago. She denied any joint pain, hair loss, oral ulcers, nasal ulcers, rash on the face, photosensitivity, discoloration of finger tips in cold weather, hemoptysis, or shortness of breath. Examination revealed tender retiform purpura in the hand and tender retiform purpura with hemorrhagic bulla in the legs. There were no skin lesions on the other parts of the body. Other system examination was unrevealing. Her initial laboratory results showed mild hypochromic microcytic anemia with a hemoglobin of 10.9 g/dL, with evidence of iron deficiency in the iron panel. The white blood cell count of 4300/mm^3 with a neutrophil count of 2600/mm^3 and platelet count was 212 000/mm^3. Serum electrolytes, renal and liver function tests, and coagulation profile were normal. Urine analysis showed microscopic hematuria with red blood cells of 5–15 with mild proteinuria. There was no evidence of hepatitis B infection and the rapid plasma reagin was negative. HIV serology 1 month ago and was negative. Her urine toxicology was positive for cocaine. Levamisole levels were not done. The differentials were cocaine or levamisole-induced vasculitis, ANCA-associated vasculitis, cryoglobulinemic vasculitis related to hepatitis C, and connective tissue disease-related vasculitis. A vasculitic panel revealed high levels of anti-PR3 antibody and anti-MPO antibody with a p-ANCA pattern. Her cryoglobulins were negative. Further autoimmune work-up showed a positive antinuclear antibody (ANA) with a titer of 1:80 and homogenous pattern. The rheumatoid factor (RF) and anticardiolipin IgM antibody were also positive. Anti-Smith antibody, anti-double-stranded DNA antibody (ds DNA antibody), anti-citrullinated protein antibody (Anti CCP antibody), anti-SSA antibody, anti-SSB antibody, and anticardiolipin IgG were negative. There was decreased C3 with normal C4 levels. ESR was 53 mm/h and C-reactive protein 65.9 mg/L (normal range 0–4.9). A vasculitic panel in 2010 revealed a positive atypical p-ANCA with negative anti-proteinase 3 antibody (PR3 antibody) and anti-myeloperoxidase antibody (MPO antibody). However, in 2013, the patient had developed anti-PR3 antibody but had negative anti-MPO antibody. ANCA pattern on immunofluorescence was not done in 2013. During this presentation, the patient had a very high level of anti-PR3 antibody and went on to develop anti-MPO antibody with a p-ANCA pattern. However, she did not demonstrate a c-ANCA pattern. Her skin biopsy revealed vasculitis with fibrin thrombi. She was treated with steroids during this admission and the skin lesions improved significantly. She was counseled on cessation of cocaine to prevent recurrent similar skin lesions.*

• *A 50-year-old woman presented with a 3-day history of a progressive, painful, non-blanching, purpuric rash (retiform purpura) with areas of necrosis and bullae formation involving her face, trunk, extremities, and oral and nasal mucosa. She reported a history of cocaine use, and urine toxicology screening was positive for both cocaine and levamisole by liquid chromatography–tandem mass spectrometry. Laboratory findings included leukopenia and an elevated erythrocyte sedimentation rate (67 mm/h). Antinuclear antibody and antineutrophil cytoplasmic antibody (ANCA) testing was positive with elevated antimyeloperoxidase and antiproteinase 3. An anticardiolipin antibody assay was negative. She was diagnosed with levamisole-induced vasculitis given the typical features of diffuse purpuric lesions (including the helical rims of the ears) and associated ANCA positivity in the appropriate epidemiologic context. Intravenous dexamethasone (4 mg/day for 7 days) was initiated, which halted progression of skin lesions. She was transferred to a burn unit where she received surgical debridement of the necrotic tissue and skin grafting [20A].*

Vasculitis without cutaneous involvement has been described [21A].

• *A 43-year-old homeless male presented with several weeks history of weight loss, bilateral burning foot pain, and overall weakness that had progressed to an inability to walk. His past medical history included admission to a hospital 2 years prior with acute kidney injury secondary to rhabdomyolysis, with a serum creatinine of 1.5 mg/dL on discharge. The social history was significant for crack cocaine use. On admission, he appeared cachectic and had a temperature of 38.7 °C. On neurological exam, he had impaired soft touch sensation bilaterally up to the ankles and diffuse weakness. There were no skin abnormalities. The creatinine on admission was 3.93 mg/dL, and the BUN was 55 mg/dL. A globulin gap was present with a total protein of 6.7 g/dL and albumin of 1.4 g/dL. Urinalysis demonstrated moderate protein and blood, with a spot protein–creatinine ratio of 1:55 mg/mg. There was no peripheral eosinophilia. Microscopic urinalysis showed granular casts. His urine tested positive for eosinophils. Cocaine metabolites were found on urine toxicology. HIV, anti-nuclear and anti-glomerular basement membrane antibodies, RPR, and hepatitis B and C serologies were negative. There were no abnormal bands on serum or urine protein electrophoresis. ANCA were strongly positive at 1:5120 with a perinuclear staining pattern and myeloperoxidase reactivity at 76 AU/mL. Kidney biopsy specimen had a total of 21 glomeruli, out of which only two were globally sclerotic. The majority of* glomeruli showed pauci-immune necrotizing crescentic glomerulonephritis. A prominent plasma cell-rich tubulointerstitial nephritis was also present. Based on his laboratory findings and renal biopsy, a diagnosis of microscopic polyangiitis was considered, but levamisole-induced ANCA vasculitis remained a likely possibility given his history of cocaine use. The presence of interstitial nephritis on biopsy was felt to explain the eosinophils in his urine, a finding previously reported in cocaine users. He was treated with pulse methylprednisolone 1000 mg for 3 days and 600 mg of IV cyclophosphamide. His creatinine peaked to 7.21 mg/dL during hospitalization but stabilized at 6.25 mg/dL after treatment. The patient was counselled on abstaining from cocaine and was discharged on 40 mg of prednisone per day with instructions to follow-up for monthly cyclophosphamide injections at renal clinic. The patient was readmitted 1 month later with increasing lower extremity swelling and pain. He had been off prednisone since discharge and had ongoing crack-cocaine use. Renal function had declined, reaching serum creatinine of 8.8 mg/dL. He was treated with cyclophosphamide and prednisone, and his fluid status and electrolyte abnormalities were corrected. Renal function did not improve with treatment, and hemodialysis was initiated.

Immune complex glomerulonephritis secondary to levamisole has been reported [22A].

- A 40-year-old Caucasian male presented to the emergency room with 1-week history of progressive shortness of breath on exertion. He also complained of palpitations, fatigue, and orthopnea. There was a history of progressive lower extremity swelling for the last 3 weeks and multiple painful ulcerations on his tongue and in his mouth for 2 weeks. History was also notable for multiple joint pains for 6 months. He was diagnosed with Lyme's disease and was treated with high dose doxycycline for 2 months. Two months prior to admission, he noticed diffuse non-itchy rash on his chest, back, abdomen, arms, and legs that subsequently resolved. One month prior to admission, he noticed decreased urine output and dark colored urine. There was no history of fever, chills, weight loss, night sweats, cough, chest pain, or hemoptysis. He denied having any dry eyes, oral ulcers, photosensitivity, abdominal pain, hematuria, dysuria, or neurologic symptoms. Medications included doxycycline and ibuprofen. He had history of long-standing tobacco abuse, alcohol use, and regular cocaine use. He denied having any tattoos, sick contacts, recent travel, or environmental or occupational exposure. On examination, he was afebrile, tachycardic, tachypneic, and hypoxic on room air. The tongue had hyperkeratotic, hyperpigmented papules. There were scattered erythematous maculopapular lesions on the chest. He had bilateral lower extremity edema with skin changes suggestive of chronic venous stasis and prominent symmetric synovitis of metacarpophalangeal

and wrist joints. Chest auscultation revealed diffuse rales bilaterally. Cardiovascular, abdominal, and neurologic examinations were unremarkable. Notable lab abnormalities included anemia and severe azotemia with multiple electrolyte abnormalities. Urinalysis showed significant hematuria and proteinuria. Urine protein/creatinine ratio was 4.7. Acute phase reactants ESR and CRP were elevated. BNP and PTH were also elevated. Rheumatologic testing revealed borderline ANA, positive atypical p-ANCA (1:640), and positive anti-myeloperoxidase antibodies. Complement levels (C3 and C4) were low. The remainder of the rheumatologic work-up was negative. Chest X-ray showed pulmonary edema. Urine screen for drugs returned positive for cocaine and levamisole. Kidney biopsy showed diffuse tubulointerstitial fibrosis with the majority of glomeruli globally sclerosed. Few intact glomeruli showed mesangial proliferation and immune complex deposition consisting of IgG, IgM, and complement in mesangial and endocapillary distribution. It was consistent with immune-mediated glomerulonephritis. Skin biopsy of the rash was consistent with leukocytoclastic vasculitis. Given the clinical, laboratory, and pathologic findings, a diagnosis of ANCA-associated systemic vasculitis and immune complex-mediated glomerulonephritis were secondary to levamisole/cocaine use was made.

- A 49-year-old Caucasian man who was a regular user of intravenous drugs and infected with the hepatitis C virus (HCV) was diagnosed with microcytic anemia; he had purple skin with ANCA-positive pseudovasculitis from levamisole use (prior skin biopsy). He was admitted with acute oligoanuric renal failure and macroscopic hematuria, and with the appearance of new skin-necrotic lesions on his nose, trunk and extremities. The patient confirmed that the last parenteral cocaine consumption had been 3–4 days before. Further testing showed evidence of renal failure with serum creatinine levels of 7.09 mg/dL, 263 mg/dL for urea and 5.5 mEq/L for potassium. Elevated serum acute phase reactants were also observed. Serial blood cultures revealed methicillin-resistant Staphylococcus aureus (MRSA). Prothrombotic parameters were elevated with a D-dimer value of 5825 ng/mL. Other test results were: hemoglobin: 8.9 g/dL; mean corpuscular volume: 76 fL; platelet count: $65 \times 10^3/\mu L$; and LDH: 766 U/L. Serum immunological parameters were as follows: 52 mg/dL for C3; 7 mg/dL for C4; ANCA antibodies were positive with a perinuclear staining pattern (1:1280); myeloperoxidase (MPO)-ANCA and proteinase 3 (PR3)-ANCA antibodies were positive (56.4 and 47.10 U/mL, respectively), and anti-glomerular basement membrane antibodies were negative. After recovering diuresis, a proteinuria of 1.35 g/24 h was reported and dysmorphic erythrocytes and cell casts were also observed in the urinary sediment. An abdominal ultrasound showed kidneys with normal cortico-medullary differentiation and a minimal amount of free fluid in the pelvis with no other pathological findings. Transthoracic echocardiography (TTE) was negative for endocarditis. Physical examination revealed tense ascites of unknown origin, whilst the subsequent peritoneal biopsy showed vasculopathy (peritoneal thrombotic vasculitis) of probable toxic origin. The kidney biopsy, at which time the serum creatinine level was 2.79 mg/dL and for urea 87 mg/dL, showed membranous nephropathy with cellular crescents. The patient was treated with boluses of methylprednisolone (500 mg/day) for 3 days. Thereafter, methylprednisolone was changed to prednisone 40 mg/day (1 mg/kg/day). A total of 17 sessions of hemodialysis via jugular vein catheter were needed. Skin lesions and renal function improved significantly 10 days after starting treatment, in conjunction with the withdrawal from cocaine consumption, and there were residual scars. Both blood and urine cultures were negative after treatment with daptomycin for 15 days (4 mg/kg/48 h, in conjunction with the days free of dialysis). At the 3-month follow-up (after decreasing doses of prednisone and without toxic consumption of levamisole), the skin lesions had subsided, and stable analytical parameters were seen both for anemia (Hb: 10.2 g/dL) and renal function (creatinine: 1.98 mg/dL; glomerular filtration rate using the CKD-EPI: 20–30 mL/min; proteinuria <1 g/24 h) [23A].

- A 47-year-old male was referred for management of kidney failure and nephrotic syndrome. Two years earlier, he presented with self-limited skin lesions in the right flank and earlobes, and laboratory testing revealed neutropenia, positive ANA and ANCA. In the current presentation, he reported a history of nocturia, dark urine, intermittent edema and joint pains. He denied consumption of any toxic medication. Physical examination was unremarkable. Laboratory results were: hemoglobin 9.2 g/dL, leukocytes 3.190/μL (neutrophils 54.6%), platelets 248 000/μL, APTT 41.7 min, Cr 2.66 mg/dL, 2.9 g albumin/dL. Rheumatoid factor and thyroid hormones were within normal limits. ANA was positive, and anti-DNA negative, lupus anticoagulant positive, anticardiolipin IgG negative, IgM 18.8 MPL/mL (positive > 18 MPL/mL), cryoglobulins negative, c-ANCA negative, and p-ANCA positive. HLA B27 were negative. Serology test for hepatitis B and C, and HIV was negative. Chest X-ray, echocardiogram and CT of the abdomen were normal. Urine toxicology for cocaine showed 60–100 sediment erythrocytes per field with 20–30% of dysmorphic 6–12 leukocytes per field, negative culture, proteinuria 7680 mg/24 h with nonselective glomerular pattern. Renal biopsy showed 27 glomeruli; 3 ischemic changes, one with a fibrous crescent and the rest of the capillary tuft segmental necrosis. The patient was administered methylprednisolone (1.5 g IV), cyclophosphamide (750 mg IV) and oral prednisone 60 mg/day, in a tapering pattern. One month later, serum creatinine had returned to normal [24A].

Two cases of thrombotic vasculopathy (one of which was fatal) because of cocaine contaminated with levamisole have also been reported in Mexico [25A].

- A 31-year-old female with a history of cocaine abuse presented with purple spots on her pinnae. Skin biopsy results suggested a diagnosis of necrotizing infectious chondritis. Histological examination showed thrombotic vascular and intravascular papillary endothelial hyperplasia. The blood count was normal; HIV, antinuclear antibodies (ANA), rheumatoid factor and the panel of viral hepatitis were negative. She was treated with corticosteroids and had a complete recovery.
- A 38-year-old male with a 20-year history of cocaine abuse presented with a 6-month history of recurring fever, arthralgia, myalgia and skin lesions. One week after the last cocaine inhalation, he developed purple retiform rash, atrophic plaques and ulcers with sores on cheeks, auricles and legs. He underwent skin biopsy for suspected lupus erythematosus and antiphospholipid syndrome. Biopsy results showed multiple newly formed vessels, fibrosis and intraluminal thrombi in small vessels without vasculitis. Laboratory studies showed neutrophils 600/μL, hemoglobin 4.5 g/dL, platelets 450 000/μL, and normal clotting times and complement. ANA and anti-DNA titers were negative. The patient discharged himself but was admitted to another hospital within 48 h, where he died of apparent diffuse alveolar hemorrhage.

MEBENDAZOLE

See SEDA-35, 565; SEDA-36, 457; SEDA-37, 367.

OXANTEL PAMOATE

Dose-Comparison Study

The efficacy and safety of six different disease of oxantel pamoate (5–30 mg/kg) in the treatment of *Trichuris trichiura* in school-aged children have been evaluated in a single-blind trial including 350 children [26C]. The most common adverse events reported were abdominal cramps (2%). There were no significant differences in the frequency of adverse events across groups based on doses. No serious adverse events were reported.

PRAZIQUANTEL

Dose Comparison Studies

The impact of single versus double dose praziquantel (40 mg/kg/day) on cure rates, egg reduction rates and re-infection rates have been evaluated in a randomized trial including 1017 children aged 1–5 years [27C]. No serious adverse events were reported.

Placebo-Controlled Studies

The efficacy and safety of praziquantel (30 mg/kg) for the treatment of schistosomiasis in pregnancy had been assessed in a randomized trial including 370 women [28C]. Severe adverse events reported were headache, fever and fatigue (5 with praziquantel versus 2 with placebo). There were no significant differences in the rates of abortion, intrauterine deaths or congenital anomalies between groups.

Cholangiocarcinoma

The association between praziquantel administration and the risk of cholangiocarcinoma has been evaluated in a hospital-based case–control study of 210 incident cases and 840 matched controls [29C]. Potential confounders including history of eating of raw fish, family history of cancer, and level of education were adjusted for. Compared with controls, subjects who used praziquantel once, twice, or more than twice likely to develop cholangiocarcinoma: OR 1.49 (95% CI: 1.02–2.20), 1.82 (95% CI: 0.92–3.60), and 2.30 (95% CI: 1.20–4.40), respectively. Additional praziquantel usage increased the odds of developing cholangiocarcinoma by 23.0% (OR: 1.23; 95% CI: 1.07–1.43).

TRIBENDIMIDINE

See SEDA-35, 565; SEDA-36, 457; SEDA-37, 367.

References

[1] Speich B, Ali SM, Ame SM, et al. Efficacy and safety of albendazole plus ivermectin, albendazole plus mebendazole, albendazole plus oxantel pamoate, and mebendazole alone against Trichuris trichiura and concomitant soil-transmitted helminth infections: a four-arm, randomised controlled trial. Lancet Infect Dis. 2015;15(3):277–84 [C].

[2] Thomsen EK, Sanuku N, Baea M, et al. Efficacy, safety, and pharmacokinetics of coadministered diethylcarbamazine, albendazole, and ivermectin for treatment of Bancroftian filariasis. Clin Infect Dis. 2016;62(3):334–41. pii: civ882. [c].

[3] Tafatatha TT, Ngwira BM, Taegtmeyer M, et al. Randomised controlled clinical trial of increased dose and frequency of albendazole and ivermectin on Wuchereria bancrofti microfilarial clearance in northern Malawi. Trans R Soc Trop Med Hyg. 2015;109(6):393–9 [c].

[4] Kar SK, Dwibedi B, Kerketa AS, et al. A randomized controlled trial of increased dose and frequency of albendazole with standard dose DEC for treatment of Wuchereria bancrofti microfilaremics in Odisha, India. PLoS Negl Trop Dis. 2015;9(3):e0003583 [c].

[5] Aksoy EK, Koklu S. Albendazole-induced cirrhosis decompensation and pancytopenia. Ann Pharmacother. 2015;49(8):945–6 [A].

[6] Koca T, Akcam M. Albendazole-induced autoimmune hepatitis. Indian Pediatr. 2015;52(1):78–9 [A].

[7] Ortonobes Roig S, López García B, Solano Luque MF, et al. Haematological toxicity during treatment with albendazole. [Article in Spanish]. Enferm Infecc Microbiol Clin. 2016;34(5):326–7. pii: S0213-005X(15)00288-8. [A].

[8] Hogan J, Dehoux L, Niel O, et al. Hemolytic anemia and irreversible kidney and brain injuries after accidental intravenous injection of albendazole suspension in an infant. Clin Toxicol (Phila). 2016;54(1):72–3 [A].

[9] Pawluk SA, Roels CA, Wilby KJ, et al. A review of pharmacokinetic drug-drug interactions with the anthelmintic medications albendazole and mebendazole. Clin Pharmacokinet. 2015;54(4):371–83 [M].

[10] Ittyachen AM, Jose MB, Benjamin JR. A case of recurrent agranulocytosis due to levamisole. Indian J Pharmacol. 2015;47(5):565–6 [A].

[11] Patnaik S, Balderia P, Vanchhawng L, et al. Is levamisole-induced vasculitis a relegated diagnostic possibility? A case report and review of literature. Am J Case Rep. 2015;16:658–62 [A].

[12] Chung C, Tumeh PC, Birnbaum R, et al. Characteristic purpura of the ears, vasculitis, and neutropenia—a potential public health epidemic associated with levamisole-adulterated cocaine. J Am Acad Dermatol. 2011;65(4):722–5 [A].

[13] Vosoughi R, Schmidt BJ. Multifocal leukoencephalopathy in cocaine users: a report of two cases and review of the literature. BMC Neurol. 2015;15(1):208 [A].

[14] Ramesh S, Sobti D, Mancini R. Eyelid necrosis and secondary cicatricial ectropion secondary to levamisole-associated vasculitis. Ophthal Plast Reconstr Surg. 2015; http://dx.doi.org/10.1097/IOP.0000000000000568 [A].

[15] Ogunbameru A, Jandali M, Issa A, et al. Acute pancreatitis as initial presentation of cocaine-induced vasculitis: a case report. JOP. 2015;16(2):192–4 [A].

[16] Martinez E, Alvi R, Venkatram S, et al. Recurrent febrile neutropenia and thrombocytopenia in a chronic cocaine user: a case of levamisole induced complications. Case Rep Crit Care. 2015;2015:303098 [A].

[17] Dherange PA, Beatty N, Al-Khashman A. Levamisole-adulterated cocaine: a case of retiform purpura, cutaneous necrosis and neutropenia. BMJ Case Rep. 2015;2015. http://dx.doi.org/10.1136/bcr-2015-211768 pii: bcr2015211768. [A].

[18] Reynolds 2nd FH, Hong MW, Banks SL. Extensive skin necrosis from suspected levamisole-contaminated cocaine. Cutis. 2015;96(3):E15–7 [A].

[19] Yogarajah M, Pervil-Ulysse M, Sivasambu B. Cocaine-induced delayed recurrent vasculitis: a 4-year follow-up. Am J Case Rep. 2015;16:310–4 [A].

[20] Hahn E, Bogoch II. Levamisole-induced vasculitis in a cocaine user. J Rheumatol. 2015;42(10):1924–5 [A].

[21] Baptiste GG, Alexopoulos AS, Masud T, et al. Systemic levamisole-induced vasculitis in a cocaine user without cutaneous findings: a consideration in diagnosis. Case Rep Med. 2015;2015:547023 [A].

[22] Garg L, Gupta S, Swami A, et al. Levamisole/cocaine induced systemic vasculitis and immune complex glomerulonephritis. Case Rep Nephrol. 2015;2015:372413 [A].

[23] Roca-Argente L, Moll-Guillen JL, Espí-Reig J, et al. Membranous glomerulonephritis and cellular crescents induced by levamisole-adulterated cocaine abuse: a case report. Ann Transl Med. 2015;3(18):271 [A].

[24] Sirvent AE, Enríquez R, Andrada E, et al. Necrotising glomerulonephritis in levamisole-contaminated cocaine use. Nefrologia. 2016;36(1):76–8. pii: S0211–6995(15)00193-9. [A].

[25] Martínez-Velasco MA, Flores-Suárez LF, Toussaint-Caire S, et al. Thrombotic vasculopathy probably associated with cocaine contaminated with levamisole: report of 2 cases. [Article in Spanish]. Rev Med Inst Mex Seguro Soc. 2015;53(1):98–101 [A].

[26] Moser W, Ali SM, Ame SM, et al. Efficacy and safety of oxantel pamoate in school-aged children infected with Trichuris trichiura on Pemba Island, Tanzania: a parallel, randomised, controlled, dose-ranging study. Lancet Infect Dis. 2016;16(1):53–60 [C].

[27] Nalugwa A, Nuwaha F, Tukahebwa EM, et al. Single versus double dose praziquantel comparison on efficacy and schistosoma mansoni re-infection in preschool-age children in Uganda: a randomized controlled trial. PLoS Negl Trop Dis. 2015;9(5): e0003796 [C].

[28] Olveda RM, Acosta LP, Tallo V, et al. Efficacy and safety of praziquantel for the treatment of human schistosomiasis during pregnancy: a phase 2, randomised, double-blind, placebo-controlled trial. Lancet Infect Dis. 2016;16(2):199–208. pii: S1473-3099(15)00345-X. [C].

[29] Kamsa-Ard S, Luvira V, Pugkhem A, et al. Association between praziquantel treatment and cholangiocarcinoma: a hospital-based matched case-control study. BMC Cancer. 2015;15:776 [C].

30

Vaccines

K.M. Damer*,[1], C.M. Jung*,[†]

*Butler University College of Pharmacy and Health Sciences, Indianapolis, IN, USA
[†]Eskenazi Health, Indianapolis, IN, USA
[1]Corresponding author: kmdamer@butler.edu

Abbreviations

9vHPV	9-valent human papillomavirus vaccine
aP	acellular pertussis
bHPV	bivalent human papillomavirus vaccine
DTaP	diphtheria + tetanus toxoids + acellular pertussis vaccine
HBV	hepatitis B virus
Hib	*Haemophilus influenzae* type b
HPV	human papillomavirus
HPV4	quadrivalent human papillomavirus vaccine
IIV	inactivated influenza vaccine
IPV	inactivated poliovirus vaccine
JE vaccine	Japanese encephalitis vaccine
LAIV	live attenuated influenza vaccine
MCV4	quadrivalent (serogroups A,C,W,Y) meningococcal conjugate vaccine
MenB	*Neisseria meningitidis* serogroup B
MenC	*Neisseria meningitidis* serogroup C
MMR	measles + mumps + rubella vaccine
MMRV	measles + mumps + rubella + varicella vaccine
PCV13	13-valent pneumococcal conjugate vaccine
PCV7	7-valent pneumococcal conjugate vaccine
PPSV23	23-valent pneumococcal polysaccharide vaccine
Td	diphtheria + tetanus toxoids vaccine
Tdap	tetanus toxoid + diphtheria toxoid + acellular pertussis vaccine
VZV	varicella zoster virus
wP	whole-cell pertussis
YF	yellow fever

GENERAL [SEDA-36, 465]

A consistent approach to the classification of adverse events following immunization (AEFI) is important for the determination of actual causality related to the adverse event. The Clinical Immunization Safety Assessment (CISA) Network defined terminology to be used in describing the causality of an AEFI which the World Health Organization (WHO) has similarly adopted [1H,2H]. In summary, it is the recommendation of the CISA network to categorize AEFI as "consistent with", "inconsistent with", or "indeterminate". Additional details on the approach to determining how AEFI should be categorized with these terms have previously been described and readers should refer to the SEDA volume 36 for the detailed descriptions of definitions and criteria. A universal method to classifying AEFI is important to conveying correct education on vaccination to patients and vital to ensuring immunization practices are maintained as a major public health initiative. Although not uniformly reported in the current literature, authors are encouraged to adopt the recommended classification system in order to more appropriately categorize AEFI in the future.

Viral Vaccines

Hepatitis B Vaccine [SED-15, 3565, 3566, 3568; SEDA-37, 383]

SUSCEPTIBILITY FACTORS

Immunocompromised: Human Immunodeficiency Virus (HIV) Patients with HIV are known to have a lower response to hepatitis B virus (HBV) vaccination than non-HIV infected individuals. A parallel group, randomized controlled trial studied the effect of standard or double-dose HBV vaccination in HIV-positive patients previously unresponsive to HBV vaccination. Eligible patients first received a 20-mcg booster to validate vaccine non-responsiveness. Of 411 individuals receiving the booster, 218 had an appropriate immune response. Non-responders were randomized to receive either 20 or 40 mcg HBV vaccine at 0, 4, and 24 weeks. All patients included had a CD4 count greater than 200 cells/µL. The double-dose vaccine did not provide additional benefit 4 weeks after completion of the vaccination series compared to the single-dose vaccine. Adverse events in this study were similar between groups, showing that additional antigen did not significantly impact the presence of adverse effects [3C].

INTERACTIONS

Drug–Drug Interactions Hepatitis A and B are common vaccine-preventable diseases acquired through international travel. Vaccination is recommended for any travelers to an area where hepatitis A or B is moderately to highly endemic. Similarly, meningococcal vaccination is recommended for travelers to endemic areas of disease, typically parts of Africa or Asia. Alberer and colleagues studied the immunogenicity of an accelerated vaccination schedule, which combined hepatitis A, hepatitis B, and meningococcal administration. Subjects were randomized to one of three groups: hepatitis A and B alone on days 1, 8, and 29, hepatitis A and B with quadrivalent meningococcal vaccine (MenACWY-CRM) on day 1, followed by hepatitis A and B on days 8 and 29, or MenACWY-CRM alone on day 1. The combination of hepatitis A, hepatitis B, and MenACWY-CRM was non-inferior to administration with hepatitis A and B or MenACWY-CRM alone. Adverse effects were mild and similar between groups. The most common adverse effects were headache, nasopharyngitis, and fatigue. This study suggests an accelerated schedule with concomitant administration of hepatitis A, hepatitis B, and MenACWY-CRM is an effective and safe strategy for vaccination in individuals wishing to travel [4C].

Human Papillomavirus Vaccine [SEDA-35, 574; SEDA-36, 466; SEDA-37, 384]

GENERAL

The safety of human papillomavirus (HPV) vaccines is still an on-going concern for many, resulting in non-adherence to vaccination recommendations. A review of safety reports in pre- and post-licensure data revealed that both the bivalent and quadrivalent vaccines are well tolerated and safe in most instances. The most common adverse events tend to be injection-site reactions. Serious adverse events occur similarly to control groups. On-going education to the public should occur to promote the benefits of vaccination with the contrasted risk of non-vaccination [5R].

ORGANS AND SYSTEMS

Nervous System: Autonomic Dysfunction Postural orthostatic tachycardia syndrome (POTS) has been described previously. Brinth and colleagues conducted a study with 35 women to characterize the prevalence of POTS. All women were referred to the clinic for orthostatic intolerance, fatigue, headache, and cognitive dysfunction following vaccination with quadrivalent HPV (HPV4) vaccine. A 60% prevalence of POTS was found

in the study. On-going data are needed to assess causality [6c]. A retrospective review by the same authors concluded symptoms of POTS were consistent amongst the study subjects and consistent with previously described cases [7c].

Nervous System: Abnormal Peripheral Sympathetic Response A review of 40 Japanese girls with various symptoms after HPV vaccination was conducted to characterize the causes of neurological manifestations. Of the 40 girls, 18 were diagnosed with complex regional pain syndrome (CRPS). Thirteen of these cases had a dual diagnosis of orthostatic hypotension (OH), orthostatic dysregulation (OD), or POTS with CRPS. Three cases were due to OH alone, seven due to OD alone, and one due to POTS alone. There were 11 cases diagnosed due to another cause [8A].

Nervous System: Multiple Sclerosis A review of national registries in Denmark and Sweden assessed the diagnoses of multiple sclerosis or other demyelinating diseases in females ages 10–44 years following HPV4 vaccination. No increased risk of multiple sclerosis or other demyelinating diseases was found amongst 789 082 women who had received 1 927 581 doses of vaccine [9C].

SECOND-GENERATION EFFECTS

Pregnancy Two reviews of the Vaccine Adverse Event Reporting System (VAERS) database were conducted to assess adverse effects following vaccination during pregnancy. The first review was specifically conducted to assess chorioamnionitis risk after vaccination during pregnancy. Of the 31 reports submitted, eight patients had received HPV4 only and one patient received HPV4 and tetanus–diphtheria–acellular pertussis (Tdap) vaccines. Other administered vaccines were influenza, measles–mumps–rubella (MMR), varicella, and hepatitis B. Investigators concluded there was no safety concern regarding vaccination during pregnancy and the risk of chorioamnionitis [10c]. The second review was specific to VAERS reports after HPV4 administration during pregnancy. Those reviewed were non-manufacturer reports and a total of 147 reports were assessed. The HPV4 vaccine was given during the first trimester in most cases. Seventy percent of reports did not describe an adverse effect and the primary reason for report was vaccination during pregnancy. Pregnancy-related adverse effects were most commonly spontaneous abortion (10.2%) and elective termination (4.1%). Fever was the most common non-pregnancy-related adverse effect. Two birth defects were reported which included an infant born without both lower limbs and an infant with total anomalous pulmonary venous return. Both infants were exposed to other vaccines during gestation. No new adverse effects were identified [11A].

A similar review of the post-marketing prenatal vaccine exposure registry was conducted. The registry was a manufacturer-sponsored initiative. The review found that spontaneous abortion and birth defects did not occur more frequently in vaccinated individuals than the general population [12A]. Additionally, a follow-up study of individuals included in the Costa Rica HPV Vaccine Trial was conducted. Women in the study received either bivalent HPV vaccine (bHPV), hepatitis A vaccine (indicated as placebo), or were unvaccinated. The primary endpoint was miscarriage within 20 weeks gestation. Secondary endpoints included total number of conceived pregnancies and live births. The miscarriage rates for women exposed to bHPV vaccine, hepatitis A vaccine, and unvaccinated women were 13.3%, 12.6%, and 13.6%, respectively. For women with conception within 90 days of bHPV vaccination, the miscarriage rate was 13.1%. There was no difference between secondary endpoints. Bivalent HPV vaccine does not increase the risk of miscarriage according to this study, but continued adverse event report monitoring is encouraged [13C]. Considering the observed data, HPV vaccine has a low risk of adverse events if given during pregnancy.

SUSCEPTIBILITY FACTORS

Autoimmune Disease A review of literature on HPV vaccination in the setting of autoimmune diseases was conducted to determine the safety and efficacy of vaccination in this population. Studies for review were available for autoimmune diseases limited to juvenile idiopathic arthritis (JIA), inflammatory bowel disease (IBD), and systemic lupus erythematosus (SLE). None of the studies found any safety concerns with HPV vaccination in these conditions and the vaccine was found to be effective. On-going data are needed in the setting of immunosuppression, particularly with transplantation [14M].

DRUG ADMINISTRATION

Drug Dosage Regimens Gilca and colleagues previously studied a two-dose alternative vaccination schedule with HPV4 vaccine. A follow-up study to assess the immunogenicity and safety of a booster dose of either bHPV or HPV4 3 years after vaccination in the previous study population was conducted. Both vaccines produced an increase in antibody response, but the degree varied based on vaccine type. Interestingly, pre-booster antibody titers in this study showed a lasting immune response to the two-dose alternative schedule. Pain at the injection site was the most common adverse reaction in both groups. Pain and swelling were more common in the bHPV group. There were no serious adverse events (SAE) reported during the 1-month follow-up period [15C].

INTERACTIONS

Drug–Drug Interactions Schilling and colleagues studied the antibody response and safety of concomitant administration of 9-valent HPV (9vHPV) with quadrivalent meningococcal conjugate vaccine (MCV4) and Tdap vaccines. Participants were 11–15-year-old boys and girls. Coadministration of the vaccines was found to be non-inferior in producing an immune response compared to the vaccines being administered separately. A statistical difference in swelling at the 9vHPV injection site was observed in the coadministration group. Pain and erythema at both injection sites was not significantly different. Four subjects had SAEs, but none were deemed vaccine-related. Two subjects discontinued the study due to an adverse event (AE). Overall, coadministration of the three vaccines was found to be a safe and effective practice [16C].

Influenza Vaccines [SED-15, 3565, 3568; SEDA-35, 574; SEDA-36, 467; SEDA-37, 385]

GENERAL

The World Health Organization (WHO) recently published a report of global influenza activity and recommendations for the composition of influenza vaccines for the upcoming 2016–2017 northern hemisphere influenza season. Activity from Africa, the Americas, Asia, Europe, and Oceania indicated co-circulation of the 2009 pandemic strain of influenza A (H1N1)pdm09, A (H3N2), and influenza B viruses, with a predominance of A (H1N1)pdm09. In addition, during the reporting period five human cases of A (H5N6), two A (H5N1), 44 A (H9N2), three A (H1N1) v, and one case of A (H3N2)v were reported. The antigenic characteristics of the circulating influenza viruses provide support for continued study of current and new vaccine formulations to continue prevention efforts [17S].

ORGANS AND SYSTEMS

Cardiovascular The incidence of myocarditis/pericarditis following immunization has been studied following smallpox (SPX) vaccination. A recent multicenter, prospective, observational cohort study was conducted to assess the incidence of new onset cardiac symptoms, clinical myocarditis/pericarditis, and cardiac specific troponin (cTnT) increases in healthy, active subjects following either live attenuated SPX vaccine or inactivated influenza virus (IIV) vaccine. Enrolled subjects consisted of healthy, active persons presenting for military readiness and/or preventative healthcare requirements in the United States. Significant baseline differences between the groups revealed a higher percentage of male subjects in the SPX vaccine group ($p < 0.001$), subjects were younger ($p < 0.001$), 53.7% of subjects were current or recent smokers ($p < 0.001$), and a smaller percentage had physical limitations ($p < 0.001$). It is also noteworthy that the number of subjects differed significantly between the two groups ($n = 1081$ in the SPX group versus 189 in the IIV group). There was a significantly higher incidence of new onset cardiac symptoms following SPX vaccine (10.6%) compared to IIV vaccine (2.6%, $p < 0.001$). The most commonly reported cardiac symptoms were chest pain (8% versus 1.6% in the SPX and IIV groups, respectively) and dyspnea on exertion (4% versus 0% in the SPX and IIV groups, respectively). Thirty-one subjects in the SPX cohort experienced elevations in cTnT levels post vaccination that met criteria for subclinical myocarditis/pericarditis. Zero subjects who received the IIV vaccine had cases of clinical or subclinical myocarditis/pericarditis, in contrast to five cases of new onset clinical myocarditis/pericarditis among the SPX cohort. All clinical and subclinical signs and symptoms of myocarditis/pericarditis resolved spontaneously with conservative management. The calculated relative risk of clinical myocarditis/pericarditis following SPX vaccine was 214-fold higher than previously published studies. The study results suggest an association between SPX vaccination and myocarditis/pericarditis; this association did not present itself among the IIV cohort. Limitations of the study included the size of the IIV cohort, the need to validate the definition of subclinical myocarditis/pericarditis, and a specific study population. The authors concluded that the results provide evidence that further study of post-licensure AE surveillance to better characterize and quantify AEFI [18C].

Immunologic In general, influenza vaccines induce mild to moderate and typically transient inflammatory responses that may correspond with subjective local and systemic AEs reported by patients. A study of 56 women (28 pregnant and 28 non-pregnant) took place at one medical center during the 2011–2012 influenza season in the United States to assess serum pro-inflammatory markers at baseline and days 1, 2, and 3 following receipt of trivalent IIV (IIV3). Pro-inflammatory markers measured included interleukin (IL)-6, tumor necrosis factor (TNF)-α, IL-8, IL-1β, and macrophage migration inhibitory factor (MIF). The most common local reaction reported was mild arm soreness 1 day after vaccination ($n = 31$; 55%). Five women reported being very sore 1 day after vaccination (3 pregnant and 2 non-pregnant). The majority of subjects reported zero systemic reactions ($n = 44$; 78.6%). Ten women reported systemic reactions (mild = 6 and moderate = 4), which consisted of headache ($n = 3$), sleepiness/tired ($n = 2$), nausea ($n = 2$), sore throat ($n = 2$), dizziness ($n = 1$), mild achiness ($n = 1$), and mild fever ($n = 1$). There were no significant differences in local ($p = 0.42$) or systemic ($p = 0.49$) reactions based on pregnancy status. In addition, pregnant and non-pregnant women demonstrated similar systemic inflammatory responses after vaccination. Subjects who reported a very sore arm had higher TNF-α 1 day after vaccination compared to subjects with mild or no soreness, respectively ($p < 0.03$, $p < 0.03$). Women who reported a very sore arm also had higher MIF level 2 days after vaccination compared to women with mild ($p = 0.01$) or no ($p = 0.04$) arm soreness. Subjects who went on to report systemic reactions had higher IL-6 levels at baseline and higher MIF levels 2 days after vaccination compared to those subjects who did not report systemic reactions ($p = 0.055$ and $p = 0.03$, respectively). The results indicate that subjective local and systemic reactions correspond with biological markers of inflammatory response to IIV3 vaccination. This was a small study and the generalizability is limited due to the subject population included [19c].

Anaphylaxis following vaccination is a rare but potentially fatal event. The study of allergic reactions, including anaphylaxis, following IIV is of particular interest given the potential for a small amount of egg albumin contamination during the manufacturing process of egg-based products. One manufacturer in Japan reported an increased number of anaphylaxis cases following IIV. It was noted that there was one difference between the vaccines administered; the vaccine from this one manufacturer contained a different preservative (2-phenoxyethanol or 2-PE). Nineteen children who had a diagnosis of anaphylaxis (four with history of egg allergy, but not anaphylaxis) and two control groups (10 age-matched controls with egg allergy and 15 without egg allergy) were studied to investigate the possible cause(s) of anaphylaxis. Levels of IgE specific to vaccine components and CD203c expression on basophils were measured in all subjects. Results indicated higher levels of vaccine-specific IgE in the anaphylaxis group compared to the egg allergy and non-egg allergy control groups ($p < 0.001$ and $p < 0.005$, respectively). There was no IgE binding to excipients used in the vaccines. Levels of vaccine-induced expression of CD203c in basophils were significantly higher in the anaphylaxis group compared to the egg allergy and non-egg allergy controls ($p < 0.001$ and $p < 0.01$, respectively) at higher vaccine dilutions. The findings seem to suggest that the allergy experienced by the anaphylaxis group subjects may be related to a vaccine component but not the egg albumin. Three subjects in the anaphylaxis group did receive IIV the following season that included a different preservative (thimerosal) and no subject experienced anaphylaxis. The noted AEs included two subjects with extensive local swelling and one with mild cough. No direct causal relationship was proven during the study, but further study is warranted to continue the efforts is assessing the mechanisms and potential causes of severe allergic reactions, such as anaphylaxis following vaccination [20c].

A recombinant trivalent IIV (RIV3) was licensed in the United States in January 2013. It is the first completely egg-free influenza vaccine and is recommended for individual with a history of egg allergy (including severe reactions). The US Food and Drug Administration (FDA) recently examined AEs reported to the VAERS database between January 2013 and July 2014 to evaluate cases of allergic and anaphylactic reactions when RIV3 was the primary vaccine. Eighteen reports of AEs following receipt of RIV3 were received in the study period. The level of detail provided in the report varied. Twelve of those reports were consistent with acute hypersensitivity reactions following RIV3 vaccination. Three cases met the Brighton Collaboration case definition for level 2 anaphylaxis. All of the reports were in women aged 36–57 years of age. Ten of the 12 patients reported a history of allergies to eggs or previous reaction to other influenza vaccines. No concomitant vaccines were administered at the time of RIV3 vaccination. No fatalities or hospitalizations were reported in the database. The limitations of data retrieved from the VAERS system were discussed by the author, including heterogeneity in the detail of reports from a variety of reporters, the possibility of reporting bias, the inability to determine a causal relationship with RIV3 and the reactions, the lack of comparisons, etc. However, the results of this small collection of AEs may suggest that allergic reactions following influenza vaccination may not always be related to egg proteins. The package insert was updated for RIV3 to include this postmarketing data. Continued study will be necessary to further characterize and quantify AEs following vaccination with RIV3 [21A].

A 75-year-old female developed swelling, high fever, and malaise following vaccination with IIV (exact vaccine not reported) on three occasions. Following the third vaccination, the patient developed spontaneous skin lesions on the left arm and several occurrences of fever. She also demonstrated induration and swelling at the injection site. A skin biopsy revealed inflammatory infiltrate of lymphoid mononuclear cells, eosinophils, and plasma cells. Large-sized lymphoid mononuclear cells expressed CD3, CD8, granzyme B and Ki-67. Further testing revealed the presence of Epstein-Barr virus (EBV) in the large-sized lymphoid cells. Radiotherapy was utilized, which resulted in complete resolution. The presentation and data suggest that influenza vaccine-specific lymphocytes and EBV-positive CD8+ T cells may have been involved in the reaction of this patient. No direct causality assessment was reported by the authors [22A].

Musculoskeletal Appropriate injection technique is vital for the administration of vaccines. Aside from the common AEs associated with vaccination, additional reactions secondary to improper depth or location may result. Three cases of frozen shoulder (adhesive capsulitis) were reported in patients following receipt of pneumococcal ($n=1$) or IIV ($n=2$) vaccine. All three patients experienced shoulder stiffness, pain, and a decreased range of motion beginning the day of or day after vaccination. The diagnosis of frozen shoulder was made by clinical presentation of stiffness and pain with an absence of radiological, laboratory, and history supportive of other diagnoses. All three patients received recommendations for physical therapy and non-steroidal anti-inflammatory agents (NSAIDS), and two of the three patients received injections of a corticosteroid. The treatments recommended represented common therapy for frozen shoulder of different etiology. These reports cannot suggest a causal relationship between pneumococcal or influenza vaccine and frozen shoulder; however, the acute onset of symptoms following recent administration of the vaccines creates a possible association. This report strengthens the recommendation to ensure proper injection technique is utilized to prevent any potential AE related to vaccination [23A].

Nervous System Acute disseminated encephalomyelitis (ADEM) is an inflammatory demyelinating disease that is characterized by acute onset and rapid progression involving multifocal neurological signs, demyelinating lesions on brain magnetic resonance imaging (MRI), and potentially abnormal cerebrospinal fluid (CSF) protein. A 27-year-old previously healthy male was admitted 6 days after receipt of IIV vaccine with fever, vomiting, headache, blurred vision, nuchal pain, and fluctuating alertness. He was initially treated for suspected bacterial meningitis but did not improve on antibiotic therapy. He developed progressive weakness in all four limbs 8 days following vaccination with IIV vaccine until he was unable to walk. In addition, he developed urinary retention, constipation, and paresthesia over the trunk and legs. His CSF contained 100% lymphocytes and an elevated protein level. Brain MRI revealed brain and spinal cord lesions. The MRI lesion findings were indicative of ADEM. Infectious and autoimmune evaluations were negative. The patient received corticosteroids and intravenous immunoglobulin (IVIG). Upon completion of therapy, the patient achieved clinical remission. The authors assessed causality using criteria define by the WHO and deemed the patient's ADEM as possibly related to the IIV vaccine. Given the potential negative outcomes associated with ADEM, it is critical to advocate for thorough evaluations of patients presenting with neurological symptoms following vaccination [24A].

Chronic fatigue syndrome/myalgic encephalomyelitis (CFS/ME) is a debilitating disorder that is characterized by severe fatigue of unknown origin. A study conducted in Norway examined the risk of CFS/ME in relationship to subjects who either received monovalent influenza A (H1N1)pdm09 vaccine adjuvanted with adjuvant system 03 (AS03) (Pandemrix®) or who had influenza infection. The study population was the entire population of Norway and national databases were utilized to assess incidence of vaccination and infection. Between 2009 and 2012, 3737 cases of CFS/ME were registered. The overall rate of CFS/ME was 2.08 per 100 000 person-months. The adjusted HR of CFS/ME following influenza infection was 2.04 (95% CI: 1.78–2.33) and was 0.97 (95% CI: 0.91–1.04) following vaccination. Therefore, there was no evidence of an association between Pandemrix® and CFS/ME. Limitations of the study include the potential for missing data or misclassification of information provided in the national databases. In addition, this study was conducted in one country [25MC].

Fever and febrile seizures or convulsions remain an important area of study following vaccine administration. A systematic review recently examined data from randomized, non-randomized/observational, and unpublished studies between 2005 and 2012 to assess the incidence of fever, febrile seizure, and SAEs following receipt of IIV3. The systematic review was conducted in response to an increase in reporting of fever and febrile seizures in young (<5 years) Australian children, particularly after receipt of IIV from one manufacturer (CSL Biotherapies) and increased reporting of febrile seizures in the United States following IIV with or without concomitant vaccines [26M,27C,28r,29C]. Overall, results of the analyses performed indicated that SAEs following IIV were uncommon. Randomized and non-randomized studies reported rates of fever (≥38 °C) for children 6 months to 17 years ranging from 0.4% to 16.9% following IIV3 for all manufacturers, except CSL Biotherapies. Higher rates of fever were noted among subjects who received adjuvanted vaccines. Markedly higher fever rates were reported in the two published studies describing the bioCSL IIV vaccines; pooled estimates ranged from 5% to 39.5% with the highest percentages reported among children aged 6–35 months (39.5%, 95% CI: 28.4–51.4) and 3–8 years (27%, 95% CI: 21–33.8) [26M]. Brady and colleagues reported an incidence of 58.5% for fever in children aged 6 months to <3 years following the first dose of CSL's IIV3 compared to Fluzone® (37.3%); subjects who received CSL's IIV3 were 2.73 times as likely to develop fever compared to Fluzone® (95% CI: 1.89–3.94) [27C]. Calculation of febrile seizure rates from the systematic review was limited by the heterogeneity of the methods/design, controls, and definitions utilized by all included studies. However, the calculated rate of febrile seizures for the randomized controlled trials was 1.1 per 1000 children 6 to <72 months of age vaccinated with a non-adjuvanted IIV3 vaccine. These findings highlight the potential for differing event incidences based on manufacturer and emphasize the importance for continued vigilance regarding the study of the ever-changing influenza vaccines, particularly in young children [26M].

Guillain-Barré syndrome (GBS) is an acute, autoimmune condition of the peripheral nerves that is characterized by muscle weakness and loss of reflexes. The exact causes of GBS are unknown, but the syndrome has been associated with infections of the gastrointestinal tract as well as respiratory tract, including influenza. It is theorized that GBS may be triggered by antigenic stimulation, which results in demyelination and damage to the peripheral nerves. A meta-analysis was conducted to assess the risk of GBS with different influenza vaccines from January 1977 to April 2014. Thirty-nine studies were included, involving seasonal influenza vaccine in 22 and pandemic H1N1 vaccines in 16. The statistical analysis demonstrated that 6 out of the 22 seasonal influenza studies and 7 of the 16 pandemic H1N1 vaccine studies discovered a statistically significant difference in the risk of GBS associated with the influenza vaccine studied. The heterogeneity among the study designs, populations and vaccines included, and statistical analysis undertaken by each study should be considered. In addition, the authors did not consider the quality of the studies included in this meta-analysis. While this meta-analysis indicates an association between influenza vaccines and GBS, this does not correlate with previously published studies and the results should be carefully considered. Further study regarding the possible connection between GBS and influenza vaccination is warranted to more thoroughly describe this possible association [30M].

Narcolepsy is a chronic sleep disorder caused by hypothalamic hypocretin deficiency. It is suspected to have an autoimmune etiology. Narcolepsy is rare, with an estimated incidence of 0.74–1.37 cases per 100 000 person/years. The association of the monovalent influenza A (H1N1)pdm09 adjuvanted with AS03 vaccine (Pandemrix®) and narcolepsy continues to undergo extensive study. The Pandemrix® vaccine was primarily used in European countries during the 2009–2010 pandemic. As of July 2014, over 1000 reports of narcolepsy can be found in the EUDRAVIGILANCE database (many of which may represent duplicates due to the ability of a variety of reporters). An extensive research initiative has taken place in Sweden with studies concluded that a three to fourfold increased risk of narcolepsy exists among subjects ≤20 years who received Pandemrix® compared to those who did not [31H]. A number of questions and theories are being examined in order to determine the nature of the association between the vaccine and narcolepsy. Hypotheses under consideration include a dysregulation of the immune system potentially associated with the adjuvant (AS03), molecular mimicry with hypocretin, genetic predisposition, and the potential for natural infection exposure impacting narcolepsy development. While a great number of studies are being performed, limitations of such studies have been extensive and have been yet unsuccessful in characterizing this association. Further research is critical to validate this association and characterize the mechanism of narcolepsy development in subjects exposed to the Pandemrix® vaccine [31H,32H].

Increased study and concern for neurological conditions and their potential association with influenza A (H1N1)pdm09 vaccines has lead to examination of a number of AEFI. A study conducted in Quebec, Canada examined AEFI characterized as paresthesia in subjects aged 18–64 years with an onset within 72 hours of vaccination. Data were extracted from the Quebec VAERS systems; healthcare professionals are required to report unusual clinical problems potentially associated with vaccination. Subjects were also interviewed with a standard questionnaire regarding their experience, this occurred 6–8 months following the reported reaction. A total of 328 paresthesia cases were reported, the majority of cases were in females (81%), and the overall rate was 7.5 cases per 100 000 doses administered. Most cases (97%) reported receiving the AS03 adjuvanted H1N1 vaccine. Symptom onset occurred quickly after vaccination (15 minutes to 2 hours). Paresthesia was most commonly described as numbness (86%) or prickling/tingling (66%); however; pain was reported by 58% of subjects. Visual problems were reported in 14% of subjects and speaking problems in 15% of subjects. Overall, paresthesia represented the third most commonly report AEFI reported in the Quebec VAERS systems following vaccination with AS03 adjuvanted H1N1pdm09 vaccine. Symptoms subsided within 1 week for ~40% of the subjects but persisted up to ≥6 months in a number of subjects. The results cannot confirm a causal relationship between the vaccine and paresthesia but does demonstrate temporal association. Further investigation will improve understanding of the association as a possible AEFI following vaccination [33C].

A 41-year-old man presented with headache, leg paresthesia, and sensory loss two of 2 months duration 2 months following vaccination with monovalent influenza A (H1N1)pdm09 vaccine (specific vaccine not indicated). The patient had a history of psoriasis, diagnosed 9 years earlier. The patient had received yellow fever (YF) vaccine 16 months prior to the onset of neurologic symptoms. Noted reactions following YF vaccine included myalgia, arthralgia, fatigue, xerostomia, and vomiting for 8 days following vaccination. Following H1N1 vaccine, the patient's neurologic symptoms (occipital headache, xerostomia, paresthesia of both legs, and loss of transient vibratory sensation in both thighs) persisted and further evaluation was performed which included hospital admission, blood, immunoglobulin, liver, and muscle enzyme evaluation, autoimmune markers, bacterial and parasitic testing, and brain and spinal cord imaging. Based upon the clinical symptoms and MRI findings, the patient was diagnosed with transverse myelitis. He was treated with corticosteroids and azathioprine for 3 months and achieved total remissions of all neurological symptoms. Follow-up imaging at 7 months did not reveal any signs of demyelinating lesions. Given the patient's

response to treatment, previous history, and recent receipt of H1N1 vaccine, the authors concluded that the symptoms suggest an immune-mediated reaction to the vaccine, or potentially an adjuvant used in the vaccine. However, the specific vaccine was not described in the report, nor was a formal causality assessment. Neurological symptoms have been reported following influenza vaccination previously and this report indicates further need for study and assessment of such symptoms to better characterize any association between symptoms and vaccination [34A].

Skin A 48-year-old man presented to a contact dermatitis clinic after he developed an acute erythematous, excoriated dermatitis on his neck, anterior chest, shoulders, antecubital fossa, and forearms with severe pruritus that began 48 hours following vaccination with IIV vaccine (Agriflu®). The patient was treated with two courses of corticosteroids and an oral antibiotic and his symptoms resolved completely. The patient's history revealed a similar pattern of dermatitis on his forearms that developed after he was working with plywood and pressure-treated lumber. He had also been using a topical lotion containing imidazolidinyl urea at the time. The Agriflu® vaccine contains formaldehyde, which is used during the manufacturing process. The patient had previously been exposed and likely sensitized to formaldehyde and formaldehyde-releasing preservatives in the plywood and his topical lotion. The patient was skin patch tested with positive results for reactions to formaldehyde and four of the formaldehyde-releasing preservatives, including imidazolidinyl urea. Systemic contact dermatitis may present in patterns of flare-up at previously affected sites. This case represents a patient with a systemic contact dermatitis at previously affects site (his forearms) in addition to new sites (neck and anterior chest). It is the authors' conclusion that the patient experienced the case of dermatitis from the formaldehyde contained in the IIV vaccine. Awareness of all patient hypersensitivity reactions, including any potential excipients included in vaccines, is valuable information that may lead to a recommendation for an alternative agent to prevent future reactions [35A].

Pityriasis lichenoides (PL) is a group of inflammatory cutaneous diseases and there are three subtypes recognized. Pityriasis lichenoides et varioliformis acuta (PLEVA) typically consists of erythematous macules smaller than 5 mm, which evolve into papules with thin micaceous desquamation, in addition systemic manifestations are uncommon. A 12-year-old male patient presented 5 days following influenza vaccination (exact product unknown) with multiple pruritic erythematous papules (2–4 mm) on the trunk, abdomen, and limbs. He did not initially demonstrate systemic reactions and was diagnosed with chickenpox based on his lack of history of the infection. However, his symptoms progressed to include fever, tachycardia, moderate dehydration, vomiting, and prostration, which led to hospital admission. His laboratory values indicated leukocytosis, elevated C-reactive protein, negative infectious etiology evaluation, and histopathological exam revealing extensive lymphocytic inflammatory infiltrate invading the epidermis. A diagnosis of PLEVA was made according to the clinical presentation and histopathological data. The patient was treated with a corticosteroid and oral antibiotic. Nearly complete remission of lesions was obtained after 3 months. Extrinsic antigens, such as contained in vaccines, may trigger PLEVA. The authors concluded that the probable cause of PLEVA in this patient was influenza vaccination. The PL subtypes may be mistaken for chickenpox and this report encourages education and in-depth examinations to ensure appropriate diagnoses [36A].

Urinary Tract A 60-year-old African-American female presented to the emergency department 2 weeks after she received the 2009 monovalent influenza A H1N1pdm09 vaccine. Soon after vaccination, she developed fever, nausea and vomiting, and lower extremity edema. Her history included bronchial asthma. Her initial serum creatinine was 10.3 mg/dL 1 day prior to the emergency department visit, which was 9.93 mg/dL upon emergency department presentation. Additional manifestations upon admission included elevated blood pressure (220/100 mm Hg), 3+ pitting edema of the lower extremities, a total protein of 4.5 g/dL, and a serum albumin of 2.2 g/dL. The patient's serum creatinine 3 months prior to this event was normal at 0.9 mg/dL. Infectious and autoimmune work-ups were negative/normal. A kidney biopsy demonstrated patchy edema and mild to moderate inflammatory cell infiltrate composed of mononuclear cells with many eosinophils. The findings were consistent with stage I membranous nephropathy (MN) and acute interstitial nephritis (AIN). The patient was treated with diuretics, anti-hypertensive agents, and corticosteroids with normalization of serum creatinine. The patient did suffer a relapse upon discontinuation of the steroid therapy; however, when reinitiated for a longer duration of therapy, the patient achieved and maintained a full recovery. No formal causality assessment was discussed by the authors; however, the timeline between influenza vaccination and symptoms onset creates a temporal relationship and warrants further investigation to establish the association and pathogenesis of this reaction [37A].

SECOND-GENERATION EFFECTS

Pregnancy Continued study of the reactogenicity of influenza vaccine in pregnant women remains important given the potential antigenic alterations of the vaccines from year to year. An observational study conducted in Australia utilized short message service (SMS) to compare AEFI of the same type of IIV3 vaccine among pregnant and non-pregnant female healthcare workers of similar age. At least one AEFI was reported in 13% of pregnant women and 17.3% of non-pregnant healthcare workers ($p = 0.34$). The most common reactions reported were local reactions (4.5% and 7.3%) of pregnant and non-pregnant women, respectively ($p = 0.13$). Systemic reactions were similar between the two groups; however, fever and headache were more frequently reported among non-pregnant healthcare workers (5.8% versus 1.6% and 4.7% versus 2.9% for fever and headache, respectively. No SAEs related to the vaccine were reported. The limitations of this study included the observational nature of the study and potential for reporting bias. In addition, the non-pregnant female healthcare works are not likely the most appropriate comparator for this population. Overall, the results indicated that SMS may provide AEFI data in this population and pregnant women reported similar rates of side effects compared to non-pregnant women of similar age [38C].

A systematic review of published studied attempted to characterize the effects of influenza vaccination during pregnancy related to fetal death, spontaneous abortion, and congenital malformation outcomes. Of the 19 studies from multiple countries included in the review, there was significant heterogeneity with regard to study design, definitions of outcomes, vaccine products provided, and potential confounders encountered. For example, women vaccinated in the first trimester were underrepresented in the review. The results did not indicate an association between maternal vaccination with influenza vaccine and increased risk of fetal death, spontaneous abortion, or congenital malformation, but the observational design and clinical and methodological heterogeneity lead to significant potential for bias and the inability to state definitive conclusions [39M].

A retrospective cohort study was conducted in Italy to evaluate maternal and fetal outcomes following vaccination with a monovalent influenza A (H1N1)pdm09 vaccine during the second or third trimester. Regional databases and registries were utilized to access patient data following vaccination and up to the first 6 months of life for newborns. Maternal outcomes assessed included hospital admissions with a primary or secondary diagnosis of influenza, pneumonia, gestational hypertension, eclampsia, gestational diabetes, thyroid disease, or anemia. Fetal and neonatal outcomes assessed included stillbirth, preterm birth (<37 weeks' gestation), very preterm birth (<32 weeks' gestation), low birth weight (<2500 g), very low birth weight (<1500 g), low 5-minute Apgar score (<7), and presence of any congenital malformation (at birth or hospital admission within 6 months of birth). Of the 2003 vaccinated women included, nearly half were vaccinated during the second trimester (45.3%) and the remainder during the third trimester (54.7%). The overall vaccine coverage rate was very low (2%). Compared to the 98 329 unvaccinated pregnant women used as comparators, vaccinated pregnant women had more frequently reported pre-existing health-risk conditions as evidenced by hospital admissions in the 12 months prior to pregnancy (1.4% versus 0.8%, $p = 0.008$). Results did not reveal any statistically significant association between vaccination with the pandemic influenza A (H1N1)pdm09 vaccine and adverse outcomes. However, an increased risk of limb congenital malformation, diagnosed in the first 6 months of life was observed in the vaccinated group (adjusted HR = 2.35, 95% CI: 0.84–6.58, $p = 0.105$). Noted limitations include the study sample size, calculations utilized for age, pre-existing health-care risk condition identification, and lack of inclusion of women vaccinated in the first trimester. Further study is warranted in a multicenter setting [40MC].

Chorioamnionitis is a serious infection that may affect term and pre-term pregnancies. There are a significant number of risk factors that have been associated with chorioamnionitis. A review of the VAERS reporting system over a 24-year timespan was conducted to assess reports of chorioamnionitis after receipt of any vaccine in the United States to determine if a potential safety concern exists and warrants further investigation. The potential limitations of VAERS-reported data were reviewed by the authors, including the passive nature of the system that may lead to bias, the acceptance of a report from anyone, the potential inconsistency of included reports, and the lack of any causality assessment. The review discovered 31 cases of chorioamnionitis during the study period documented following a variety of vaccines. The most common vaccines included in reports were monovalent 2009 influenza A (H1N1)pdm09 (32%), HPV4 (29%), and Tdap (26%) vaccines. Fifty-eight percent of the reports indicated at least one risk factor for chorioamnionitis. Adverse outcomes reported included nine fetal deaths, 22 live births (6 pre-term and 16 term), two postpartum hemorrhage, and one maternal intensive care unit admission. Of the six pre-term births, two resulted in infant deaths. Overall, the review noted that chorioamnionitis was a "very" infrequently reported in the VAERS database and did not signify a safety concern based on this review over 24 years. Continued studied will occur to assess the safety of vaccination [10c].

The safety of concomitant administration of vaccines in pregnancy is becoming a more prominent question given the recommendations for IIV and Tdap during pregnancy. A review of seven participating sites of the Vaccine Safety Datalink (VSD) in the United States sought to assess the risk of medically attended acute AEs or adverse birth outcomes in pregnant women who either received concomitant IIV and Tdap compared to those who received the vaccines sequentially between 2007 and 2013. Overall, AEs were rare and there were no differences between women receiving IIV and Tdap concomitantly compared to sequentially with regard to medically attended fever and any acute event within 3 or 7 days after vaccination. In addition, no differences were noted in the birth outcomes of pre-term delivery ($p = 0.54$), low-birth-weight ($p = 0.34$), and small for gestational age ($p = 0.92$) neonates born to women receiving concomitant compared to sequential IIV and Tdap vaccines. It is important to note that no causality assessment was performed during the study. Additional limitations include the inclusion of only medically attended AEs, the presence of potential confounders, the exclusion of non-live births, the inclusion of only insured women, and lack of long-term follow-up of infants. Overall, results support the concomitant administration of IIV and Tdap vaccines in pregnant women [41MC].

SUSCEPTIBILITY FACTORS

Disease: Duchenne Muscular Dystrophy (DMD) Preventing respiratory infections in patients with Duchenne muscular dystrophy (DMD) is significantly important based upon the pathogenesis of the disease state and potential complications resulting from infections, such as influenza. Vaccination against influenza annually is recommended for this patient population; however, limited published data exist with regard to the safety and efficacy of influenza vaccine in patients with DMD. A small study was conducted with 44 patients with DMD compared to 41 healthcare worker control subjects. All subjects received one dose of monovalent, un-adjuvanted, inactivated, split influenza A (H1N1)pdm09 vaccine subcutaneously. All reported reactions were mild in severity. Both local and systemic reactions were more common on the healthcare work control subjects compared to the DMD patients. Redness was the most commonly reported local reaction in 27% of DMD patients versus 41% of controls ($p = 0.170$) and pain was noted in 5% of DMD patients compared to 32% of controls ($p = 0.001$). Malaise was the most commonly reported systemic reaction in 20% of the control subjects compared to 0% of the DMD patients ($p = 0.002$). Fever of $\geq 37.5\,°C$ was noted in 5% of DMD patients versus 10% of controls ($p = 0.432$). The method for collection of AEs was self-reporting via a questionnaire; this may have introduced information bias and affected results. The capability of DMD patients to elicit inflammatory responses may have also impacted the results; this remains unclear. The study also took place in one hospital setting and included a small number of DMD patients who were not immunosuppressed with corticosteroids, which may limit generalizability [42c].

Disease: Systemic Lupus Erythematosus (SLE) Systemic lupus erythematosus (SLE) is an autoimmune disease that may affect a number of organs and impair immunity. The immune response and safety of influenza vaccine has remained under debate and consideration based upon previously published works. A recent meta-analysis reported findings from 17 cohort studies and one abstract from 1978 to 2013 conducted in eight countries regarding the immunogenicity and safety of influenza vaccine in SLE patients. The influenza antigens included in study vaccines were trivalent (H1N1, H3N2, and influenza B), bivalent (H1N1 and H3N2), or monovalent (H1N1). Safety data indicated that all side effects were mild and transient and the rate of side effects in SLE patients was not significantly higher compared to the general population, although side effects were numerically higher in SLE patients compared to healthy controls. The OR for side effects was 3.24 (95% CI: 0.62–16.67). Among the 1966 SLE patients examined in the meta-analysis, 32 had mild SLE exacerbations and five had serious side effects, including two hospitalization, two severe SLE exacerbations, and one death. Most of the serious AEs could not be attributed to vaccination with influenza vaccine. The authors concluded that influenza vaccine was not detrimental to patients with a low-moderate SLE disease score or stable disease based on the studies evaluated. In addition, it did not appear that influenza vaccine exacerbated SLE based on the analysis. The overall conclusion supported the use of influenza vaccination practices in SLE patients in a pandemic setting in order to prevent complications of a severe infection. Further study is required to expand the practice of influenza vaccination in the SLE population [43M].

DRUG ADMINISTRATION

Drug Formulations Quadrivalent inactivated influenza vaccines (IIV4) have been incorporated into the seasonal vaccination recommendations. A large, phase III, randomized, controlled, multicenter trial was conducted in Australia and the Philippines to assess the safety of IIV4 in children aged 9–17 years and adults aged 18–60 years compared to IIV3 vaccine. Reactions were similarly reported between subjects receiving IIV4 and IIV3. In adult subjects, 61.2% and 57.1% reported local or systemic reactions in the IIV4 and IIV3 groups, respectively. In children, 66.6% and 67.3% of subjects reported local or systemic reactions, respectively. Pain at the injection site was the most frequently reported local reaction, while headache, malaise, and myalgia were the most common systemic reactions. The majority of reactions were mild or moderate in severity. Two reactions occurred within 30 minutes of vaccination, one adult with urticaria (IIV4) and one with cough (IIV3); both subjects recovered and completed the study. Thirteen SAEs were reported in IIV4 subjects and none were related to the vaccine. No AEs of interested or deaths were reported during the study period. The results support the safety and tolerability of IIV4 vaccines in children and adults aged 9–60 years [44MC].

Several influenza viruses are labeled with pandemic potential for a variety of reasons and preparation tactics including vaccination preparation must be considered to prevent morbidity and mortality. Influenza A (H2N2) has been associated with pandemics of the past and continues to be studied in order to prepare for potential pandemics of the future. A phase I, double-blind, randomized, placebo-controlled study was conducted assessing safety and immunogenicity of two doses 28 days apart of a live attenuated influenza vaccine (LAIV) containing a monovalent strain of influenza A/17/California/66/395 (H2N2) in healthy adults in Russia. Local reactions were reported in four (14.3%) of vaccinated subjects after the first dose, but zero after the second dose of LAIV H2N2. Systemic reactions were similarly reported among subjects in the LAIV H2N2 subjects compared to the placebo subjects. Reactions were reported 46.4% after dose one and 32.1% after dose two for LAIV subjects versus 50% after dose one and 20% after dose two for placebo subjects. The most common systemic reaction was fever (42.9% after dose one and 14.3% after dose two) in the LAIV H2N2 group. All reported reactions were classified as mild. Additional AEs reported after receipt of LAIV H2N2 vaccine included laboratory abnormalities. Two cases of moderate increased alanine aminotransferase (one after each dose), one case of increased bilirubin, and one case of increased glucose occurred after dose two in the LAIV group. One case of moderately elevated bilirubin occurred in the placebo group after dose one. Overall, the LAIV H2N2 vaccine was well tolerated and safe and was not associated with any SAEs during this study which supports continued examination of this drug formulation for pandemic preparedness [45c].

Additional influenza A subtypes under consideration for pandemic potential include the H9N2 subtype. A phase I/II, randomized, double-blind study was performed to assess safety and immunogenicity of various dosages of two doses 21 days apart of a Vero cell culture-derived whole-virus influenza A (H9N2) vaccine in health adults aged 18–49 years. The most commonly reported local reactions were pain and tenderness at the injection site. The rates of injection site reactions were lower at lower doses (3.75 and 7.5 mcg) of the vaccine (16.1–18.2% after dose one and 13.2–15.1% after the second dose) compared to higher doses (15, 30, and 45 mcg). Systemic reactions were comparable across all study groups and ranged from 12.5% to 25.9% after the first dose and 5.6% to 13% after the second dose. Headache and fatigue were the most frequently reported reactions. Zero subjects reported a fever after the first dose and only one after the second dose (45 mcg dose subject). No vaccine-related SAEs were reported. Overall, the vaccine was considered safe and well tolerated across all dosage groups and comparable to previously reported data with H5N1 and H1N1 studies [46C].

Drug Additives The first oil-in-water, squalene-based emulsion to be used as a vaccine adjuvant was MF-59. The first MF-59 adjuvanted influenza vaccines licensed for use occurred in Europe in 1997. The safety of MF-59 adjuvanted vaccines has been studied in children, adults, and pregnant women. Such studies have sited minimal difference with regard to local reactions of redness, swelling, and tenderness among children and only slightly more frequent local reactions among elderly adults compared to non-adjuvanted IIV vaccines. No significant differences were noted for risk of GBS, anaphylaxis, demyelinating disorders, idiopathic thrombocytopenic purpura, or vasculitis as reported in a post-licensure review in Italy. Finally, no significant differences were observed in the pregnancy and neonatal outcomes of preeclampsia, spontaneous abortion, stillbirth, neonatal death, or congenital malformation in a previously published meta-analysis. This review supports the consideration of further study and utilization of MF-59 as a vaccine adjuvant [47r].

Drug Administration Route: Intradermal Due to the prevalence data indicating the co-circulation of the two influenza B virus lineages, incorporation of both lineages into IIV4 vaccines was introduced in the United States during the 2013–2014 influenza season for adults aged 18–64 years. A phase III, randomized, double-blind, active-controlled trial examined the safety and immunogenicity of the intradermal quadrivalent inactivated influenza vaccine (IIV4-ID) compared to two IIV3-ID products. Pain and pruritus were the most frequently reported local reactions and myalgia, headache, and malaise were the most commonly reported systemic reactions. The rates of injection-site pain and pruritus were higher among the younger adults in the study (18–49 years) for both IIV4-ID and IIV3-ID subjects. Headache was reported in 3.2% of the IIV4-ID pooled subjects compared to 2.1% of the pooled IIV3-ID subjects. Previous influenza vaccination appeared to have little effect on the reactogenicity of IIV4-ID. Six SAEs were reported during the study but zero events were considered vaccine related. One death occurred that was unrelated to the study vaccines. Results indicate a comparable safety profile of IIV4-ID to two IIV3-ID products in this patient population [48C].

Drug Dosage Regimens A number of significant research questions have been generated following the 2009–2010 influenza A (H1N1) pandemic. Research continues to answer such questions regarding the safety and immunogenicity of various dosages, dose frequencies, and adjuvant inclusion. In addition, the profound impact on morbidity and mortality of children during a pandemic heightens the importance for study in this population. Knuf and colleagues have reported results from two studies to provide support of the further study and use of monovalent MF-59 adjuvanted H1N1pmd09 vaccines manufactured via egg-based production as well as cell-derived methods in children aged 6 months to 17 years. Reactions were similar to previously published studies and demonstrated slightly higher rates of reactions following adjuvanted vaccines compared to non-adjuvanted formulations as well as improved immunogenicity. The higher doses of the MF-59 adjuvant were associated with increased rates of AEs reported. The study performed in children aged 3–17 years did not report any SAEs related to the study vaccine [49C]. Whereas, the study of the cell-derived vaccine conducted in children aged 6 months to 17 years did conclude that three SAEs were possibly related to the study vaccine. The events included a case of multiple seizure episodes 98 days following vaccination, vomiting in one subject 26 days after vaccination, and one case of febrile convulsion 10 days following vaccination [50C]. Dosing considerations remain, however, the safety of MF-59 adjuvanted egg-based and cell-derived formulations appear generally well tolerated among this population.

In response to the significant number of avian influenza A (H5N1) cases documented between 2003 to present, consideration and study of H5N1 vaccines is necessary in order to continue appropriate prevention efforts as well as prepare for the significance of the potential future impact of this virus. A phase II trial provided safety data in children aged 3–9 years who received one of three formulations of influenza A (H5N1) vaccine compared to subjects receiving IIV3. More recently, an extension of this trial was conducted to assess safety data 24 months after vaccination. The authors reported no apparent differences in frequency or severity of AEs between those subjects who received influenza A (H5N1) vaccine versus IIV3 and concluded that the H5N1 formulations presented a clinically acceptable safety profile [51C]. The results of this trial encouraged further study of the H5N1 vaccines in younger children given the increased risk of morbidity and mortality if this population were to present with natural infection due to influenza A (H5N1). Therefore, a phase II/III, placebo-controlled trial was conducted in three countries to asses a two-dose regimen of influenza A (H5N1) vaccine containing one of the formulations previously studied in children 3–9 years (inactivated, split-virion H5N1 influenza with 1.9 mcg of hemagglutinin antigen [HA] adjuvanted with AS03$_B$ [5.93 mg tocopherol]) in children aged 6 months to 17 years. The frequencies of local symptoms following vaccination with the first and second doses were 58.8% and 51.4%, respectively in the H5N1 group compared to 23.4% and 19.6% in placebo group, respectively. Pain at the injection site was the most commonly reported symptom in 67.2% of H5N1 subjects and 30.1% of the placebo subjects. In children less than 6 years, irritability/fussiness and drowsiness were the most commonly reported general symptoms reported in 43.5% and 34.4%, respectively, in the H5N1 group and 32.8% and 23.8%, respectively, in the placebo group. Rates of fever in the 6- to 35-month groups were 22.4% and 16.4%, respectively, in the H5N1 and placebo groups. Rates of fever were lower in the H5N1 groups of older children. There were no study withdrawals due to AE or SAEs. One incidence of febrile convulsion was reported in the H5N1 group but this was not considered vaccine related. No cases of narcolepsy were observed, which is pertinent given the reports included elsewhere in this chapter regarding the influenza A (H1N1)pdm09 vaccine adjuvanted with AS03 and the potential link to narcolepsy [52C].

The currently available H5N1 vaccines have undergone continued study to ascertain the safety and most appropriate dosage formulation and regimen for various populations of susceptible patients. A phase IV, randomized, open-label study was conducted in Korea in adults aged 18–60 years with two doses 21 days apart of the H5N1 inactivated virion recombinant vaccine containing 3.75 mcg of HA and adjuvanted with AS03 containing 11.86 mg of tocopherol compared to IIV3. Pain was the most common local symptom reported, which occurred at a rate of 88.1% after the first and second doses of H5N1 vaccine. Overall, the frequency of pain was 95.2% in the H5N1 group (first and second doses combined) compared to 68.1% in the IIV3 group. Muscle aches and fatigue were the most commonly reported general symptoms occurring in 73.8% and 64.3%, respectively, of subjects in the H5N1 group compared to 27.7% and 29.8%, respectively, of the IIV3 group subjects. No increase in incidence of general symptoms was noted after the first and second doses of H5N1 vaccine. One subject in the H5N1 group reported three SAEs, which were not related to the vaccine. No SAEs were reported in the IIV3 group. The study results supported further study and use of the H5N1 vaccine in this patient population [53C].

Remaining questions and concerns regarding the preparedness for potential pandemic producing influenza strains such as H5N1 include the safety and immunogenicity of stockpiled vaccine. A phase II study recently examined two doses 21 days apart of a H5N1 inactivated, split-virion influenza vaccine containing 3.75 mcg HA of influenza A/Indonesia/5/2005 adjuvanted with AS03 containing 11.86 mg of tocopherol in adults aged 18–64 years. The bulk antigen was manufactured in 2007 and the adjuvant was created in 2009. The study was initiated in 2011 and the two products were mixed together prior to administration to subjects. The most common injection site reaction was pain reported in 91% of subjects (89.9% after the first dose and 77.9% after the second dose). Swelling and redness were reported in 15.4% and 9% of subjects, respectively. The most common general

symptoms were fatigue, muscle aches, and headache, reported in 44.9%, 39.7%, and 35.9%, respectively. Seven subjects reported eight AEs considered related to the vaccine and the reactions included dryness at the injection site, injection site hematoma, injection pruritus, dysgeusia, pruritus, and pruritic rash. No SAEs were considered related to the study vaccine. The results of this study support the consideration for stockpiling of antigen (subtype but not strain-matched) and adjuvant as the results did not indicate a compromise to immune response or the reactogenicity of the vaccine [54c].

Japanese Encephalitis [SEDA-35, 575; SEDA-36, 475; SEDA-37, 393]

GENERAL

The WHO updated their previous 2006 recommendations on Japanese encephalitis (JE) vaccine. Where JE is a concern, mainly South-East Asia and Western Pacific areas, routine vaccination should be integrated into the immunization schedules. Three types of vaccine are preferred, which include inactivated Vero cell-derived vaccine, live-attenuated vaccine, and live recombinant vaccine. Due to a less favorable safety profile, inactivated mouse brain-derived vaccines should be replaced with one of the three newer, preferred vaccines. The WHO reviewed the safety of the three preferred vaccine types and found favorable side effect profiles [55S].

DRUG ADMINISTRATION

Drug Formulations A meta-analysis compared study results on the immunogenicity and safety in infants and children less than 2 years of three JE vaccines: inactivated Vero cell-derived vaccine (JEV-I(Vero)), inactivated primary hamster kidney cell-derived vaccine (JEV-I(PHK)), and live-attenuated vaccine (JEV-L). Safety profiles for all three vaccines were favorable. The immunogenicity of JEV-I(PHK) was found to be less than JEV-I (Vero) and JEV-L [56M].

DRUG ADMINISTRATION

Drug Dosage Regimens An accelerated regimen of JE vaccine in combination with rabies vaccine was studied for immunogenicity and safety. The accelerated combination was compared to a standard vaccination schedule of combined vaccine as well as both vaccine components alone. A Vero cell-derived inactivated JE vaccine was utilized in this study. Non-inferiority of the accelerated schedule was established in the study. Adverse effects occurred in 79–85% of patients between groups. Most common side effects included injection site pain. The most common systemic reactions were fatigue and headache. Severe reactions were uncommon, but reported by eight patients. One patient experienced eyelid edema and generalized pruritus following JE vaccination, likely related to vaccination. The most common possible or probable side effect related to vaccination was nasopharyngitis [57C].

Measles–Mumps–Rubella (MMR) Vaccine [SED-15, 3555, 3566, 3567, 3569; SEDA-35, 575; SEDA-36, 473; SEDA-37, 391]

ORGANS AND SYSTEMS

Psychiatric Autism spectrum disorders (ASD) have been a public concern following MMR vaccination, despite the substantial medical literature finding no link between MMR vaccination and ASD. Various studies have suggested that younger siblings of children with ASD are less likely to complete the MMR vaccination series than their older siblings or children without ASD. A retrospective cohort study sought to describe the occurrence of ASD in younger siblings of children with ASD after MMR vaccination. Unadjusted and adjusted relative risk values were reported for MMR vaccination and ASD at ages two through 5 years. Following one dose of MMR vaccine, there were no significant differences in ASD occurrence at any age for younger siblings of a child with or without ASD. Following two doses of MMR vaccine at age five, the unadjusted risk ratios were significantly different in both groups. However, when adjusted for covariates such as birth year, sex, race/ethnicity, there were no significant differences in occurrence of ASD in either group [58C].

Body Temperature A retrospective review of febrile seizure episodes was conducted to determine the relative incidence and vaccine-attributable risk of febrile seizures after MMR or varicella vaccination. The study found a significantly higher risk of febrile seizure following the first dose of MMR 5–12 days after vaccination. There was no significantly different risk in the 13–30-day period. The varicella vaccination was not found to have a significant risk of febrile seizures in this study [59c].

Measles–Mumps–Rubella–Varicella (MMRV) Vaccine [SEDA-35, 575; SEDA-36, 474, SEDA-37, 391]

GENERAL

A cohort study of children aged 12–23 months was conducted to determine the risk of additional safety concerns following MMR and varicella zoster virus vaccines (MMR + V) administered separately versus the combination MMRV vaccination. No increased risk of acute disseminated encephalomyelitis, anaphylaxis, arthritis, ataxia, immune thrombocytopenia purpura, Kawasaki disease, or meningitis/encephalitis was found. There was a twofold increased risk for seizure in the 7–10-day period post-vaccination for the MMRV recipients. No new safety concerns were identified [60MC].

ORGANS AND SYSTEMS

Infection Risk An 18-month, previously health child was diagnosed with measles 7 days after vaccination with MMRV vaccine. The child was admitted for further evaluation on day 13 post-vaccination due to the persistence of symptoms. The child had a positive throat swab for measles, influenza A (H3N2), and respiratory syncytial virus. The measles virus was determined to be the vaccine strain through genome sequencing. The child's symptoms persisted for 17 days, after which a full recovery was made. Throat swabs continued to be positive through day 25 and had cleared by day 28 [61A].

Body Temperature A meta-analysis of 39 trials reviewed the risk of febrile seizures following vaccination with MMR + V, MMR, and MMRV. A twofold increase in risk for febrile seizure or seizure was found amongst children 10–24 months following MMRV vaccination between 7 and 10 days or 5 and 12 days. No other significant risks were found. This study adds to the body of evidence that febrile seizures are more frequently reported with MMRV vaccination [62M].

Death A 13-month-old female died following complications from severe combined immunodeficiency (SCID), multiple infections from vaccine-derived viruses, and nosocomial adenovirus pneumonia. The girl was vaccinated with MMRV and hospitalized 4 weeks later. She was diagnosed with SCID at that time, related to adenosine deaminase deficiency. On presentation, she had a generalized rash consistent with an active varicella infection. Sputum cultures and polymerase chain reaction confirmed diagnoses of varicella, measles, mumps, and rubella. Post-mortem assessment concluded the infections were from vaccine-derived strains. This case emphasizes the importance of consideration for immunodeficiency syndromes prior to vaccination with live-attenuated vaccines [63A].

Drug–Drug Interactions Routine vaccination against measles, mumps, rubella, varicella, poliomyelitis, diphtheria-tetanus-pertussis, HBV, and *Haemophilus influenzae* type b (Hib) are common practice throughout the globe. Combination vaccines may help to increase vaccination rates and potentially decrease stress/pain associated with multiple injections. A study conducted in Germany and Italy evaluated the concomitant administration of MMRV (ProQuad®) with hexavalent diphtheria-tetanus-acellular pertussis, HBV, inactivated poliovirus (IPV), Hib (DTaP-HBV-IPV/Hib [Infanrix hexa®]) in children ≥12 to <24 months of age (Group 1) compared to children who received only ProQuad® (Group 2) or only Infanrix hexa® (Group 3). Most subjects in each of the three groups experienced at least one local injection-site AEs or systemic AE (90.5%, 72.6%, and 84.1%). The intensity of the local reactions was largely mild or moderate in nature. Increases in temperature ($\geq$39.4 °C) were comparable between Groups 1 and 3 (3.2% and 3.8%) and Groups 1 and 2 (16.4% and 14.6%). Two cases of febrile convulsions occurred in subjects in Group 1 during the study period. Neither was deemed related to the study vaccine. The first occurred in a subject 33 days post vaccination and the second occurred in a subject 2 days post vaccination with two concomitant infections. The authors concluded that the concomitant administration of ProQuad® with a hexavalent vaccine did not adversely affect the safety or the immunogenicity results of either vaccine and advocated for further co-administration [64C].

Poliovirus Vaccines [SED-15, 3567]

GENERAL

The recommendation to replace trivalent oral polio vaccine (tOPV) with bivalent OPV following an initial dose of IPV was made to eliminate the exposure to type 2 poliovirus. Polio cases due to wild-type poliovirus type 2 have been non-existent for almost two decades; however, complications due to vaccine-related type 2 virus still occur. The United States has been using an IPV-alone vaccination schedule since 2000. Data supporting the combination regimen of bOPV-IPV are lacking. Concern also exists regarding the worldwide acceptance of IPV. An analysis of VAERS data was completed to characterize AEs due to IPV between 2000 and 2012. A total of 41 792 AEs were reported during this time, with 36 946 (88%) being non-serious and 4050 (10%) being non-fatal serious. A total of 796 deaths (2%) occurred. The majority of reports occurred in children less than 7 years while most non-fatal serious adverse events and deaths occurred in infants 12 months and younger. Only 0.5% of the reports were for IPV given alone without other vaccinations. These reports consisted of three deaths and eight non-fatal serious events. IPV was determined to have a suitable safety profile and there was no identification of new safety concerns [65M].

SUSCEPTIBILITY FACTORS

Immunocompromised: HIV A 40% reduced dose of IPV administered intradermally (ID) was studied in HIV patients. Comparator groups received either standard dose IPV or 40% reduced dose intramuscularly (IM) or a 20% reduced dose IPV intradermally. Included patients had an HIV viral load < 400 copies/mL. All groups were non-inferior to the standard dose of IM IPV in antibody response. Adverse events were similar between groups, although the ID group had higher rates of itching or redness at the injection site [66C].

DRUG ADMINISTRATION

Drug Formulations A surveillance study was conducted assessing vaccine-related AEs reported by the French armed forces between 2011 and 2012. The rate of AEs per 100 000 doses of Tdap-IPV (Repevax®) was 106.1 (95% CI: 82.4–134.5). Rates per 100 000 doses of local, regional, and systemic AEs were 45.2 (30.3–55.0), 17.2 (8.6–30.7), and 35.9 (22.8–53.8), respectively. One unexpected AE of Guillain-Barré syndrome occurred in a patient 21 days after vaccination with dTap-IPV and typhoid vaccine. Two cases of persistent pain lasting more than 2 weeks occurred as well. Three patients had fainting spells; all of these patients received Tdap-IPV with MMR, yellow fever, or typhoid vaccine [67MC].

Drug Dosage Regimens A Chilean study randomized infants to receive one of three poliovirus vaccination schedules beginning at 8 weeks of age: IPV-bOPV-bOPV, IPV-IPV-bOPV, or IPV-IPV-IPV. The bOPV-containing schedules were non-inferior to the IPV-alone schedule in producing an appropriate immune response. There were no differences in the occurrence of SAEs amongst the groups. One serious event of intestinal intussusception was determined to be indeterminately vaccine-related [68C].

Varicella Vaccine and Herpes Zoster Vaccine [SEDA-36, 474; SEDA-37, 391]

ORGANS AND SYSTEMS

Immunologic A case–control study of VAERS reports investigated the risk of autoimmune events after zoster vaccination. Vaccination with tetanus toxoid served as the control. There was a significant risk of alopecia (OR 2.2, $p = 0.015$) and arthritis (OR 2.7, $p < 0.001$) in the zoster group. There was no significant difference in risk for Guillain-Barré syndrome, multiple sclerosis and optic neuritis, SLE, thrombocytopenia, or vasculitis [69c].

Infection Risk A case of herpes zoster was diagnosed in a 17-month old, previously healthy boy. The boy was vaccinated 37 days prior to presentation with varicella zoster virus (VZV) vaccine. He presented with lesions following two dermatomes. A positive VZV polymerase chain reaction confirmed the diagnosis. Upon serotyping through the VZV Identification Program, the vaccine VZV strain was identified. The patient was not treated with antiviral therapy due to improvement in his clinical condition. This is a second recent case report of herpes zoster following VZV vaccination; however, this complication remains rare in pediatric patients [70A].

Death A mid-60s aged man with a history of non-Hodgkin's lymphoma in remission and diffuse large B-cell lymphoma (DLBCL) and stem-cell transplant

(SCT) received MMR, hepatitis, and varicella vaccines. The patient was 4 years from his SCT and was diagnosed with recurrent DLBCL limited to the lymph nodes a year prior to vaccination. Three months after vaccination, the patient developed a rash consistent with herpes zoster on his forehead. He was treated with valacyclovir. The patient continued to have recurrent episodes of herpes zoster and gradual functional and clinical decline. The patient was diagnosed with hemophagocytic lymphohistiocytosis 7 months after vaccination. He had multiple scans and biopsies confirming his DLBCL was stable. He also continued to have skin lesions throughout this time that were positive for VZV. After multi-organ failure, the patient was admitted to hospice and died 3 days later, a total of 9 months after vaccination. The VZV sample was confirmed to be the vaccine strain through the VZV Identification Program. Disseminated herpes zoster was determined to be the most likely cause of death in this patient compared to his stable DLBCL [71A].

SUSCEPTIBILITY FACTORS

Ethnicity Herpes zoster vaccine is not well studied in Asian populations. A study of the immunogenicity and safety of herpes zoster vaccine was conducted in healthy Taiwanese adults. Adverse effects were similar to previous studies. No new concerns were identified. Appropriate immune responses occurred in patients 4 weeks following vaccination [72C].

Immunosuppression Six pediatric patients with juvenile idiopathic arthritis on biologic therapy were vaccinated with VZV vaccine. Patients were between 2.5 and 7 years of age. Three patients were treated with etanercept, two with tocilizumab, and one with infliximab. There were no serious side effects noted during the 3-month follow-up period and none of the children experienced varicella infection during this time. One patient had a mild case of varicella 4 months after the second vaccination, but this was likely due to low protective antibody levels against VZV according to serologic testing [73A].

A prospective, double-blinded, placebo-controlled study investigated the immunogenicity and safety of herpes zoster vaccination in patients receiving chronic corticosteroid therapy at doses ≥5 mg/day. Of 295 subjects, 40% experienced an AE in the herpes zoster group compared to 30% in the placebo group. The majority of this difference was accounted for by an increase in injection-site reactions in the herpes zoster group. Six deaths occurred during the study, but none were vaccine related. Side effects were otherwise consistent with previous studies of herpes zoster in healthy populations. Of the four herpes zoster-like reported rashes (three in the herpes zoster group), none were found to be the vaccine

strain. The vaccine was also found to be sufficiently immunogenic at 6 weeks post-vaccination [74C].

A review of the VSD was conducted to assess risk of herpes zoster and disseminated disease in patients taking immunosuppressant medications. Immunosuppressants included corticosteroids disease-modifying anti-rheumatic drugs (DMARDs), and oral antirejection drugs. Patients' currently receiving immunosuppressant therapy had an increased risk of herpes zoster within 42 days post-vaccination compared to individuals remotely on immunosuppressant therapy [75c]. Overall, current data suggest a relatively acceptable safety profile when varicella or herpes zoster vaccine are administered to patients receiving various immunosuppressive therapies.

DRUG ADMINISTRATION

Drug Administration Route A prospective study between IM and subcutaneous administration of herpes zoster vaccine found IM administration resulted in a similar immune response as subcutaneous administration. Adverse effects were observed less in the IM group, with less injection-site reactions as compared to the subcutaneous group. This study supports the choice for the IM administration route [76C].

Yellow Fever Vaccine [SEDA-35, 577; SEDA-36, 475; SEDA-37, 392]

ORGANS AND SYSTEMS

Death Viscerotropic disease is a known, although rare, risk associated with vaccination with yellow fever (YF) vaccine. In eight observational studies of 437 million doses of YF vaccine, 72 people had viscerotropic disease associated with YF vaccination [77S]. A recent case report highlights a previously healthy woman in her 60s who was admitted 6 days after receipt of YF vaccine. She presented with symptoms of malaise, dyspnea, vomiting, and diarrhea lasting 3–5 days. The woman had leukopenia, thrombocytopenia, hypokalemia, and hypocalcemia, and developed acute respiratory failure requiring mechanical ventilation on hospital day 1. Three days into admission, the patient died from complications of cardiogenic shock and acute renal failure. Post-mortem, the patient was found to have a thymoma and laboratory testing consistent with myasthenia gravis. She also had tissue and serum samples that were positive for vaccine-strain YF virus. The patient met criteria for YF vaccine-associated viscerotropic disease of definite causality. Both the patient's age and undiagnosed thymic disease increased her risk of YF vaccine-associated viscerotropic disease [78A].

SUSCEPTIBILITY FACTORS

Immunosuppression A 63-year-old female on adalimumab was inadvertently given YF vaccine. The patient had Crohn's disease since 16 years of age and had been in remission for 8 years prior to receipt of the vaccination. She had been on adalimumab for 3 of those years before vaccination. The patient was vaccinated for purposes of travel to a YF endemic area. She experienced no adverse effects following vaccination. She was advised not to take her next dose of adalimumab, which was due 4 days after vaccination. She resumed treatment with adalimumab on day 35 post-vaccination due to increasing loose bowel movements per her gastroenterologist. Antibody titers remained positive up to 2 years post-vaccination [79A].

Bacterial Vaccines

Meningococcal Vaccines [SEDA-36, 476; SEDA-37, 393]

GENERAL

Invasive meningococcal disease (IMD) remains a significant threat to global public health. *Neisseria meningitidis* serogroups A, B, C, W-135, X, and Y are associated with high virulence in humans. The significance and severity of IMD infections are associated with global distribution, the organism's antigenic variability, the potential for epidemics, rapid progression, risk of mortality (10–15%) and disabling sequelae (up to 19%). *Neisseria meningitidis* serogroup A demonstrates continued predominance in Africa where the WHO continues vaccination campaigns, and serogroup B (MenB) accounts for a significant number of IMD infections in North America, Europe, Australia, and New Zealand [80H]. A number of meningococcal vaccines remain available that include various combinations of serogroups A, C, Y, and W-135. Recently, two MenB vaccines have been approved. The 4CMenB (Bexsero®) vaccine is licensed in the United States, European Union, Canada, Australia, and other countries and the MenBFHbp or bivalent recombinant lipoprotein 2086 [rLP2086] (Trumemba®) vaccine is licensed in the United States [80H,81S].

DRUG ADMINISTRATION

Drug Formulations Formulating the new MenB vaccines has required extensive study. The 4CMenB vaccine (Bexero®) formulation was examined in a phase II study to assess the safety and reactogenicity of the final formulation of the vaccine, in particular the outer membrane vesicle (OMV) component dose. Two-month-old infants were enrolled to receive either the licensed formulation of 4CMenB, recombinant MenB (rMenB) vaccine that did not contain OMV, rMenB plus ¼ OMV, rMenB plus ½ OMV, or ½ 4CMenB vaccine as a three dose primary series with a booster dose at 12 months. A majority of subjects experiences at least one AE. The lowest rates were among those who received the rMenB vaccine formulation, but it was noted that the difference in dose of OMV did not result in a meaningful decrease in reactions. The most frequent local reaction was injection site

tenderness, which occurred in 53–67% of subjects receiving a vaccine with OMV compared to only 29% of subjects in the rMenB group. Local reactions did increase with the number of doses received, the highest rate at dose four at 12 months of age. It was evident that the presence of OMV was also associated with fever. Thirteen percent of rMenB subjects experienced fever after the first dose compared to 33–53% of subjects who received OMV-containing vaccine. Other systemic reactions also occurred in a smaller number of subjects compared to those who received an OMV-containing vaccine. Six to 11% of subjects reported a SAE during the primary series and 3–9% after the booster dose. Only three SAEs were deemed possibly related to the study vaccine, one case of vomiting, somnolence, and an extensive area of erythema following vaccination. All SAEs resolved without complication. Four seizures were reported in three subjects during the study. None were temporally associated with study vaccination and were considered to be unrelated to the vaccine. While local and systemic reactions were increased with the inclusion of OMV in the vaccine, omission was associated with an undesirable decrease in immunogenicity. The authors concluded that the study results supported the continued utilization and study of the licensed formulation of 4CMenB vaccine [82C].

A meningococcal vaccine that provides protection against all significant serogroups represents a continued unmet public health need. Recently, two formulations of a meningococcal ABCWY vaccine were evaluated in a phase II, randomized, controlled trial. The two formulations included glycoconjugate components of serogroups ACWY and recombinant serogroup B proteins and OMV components. The formulations differed only in the amount of OMV incorporated into the vaccine (25 mcg versus 6.25 mcg), indicated as ABCWY+OMV and ABCWY+¼OMV. The new formulations were compared to a currently recommended conjugate quadrivalent vaccine, MenACWY-CRM (Menveo®), and 4CMenB (Bexsero®). The study included subjects aged 10–25 years in the United States and Poland. The relationship of any reported AEs were described by the authors as not related, possibly related, or probably related to the study vaccine. The most common solicited local reaction was injection site pain, which was reported by 84–90% of subjects in the ABCWY and 4CMenB groups versus 27% in the MenACWY-CRM group. Rates of injection site pain did decrease in the ABCWY groups following the second vaccination (73–83%) but increased in the MenACWY-CRM group (42%). The most common systemic reactions included myalgia (49–52% versus 26%), fatigue (23–36% versus 22%), and headache (23–32% versus 20%). Overall, 8–13% of subjects in the ABCWY and 4CMenB groups reported unsolicited AEs that were deemed possibly related to study vaccine. The most common events were injection site induration (2–6%), injection site pain (1–4%), and headache (1–3%). Two subjects in the 4CMenB group reported unsolicited AEs that included generalized lymphadenopathy and convulsion that developed 6 and 60 days following the first vaccination, the former was judged as possibly related to the study vaccine. One to 3% of subjects reported an SAE, none were related to the study vaccine. No deaths were reported during the study period [83C].

Drug Dosage Regimens The immunogenicity and safety of the newly approved MenB vaccines remains a focus of continued study. A study published in 2012 demonstrated the immunogenicity and safety of three dosing cohorts of the bivalent rLP2086 vaccine. Immunogenicity and AE results lead the investigators to suggest that the 120 mcg dose would be the optimal dose for future trials. The majority of local and systemic AEs were mild to moderate in nature. One SAE was considered related to the study vaccine. A 13-year-old male subject experienced sudden onset of severe headache and vomiting nearly 50 minutes after receiving the third dose of the 200 mcg vaccine dose. The subject developed a rash and a hypotensive episode that resulted in the receipt of one dose of adrenaline. The subject recovered and was discharged the next day. The study investigator diagnosed this reaction as anaphylaxis and this resulted in a study pause. The study resumed with an optional longer window for receipt of the third dose from 6 months to 6–9 months. An increased incidence of solicited AEs in the 200 mcg dose group in conjunction with no observable dose-proportional increase in immune response supports the continued study and utilization of the 120 mcg dose vaccine [84C].

Vesikari and colleagues recently evaluated the serum bactericidal responses of two or three dose regimens of the bivalent rLP2086 vaccine (Trumemba®) in a phase two study in healthy adolescents (11–<19 years) from seven countries. Subjects either received bivalent rLP2086 vaccine in a two or three dose regimen or placebo. During the vaccination phase of the study, 35.5–37.5% of subjects reported ≥1 AE across all study groups. The most common AE was nasopharyngitis (5.5–10.1%). Pain at the injection site was the most common local reaction and most cases were mild or moderate. Other common local reactions included redness and swelling, which were also mild to moderate in severity. The most common systemic events were headache and fatigue. SAEs considered to be related to the study vaccine, the SAEs included headache, injection-site pain, pyrexia, vomiting, and injection-site swelling. There was no increase in AEs with subsequent dosing. No deaths were reported during the study period. The authors concluded that a two or three dose regimen yielded robust immunogenicity results and both were generally well tolerated in healthy adolescents [85C].

The 4CMenB vaccine (Bexsero®) dosing regimen also continues to be evaluated. A phase IIb/III study published by Santolaya and colleagues evaluated various dosing regimens of 4CMenB vaccine in healthy adolescents (11–17 years) in Chile. The regimens included a priming of one-dose, two doses at 1 or 2 months apart, three doses once month apart, or placebo. A second phase consisted of receiving a fourth dose or placebo. The authors concluded that a two-dose regimen would be preferable. The majority of AEs were mild to moderate in severity and resolved in a few days after vaccination. The most commonly reported local reaction was pain, which was reported in 86% of 4CMenB recipients compared to 60% of placebo recipients. The most common systemic reaction was malaise in 51% of 4CMenB versus 30% of placebo subjects. One SAE led to study discontinuation in a subject who experienced a vasovagal reaction and convulsion immediately after a first dose of 4CMenB. The subjects had a paternal history of epilepsy. The investigator deemed the reaction to be related to the vaccination procedure and not the actual vaccine. Two cases of juvenile arthritis were assessed as possibly and probably related to the 4CMenB vaccine. The cases were reported 170 and 198 days after the third of three doses of the study vaccine, respectively. All other SAEs were deemed unrelated to the study vaccine [86C].

Further study continues regarding the dosing regimens for adolescents. A recent phase III study examined the two-dose regimen (administered 1 month apart) of two lots of 4CMenbB in health adolescents aged 11–17 years. Both lots produced similar safety profiles and were generally well tolerated. Most local and systemic reactions were mild to moderate in severity. The most frequent local reaction reported was pain 96% and 98%. The most frequent systemic reaction was myalgia (59% and 68%), followed by headache (44% and 51%), and fatigue (44% and 49%) in lot one and two, respectively. Fever was infrequently reported (5% and 3%) in lot one and two subjects. No deaths or SAEs were noted by the authors [87C].

INTERACTIONS

Drug–Drug Interactions The addition of vaccines to infant and child immunization schedules often necessitates simultaneous administration; therefore, both safety and immunogenicity data must be demonstrated in order to support concomitant administration. A recent study examined the coadministration of quadrivalent meningococcal vaccine conjugated to tetanus toxoid, MenACWY-TT, in toddlers who had previously received meningococcal serogroup C and Y combined with Hib conjugate vaccine (HibMenCY-TT) as their primary series. The two-treatment group either received the MenACWY-TT vaccine coadministered with the fourth dose of the DTaP vaccine at 15–18 months or administered at 12–15 months with administration of the DTaP vaccine at 15–18 months. The most frequently reported local and general AEs were comparable and included injection site pain, redness and irritability/fussiness.

Three SAEs reported in two subjects that were considered to be vaccine-related. One case of a "floppy" infant was reported 47 days post vaccination in the co-administration group. The condition resolved in 2 days. One case of convulsion occurred 65 days after the first dose of the primary series vaccine HibMenCY-TT; the condition resolved but the infant later died of sudden infant death syndrome 89 days post dose. Three other deaths occurred during the study period, but none of them were considered vaccine related [88C].

Given the recent availability of two MenB vaccines, the question regarding safe concomitant administration with routine vaccines must be considered in order to continue to optimize vaccination efforts. A phase II, randomized, placebo-controlled, single-blinded study conducted in three countries examined the concomitant administration of bivalent rLP2086 vaccine with a booster dose of DTaP/IPV vaccine compared to subjects receiving saline plus DTaP/IPV. In terms of safety, 37.4% and 40.2% of study subjects reported ≥1 AE during the vaccination phase in the concomitant rLP2086/DTaP/IPV and saline plus DTaP/IPV groups, respectively. The most common AEs were nasopharyngitis, pharyngitis, and upper respiratory tract infections. The most common local reactions were injection-site pain, swelling, and redness. Most cases were mild to moderate in severity. One subject in the rLP2086/DTaP/IPV group did withdraw from the study due to moderate pain and swelling at the injection site. Headache and fatigue were the most common systemic events after any vaccination. The most common SAE was appendicitis, which occurred in three participants and was deemed not related to the study vaccine. One death occurred during the study period that was not related to the study vaccine [89C].

The safety of administering the 4CMenB vaccine with routine infant vaccinations has also been evaluated. In a large, multicenter, phase III trial, investigators administered a primary dose of 4CMenB vaccine with concomitant DTaP/IPV/HBV/Hib (Infanrix Hexa®) and seven-valent pneumococcal conjugate vaccine (PCV7) at 2, 4, and 6 months and then a booster dose concomitantly with MMRV vaccine at 12 months to examine immunogenicity and safety. Subjects either received 4CMenB plus routine vaccines, routine vaccines alone, or routine vaccines plus meningococcal serogroup C (MenC) conjugate vaccine as the primary series. During the booster phase, subjects received 4CMenB plus MMRV or 4CMenB alone with receipt of MMRV 1 month later. All safety data were pooled for all doses. The most frequent local reactions were tenderness, erythema, induration, and swelling. The most common systemic reaction during the primary phase was fever. Rectal temperatures ≥38.5 °C were reported in 65.3% of 4CMenB recipients within 6 hours of vaccination, 32.2% of subjects who received routine

vaccines alone, and 33.7% of recipients who received MenC vaccine plus routine vaccines. After the booster dose, 31.6% and 30.6% of subjects reported a temperature of ≥38 °C within 6 hours of vaccination in the 4CMenB and 4CMenB plus MMRV groups, respectively. Two cases of febrile seizures occurred in subjects who received 4CMenB and were assessed by the investigators as probably related to the vaccine. The seizures occurred within 24 hours of receipt of the 4CMenB plus routine vaccines. Two additional cases of seizures were reported as leg convulsions and jerking right arm movements occurred the same day as the first dose of 4CMenB plus routine vaccines and were deemed possibly related to the 4CMenB vaccine. Four cases of suspected Kawasaki disease were reported during the primary phase of the study. Three cases were confirmed and one remained unconfirmed. The cases occurred at 3, 7, and 14 weeks after receipt of 4CMenB vaccine. The authors did not provide a final assessment of the relationship between the receipt of 4CMenB and the cases of Kawasaki disease; causality is unclear but a possible association with the vaccine could not be ruled out. Overall, 17 SAEs (one with routine vaccines only and 16 with 4CMenB plus routine vaccines) were deemed vaccine related during the primary phase. After the booster dose, two SAEs were deemed possibly related to vaccination with 4CMenB plus MMRV vaccine. The authors concluded that the concomitant administration of 4CMenB plus routine vaccines resulted in robust immune response and there appeared to be no clinically meaningful immunological interference with co-administration. In addition, an additive effect in regards to reactogenicity was noted among subjects who received 4CMenB plus routine vaccines, which indicates a need for further study to characterize the impact of this observation [90MC].

An extension of this phase III trial was recently published, which sought to describe safety and the persistence of antibody response 12 months after the booster (fourth) dose in toddlers who had previously received a three-dose series at 2, 4, and 6 months of age (Group I). This group of toddlers was compared to groups that previously received routine vaccines alone during the primary phase and then either 4CMenB plus MMRV at 12 months and 4CMenB at 14 months (Group IIa) or MMRV at 12 months and 4CMenB at 13 and 15 months (Group IIb). Groups IIa and IIb received a third dose 12 months after their second dose. The final group consisted of toddlers who were 4CMenB naïve who received two doses of 4CMenB at 24 and 26 months (Group III). No SAEs or deaths were reported during the extension study. One subject withdrew from the study due to an AE that was unrelated to the study vaccine. The most common local reactions were erythema (58–77%) and tenderness at the injection site. Tenderness was reported in 56–57% of toddlers after the first dose at 12 or 13 months of age, 66–67% after the second dose, and 94% after the third dose. The most frequently reported systemic reactions were irritability, sleepiness, change in eating habits, and unusual crying. The majority of cases were mild to moderate and all resolved without complications. Fevers were reported in 37% of toddlers in Group IIa and 46% in Group IIb after the first vaccine. Fever rates were lower in the older children receiving their first doses (Group III). The noted trend was an increase in local reactions with age but a lower rate of systemic reactions. The authors concluded that the presence of OMV may enhance the reactogenicity of the vaccine and the OMV dose to body weight proportion may potentially explain the trends in AEs [91C].

Pertussis Vaccines (Including Diphtheria-Tetanus-Acellular/Whole-Cell Pertussis-Containing Vaccines) [SED-15, 3555, 3562; SEDA-35, 573; SEDA-36, 478; SEDA-37, 396]

GENERAL

The WHO recently published a position paper pertaining to pertussis vaccines. The position paper provided a review of pertussis vaccines in regards to reported immunogenicity, efficacy, and safety of both whole-cell pertussis (wP) and acellular pertussis (aP) vaccines. Vaccines containing pertussis antigens typically contain a number of other components (e.g. diphtheria, tetanus, HiB, HBV, etc.). Whole-cell pertussis-containing vaccines are only recommended for use during the primary vaccination series and are associated with minor local and systemic reactions (redness, swelling, induration, fever, and agitation). Local reactions tend to increase with age and the number of vaccinations. Therefore, wP vaccines are not recommendation in children ≥7 years of age, adolescents, or adults. Acellular pertussis-containing vaccines may also be used for the primary series and aP vaccines are the recommended pertussis vaccine for older children, adolescents, and adults due to the available data and increased risk of reactogenicity with wP vaccines. Rates and severity of local reactions tend to also increase with the number of doses of DTaP and transient, painless swelling has been reported in children receiving booster doses of DTaP vaccines. Combination vaccines are not associated with an increase in SAEs, but may cause slightly more frequent minor reactions (e.g. redness). In addition, the concomitant administration of pertussis-containing vaccines is generally recommended with other routine vaccinations. Multiple vaccinations may result in slightly increased AEs compared to the pertussis-containing vaccine alone, but this risk is generally outweighed by the benefits of providing this important disease prevention strategy, particularly given the seemingly resurgence of pertussis cases across the globe [92S].

ORGANS AND SYSTEMS

Nervous System The debate regarding the controversial association between pertussis-containing vaccines and the development of neurologic AEs continues. A recent study by Lateef and colleagues reviewed records of 165 claims submitted to the National Vaccines Injury Compensation Program (VICP) with designated injuries of "seizures" and/or "encephalopathy" believed to be caused by a vaccine in children less than 2 years of age. Eighty percent of the claims implicated DTwP vaccines (61%) or DTaP (19.3%) vaccines, indicating that wP containing vaccines were four times more often implicated compared to aP containing vaccines [93C]. Currently, the data suggest that a temporal association may exist between the receipt of a pertussis-containing vaccine and neurologic AEs; however, temporal association is not causality and a number of limitations exist in the currently available data sets [94r,95r]. The current review of VICP data indicated that 79% of subjects had a neuroimaging study, 51% had a documented metabolic work-up, and only 19% had any genetic testing completed. In addition, a number of subjects had "unknown" details related to their AE [93C]. The WHO echoes this lack of causality conclusion as repeated studies have failed to confirm causality, particularly given the advances in diagnostic tools [92S]. Practitioners are encouraged to complete a thorough examination, imaging, metabolic, and potentially genetic assessment of patients with the development of seizures and/or encephalopathy following vaccination to determine a comprehensive diagnosis and avoid further potential loss of public confidence in vaccinations [93C,94r]. Finally, the possibility of children developing encephalopathy during the natural course of pertussis infection has been estimated at six times more frequently reported compared to those patients who were immunized [93C].

SECOND-GENERATION EFFECTS

Pregnancy In 2012, the Advisory Committee on Immunization Practices (ACIP) began recommending the administration of tetanus–diphtheria–acellular pertussis (Tdap) vaccine for all pregnant women in the United States during each pregnancy regardless of prior immunization status. A recent retrospective study of seven VSD sites was completed to evaluate medically attended acute adverse effects in mothers and birth outcomes in neonates between women who received a prior tetanus-containing vaccine less than 2 years, between 2 and 5 years, and greater than 5 years before the receipt of Tdap during their pregnancy. Overall, adverse events after vaccination were rare and no statistically significant difference was noted in fever, allergic reactions, or local reactions among the three groups studied. No cases of anaphylaxis, Arthus reactions, or Guillain-Barré syndrome were reported. No statistically significant difference in adverse birth outcomes was noted among the three groups. Birth outcomes evaluated included preterm delivery, small for gestational age, and low-birth-weight. The authors concluded that no differences in acute adverse events in mothers or birth outcomes in neonates noted regardless of the length of time since the prior tetanus-containing vaccine. There are notable limitations to this study. The study included only medically attended acute events, which are typically rare. In addition, the subjects included were all from the United States and were all insured throughout the study period; this may limit the generalizability to other country populations and even those in the United States are uninsured. Finally, a limited number of birth outcomes were evaluated. Additional study is warranted with regard to the type and quantity of AEs in pregnant women receiving multiple doses of tetanus-containing vaccines given the recent recommendations from ACIP [96MC].

SUSCEPTIBILITY FACTOR

Ethnicity A phase IV, open-label study of the combination DTaP-HBV-IPV/Hib (Infanrix Hexa®) vaccine was conducted in Canadian Aboriginal and non-Aboriginal infants aged 6–12 weeks. Enrolled subjects received study vaccine at 2, 4, and 6 months of age. Routine vaccinations (e.g. rotavirus, pneumococcal conjugate vaccine, and meningococcal C conjugate) were permitted during the study period. Medically attended adverse events were higher in the Aboriginal group of infants compared to the non-Aboriginal group (23.2% versus 17%), but most of the events were not vaccine-related. Five SAEs were reported among the Aboriginal subjects, only a SAE of fever was deemed possibly related to the study vaccine as the onset occurred shortly after vaccination. Specific details regarding AEs were limited in the study document. This information paired with the small number of patients included leads to questionable generalizability for all Aboriginal infants at this time [97c].

DRUG ADMINISTRATION

Drug Formulations In efforts to further enhance immunization coverage, combination vaccines continue to undergo study to assess safety. A pentavalent combination vaccine containing DTwP-HBV plus Hib (Pentavac®) was compared to DTwP-HBV plus Hib (Tritanrix-HB® combined with Hiberix® just prior to injection) to assess safety. Tenderness was the most common local reaction and was reported in 35.9% of Pentavac® subjects and 33.6% of Tritanrix-HB plus Hib subjects. Other local reactions included swelling, redness, and induration. Most reactions were mild and all resolved without sequelae. No significant differences were noted between the two groups. Of the 149 unsolicited events reported in the Pentavac® group, eight were considered possibly and probably related to the study vaccine. The events included

vomiting, fever, irritability, and induration, swelling (two), and tenderness (two), respectively. Two events of the 92 reported in the Tritanix-HB plus Hib group were considered possibly and very likely related to the study vaccine; the events included sneezing and rash. Six SAEs and one death were reported during the study period, none of which were related to the study vaccines. The continued study of combination vaccines appears warranted based on the general tolerability reported in the study, particularly in regards to the DTwP component in this time of pertussis resurgence [98C].

An investigational hexavalent vaccine containing DTaP-IPV-Hib-HepB was recently studied in the United States to determine immunogenicity, safety, and tolerability. Healthy infants received with DTaP-IPV-Hib-HepB, PCV13, and rotavirus (RV) at 2, 4, and 6 months (Group 1) or DTaP-IPV/Hib, PCV13, RV at 2, 4, and 6 months plus HepB at 2 and 6 months (Group 2). The investigational hexavalent vaccine produced a robust immune response. In general, AEs were similarly reported in both groups, 95.5% and 93.4% of subjects in Group 1 and Group 2 reported at least one AE. Noted exceptions include more common reporting of decreased appetite in Group 1 (48.9%) compared to Group 2 (43.4%) and larger number of subjects' parents reporting fever in Group 1 (47.4%) compared to Group 2 (34.4%). There was no vaccine-related fever SAEs as determined by the investigators. Most AEs were mild to moderate in nature. Reports of at least one SAE occurred in 5.4% of subjects in Group 1 and 6.4% of those in Group 2. One subject in each group died during the study period, but neither death was considered related to the study vaccinations. Further consideration of the hexavalent vaccine for infants is warranted to potentially improve vaccine coverage and decrease the number of separate injections [99C].

Drug Dosage Regimens Neither natural pertussis infection nor vaccination results in lifelong immunity from pertussis. This information, paired with the seemingly resurgence of pertussis cases around the globe, vaccination strategies continue to be questioned and studied to determine the optimal schedule to provide protection for all susceptible persons. Kovac and colleagues conducted a phase IV study to examine a decennial booster of Tdap with inactivated poliovirus vaccine (Tdap-IPV) 10 years after the receipt of a booster of either Tdap-IPV (Boostrix-Polio®), Tdap plus IPV (Boostrix® plus Poliorix®, or tetanus–diphtheria (Td)-IPV (Revaxis®)) in two countries. The decennial booster resulted in favorable immunogenicity results for all antigens tested. Local AEs were reported in 71.6%, 75%, and 72.2% of subjects in the Tdap-IPV, Tdap plus IPV, and Td-IPV groups, respectively. Pain was the most frequently reported local AE, reported in at least 62.7% of all subjects. Fatigue was the most frequently reported general AE, which was reported in at least 18.5% of subjects across all groups. No cases of fever >39 °C were recorded during the study. No SAEs occurred during the study and no subjects withdrew from the study due to an AE. Overall, the decennial booster dose of Tdap-IPV was well tolerated. The safety results paired with the positive immunogenicity results support consideration of a decennial booster to potentially increase coverage against pertussis as well as tetanus among adults [100C].

Booster dosage regimens were also studied in a combined phase II/IV trial in Swedish children and adolescents. Children previously studied and vaccinated with DTaP as a three-dose primary infant series were invited to participate in a booster study to receive Tdap (either combined with IPV or administered separately) at age five and then to receive Tdap or a monocomponent pertussis vaccine (Tdap1) 10 years later at age 14–15 years. The 5-year-old children who received Tdap-IPV combined were noted to have higher rates of general and local symptoms compared to children who received Tdap plus IVP separately. Noted reactions included temperature >38 °C (11.3% versus 6.1%) and moderate-severe or severe redness or swelling and pain (RR 2.3, 95% CI 1.2–4.7). In the adolescent group, nine subjects reported staying home from school due to severe pain following receipt of the Tdap vaccine compared to one subject in the Tdap1 group, this finding was statistically significant. No statistically significant differences were noted in regards to safety between the groups. An additional comparison was made between the subjects who received the Tdap booster at age five and the same vaccine (Tdap) at age 14–15 years. The only significant differences reported were moderate pain (43.4% as adolescence versus 12.9% as children) and itching (0% versus 18.8%). The study findings are consistent with observations noting an increase in pain and potentially mild local reactions with subsequent doses of Tdap [101C].

A decennial Tdap booster dose was also studied as a phase IV extension study of young adults in Belgium who had received their primary series with DTwP and a booster of Tdap (containing either 0.5, 0.3, or 0.133 mg of aluminum) at 10–18 years of age. Subjects who completed the original study were invited to participate in the extension study and were assessed at 8.5 and 10 years after the first booster dose. Enrolled participants received a second booster dose containing the same dose of aluminum as previously received, with the exception of the 0.133 mg group who received 0.5 mg aluminum at the time of the second booster dose. Pain was the most common local reaction most frequently reported (87.1–92.3% across all groups). The most frequent systemic reaction was fatigue (31.5–35.5% across all groups). Fever was reported in one participant in each group (<2%). No SAEs were reported during the study period. The reported local and systemic symptoms were similar of lower than observed following the first booster dose 10 years prior. The dose of aluminum did not appear to have a significant effect on reactogenicity or safety of the decennial booster dose [102C].

INTERACTIONS

Drug–Drug Interactions Adolescents are target populations for an increasing number of vaccines. Concomitant administration remains an important area of study to determine and hopefully ensure continued vaccination practices and coverage by potentially decreasing the number of visits required to administer recommended vaccines. An evaluation of 9vHPV (Gardasil-9®) vaccine administered concomitantly with Tdap-IPV (Repevax®) was conducted in six countries in healthy adolescents aged 11–15 years. Subjects either received both vaccines concomitantly with the first dose of the 9vHPV series (Group A) or received 9vHPV and then Tdap-IPV 1 month later (Group B). A higher number of subjects in Group A reported erythema (8.2%) and swelling (13%) at the 9vHPV injection site compared to the subjects in Group B (5.7% and 8.2%). Subjects in Group A also reported a higher proportion of erythema (26.9%) and swelling (39.4%) at the Tdap-IPV site compared to Group B (21.7% and 31.3%). The risk difference between the groups for swelling at the injection site was statistically significant ($p = 0.006$). Most of the swelling was mild or moderate in severity. Headache was the most common systemic AE reported and this was more common in Group A (25.1%) compared to Group B (21.4%) with a risk difference of 3.7% (95% CI −1.4 to 8.8). Nine subjects reported a SAE but none were vaccine-related. No subjects withdrew from the study due to an AE and no deaths were reported during the study period. Concomitant administration of 9vHPV and Tdap-IPV appeared to be generally well tolerated and immunogenicity results met non-inferiority criteria set by the investigators [103C].

Pneumococcal Vaccines [SED-15, 3562; SEDA-36, 477]

SUSCEPTIBILITY FACTORS

Age: Adults and Elderly Adults Streptococcus pneumoniae is a leading cause of invasive pneumococcal diseases (IPD) and community acquired pneumonia (CAP) in the elderly. Prevention of such diseases is of public health importance due to the significant impact of morbidity and mortality rates associated with these infections. The 13-valent pneumococcal conjugate vaccine (PCV13) vaccine has been studied in infants, children, and adults, and review of the immunogenicity and safety of PCV13 in elderly patients continues. Safety and immunogenicity of PCV13 was studied in an open-label trial in a 23-valent pneumococcal polysaccharide vaccine (PPSV23) naïve group of subjects ≥50 years of age in Mexico. The two study groups were stratified by age (50–64 years and ≥65 years). The majority of local and systemic reactions were mild to moderate in nature. Pain at the injection site was the most common local reaction, reported in 75.5% and 60.6% of the subjects in the 50–64 years and ≥65 years subjects, respectively ($p = 0.007$). Muscle and joint pain, fatigue, and headache represented the most commonly reported systemic reactions. Muscle pain and headache were statistically significantly higher in the 50–64 years group (60.5% and 43.9%, $p = 0.006$ and 44.3% and 32.6%, $p = 0.049$, respectively). Fever, in contrast, was more commonly reported in subjects ≥65 years (10.2% versus 2.4%, $p = 0.012$). Only two SAEs were reported and neither was related to study vaccine. No deaths occurred and no subjects withdrew due to an AE. Overall, PCV13 demonstrated robust immune responses and a well-tolerated safety profile in this study population [104C].

At present, a variety of pneumococcal vaccination schedules exist for adults and the elderly and continued study remains underway to investigate the tolerance of these vaccines in adults of various ages. An observational study was performed in subjects ≥70 years of age in Italy to assess safety and tolerability of PCV13. The study enrolled 871 subjects for their response to a single dose of PCV13. Subjects were excluded if they received PPSV23 vaccine within the previous year. At least one local reaction was reported in 31.6% of subjects, reactions were typically mild in nature. Injection site pain was the most commonly reported reaction (27.4%). The most common systemic reactions were muscle pain (11.6%), fatigue (10.7%), and headache (9.9%). Two SAEs were reported, one case of a subject who developed CAP 29 days following vaccination and was deemed possibly related to the study vaccine. The authors noted that the rates of AEs in this observational study were lower than those previously reported in elderly patients, limitations in the study design and data collection methods may help explain the results [105C].

Autoimmune Disease: Juvenile Idiopathic Arthritis It is unclear whether anti-tumor necrosis factor alpha (TNF-α) affect the response to pneumococcal vaccination. A small population of subjects aged 5–18 years with polyarticular juvenile idiopathic arthritis (JIA) was observed for 1 year following receipt of PPSV23 vaccine. Subjects were either treated with a stable dose of methotrexate (Group 2, $n = 10$) or refractory to methotrexate and initiated on TNF-α therapy with etanercept (Group 1, $n = 17$). Details regarding the safety and tolerance of the vaccine were somewhat limited in the study report. It was noted that one subject in Group 2 reported a mild local reaction of redness and swelling at the injection site. Other AEs reported included upper respiratory tract infections,

reported in 60% of subjects in Group 1 and 30% of subjects in Group 2 ($p = 0.12$). One SAE was reported in a subject in Group 1, which was documented as invasive pneumococcal diseases with bacterial pneumonia requiring hospitalization 5 months after vaccination. The authors provided no specific causality relationship assessment. The primary limitation of this study was the small sample size, although it appeared that the small number of subjects in both groups produced comparable immune responses [106c].

Hematologic Disease: Sickle Cell Disease Due to an increased risk of pneumococcal disease, it is recommended that patients with sickle cell disease (SCD) receive additional doses of pneumococcal vaccine to prevent infection. A recently published case series described local and systemic SAEs that occurred in five subjects following vaccination with PPSV23 vaccine. Subjects ranged in age from 2 to 22 years. Presenting symptoms included erythema, edema, fever, leukocytosis, and pain. Fever and hospital admission was more common in the younger subjects (2, 3, and 6 years). Two subjects received pneumococcal vaccines 6 weeks and 4 months prior to the PPSV23 dose in question and two subjects received concomitant meningococcal vaccines. The authors also reviewed the VAERS database and reported findings related to SCD patients. Of the 123 vaccine-related AEs included in the database, 76 (62%) were related to PPSV23, which represented the most common vaccine-related AE in SCD patients. The authors concluded with recommendations to ensure the appropriate timeframe of pneumococcal vaccination and consider avoiding concomitant vaccines in patients with SCD [107A].

Immunocompromised: Allogeneic Hematopoietic Stem Cell Transplant Allogeneic hematopoietic stem cell transplant (HSCT) patients are at a significantly higher risk of pneumococcal infections and IPD compared to the general population. An open-label study examined the immunogenicity and safety of a four-dose PCV13 series following allogeneic HSCT in children ≤2 years. The first three doses were administered 1 month apart and the final dose was administered 6 months later. Subjects also received a dose of PPSV23 1 month after the final dose of PCV13. In general, local reactions were more common in pediatric patients compared to adult patients whereas systemic reactions were more similar between the groups with the exception of fever, which was more common in the pediatric patients. Local and systemic reactions were more frequently reported after PCV13 dose four. The investigators concluded that six SAEs were possibly related to the study vaccine. The events included a case of facial diplegia, injection-site erythema and pyrexia, two cases of autoimmune hemolytic anemia, one Guillain-Barré syndrome, and one cellulitis case. In addition, one case of bilateral pneumonia 36 days after PCV13 dose three was deemed possibly related to the vaccine in terms of suspected lack of efficacy. Fifty-one AEs led to study withdrawal and 14 deaths occurred. Most study withdrawals were due to disease relapse or complications of HSCT. No deaths were related to the study vaccines [108C].

Immunocompromised: HIV Examining immune response and safety of pneumococcal vaccines in patients with HIV remains of significant importance due to the substantial risk of IPD among HIV-infected children and adults. Even with the advent and increased utilization of antiretroviral therapy, this population remains at approximately 20- to 40-fold greater risk of IPD compared to healthy patients. The immune response of PPSV23 vaccine has come into question in patients with HIV but remains a recommended vaccine for this population in the United States and many other countries. A phase III, open-label, single-arm study was conducted in HIV-infected adults (≥18 years of age) in the United States with a history of receipt of at least one PPSV23 vaccination to assess the immunogenicity and safety of a three-dose series of PCV13 administered 6 months apart. Nearly half (48.6%) of the subjects enrolled had received one previous dose of PPSV23 and 51.4% of subjects had received ≥2 doses. A robust immune response was noted, particularly following the first dose of PCV13 vaccine. The majority of local reactions were mild and pain at the infection was the most frequently reported reaction after each of the three doses (78.8–81.9%). Subjects who had received ≥2 doses of PPSV23 in the past reported redness and swelling more frequently following dose three (12.3% and 13.6%, respectively) compared to those subjects who had only received one dose (6.3% and 8.3%, respectively). The most common systemic events were fatigue, headache, and new generalized muscle pain. The events of fatigue, headache, and vomiting tended to be higher in subjects who had previously received ≥2 doses of PPSV23 vaccine (62%, 51.9%, and 14.8%, respectively) compared to those subjects who had only received one previous dose (48.5%, 40%, and 6.3%, respectively). Overall, AEs were reported in 63.5% of subjects. No vaccine-related SAEs were reported and no deaths occurred during the study period. The authors concluded that receipt of PCV13 vaccine after PPSV23 vaccine resulted in functional immune response. It was noted that the administration of additional doses of PCV13 might have limited impact [109C].

A similar phase III, open-label study recently examined the safety and immunogenicity of PCV13 vaccine among pneumococcal vaccine naïve HIV-infected children and adults aged ≥6 years in South Africa and Romania. Subjects received three doses of PCV13 1 month apart followed by one dose of PPSV23 1 month after the last dose of PCV13. As described in the study above, a significant immune response to the vaccine was observed, particularly following the first dose of PCV13 vaccine. The majority of local reactions were mild to moderate in severity and pain at the infection site was the most frequently reported event (61.5–70.3%). The most common systemic reactions were muscle pain (42.4–55.8%), fatigue (36.1–53.5%), and headache (39.1–50.5%). Most systemic reactions were mild to moderate in severity and decreased in frequency with each subsequent dose of PCV13. Fever of ≥40 °C was reported in only one subject following PCV13 dose three. Nine SAEs were reported in eight subjects. The most common were infections or infestations; none of the SAEs were considered related to the study vaccine. One death occurred but was not related to PCV13 vaccine. The authors concluded with support for the administration of one dose of PCV13 vaccine in HIV-infected children and adults. Sequencing of PCV13 and PPSV23 vaccinations will depend upon the patient's history of pneumococcal vaccine exposure [110C].

DRUG ADMINISTRATION

Drug Formulations The conjugate pneumococcal vaccines have demonstrated significant impact on the incidence and outcomes associated with IPD infections associated with the serotypes included in available vaccines. Continued surveillance of circulating serotypes and inclusion of such serotypes in conjugated vaccines may further enhance protection and decrease pneumococcal disease burden. The safety and immunogenicity of an investigational 15-valent pneumococcal conjugate (PCV15) vaccine was studied in a small, randomized, double-blind, multicenter trial in healthy adults aged 18–45 years in the United States. Subjects either received a single dose of PCV15 or PCV7. The majority of AEs were mild to moderate and transient in nature. The most common injection-site reactions reported among the PCV15 and PCV7 subjects were pain (90% and 80%), swelling (50% and 23.3%), erythema (33.3% and 13.3%), and nodule (26.7% and 16.7%). The most common systemic reactions reported by subjects in the PCV15 and PCV7 groups were myalgia (63.3% and 36.7%), fatigue (46.7% and 33.3%), arthralgia (20% and 10%), and fever (16.7% and 3.3%). A higher number of injection-site and systemic reactions were reported in the PCV15 group (90% and 80%, respectively) compared to the PCV7 group (80% and 60%, respectively), but these differences were not statistically significant. No vaccine-related SAEs or deaths were reported during the study period. Overall, the investigational PCV15 vaccine demonstrated an acceptable safety profile and immune responses based on this small sample size. Further study on a larger scale will determine the place for the vaccine in prevention strategies for pneumococcal diseases [111c].

The investigational PCV15 was also recently studied in a small, randomized, double-blind, multicenter trial in healthy toddlers (12–15 months of age) who were previously vaccinated with PCV7 in the United Sates and Finland. Included subjects either received aluminum-adjuvanted PCV15, non-adjuvanted PCV15, or PCV7 to assess immunogenicity and safety. The majority of AEs were mild to moderate in intensity. Pain was the most common injection-site AE, reported in 57.6% of adjuvanted PCV15 subjects, 57.1% of non-adjuvanted PCV15 subjects, and 35.7% of PCV7 subjects. The most common systemic AEs were fatigue, myalgia, fever, and irritability. Subjects in the PCV7 had reported systemic AEs in a lower frequency compared to both PCV15 groups. Subjects in the adjuvanted PCV15 group reported higher rates of myalgia (30.3%), irritability (18.2%), or fever (24.2%) compared to the non-adjuvanted (28.6%, 7.1%, and 7.1%, respectively) and PCV7 (3.6%, 7.1%, and 7.1%, respectively) groups. A higher number of injection-site and systemic AEs were reported in the adjuvanted PCV15 group (72.7% and 93.9%, respectively) and non-adjuvanted PCV15 group (64.3% and 85.7%, respectively) compared to the PCV7 group (57.1% and 82.1%, respectively); however, these differences were not statistically significant. No vaccine-related SAEs or study withdrawals were reported. One subject in the adjuvanted PCV15 group reported a febrile convulsion 10 days after vaccination; this was deemed unrelated to the study vaccine and likely related to the concomitant MMR vaccine received by the subject on day 1. The authors concluded that PCV15 vaccines were generally well tolerated and had comparable safety profiles to PCV7. The higher incidences of local and systemic AEs are consistent with previous reports related the adjuvanted and higher-valency vaccines. The small sample size of the study must also be considered when interpreting AE data [112c].

A number of countries have implemented the recommendation of vaccination against pneumococcal diseases with conjugated vaccines due to the demonstrated immunogenicity and general tolerability. However, the study of PPSV23 vaccine continues and results may benefit those countries continuing to utilize PPSV23 vaccine to protect against pneumococcal diseases. A randomized, double-blinded, parallel-controlled study was conducted in subjects aged 2–70 years in China. Subjects either received the licensed PPSV23 vaccine (Group C) or a "tested" PPSV23 vaccine (Group T). There was no significant difference in the number of subjects reporting an AE during the study period ($p = 0.3533$). The most common local AE was pain after vaccination, occurring in 15.83% of subjects in Group T and 16.33% in Group C ($p = 0.8752$). Other common local reactions included swelling and redness following vaccination. Most local reactions were mild in intensity. The most common

general AE was fever, reported in 8.83% of subjects in Group T and 9.83% in Group C ($p = 0.6199$). Other general AEs included myalgia and headache. Most general reactions were mild in nature as well. One SAE was reported but was not related to the study vaccines. The authors concluded with support of the "tested" PPSV23 vaccine for wider use in the Chinese population [113C].

Drug Additives Polysorbate 80 (P80) is a nonionic detergent that is used to solubilize proteins and widely used in injectable medications, including certain vaccines. Polysorbate 80 was not included in PCV7 vaccine but was studied for the final formulation of PCV13 in order to create a more robust manufacturing process. A phase III, parallel group, randomized, active-controlled, double-blind trial was conducted in Poland to assess the safety and immunogenicity of PCV13 + P80 versus PCV13 without P80 in healthy infants (42–98 days at enrollment) as a three-dose series. Concomitant vaccines were permitted during the study and included DTaP-IPV-Hib (Pentaxim®), HBV vaccine (Engerix-B®), and MMR (Priorix®). The majority of local reactions were mild in nature. The incidence of local reactions was significantly lower in PCV13 + P80 compared to PCV13 without P80 after doses one and two ($p = 0.0017$ and $p = 0.024$, respectively). There were no instances when the rates of local reactions were significantly greater in the PCV13 + P80 group versus the PCV13 without P80 group. Systemic reactions were similarly reported between the two study groups. There was a statistically significantly lower incidence of decreased appetite after dose two ($p = 0.0450$) and increased sleep after the toddler dose ($p = 0.010$) in the PCV13 + P80 group compared to the PCV13 without P80 group. Fever was mild to moderate in severity as well, no subjects reported severe (>40 °C) in either group. Other AEs reported were mild or moderate in severity, consisted of childhood illnesses, and were considered unrelated to the study vaccines. One SAE was considered related to the study vaccine in the PCV13 without P80 group, which was a case of bronchitis that occurred during the infant series of vaccination. No SAEs were considered related to the vaccine after the toddler dose in either group. Of note, subjects in the two groups represented a homogeneous study population, therefore; results may not be entirely generalizable. No apparent safety concerns surfaced during this study, which supports the inclusion of P80 into the PCV13 vaccine to help ensure consistent manufacturing processes [114C].

Drug Dosage Regimens Conjugate pneumococcal vaccines continue to undergo study and consideration and one area of recent study pertains to the possible use of conjugate vaccines for "catch-up" vaccinations. A phase IV, open-label, single-center study was conducted in healthy Chinese children aged 121 days to <72 months to assess safety and immunogenicity of catch-up dosing strategies for PCV7 vaccine. Children aged 121 to <212 days received four doses of PCV7, 212 days to <12 months received three doses, 12 to <24 months received two doses, and 24 to <72 months received one dose either 28–42 days apart (two younger subject groups) or 56–70 days apart (12- to <24-month group). Interestingly, only 13 AEs were reported in a study population of over 400. The number of events reported per group was four each (121 to <212 days and 212 days to <12 months), three (12 to <24 months), and one (24 to <72 months). One subject in the 12- to <24-month group had two reported AEs. The most common AE was fever (nine events). The majority of AEs were mild to moderate in intensity. Two subjects reported SAEs, which included one subject with a case of enteritis and one subject with cases of gastroenteritis, respiratory failure, and circulatory collapse. The latter subject died. None of the SAEs or the death were related to the study vaccine. The results indicate that the PCV7 vaccine was well tolerated in this study population. However, the low incidence of AEs described may require further examination with regard to the definitions utilized for AE, SAE, and reporting structures [115C].

Catch-up vaccination strategies have also been studied with the use of PCV13 vaccine. A phase III, open-label, multicenter study performed in Poland evaluated the safety and immune responses of PCV13 among healthy children aged 7 to <72 months who were naïve to pneumococcal vaccination. Subjects were grouped according to age, Group 1 consisted of children aged 7 to <12 months, Group 2 subjects were 12 to <24 months, and Group 3 subjects were 24 to <72 months. The dosing schedule was based on the PCV7 catch-up schedule, Group 1 received three doses (28–42 days apart), Group 2 received two doses (56–70 days apart), and Group 3 received one dose. Reported local and systemic reactions were mainly mild to moderate in severity. Local tenderness was reported in 15.2%, 43.7%, and 42.3% of subjects in Groups 1, 2, and 3, respectively. This represented a trend toward great tenderness in the older children. However, this trend was not observed with swelling and redness. Swelling was reported in 36%, 44.5%, and 36.9% of subjects in Groups 1, 2, and 3, respectively. Redness was reported in 48.8% in Group 1, 70% in Group 2, and 50% in Group 3. In general, fewer systemic reactions were reported in subjects in Group 3 (older children). Mild fever ($\geq 38\,^{\circ}C$ to $\leq 39\,^{\circ}C$) was noted in 3.4–8.1% of Group 1 subjects, 3.7–5.1% of Group 2 subjects, and 0.7% of Group 3 subjects. Twelve SAEs were reported which were characterized as infections, infestations, or gastrointestinal disorders. No SAEs were related to the study vaccine, no subjects withdrew secondary to an SAE, and no deaths occurred during the study period.

The study population was homogenous in nature, but overall, results of the study support the continued study and potential utilization of PCV13 for catch-up vaccination schedules in children naïve to pneumococcal vaccine [116C].

References

[1] Halsey NA, Edwards KM, Dekker CL, et al. Algorithm to assess causality after individual adverse vents following immunization. Vaccine. 2012;30(39):5791–8 [H].

[2] Tozzi AE, Asturias EJ, Balakrishnan MR, et al. Assessment of causality of individual adverse events following immunization (AEFI): a WHO tool for global use. Vaccine. 2013;31(44):5041–6 [H].

[3] Rey D, Piroth L, Wendling MJ, et al. Safety and immunogenicity of double-dose versus standard-dose hepatitis B revaccination in non-responding adults with HIV-1 (ANRS HB04 B-BOOST): a multicenter, open-label, randomised controlled trial. Lancet Infect Dis. 2015;15(11):1283–91 [C].

[4] Alberer M, Burchard G, Jelinek T, et al. Immunogenicity and safety of concomitant administration of a combined hepatitis A/B vaccine and a quadrivalent meningococcal conjugate vaccine in healthy adults. J Travel Med. 2015;22:105–14 [C].

[5] Stillo M, Santisteve PC, Lopalco PL. Safety of human papillomavirus vaccines: a review. Expert Opin Drug Saf. 2015;14(5):697–712 [R].

[6] Brinth LS, Pors K, Theibel AC, et al. Orthostatic intolerance and postural tachycardia syndrome as suspected adverse effects of vaccination against human papillomavirus. Vaccine. 2015;33:2602–5 [c].

[7] Brinth L, Theibel AC, Pors K, et al. Suspected side effects to the quadrivalent human papilloma vaccine. Dan Med J. 2015;62(4): A5064 [c].

[8] Kinoshita T, Abe R, Hineno A, et al. Peripheral sympathetic nerve dysfunction in adolescent Japanese girls following immunization with the human papillomavirus vaccine. Intern Med. 2014;53:2185–200 [A].

[9] Scheller NM, Svanström H, Pasternak B, et al. Quadrivalent HPV vaccination and risk of multiple sclerosis and other demyelinating diseases of the central nervous system. JAMA. 2015;313(1):54–61 [C].

[10] Datwani H, Moro P, Harrington T, et al. Chorioamnionitis following vaccination in the Vaccine Adverse Event Reporting System. Vaccine. 2015;33:3110–3 [c].

[11] Moro PL, Zheteyeva Y, Lewis P, et al. Safety of quadrivalent human papillomavirus vaccine (Gardasil®) in pregnancy: adverse events among non-manufacturer reports in the Vaccine Adverse Event Reporting System, 2006–2013. Vaccine. 2015;33:519–22 [A].

[12] Goss MA, Lievano F, Buchanan KM, et al. Final report on exposure during pregnancy from a pregnancy registry for quadrivalent human papillomavirus vaccine. Vaccine. 2015;33:3422–8 [A].

[13] Panagiotou OA, Befano BL, Gonzalez P, et al. Effect of bivalent human papillomavirus vaccination on pregnancy outcomes: long term observational follow-up in the Costa Rica HPV Vaccine Trial. BMJ. 2015;351:h4358 [C].

[14] Pellegrino P, Radice S, Clementi E. Immunogenicity and safety of the human papillomavirus vaccine in patients with autoimmune diseases: a systematic review. Vaccine. 2015;33:3444–9 [M].

[15] Gilca V, Sauvageau C, Boulianne N, et al. The effect of a booster dose of quadrivalent or bivalent HPV vaccine when administered to girls previously vaccinated with two doses of quadrivalent HPV vaccine. Hum Vaccin Immunother. 2015;11(3):732–8 [C].

[16] Schilling A, Macias Parra M, Gutierrez M, et al. Coadministration of a 9-valent human papillomavirus vaccine with meningococcal and Tdap vaccines. Pediatrics. 2015;136:e563–72 [C].

[17] Recommended composition of influenza virus vaccines for use in the 2016–2017 northern hemisphere influenza season. Wkly Epidemiol Rec. 2016;91(10):121–32 [S].

[18] Engler RJM, Nelson MR, Collins LC, et al. A prospective study of the incidence of myocarditis/pericarditis and new onset cardiac symptoms following smallpox and influenza vaccination. PLoS One. 2015;10(3):1–18 [C].

[19] Christian LM, Porter K, Karlsson E, et al. Proinflammatory cytokine responses correspond with subjective side effects after influenza virus vaccination. Vaccine. 2015;33:3360–6 [c].

[20] Nagao M, Fujisawa T, Ihara T, et al. Highly increased levels of IgE antibodies to vaccine components in children with influenza vaccine-associated anaphylaxis. J Allergy Clin Immunol. 2016;137:861–7 [c].

[21] Woo EJ. Allergic reactions after egg-free recombinant influenza vaccine: reports to the US vaccine adverse event reporting system. Clin Infect Dis. 2015;60(5):777–80 [A].

[22] Himuro Y, Miyagawa F, Fukumoto T, et al. Hypersensitivity to influenza vaccine in a case of Epstein-Barr virus-associated T-lymphoproliferative disorder. Br J Dermatol. 2015;172:1686–8 [letter] [A].

[23] Saleh ZM, Faruqui S, Foad A. Onset of frozen shoulder following pneumococcal and influenza vaccinations. J Chiropr Med. 2015;14:285–9 [A].

[24] Andrade SD, Andrade MG, Santos PJ, et al. Acute disseminated encephalomyelitis following inactivated influenza vaccination in the Brazilian Amazon: a case report. Rev Soc Bras Med Trop. 2015;48(4):498–500 [A].

[25] Magnus P, Gunnes N, Tveito K, et al. Chronic fatigue syndrome/myalgic encephalomyelitis (CFS/ME) is associated with pandemic influenza infection, but not with an adjuvanted pandemic influenza vaccine. Vaccine. 2015;33:6173–7 [MC].

[26] Li-Kim-Moy J, Yin JK, Rashid H, et al. Systematic review of fever, febrile convulsions and serious adverse events following administration of inactivated trivalent influenza vaccines in children. Euro Surveill. 2015;20(24):1–20 [M].

[27] Brady RC, Hu W, Houchin VG, et al. Randomized trial to compare the safety and immunogenicity of CSL Limited's 2009 trivalent inactivated influenza vaccine to an established vaccine in the United States children. Vaccine. 2014;32:7141–7 [C].

[28] Effler PV, Kelly HA. bioCSL Limited's 2009 clinical trial to assess the immunogenicity and safety of trivalent influenza vaccine in US children raises concern. Vaccine. 2015;33:5492 [letter] [r].

[29] Kawai AT, Martin D, Kulldorff M, et al. Febrile seizures after 2010–2011 trivalent inactivated influenza vaccine. Pediatrics. 2015;136(4):e848–55 [C].

[30] Arias LH, Sanz R, Sáinz M, et al. Guillain-Barré syndrome and influenza vaccines: a meta-analysis. Vaccine. 2015;33:3772–8 [M].

[31] Feltelius N, Persson I, Ahlqvist-Rastad J, et al. A coordinated cross-disciplinary research initiative to address an increased incidence of narcolepsy following the 2009-2010 Pandemrix vaccination programme in Sweden. J Intern Med. 2015;278:335–53 [H].

[32] Sturkenboom M. The narcolepsy-pandemic influenza story: can the truth ever be unraveled? Vaccine. 2015;33S:B6–B13 [H].

[33] De Serres G, Rouleau I, Skowronski DM, et al. Paresthesia and sensory disturbances associated with 2009 pandemic vaccine receipt: clinical features and risk factors. Vaccine. 2015;33:4464–71 [C].

[34] Austin A, Tincani A, Kivity S, et al. Transverse myelitis activation post-H1N1 immunization; a case of adjuvant induction? Isr Med Assoc J. 2015;17:120–2 [A].

[35] Kuritzky LA, Pratt M. Systemic allergic contact dermatitis after formaldehyde-containing influenza vaccination. J Cutan Med Surg. 2015;19(5):504–6 [A].

[36] Castro BA, Pereira JM, Meyer RL, et al. Pityriasis lichenoides et varioliformis acuta after influenza vaccine. An Bras Dermatol. 2015;90(3 Suppl 1):S181–4 [A].

[37] Patel C, Shad HH. Membranous nephropathy and severe acute kidney injury following influenza vaccination. Saudi J Kidney Dis Transpl. 2015;26(6):1289–93 [A].

[38] Regan AK, Tracey L, Blyth CC, et al. A prospective cohort study comparing the reactogenicity of trivalent influenza vaccine in pregnant and non-pregnant women. BMC Pregnancy Childbirth. 2015;15:61–7 [C].

[39] McMillan M, Porritt K, Kralik D, et al. Influenza vaccination during pregnancy: a systematic review of fetal death, spontaneous abortion, and congenital malformation safety outcomes. Vaccine. 2015;33:2108–17 [M].

[40] Fabiani M, Bella A, Rota MC, et al. A/H1N1 pandemic influenza vaccination: a retrospective evaluation of adverse maternal, fetal, and neonatal outcomes in a cohort of pregnant women in Italy. Vaccine. 2015;33:2240–7 [MC].

[41] Sukumaran L, McCarthy NL, Kharbanda EO, et al. Safety of tetanus toxoid, reduced diphtheria toxoid, and acellular pertussis and influenza vaccination in pregnancy. Obstet Gynecol. 2015;126:1069–74 [MC].

[42] Saito T, Ohfuji S, Matsumura T, et al. Safety of a pandemic influenza vaccine and the immune response in patients with Duchenne muscular dystrophy. Intern Med. 2015;54:1199–205 [c].

[43] Liao Z, Tang H, Xu X, et al. Immunogenicity and safety of influenza vaccination in systemic lupus erythematosus patients compared with health controls: a meta-analysis. PLoS One. 2016;11(2):e0147856 [M].

[44] Cadorna-Carlos JB, Nolan T, Borja-Tabora CF, et al. Safety, immunogenicity, and lot-to-lot consistency of a quadrivalent inactivated influenza vaccine in children, adolescents, and adults: a randomized, controlled, phase III trial. Vaccine. 2015;33:2485–92 [MC].

[45] Isakova-Sivak I, Stukova M, Erofeeva M, et al. H2N2 live attenuated influenza vaccine is safe and immunogenic for healthy adult volunteers. Hum Vaccin Immunother. 2015;11(4):970–82 [c].

[46] Aichinger G, Grohmann-Izay B, van der Velden MV, et al. Phase I/II randomized double blind study of the safety and immunogenicity of a nonadjuvated vero cell culture-derived whole-virus H9N2 influenza vaccine in health adults. Clin Vaccine Immunol. 2015;22(1):46–55 [C].

[47] Black S. Safety and effectiveness of MF-59 adjuvanted influenza vaccines in children and adults. Vaccine. 2015;33S:B3–5 [r].

[48] Gorse GJ, Falsey AR, Ozol-Godfrey A, et al. Safety and immunogenicity of a quadrivalent intradermal influenza vaccine in adults. Vaccine. 2015;33:1151–9 [C].

[49] Knuf M, Leroux-Roels G, Rümke HC, et al. Safety and immunogenicity of an MF-59-adjuvanted A/H1N1 pandemic influenza vaccine in children from three to seventeen years of age. Vaccine. 2015;33:174–81 [C].

[50] Knuf M, Leroux-Roels G, Rümke H, et al. Immunogenicity and safety of cell-derived MF59-adjuvanted A/H1N1 influenza vaccine for children. Hum Vaccin Immunother. 2015;11(2):358–76 [C].

[51] Díez-Domingo J, Baldó JM, Planelles-Catarino MV, et al. Phase II, randomized, open, controlled study of AS03-adjuvanted H5N1 pre-pandemic influenza vaccine in children aged 3 to 9 years: follow-up of safety and immunogenicity persistence at 24 months post-vaccination. Influenza Other Respir Viruses. 2015;9(2):68–77 [C].

[52] Kosalaraska P, Jeanfreau R, Frenette L, et al. AS03B-adjuvanted H5N1 influenza vaccine in children 6 months through 17 years of age: a phase 2/3 randomized, placebo-controlled observer-blinded trial. J Infect Dis. 2015;211:801–10 [C].

[53] Izurieta P, Kim WJ, Wie SJ, et al. Immunogenicity and safety of an AS03-adjuvanted H5N1 pandemic influenza vaccine in Korean adults: a phase IV, randomized, open-label, controlled study. Vaccine. 2015;33:2800–7 [C].

[54] Godeaux O, Izurieta P, Madariaga M, et al. Immunogenicity and safety of AS03$_A$-adjuvanted H5N1 influenza vaccine prepared from bulk antigen after stockpiling for 4 years. Vaccine. 2015;33:2189–95 [c].

[55] Japanese encephalitis vaccines: WHO position paper, February 2015. Wkly Epidemiol Rec. 2015;90(9):69–88 [S].

[56] Wang SY, Cheng XH, Li JX, et al. Comparing the immunogenicity and safety of 3 Japanese encephalitis vaccines in Asia-Pacific area: a systematic review and meta-analysis. Hum Vaccin Immunother. 2015;11(6):1418–25 [M].

[57] Jelinek T, Burchard GD, Dieckmann S, et al. Short-term immunogenicity and safety of an accelerated pre-exposure prophylaxis regimen with Japanese encephalitis vaccine in combination with a rabies vaccine: a phase III, multicenter, observer-blind study. J Travel Med. 2015;22:225–31 [C].

[58] Jain A, Marshall J, Buikema A, et al. Autism occurrence by MMR vaccine status among US children with older siblings with and without autism. JAMA. 2015;313(15):1532–40 [C].

[59] Macartney KK, Gidding HF, Trinh L, et al. Febrile seizures following measles and varicella vaccines in young children in Australia. Vaccine. 2015;33:1412–7 [c].

[60] Klein NP, Lewis E, Fireman B, et al. Safety of measles-containing vaccines in 1-year-old children. Pediatrics. 2015;133(2): e321–9 [MC].

[61] Tramuto F, Dones P, D'Angelo C, et al. Post-vaccine measles in a child with concomitant influenza, Sicily, Italy, March 2015. Euro Surveill. 2015;20(20):1–4. pii: 21134; [A].

[62] Ma SJ, Xiong YQ, Jiang LN, et al. Risk of febrile seizure after measles-mumps-rubella-varicella vaccine: a systematic review and meta-analysis. Vaccine. 2015;33:3636–49 [M].

[63] Woo EJ. Letter to the editor: fatal varicella due to the vaccine-strain varicella-zoster virus. Hum Vaccin Immunother. 2015;11(3):679 [A].

[64] Deichmann KA, Ferrera G, Tran C, et al. Immunogenicity and safety of a combined measles, mumps, rubella and varicella live vaccine (ProQuad®) administered concomitantly with a booster dose of a hexavalent vaccine in 12–23 month-old infants. Vaccine. 2015;33:2379–86 [C].

[65] Iqbal S, Shi J, Seib K, et al. Preparation for global introduction of inactivated poliovirus vaccine: safety evidence from the US Vaccine Adverse Event Reporting System, 2000–12. Lancet Infect Dis. 2015;15:1175–82 [M].

[66] Troy S, Kouiavskaia D, Siik J, et al. Comparison of the immunogenicity of various booster doses of inactivated polio vaccine delivered intradermally versus intramuscularly to HIV-infected adults. J Infect Dis. 2015;211:1969–76 [C].

[67] Mayet A, Duron S, Meynard JB, et al. Surveillance of adverse events following vaccination in the French armed forces, 2011–2012. Public Health. 2015;129:763–8 [MC].

[68] O'Ryan M, Bandyopadhyay AS, Villena R, et al. Inactivated poliovirus vaccine given alone or in a sequential schedule with bivalent oral poliovirus vaccine in Chilean infants: a randomised, controlled, open-label, phase 4, non-inferiority study. Lancet Infect Dis. 2015;15:1273–82 [C].

[69] Lai YC, Yew YW. Severe autoimmune adverse events post herpes zoster vaccine: a case-control study of adverse events in a national database. J Drug Dermatol. 2015;14(7):681–4 [c].

[70] Kim M, Juern A, Paley S, et al. Vaccine-associated herpes zoster. J Pediatr. 2015;167:494 [A].

[71] Bhalla P, Forrest GN, Gershon M, et al. Disseminated, persistent, and fatal infection due to the vaccine strain of varicella-zoster virus in an adult following stem cell transplantation. Clin Infect Dis. 2015;60(7):1068–74 [A].

[72] Yao CA, Chen LK, Huang KC. The immunogenicity and safety of zoster vaccination in Taiwanese adults. Vaccine. 2015;33:1515–7 [C].

[73] Toplak N, Avcin T. Long-term safety and efficacy of varicella vaccination in children with juvenile idiopathic arthritis treated with biologic therapy. Vaccine. 2015;33:4056–9 [A].

[74] Russell AF, Parrino J, Fisher CL, et al. Safety, tolerability, and immunogenicity of zoster vaccine in subjects on chronic/maintenance corticosteroids. Vaccine. 2015;33:3129–34 [C].

[75] Cheetham TC, Marcy SM, Tseng HF, et al. Risk of herpes zoster and disseminated varicella zoster in patients taking immunosuppressant drugs at the time of zoster vaccination. Mayo Clin Proc. 2015;90(7):865–73 [c].

[76] Diez-Domingo J, Weinke T, Garcia de Lomas J, et al. Comparison of intramuscular and subcutaneous administration of a herpes zoster live-attenuated vaccine in adults aged ≥50 years: a randomised non-inferiority clinical trial. Vaccine. 2015;33:789–95 [C].

[77] Staples JE, Bocchini JA, Rubin L, et al. Yellow fever vaccine booster doses: recommendations of the Advisory Committee on Immunization Practices, 2015. MMWR Morb Mortal Wkly Rep. 2015;64(23):647–50 [S].

[78] DeSilva M, Sharma A, Staples E, et al. Fatal yellow fever vaccine-associated viscerotropic disease—Oregon, September 2014. MMWR Morb Mortal Wkly Rep. 2015;64(10):279–81 [A].

[79] Nash ER, Brand M, Chalkias S. Yellow fever vaccination of a primary vaccine during adalimumab therapy. J Travel Med. 2015;22(4):279–81 [A].

[80] Leca M, Bornet C, Montana M, et al. Meningococcal vaccines: current state and future outlook. Pathol Biol. 2015;63:144–51 [H].

[81] MacNeil JR, Rubin L, Folaranmi T, et al. Use of serogroup B meningococcal vaccines in adolescents and young adults: recommendations of the advisory committee on immunization practices, 2015. Morb Mortal Wkly Rep. 2015;64(41):1171–6 [S].

[82] Esposito S, Prymula R, Zuccotti GV, et al. A phase 2 randomized controlled trial of a multicomponent meningococcal serogroup B vaccine, 4CmenB, in infants (II). Hum Vaccin Immunother. 2014;10(7):2005–14 [C].

[83] Block SL, Szenborn L, Daly W, et al. A comparative evaluation of two investigational meningococcal ABCWY vaccine formulations: results of a phase 2 randomized, controlled trial. Vaccine. 2015;33:2500–10 [C].

[84] Richmond PC, Marshall HS, Nissen MD, et al. Safety, immunogenicity, and tolerability of meningococcal serogroup B bivalent recombinant lipoprotein 2086 vaccine in healthy adolescents: a randomized, single-blind, placebo-controlled, phase 2 trial. Lancet Infect Dis. 2012;12:597–607 [C].

[85] Vesikari T, Ostergaard L, Diez-Domingo J, et al. Meningococcal serogroup B bivalent rLP2086 vaccine elicits broad and robust serum bactericidal responses in healthy adolescents. J Pediatric Infect Dis Soc. 2016;5(2):152–60 [C].

[86] Santolaya ME, O'Ryan ML, Valenzuela MT, et al. Immunogenicity and tolerability of a multicomponent serogroup B (4CMenB) vaccine in healthy adolescent in Chile: a phase 2b/3 randomized, observer-blind, placebo-controlled study. Lancet. 2012;379:617–24 [C].

[87] Perrett KP, McVernon J, Richmond PC, et al. Immune responses to a recombinant, four-component, meningococcal serogroup B vaccine (4CMenB) in adolescents: a phase III,

randomized, multicenter, lot-to-lot consistency study. Vaccine. 2015;33:5217–24 [C].

[88] Leonardi M, Latiolais T, Sarpong K, et al. Immunogenicity and reactogenicity of Infanrix when co-administered with meningococcal MenACWY-TT conjugate vaccine in toddlers primed with MenHibrix and Pediarix. Vaccine. 2015;33:924–32 [C].

[89] Vesikari T, Wysocki J, Beeslaar J, et al. Immunogenicity, safety, and tolerability of bivalent rLP2086 meningococcal group B vaccine administered concomitantly with diphtheria, tetanus, and acellular pertussis and inactivated poliomyelitis vaccines to health adolescents. J Pediatric Infect Dis. 2016;5(2):180–7 [C].

[90] Vesikari T, Esposito S, Prymula R, et al. Immunogenicity and safety of an investigational multicomponent, recombinant, meningococcal serogroup B vaccine (4CMenB) administered concomitantly with routine infant and child vaccinations: results of two randomized trials. Lancet. 2013;381:825–35 [MC].

[91] Vesikari T, Prymula R, Merrall E, et al. Meningococcal serogroup B vaccine (4CMenB): booster dose in previously vaccinated infants and primary vaccination in toddlers and two-year-old children. Vaccine. 2015;33:3850–8 [C].

[92] Pertussis vaccines: WHO position paper. Wkly Epidemiol Rec. 2015;90(35):433–60 [S].

[93] Lateef TM, Johann-Liang R, Kaulas H, et al. Seizures, encephalopathy, and vaccines: experience in the national vaccine injury compensation program. J Pediatr. 2015;166:576–81 [C].

[94] De St Maurice A, Edwards KM. Post-licensure monitoring to evaluate vaccine safety. J Pediatr. 2015;166(3):513–5 [letter] [r].

[95] Long S. Explaining alleged pertussis vaccine associated neurologic disorders. J Pediatr. 2015;166(3):509 [letter] [r].

[96] Sukumaran L, McCarthy N, Kharbanda EO, et al. Association of Tdap vaccination with acute events and adverse birth outcomes among pregnant women with prior tetanus-containing immunizations. JAMA. 2015;314(15):1581–7 [MC].

[97] Scheifele DW, Ferguson M, Predy G, et al. Immunogenicity and safety of 3-dose primary vaccination with combined DTPa-HBV-IPV/Hib vaccine in Canadian Aboriginal and non-Aboriginal infants. Vaccine. 2015;33:1897–900 [c].

[98] Dalvi S, Kullkarni PS, Phadke MA, et al. A comparative clinical study to assess safety and reactogenicity of a DTwP-HepB+Hib vaccine. Hum Vaccin Immunother. 2015;11(4):901–7 [C].

[99] Marshall GS, Adams GL, Leonardi ML, et al. Immunogenicity, safety, and tolerability of a hexavalent vaccine in infants. Pediatrics. 2015;136(2):e323–32 [C].

[100] Kovac M, Rathi N, Kuriyakose S, et al. Immunogenicity and reactogenicity of a decennial booster dose of a combined reduced-antigen-content diphtheria-tetanus-acellular pertussis and inactivated poliovirus booster vaccine (dTpa-IPV) I health adults. Vaccine. 2015;33:2594–601 [C].

[101] Carlsson RM, Gustafsson L, Hallander HO, et al. Two consecutive randomized controlled pertussis booster trials in children initially vaccinated in infancy with an acellular vaccine: the first with a five-component Tdap vaccine to 5-year old and the second with five-or monocomponent Tdap vaccines at age 14–15 years. Vaccine. 2015;33:3717–25 [C].

[102] Vandermeulen C, Theeren H, Rathi N, et al. Decennial administration in young adults of a reduced-antigen content diphtheria, tetanus, acellular pertussis vaccine containing two different concentrations of aluminum. Vaccine. 2015;33:3026–34 [C].

[103] Kosalaraksa P, Mehlsen J, Vesikari T, et al. An open-label, randomized study of a 9-valent human papillomavirus vaccine given concomitantly with diphtheria, tetanus, pertussis, and poliomyelitis vaccines to healthy adolescents 11–15 years of age. Pediatr Infect Dis J. 2015;34:627–34 [C].

[104] Tinoco JC, Juergens C, Ruiz GM, et al. Open-label trial of immunogenicity and safety of a 13-valent pneumococcal conjugate vaccine in adults ≥50 years of age in Mexico. Clin Vaccine Immunol. 2015;22(2):185–92 [C].

[105] Durando P, Rosselli R, Cremonesi I, et al. Safety and tolerability of 13-valent pneumococcal conjugate vaccine in the elderly. Hum Vaccin Immunother. 2015;11(1):172–7 [C].

[106] Aikawa NE, França ILA, Ribeiro AC, et al. Short and long-term immunogenicity and safety following the 23-valent polysaccharide pneumococcal vaccine in juvenile idiopathic arthritis patients under conventional SMARDS with or without anti-TNF therapy. Vaccine. 2015;33:604–9 [c].

[107] Han J, Kemiki O, Hsu LL, et al. Adverse reactions to pneumococcal vaccine in pediatric and adolescent patients with sickle cell disease. Pharmacotherapy. 2015;35(7):696–700 [A].

[108] Cordonnier C, Ljungman P, Juergens C, et al. Immunogenicity, safety, and tolerability of 13-valent pneumococcal conjugate vaccine followed by 23-valent pneumococcal polysaccharide vaccine in recipients of allogeneic hematopoietic stem cell transplant aged ≥2 years: an open-label study. Clin Infect Dis. 2015;61(3):313–23 [C].

[109] Glesby MJ, Watson W, Brinson C, et al. Immunogenicity and safety of 13-valent pneumococcal conjugate vaccine in HIV-infected adults previously vaccinated with pneumococcal polysaccharide vaccine. J Infect Dis. 2015;212:18–27 [C].

[110] Bhorat AE, Madhi SA, Laudat F, et al. Immunogenicity and safety of the 13-valent pneumococcal conjugate vaccine in HIV-infected individuals naïve to pneumococcal vaccination. AIDS. 2015;29:1345–54 [C].

[111] McFetridge R, Meulen AS, Folkerth SD, et al. Safety, tolerability, and immunogenicity of 15-valent pneumococcal conjugate vaccine in healthy adults. Vaccine. 2015;33:2793–9 [c].

[112] Meulen AS, Vesikari T, Malacaman EA, et al. Safety, tolerability and immunogenicity of 15-valent pneumococcal conjugate vaccine in toddlers previously vaccinated with 7-valent pneumococcal conjugate vaccine. Pediatr Infect Dis J. 2015;34:186–94 [c].

[113] Li G, Liang Q, Shi J, et al. Safety and immunogenicity of 23-valent pneumococcal polysaccharide vaccine in 2 to 70 year old healthy people in China: a phase III double blind, randomized clinical trial. Hum Vaccin Immunother. 2015;11(3):699–703 [C].

[114] Gadzinowski J, Tansey SP, Wysocki J, et al. Safety and immunogenicity of a 13-valent pneumococcal conjugate vaccine manufactured with and without polysorbate 80 given to healthy infants at 2, 3, 4, and 12 months of age. Pediatr Infect Dis J. 2015;34:180–5 [C].

[115] Li R, Huang L, Mo S, et al. Safety, tolerability, and immunogenicity of 7-valent pneumococcal conjugate vaccine in older infants and young children in China who are naïve to pneumococcal vaccination: results of a phase 4 open-label trial. Vaccine. 2015;33:3580–5 [C].

[116] Wysocki J, Brzostek J, Szmańksi H, et al. Immunogenicity and safety of a 13-valent pneumococcal conjugate vaccine administered to older infants and children naïve to pneumococcal vaccination. Vaccine. 2015;33:1719–25 [C].

31

Blood, Blood Components, Plasma, and Plasma Products

Alison Brophy*,†,1, *Yekaterina Opsha**,†, *Maria Cardinale**,‡

*Ernest Mario School of Pharmacy, Rutgers, The State University of New Jersey, Piscataway, NJ, USA
†Saint Barnabas Medical Center, Livingston, NJ, USA
‡Saint Peter's University Hospital, New Brunswick, NJ, USA
1Corresponding author: aabrophy@pharmacy.rutgers.edu

ALBUMIN AND DERIVATIVES
[SED-15, 54; SEDA-35, 583; SEDA-36, 483; SEDA-37, 403]

Scandinavian guidelines for resuscitation released in 2015 recommend the use of crystalloids over colloids including starches, albumin, and gelatin for resuscitation of critically ill patients with sepsis and trauma. This is based on meta-analysis review and GRADE methodology [1M].

Albumin [SED-15, 54; SEDA-35, 583; SEDA-36, 483; SEDA-37,403]

Several reviews discuss the reporting of meta-analysis demonstrating lack of mortality benefit for albumin in sepsis resuscitation but the potential of alternative benefits. Immunomodulation, oncotic pressure, and effect on acid–base equilibrium are all effects of albumin [2r, 3r].

Hematologic

The ALIAS study analyzed the use of albumin for stroke treatment in a total of 800 patients; a subgroup of 41 individuals experienced symptomatic intracranial hemorrhage. The odds ratio with albumin therapy was 2.15 (95% CI 1.08–4.25) [4C]. An in vitro evaluation of whole-blood samples with 4% albumin or normal saline found an increase in time to clotting with a decrease in clot firmness, suggesting that albumin impairs fibrinogen activity [5c].

Renal

In a retrospective 510 center US study comparing over 1 million patients with knee or hip arthroplasty, patients who received albumin perioperative resuscitation were found to have increased risk of renal failure with an odds ratio of 1.56 (95% CI 1.36–1.78) [6MC].

Conversely, a study of 22 patients with cirrhosis and either acute kidney injury (AKI) or refractory ascites administered 30–60 g per day of albumin for 3–4 days showed improvement in renal blood flow and hemodynamics. It was postulated by the authors that this improvement was most likely due to reduced oxidative stress, reduction in sympathetic tone, and endotoxemia [7c].

In a similar study, 193 cirrhotic patients with infections other than bacterial peritonitis received albumin 1.5 g/kg on Day 1 and 1 g/kg on Day 3. The occurrence of renal failure was delayed in these patients compared to the control patients (29 days versus 11.7 days, respectively, $p = 0.018$) [8c].

Multi-Organ Failure

Liver transplant recipients who received 100 g per day of albumin post-operatively for 7 days were found to have a lower Sequential Organ Failure Assessment scores than the control patients (11.0 versus 13.4, respectively, $p < 0.001$). The study was a retrospective analysis of 15 hypo-albuminemic patients undergoing liver transplants with 15 matched controls [9c].

Drug Dosage Regimens

Evaluation of a reduced albumin dosing regimen for large volume paracentesis in 937 procedures found no difference in rate of complications included hemodynamic instability and renal failure. In the reduced dose group the maximum albumin administered was 50 g. This was compared to 12.5 g per liter as a historical control [10C].

Drug Overdosage

A unique use of albumin as a drug was employed in an 86-year-old woman with phenytoin toxicity. The patient's total serum level was 32 µmol/L and free level of 15.1 µmol/L. The patient was hemodynamically unstable and administered 25 g of 5% albumin over 4 hours. Her consciousness and blood pressure improved and the free level decreased to 8 µmol/L with a total level of 44 µmol/L. Binding of phenytoin by albumin prevented further toxicity and allowed drug metabolism and removal by improved hemodynamics [11A].

BLOOD TRANSFUSION [SEDA-15, 529; SEDA-35, 583, SEDA-36, 483; SEDA-37, 404]

Erythrocytes

Red blood cell (RBC) transfusions are administered to prevent anemia-related hypoxia when treating the cause of anemia is either inadequate or not possible [12r]. In an analysis from the National Healthcare Safety Network (NHSN) Hemovigilance Module, 5136 adverse reactions from a total of 1346 facility-months and 1 225 496 RBC units transfused were reported from 2010 to 2012. The rate of adverse reactions following RBC transfusions was reported as 205.5 per 100 000 transfused units. The most commonly reported adverse events were allergic reactions (46.8%, of which 7.1% were severe or life threatening), followed by febrile nonhemolytic reactions (36.1%). Higher rates of adverse reactions were seen with apheresis compared to whole-blood derived units, but similar rates were seen regardless of irradiation or leukoreduction [13MC].

In another report, hemovigilance data were analyzed from 17 countries between 2010 and 2013 [14MC]. Allergic reactions were reported in 11 patients per 100 000 units transfused; febrile nonhemolytic transfusion reactions (FNHTR) occurred in 26 patients per 100 000 units, and hypotension occurred with 2 per 100 000 units. Allergic reactions occurred at a significantly greater rate in the United States compared to other developed countries (53.61 per 100 000 compared to 9.7 per 100 000) and FNHTR occurred most commonly in the Netherlands, New Zealand, and the United States. FNHTR appeared to occur more often with leukoreduced products compared to nonleukoreduced products. Acute transfusion-related pain was also reported by the Swedish hemovigilance program at a rate of one per 100 000 transfused units [14MC].

Respiratory

Transfusion-related acute lung injury (TRALI) is typically regarded as a major cause of transfusion-related death. It is characterized by acute hypoxia and bilateral infiltrates on chest radiograph within 6 hours of transfusion, and is typically managed by supportive care [15C]. In the international hemovigilance report by Rogers and colleagues, TRALI was reported at a rate of 0.35 per 100 000 units transfused [14MC]. A retrospective cohort study described outcomes in 3379 adult patients undergoing noncardiac surgery that received allogenic RBC transfusions before and after TRALI mitigation strategies were implemented including universal leukoreduction and male-only plasma donation. The overall rate of TRALI occurring within 6 hours of transfusion was 1.3% (45 out of 3379) and included both definite and possible TRALI cases. The composite rate of TRALI was similar before and after implementation of the aforementioned mitigation strategies (1.3% vs. 1.4%) and the risk of TRALI occurrence increased with increasing transfusion volumes ($p < 0.001$). Importantly, patients with TRALI had a significantly longer median intensive care unit length of stay, hospital length of stay, and in-hospital mortality, with an odds ratio of 15.6 (95% CI: 7.9–30.8) for death compared to non-TRALI controls [15C].

The impact of TRALI is poorly described in pediatric patients. In a retrospective cohort study, all admissions to the pediatric intensive care unit at a single institution were screened for onset of TRALI using consensus criteria over a 4-year period. TRALI developed in 21 of 304 transfused patients (6.9%). Risk factors for TRALI included mechanical ventilation, sepsis, and a high Pediatric Risk of Mortality III score. TRALI was associated with an increased mortality rate (76.2% vs. 11.3%, $p < 0.001$) and longer duration of mechanical ventilation (183 hours vs. 25 hours, $p < 0.002$) compared with transfused control patients [16C].

Pneumonia has also been described following RBC transfusion. A multicenter retrospective study was performed on 16 182 patients undergoing coronary artery bypass grafting (CABG) in Michigan between 2011 and 2013. Using a multivariable logistic regression, this study found a significant association between RBC transfusion and pneumonia (odds ratio of 3.4, $p < 0.001$). In addition, the risk of developing pneumonia increased as the number of transfused units increased [17MC].

Nervous System

A retrospective analysis of patients undergoing CABG and valve surgery at three European University Hospitals aimed to determine the relationship between RBC transfusion and post-operative stroke using logistic regression and a propensity score analysis. Of the 14 956 patients analyzed, 6419 received RBC transfusions at a mean of 1.3 ± 2.4 units. Transfused patients had a higher rate of stroke (1.6% vs. 0.5%, $p < 0.001$) and stroke/transient ischemic attack (TIA) (2.6% vs. 0.8%, $p < 0.001$) compared to non-transfused controls, and the incidence increased with increasing number of transfused units. In addition, transfused patients had a higher in-hospital mortality (3.9% vs. 0.6%, $p < 0.001$), as well as longer length of stay and intensive care unit length of stay. On regression analysis, RBC transfusion was identified as an independent risk factor for post-operative stroke or stroke/TIA [18MC].

Electrolyte Imbalance

A prospective observational study of 125 medical intensive care unit patients receiving washed RBC transfusions demonstrated a 4% (5/125) incidence of serum potassium greater than or equal to 5.5 mEq/L. Multivariate logistic regression showed a linear correlation between duration of blood storage prior to transfusion and serum potassium levels. Importantly, one patient experienced cardiac arrest after transfusion of seven units and a serum potassium of 9 mEq/L [19C].

Fluid Balance

Transfusion-associated circulatory overload (TACO) occurred in three patients per 100 000 units transfused according to international hemovigilance programs; however, when utilizing published frequency rates from active surveillance, the pooled rate of TACO was found to be 368 per 100 000 transfusions [14]. In another retrospective cohort study of noncardiac surgery patients that received autologous or allogenic transfusions, there was a 2.7% incidence (90 patients out of 3322) of TACO in patients that received only RBC transfusions and no other blood types [20C].

Hematologic

In hemovigilance data, hemosiderosis (iron overload) was reported by France and Spain at a rate of 0.3 per 100 000 transfused units. In addition, acute hemolytic reactions were reported in one per 100 000 and delayed hemolytic reactions in 2 per 100 000 transfused units. Delayed serologic transfusion reactions were reported at a rate of 24.6 per 100 000 units, and post-transfusion purpura occurred at a rate of 0.08 per 100 000 [14MC]. In a prospective, observational study of 100 critically ill children, RBC transfusions were associated with a variable response in markers of hemolysis, including indirect bilirubin, free hemoglobin, haptoglobin, serum iron and non-transferrin-bound iron at 4 hours post-transfusion. In a subset of patients ($n = 21$) who experienced an increase in indirect bilirubin, an acute phase response (increased C-reactive protein) was observed that was independent of the duration of RBC storage, suggesting that other unknown factors may be responsible for the variability in the amounts of hemolysis observed [21c]. Lastly, a retrospective review of 220 adult patients with sickle cell disease that received transfusions revealed 23 delayed hemolytic transfusion reactions occurring in 17 patients. The mean time from transfusion to reaction was 10.1 ± 5.4 days, and the reactions were characterized by fever, pain, and hemoglobinuria. Five of the reactions required treatment with immunosuppressive therapy. Importantly, a large proportion of reactions were initially misdiagnosed as vaso-occlusive crisis [22c].

Immunologic

Transfusion-associated graft-versus-host disease (TA-GVHD) is infrequently associated with blood transfusions, but is often fatal when it occurs. Recipient immune status, blood component characteristics, and the donor-recipient Human Leucocyte Antigen (HLA) relationship are likely involved in predisposing a transfused patient to TA-GVHD, but the specific roles of these risk factors remain to be elucidated. Currently, irradiation of blood products is one strategy that is often employed, but this practice is not without practical limitations, and may result in cellular damage. A systematic review was performed of 348 unique cases of TA-GVHD reported in the literature. Of the 348 cases, 133 (38.2%) were due to RBC transfusion. The majority of cases were attributed to cellular blood components stored for less than 10 days that were neither leukoreduced or irradiated as 50.9% of cases were immune-competent and did not meet current guideline-recommended indications for component irradiation. Symptoms included fever, rash, liver enzyme elevation, pancytopenia, diarrhea, or bone marrow aplasia and they first appeared a median of 11 days (IQR, 8–14 days; range, 1–198 days) post-transfusion. Immunosuppressive therapy was supplied to 50.3% of cases with a mortality rate of an overwhelming 89.7%. The results of this review deemphasize the role of recipient immunodeficiency and demonstrate that the greatest contributor to the risk of TA-GVHD appears to be the introduction of viable donor lymphocytes to the host. HLA typing was available for only 84 cases, leading the authors to conclude that due to potential bias, the role of donor-recipient HLA similarity in the development of TA-GVHD remains unclear [23M].

Infection Risk

The risk of viral transmission with blood transfusions has decreased significantly due to advancements in donor selection and screening [12r]. There were no viral infections reported out of more than more than 1.2 million transfused units in the NHSN report, and only 4 bacterial infections were reported [13MC].

Death

A systematic review of six trials including 2722 patients undergoing hip fracture surgery and randomized to a liberal or restrictive strategy did not observe a difference between either strategy in 30-day or 60-day mortality. In the largest trial (2016 patients), 60% had pre-existing cardiovascular disease. In addition, no difference was found between strategies in terms of thromboembolism, respiratory infection, wound infection, or new congestive heart failure, but there was a decreased incidence of myocardial infarction in the liberal group compared to the restrictive group (RR: 0.59, 95% CI: 0.36–0.96). These results, however, were based on low-quality evidence due to protocol violations, baseline imbalances, and lack of blinding of study personnel [24M].

In a retrospective analysis of acute non-variceal upper gastrointestinal bleeding, all hospital admissions in Denmark with hemostatic endoscopic interventions in either the stomach or duodenum were identified. This analysis included 5107 patients from 2011 to 2013 with a median age of 74 years and a median of 2 endoscopic interventions per admission. The number of units of RBC transfused was identified as an independent predictor of re-endoscopy (OR: 1.08, 95% CI: 1.06–1.09) and 30-day mortality (OR 1.04, 95% CI: 1.01–1.06). This study also found that a high ratio of transfusions of RBC to fresh frozen plasma to platelets (1:1:1) reduced the need for re-endoscopy but, at the same time, increased mortality. The conclusions of this study are limited by the inability to assess severity of hemorrhage, as patients receiving more transfusions likely had the greatest risk of death because they were more critically ill [25MC].

Red Blood Cell Storage Age

In a meta-analysis of eight randomized controlled trials, a trend toward decreased mortality with stored RBCs was observed (OR: 0.91, 95% CI: 0.78–1.05). In a subset of observational studies that included intensive care unit, cardiac surgery, and trauma patients, the use of stored RBCs may have been correlated with increased mortality and possibly increased infection risks. However, due to the lack of high-quality evidence, the authors of this analysis cautioned that it would be premature to make conclusions on the safety of stored RBC transfusions based on currently available literature. In addition, they did not report the age of RBCs at the time of transfusion in the studies that were analyzed [26M]. A secondary analysis was performed on a randomized trial that enrolled 200 patients comparing erythropoietin or placebo for severe traumatic brain injury. In the 125 patients that received at least one transfusion of RBCs, no association was observed between RBC age and jugular venous oxygen saturation, brain tissue oxygenation, Glasgow Outcome Scale at 6 months, or mortality at 6 months [27c].

Prior Transfusion History

Data from standardized hemovigilance reporting programs in five reporting hospitals in Japan demonstrated that among 7594 RBC units transfused between January 2010 and December 2011, the incidence of adverse transfusion reactions of any severity was significantly higher on first transfusions (1.08%) compared to subsequent (0.69%) transfusion ($p = 0.0004$). This was especially true for FNHTR and allergic reactions. The authors concluded that there are risks of adverse reactions with the first transfusion as well as with subsequent transfusions [28MC].

Granulocytes

Granulocytes are white blood cells that contain granules and are essential elements of a functioning immune system. The most common subtype of granulocytes is neutrophils, which provide a critical line of defense against bacterial and fungal infections. Severe neutropenia (defined as an absolute neutrophil count less than 500 cells/pL) increases the risk of severe infection and is often an inevitable side effect of chemotherapy [29M]. Granulocyte transfusions have been used for decades in patients with severe neutropenia and severe infections that are inadequately responsive to antimicrobial therapy as well as patients with functionally defective neutrophils [30R].

Major Review

In a Cochrane review of 11 trials containing 653 neutropenic patients that received prophylactic granulocyte transfusions, there was insufficient evidence to observe a difference in serious adverse effects when compared to patients that did not receive granulocyte transfusions. There was also insufficient evidence to report a difference in all-cause mortality and mortality due to infection at 30 days in patients that received prophylactic granulocyte transfusions compared to those that did not. However, this analysis did observe a decreased number of people with infections over 30 days with intermediate-dose granulocyte transfusions (1.0×10^{10} to 4.0×10^{10} granulocytes per day) that was not observed with low-dose granulocyte transfusions when compared to no transfusion, suggesting a dose-dependent effect; however, this was based on low-quality evidence [29M]. A review of granulocyte transfusions published in the *Journal of Intensive Care Medicine* revealed that this therapy is generally well tolerated with mild to moderate fever and chills occurring in 10–20% of transfusions. Infections such as cytomegalovirus (CMV) as well as graft-versus-host disease have also been reported in recipients. Pulmonary complications, including dyspnea, hypoxia, and pulmonary infiltrates, have been reported within a few hours of transfusion in 5–10% of patients [30R]. In addition, a systematic review of 23 cases of granulocyte transfusions for patients with invasive *Fusarium* infection revealed two cases of pulmonary failure and death that was possibly due to the transfusion [31c].

Renal

Hydroxyethyl starch (HES) is the most common red blood cell sedimentation agent used to purify neutrophil collections for granulocyte transfusions. HES is a volume expander that carries a black box warning for increased risk of mortality and renal failure in critically ill patients, including patients with sepsis, and has been associated with increased bleeding risk. Because granulocyte transfusions contain relatively low levels of HES, and HES-related toxicities have not been reported in granulocyte recipients, HES is expected to play a minimal role in adverse events attributable to granulocyte transfusions. However, caution should be exercised, especially in critically ill patients [32r].

Platelets

Observational Studies

In 2015, the AABB (American Association of Blood Banks) published clinical practice guidelines on the use of platelet transfusions. The guidelines list febrile reactions (1 in 14 transfusions), allergic reactions (1 in 50), and bacterial sepsis (1 in 75000) as the most common adverse reactions of platelet transfusions [33R]. Hemovigilance data (2010–2012) from the National Healthcare Safety Network Hemovigilance Module revealed that compared to other blood components, platelets were associated with the highest rate of adverse events (421.7 out of 100000 units transfused). Reactions occurred slightly more frequently with apheresis compared to whole blood-derived, with non-irradiated compared to irradiated, and with leukoreduced compared to nonleukoreduced transfusions [34MC]. A registry of 6745 consecutive patients undergoing coronary artery bypass grafting (CABG) in Denmark demonstrated that, after propensity matching and adjusting for red blood cell and fresh frozen plasma transfusion, there was no difference in mortality or stroke, although platelet transfusions were still associated with an increased need for coronary angiography (adjusted OR: 2.34, 95% CI: 1.15–4.76) [35MC]. In a Cochrane review of seven randomized controlled trials, a therapeutic-only platelet transfusion strategy increased the risk of bleeding when compared to a prophylactic platelet transfusion strategy in patients with thrombocytopenia due to myelosuppressive chemotherapy or stem cell transplantation. There was no difference in the occurrence of transfusion reactions between the two strategies [36M]. In another retrospective study of noncardiac surgery patients, transfusion-associated circulatory overload (TACO) was reported at a rate of 2 out of 89 platelet transfusions (2.2%) [37C]. In an analysis of 5034 platelet transfusions given to 1102 patients in the multicenter Platelet Dose study, high-dose platelet transfusions (4.4×10^{11} platelets/m^2) were associated with a higher rate of adverse events. The most common adverse events were fever (6.6% of transfusions), allergic reactions (1.9%), sinus tachycardia (1.8%), and rigors or chills (1.1%) [38MC].

Strategies to Improve Platelet Transfusion Safety

A photochemical treatment process using amotosalen and UVA light (INTERCEPT™ Blood System) to inactive infectious contaminants of blood products has been in 20 countries since 2002 and appears to be well tolerated based on 7 years of hemovigilance reporting [39MC]. Utilizing male-only donors is recommended to reduce the titers of anti-HLA antibodies in donor blood and decrease the rate of transfusion-associated acute lung injury (TRALI). Biological response modifiers (BRMs), such as pro-inflammatory cytokines, seem to increase with increase age of the platelet concentrates and have been shown to be associated with certain adverse events. Attempts have been made to selectively remove BRMs, but this practice is considered experimental [40R].

BLOOD SUBSTITUTES [SEDA-35, 586; SEDA-36, 485; SEDA-37, 406]

Hemoglobin-Based Oxygen Carriers [SEDA-35, 586; SEDA-36, 48; SEDA-37, 406]

Cardiovascular

In a review focused on the regulatory evaluation of hemoglobin-based oxygen carriers (HBOC) by the FDA, the authors discuss different in rates of adverse events including cardiovascular ischemia and hypertension. Binding of nitric oxide (NO) varies between HBOC products and, therefore, vasoactivity differs between agents. The methodology of previous meta-analyses is also questioned due to the lack of regulatory approval for these agents [41R].

Drug Formulations

Four novel HBOC products with the addition of bioactive particles, for example nitroxide moieties, to mitigate side effects currently under investigation were reviewed. The new formulations discussed propose to decrease NO scavenging and interactions with endothelial cells, thereby decreasing HBOC-induced vasoconstriction. This review also discusses FDA regulatory decisions based on flawed meta-analysis methodology, the potential role of HBOC in developing countries and organ transport during transplantation [42R].

Plasma and Plasma Products [SEDA-35, 586, SEDA-36, 486, SEDA-37, 407]

Alpha1-Antitrypsin

It has been known for a long time in clinical practice that alpha1 antitrypsin (AAT) has broad anti-inflammatory and immunomodulating properties. It is also a known fact that deficiency in this protein (which seems to exhibit protective properties on the lungs) can lead to very common genetic respiratory disorders. The objective of one particular German study was to provide an overview of some research highlights surrounding AAT use in respiratory disease and discuss any new adverse events with the experience of the use of this protein during the past 25 years. A small proportion of adverse effects, such as dyspnea and headache, were reported to be mild and could be readily managed [43R]. Previous reports indicated that these side effects were mild in nature; however, current literature suggests that they may be more moderate-severe than previously thought. Since this product is derived from human plasma, it carries the potential risk of transmitting other infectious agents like viruses and has been recently reported to cause severe hypersensitivity [44M].

C1 Esterase Inhibitor Concentrate

Observational Studies

Hereditary angioedema (HAE) due to C1 esterase inhibitor (HAE-C1-INH) deficiency is a rare genetic disorder which frequently manifests as recurrent episodes of skin swellings, abdominal pain, and potentially fatal laryngeal edema. Prophylaxis with twice-weekly intravenous injections of plasma-derived C1-inhibitor (pdC1-INH) has been established as an effective treatment. Subcutaneous (SC) administration of this agent however has not been adequately studied in patients with HAE. An open-label, dose ranging, cross-over study (COMPACT Phase II) was conducted in 18 patients with type I or II HAE to determine the overall efficacy, safety and tolerability of this agent administered via the SC route. Patients received two of twice-weekly doses of 1500, 3000, or 6000 IU SC for 4 weeks. All doses were well tolerated. Several patients reported to have mild-moderate local site reactions and some noted to have pain and swelling at the injection site [45c].

Another active surveillance study sought to evaluate the safety and clinical usage patterns of pasteurized C1-inhibitor concentrate with a specific interest in thromboembolic events. Registry data for a span of 3 years were obtained and evaluated in May of 2013. The registry contained information regarding the use of pasteurized C1-inhibitor concentrate (Berinert) from 27 US and 4 EU sites. A total of 135 subjects and 3196 infusions were evaluated and a total of 299 adverse events were reported, for an overall rate of 0.09 events per infusion. Only two thromboembolic events were reported, both in patients with prothrombotic risk factors. Hence, this particular surveillance study found no evidence to suggest the causative risk for thromboembolic events and the studied product [46C].

Fixed Dose Study

Another open-label study sought to evaluate the efficacy and safety of C1-INH (50 IU/kg) for the treatment of multiple HAE attacks. The study evaluated a total of 44 patients and reported that the agent was well tolerated. There were no discontinuations due to adverse events. No thrombotic or anaphylactic events were reported, and repeat C1-INH treatments were not associated with neutralizing anti-C1-INH antibodies [47c]. Similar results were found in the Canadian guidelines for the treatment of hereditary angioedema attacks. The guideline states that the agent is well tolerated and the most frequent adverse events seen with its use is lightheadedness/headache, fever, and rash at the injection site [48R]. Similar results were also discussed in a review article by Riedl with headaches being the most common adverse event and some previously less described adverse events of vertigo, pneumonia, urosepsis (two episodes) and itching of the lips and soft palate with no signs of a systemic allergic reaction [49R].

Agent Specific Safety Evaluation (Ruconest®)

Ruconest® is a highly purified recombinant human C1-INH which is now approved for use in Europe, Israel and the Untied States. In the 10 completed clinical studies a total of 236 subjects have received a total of nearly one thousand administrations of Ruconest®. Safety data analyses demonstrated that Ruconest® at doses of up to 100 U/kg is generally safe and well tolerated. No safety concerns related to hematology, urinalysis, vital signs or ECG parameters were noted. No thromboembolic events or increased risk of thromboembolism were reported. No patients experienced a treatment-emergent adverse event that required discontinuation of medication. The most common adverse reactions ($\geq 2\%$) reported in all clinical trials were headache (9%), nausea (2%) and diarrhea with 2% event rate [50R].

Pediatric Population

Similar results (as previously stated) were observed in 9 pediatric patients treated with C1-INH for acute angioedema attacks who had hereditary angioedema (HAE). The safety results were similar to above and stated that doses ranging from 500 to 1500 IU were well tolerated in this population [51c].

Cryoprecipitate

Cryoprecipitate was originally developed as a therapy for patients with antihaemophilic factor deficiency or hemophilia A and has been used for nearly 50 years. Cryoprecipitate is now most commonly used to replenish fibrinogen levels in patients with acquired coagulopathy (e.g. hemorrhage including cardiac surgery, trauma, organ transplantation, or obstetric hemorrhage).

This agent is a blood product that is manufactured from fresh frozen plasma. It contains a subset of coagulation factors namely: fibrinogen (minimum of 150 mg/unit), factor VIII, von Willebrand factor, and factor XIII. Currently, cryoprecipitate is used to treat hypofibrinogemeia. Typical adverse events associated with the administration of cryoprecipitate include transmission of infectious diseases, transfusion-associated circulatory overload (TACO), and transfusion-related acute lung injury (TRALI) [SEDA-36, 407]. This agent has been withdrawn from many European countries because of safety concerns such as the transmission of pathogens. Instead, commercial fibrinogen preparations are available for fibrinogen replacement therapy. Nevertheless, cryoprecipitate remains available for hemostatic therapy in several countries, including the USA and Canada [52R].

Pediatric Transfusion Reactions

One of the first studies to evaluate the rates and reaction types post-transfusion administration in pediatric patient population was recently conducted at Vanderbilt University Medical Center (VUMC) between the period of January 1, 2011, and February 1, 2013. The report consisted of both adult and pediatric data and consisted of transfusions from platelets, plasma and red blood cells. In both adult and pediatric populations, transfusion reactions were most commonly associated with platelet transfusion, followed by RBC, and then plasma transfusions. Within the pediatric population, subset analysis identified multiple differences when compared to the adult population including an increased incidence of allergic transfusion reactions (2.7/1000 vs. 1.1/1000, respectively, $p < 0.001$), febrile nonhemolytic transfusion reactions (1.9/1000 vs. 0.47/1000, respectively, $p < 0.001$), and hypotensive transfusion reactions (0.29/1000 vs. 0.078/1000, respectively, $p < 0.05$). Interestingly, while the reaction incidence was the same between sexes in adults, in pediatric patients, reactions were more common in male patients (7.9/1000 pediatric males vs. 4.3/1000 pediatric females, $p < 0.01$). This data provided interesting insights into the potential clinical trends of transfusion reactions amongst pediatric patients [53R].

Similar results are found in the adult transfusion data with febrile nonhemolytic reactions (36.1%) being the most common type of a reaction reported [54R].

Fresh Frozen Plasma [SEDA-35, 587; SEDA-36, 486, SEDA-37, 408]

Systemic Review in Cardiovascular Surgery

A Cochrane review was performed to assess the risk of mortality for patients undergoing cardiovascular surgery who received fresh frozen plasma (FFP). The authors evaluated the use of FFP both for therapeutic and prophylactic use in all age categories (neonates, children and adults). A total of 15 trials with over 750 participants were evaluated. There were no reported adverse events attributable to FFP transfusion, although there was a significant increase in the number of patients requiring red cell transfusion who received FFP [55R]. Similar findings were reported in the most recent transfusion guidelines [56S].

PLASMA SUBSTITUTES [SEDA-35, 587; SEDA-36, 487; SEDA-37, 408]

Dextrans [SEDA-15, 1082; SEDA-35, 587; SEDA-36, 487; SEDA-37, 408]

Observational Studies

A Danish retrospective cohort study of intensive care septic shock patients receiving either dextran-70 ($n = 91$) or crystalloids ($n = 150$) for resuscitation evaluated the mortality and use of these continuous renal replacement therapies (CRRT). The 90-day mortality was 42% versus 35% in patients treated with dextran and crystalloids, respectively, $p = 0.08$. There was a significant difference in the use of CRRT between dextran and crystalloids: 48% versus 23%, $p = 0.004$. There were also more major bleed events in the dextran group 32% versus 15%, $p = 0.004$ [57c].

Etherified Starches [SEDA-15, 1237; SEDA-35, 587; SEDA-36, 487; SEDA-37, 408]

Renal

In a retrospective 510 center US study comparing over 1 million patients with knee or hip arthroplasty, patients who received 6% hydroxyethyl starch (HES) perioperative resuscitation were found to have increased risk of renal failure with an odds ratio of 1.23 (95% CI 1.13–1.34) [58C]. Increased risk of acute kidney injury (AKI) was also found in a retrospective study of 99 liver transplant recipients who received 6% HES compared to 50 recipients who received albumin with an odds ratio at

7 days of 2.94, 95% CI, 1.13–7.7, $p = 0.027$ [59C]. In deceased donor kidney transplants, donors receipt of HES lead to prolonged kidney injury in the recipients. In those whose donors received 200/0.6 HES, the creatinine level was significantly higher even 7 years after transplant then in recipients whose donors received 130/0.4 HES, $p = 0.05$ [60r]. A *post-hoc* analysis of a Scandinavian study comparing HES resuscitation with lactated ringers in 798 septic patients demonstrated more patient received renal replacement therapy within 5 days when treated with HES, $p = 0.03$. Patients treated with HES also had a higher stage of AKI after 5 days, $p = 0.03$ [61C].

Hematologic

A randomized prospective study compared administration of 6% 130/0.4 HES with saline in patients undergoing radical prostatectomy. No difference in nephrotoxicity was found but the HES group had a greater blood loss (1250 mL with HES versus 750 mL with saline) [62c]. In a meta-analysis of 13 randomized studies with 1156 pediatric patients receiving HES for volume expansion, HES was found to decrease blood platelet count and increase length of ICU stay but did not have statistically significant effects on mortality or creatinine levels [63M].

Fluid Balance

A retrospective review of more than 1400 pediatric patients undergoing cardiac surgery compared administration of 6% HES with human albumin for volume replacement. Administration of HES was associated with a decreased need for blood products and less fluid accumulation following cardiopulmonary bypass surgery [64C].

Immunologic

A study of 30 patients undergoing CABG and receiving treatment with crystalloid, HES, or gelatin evaluated immunologic markers after anesthesia and postoperatively. HES treatment was associated with lower levels of IL-9 and higher levels of TNF-α and IL-10. The ratio of CD4+:CD8+ cells showed a smaller reduction in patients treated with HES than with the other treatments. These results represent potentially less immunosuppression with HES [65c].

Death

A meta-analysis evaluating the use of HES versus other fluids for non-septic ICU patients included 22 studies with over 6064 patients. No difference was found in mortality, renal replacement therapy, bleeding, or transfusion but the studies were of small sample size with poor quality [66M].

Gelatin [SEDA-35, 584; SEDA-36, 487; SEDA-37, 409]

Immunologic

Two separate case reports of pediatric patients with hypersensitivity reactions to topical hemostatic products containing gelatin are reported. A 9-year-old boy with history of hypersensitivity reactions and asthma undergoing spinal instrumentation for kyphosis received Floseal (Baxter Healthcare Corp, Hayward, Calif), combination of gelatin granules with pooled human thrombin. Within minutes of injection through screw holes, the patient developed hypotension that was unresponsive to 4 doses of epinephrine and became pulseless requiring 1 minute of chest compressions before the return of spontaneous circulation. The patient was administered vasopressors, methylprednisolone, fluids and transferred to intensive care. IgE levels for bovine gelatin and bovine protein were elevated. It was also determined that the patient had previous less severe reactions to Floseal and gelatin containing vaccines [67A]. A 2-year-old girl under general anesthesia for dental treatment, including ionomer restoration, stainless-steal crown placement and extractions received packing with Gelfoam (gelatin sponges) for hemostatic effect. Within 2 minutes, hypotension and bradycardia unresponsive to fluids and atropine developed. Peripheral pulses were absent but a weak carotid pulse was palpable and T wave inversions were present on EKG. Periorbital and lip edema along with a rash on the back were also noted. The patient was administered epinephrine, diphenhydramine and hydrocortisone and was able to be extubated in the post-anesthesia care unit. Skin testing performed, including all intraoperative medications, was positive only for Gelfoam [68A].

GLOBULINS

IMMUNOGLOBULINS [SEDA-15, 1719; SEDA-35, 588; SEDA-36, 488; SEDA-37, 409]

Intravenous Immunoglobulin (IVIG)

Adverse events are reported to occur in 10–30% of IVIG infusions and range from infusion-related reactions to thrombotic events and acute kidney injury (AKI) [69R]. A retrospective study was conducted of critically ill adults receiving IVIG or plasmapheresis for various indications; of the 59 patients who received IVIG, renal dysfunction possibly due to IVIG occur in 6.8%, and transfusion reactions occurred in 8% [70c]. Another retrospective study of adverse reactions in 244 patients (152 were ≥60 years old) treated for various neurological conditions, the overall relative risk of adverse events was not increased in elderly patients, but there was a higher incidence of hypertension (RR: 1.38, 95% CI: 1.41–5.29). In patients ≥60 years old, sucrose-free IVIG administration and total daily dose ≥35 g were associated with adverse reactions [71C].

Anaphylaxis is a rare but serious side effect of IVIG infusion and usually attributed to the IgA content of the solution and the anti-IgA antibody in the patient's serum [72r]. In one case report, a 26-year-old female with myasthenic crisis developed tachypnea and hypoxia 2 hours after her first dose of IVIG. After symptomatic improvement with oxygenation, her respiratory status deteriorated again following her second dose and again following her third dose [73A]. An additional case describes a paradoxical exacerbation of symptoms and increased vermeil in a patient that received high-dose IVIG (Venital) for parvovirus-associated chronic fatigue syndrome. The mechanism of this reaction is unclear [74A].

Cardiovascular

Transient hypertension has been reported during IVIG infusion but the evidence is mostly limited to case reports and the mechanism is poorly described [75A]. Thromboembolic events are reported in 0.5–15% of patients that receive IVIG [76MC]. In a large, retrospective cohort study of a Medicare database ($N = 10759$, propensity-matched), patients treated for chronic lymphocytic leukemia or multiple myeloma with IVIG demonstrated a transient increased risk of arterial thrombosis during the day of IVIG infusion and the following day (HR: 3.40, 95% CI: 1.25–9.25). The risk declined over the remainder of the 30-day treatment period. The absolute risk of arterial thrombosis over a 1-year period attributable to IVIG was estimated as 0.7% (95% CI: −0.2% to 2%, number needed to harm: approximately 150) while the risk for venous thrombosis was not statistically different between groups. The authors state that the arterial thrombosis risk may have been higher in older patients [76MC]. Other reports have also demonstrated that arterial thrombosis is four times more common than venous thrombosis and typically occurs 4–24 hours after the infusion. These patients typically have other cardiovascular risk factors for thrombosis such as increased blood viscosity [77A].

A case report described an incident occurring in May 2008 where six patients in China died after receiving IVIG products from a specific lot. It was determined that an unusually high level of aggregates and microparticles contained in this particular lot led to a blockage of the pulmonary circulation and contributed to the fatalities [78c].

Two cases of sudden cardiac death were reported in pediatric heart transplant recipients. Both patients had known graft coronary artery disease and became unresponsive during or within 2 hours of a scheduled IVIG infusion [79r].

Finally, two cases of supraventricular tachycardia in newborn patients were reported during IVIG infusion to treat hemolytic disease. Although cause and effect could not be confirmed, the authors recommend cardiorespiratory monitoring in neonatal patients [80A].

Nervous System

The incidence of headache due to IVIG is reported as 2–75% based on clinical trials. Some strategies used to mitigate the headaches include switching to another immunoglobulin, if possible, as well as prophylactic treatment with acetaminophen, NSAIDs, or corticosteroids, and reduction of the infusion rate [81R].

Hematologic

A retrospective review identified five pediatrics patients with apparent IVIG-related hemolytic anemia when treated for Kawasaki's disease. All five patients required red blood cell transfusions and all patients had positive direct antiglobulin testing and laboratory markers of hemolysis [82c]. Another case of a neonatal patient treated for erythroblastosis fetalis is described in which increased hemolysis occurred following each of two doses of IVIG (Privigen 10%) [83r]. An analysis of reports of hemolysis to IVIG manufacturers over the last 10 years revealed that hemolysis occurred most commonly at doses exceeding 0.5 g/kg, in all age groups, and is not correlated with hemagglutinin exposure. In this analysis, the onset of hemolysis was a median of 36 hours after administration and 58% of patients with hemolysis required transfusion [84C]. A review of the literature reveals that patients with non-O blood group and underlying inflammatory or immune-mediated disorders receiving high doses of IVIG are at highest risk of hemolysis [85R].

Drug Formulations

Differences in IVIG purification methods by manufacturers lead to various isoagglutinin retention within the various IVIG products [86r]. Concerns that liquid immune globulins may be associated with more hemolysis than lyophilized immune globulins due to differences in isohemagglutinin content were addressed in another large study of a manufacturer's database. However, hemolysis was similar with the two formulations (0.27 cases per 1 million grams of Gammagard liquid versus 0.33 cases per 1 million grams of Gammagard S/D) [87C]. In a systematic review of head to head trials comparing IVIG products, only two studies were identified and no difference was found in morbidity or tolerance between studied formulations; however, the literature comparing products is very scarce [88M]. Lastly, in a prospective study of 20 patients that initially received 5% IVIG followed by 10% IVIG, there was no difference in side effects reported by the patients via a questionnaire [89r].

Subcutaneous Immunoglobulin (SCIG)

Observational Studies

In a prospective, multicenter observational study of 50 patients with primary immunodeficiency, patients were transitioned from other immunoglobulin products including IVIG to 16% SCIG (Vivaglobin®) and followed for 24 months. In this study, the rate of severe bacterial infection was 0.056 per patient/year. Skin reactions occurred in 28% of the patients and three patients discontinued therapy after an infusion-site reaction [90c]. A second study assessed patients with chronic inflammatory demyelinating polyradiculoneuropathy or multifocal motor neuropathy who were switched from stable IVIG therapy (Privigen® 10%) to SCIG (Hizentra® 20% or Gammanorm® 16.5%). Using a satisfaction questionnaire, the patients reported an improvement in nausea and headache, neutropenia, treatment wearing-off fluctuations, allergy, and time off from work [91c]. In a single center, open-label study, 16% SCIG (Vivaglobin®) was compared to 20% SCIG (Hizentra®) in 32 patients with primary antibody deficiency who were clinically stable and receiving Vivaglobin® for at least 6 months. Eligible patients were given Vivaglobin® for an additional 8 weeks followed by 24 weeks of Hizentra®. The median steady state IgG levels were similar between both products. Local site reactions occurred at injection site at a higher rate with Vivaglobin® with edema and pain most commonly reported while tolerability of Hizentra® improved over time [92c]. In a study of patients receiving either SCIG or IVIG for neurological disorders, headache and nausea were less severe with SCIG compared to IVIG [93c]. Lastly, in a retrospective review of 19 cases from 8 centers treated with SCIG for inflammatory myopathies for a median of 18.8 months, treatment was relatively safe, with mild headaches, skin reactions, myalgias, and pain as the most common adverse effects [94c].

Anti-D Immunoglobulin

Major Reviews

The Society of Obstetrics and Gynecology published guidelines for the management of a pregnant trauma patient using GRADE methodology. Two III B recommendations included administration of anti-D immunoglobulin to all Rh-negative pregnant trauma patients and quantification of maternal-fetal hemorrhage using Kleihauer-Betke test to determine the need for additional doses [95R].

A Cochrane review of two trials with more than 4500 patients comparing anti-D administration to no treatment found no difference in rate of neonatal jaundice or adverse effects from treatment [96R].

Infection Risk

The risk of infection from anti-D immunoglobulin is mitigated by multiple processes: nanofiltration, screening for viruses, use of detergents, chemical degradation by pH modification, and enzymatic inactivation. The risk of prion disease, variant Creutzfeldt-Jakob disease, is minimal due to infection control processes. A review article highlights the minimal risk of side effects other than infection such as malaise, fever, hypersensitive and injection site reactions [97R].

Drug Dosage

An editorial highlights the risk of underdosing anti-D immunoglobulin in pregnant patients due to increasing rates of obesity. The authors indicate using an estimated total blood volume of 5000 mL may no longer be appropriate and place infants at risk of hemolytic disease due to underdosing [98r].

COAGULATION PROTEINS [SEDA-34, 518; SEDA-36, 493, SEDA-37, 411]

Factor I

Fibrinogen (factor I) concentrate may be either plasma-derived or a recombinant product. It is the final protein in the common coagulation cascade.

Safety of Fibrinogen Concentrate

A database review encompassed fibrinogen safety data from January 1986 to December 2013 with a total of 383 adverse drug reactions (ADRs) in 106 cases (approximately 1 per 6200 standard doses). The adverse events included hypersensitivity reactions in 20 cases, possible thromboembolic events in 28 cases, and suspected virus transmission in 21 cases. This assessment indicates that fibrinogen concentrate has few ADRs and a low thromboembolic event rate although it is noted that one of the biggest limitations in this type of data is under-reporting of ADRs [99M].

Fibrinogen Use in Postpartum Hemorrhage

A prospective, randomized, double-blind placebo-controlled trial evaluating the safety and efficacy of fibrinogen concentrate or placebo (isotonic saline) for postpartum hemorrhage management is currently ongoing and is scheduled to enroll a total of 60 females. The trial has no safety concerns to report at this time [100c].

Factor II

A wide variety of topical agents are approved as potential therapies in the maintenance of hemostasis during surgical procedures. Topical thrombin stimulates platelet aggregation and its use was specifically addressed in upper extremity surgical procedures. The product can be applied as spray, solution or a powder. Regardless of the form, the product is reported to be well tolerated and has shown to be clinically efficacious in various orthopedic procedures [101r]. Of note, topical thrombin may be either from a bovine or recombinant source.

FACTOR VIIa [SEDA-35, 592; SEDA-36, 493, SEDA-37, 412]

Observational Studies

Severe perioperative bleeding during a cardiac surgery is a major (but usually rare) complication. The use of recombinant factor VIIa (rFVIIa) for management of perioperative bleeding in HeartMate II was evaluated in 57 recipients. Among several indicators, chest tube drainage was a marker used to evaluate efficacy and 30-day incidence of thromboembolic events was used to assess safety. The authors concluded that there were no 30-day thromboembolic events to report in those patients who received rFVIIa which was considered a very positive finding [102c]. Similar conclusions were made by Matino et al. while investigating the use of rFVIIa for the treatment of acute bleeding episodes in people with hemophilia [103R].

FACTOR VIII [SEDA-35, 592; SEDA-36, 494, SEDA-37, 412]

Hemophilia A and B

Hemophilia A and B are hereditary hemorrhagic disorders characterized by the deficiency or dysfunction of coagulation protein factors VIII and IX, respectively. Current treatment relies on replacement therapy with clotting factors, either at the time of bleeding (on demand) or as part of a prophylactic schedule. One of the major complications of this therapy is the development of neutralizing antibodies (inhibitors) which commonly occurs in hemophilia type A. Treatment might improve considerably with the availability of new modified drugs; however, some reported shortcomings of currently available therapies are short half-lives requiring frequent administrations, modes of administration (subcutaneous versus IV), neutralizing antibodies formation and dosing frequency [104r,105H].

Eloctate®

Eloctate®, a recombinant factor VIII fusion protein with an extended half-life, is reported to be effective in preventing and controlling bleeding in patients with severe hemophilia A. The extended half-life reduces the number of doses required for routine prophylaxis which could improve adherence and, to date, Eloctate® has not been associated with formation of neutralizing antibodies. According to the manufacturing company, the most frequently reported adverse reactions in clinical studies were headache, join/muscle pain, rash and general discomfort which occurred in 2 patients (0.9%), and abdominal pain with lower back pain which was reported by one patient (0.4%). Eloctate® is currently indicated in adults and children with hemophilia A for on-demand and prophylactic treatment option in this patient population [106S].

FACTOR IX [SEDA-35, 592; SEDA-36, 494, SEDA-37, 412]

Factor IX Gene Therapy

A new study evaluated long-term safety and efficacy of Factor IX gene therapy in hemophilia B patients where gene therapy that is mediated by a novel adeno-associated virus serotype 8 vector has been shown to raise factor IX levels. The authors sought to evaluate if patients with severe hemophilia B can benefit from gene therapy to raise factor IX levels and decrease rates of bleeding. The effects were found to be clinically positive with a significant decrease in rates of acute bleeding episodes with no reported acute or late toxic effects. The only transiently observed effect reported was an increase in the mean alanine aminotransferase (ALT) level which occurred between week 7 and week 10 in 67% of patients (4/6). This effect was reported to resolve over the next 5 days after prednisolone treatment [107c].

PROTHROMBIN COMPLEX CONCENTRATE [SEDA-35, 518; SEDA-36, 494, SEDA-37, 412]

There are three main types of Prothrombin Complex Concentrates (PCC) that are available on the market worldwide. The first type is an activated-PCC which contains activated forms of factors II, VII, IX, and X. Activated PCCs are used for bypass therapy in hemophilia patients who have developed inhibitor antibodies. The second type is a 4-factor PCC which contains non-activated forms of factors II, VII, IX, and X. The third type is a 3-factor PCC containing non-activated forms of factors II, IX, and X (while lacking factor VII). The 3- and 4-factor non-activated PCCs are most often used for anticoagulation reversal and severe hemorrhage in clinical practice.

Cardiac Surgery

An observational study evaluated a total of 3454 cardiac surgeries performed between January 2005 and December 2013 to investigate the efficacy and safety of PPC as a first-line treatment option as a replacement to fresh frozen plasma (FFP) administration. A one-to-one score matched analysis with 225 pairs of patients was evaluated (PCC mean dose of 1500 IU vs FFP mean dose of 2 units). A clinically significant finding indicated that PCC was associated with significantly less 24-hour postoperative blood loss (836 ± 1226 mL vs. 935 ± 583 mL, $p < 0.0001$) and significantly less red blood cell (RBC) transfusions (odds ratio (OR) 0.50; 95% confidence interval [CI] 0.31–0.80). However, patients receiving PCC had an increased risk of post-operative AKI (OR 1.44, 95% CI 1.02–2.05) and renal replacement therapy (OR 3.35, 95% CI 1.13–9.90). The reported hospital mortality was unaffected [108C].

Mechanical Heart Valve and Warfarin Reversal

A safety and efficacy comparison study was conducted between FFP and PCC for the use of INR reversal in patients with a mechanical heart valve requiring interventional procedures. A total of 50 patients (25 in each arm) were randomized to receive either PCC or FFP. The authors concluded that there was no significant difference between the two groups in hemoglobin and hematocrit before and during a 48-hour period after administration of either of the two agents. With regards to safety, there were no reports of hemorrhage in either of the groups. However, the authors concluded that PCC offers a number of advantages over FFP, including lower infusion volumes (this is a better option for patients with valvular heart disease), rapid reconstitution, immediate availability and lack of blood group specificity [109c]. In a Cochrane review of 4 randomized controlled trials (RCTs) evaluating the use of PCC vs FFP for reversal therapy, both products were very similar in their safety and efficacy profiles. This meta-analysis concluded that there was no difference in mortality rates when using either of these therapies and no statistical difference was seen in any further transfusion requirements. The current systematic review of RCTs does not support the routine use of PCC over FFP [110R].

von WILLEBRAND FACTOR (VWF)/ FACTOR VIII CONCENTRATES [SEDA-35, 594; SEDA-36, 494, SEDA-37, 413]

Drug Formulations

FDA approved Vonvendi®, a von Willebrand factor (recombinant), for use in adults 18 years of age and older who have von Willebrand disease (VWD) in December of 2015. Vonvendi® is the first FDA-approved recombinant von Willebrand factor and is approved for the on-demand (as needed) treatment and control of bleeding episodes in adults diagnosed with VWD. According to the FDA, "The safety and efficacy of Vonvendi were evaluated in two clinical trials of 69 adult participants with VWD. These trials demonstrated that Vonvendi was safe and effective for the on-demand treatment and control of bleeding episodes from a variety of different sites in the body. No safety concerns were identified in the trials. The most common adverse reaction observed was generalized pruritus" [111S,112H].

ERYTHROPOIETIN AND DERIVATIVES [SEDA-35, 594; SEDA-36, 494, SEDA-37, 413]

Systematic Reviews

Epoetin alfa (EPO) and darbepoetin alfa (DPO) are erythropoiesis-stimulating agents (ESAs) that are widely and interchangeably used for the treatment of anemia in patients with advanced chronic kidney disease and end-stage renal disease. The following systematic review summarizes key safety findings of 9 randomized controlled trials with 2024 patients who required treatment with these agents for anemia. The authors found no significant difference in mortality between patients randomly assigned to EPO vs DPO [113M].

Cardiovascular

A systematic review evaluated 9 studies conducted over the last 60 years to determine the efficacy and safety of ESAs for the treatment of anemia in patients with systolic heart failure. All studies examining hematological parameters found a statistically significant increase in hemoglobin levels with active treatment versus placebo. According to the authors "a non-significant trend for decreased mortality in patients treated with darbepoetin with a similar adverse event profile compared to placebo was shown in one study; however, the largest trial to date showed no benefit in all-cause mortality or heart failure-related hospitalizations with the use of ESAs." Additionally, a statistically significant increase in the number of cerebrovascular events and thrombotic events was found [114R,115r].

Renal

According to Vlachopanos et al., "delayed graft function (DGF) due to ischemia-reperfusion injury is a major early complication of kidney transplantation (KT). Recombinant human erythropoietin (rHuEPO) has been shown to exert nephroprotective action in animal models." A meta-analysis was conducted to explore the impact of rHuEPO on DGF in kidney transplant patients.

The safety findings are consistent with what was previously reported in the literature in regards to the use of EPO. Perioperative, high-dose EPO administration does not prevent delayed graft function in deceased donor kidney transplant. Furthermore, it is associated with higher systolic blood pressure leading to safety concerns [116E].

Drug Formulations

Biosimilars are therapeutic products exhibiting comparable quality, safety and efficacy to an existing product, the patent of which has typically expired. To date, the observed post-marketing safety experience with epoetin zeta (biosimilar product) is consistent with the known profile of epoetin alfa (Hospira) [117M].

THROMBOPOIETIN AND RECEPTOR AGONISTS [SED-15, 3409; SEDA-36, 495; SEDA-37, 414]

Eltrombopag is an oral thrombopoietin receptor agonist which stimulates platelet production by differentiation of the megakaryocyte precursors and proliferation of progenitor cells. Clinical uses of the drug continue to expand to include hepatitis associated thrombocytopenia, MDS, stem cell transplant and pediatric patients. Common side effects include thromboembolic events, liver function test elevations, and potentially myelofibrosis [118r]. Romiplostim is a peptide antibody that binds to the THPO receptor to stimulate megakaryocyte colon forming cells. This is a subcutaneous injectable drug. It has similar risks for thromboembolism and myelofibrosis [119c].

Ear, Nose, and Throat

The PETIT 2 study for eltrombopag in children with chronic immune thrombocytopenia included a total of 92 patients. The highest reported adverse events in the treatment group included nasopharyngitis, rhinitis, upper respiratory tract infection and cough. Two patients withdrew from the study for elevated liver function tests [120c].

Cardiovascular

A case series of 5 patients with HIV-associated immune thrombocytopenic purpura described the use of romiplostim and eltrombopag as effective for salvage therapy. However, two patients experienced thromboembolic complications which may or may not be secondary to TBO use: a 43-year-old African American female with significant cardiac history died from myocardial infarction during treatment with eltrombopag and a 32-year-old male who underwent lumbar surgery on romiplostim suffered cardiac arrest secondary to presumed pulmonary embolism [121A]. A study evaluating

51 patients who switched from romiplostim to eltrombopag found that 9.8% of patients experienced a grade 3–4 adverse event. Two patients experienced strokes, an 83-year-old male after 5 months of treatment, and a 56-year-old female after 12 months of treatment [122c].

Hematologic

A retrospective analysis of data from 13 studies for safety of TBO's in patients over age 65 demonstrated numerical but not statistically significant increases in grade 3 or higher bleeding events and thromboembolic complications compared to placebo [123C]. A case report of a 65-year-old man with refractory immune thrombocytopenic purpura demonstrated profound rebound thrombocytopenia after receiving romiplostim 4 mcg/kg for 3 days. The platelet count fell to $9 \times 10^9/L$ and the patient experienced epistaxis. Romiplostim was reinstated at 5 mcg/kg with recovered. A second time the patient missed a scheduled dose again and platelets fell to $23 \times 10^9/L$ with reinstitution and recovery. The repeated nature of the reaction indicates the profound rebound thrombocytopenia was associated with omission of romiplostim treatment [124A].

Urinary Tract

In a retrospective review of 18 patients with thrombocytopenia who received romiplostim at therapeutic dose, before surgical procedures, 1 patient was found to have a Foley catheter clot after surgery and 4 post-operative bleed events were reported [125c].

Drug Dosage Regimens

A post-hoc analysis of patient self-administered subcutaneous romiplostim compared to healthcare practitioner administered romiplostim found a lower rate of serious adverse events in the self-administered group. Reported adverse events included headache, contusion, epistaxis, fatigue, nasopharyngitis, arthralgia, petechiae, and cough [126C].

TRANSMISSION OF INFECTIOUS AGENTS THROUGH BLOOD DONATION [SEDA-34, 521; SEDA-35, 596; SEDA-36, 495; SEDA-37, 414]

Bacteria

In a French hemovigilance study, transfusion transmitted bacterial infections (TTBI) were identified at a rate of 2.45, 24.7, and 0.39 per million components for red blood cells, platelet concentrates and fresh frozen plasma, respectively. The incidence of severe or fatal TTBI was 13.4 and 5.14 per million units of platelets. Gram-positive bacteria were isolated in 66.7% of the cases and gram negative bacteria in 33.3% of the cases [127C].

An elderly man with chronic myelogenous leukemia, previously splenectomized, was transfused 2 buffy coat platelet pools. Four hours after transfusion, the patient presented with fever, nausea, shortness of breath, and hypotension. Blood cultures were positive for staphylococci. He developed septic shock and lactic acidosis with lactate of 9.6 and died less than 48 hours after transfusion. The platelet pools were positive for the same strain of coagulase negative staphylococci epidermidis as in the patient blood and it was determined the bacteria was found in the buffy coat fractions. Prior to transfusion, the units were tested with BacT/ALEART screening and found negative. This is a false negative leading to a fatal event [128A].

Virus

Risk of Dengue fever in the Nuevo Leon State of Mexico led to seroprevalence testing between the years of 2010 and 2012 when between 2% and 6% of blood donors were antibody positive [129r].

A case report of dengue transmission to a 37-year-old female neurosurgical patient was reported from a tertiary care center in Singapore during a dengue outbreak. The donor presented with symptoms 2 days after donation and the infection was confirmed using donor and receipt viral nucleotide sequences. The patient experienced prolonged hospitalization and thrombocytopenia [130A].

A 27-year-old Japanese woman being treated for acute promyelocytic leukemia developed hepatitis E viral genotype 3 infection 7 months after transfusion with contaminated blood products. The viral nucleotide sequence of the donor product and recipient was very similar. Another recipient received a similar contaminated product but did not develop symptomatic infection. The authors hypothesized the immunosuppressing chemotherapy, including all-*trans* retinoic acid (ATRA), prevented the first patient from clearing the virus, thereby leading to development of the hepatitis infection [131A].

Hepatitis E virus was considered responsible for elevated liver function tests and episodes of fatigue in a 61-year-old male patient with transfusion-dependent beta thalassemia. The patient received regular red blood cell transfusions and consumed wild game. No blood product samples were available to confirm transfusion-associated transmission [132A].

STEM CELLS [SEDA-35, 597; SEDA-36, 496; SEDA-37, 415]

Hematopoietic stem cell transplant (HSCT) is a curative treatment for several hematological disorders. Risk factors for long-term adverse effects following allogeneic HSCT include co-morbid conditions and patient characteristics (e.g. age), pre-transplant cancer treatment, conditioning regimen, stem cell source, donor characteristics, and graft-versus-host disease (GVHD) prophylaxis [133R]. In a large study of registry data of more than 26000 patients from over 500 transplant centers between 1995 and 2007, a multivariate analysis showed an increased incidence of chronic GVHD (cGVHD) in more recent years (odds ratio: 1.19, $p < .0001$), even when adjusting for donor type, graft type, or conditioning intensity. The major causes of death in this study were relapse of disease (33%), infection (17%), organ failure (13%), and GVHD (13%) [134MC]. Neurologic complications are reported in 30–80% of allogenic HSCT recipients, and are frequently complications of cGVHD. For example, myositis is reported to occur in 7.6% of patients with cGVHD, and myasthenia gravis has also been reported. Guillain-Barré syndrome and peripheral neuropathy have also been reported to occur in HSCT at a rate of 1–2%, but it is unknown whether this is a manifestation of cGVHD [135R]. Other effects include loss of bone density, obstructive pulmonary disease, and secondary malignancy [133R].

Endocrine

Endocrine disorders associated with HSCT include metabolic syndrome, diabetes, and gonadal failure [133R]. Case reports of various thyroid disorders, including hypothyroidism or hyperthyroidism, have been reported [136c]. Cataract development has also been linked to HSCT. In a prospective study of 271 childhood leukemia survivors, the cumulative incidence of cataracts affecting quality of life 15 years after a total body irradiation conditioning regimen was 78%. This study identified high cumulative steroid doses as a risk factor for cataracts [137C].

Transplant-associated thrombotic microangiopathy (TA-TMA) is caused by endothelial damage, platelet activation due to cytokine release following HSCT [137C]. Microvascular thrombosis may lead to injury to vital organs, such as the lungs or kidney [138R]. In young adults, TA-TMA is reported at an incidence of 0–74% [138]. In one prospective study of 100 pediatric patients receiving HSCT, 32 patients (32%) were diagnosed with TA-TMA [139c]. Treatment of TA-TMA typically consists of pharmacologic agents such as rituximab or vincristine, or therapeutic plasma exchange [138R]. In addition, in analysis of 533 patients undergoing allogenic HSCT from a single institution, 19 patients (3.6%) developed autoimmune hemolytic anemia a median of 202 days after transplant, which was associated with a higher mortality rate [140C].

Hepatobiliary

Liver-related complications can affect up to 80% of patients following HSCT and are associated with a tremendous increase in mortality. In fact, total bilirubin between 4 and 7 mg/dL within 100 days of HSCT is associated with a non-relapse mortality rate of 50% [141R]. Interestingly, one retrospective study of 160 children undergoing allogenic HSCT found that heparanase (HPSE) single-nucleotide polymorphisms (SNPs) were independent risk factors for sinusoidal obstruction syndrome. The authors recommend further evaluation of this link in subsequent trials [142c].

Cardiovascular

Patients receiving HSCT are at an increased risk of atrial fibrillation with an incidence of 7–27%. Risk factors include advanced age, weight gain, elevated creatinine, diastolic dysfunction, or mediastinal radiation [143R]. A long-term cross-sectional study included 15 patients that received autograft transplants and three that received allogeneic grafts at a median age of 9.8 years and followed these patients for 18.2 years. All patients received anthracyclines in their primary treatment. At the end of the study period, patients in this analysis had normal cardiac function, but when compared to healthy controls, they had reduced systolic longitudinal and diastolic left ventricular function, as well as reduced right ventricular function [144c].

Filtration

It has been suggested that clumped cellular debris, sometimes visible in stem cell products, may be responsible for transient respiratory symptoms that occur during infusion. One study demonstrated that filtration can be performed without decreasing the number of viable stem cells within the product [145c].

References

[1] Perner A, Junttila E, Haney M, et al. Scandinavian clinical practice guidelines on choice of fluid resuscitation of critically ill patients with acute circulatory failure. Acta Anaesthesiol Scand. 2015;59:274–85 [M].

[2] Caironi P, Langer T, Gattinoni L. Albumin in critically ill patients: the ideal colloid? Curr Opin Crit Care. 2015;21:302–8 [r].

[3] Das U. Albumin infusion for the critically ill—is it beneficial and if so why and how? Crit Care. 2015;19:156 [r].

[4] Ginsberg MD, Hill MD. Symptomatic intracranial hemorrhage in the ALIAS multicenter trial: relationship to endovascular thrombolytic therapy. Int J Stroke. 2015;10(4):494–500 [C].

[5] Pathirana S, Wong G, Williams P, et al. The effects of hemodilution with albumin on coagulation in vitro as assessed by rotation thromboelastometry. Anaesth Intensive Care. 2015;43(2):187–92 [C].

[6] Opperer M, Poeran J, Rasul R, et al. Use of perioperative hydroxyethyl starch 6% and albumin 5% in elective joint arthroplasty and association with adverse outcomes: retrospective population based analysis. BMJ. 2015;350:h1567 [MC].

[7] Garcia-Martinez R, Noiret L, Sen S, et al. Albumin infusion improves renal blood flow autoregulation in patients with acute decompensation of cirrhosis and acute kidney injury. Liver Int. 2015;35(2):335–43 [c].

[8] Thevenot T, Bureau C, Oberti F, et al. Effect of albumin in cirrhotic patients with infection other that spontaneous bacterial peritonitis, a randomized trial. J Hepatol. 2015;62:822–30 [c].

[9] Ertmer C, Kampmeier TG, Wolters TVH, et al. Impact of human albumin infusion on organ function in orthotopic liver transplantation—a retrospective matched-pair analysis. Clin Transplant. 2015;29:67–75 [c].

[10] Jonhson KB, Mueller JL, Simon TG, et al. Reduced albumin dosing during large-volume paracentesis is not associated with adverse clinical outcomes. Dig Dis Sci. 2015;60:2190–5 [C].

[11] Tatlow D, Poothencheri S, Bhangal R, et al. Novel method for rapid reversal of drug toxicity: a case report. Clin Exp Pharmacol Physiol. 2015;42(4):389–93 [A].

[12] Muller MM, Geisen C, Zacharowski K, et al. Transfusion of packed red cells: indications, triggers and adverse events. Dtsch Arztebl Int. 2015;112:507–18 [r].

[13] Harvey AR, Basavaraju SV, Chung K, et al. Transfusion-related adverse reactions reported to the National Healthcare Safety Network Hemovigilance Module, United States, 2010 to 2012. Transfusion. 2015;55:709–18 [MC].

[14] Rogers MAM, Rohde JM, Blumberg N. Haemovigilance of reactions associated with red blood cell transfusion: comparison across 17 countries. Vox Sang. 2016;110(3):266–77 [MC].

[15] Clifford L, Jia Q, Subramanian A, et al. Characterizing the epidemiology of postoperative transfusion-related acute lung injury. Anesthesiology. 2015;122:12–20 [C].

[16] Mulder HD, Augustijn QJJ, van Woensel JB, et al. Incidence, risk factors, and outcome of transfusion-related acute lung injury in critically ill children: a retrospective study. J Crit Care. 2015;30(1):55–9 [C].

[17] Likosky DS, Paone G, Zhang M, et al. Red blood cell transfusions impact pneumonia rates after coronary artery bypass grafting. Ann Thorac Surg. 2015;100:794–801 [MC].

[18] Mariscalco G, Biancari F, Juvonen T, et al. Red blood cell transfusion is a determinant of neurological complications after cardiac surgery. Interact Cardiovasc Thorac Surg. 2015;20(2):166–71 [MC].

[19] Raza S, Baig MA, Chang C, et al. A prospective study on red blood cell transfusion related hyperkalemia in critically ill patients. J Clin Med Res. 2015;7(6):417–21 [C].

[20] Clifford L, Jia Q, Yadav H, et al. Characterizing the epidemiology of perioperative transfusion-associated circulatory overload. Anesthesiology. 2015;122(1):21–8 [C].

[21] Vidler JB, Gardner K, Amenyah K, et al. Delayed haemolytic transfusion reaction in adults with sickle cell disease: a 5-year experience. Br J Haematol. 2015;169(5):746–53 [c].

[22] L'Acqua C, Bandyopadhyay S, Francis RO, et al. Red blood cell transfusion is associated with increased hemolysis and an acute phase response in a subset of critically ill children. Am J Hematol. 2015;90(10):915–20 [c].

[23] Kopolovic I, Ostro J, Tsubota H, et al. A systematic review of transfusion-associated graft-versus-host disease. Blood. 2015;126(3):406–14 [M].

[24] Brunskill SJ, Millette SL, Shokoohi A, et al. Red blood cell transfusion for people undergoing hip fracture surgery. Cochrane Database Syst Rev. 2015;4:CD009699. http://dx.doi.org/10.1002/14651858.CD009699.pub2 [M].

[25] Fabricius R, Svenningsen P, Hillingsø J, et al. Effect of transfusion strategy in acute non-variceal upper gastrointestinal bleeding: a nationwide study of 5861 hospital admissions in Denmark. World J Surg. 2016;40(5):1129–36 [MC].

[26] Ng MSY, Ng ASY, Chan J, et al. Effects of packed red blood cell storage duration on post-transfusion clinical outcomes:

a meta-analysis and systematic review. Intensive Care Med. 2015;41:2087–97 [M].

[27] Yamal J, Benoit JS, Doshi P, et al. Association of transfusion red blood cell storage age and blood oxygenation, long-term neurologic outcome, and mortality in traumatic brain injury. J Trauma Acute Care Surg. 2015;79:843–9 [c].

[28] Kato H, Nakayama T, Uruma M, et al. A retrospective observational study to assess adverse transfusion reactions in patients with and without prior transfusion history. Vox Sang. 2015;108:243–50 [MC].

[29] Estcourt LJ, Stanworth S, Doree C, et al. Granulocyte transfusions for preventing infections in people with neutropenia or neutrophil dysfunction. Cochrane Database Syst Rev. 2015;6: CD005341 [M].

[30] Marfin AA, Price TH. Granulocyte transfusion therapy. J Intensive Care Med. 2015;30(2):79–88 [R].

[31] Kadri SS, Remy KE, Strich JR, et al. Role of granulocyte transfusions in invasive fusariosis: systematic review and single-center experience. Transfusion. 2015;55:2076–85 [c].

[32] Ambruso DR. Hydroxyethyl starch and granulocyte transfusions: considerations of utility and toxicity profile for patients and donors. Transfusion. 2015;55:911–8 [r].

[33] Kaufman RM, Djulbegovic B, Gernsheimer T, et al. Platelet transfusion: a clinical practice guideline from the AABB. Ann Intern Med. 2015;162:205–13 [R].

[34] Harvey AR, Basavaraju SV, Chung K, et al. Transfusion-related adverse reactions reported to the National Healthcare Safety Network Hemovigilance Module, United States, 2010 to 2012. Transfusion. 2015;55:709–18 [MC].

[35] Kremke M, Hansen MK, Christensen S, et al. The association between platelet transfusion and adverse outcomes after coronary artery bypass surgery. Eur J Cardiothorac Surg. 2015;48(5):e102–9 [MC].

[36] Crighton GL, Estcourt LJ, Wood EM, et al. A therapeutic-only versus prophylactic platelet transfusion strategy for preventing bleeding in patients with haematological disorders after myelosuppressive chemotherapy or stem cell transplantation. Cochrane Database Syst Rev. 2014;9:CD010981. http://dx.doi.org/10.1002/14651858.CD010981.pub2 [M].

[37] Clifford L, Jia Q, Yadav H, et al. Characterizing the epidemiology of perioperative transfusion-associated circulatory overload. Anesthesiology. 2015;122(1):21–8 [C].

[38] Kaufman RM, Assmann SF, Triulzi DJ, et al. Transfusion-related adverse events in the platelet dose study. Transfusion. 2015;55:144–53 [MC].

[39] Knutson F, Osselaer J, Pierelli L, et al. A prospective, active haemovigilance study with combined cohort analysis of 19,175 transfusions of platelet components prepared with amotosalen-UVA photochemical treatment. Vox Sang. 2015;109:343–52 [MC].

[40] Garraud O, Cognasse F, Tissot JD, et al. Improving platelet transfusion safety: biomedical and technical considerations. Blood Transfus. 2016;14(2):109–22 [R].

[41] Mackenzie CF, Pitman AN, Hodgson RE, et al. Are hemoglobin-based oxygen carriers being withheld because of regulatory requirement for equivalence to packed red blood cells? Am J Ther. 2015;22:e115–21 [R].

[42] Njoku M, St Peter D, Mackenzie CF. Haemoglobin-based oxygen carriers: indications and future applications. Br J Hosp Med. 2015;76(2):78–83 [R].

[43] Teschler H. Long-term experience in the treatment of alpha-1 antitrypsin deficiency: 25 years of augmentation therapy. Eur Respir Rev. 2015;24:46–51 [R].

[44] Zuo L, Pannel BK, Zhou T, et al. Historical role of alpha-1 antitrypsin in respiratory and hepatic complications. Gene. 2016;16:6–8 [M].

[45] Zuraw BL, Cicardi M, Longhurst HJ, et al. Phase II study results of a replacement therapy for hereditary angioedema with

subcutaneous C1-inhibitor concentrate. Allergy. 2015;70(10):1319–28 [c].

[46] Busse P, Bygum A, Edelman J, et al. Safety of C1-esterase inhibitor in acute and prophylactic therapy of hereditary angioedema: findings from the ongoing international Berinert patient registry. J Allergy Clin Immunol Pract. 2015;3(2):213–9 [C].

[47] Li HH, Moldovan D, Bernstein J, et al. Recombinant human-C1 inhibitor is effective and safe for repeat hereditary angioedema attacks. J Allergy Clin Immunol Pract. 2015;3(3):417–23 [c].

[48] Rapid response report. C1 Esterase inhibitors for prophylaxis against hereditary angioedema attacks: a review of the clinical effectiveness, cost-effectiveness and guidelines. Ottawa (ON): Canadian Agency for Drugs and Technologies in Health; 2015. p. 1–26 [R].

[49] Riedl M. Recombinant human C1 esterase inhibitor in the management of hereditary angioedema. Clin Drug Investig. 2015;35:407–17 [R].

[50] Moldovan D, Bernstein JA, Cicardi M. Recombinant replacement therapy for hereditary angioedema due to C1 inhibitor deficiency. Immunotherapy. 2015;7(7):739–52 [R].

[51] Lumry W, Soteres D, Gower R, et al. Safety and efficacy of C1 esterase inhibitor for acute attacks in children with hereditary angioedema. Pediatr Allergy Immunol. 2015;26(7):674–80 [c].

[52] Nascimento B, Goodnough T, Levy JH. Cryoprecipitate therapy. Br J Anaesth. 2014;113(6):922–34 [R].

[53] Oakley FG, Woods M, Arnold S, et al. Transfusion reactions in pediatric compared with adult patients: a look at rate, reaction type, and associated products. Transfusion. 2015;55(3):563–70 [R].

[54] Harvey AR, Basavaraju SV, Chung KW, et al. Transfusion-related adverse reactions reported to the National Healthcare Safety Network Hemovigilance Module, United States, 2010 to 2012. Transfusion. 2015;55(4):709–18 [R].

[55] Desborough M, Sandu R, Brunskill S, et al. Fresh frozen plasma for cardiovascular surgery. Cochrane Database Syst Rev. 2015;7: CD007614. http://dx.doi.org/10.1002/14651858.CD007614.pub2 [R].

[56] Murphy M, Allard S, Blackwell D, et al. Blood transfusion: summary of NICE guidance. BMJ. 2015;351:h5832 [S].

[57] Rasmussen AM, Jakobsen R, Strøm T, et al. More complications in patient with septic shock treated with dextran compared to crystalloids. Dan Med J. 2015;62(2):A5018 [c].

[58] Opperer M, Poeran J, Rasul R, et al. Use of perioperative hydroxyethyl starch 6% and albumin 5% in elective joint arthroplasty and association with adverse outcomes: a retrospective population based analysis. BMJ. 2015;30:h1567 [C].

[59] Hand WR, Whiteley JR, Epperson TI, et al. Hydroxyethyl starch and acute kidney injury in orthotopic liver transplantation: a single-center retrospective review. Anesth Analg. 2015;120:619–26 [C].

[60] Blasco V, Colavolpe JC, Antonini F, et al. Long-term outcome in kidney recipients from donors treated with hydroethylstarch 130/0.4 and hydroxyethylstartch 200/0/6. Br J Anaesth. 2015;115(5):798 [r].

[61] Muller RB, Haase N, Lange T, et al. Acute kidney injury with hydroxyethyl starch 130/0.42 in severe sepsis. Acta Anaesthesiol Scand. 2015;59(3):329–36 [C].

[62] Pinholt Kancir AS, Johansen JK, Ekeloef NP, et al. The effect of 6% hydroxyethyl starch 130/0.4 on renal function, arterial blood pressure and vasoactive hormones during radical prostatectomy: a randomized controlled trial. Anesth Analg. 2015;120:608–18 [c].

[63] Li L, Li Y, Xu X, et al. Safety evaluation on low-molecular-weight hydroxyethyl starch for volume expansion therapy in pediatric patients: a meta-analysis of randomized controlled trial. Crit Care. 2015;19:79 [M].

[64] Van der Linden P, Dumoulin M, Van Lerberghe C, et al. Efficacy and safety of 6% hydroxyethyl starch 130/0.4 for perioperative

volume replacement in children undergoing cardiac surgery: a propensity-matched analysis. Crit Care. 2015;19:87 [C].

[65] Ozturk T, Onur E, Cerrahoglu M, et al. Immune and inflammatory role of hydroxyethyl starch 130/0.4 and fluid gelatin in patients undergoing coronary surgery. Cytokine. 2015;74:69–75 [c].

[66] He B, Xu B, Xu X, et al. Hydroxyethyl starch versus other fluids for non-septic patients in the intensive care unit: a meta-analysis of randomized controlled trials. Crit Care. 2015;19:92 [M].

[67] Agarwal NS, Spalding C, Nassef M. Life-threatening intraoperative anaphylaxis to gelatin in Floseal during pediatric spinal surgery. J Allergy Clin Immunol Pract. 2015;3(1):110–1 [A].

[68] Ji J, Barrett EJ. Suspected intraoperative anaphylaxis to gelatin absorbable hemostatic sponge. Anesth Prog. 2015;62:22–4 [A].

[69] Wang J, McQuilten ZK, Wood EM, et al. Intravenous immunoglobulin in critically ill adults: when and what is the evidence? J Crit Care. 2015;30:652e9–652e16 [R].

[70] Clark SL, Rabinstein AA. Safety of intravenous immunoglobulin and plasma exchange in critically ill patients. Neurol Res. 2015;37(7):593–8 [c].

[71] Lozeron P, Theaudin M, Denier C, et al. Safety of IVIg in the elderly treated for a dysimmune neuromuscular disease. Muscle Nerve. 2015; [Epub ahead of print] [C].

[72] Jain RS, Agrawal R, Kumar S, et al. Anaphylaxis with intravenous immunoglobulin: a time for introspection. Am J Emerg Med. 2015;33(9):1332.e1–2 [r].

[73] Reddy DR, Guru PK, Blessing MM, et al. Transfusion-related acute lung injury after IVIG for myasthenic crisis. Neurocrit Care. 2015;23(2):259–61 [A].

[74] Attard L, Bonvicini F, Gelsomino F, et al. Paradoxical response to intravenous immunoglobulin in a case of Parvovirus B19-associated chronic fatigue syndrome. J Clin Virol. 2015;62:54–7 [A].

[75] Kissel M, Phoon CK, Kahn PJ. Hypertension during intravenous immune globulin infusion for Kawasaki's disease: an underreported phenomenon? Clin Pediatr (Phila). 2015;54(5):491–3 [A].

[76] Ammann EM, Jones MP, Link BK, et al. Intravenous immune globulin and thromboembolic adverse events in patients with hematologic malignancy. Blood. 2016;127(2):200–7 [MC].

[77] Flannery MT, Humphrey D. Deep venous thrombosis with pulmonary embolism related to IVIG treatment: a case report and literature review. Case Rep Med. 2015;2015:971321 [Epub 2015 May 19] [A].

[78] Yu CF, Hou JF, Shen LZ, et al. Acute pulmonary embolism caused by highly aggregated intravenous immunoglobulin. Vox Sang. 2016;110(1):27–35 [c].

[79] Dorwart E, McDonald N, Maeda K, et al. IVIG and graft coronary artery disease: a potentially deadly combination in pediatric heart transplant recipients. Pediatr Transplant. 2015;19:130–1 [r].

[80] Tufekci S, Coban A, Bor M, et al. Cardiac rhythm abnormalities during intravenous immunoglobulin G (IVIG) infusion in two newborn infants: coincidence or association? Clin Case Rep. 2015;3(9):731–4 [A].

[81] Thornby KA, Henneman A, Brown DA. Evidence-based strategies to reduce intravenous immunoglobulin-induced headaches. Ann Pharmacother. 2015;49(6):715–26 [R].

[82] Luban NL, Wong ED, Lobo RH, et al. Intravenous immunoglobulin-related hemolysis in patients treated for Kawasaki disease. Transfusion. 2015;55:S90–4 [c].

[83] Christensen RD, Ilstrup SJ, Baer VL, et al. Increased hemolysis after administering intravenous immunoglobulin to a neonate with erythroblastosis fetalis due to Rh hemolytic disease. Transfusion. 2015;55:1365–6 [r].

[84] Berg R, Shebl A, Kimber MC, et al. Hemolytic events associated with intravenous immune globulin therapy: a qualitative analysis of 263 cases reported to four manufacturers between 2003 and 2012. Transfusion. 2015;55:S36–46 [C].

[85] Padmore R. Possible mechanisms for intravenous immunoglobulin-associated hemolysis: clues obtained from review of clinical case reports. Transfusion. 2015;55:S59–64 [R].

[86] Scott DE, Epstein JS. Hemolytic adverse events with immune globulin products: product factors and patient risks. Transfusion. 2015;55:S2–5 [r].

[87] Berg R, Jacob D, Fuellenhals E. Hemolytic events after the administration of lyophilized versus liquid immune globulin: an analysis of a single manufacturer's safety database. Transfusion. 2015;55:1847–54 [C].

[88] Buehler AM, Flato UP, Ferri CP, et al. Is there evidence for recommending specific intravenous immunoglobulin formulations? A systematic review of head-to-head randomized controlled trials. Eur J Pharmacol. 2015;747:96–104 [M].

[89] Rappold LC, Denk K, Enk AH, et al. Comparison of high-dose intravenous immunoglobulin (IVIG) in a 5% and a 10% solution does not reveal a significantly different spectrum of side-effects. J Eur Acad Dermatol Venereol. 2015; [Epub ahead of print] [r].

[90] Vultaggio A, Azzari C, Milito C, et al. Subcutaneous immunoglobulin replacement therapy in patients with primary immunodeficiency in routine clinical practice: the VISPO prospective multicenter study. Clin Drug Investig. 2015;35(3):179–85 [c].

[91] Markvardsen LH, Ingelise C, Andersen H, et al. Heacache and nausea after treatment with high-dose subcutaneous versus intravenous immunoglobulin. Basic Clin Pharmacol Toxicol. 2015;117(6):409–12 [c].

[92] Niebur HB, Duff CM, Shear GF, et al. Efficacy and tolerability of 16% subcutaneous immunoglobulin compared with 20% subcutaneous immunoglobulin in primary antibody deficiency. Clin Exp Immunol. 2015;181:441–50 [c].

[93] Hadden RDM, Marreno F. Switch from intravenous to subcutaneous immunoglobulin in CIDP and MMN: improved tolerability and patient satisfaction. Ther Adv Neurol Disord. 2015;8(1):14–9 [c].

[94] Cherin P, Belizna C, Cartry O, et al. Long-term subcutaneous immunoglobulin use in inflammatory myopathies: a retrospective review of 19 cases. Autoimmun Rev. 2016;15(3):281–6 [c].

[95] Jain V, Chari R, Maslovitz S, et al. Guidelines for the management of a pregnant trauma patient. J Obstet Gynaecol Can. 2015;37(6):553–71 [R].

[96] McBain RD, Crowther CA, Middleton P. Anti-D administration in pregnancy for preventing Rhesus alloimmunisation. Cochrane Database Syst Rev. 2015;3:9 [R].

[97] Aitken SL, Tichy EM. RhoD immune globulin products for prevention of alloimmunization during pregnancy. Am J Health Syst Pharm. 2015;72:267–76 [R].

[98] Pham HP, Margues MB, Williams LA. Rhesus immune globulin dosing in the obesity epidemic era. Arch Pathol Lab Med. 2015;139:1084 [r].

[99] Solomon C, Groner A, Ye J, et al. Safety of fibrinogen concentrate: analysis of more than 27 years of pharmacovigilance data. Thromb Haemost. 2015;113(4):759–71 [M].

[100] Aawar N, Alikhan R, Bruynseels D, et al. Fibrinogen concentrate versus placebo for treatment of postpartum haemorrhage: study protocol for a randomized controlled trial. Trials. 2015;16(169):1–11 [c].

[101] Wasilko S, Quinlan N, Shafritz A. Topical hemostatic agents and their role in upper extremity surgery. J Hand Surg Am. 2015;40(3):602–4 [r].

[102] Karimi A, Daigle SS, Smith WB, et al. Efficacy and safety of recombinant factor VII as rescue for severe perioperative bleeding in heartmate II recipients. J Card Surg. 2015;30(6):500–55 [c].

[103] Matino D, Makris M, Dwan K, et al. Recombinant factor VIIa concentrate versus plasma-derived concentrates for treating acute bleeding episodes in people with haemophilia and inhibitors. Cochrane Database Syst Rev. 2015;12:CD004449. http://dx.doi.org/10.1002/14651858.CD004449.pub4 [R].

[104] Peyvandi F, Garagiola I, Young G. The past and future of haemophilia: diagnosis, treatments and its complications. Lancet. 2016;388:187–97 [r].

[105] Carcao M, Re W, Ewenstein B. The role of previously untreated patient studies in understanding the development of FVIII inhibitors. Haemophilia. 2016;22(1):22–31 [H].

[106] Eloctate for hemophilia A. Med Lett Drugs Ther. 2015;57(1479):143–4 [S].

[107] Nathwani AC, Reiss UM, Tuddenham EG, et al. Long term safety and efficacy of factor IX gene therapy in hemophilia B. N Engl J Med. 2014;371(21):1994–2004 [c].

[108] Cappabianca G, Mariscalco G, Biancari F. Safety and efficacy of prothrombin complex concentrate as first-line treatment in bleeding after cardiac surgery. Crit Care. 2016;20(1):5 [C].

[109] Farsad BF, Golpira R, Najafi H, et al. Comparison between PCC and FFP for the urgent reversal of warfarin in patients with mechanical heart valve in a tertiary care cardiac center. Iran J Pharm Res. 2015;14(3):877–85 [c].

[110] Johansen M, Wikkelso A, Lunde J, et al. Prothrombin complex concentrate for reversal of vitamin K antagonist treatment in bleeding and non-bleeding patients. Cochrane Database Syst Rev. 2015;7:CD010555. http://dx.doi.org/10.1002/14651858.CD010555.pub2 [R].

[111] FDA News Release. FDA approves first recombinant von Willebrand factor to treat bleeding episodes; 2015. [S].

[112] Zheng XL. ADAMTS13 and von Willebrand factor in thrombotic thrombocytopenic purpura. Annu Rev Med. 2015;66:211–25 [H].

[113] Wilhelm-Lee ER, Winkelmayer WC. Mortality risk of darbepoetin alfa versus epoetin alfa in patients with CKD: systematic review and meta-analysis. Am J Kidney Dis. 2015;66(1):69–74 [M].

[114] Lindguist DE, Cruz JL, Brown JN. Use of erythropoiesis-stimulating agents in the treatment of anemia in patients with systolic heart failure. J Cardiovasc Pharm Ther. 2015;20(1):59–65 [R].

[115] Mastromarino V, Musumeci MB, Conti E, et al. Erythropoietin in cardiac disease: effective or harmful? J Cardiovasc Med. 2014;14(12):870–8 [r].

[116] Vlachopanos G, Kassimatis TI, Agrafiotis A. Perioperative administration of high-dose recombinant human erythropoietin for delayed graft function prevention in kidney transplantation: a meta-analysis. Transpl Int. 2015;28(3):330–40 [E].

[117] Mauricette M, Losem C. Biosimilar epoetin zeta in oncology and haematology: development and experience following 6 years of use. Acta Haematol. 2016;135:44–52 [M].

[118] Merli P, Strocchio L, Vinti L, et al. Eltrombopag for the treatment of thrombocytopenia-associated disorders. Expert Opin Pharmacother. 2015;16(14):2243–56 [r].

[119] Brierley CK, Steensma DP. Thrombopoiesis-stimulating agents and the myelodysplastic syndromes. Br J Haematol. 2015;169:309–23 [r].

[120] Grainger JD, Locatelli F, Chotsampancharoen T, et al. Eltrombopag for children with chronic immune thrombocytopenia (PETIT2): a randomized, multicenter, placebo-controlled trial. Lancet. 2015;386:1649–58 [c].

[121] Kowalczk M, Rubinstein PG, Aboluafia DM. Initial experience with the use of thrombopoetin receptor agonists in patients with refractory HIV-associated immune thrombocytopenic purpura: a case series. J Int Assoc Provid AIDS Care. 2015;14(3):211–6 [A].

[122] Gonzales-Porras JR, Mingot-Castellano ME, Andrade MM, et al. Use of eltrombopag after romiplostim in primary immune thrombocytopenia. Br J Haematol. 2015;169:111–6 [c].

[123] Michel M, Wasser J, Godeau B, et al. Efficacy and safety of the thrombopoietin receptor agonist romiplostim in patients aged >65 with immune thrombocytopenia. Ann Hematol. 2015;94:1973–80 [C].

[124] Choe MJ, Packer CD. Severe romiplostim-induced rebound thrombocytopenia after splenectomy for refractory ITP. Ann Pharmacother. 2015;49(1):140–4 [A].

[125] Marshall AL, Goodarszi K, Kuter DJ. Romiplostim in the management of the thrombocytopenic surgical patient. Transfusion. 2015;55:2505–10 [c].

[126] Selleslag D, Bird R, Altomare I, et al. Impact of self-administration of romiplostim by patient with chronic immune thrombocytopenia compare with administration by healthcare provided. Eur J Haematol. 2015;94(2):169–76 [C].

[127] Lafeuillade B, Eb F, Ounnoughene N, et al. Residual risk and retrospective analysis of transfusion-transmitted bacterial infection reported by the French national hemovigilance network from 2000 to 2008. Transfusion. 2015;55:636–46 [C].

[128] Kou Y, Pagotto F, Hannach B, et al. Fatal false-negative transfusion infection involving a buffy coat platelet pool contaminated with biofilm-positive Staphylococcus epidermidis: a case report. Transfusion. 2015;55:2384–9 [A].

[129] Arellanos-Soto D, Cruz VBdl, Mendoza-Tavera N, et al. Constant risk of dengue virus infection by blood transfusion in an endemic area in Mexico. Transfus Med. 2015;25:122–4 [r].

[130] Oh HB, Muthu V, Daruwall ZJ, et al. Bitten by a bug or a bag? Transfusion-transmitted dengue: a rare complication in the bleeding surgical patient. Transfusion. 2015;55:1655–61 [A].

[131] Fuse K, Matsuyama Y, Moriyama M, et al. Late onset post-transfusion hepatitis E developing during chemotherapy for acute promyelocytic leukemia. Intern Med. 2015;54:657–66 [A].

[132] Sayani F, Goldberg D, Slaven L, et al. Hepatitis E infection in a patient with transfusion-dependent β thalassemia. Am J Hematol. 2015;90(3):E50–1 [A].

[133] Mosesso K. Adverse late and long-term treatment effects in adult allogeneic hematopoietic stem cell transplant survivors. Am J Nurs. 2015;115(11):22–34 [R].

[134] Arai S, Arora M, Wang T, et al. Increasing incidence of chronic graft-versus-host disease in allogeneic transplantation: a report from the Center for International Blood and Marrow Transplant Research. Biol Blood Marrow Transplant. 2015;21:266–74 [MC].

[135] Ruzhansky KM, Brannagan TH. Neuromuscular complications of hematopoietic stem cell transplantation. Muscle Nerve. 2015;52:480–7 [R].

[136] Sag E, Ginc N, Alikasifoglu A, et al. Hyperthyroidism after allogeneic hematopoietic stem cell transplantation: a report of four cases. J Clin Res Pediatr Endocrinol. 2015;7(4):349–54 [c].

[137] Horwitz M, Auquier P, Barlogis V, et al. Incidence and risk factors for cataract after haematopoietic stem cell transplantation for childhood leukaemia: an LEA study. Br J Haematol. 2015;168(4):518–25 [C].

[138] Kim SS, Patel M, Yum K, et al. Hematopoietic stem cell transplant-associated thrombotic microangiopathy: review of pharmacologic treatment options. Transfusion. 2015;55:452–8 [R].

[139] Dandoy CE, Davies SM, Hirsch R, et al. Abnormal echocardiography 7 days after stem cell transplantation may be an early indicator of thrombotic microangiopathy. Biol Blood Marrow Transplant. 2015;21(1):113–8 [c].

[140] Wang M, Wang W, Abeywardane A, et al. Autoimmune hemolytic anemia after allogeneic hematopoietic stem cell transplantation: analysis of 533 adult patients who underwent transplantation at King's College Hospital. Biol Blood Marrow Transplant. 2015;21(1):60–6 [C].

[141] Norvell JP. Liver disease after hematopoietic cell transplantation in adults. Transplant Rev (Orlando). 2015;29(1):8–15 [R].

[142] Seifert C, Wittig S, Arndt C, et al. Heparanase polymorphisms: influence on incidence of hepatic sinusoidal obstruction syndrome in children undergoing allogeneic hematopoietic stem cell transplantation. J Cancer Res Clin Oncol. 2015;141:877–85 [c].

[143] Mathur P, Paydak H, Thanendrarajan S, et al. Atrial fibrillation in hematologic malignancies, especially after autologous hematopoietic stem cell transplantation: review of risk factors, current management, and future directions. Clin Lymphoma Myeloma Leuk. 2016;16(2):70–5 [R].

[144] Genberg M, Öberg A, Andrén B, et al. Cardiac function after hematopoietic cell transplantation: an echocardiographic cross-sectional study in young adults treated in childhood. Pediatr Blood Cancer. 2015;62:143–7 [c].

[145] Paulson K, Gilpin SG, Shpiruk TA, et al. Routine filtration of hematopoietic stem cell products: the time has arrived. Transfusion. 2015;55:1980–4 [c].

32

Vitamins, Amino Acids, and Drugs and Formulations Used in Nutrition

Deepa Patel*, Christopher S. Holaway*, Sonia Thomas*, Harish Parihar*, Zhiqian Wu†, Skye Bickett‡, Vicky V. Mody†,1

*Department of Pharmacy Practice, PCOM School of Pharmacy, Suwanee, GA, USA
†Department of Pharmaceutical Sciences, PCOM School of Pharmacy, Suwanee, GA, USA
‡Medical Librarian. Assistant Director of Library Services, PCOM, Suwanee, GA, USA
1Corresponding author: vickymo@pcom.edu

VITAMIN A (CAROTENOIDS) [SED-15, 3642; SEDA-32, 607; SEDA-33, 691; SEDA-34, 531; SEDA-35, 607, SEDA-36, 503]

Acute Coronary Syndrome

Case Report

A case of acute coronary syndrome manifesting as an adverse effect of all-*trans* retinoic acid in a lady with acute promyelocytic leukemia who had no other risk factors for cardiovascular disease [1A]. Despite this case, these rare instances of all-*trans* retinoic acid associated acute myocardial ischemia recorded in the literature [2C,3R,4M]. A 42-year-old female presented with a 10-day history of menorrhagia, multiple bruises, and fatigue. She had multiple ecchymotic patches, petechiae, and bilateral retinal hemorrhages [1A]. Her hemoglobin was 10.4 g/dL, WBC count was 5900/mm³, and platelet count was 31 000/mm³. Peripheral smear revealed numerous promyelocytes, some with Auer rods. Serum fibrinogen level was 247 mg/dL (range: 180–350 mg/dL), and prothrombin time (international normalized ratio) (PT INR) was prolonged; there was no clot formation for >120 seconds. Activated partial thromboplastin time (aPTT) was prolonged (>50 seconds). Diagnosis of APL was made, intermediate risk with variant form of PML-RARα, and disseminated intravascular coagulation (DIC). Treatment protocol with ATRA 45 mg/m² body and

arsenic trioxide (ATO) 0.15 mg/kg/day as was initiated. Here coagulation profile returned to normal after 9 days of therapy, with no evidence of APL differentiation syndrome (APL-DS). On 10th day after commencement of treatment with ATRA, she had sudden onset of retrosternal pain and dyspnea with high pulse rate (100 beats per minute). The case was assigned to the adverse reaction to ATRA based on the Naranjo Adverse Drug Reaction (ADR) Probability Scale. Induction therapy was continued with single-agent ATO and the patient was further not rechallenged with ATRA to avoid any life-threatening complications.

Atrioventricular Block

Case Report

A case of complete atrioventricular block with ventricular asystole and recurrent atrioventricular blocks due to all-*trans* retinoic acid (ATRA) was reported by Shinh and Wu [5A]. The authors report the case of a 57-year-old man with acute promyelocytic leukemia on induction therapy with ATRA. Two weeks following ATRA the patient developed seizures with altered consciousness followed by complete atrioventricular block (CAVB) next day. Patient was resuscitated but suffered recurrent CAVB even after ATRA discontinuation. ATRA treatment was then continued with reduced dosage, leading to a high-degree atrioventricular block. ATRA therapy was the completely discontinued and the patient completely recovered without any recurrent episode of cardiovascular event. The authors suggested an infra-Hisian block with possible ATRA dose–response relationship based on the ECG changes.

Genital Vasculitis

Case Report

Acute promyelocytic leukaemia (APL) accounts for 10% of acute myeloid leukaemia (AML) cases and is one of the curable haematological malignancies managed by all-trans-retinoic-acid (ATRA). Authors have observed over 3 cases of genital vasculitis of 124 cases they have managed in 10 years (2.4%) [6A]. A 50-year-old man, farmer by occupation, with a diagnosis of acute promyelocytic leukaemia (APL) received all-trans-retinoic-acid therapy [ATRA ($45 \, mg/m^2$) and ATO (0.15 mg/kg)]. On the eighth day of therapy he developed painless, punched out scrotal ulcers. In another case a 17-year-old girl was treated with ATRA for the management of APL. On the ninth day girl developed painful redness and swelling of both labia majora. A diagnosis of vasculitic lesions secondary to ATRA was established in both cases. In both cases, prednisolone (1 mg/kg × 14 days)/amoxicillin (1 g/dL × 7 days) was used along with ATRA with which the lesions started healing.

Hypercalcemia

Case Report

A case report of a 4-year-old boy was presented to the ER with a 2-week history of pyrexia, weight loss, and right hip pain was reported by Chen et al. [7A]. The patient was diagnosed with high-risk stage IV neuroblastoma. 13-cis-retinoic acid was commenced at $160 \, mg/m^2/day$ with a view to immunotherapy. However, after 5 days the patient showed signs of muscle weakness and dry facial skin. Moreover, his calcium level was 3.49 mmol/L (grade 4 hypercalcemia) with normal creatinine, vitamin D levels were within normal range (25-OH-D 25 nmol/L) and PTH was appropriately suppressed at <1 pmol/L (normal range, 1.6–7.5). 13-cis-RA was discontinued. The hypercalcemia was managed with intravenous pamidronate 1 mg/kg as furoseminde was found to be ineffective after 48 hours. It was stated that while using a high dose of 13-cis-retinoic acid therapy in children with high-risk neuroblastoma, clinicians need to be aware of the associated risk of hypercalcemia [7A].

Hypersensitivity Reactions

Case Report

First case of delayed hypersensitivity induced by lipoic acid was reported by Rizzi et al. [8A]. A 34-year-old patient, suffering from shoulder pain due to cervical disc herniation, was treated with Dianural®, oral etoricoxib (Tauxib®) 60 mg, intramuscular diclofenac (Voltaren®) 75 mg, and oral naproxen (Synflex®) 550 mg. After 10 days of treatment she developed a pruritic maculopapular rash on the face and scalp. All the medications were stopped and oral corticosteroids were used for 2 days. Diagnostic workup was performed 4 months later. Prick tests were performed as recommended by European Network for Drug Allergy (ENDA) with Dianural®, etoricoxib, diclofenac, naproxen, saline (negative control), and histamine (positive control). The results were recorded after 20 min and gave negative results for etoricoxib, diclofenac, naproxen, and saline (negative control) and positive for Dianural® after 20 min. Further patch test was done with the individual constituents of the dietary supplement Dianural®. Of all the dietary constituents LA gave a strong positive reaction on the test subject. However, to confirm that LA was responsible for hypersensitivity reactions additional 12 healthy subjects with no history of contact dermatitis and/or drug hypersensitivity were used as control and they showed negative result for LA patch test. The results obtained with the LA patch test were conclusive of a cell-mediated, type IV allergic reaction.

Hypervitaminosis

Case Report

A case report that describes how hypervitaminosis A causes portal hypertension and can lead to liver damage [9A]. A 54-year-old man reported to the ER with a 1-month history of edema in the lower legs and a 1-week history of abdominal pain. Patient was not taking any prescription except a probiotic supplement and 100 IU of vitamin A daily. However, 6 months prior to admission he used high doses of vitamin A daily and his daily doses of vitamin A ranged from 7000 to 1 367 000 IU but decreased to 100 IU 14 days before admission as he was following some weight regimen. Liver-biopsy suggested that hepatotoxicity induced by vitamin A. Other potential side effects of vitamin A anorexia, dry skin on his legs, nail fractures, and hair loss were also reported by the patient.

Pseudotumour Cerebri

Case Report

A 17-year-old girl presented with a 2-week history of increasingly severe generalized headache that was worse on waking, with blurring of vision and transient visual obscurations [10A]. Her ophthalmic examination revealed no cause for optic disc swelling and the exam was otherwise normal. She was diagnosed with a pseudotumour cerebri.

VITAMINS OF THE B GROUP
[SED-15, 2700; SEDA-32, 608; SEDA-33, 693; SEDA-34, 531; SEDA-35, 607; SEDA-36, 504]

Cobalamins (Vitamin B12)

A Man with Purple Urine

Case Report

Cellular hypoxia occurs when oxidative phosphorylation becomes inhibited by cyanide poisoning. Hydroxyocobalamin chelates with cyanide forming cyanocobalamin (vitamin B_{12}) causing it to be expelled in the urine. Hydroxyocobalamin-induced chromaturia was seen in the healthy volunteers who were given an hydroxyocobalamin. These volunteers presented with extremely dark red urine. Other noted common side effects were reddening of skin, allergic reactions, headache, and erythema at injection site [11A].

Anaphylactic Reaction

Case Report

There are two compounds used to treat vitamin B12 deficiency, hydroxycobalamin and cyanocobalamin. Positive skin tests with the vitamin indicate a probable IgE-mediated hypersensitivity. In 1993 a 37-year-old male patients had urticaria 1 hour after receiving intramuscular hydroxycobalamin. The same incidence occurred in the patient in 2010 where he yet again developed an allergic reaction of urticaria 1 hour after receiving an intramuscular injection of hydroxycobalamin. An allergist performed tests with all results coming back negative; eventually the patient was placed on cyanocobalamin and did not suffer any allergic reactions. All allergic reactions were due to the hydroxycobalamin and were all confined to the skin [12A].

Women With Red Urine: Hydroxyocobalamin-Induced Chromaturia

Case Report

Hydroxyocobalamin is used in patients with cyanide toxicity since it binds to cyanide and forms the molecule cyanocobalamin which is then excreted through the kidneys. An estimated dose of 4 g of hydroxyocobalamin is used for cyanide toxicity. Adverse effect of red urine (chromaturia) was noted in a 92-year-old African-American woman who suffered from smoke inhalation and cyanide poisoning after a house fire [13A]. The red urine is harmless and resolves within a few days to weeks, but it may alter lab values such as creatine, iron, magnesium, liver enzymes, coagulation measurements and urine results. It also creates a false alarm within dialysis machines by making it seem like a blood leak as has occurred and therefore shuts down the machine [13A].

FOLIC ACID

Anaphylactic Shock

Case Report

A 53-year-old woman presented with anaphylactic shock 10 min after oral intake of oral intake of folic acid, prednisone, vitamin B1, and B6, complex, and a complex of activated charcoal (140 mg), magnesium oxide (180 mg), and simethicone (45 mg) [14A]. These symptoms were very mild (pruritus, flush, diarrhea, and need to lie down to recover) when this polypharmacy regimen was taken on previous day. Patient had a long history of chronic urticaria treated with antihistamines on demand (thus complicating the interpretation of skin test results), and asthma during childhood. The folic acid solution showed positive result for the skin prick test, while rest of all the medication and vitamins were negative on prick test. The authors hypothesize an IgE-mediated reaction to synthetic folic acid suggesting the need to additional testing of vitamin supplements or other fortified foods should be done to when there is a case of anaphylactic reactions on patients taking them [14A].

Skin Cancer

Prospective Study

Donnenfeld et al. did prospective study to investigate the association between dietary folate intake and increased risk of overall skin cancer, nonmelanoma skin cancer, and basal cell carcinoma [15A]. The study included 5880 participants who completed at least six

24-h dietary records during the first 2 years of the study. After a median follow-up of 12.6 years, 144 incident skin cancers were diagnosed. Hence, authors concluded that the dietary folate intake was associated with increased risk of overall skin cancer. However, no conclusive evidence is available to elucidate the mechanistic hypotheses for these results.

Asthma

Meta Analysis

A case–control study which includes 150 onset infant asthma cases and 212 controls was compared with a meta-analysis involving 14 438 participants [16C]. A high dose of folic acid for mother during pregnancy was associated with an increased risk of infant asthma, whereas supplementation with a relatively low dose was associated with a decreased risk of infant asthma. These authors report that high-dose folic acid levels can trigger asthma and these findings should be further investigated in a large population.

Retrospective Study

Retrospective study was conducted for 100 000 Medicaid patients to evaluate association of folic acid exposure and asthma [17M]. Categorized women were distributed into exposure groups based on prescription filling centered around the first trimester: no folic acid prescription exposure, exposure in first trimester only, exposure after first trimester, and exposure in first trimester and beyond. Children born to women with no folic acid prescription exposure and children born to women with exposures in the first trimester only or first trimester and beyond were compared. It was found that the children born to women first trimester and beyond had increased relative odds of asthma (adjusted OR = 1.2, 95% CI = 1.1–1.3, 95% CI = 1.2–1.3); however, no association was seen in children born to women exposed after the first trimester.

Hopantenic Acid (Pantogram)

Skin

Case Report

An 8-year-old female presented with pruriginous pustular lesions, pustule remnants and thin scales over an erythematous and eczematous areas on the face and neck 2 days following application of a cream containing dexpanthenol [18A]. The cream had been used as a moisturizer. There was no fever, systemic symptoms or positive laboratory tests. Complete blood count, routine biochemistry including hepatic and renal function test, thyroid function tests and erythrocyte sedimentation rate were within normal limits. Topical corticosteroids were administered and complete resolution of the lesions was achieved. To the author's knowledge, this is the first case reported that is diagnosed as pustular irritant contact dermatitis caused by dexpanthenol.

RIBOFLAVIN

Arsenic-Related Keratotic Skin Lesions

Meta-Analysis

In this study the meta-analysis of 54 913 participants in all included 14 trials, all double-blinded, with a mean age ranging from 52 to 68.9 years [19R]. All trials has combined intervention with B vitamins, except one study which had only folic acid as the intervention. In the study reporters noted a reduction in overall stroke events resulting from lowered homocysteine levels following B vitamin supplementation (RR, 0.93; 95% CI, 0.86–1.00; $P = 0.04$). However, the findings showed that taking vitamin B supplements did not reduce the severity of strokes or the risk of death.

The researchers found that a supplemental form of folate (vitamin B9), a vitamin frequently found in fortified cereals, actually reduced the effect of vitamin B on the risk of stroke. The effect of B vitamins supplementation is influenced by many factors such as status of absorption, response to vitamin supplementation, the existence of chronic kidney disease, or high blood pressure. The study revealed that patients with chronic kidney disease reported decreased glomerular filtration rate with B vitamin supplements.

As for analyses specific to vitamin B12, the report did not find significant benefit for reduction of stroke events in subgroups according to intervention dose, reduction of homocysteine level, or baseline blood vitamin B12 concentration [19R].

Vitamin B6 (Pyridoxine)

Dermatitis

Case Report

A case report of a 53-year-old female developing rosacea-like dermatitis [20A]. The association was linked to the combination of isoniazid and pyridoxine, which she was receiving along with rifampin for treatment of pulmonary tuberculosis

Diarrhea and Emesis

Case Report

A 50-year-old Caucasian woman was admitted to hospital with intermittent diarrhea, emesis, and increasingly brown-colored skin, mainly the in light-exposed areas, after biliopancreatic diversion for obesity treatment [21A]. Differential diagnoses were ruled out, but laboratory analysis reveals unusual high pyridoxine serum levels (vitamin B6). History revealed the intake of 300 mg of vitamin B6 per day over 6 months as described by her general practitioner. All symptoms disappeared after the discontinuation of vitamin B6 supplementation.

GI Distress

Randomized Trials

The impact of metadoxine (pyrrolidone carboxylate of pyridoxine) administration on the 3- and 6-month survival in patients with severe alcoholic hepatitis was evaluated [22A]. The open label clinical trial randomized 135 patients into one of four groups: prednisone, prednisone and metadoxine, pentoxyphylline, or pentoxyphylline and metadoxine. Patients who received combination therapy with metadoxine were more likely maintain abstinence than those who received monotherapy with either prednisone or pentoxyphylline. The occurrence of adverse effects was similar in all of the groups, principally consisting of epigastric burning, nausea and vomiting, leading to 12 patients dropping out of the study. Serious adverse effects were not reported in any of these groups [22A].

PANTOTHENIC ACID

Skin

Case Report

Two cases of contact dermatitis due to dexpanthenol derivative of pantothenic acid have been reported [23A]. The first patient who was being treated for stasis dermatitis of the lower limb, whereas the second patient was treated for basal cell carcinoma symptoms. Both of them developed allergic symptoms upon local application of the agent dexpanthenol which was confirmed by patch testing. The symptoms however resolved after withdrawal of dexpanthenol and administration of antiinflammatory agents. Hence it should be noted that the use of topical agents containing dexpanthenol is associated with the risk of allergic contact dermatitis.

Tetrahydrobiopterin and Sapropterin

Placebo-Controlled Study

Tetrahydrobiopterin and Sapropterin are relatively safe and in 16-week a placebo-controlled randomized, double-blind study conducted to evaluate the efficacy of tetrahydrobiopterin (BH4), authors found that only mild adverse effects such as irritability, sleep difficulty, repetitive behavior, hyperactivity, and transient viral rash were observed as compared to the control [24C].

Systematic Reviews

The efficacy and safety of sapropterin dihydrochloride in lowering phenylalanine concentration in patients with phenylketonuria have been systematically reviewed in many literature [25M,26M]. Sapropterin has been found to be very safe and no serious adverse events were associated with the use of sapropterin on the short-term [26M].

Thiamine

Randomized, Double-Blind Study

Manzardo et al. evaluated the efficacy of benfotiamine for treatment of severe alcohol dependence in 120 participants [27C]. In this randomized, double-blind study they found that benfotiamine was well tolerated and without any serious adverse events.

Anaphylaxis

Case Report

Juel and coworkers reported a case of a 44-year-old alcohol-intoxicated man presented to the ER due to non-localised pain in the chest and abdomen. Patient was given 300 mg of thiamine hydrochloride (IV). Based on his history, patient had been given this drug many times in the past without any problems. Shortly, the patient was found unresponsive and hyperventilating with abnormal sinus rhythm. Epinephrine was given and the patient was intubated and sinus rhythm was re-established shortly. The authors concluded clinicians should be aware anaphylactic reactions due to thiamine.

Angioneurotic Oedema

A 47-year alcoholic patient was hospitalized for alcohol dependency syndrome. She was prescribed thiamine during the process of detoxification as a prophylaxis against Wernicke–Korsakoff encephalopathy [28A]. The patient responded well for 6 days and on seventh day she developed sudden onset bilateral lower limb swelling, more remarkable below the skin surface of the left leg. Oedema was mildly painful but spread out rapidly to the upper two-thirds of the leg. Erythema was evident [28A]. The patient found it 'difficult to put her shoes on', and she 'had to drag her left leg as it was heavy'. Thiamine was stopped and her symptoms resolved in 4 days. After 18 months the patient had a relapse and was readmitted alcohol dependency syndrome. Thiamine was prescribed for during the process of detoxification. Her symptoms of oedema recurred with slight pain, marked redness and inability to walk recognizing it as an allergic reaction, the patient self-discontinued thiamine, and symptoms resolved over a period of 2 days.

VITAMIN C (ASCORBIC ACID) [SED-15, 351; SEDA-32, 611; SEDA-33, 694; SEDA-34, 531; SEDA-35, 609; SEDA-36, 508]

Case Report

A 69-year-old woman presented with acute kidney failure of unknown cause that required dialysis. Kidney biopsy revealed the diagnosis of oxalate nephropathy [29A]. The patient had several risk factors for oxalate nephropathy which included high-dose oral vitamin C intake in addition to history of Roux-en-Y gastric bypass for weight loss, and chronic kidney disease. This presentation of risk factors for oxalate nephropathy is relevant to patients consuming vitamin C supplementation use after gastric bypass surgery.

VITAMIN D ANALOGUES [SED-15, 3669; SEDA-32, 612; SEDA-33, 695; SEDA-34, 532; SEDA-35, 609; SEDA-36, 508]

Hypercalcemia

Case Report

A 1-year-old child was brought to ER with onset vomiting, irritable, anxious, lethargic, slow skin pinch, and dry oral mucosa conforming to severe dehydration [30R]. Furthermore, investigations revealed hypercalcemia (15.3 mg/dL) and marginally low serum phosphate levels. Patient had a history of calcium and vitamin D3 supplementation and as a baby, periodic injections for alleged bowlegs and calcium supplementation. Oral calcitriol 60 000 units were added 4 months back on weekly basis after an upper respiratory tract injection. Hypercalcemia and hypertension were quickly associated as the side effects of Vitamin D overdose and detoxification therapy were initiated and low calcium and no vitamin D diet were initiated.

Case Report

Hypercalcemia can occur secondary to hyperparathyroidism or malignancy. A 22-year-old weightlifter was diagnosed with hypertension during routine medical examination [31A]. Patient reported to consume over the counter multivitamin pills containing vitamin A and D. Metastatic calcification in the pancreas, GFR of 53.7 mL/min (85–125), hypercalciuria (24 hours urine test) and suppressed PTH levels and toxic levels of 25 (OH) D_3 were noted. The patient was asked to stop taking any vitamin supplements, increase fluid intake and daily dose of furosemide and amlodipine tablets were initiated. Two months later showed his serum calcium levels had normalized; however, serum creatinine still remained elevated.

VITAMIN E (TOCOPHEROL) [SED-15, 3677; SEDA-32, 612; SEDA-33, 696; SEDA-34, 533; SEDA-35, 610; SEDA-36, 515]

Fat Embolism Syndrome (FES)

Case Report

The number of cosmetic surgeries has increased Mexico. Medicinal agents such as injectable oil, which can cause disfigurement or death, have been used [32A]. This is a case of fat embolism syndrome (FES) caused by injections of vitamin E (tocopherol) which were used to increase the volume of the buttocks. Gas chromatograph and Mass Spectrophotometry was used to confirm the FES caused by injections of vitamin E.

Case Report

Three cases of lipogranuloma after liquid vitamin E injection for lip augmentation were reported [33A]. The vitamin was extracted from capsules and injected by uncertified personnel. All patients develop edema at the injected area right after the procedure, and swelling became more prominent a week later. One patient also reported with swelling surrounding perioral skin, nose, face, and the neck leading to the difficulty to open her mouth, pruritus, burning sensation, and fever.

VITAMIN K ANALOGUES [SED-15, 3681; SEDA-34, 533; SEDA-35, 610; SEDA-36, 515]

Mild Hypotension: Cardiovascular

Case Report

A patient with the history of coronary artery disease (CAD) and benign prostatic hyperplasia. He was prescribed menaquinone 100 μg daily [34A]. However, after taking the first dose of menaquinone, the patient experienced sudden weakness and dizziness. Three days after menaquinone ingestion, his blood pressure dropped to (100/60 mmHg) with symptoms of generalized weakness and dizziness, at which point menaquinone was discontinued and his blood pressure returned to normal. The menaquinone therapy was restarted after 10 days. During this therapy patient showed similar adverse effects indicating that menaquinone was probably responsible for this specific adverse reaction.

AMINO ACIDS [SED-36, 516]

Arginine

Randomized trials

A study evaluating whether supplementation with arginine, zinc and antioxidants within a high calorie, high protein formula improves healing of pressure ulcers was performed in 200 adult patients with stage II, III and IV pressure ulcers [35C]. All patients in the intervention arm ($n = 101$) received 1.5 g per 100 mL of arginine (total dose 400 mL daily). Other notable differences in formulas included more zinc, selenium, vitamin E and vitamin C in the intervention group. The study found that among malnourished patients with pressure ulcers, 8 weeks of supplementation improved pressure ulcer healing. Gastrointestinal intolerance was reported in a total of five patients. However, two patients in experimental group complained of dyspepsia and diarrhea [35C]. No other treatment-related serious adverse events occurred.

Case Report

A 12-year-old girl developed chest pain and sore throat, 2 days after treatment for small stature with one oral capsule of 500 mg L-Arginine at night. She took the capsules lying down with very little water [36A]. A shallow circumferential ulcer in her middle third and small ulcers in the distal third of the oesophagus were identified by endoscopy. The patient recovered after 7 days of treatment with analgesics and discontinuation of L-Arginine. This case is the first time that L-Arginine induced oesophageal ulcer is reported.

Glutamine

Hyperammonemic Encephalopathy

Case Report

A 52-year-old female with history of weight loss of 30 kg, total pancreatectomy, multiple laparotomies was transferred to ICU, and septic shock with coagulopathy developed followed by altered mental status and myoclonus [37A]. Cerebral edema was verified with brain CT, and blood test showed hyperammonemia with ammonia level of 271 μmol/L (reference: 11–48 μmol/L). For the 3 days prior to referral, she had been given enteral glutamine supplementation (30 g/day), and total daily nitrogen intake during the 3 days of glutamine supplement was 13, 17, and 21 g, respectively. At admission, she was comatose (GCS scale 3) with normal vital signs. Lab tests showed increased total and direct bilirubin (107 and 70.6 μmol/L). Plasma amino acid analysis showed significant elevation of glutamine, alanine, asparagine, lysine, proline, and glycine and normal levels of most essential amino acids. A protein restriction and two ammonia scavenger drugs sodium benzoate and phenylacetate were initiated to correct urea cycle defect induced by excessive elevated glutamine, alanine, and asparagine. The protein and nitrogen intake was stopped for first 2 days in ICU, and nitrogen intake restarted as 4 g on day 3 and 6 g on day 4 and 5. Her ammonia and glutamine levels were decreased along with improvement of neurologic status. Enzymatic analysis of liver biopsy showed 50% reduction of carbamolyphosphate synthase (CPS) activity; low CPS activity leads in elevated glutamine and ammonia in blood. After increasing protein intake, a decreased level of consciousness, hemiparesis, and non-convulsive status epilepticus occurred, and her plasma glutamine (2230 μmol/L) was increased with normal ammonia level (22 μmol/L). To manage rebound plasma glutamine, protein intake was restricted and sodium benzoate was administered. Seven week later, the patient was discharged without any neurologic deficits.

Systematic Reviews

In a meta analysis reviewing 32 RCTs with a total of 3696 patients receiving either glutamine (GLN) via parenteral, enteral or no nutrition support [38M]. Daily dose of GLN did not affect the endpoints of ICU mortality and rate of infection, but a duration of supplementation >5 days was associated with a significant reduction of infection morbidity.

A protective effect of GLN on hospital mortality and occurrence of infections was more evident when given parenterally and in less critically ill patients (APACHE II score ≤ 15), even though the number of studies and subjects analyzed in this last cohort was extremely limited. The results of this meta-analysis did not recommend glutamine supplementation in critically ill patients. However, in case of patients with APACHE II score < 15 who required glutamine supplementation, parental glutamine administration for more than 5 days might produce a protective effect on hospital mortality and a reduced occurrence of infections in hospitalized.

Post Hoc Analysis

High-dose glutamine is associated with increased mortality in critically ill patients with multiorgan failure [39C]. To evaluate the effect of dosing on the mortality a post hoc analysis of a randomized trial was conducted in 40 intensive care units in North America and Europe. In all, 1223 mechanically ventilated adult patients with multiorgan failure were randomly grouped into four different groups. Each group received either glutamine, antioxidants, both glutamine and antioxidants, or placebo administered separately from the artificial nutrition. The 28-day mortality was compared for each of the three active arms, glutamine alone, antioxidants alone, and glutamine+antioxidants in reference to placebo. The results indicated that the 28-day mortality rates in the placebo, antioxidant, glutamine, and glutamine +antioxidant were 25%, 29%, 32%, and 33%, respectively. After adjusting for prespecified baseline covariates, the adjusted odds ratio of 28-day mortality vs placebo was 1.5 (95% CI, 1.0–2.1, $P=0.05$), 1.2 (0.8–1.8, $P=0.40$), and 1.4 (0.9–2.0, $P=0.09$) for glutamine, antioxidant, and glutamine plus antioxidant arms, respectively. Thus the results indicated that the early provision of high-dose glutamine may be associated with increased mortality in critically ill patients with multiorgan failure.

ENTERAL NUTRITION [SED-15, 1221; SEDA-33, 700; SEDA-34, 536; SEDA-35, 611; SEDA-36, 522]

Respiratory Complications and Regurgitation

Randomized Clinical Trial

Stroke patients usually rely on enteral nutrition (EN) [40C]. Unfortunately, regurgitation and respiratory complications have been noted in those patients. Gastric residual volume (GRV) plays an important role in defining the infusion rate of the EN; hence, measuring GRV can be critical and can be correlated to respiratory complications and regurgitation in stroke patients. GRV is defined as the fluid remaining in the stomach at a point in time during enteral nutrition feeding. Hence to evaluate the effect of GRV on the EN a randomized controlled trial to evaluate the incidence of regurgitation and aspiration was conducted on 210 patients with severe stroke undergoing EN therapy. These patients were randomly assigned into two groups. For treatment group the infusion rate was

regulated based on their GRV which was evaluated every 4 hours. Similarly the initial infusion rate for the treatment group was defined according to the total volume to be infused. Whereas, the patients in the control group were not monitored for their GRV and their target infusion volume was reached within 72 hours. The incidence of reflux and aspiration was recorded in both groups. The results showed that the incidences of regurgitation and aspiration were significantly higher in the control group (18.8% and 17.5%, respectively) as compared to the control group (6.3% and 7.9%, respectively). Thus the authors concluded that adjusting infusion rate based on GRV could reduce the incidence of respiratory complications.

PARENTERAL NUTRITION [SED-15, 2700; SEDA-32, 613; SEDA-33, 697; SEDA-34, 533; SEDA-35, 611; SEDA-36, 516]

Catheter-Related Bloodstream Infections

Observational Study

An observational, retrospective study of 225 patients of home parenteral nutrition (HPN) therapy to identify risk factors associated with catheter-related bloodstream infections in this patient population was conducted. In total, 111 of 225 patients (49%) developed complications while receiving HPN (incidence=5.06 episodes/1000 catheter days) [41M]. Complications were defined as any cause that led to either premature discontinuation of HPN therapy or catheter replacement. Sixty-eight of 225 patients (30%) required catheter removal for CR-BSI (incidence=3.10 episodes/1000 catheter days). Independent predictors of line removal specifically due to infection included anticoagulant use, ulcer or open wound, and Medicare or Medicaid insurance. The following risk factors were associated with catheter-associated complications and/or CR-BSI: the presence of ulcers, the use of systemic anticoagulants, public insurance (Medicare or Medicaid), and patient age. Independent predictors of line removal for any complication included age and anticoagulant use. The authors concluded that catheter-related complications were extremely common in patients receiving HPN and as such, healthcare providers caring for individuals who require home TPN should be aware of risk factors for complications.

References

[1] Govind Babu K, Lokesh KN, Suresh Babu MC, et al. Acute coronary syndrome manifesting as an adverse effect of All-trans-retinoic acid in acute promyelocytic leukemia: a case report with review of the literature and a spotlight on management. Case Rep Oncol Med. 2016;2016:9. http://dx.doi.org/10.1155/2016/2829142 [A].

[2] De Botton S, Dombret H, Sanz M, et al. Incidence, clinical features, and outcome of all trans-retinoic acid syndrome in 413 cases of newly diagnosed acute promyelocytic leukemia. Blood. 1998;92(8):2712–8 [C].

[3] Avvisati G, Tallman MS. All-trans retinoic acid in acute promyelocytic leukaemia. Best Pract Res Clin Haematol, 2003;16(3):419–32. http://dx.doi.org/10.1016/S1521-6926(03) 00057-4 [R].

[4] Montesinos P, Bergua JM, Vellenga E, et al. Differentiation syndrome in patients with acute promyelocytic leukemia treated with all-trans retinoic acid and anthracycline chemotherapy: characteristics, outcome, and prognostic factors. Blood. 2009;113(4):775–83. http://dx.doi.org/10.1182/blood-2008-07-168617 [M].

[5] Shih CH, Wu HB. All-trans retinoic acid-induced, life-threatening complete atrioventricular block, J Chin Med Assoc. 2015;78(5):316–9. http://dx.doi.org/10.1016/j.jcma.2014.05.018. PubMed PMID: 25726499 [A].

[6] Yanamandra U, Khadwal A, Nahar Saikia U, et al. Genital vasculitis secondary to all-trans-retinoic-acid, BMJ Case Rep. 2016;2016. http://dx.doi.org/10.1136/bcr-2015-212205. PubMed PMID: 26791116 [A].

[7] Chen SC, Murphy D, Sastry J, et al. Predicting, monitoring, and managing hypercalcemia secondary to 13-cis-retinoic acid therapy in children with high-risk neuroblastoma. J Pediatr Hematol Oncol. 2015;37(6):477–81. http://dx.doi.org/10.1097/MPH.0000000000000362. PubMed PMID: 26056798 [A].

[8] Rizzi A, Nucera E, Buonomo A, et al. Delayed hypersensitivity to α-lipoic acid: look at dietary supplements. Contact Dermatitis. 2015;73(1):62–3. http://dx.doi.org/10.1111/cod.12393 [A].

[9] Beste LA, Moseley RH, Saint S, et al. Clinical problem-solving. Too much of a good thing. N Engl J Med. 2016;374(9):873–8. http://dx.doi.org/10.1056/NEJMcps1405984. PubMed PMID: 26962907 [A].

[10] Benzimra JD, Simon S, Sinclair AJ, et al. Sight-threatening pseudotumour cerebri associated with excess vitamin A supplementation. Pract Neurol. 2015;15(1):72–3. http://dx.doi.org/10.1136/practneurol-2014-000934 [A].

[11] Hudson M, Cashin BV, Matlock AG, et al. A man with purple urine. Hydroxocobalamin-induced chromaturia. Clin Toxicol (Phila). 2012;50(1):77. http://dx.doi.org/10.3109/15563650.2011.626782. PubMed PMID: 22115054 [A].

[12] Djuric V, Bogic M, Popadic AP, et al. Anaphylactic reaction to hydroxycobalamin with tolerance to cyanocobalamin. Ann Allergy Asthma Immunol. 2012;108(3):207–8. http://dx.doi.org/10.1016/j.anai.2011.12.009. PubMed PMID: 22374207 [A].

[13] Geraci MJ, McCoy SL, Aquino ME. Woman with red urine: hydroxocobalamin-induced chromaturia. J Emerg Med. 2012;43(3):e207–9. http://dx.doi.org/10.1016/j.jemermed.2011.03.012. PubMed PMID: 21530137 [A].

[14] Schrijvers R, Chiriac AM, Demoly P. Allergy workup for suspected folic acid hypersensitivity. J Investig Allergol Clin Immunol. 2015;25(3):233–6. PubMed PMID: 26182697 [A].

[15] Donnenfeld M, Deschasaux M, Latino-Martel P, et al. Prospective association between dietary folate intake and skin cancer risk: results from the supplémentation en vitamines et minéraux antioxydants cohort. Am J Clin Nutr. 2015;102(2):471–8. http://dx.doi.org/10.3945/ajcn.115.109041 [A].

[16] Yang L, Jiang L, Bi M, et al. High dose of maternal folic acid supplementation is associated to infant asthma. Food Chem Toxicol. 2015;75:88–93. http://dx.doi.org/10.1016/j.fct.2014.11.006 [C].

[17] Veeranki SP, Gebretsadik T, Mitchel EF, et al. Maternal folic acid supplementation during pregnancy and early childhood asthma. Epidemiology. 2015;26(6):934–41. http://dx.doi.org/10.1097/EDE.0000000000000380. PubMed PMID: 26360371 [M].

[18] Gulec AI, Albayrak H, Uslu E, et al. Pustular irritant contact dermatitis caused by dexpanthenol in a child. Cutan Ocul Toxicol. 2015;34(1):75–6. http://dx.doi.org/10.3109/15569527.2014.883405. PubMed PMID: 24506320 [A].

[19] Melkonian S, Argos M, Chen Y, et al. Intakes of several nutrients are associated with incidence of arsenic-related keratotic skin lesions in Bangladesh. J Nutr. 2012;142(12):2128–34. http://dx.doi.org/10.3945/jn.112.165720 [R].

[20] Rezakovic S, Mokos ZB, Pastar Z. Pyridoxine induced rosacea-like dermatitis. Acta Clin Croat. 2015;54(1):99–102. PubMed PMID: 26058251 [A].

[21] Cupa N, Schulte DM, Ahrens M, et al. Vitamin B6 intoxication after inappropriate supplementation with micronutrients following bariatric surgery, Eur J Clin Nutr. 2015;69(7):862–3. http://dx.doi.org/10.1038/ejcn.2015.83. PubMed PMID: 26039319 [A].

[22] Higuera-de la Tijera F, Servin-Caamano AI, Serralde-Zuniga AE, et al. Metadoxine improves the three- and six-month survival rates in patients with severe alcoholic hepatitis, World J Gastroenterol. 2015;21(16):4975–85. http://dx.doi.org/10.3748/wjg.v21.i16.4975. PubMed PMID: 25945012 PMCID: PMC4408471. [A].

[23] Fernandes S, Macias V, Cravo M, et al. Allergic contact dermatitis caused by dexpanthenol: report of two cases, Contact Dermatitis. 2012;66(3):160–1. http://dx.doi.org/10.1111/j.1600-0536.2011.02005.x. PubMed PMID: 22320671 [A].

[24] Klaiman C, Huffman L, Masaki L, et al. Tetrahydrobiopterin as a treatment for autism spectrum disorders: a double-blind, placebo-controlled trial. J Child Adolesc Psychopharmacol. 2013;23(5):320–8 [C].

[25] Somaraju UR, Merrin M. Sapropterin dihydrochloride for phenylketonuria, Cochrane Database Syst Rev. 2010;(6):CD008005. http://dx.doi.org/10.1002/14651858. pub2. PubMed PMID: CD008005 [M].

[26] Longo N, Arnold GL, Pridjian G, et al. Long-term safety and efficacy of sapropterin: the PKUDOS registry experience. Mol Genet Metab. 2015;114:557–63. http://dx.doi.org/10.1016/j.ymgme.2015.02.003 [M].

[27] Manzardo AM, He J, Poje A, et al. Double-blind, randomized placebo-controlled clinical trial of benfotiamine for severe alcohol dependence. Drug Alcohol Depend. 2013;133(2):562–70. http://dx.doi.org/10.1016/j.drugalcdep.2013.07.035 [C].

[28] Osman M, Casey P. Angioneurotic oedema secondary to oral thiamine. BMJ Case Rep. 2013;2013:1–2. http://dx.doi.org/10.1136/bcr-2013-200558. PubMed PMID: 24051148 PMCID: PMC3794222. [A].

[29] Sunkara V, Pelkowski TD, Dreyfus D, et al. Acute kidney disease due to excessive vitamin C ingestion and remote Roux-en-Y gastric bypass surgery superimposed on CKD. Am J Kidney Dis. 2015;66(4):721–4. http://dx.doi.org/10.1053/j.ajkd.2015.06.021 [A].

[30] Nimesh M, Singh P, Jhamb U, et al. An unsuspected pharmacological vitamin D toxicity in a child and its brief review of literature. Toxicol Int. 2015;22(1):167–9. http://dx.doi.org/10.4103/0971-6580.172284. PubMed PMID: 26862282 PMCID: PMC4721169. [R].

[31] Menon A, Sharma ML, Kumrah N, et al. Hypercalcemia in a weight lifter on nutritional supplements. Turk J Endocrinol Metab. 2015;19(1):31–3 [A].

[32] Mendoza-Morales RC, Camberos-Nava EV, Luna-Rosas A, et al. A fatal case of systemic fat embolism resulting from gluteal injections of vitamin E for cosmetic enhancement. Forensic Sci Int. 2016;259:e1–4. http://dx.doi.org/10.1016/j.forsciint.2015.11.012. PubMed PMID: 26704422 [A].

[33] Kamouna B, Darlenski R, Kazandjieva J, et al. Complications of injected vitamin E as a filler for lip augmentation: case series and therapeutic approach. Dermatol Ther. 2015;28(2):94–7. http://dx.doi.org/10.1111/dth.12203 [A].

[34] Teperikidis E. Hypotension associated with menaquinone, Am J Health Syst Pharm. 2012;69(15):1307–9. http://dx.doi.org/ 10.2146/ajhp110235. PubMed PMID: 22821789 [A].

[35] Cereda E, Klersy C, Serioli M, et al. A nutritional formula enriched with arginine, zinc, and antioxidants for the healing of pressure ulcers: a randomized trial, Ann Intern Med. 2015;162(3):167–74. http://dx.doi.org/10.7326/M14-0696. PubMed PMID: 25643304 [C].

[36] Marín Pineda R, Aguilera MdL Rodríguez, Leyva Bohórquez PdC. Úlcera esofágica inducida por L-arginina: informe de un caso, Endoscopia. 2015;27(2):84–6. http://dx.doi.org/10.1016/j. endomx.2015.07.001 [A].

[37] Cioccari L, Gautschi M, Etter R, et al. Further concerns about glutamine: a case report on hyperammonemic encephalopathy, Crit Care Med. 2015;43(10):e458–60. http://dx.doi.org/10.1097/CCM.0000000000001151. PubMed PMID: 26035146 [A].

[38] Oldani M, Sandini M, Nespoli L, et al. Glutamine supplementation in intensive care patients: a meta-analysis of randomized clinical trials. Medicine (Baltimore). 2015;94(31):e1319. http://dx.doi.org/ 10.1097/MD.0000000000001319. PubMed PMID: 26252319 PMCID: PMC4616616. [M].

[39] Heyland DK, Elke G, Cook D, et al. Glutamine and antioxidants in the critically ill patient: a post hoc analysis of a large-scale randomized trial. JPEN J Parenter Enteral Nutr. 2015;39(4):401–9. http://dx.doi.org/10.1177/0148607114529994. PubMed PMID: 24803474 [C].

[40] Chen S, Xian W, Cheng S, et al. Risk of regurgitation and aspiration in patients infused with different volumes of enteral nutrition. Asia Pac J Clin Nutr. 2015;24(2):212–8. http://dx.doi.org/10.6133/apjcn.2015.24.2.12. PubMed PMID: 26078237 [C].

[41] Durkin MJ, Dukes JL, Reeds DN, et al. A descriptive study of the risk factors associated with catheter-related bloodstream infections in the home parenteral nutrition population. JPEN J Parenter Enteral Nutr. 2015;40:1006–13. http://dx.doi.org/ 10.1177/0148607114567899. PubMed PMID: 25596210 PMCID: PMC4504831. [M].

33

Drugs That Affect Blood Coagulation, Fibrinolysis and Hemostasis

Jason Isch*,1, Diane Nguyen†, Asima N. Ali‡,§

*PGY2 Ambulatory Care, Saint Joseph Health System, Mishawaka, IN, USA
†Department of Pediatrics, Baylor College of Medicine, Houston, TX, USA
‡Campbell University CPHS, Buies Creek, NC, USA
§Wake Forest Baptist Health—Internal Medicine OPD Clinic, Winston-Salem, NC, USA
1Corresponding author: jason.isch@sjrmc.com

EDITORS NOTE

The clotting factors and anti-coagulant proteins are included in chapter "Blood, blood components, plasma, and plasma products" by Brophy et al.

COUMARIN ANTICOAGULANTS [SEDA-35, 617; SEDA-36, 529; SEDA-37, 419]

A review examines the increased risk of ischemic stroke while initiating warfarin in patients with atrial fibrillation [1r]. The author recommends considering bridging therapy with heparin or use of a novel anticoagulant in high-risk patients.

Cardiovascular

A retrospective cohort study looked at the incidence of breast arterial calcification (BAC) using screening mammograms to examine the effect of warfarin on medial arterial calcification [2C]. 637 patients were identified as having received warfarin out of the 16 555 women with screening mammograms. In mammograms performed after initiation of warfarin therapy, the prevalence of arterial calcification was 50% greater than in the control mammograms (39.0% versus 25.9%; $p < 0.0001$). The effect of warfarin was dependent on the duration of therapy, with a nonsignificant 25% increase in the prevalence of arterial calcification after less than 1 year (mean duration, 0.48 ± 0.02), a 67% increase between 1 and 5 years

(mean duration, 0.48 ± 0.1), and a 74% increase beyond 5 years (mean duration, 11.4 ± 0.5). Further prospective studies will be required to confirm the evidence that warfarin promotes vascular calcification.

A 63-year-old African American female on warfarin therapy for mechanical aortic valve replacements presented with multiple painful, violaceous nodules on her lower extremities [3A]. She was initiated on treatment with intravenous sodium thiosulfate, 12.5 g thrice weekly and increased to 25 g thrice weekly with significant improvement of the skin ulcers. Current studies are currently identifying the effect of vitamin K1 supplementation on progression of coronary and aortic calcification.

A study found that 10 patients diagnosed with metastatic cancer developed venous limb gangrene after warfarin was initiated for treatment of DVT [4A]. Warfarin-induced venous gangrene affected the limb with DVT in each of the cases and featured platelet fall after stopping heparin and supratherapeutic INR.

Hematologic

A retrospective analysis of patients enrolled in the WARCEF trial found that predictors of major bleeding differed between patients receiving warfarin and aspirin [5R]. The study confirmed that HAS-BLED and OBRI can be used to predict major bleeding in patients with HFrEF who are in sinus rhythm. OBRI scores of 0 or 1 reduced the risk of ischemic stroke, but did not increase the risk of major bleeding.

A systematic review evaluated the incidence of delayed intracranial hemorrhage in elderly Americans on warfarin [6M]. The reviewed studies revealed a low rate of delayed hemorrhage among patients on warfarin with minor head injuries.

A prospective cohort study ($n = 1273$) assessed whether the interaction of INR and lower estimated glomerular filtration rate (eGFR) increased hemorrhage risk and also evaluated whether patients with lower eGFRs experienced slower anticoagulation reversal [7MC]. In patients with eGFR < 60 mL/min/1.73 m^2 ($n = 454$, 35.7%), there were 137 hemorrhages in 119 patients in over 1802 person-years of follow-up (incidence rate, 7.6 [95% CI, 5.4–8.9]/100 person-years). Patients with lower eGFRs had a higher frequency of INR ≥ 4 ($p < 0.001$). Risk of hemorrhage was affected significantly by eGFR–INR interaction. At INR < 4, there was no difference in hemorrhage risk by eGFR ($p \geq 0.4$). At INR ≥ 4, patients with eGFRs of 30–44 and <30 mL/min/1.73 m^2 had 2.2-fold (95% CI, 0.8–6.1; $p = 0.1$) and 5.8-fold (95% CI, 2.9–11.4; $p > 0.001$) higher hemorrhage risks, respectively, versus those with eGFRs ≥ 60 mL/min/1.73 m^2. In the reversal cohort, patients with eGFRs < 45 mL/min/1.73 m^2 experienced slower anticoagulation reversal as assessed by INR ($p = 0.04$) and PIVKA-II level ($p = 0.008$) than those with eGFRs ≥ 45 mL/min/1.73 m^2. The authors concluded that patients with lower eGFRs have higher hemorrhage risk at INR ≥ 4 and hemorrhage risk is prolonged in this population.

A retrospective cohort study reviewed the association between kidney function and major bleeding in older adults with atrial fibrillation starting warfarin [8c]. Of 12 403 participants aged 66 years or older, 45% had an eGFR < 60 mL/min/1.73 m^2. Overall, 1443 (11.6%) experienced a major bleeding episode over a median follow-up of 2.1 years. During the first 30 days of warfarin treatment, unadjusted and adjusted rates of major bleeding were higher at lower eGFR ($p < 0.001$ and 0.001, respectively). Adjusted bleeding rates per 100 person-years were 63.4 (95% CI 24.9–161.6) in participants with eGFR < 15 mL/min/1.73 m^2 compared with 6.1 (1.9–19.4) among those with eGFR > 90 mL/min/1.73 m^2 (adjusted incidence rate ratio 10.3, 95% CI 2.3–45.5). Across all eGFR categories, adjusted rates of major bleeding were consistently higher during the first 30 days of warfarin treatment compared with the remainder of follow-up. Gastrointestinal bleeding rates largely increased (3.5-fold greater in eGFR < 15 mL/min/1.73 m^2 compared with ≥ 90 mL/min/1.73 m^2), while intracranial bleeding was not increased with worsening kidney function. The authors conclude that the risk of warfarin treatment should be weighed against the potential benefits based on the presence of comorbidities and bleeding risk amount patients with reduced kidney function especially during the first 30 days of treatment.

Another retrospective cohort study analyzed the rate of intracranial bleeding in patients with minor or minimal head injuries in association with clinical features and INRs for patients on warfarin therapy [9c]. Of the 176 patients enrolled, 28 (15.9%) were found to have intracranial bleeding. The rates of intracranial bleeding in the minor and minimal head injury groups were 21.9% and 4.8%, respectively. There was no significant difference in INR between patients with and without intracranial bleeding. The authors conclude that CT scans should be ordered for anticoagulated patients with head injuries whenever possible.

Urinary Tract

A 56-year-old man developed gross hematuria and severe acute kidney injury (AKI) necessitating hemodialysis, following a supra-therapeutic INR level [10A]. Renal pathology obtained from the patient revealed extensive intratubular obstruction with red blood cell casts. Warfarin was temporarily discontinued, and the patient did not require long-term dialysis. Warfarin-related nephropathy (WRN) is a newly recognized complication of warfarin, especially in patients with chronic kidney disease.

Death

An editorial described two case reports of patients diagnosed with idiopathic pulmonary fibrosis (IPF) passing away after being initiated on warfarin [11r]. A 77-year-old man with IPF was diagnosed with atrial fibrillation and initiated on warfarin. After 1 month of therapy, the patient began to complain of progressive dyspnea with dry cough and was hospitalized. He was discharged with a slight clinical improvement on prednisone 80 mg/day, but 3 days after withdrawal of corticosteroids, he was readmitted. HRCT showed no pulmonary embolism, but did show bilateral ground-glass opacities. Dyspnea continued to worsen. Patient died on Day 5 after readmission. A 64-year-old man with IPF was diagnosed with a DVT and was initiated on warfarin. After 1 month of therapy was initiated, the patient presented to the ED with rapid worsening of dyspnea. A new HRCT showed bilateral ground-glass opacities without pulmonary embolism. Prednisolone 500 mg/day was started without benefit. The patient was intubated at Day 3 and died at Day 6. The proposed mechanism for the increased mortality of warfarin in patients with IPF is due to the activation of the coagulation cascade as well as the inhibition of vitamin K-dependent synthesis of protein C. The author strongly recommends the prohibition of warfarin in patients with IPF in favor of other direct thrombin inhibitors.

Genetic Factors

A review article looked at studies analyzing the pharmacogenetics of warfarin [12R]. Current evidence does not support genetic testing to guide warfarin dosing. Future recommendations will be largely based on the results of a current randomized controlled trial that will be completed in the near future.

In a Croatian study of 186 patients, VKORC1 polymorphisms were analyzed to determine the impact they had on warfarin therapy [13C]. VKORC1—1173C > T and VKORC1—1639G > A were analyzed using real-time PCR. The study found statistically significant differences between variant-allele carriers and wild-type patients. Patients homozygous for variant-allele patients were more likely to experience a bleeding event ($p < 0.001$) and were also more likely to experience over-anticoagulation during the first 30 days of therapy ($p = 0.040$). The study suggests implementation of VKORC1 genotyping before the start of warfarin therapy.

Drug–Drug Interactions

CEFTAROLINE

A 65-year-old African American man developed an INR of >18.0 after completing 12 days of ceftaroline therapy for the treatment of cellulitis while taking warfarin therapy [14A]. The patient did not have any major bleeding events and INR levels returned to therapeutic levels after discontinuation of ceftaroline. This case report is the second to describe a probable interaction between ceftaroline and warfarin. The mechanism of the interaction is hypothesized to be due to the effect of antimicrobials on gastrointestinal flora. Further research is warranted to describe the mechanism responsible for the interaction. The report concludes that warfarin should be monitored closely for clinically significant effects on INR when given concomitantly with ceftaroline.

ELVITEGRAVIR

A 42-year-old Caucasian male experienced subtherapeutic INRs after initiation of a new antiretroviral therapy (ART) for HIV [15A]. The patient required a 60% warfarin dosage increase 3 weeks after initiation of elvitegravir/cobicistat. Elvitegravir CYP2C9 induction is usually delayed and primarily has its maximum effects within 1–2 weeks after added. Patients receiving concomitant warfarin and elvitegravir therapy should have close INR monitoring with an expected need for dose titration.

ZIDOVUDINE

A phase II metabolism trial aimed to study the modulatory effects of warfarin and its metabolites on UDP-glucuronosyltransferase (UGT) activity and to assess the potential to alter the pharmacokinetics of zidovudine (AZT) [16E]. *In vitro* studies showed that warfarin was an effective inhibitor of glucuronidation. Moreover, systemic exposure of zidovudine in rats was increased by a 1.5- to 2.1-fold upon warfarin co-administration. This study introduces a hypothetical drug interaction between warfarin and zidovudine.

HEPARINS *[SEDA-35, 618; SEDA-36, 530; SEDA-37, 419]*

Hematologic

In a review on the efficacy and safety of heparin in patients with sepsis when compared to placebo or usual care, heparin was not associated with a significantly increased risk of major hemorrhage [17M].

The risk for intracranial hemorrhage with therapeutic enoxaparin was assessed in a matched, retrospective cohort study of 293 patients with cancer with brain metastases [18C]. This study found no differences observed in the cumulative incidence of intracranial hemorrhage at 1 year in the enoxaparin and control cohorts for measurable, significant, and total intracranial hemorrhages. A 50% incidence of intracranial hemorrhage at 1 year in the melanoma and renal cell carcinoma groups was found; however, additional risk for hemorrhage attributed to low-molecular weight heparin (LMWH) was not observed.

Various studies were identified that compared or commented on the safety LMWHs to warfarin, unfractionated heparin (UFH), and other LMWHs [19C]. Tinazeparin was compared to warfarin for the treatment of acute VTE in a randomized, open-label trial and included patients with active cancer. Tinazeparin was found to be associated with a lower rate of clinically relevant non-major bleeding in comparison to warfarin (49 of 449 patients vs 69 of 451 patient, respectively; HR, 0.58 [95% CI, 0.40–0.84]).

In an observational study, enoxaparin was compared to UFH in patients with coronary heart disease and found a significantly higher average prothrombin time ($p < 0.0001$) and significantly lower incidence of hypokalemia ($p < 0.02$) [20c].

In a prospective trial, bemiparin was compared to enoxaparin for thrombophylaxis following deliveries. Some noted adverse effects in enoxaparin group were wound dehiscence, hematoma, and separation, while none of these occurred in the heparin group [21c].

In a retrospective study evaluating the safety and efficacy of LMWH use in pediatric neurosurgical patients, major and minor bleeding complications occurred in 18% (3 of 17 children) and 4% (1 of 24 children) of those receiving therapeutic and prophylactic doses, respectively [22c]. All 4 patients who experienced hemorrhagic complications had other bleeding risk factors (i.e. coagulopathies and antiplatelet medications) necessitating cautious use when present.

Musculoskeletal

Two cases of rare postpartum osteoporosis (PPO) and multiple vertebral compression factures were reported [23A]. Both were treated with enoxaparin at doses ranging 40–60 mg/day during pregnancy and shortly after delivery were diagnosed with PPO. Each patient experienced vertebral fractures 3 months and 3 weeks post-partum, respectively. Patients had no other identifiable risk factors for osteoporosis and therefore the causal relationship with low molecular heparin was suggested.

Immunologic

A 51-year-old man on hemodialysis experienced recurrent anaphylaxis due to a proposed reaction from enoxaparin use [24A]. Fondaparinux was used as safe alternative. Consideration should be given to allergy testing in patients with type I or type IV hypersensitivity reactions to rule out cross reactivity prior to treatment with fondaparinux.

Genetic Factors

A study suggests that a genetic mutation of FcγRIIa is a predisposing factor for the manifestation of HIT but the process of seroconversion may require another inducing factor [25c].

In another study, patients homozygous for the FcγRIIa 131R allele demonstrated a higher risk of thrombosis [26c].

DIRECT THROMBIN INHIBITORS [SEDA-35, 619; SEDA-36, 531; SEDA-37, 422]

Bivalirudin [SEDA-32, 633; SEDA-35, 619]

Hematologic

The BRIGHT, multicenter, randomized trial examined whether bivalirudin is superior to heparin alone and heparin with tirofiban in patients with acute myocardial infarction undergoing primary percutaneous coronary intervention (PCI) [27MC]. 2194 patients were randomized to receive bivalirudin (1.75 mg/g/h for median of 180 minutes) with post-PCI infusion, heparin alone, or heparin plus tirofiban with a post-PCI infusion. Primary endpoint was 30-day net adverse clinical events, a composite of major adverse cardiac or cerebral events, or bleeding. The net adverse clinical event occurred in 8.8% (65 of 735) who were treated with bivalirudin, 13.2% (96 of 729) who were treated with heparin (95% CI, 0.5–0.9; $p = 0.008$), and 17% (124 of 730) who were treated with heparin plus tirofiban (95% CI, 0.39–0.69; $p < 0.001$). The 30-day bleeding rate was 4.1% for bivalirudin, 7.5% for heparin, and 12.3% for heparin plus tirofiban ($p < 0.001$). There were no statistically significant differences between treatments in the 30-day rates of major adverse cardiac or cerebral events (5.0% for bivalirudin, 5.8% for heparin, and 4.9% for heparin plus tirofiban, $p = 0.74$), stent thrombosis (0.6% vs 0.9% vs 0.7%, respectively, $p = 0.77$), acquired thrombocytopenia

(0.1% vs 0.7% vs 1.1%; $p = 0.07$), or in acute (<24 hour) stent thrombosis (0.3% in each group). The authors conclude that the use of bivalirudin resulted in a decrease in net adverse clinical events compared with both heparin alone and heparin plus tirofiban, mostly due to a reduction in bleeding events with bivalirudin.

The MATRIX Antithrombin, another randomized, multicenter, controlled trial ($n = 7213$) evaluated patients with acute coronary syndrome undergoing PCI to either bivalirudin with/without post-PCI bivalirudin infusion or heparin [28MC]. The rate of major adverse cardiovascular events (10.3% and 10.9%, respectively; 95% CI, 0.81–1.09; $p = 0.44$) and the rate of net adverse clinical events (11.2% and 12.4%, respectively; 95% CI, 0.78–1.03; $p = 0.12$) were not significantly lower with bivalirudin than with heparin. Post-PCI bivalirudin infusion, as compared with no infusion, did not significantly decrease the rate of urgent target vessel revascularization, definite stent thrombosis, or net adverse clinical events (11.0% and 11.9%, respectively; 95% CI, 0.74–1.11; $p = 0.34$). The authors concluded that in patients with an acute coronary syndrome, the rates of major adverse cardiovascular events and net adverse clinical events were not significantly lower with bivalirudin than with unfractionated heparin, and the rate of net adverse events was not significantly lower with a post-PCI bivalirudin infusion.

A number of meta-analyses have evaluated the safety and efficacy of bivalirudin against heparin with/without glycoprotein IIb/IIIa inhibitor (GPI).

The first was a patient-level analysis pooling patients from the HORIZONS-AMI and EUROMAX Trials [29M]. A total of 5800 patients with acute ST-segment elevation myocardial infarction (STEMI) were randomized to bivalirudin ($n = 2889$) or heparin with/without GPI ($n = 2911$). Bivalirudin compared with heparin with/without GPI resulted in reduced 30-day rates of major bleeding (95% CI, 0.43–0.66; $p < 0.0001$), thrombocytopenia (95% CI, 0.33–0.71; $p = 0.0002$), and cardiac mortality (95% CI, 0.50–0.97; $p = 0.03$), with insignificant rates of reinfarction, ischemia-driven revascularization, stroke, and all-cause mortality. Bivalirudin resulted in increased acute (<24 hours) stent thrombosis rates (95% CI, 2.55–14.31; $p < 0.0001$), with insignificant rates of subacute stent thrombosis. Composite net adverse clinical events were lower with bivalirudin (95% CI, 0.63–0.86; $p < 0.0001$). Despite increased acute stent thrombosis, primary PCI with bivalirudin improved 30-day net clinical outcomes, with significant reductions in major bleeding, thrombocytopenia, and transfusions compared with heparin with/without GPI.

The second meta-analysis of 13 randomized, controlled trials ($n = 24\,605$) compared the 30-day safety and efficacy of bivalirudin with those of heparin with/without a GPI in patients with acute coronary syndrome

(ACS) [30M]. No significant difference in 30-day mortality or myocardial infarction rate with bivalirudin compared with heparin with/without routine GPI administration was observed. A reduction of 30-day major bleeding was noted with bivalirudin compared with heparin that was significant when GPI was routinely administered (95% CI, 0.45–0.60; $p < 0.001$) but not with provisionally administered GPI (95% CI, 0.33–1.32; $p = 0.24$). The occurrence of stent thrombosis (ST) at 30 days was significantly increased with bivalirudin compared with heparin plus routinely administered GPI (95% CI, 1.13–2.45; $p = 0.02$), but not compared with heparin plus GPI (95% CI, 0.35–12.32; $p = 0.42$). The rate of acute ST (within 24 hours) was almost 4.5-fold higher with bivalirudin compared with heparin with or without GPI, whereas the rate of subacute ST (24 hours to 30 days) did not differ significantly. The authors conclude that bivalirudin in ACS patients is associated with a significant reduction of major bleeding compared with heparin plus routinely administered GPI, but with a marked increase in ST rates compared with heparin with/without GPI.

The third meta-analysis of 17 randomized controlled trials ($n = 38096$) evaluated bivalirudin or heparin use in PCI [31M]. No significant differences in death, myocardial infarction or reinfarction, ischemia-driven revascularization, or in-stent thrombosis were observed between the 2 groups (all $p > 0.05$). Bivalirudin-based therapy showed a highly significant 34% decrease in the incidence of major bleeding (95% CI, 0.54–0.81; $p < 0.001$) and a 28% reduction in the need for blood transfusion (95% CI, 0.56–0.91; $p < 0.01$). Meta-regression analyses demonstrated that additional administration of GPI ($p = 0.01$), especially eptifibatide and tirofiban ($p = 0.001$ and $p = 0.002$, respectively), was likely to increase the major bleeding risk associated with bivalirudin. The authors concluded that bivalirudin, in comparison to heparin, is associated with a significantly lower risk of major bleeding, but the additional use of GPI may weaken this benefit.

The fourth meta-analysis of 20 randomized controlled trials ($n = 33622$) also evaluated bivalirudin versus heparin with/without GPI during PCI [32M]. Bivalirudin had significantly lower major bleeding (95% CI, 0.54–0.83) without a difference in mortality (95% CI, 0.80–1.14). With comparable GPI use, no significant difference was observed in major bleeding (pooled 95% CI, 0.82–1.10) and mortality (95% CI, 0.85–1.50). With no GPI use, bivalirudin was associated with higher mortality (95% CI, 0.83–1.65) without significant difference in major bleeding (95% CI, 0.64–1.02). The authors concluded that the effect of GPI should not be underestimated when comparing different anticoagulants during PCI. Heparin was also not to be non-inferior to Bivalirudin.

Dabigatran [SEDA-35, 620; SEDA-36, 531; SEDA-37, 422]

Respiratory

A 63-year-old man with non-valvular atrial fibrillation, who received dabigatran 150 mg twice daily for stroke prevention, was found 2 months later with a new large pericardial effusion and left pleural effusion on a pre-ablation cardiac CT angiography [33A]. Both effusions appeared sanguineous upon drainage. The patient had reported a slowly progressive dyspnea 2 weeks after starting dabigatran. It is suspected that this was secondary to the slow rate of bleeding. Microbiological studies and cytology of fluids were negative, making malignant or infectious etiology unlikely, and the absence of relevant sign and symptoms before dabigatran therapy also makes this a manifestation of systemic inflammatory or connective tissue disease unlikely. The temporal relationship between the initiation of dabigatran and the occurrence of the effusions suggests that dabigatran may be associated with sanguineous pleuro pericardial effusion.

Hematologic

A review article on the use of dabigatran for prevention and treatment of thromboembolic disorders outlines previously reported non-hemorrhagic and hemorrhagic adverse events [34R].

A propensity-matched cohort study matched dabigatran and rivaroxaban users to non-vitamin K antagonist's oral anticoagulants (VKA) (1:2 ratio) to assess the short-term risk of bleeding and arterial thromboembolic event in anticoagulant-naïve patients with non-valvular atrial fibrillation during early phase of anticoagulation therapy [35C]. There were 19713 VKA, 8443 dabigatran, and 4651 rivaroxaban users who were matched and followed for up to 90 days until outcome, death, loss to follow-up, or the end of the study inclusion year. After matching, there was no statistically significant difference in bleeding (HR, 0.88; 95% CI, 0.64–1.21) or thromboembolic events (HR, 1.10; 95% CI, 0.72–1.69) between dabigatran and VKA users. Bleeding (HR, 0.98; 95% CI, 0.64–1.51) and ischemic risk (HR, 0.93; 95% CI, 0.47–1.85) were comparable between rivaroxaban and VKA users.

A meta-analysis evaluated bleeding outcomes in elderly patients over 75 years old (see Section "Edoxaban").

Drug–Drug Interactions

ESCITALOPRAM

A 68-year-old man with a history of depression and anxiety was admitted after displaying symptoms of a depressive episode after initiating dabigatran 110 mg/day for asymptomatic atrial fibrillation for 2 weeks while on escitalopram 10 mg/day [36A]. Two years before current presentation, he also received dabigatran 110 mg/day and 3 months later was also hospitalized for depression and anxiety. Dabigatran was discontinued, and he was started on escitalopram and began to feel better after 3 weeks. During this second occurrence, no triggering life event was reported, and there was no drug history except for dabigatran and escitalopram. The medical team discontinued dabigatran, started acetylsalicylic acid 300 mg/day, and replaced escitalopram with fluvoxamine 200 mg/day. The patient recovered within 2 weeks. This case suggests possible drug interaction between dabigatran, a substrate of P-glycoprotein, and antidepressants, as dabigatran may decrease brain concentrations of antidepressant drugs.

DIRECT FACTOR XA INHIBITORS
[SEDA-35, 620; SEDA-36, 532; SEDA-37, 423]

Apixaban [SEDA-32, 635; SEDA-34, 546]

Hematologic

A meta-analysis of five randomized controlled trials compared risk of bleeding and all-cause mortality of apixaban (2.5 or 5 mg twice daily) with vitamin K antagonists in patients with atrial fibrillation, total knee replacement surgery, and venous thromboembolism ($n = 24435$) [37M]. Analysis showed that apixaban was associated with a reduced risk of any bleeding (RR, 0.73; 95% CI, 0.59–0.90) and a composite of major or clinically relevant non-major bleeding (RR 0.60; 95% CI, 0.40–0.88). Apixaban was also associated with a lower risk of intracranial bleeding (RR, 0.42; 95% CI, 0.31–0.58), whereas analyses of major and minor bleeding were inconclusive, and apixaban was associated with decreased all-cause mortality (RR, 0.89; 95% CI, 0.81–0.99).

Another meta-analysis of six randomized controlled trials examined the risk of bleeding with apixaban in patients with renal impairment ($n = 40145$) [38M]. Mild renal impairment was defined as creatinine clearance of 50–80 mL/min and moderate to severe renal impairment as creatinine clearance < 50 mL/min. The risk of bleeding with apixaban in patients with mild renal impairment was significantly less (RR, 0.80; 95% CI, 0.66–0.96) compared with conventional anticoagulants. Patients with moderate to severe renal impairment were found with a comparable risk of bleeding (RR 1.01; 95% CI 0.49–2.10).

A meta-analysis evaluated bleeding outcomes in elderly patients over 75 years old (see Section "Edoxaban").

A 55-year-old was admitted for a left atrial appendage (LAA), at which time intravenous unfractionated heparin therapy was immediately started [39A]. This was discontinued on Day 3, when apixaban 10 mg daily was initiated. On Day 8, sudden-onset right hemiparesis and aphasia

developed, and diffusion-weighted magnetic resonance imaging revealed an embolic stroke in the left frontal and occipital cerebral cortex. Intravenous tissue plasminogen activator was administered 50 minutes after symptom onset, and again, 10 hours after the final dose of apixaban. Symptoms were subsequently rapidly reversed. Apixaban has been shown to make thrombi fragile, and it is therefore necessary to monitor for thromboembolic complications after apixaban initiation for LAA thrombus.

Edoxaban [SEDA-34, 546; SEDA-35, 620]

Hematologic

Analysis from the randomized, double-blind ENGAGE AF-TIMI 48 trial correlated edoxaban dose, plasma concentration, and anti-factor Xa activity and compared safety outcomes with warfarin stratified by dose reduction [40MC]. Patients with atrial fibrillation and moderate to high risk of stroke were assigned in a 1:1:1 ratio to receive warfarin, edoxaban 60 mg daily or edoxaban 30 mg daily. Safety outcomes included major bleeding, fatal bleeding, intracranial hemorrhage, and gastrointestinal bleeding. Patients assigned to higher-dose edoxaban who had dose reductions had higher rates of stroke or systemic embolic events and major bleeding than those assigned to lower-dose edoxaban without dose reduction (1.79% vs 1.38% and 3.05% vs 1.65%). Dose reduction and lower edoxaban regimen provided greater reduction in major bleeding, fatal bleeding, and intracranial hemorrhage compared with warfarin. Gastrointestinal bleeding seemed to be comparable with warfarin.

A systematic review and meta-analysis of 11 randomized controlled trials including dabigatran, apixaban, rivaroxaban, and edoxaban evaluated the bleeding outcomes in comparisons to VKA in elderly patients over 75 years old treated for acute venous thromboembolism or stroke prevention in atrial fibrillation [41M]. A nonsignificantly higher risk of major bleeding than with VKA was observed with dabigatran 150 mg (OR, 1.18; 95% CI, 0.97–1.44) but not with the 110 mg dose. Significantly higher gastrointestinal bleeding risks with dabigatran 150 mg (OR, 1.78; 95% CI, 1.35–2.35) and dabigatran 110 mg (OR, 1.40; 95% CI, 1.04–1.90) and lower intracranial bleeding risks than VKA for dabigatran 150 mg (OR, 0.43; 95% CI, 0.26–0.72) and dabigatran 110 mg (OR, 0.36; 95% CI, 0.22–0.61) were also observed. A significantly lower major bleeding risk in comparison with VKA was observed for apixaban (OR, 0.63; 95% CI, 0.51–0.77), edoxaban 60 mg (OR, 0.81; 95% CI, 0.67–0.98), and 30 mg (OR, 0.46; 95% CI, 0.38–0.57), whereas rivaroxaban showed similar risks. The authors concluded that dabigatran was associated with a higher risk of gastrointestinal bleeding than VKA, and insufficient published data for apixaban, edoxaban, and rivaroxaban underlined that further work is needed to clarify the bleeding risks in the elderly.

Genetic Factors

Genetic analysis from the randomized, double-blind ENGAGE AF-TIMI 48 trial tested whether genetic variants can identify patients who are at increased risk of bleeding with warfarin would have a greater safety benefit with edoxaban [42MC]. Patients with atrial fibrillation ($n = 14348$) were assigned to warfarin, edoxaban 30 or 60 mg daily. Subgroup of patients were genotyped for variants in CYP2C9 and VKORC1. During the first 90 days, when compared with warfarin, treatment with edoxaban reduced bleeding more so in sensitive and highly sensitive responders than in normal responders (higher-dose edoxaban $p = 0.0066$; lower-dose edoxaban $p = 0.0036$). After 90 days, the reduction in bleeding risk with edoxaban versus warfarin was comparably beneficial across genotypes. The authors concluded that CYP2C9 and VKORC1 genotypes identify patients who are more likely to experience early bleeding with warfarin and who derive a greater early safety benefit from edoxaban compared with warfarin.

Rivaroxaban [SEDA-35, 620; SEDA-36, 532; SEDA-37, 423]

Hematologic

An observational study evaluated major bleeding in patients with non-valvular atrial fibrillation ($n = 27467$) who are treated with rivaroxaban to prevent stroke and systemic embolism [43C]. 496 major bleeding (MB) events occurred in 478 patients, an incidence of 2.86 per 100 person-years (95% CI, 2.61–3.13). Patients with MB had higher rates of hypertension, coronary artery disease, heart failure, and renal disease compared with non-MB patients Of MB patients, 63.2% were taking 20 mg, 32.2% 15 mg, and 4.6% 10 mg of rivaroxaban. Major bleeding was most commonly gastrointestinal (88.5%) or intracranial (7.5%). Fourteen died during their MB hospitalization, yielding a fatal bleeding incidence rate of 0.08 per 100 person-years (95% CI, 0.05–0.14).

A meta-analysis evaluated bleeding outcomes in elderly patients over 75 years old (see Section "Edoxaban").

INDIRECT FACTOR XA INHIBITORS [SEDA-33, 636; SEDA-34, 547; SEDA-35, 621]

Fondaparinux [SEDA-33, 718; SEDA-34, 547; SEDA-35, 621]

Hematologic

An 85-year-old woman was admitted to the orthopedic department due to hip fracture [44A]. Patient was started prior to procedure with dalteparin 5000 units/day as prophylaxis for thrombosis. On the eighth day of treatment, her platelet count fell from 163000/µL to 3000/µL. Dalteparin was stopped, and the PF4/heparin-particle gel immunoassay HIT test was strongly positive. She was started on a lower dose of fondaparinux (2.5 mg daily) because of the decreased platelet count. Four days after initiation of fondaparinux she developed bilateral deep vein thrombosis (DVT). The dose of fondaparinux was raised to 7.5 mg daily. Despite 13 days of fondaparinux treatment, her platelet count did not recover. Treatment was changed to bivalirudin and platelet count rose within 2 days from 13000/µL to 27000/µL. After 11 more days, treatment was switched back to fondaparinux, but 2 days after restarting fondaparinux, the platelet count fell again from 40000/µL to 26000/µL. The patient was restarted on bivalirudin; however, platelet count remained at only 35000/µL after 40 days. Patient was treated with 1 g/kg intravenous immunoglobulins (IVIG) for 2 days, and platelets returned to normal within 5 days. There were no reoccurrences of severe thrombocytopenia or thromboembolic complications. The authors determine that this case describes one of the rare cases of autoimmune HIT where the anti-PF4/heparin antibodies cross-reacted with PF4/fondaparinux complexes.

THROMBOLYTIC DRUGS [SEDA-35, 621; SEDA-36, 532; SEDA-37, 424]

Alteplase [SEDA-35, 621; SEDA-36, 532; SEDA-37, 424]

Hematologic

A 48-year-old patient was admitted to the emergency department because of an atraumatic right hemiplegia and aphasia [45A]. After neurological assessment, the patient was given alteplase thrombolysis at hour 3, using a dose of 0.9 mg/kg. The patient presented a dramatic neurological worsening 24 hours after hospitalization and urgent thoracoabdominal scan revealed an abundant hemoperitoneum and a splenic hematoma with venous leakage. An urgent splenectomy was performed; however, there were no further therapeutic options and the neurological status evolved to brain death. Only 6 other cases of spontaneous spleen rupture following thrombolysis for pulmonary embolism and myocardial infarction were reported in the literature.

Mouth and Teeth

A single-center retrospective study reviewed the incidence of orolingual angioedema associated with recombinant tissue plasminogen activator (rt-PA) therapy [46C]. Among 236 patients given rt-PA for acute stroke, 8 developed orolingual angioedema (3.4%). The clinical pictures ranged from localized labial edema to extensive lingual edema with respiratory distress, but in all cases, it gradually resolved with symptomatic treatment.

Streptokinase [SEDA-34, 547; SEDA-36, 533; SEDA-37, 425]

Serosae

A 54-year-old man was diagnosed with end-stage renal disease and initiated on continuous ambulatory peritoneal dialysis [47A]. Because of inadequate inflow and outflow of dialysis fluid, he was given a dose of intraperitoneal streptokinase 750 000 IU over a period of 60 minutes, and a repeat dose was given after 72 hours. After use of intraperitoneal streptokinase, there was a turbid effluent with culture showing *Staphylococcus aureus* appeared. Even after successful treatment of bacterial peritonitis, he continued to have turbid effluent, with a predominance of eosinophils in the effluent cell count. A diagnosis of eosinophilic peritonitis was made and was managed with the loratidine for 4 weeks with complete resolution.

DRUGS THAT ALTER PLATELET FUNCTION [SEDA-33, 637; SEDA-34, 547; SEDA-35, 621]

Anagrelide [SEDA-32, 637; SEDA-33, 719]

Cardiovascular

In a prospective observational single-center study, 55 patients with essential thrombocythemia were given anagrelide (ANA) and were monitored closely for cardiovascular (CV) adverse events [48c]. A total of 12 (31.6%) out of 38 patients on ANA treatment had a total of 18 CV adverse events: palpitations in 10 (26.3%), edema in 4 (10.6%), arterial hypertension in 2 (5.3%), and AMI in 2 (5.3%) patients. The rate of all CVAEs was 18.6/100 pt-years, and the rate of palpitations was 10.3/100 pt-years. The study concluded that an in-depth CV evaluation, which is recommended by EMA before and during the ANA treatment, may not be necessary to evaluate the suitability for ANA treatment, and was not able to predict the CV adverse events.

GLYCOPROTEIN IIb–IIIa INHIBITORS [SEDA-34, 548; SEDA-35, 622; SEDA-37, 426]

Abciximab [SEDA-34, 548; SEDA-35, 622; SEDA-37, 426]

A review examines the benefits and risks of using intracoronary vs intravenous abciximab in interventional cardiology [49R].

Hematologic

A 75-year-old woman was admitted with an anterior ST elevation myocardial infarction that deteriorated into ventricular fibrillation requiring prompt resuscitation, resulting in cardiogenic shock [50A]. Emergency PCI of the left anterior descending coronary artery with adjunctive abciximab and heparin resulted in adequate coronary flow, and intra-aortic balloon pump was used to support hemodynamics. She developed acute respiratory distress with opacity in four quadrants of the lung fields, difficulty with oxygenation, and hypotension within 1 hour. Emergency bronchoscopy revealed abciximab-induced alveolar hemorrhage. An emergency veno-arterial extracorporeal membranous oxygenation (ECMO) circuit was placed at the bedside, acutely improving oxygenation and hemodynamics.

Eptifibatide [SEDA-35, 622; SEDA-36, 533; SEDA-37, 426]

Hematologic

A study compared the in-hospital outcome of patients undergoing PCI across 47 hospitals and treated with eptifibatide bolus plus infusion with those treated with a catheterization laboratory—only regimen to evaluate mortality, myocardial infarction, bleeding, and need for transfusion [51MC]. In the optimally matched analysis, compared with bolus plus infusion, a catheterization laboratory—only regimen was associated with a reduction in bleeding (OR, 0.74; 95% CI, 0.58–0.93; $p=0.014$) and need for transfusion (OR, 0.70; 95% CI, 0.52–0.92; $p=0.012$), with no difference in mortality or myocardial infarction. The authors concluded that the catheterization laboratory—only eptifibatide regimen is associated with a significant reduction in bleeding complications in patients undergoing PCI.

The CLEAR-Full Dose Regimen trial was a single-arm, prospective, multisite study that evaluated the rate of symptomatic intracerebral hemorrhage (sICH) in patients with acute ischemic stroke treated with combination of full-dose recombinant tissue-type plasminogen activator (r-tPA) (0.9 mg/kg) plus eptifibatide (135 µg/kg bolus and 2-hour infusion at 0.75 µg/kg per minute) [52c]. One sICH (3.7%; 95% CI, 0.7–18) was observed within 36 hours and was comparable to the safety of full-dose r-tPA alone. The authors concluded supported proceeding with phase 3 trial evaluating full-dose r-tPA combined with eptifibatide to improve outcomes.

Tirofiban [SEDA-35, 621; SEDA-36, 533; SEDA-37, 426]

A review examines the uses and clinical trials associated with tirofiban and its place in current guidelines [53R].

Hematologic

The BRIGHT randomized, multicenter clinical trial describes tirofiban use in primary percutaneous coronary intervention. This is discussed in Section "Bivalirudin".

A study evaluated patients ($n = 508$) with ST-segment elevation myocardial infarction to assess the safety of tirofiban (bolus 10 mg/kg over 3 minutes, followed by 0.15 mg/kg/min for 36 hours) before undergoing PCI [54C]. Patients treated with tirofiban demonstrated no significant differences in composite hemorrhagic complications ($p = 0.509$), including major bleeding ($p = 0.457$), minor bleeding ($p = 0.666$), thrombocytopenia ($p = 0.963$), and blood transfusion ($p = 0.426$). Another study assessed the intracoronary tirofiban in a similar patient population ($n = 162$) and found that in-hospital major adverse cardiac events were significantly lower in the tirofiban group ($p = 0.013$) [55C].

P2Y$_{12}$ RECEPTOR ANTAGONISTS [SEDA-35, 622; SEDA-36, 533; SEDA-37, 427]

Clopidogrel [SEDA-35, 622; SEDA-36, 533; SEDA-37, 427]

Hematologic

A meta-analysis of nine trials including 25 214 patients compared the risk of major adverse cardiac events and bleeding for patients on prasugrel versus clopidogrel [56M]. In both random and fixed models, the risks of major cardiac events (MACEs) outweighed those of major bleeding (OR 7.48, 95% CI 3.75–14.94, $p < 0.0001$, random effects) and of minor bleeding (OR 3.77, 95% CI 1.73–8.22, $p = 0.009$, random effects). Results were further supported in a standard-dose clopidogrel subgroup analysis (OR 7.46, 95% CI 3.54–15.68, $p < 0.0001$, and OR 6.44, 95% CI 2.80–14.80, $p < 0.0001$, random effects, respectively). The authors concluded that despite an increase risk of bleeding with prasugrel as compared with clopidogrel treatment, the risk of MACEs far outweighed the risk of bleeding. Limitations to this study included underlying bias of trials included and clinical heterogeneity of trials.

Another meta-analysis evaluated the use of clopidogrel, aspirin, and oral anticoagulants in patients undergoing PCI [57M]. In 9 studies, 1317 patients were treated with dual antiplatelet therapy (DAPT) and 1547 were treated with triple therapy (TT). DAPT was associated with a significant reduction in major bleeding at 1 year for overall studies and for the subset of observational reports that provided adjusted data (OR 0.51, 95% CI 0.39–0.68, I^2 60% and OR 0.36, 95% CI 0.28–0.46). No increase in the risk of MACE was reported (OR 0.71, 95% 0.64–0.98). In studies that tested oral anticoagulants

(OAC) and clopidogrel versus OAC, aspirin, and clopidogrel, a significant reduction of bleeding was found (OR 0.79, 95% CI 0.64–0.98) without affecting rates of death, MI, stroke, and stent thrombosis (OR 0.90, 95% CI 0.69–1.23). The authors concluded that when compared to TT, combinations of aspirin and clopidogrel along with clopidogrel and oral anticoagulants both reduce bleeding. No difference in major adverse cardiac events was present for clopidogrel and oral anticoagulants, whereas only low-grade evidence was present for aspirin and clopidogrel.

A prospective, randomized, open-label, parallel-group study evaluated the use of high-dose clopidogrel in 1076 patients with chronic kidney disease who had clopidogrel resistance after prior percutaneous coronary intervention (PCI) [58MC]. Stent thrombosis (ST), major adverse cardiovascular events, and bleeding were analyzed after 1 month and patients in the 150 mg group had significantly lower rates of ST and MACE. There was no significant difference found in major or minor bleeding.

A 65-year-old patient with diabetic nephropathy presented to the emergency department with sudden onset right flank pain without other identifiable causes of renal laceration [59A]. The patient was diagnosed with spontaneous renal parenchymal hematoma and was considered to be associated with clopidogrel use. No other discernable causes of renal laceration could be found.

A 55-year-old man taking clopidogrel for coronary artery disease reported hematospermia after placement of a bare metal stent 6 months prior [60A]. Upon re-challenge with clopidogrel, hematospermia was seen again and therefore considered to be the most likely causative agent.

Liver

In a series of case studies, 16 patients were reported to have hepatotoxicity associated with clopidogrel use. The degree of liver injury ranged from moderate transaminase elevations to serious acute hepatitis. [61c, 62A]. In all patients observed, improvement of liver function was observed when clopidogrel was interrupted. While the mechanism is unclear, there is thought to be a direct dose-dependent toxicity and a hypersensitive dose-dependent reaction.

Infection Risk

A review article discusses the infection risks associated with clopidogrel, ticagrelor, and possibly prasugrel [63r].

Genetic Factors

A review article including 19 studies evaluated the effect of high-dose clopidogrel (600/900 mg loading dose and/or 150 mg/day maintenance dose) according to CYP2C19*2 genotypes in patients undergoing PCI

[64M]. The authors found that high-dose clopidogrel did not overcome the variability of clopidogrel antiplatelet effects between CYP2C19*2 carriers and non-carriers. Several commentaries and case reports were found discussing additional considerations when reviewing the genetic aspects of clopidogrel response and resistance [65r, 66c].

Drug–Drug Interactions

PROTON PUMP INHIBITORS (PPIs)

A propensity scored cohort study compared the risk for ischemic stroke among users of clopidogrel with individual PPIs [67MC]. Among the 325559 users of both clopidogrel and a PPI, the annual incidence of ischemic was stroke 2.4% (95% CI, 2.3–2.5). Adjusted hazard ratios did not indicate an increased rate of ischemic stroke among clopidogrel uses when compared to pantoprazole.

Prasugrel [SEDA-35, 624; SEDA-36, 535; SEDA-37, 429]

A prospective study including 143 patients found that pretreatment with prasugrel increased the need for platelet transfusions (25% vs. 12%, $p = 0.04$) compared with clopidogrel in coronary artery bypass surgery [68c].

Hematologic

An analysis including 4033 patients was conducted to identify predictors of bleeding events in patients with acute coronary syndromes, specifically patients from the A Comparisons of Prasugrel and the Time of PCI or as Pretreatment at the Time of Diagnosis in Patients with NSTEACS (ACCOAST) trial [69C]. Pretreatment with prasugrel, age, female sex, and procedural variables may predict risk in patients with NSTEMI.

Ticagrelor [SEDA-34, 541; SEDA-35, 617; SEDA-37, 429]

A review of ticagrelor's use in adults with acute coronary syndromes extensively covers associated adverse effects including bleeding and dyspnea among others [70R].

Cardiovascular

A 52-year-old male with a history of coronary bypass surgery 7 years prior experienced ticagrelor associated life-threatening complete atrioventricular block [71A]. The patient was admitted after chest pain upon slight physical exertion. On admission, his electrocardiogram showed normal sinus rhythm and complete bundle branch block with QRS width of 130 msec, while troponin levels were normal. He initially received clopidogrel and fondaparinux. Subsequently, he was found to have non ST-elevation myocardial infarction, and clopidogrel was discontinued in favor of ticagrelor. Four hours after a 180 mg ticagrelor dose, the patient experienced short episodes of complete atrioventricular block, syncope, and then a ventricular pause of 11 seconds. Patient regained consciousness and ultimately a pacemaker was implanted. Ticagrelor was discontinued, and clopidogrel was restarted without recurrence of event.

Respiratory

A report calls the need for additional studies to identify the optimal strategy in managing patients with ticagrelor-related dyspnea [72c]. The selection of replacement therapy in patients with acute coronary syndromes is not well studied.

Hematologic

A retrospective analysis of the Platelet Inhibition and Patient Outcomes (PLATO) trial found that there was no significant interaction for bleeding (PLATO major bleeding, 1.02 [95% CI 0.70–1.49] vs 1.04 [95% CI 0.95–1.14], $p = 0.938$) and other related adverse events with ticagrelor compared to clopidogrel between Asians and non-Asians [73c]. The authors conclude that further investigation, especially within the Asian population, is likely needed for result confirmation prior to extrapolation to practice.

A prospective study of one hundred patients found that ticagrelor use in real world population following PCI for ACS is associated with low risk of bleeding comparable to, if not better, than that seen in the randomized PLATO study [74c]. Within the first 30 days, there were 19 (19%) incidences of bleeding. Five patients experienced bleeding that required medical attention, two of which had gastrointestinal bleeding, while the rest presented with a hemoglobin decrease. The incidence of major bleeding was less than half when compared to PLATO (1.0% vs 2.8%) at 30 days. In contrast to the PLATO trial, they found that overall, females prescribed ticagrelor following PCI were three times more likely to bleed compared to males (10/28 (35%) vs 9/72 (12%), $p = 0.01$).This was thought to be due to heterogeneity of the patients demographics when compared to PLATO.

Drug–Drug Interaction

ATORVASTATIN

A 62-year-old woman underwent PCI following ST-elevation myocardial infarction and was discharged on ticagrelor 90 mg twice daily [75A]. Two months later, she was found to have rhabdomyolysis because of a proposed interaction between ticagrelor and high-dose atorvastatin. The interaction was suggested to be CYP3A4 mediated.

HEMOSTATIC AGENTS [SEDA-35, 624; SEDA-36, 536; SEDA-37, 430]

Protamine [SEDA-33, 727; SEDA-34, 549; SEDA-35, 625]

A study shows that protamine-induced antibodies are specific and may induce platelet activation, thereby potentially explaining the association with thromboembolic events [76c].

R15S

A new synthetic peptide, R15S, was studied and found to have comparable UFH neutralization activity *in vitro* and in rats *in vivo* [77E]. No cytotoxicity was reported at doses of 60 μg mg^{-1} or below. The authors concluded that because R15S may be safer than protamine and does not show immunogenicity, it is therefore a promising drug.

Idarucizumab

℞ *Idarucizumab, an antibody fragment, is one of the few reversal agents available for dabigatran, a direct thrombin inhibitor. Dabigatran is associated with less serious bleeding than warfarin; however, life-threatening bleeding can occur. It may also occur that a patient treated with dabigatran may require surgery or intervention, and dabigatran may increase the risk of perioperative bleeding.*

The Reversal Effects of Idarucizumab on Active Dabigatran (RE-VERSE AD) is a prospective, multicenter cohort study to determine the safety of 5 g of intravenous idarucizumab and its capacity to reverse dabigatran [78c]. The initial analysis of 90 patients showed that thrombotic event (deep vein thrombosis, pulmonary embolism, left atrial thrombus, non-ST-segment elevation myocardial infarction) occurred in 5 patients (none were receiving antithrombotic therapy when the events occurred). Other serious adverse events, including gastrointestinal hemorrhage, postoperative wound infection, delirium, right ventricular failure, and pulmonary edema occurred in 21 patients. The adverse events were related to the pre-existing patient conditions, and therefore, there were no relevant safety concerns in these 90 patients.

A randomized, placebo-controlled, double-blind, phase 1 study evaluated idarucizumab (1, 2, or 4 g 5-min infusion, or 5 g plus 2.5 g in two 5-min infusions given 1 hours apart) administered about 2 hours after the final dabigatran dose in 47 healthy male subjects [79c]. All drug-related adverse events were of mild intensity and reported in seven participants: infusion site erythema and hot flushes in, epistaxis, infusion site hematoma, and hematuria and epistaxis during dabigatran pretreatment. No serious or severe adverse events were reported, no adverse event led to discontinuation of treatment, and no clinically relevant difference in incidence of adverse events was noted between treatment groups. Authors concluded that idarucizumab reversal of dabigatran-induced anticoagulation in healthy men was well tolerated with no relevant safety concerns.

References

[1] Adhiyaman V, O'mahony K. Increased risk of ischaemic stroke while initiating warfarin in patients with atrial fibrillation. Clin Med (Lond). 2015;15(2):215 [r].

[2] Tantisattamo E, Han KH, O'Neill WC. Increased vascular calcification in patients receiving warfarin. Arterioscler Thromb Vasc Biol. 2015;35(1):237–42 [C].

[3] Bae GH, Nambudiri VE, Bach DQ, et al. Rapidly progressive nonuremic calciphylaxis in the setting of warfarin. Am J Med. 2015;128(10):e19–21 [A].

[4] Warkentin TE, Cook RJ, Sarode R, et al. Warfarin-induced venous limb ischemia/gangrene complicating cancer: a novel and clinically distinct syndrome. Blood. 2015;126(4):486–93 [A].

[5] Ye S, Cheng B, Lip GY, et al. Bleeding risk and antithrombotic strategy in patients with sinus rhythm and heart failure with reduced ejection fraction treated with warfarin or aspirin. Am J Cardiol. 2015;116(6):904–12 [R].

[6] Miller J, Lieberman L, Nahab B, et al. Delayed intracranial hemorrhage in the anticoagulated patient: a systematic review. J Trauma Acute Care Surg. 2015;79(2):310–3 [M].

[7] Limdi NA, Nolin TD, Booth SL, et al. Influence of kidney function on risk of supratherapeutic international normalized ratio-related hemorrhage in warfarin users: a prospective cohort study. Am J Kidney Dis. 2015;65(5):701–9 [MC].

[8] Jun M, James MT, Manns BJ, et al. The association between kidney function and major bleeding in older adults with atrial fibrillation starting warfarin treatment: population based observational study. BMJ. 2015;350:h246 [c].

[9] Alrajhi KN, Perry JJ, Forster AJ, et al. Intracranial bleeds after minor and minimal head injury in patients on warfarin. J Emerg Med. 2015;48(2):137–42 [c].

[10] Larpparisuth N, Cheunsuchon B, Chawanasuntorapoj R, et al. Warfarin related nephropathy: the first case report in Thailand. J Med Assoc Thai. 2015;98(2):212–6 [A].

[11] Alagha K, Secq V, Pahus L, et al. We should prohibit warfarin in idiopathic pulmonary fibrosis. Am J Respir Crit Care Med. 2015;15191(8):958–60 [r].

[12] Johnson JA, Cavallari L. Warfarin pharmacogenetics. Trends Cardiovasc Med. 2015;25:33–41 [R].

[13] Mandic D, Bozina N, Mandic S, et al. VKORC1 gene polymorphisms and adverse events in Croatian patients on warfarin therapy. Int J Clin Pharmacol Ther. 2015;53(11):905–13 [C].

[14] Farhat NM, Hutchinson LS, Peters M. Elevated International Normalized Ratio values in a patient receiving warfarin and ceftaroline. Am J Health Syst Pharm. 2016;73:56–9 [A].

[15] Goode BL, Gomes DC, Fulco PP. An unexpected interaction between warfarin and cobicistat-boosted elvitegravir. AIDS. 2015;29(8):985–6 [A].

[16] Sun H, Zhang T, Wu Z, et al. Warfarin is an effective modifier of multiple UDP-glucuronosyltransferase enzymes: evaluation of its potential to alter the pharmacokinetics of zidovudine. J Pharm Sci. 2015;104(1):244–56 [E].

[17] Zarychanski R, Abou-Setta AM, Kanji S, et al. The efficacy and safety of heparin in patients with sepsis: a systematic review and meta-analysis. Crit Care Med. 2015;43:511–8 [M].

[18] Donato J, Campigotto F, Uhlmann EJ, et al. Intracranial hemorrhage in patients with brain metastases treated with therapeutic enoxaparin: a matched cohort study. Blood. 2015;126(4):494–9 [C].

[19] Lee AYY, Kamphusien PW, Meyer G, et al. Tinazaparin vs warfarin for treatment of acute venous thromboembolism in patients with active cancer a randomized clinical trial. JAMA. 2015;314(7):677–86 [C].

[20] Ahmad A, Patel I, Asani H, et al. A comparison of enoxaparin with unfractionated heparins in patients with coronary heart disease in an emergency department in rural south Indian tertiary care teaching hospital. Indian J Pharmacol. 2015;47(10):90–4 [c].

[21] Alalaf SK, Jawad RK, Muhammed PR, et al. Bemiparin versus enoxaparin as thrombophylaxis following vaginal and abdominal deliveries: a prospective clinical trial. BMC Pregnancy Childbirth. 2015;15:72 [c].

[22] Gonda DD, Fridley J, Ryan SL, et al. The safety and efficacy of use of low molecular weight heparin in pediatric neurosurgical patients. J Neurosurg Pediatr. 2015;16:329–34 [c].

[23] Ozdemir D, Tam AA, Dirikoc A, et al. Postpartum osteoporosis and vertebral fractures in two patients treated with enoxaparin during pregnancy. Osteoporos Int. 2015;26:415–8 [A].

[24] Buonomo A, Nucera E, De Carlois S, et al. A case of heparin allergy with good tolerability to fondaparinux during pregnancy. J Investig Allergol Clin Immunol. 2015;25(3):214–6 [A].

[25] Slavik L, Svobodva G, Ulehova J, et al. Polymorphism of the Fcγ receptor II as a possible predisposing factor for heparin induced thrombocytopenia. Clin Lab. 2015;61:1027–32 [c].

[26] Rollin J, Pouplard C, Sung HC, et al. Increased risk of thrombosis in FcγRIIA 131R patients with HIT due to defective control of platelet activation by plasma IgG2. Blood. 2015;125(15):2397–404 [c].

[27] Han Y, Guo J, Zhen Y, et al. Bivalirudin vs heparin with or without tirofiban during primary percutaneous coronary intervention in acute myocardial infarction: the BRIGHT randomized clinical trial. JAMA. 2015;313(13):1336–46 [MC].

[28] Valgimigli M, Frigoli E, Leonardi S. Bivalirudin or unfractionated heparin in acute coronary syndrome. N Engl J Med. 2015;373(11):997–1009 [MC].

[29] Stone G, Mehran R, Goldstein P, et al. Bivalirudin versus heparin with or without glycoprotein IIb/IIIa inhibitors in patients with STEMI undergoing primary percutaneous coronary intervention. J Am Coll Cardiol. 2015;65(1):27–38 [M].

[30] Navarese EP, Schulze V, Andreotti F, et al. Comprehensive meta-analysis of safety and efficacy of bivalirudin versus heparin with or without routine glycoprotein IIb/IIIa inhibitors in patients with acute coronary syndrome. J Am Coll Cardiol Intv. 2015;8(1):201–13 [M].

[31] Li J, Yu S, Qian D, et al. Bivalirudin anticoagulant therapy with or without platelet glycoprotein IIb/IIIA inhibitors during transcatheter coronary interventional procedures. Medicine. 2015;94(32):1–11 [M].

[32] Huang F, Huang B, Peng Y. Heparin is not inferior to bivalirudin in percutaneous coronary intervention-focusing on the effect of glycoprotein IIb/IIIa inhibitor use: a meta-analysis. Angiology. 2015;66(9):845–55 [M].

[33] Abdallah M, Abdallah T, Rafeh N, et al. A sanguineous pleuro pericardial effusion in a patient recently treated with dabigatran. Heart Lung. 2015;44(3):209–11 [A].

[34] Enriquez A, Baranchuk A, Redfearn D, et al. Dabigatran for the prevention and treatment of thromboembolic disorders. Expert Rev Cardiovasc Ther. 2015;13(5):529–40 [R].

[35] Maura G, Blotiere P, Bouillon K, et al. Comparison of the short-term risk of bleeding and arterial thromboembolic events in nonvalvular atrial fibrillation patients newly treated with dabigatran or rivaroxaban versus vitamin K antagonists: a French nationwide propensity-matched cohort study. Circulation. 2015;132(13):1252–60 [C].

[36] Eryilmaz G, Sarcin A, Saglam E, et al. Depressive symptoms associated with dabigatran: a caser report. Psychogeriatrics. 2015;15(3):209–11 [A].

[37] Touma L, Filion K, Atallah R. A meta-analysis of randomized controlled trials of the risk of bleeding with apixaban versus vitamin K antagonists. Am J Cardiol. 2015;115:e533–41 [M].

[38] Pathak R, Pandit A, Karmacharya P, et al. Meta-analysis on risk of bleeding with apixaban in patients with renal impairment. Am J Cardiol. 2015;115:e323–7 [M].

[39] Ohyagi M, Nakamura K, Wanabe M, et al. Embolic stroke during apixaban therapy for left atrial appendage thrombus. J Stroke Cerebrovasc Dis. 2015;24(4):e101–2 [A].

[40] Ruff C, Guigliano R, Braunwald E. Association between edoxaban dose, concentration, anti-Factor Xa activity, and outcomes: an analysis of data from the randomized, double-blind ENGAGE AF-TIMI 48 trial. Lancet. 2015;385:2288–95 [MC].

[41] Sharma M, Cornelius V, Patel J, et al. Efficacy and harms of direct oral anticoagulants in the elderly for stroke prevention in atrial fibrillation and secondary prevention of venous thromboembolism: a systematic review and meta-analysis. Circulation. 2015;132:194–204 [M].

[42] Mega J, Walker J, Ruff C. Genetics and the clinical response to warfarin and edoxaban: findings from the randomized, double-blind ENGAGE AF-TIMI 48 trial. Lancet. 2015;385:2280–7 [MC].

[43] Tamayo S, Peacock F, Patel M, et al. Characterizing major bleeding in patients with nonvalvular atrial fibrillation: a pharmacovigilance study of 27,467 patients taking rivaroxaban. Clin Cardiol. 2015;38(2):63–8 [C].

[44] Tvito A, Bakchoul T, Rowe RM, et al. Severe and persistent heparin-induced thrombocytopenia despite fondaparinux treatment. Am J Hematol. 2015;90(7):675–8 [A].

[45] Sirbou R, Tissier C, Bejot Y, et al. Spontaneous splenic rupture after thrombolysis for ischemic stroke. Am J Emerg Med. 2015;33(3):478. e3–4 [A].

[46] Correia AS, Matias G, Calado S, et al. Orolingual angioedema associated with alteplase treatment of acute stroke: a reappraisal. J Stroke Cerebrovasc Dis. 2015;24(1):31–40 [C].

[47] Rathi M. Intraperitoneal streptokinase use-associated eosinophilic peritonitis. Saudi J Kidney Dis Transpl. 2015;26(1):128–31 [A].

[48] Tortorella G, Piccin A, Tieghi A, et al. Anagrelide treatment and cardiovascular monitoring in essential thrombocythemia. A prospective observational study. Leuk Res. 2015;39(6):592–8 [c].

[49] Zimarino M, Radico F, Kristensen S, et al. Intracoronary vs intravenous abciximab in interventional cardiology: a reopened question. Vascul Pharmacol. 2015;73:8–10 [R].

[50] Choi A, Blair J, Flaherty J. Abciximab-induced alveolar hemorrhage treated with rescue extracorporeal membranous oxygenation. Catheter Cardiovasc Interv. 2015;85(5):828–31 [A].

[51] Gurm H, Hosman C, Bates E, et al. Comparative effectiveness and safety of a catheterization laboratory-only eptifibatide dosing strategy in patients undergoing percutaneous coronary intervention. Circ Cardiovasc Interv. 2015;8:e001880 [MC].

[52] Adeoya O, Sucharew H, Khoury J, et al. Combined approach to lysis utilizing eptifibatide and recombinant tissue-type plasminogen activator in acute ischemic stroke-full dose regimen stroke trial. Stroke. 2015;46:2529–33 [c].

[53] King S, Short M, Harmon C. Glycoprotein IIb/IIIa inhibitors: the resurgence of tirofiban. Vascul Pharmacol. 2016;78:10–6 [R].

[54] Zhu J, Zhang T, Xie Q, et al. Effects of upstream administration of tirofiban before percutaneous coronary intervention on spontaneous reperfusion and clinical outcomes in acute ST-segment elevation myocardial infarction. Angiology. 2015;66(1):70–8 [C].

[55] Akpek M, Sahin O, Sarli B, et al. Acute effects of intracoronary tirofiban on no-reflow phenomena in patients with ST-segment elevated myocardial infarction undergoing primary percutaneous coronary intervention. Angiology. 2015;66(6):560–7 [C].

[56] Chen HB, Zhang XL, Liang HB, et al. Meta-analysis of randomized controlled trials comparing risk of major adverse cardiac events and bleeding in patients with prasugrel versus clopidogrel. Am J Cardiol. 2015;116:384–92 [M].

[57] Ascenzo F, Taha S, Moretti C, et al. Meta-analysis of randomized controlled trials and adjusted observational results of use of clopidogrel, aspirin, and oral anticoagulants in patients undergoing percutaneous coronary intervention. Am J Cardiol. 2015;115:1185–93 [M].

[58] Liang J, Wang Z, Shi D, et al. High clopidogrel dose in patients with chronic kidney disease having clopidogrel resistance after percutaneous coronary intervention. Angiology. 2015;66(4):319–25 [MC].

[59] Ozyalvacli ME, Uyeturk U, Haligioglu S, et al. Spontaneous renal parenchymal hematoma associated with clopidogrel in a patient with diabetic nephropathy. Ann Pharmacother. 2015;49(2):260–1 [A].

[60] Celik A, Gundes A, Camsari A. Hematospermia due to clopidogrel: the unknown side effect. Blood Coagul Fibrinolysis. 2015;26:113–6 [A].

[61] Pisapia R, Abdeddaim A, Mariano A, et al. Acute hepatitis associated with clopidogrel: a case report and review of the literature. Am J Ther. 2015;22:e8–e13 [c].

[62] Kapila A, Chhabra L, Locke AD, et al. An idiosyncratic reaction to clopidogrel. Perm J. 2015;19(1):74–6 [A].

[63] Kipshidze N, Platonova E, DiNicolantonio JJ, et al. Excessive long-term platelet inhibition with prasugrel or ticagrelor and risk of infection: another hidden danger? Am J Ther. 2015;22:e22–7 [r].

[64] Zhang L, Yang J, Zhu X, et al. Effect of high-dose clopidogrel according to CYP2c19*2 genotype in patients undergoing percutaneous coronary intervention—a systematic review and meta-analysis. Thromb Res. 2015;135:449–58 [M].

[65] Mendolicchio GL, Zavalloni D, Bacci Z, et al. Tailored antiplatelet therapy in a patient with ITP and clopidogrel resistance. Thromb Haemost. 2015;113:664–7 [r].

[66] Varga A, Sandor B, Nagy KK, et al. Clopidogrel resistance after renal transplantation. In Vivo. 2015;29:301–4 [c].

[67] Lenoard C, Biker W, Bresinger CM, et al. Comparative risk of ischemic stroke among users of clopidogrel together with individual proton pump inhibitors. Stroke. 2015;46:722–31 [MC].

[68] Drews S, Bollinger D, Kaiser C, et al. Prasugrel increases the need for platelet transfusions and surgical reexploration rates compared with clopidogrel in coronary artery bypass surgery. Thorac Cardiovasc Surg. 2015;63:28–35 [c].

[69] Widimsky P, Motovska Z, Bolognese L, et al. Predictors of bleeding in patients with acute coronary syndromes treated with prasugrel. Heart. 2015;101:1219–24 [C].

[70] Dhillon S. Ticagrelor: a review of its use in adults with acute coronary syndromes. Am J Cardiovasc Drugs. 2015;15:51–68 [R].

[71] Goldberg A, Rosenfeld I, Nordkin I, et al. Life-threatening complete atrioventricular block associated with ticagrelor therapy. Int J Cardiol. 2015;182:379–80 [A].

[72] Lomdardi N, Lenti MC, Matucci R, et al. Ticagrelor-related dyspnea: an underestimated and poorly managed event? Int J Cardiol. 2015;179:238–9 [c].

[73] Kang H, Clare R, Gao R, et al. Ticagrelor versus clopidogrel in Asian patients with acute coronary syndrome: a retrospective analysis from the platelet inhibition and patients outcomes trial (PLATO) trial. Am Heart J. 2015;169:899–905 [c].

[74] Subiakto I, Asrar ul Hag M, Van Gal WJ. Bleeding risk and incidence in real world percutaneous coronary intervention patients with ticagrelor. Heart Lung Circ. 2015;24:404–6 [c].

[75] Kido K, Wheeler MB, Seratnahaei A, et al. Rhabdomyolysis precipitated by possible interaction of ticagrelor with high-dose atorvastatin. J Am Pharm Assoc. 2015;55:320–3 [A].

[76] Panzer S, Schiferer A, Steinlechner B, et al. Serological features of antibodies to protamine inducing thrombocytopenia and thrombosis. Clin Chem Lab Med. 2015;53(2):249–55 [c].

[77] Zhiyun Meng TL, Zhu X, Gan H, et al. New synthetic peptide with efficacy for heparin reversal and low toxicity and immunogenicity in comparison to protamine sulfate. Biochem Biophys Res Commun. 2015;467:497–502 [E].

[78] Pollack C, Reilly P, Eikelboom J. Idarucizumab for dabigatran reversal. N Engl J Med. 2015;373(6):511–20 [c].

[79] Glund S, Stangier J, Schmohl M, et al. Safety, tolerability, and efficacy of idarucizumab for the reversal of the anticoagulant effect of dabigatran in healthy male volunteers: a randomized, placebo-controlled, double-blind phase 1 trial. Lancet. 2015;386:680–90 [c].

34

Gastrointestinal Drugs

Kirby Welston*, Dianne May[†],[1]

*AU Medical Center/University of Georgia College of Pharmacy, Augusta, GA, USA
[†]University of Georgia College of Pharmacy on Augusta University Campus, Augusta, GA, USA
[1]Corresponding author: dimay@augusta.edu

ACID-IMPACTING AGENTS

Histamine-2 Receptor Antagonists (H2RAs) [SED-15, 1629; SEDA-35, 637; SEDA-36, 545; SEDA-37, 433]

General

A systematic review of five articles investigated adverse effects of gastroesophageal reflux disease (GERD) treatments in 455 pediatric patients [1M]. Ranitidine was used in 245 children from 0 to 15 years old. Doses ranged from 2 to 15 mg/kg or an empiric dose of 45 mg. Adverse effects were reported in 59% of children in one study ($n=91$), however another study only reported adverse effects in 4% ($n=102$). Abdominal pain, diarrhea, somnolence, headache and pneumonia were most common. Another study using nizatidine 2.5–5 mg/kg reported 54.7% had at least one adverse effect. Worsening sickle cell anemia was the only serious adverse effect.

Sexual Function

A review summarized studies linking H2RAs with semen quality, assessing count, motility and morphology [2R]. Cimetidine doses $\geq$1000 mg/day for weeks to months showed mild effects on motility and morphology. Viability may be reduced with increased levels of intrasperm Ca^{2+}, possibly due to the inhibition of the Na^+/K^+ pump on the sperm membrane, stopping the efflux of Ca^{2+}. This effect has also been attributed to cimetidine. Nizatidine 150 mg/day only decreased the number of ejaculated sperm. The effects are inconclusive for famotidine and ranitidine.

Case report

• A 26-year-old female on famotidine 40 mg daily for 4 weeks for dyspepsia was prescribed tizanidine 2 mg three times daily for torticollis [3A]. Within 10 hours oftizanidine initiation, she developed cystitis symptoms including urinary frequency, severe pain, and burning. Urinalysis, urine culture and kidney function tests were normal. The metabolism of tizanidine, a CYP1A2 substrate, could be decreased due to CYP1A2 inhibition by famotidine thus increasing concentrations. Symptoms resolved after discontinuation of tizanidine.

Proton-Pump Inhibitors (PPIs) [SED-15, 2973; SEDA-35, 638; SEDA-36, 535; SEDA-37, 435]

Cardiovascular

SPECIAL REVIEW

Do PPIs cause myocardial infarction?

A retrospective, observational study evaluated the risk of myocardial infarction (MI) in GERD patients (>18 years old) receiving PPIs [4MC]. Groups were matched according to age, clopidogrel use, gender, race, length of observation, and number of unique medications in a 1:5 ratios (exposure to control). Patients were queried using data mining techniques over an 18-year time span from two independent databases. There were 70 477 patients identified with GERD and 45.9% were receiving a PPI. Mean follow-up was 2.1 years. The risk of MI was 16% higher in those taking a PPI compared with controls (adjusted OR = 1.16; 95% CI 1.09–1.24). In the prospective cohort, a twofold increase in association between cardiovascular mortality and PPI use was seen and was not limited to those on clopidogrel or those who had other cardiovascular risks; nor was it dependent on age. Only 6% of patients were on clopidogrel. An increase in cardiovascular risk was not seen in patients on H2RAs; adjusted OR = 0.93 (95% CI 0.86–1.02). Limitations include not matching patients to account for key contributing factors (e.g., dual antiplatelet therapy). Acid suppressive therapy prior to MI, especially if a PPI was written to mistakenly to treat GERD in someone actually experiencing a cardiac event, was unclear.

A case-crossover study investigated the association between PPIs and acute MI risk [5MC]. The study design allowed for controlling of time-invariant confounding and included 3490 patients (40–90 years old) hospitalized with acute MI. Prescriptions for PPIs and dispenses from a pharmacy 3 months prior to admission were collected to determine if PPI prescriptions and dispenses occurred at an increased frequency in the 3 days prior to hospitalization for acute MI (hazard period) compared with thirty 3-day periods preceding the hazard period (control periods). The analysis was stratified by MI history. Overall, the OR for those with PPI prescription written during the hazard period was 1.36 (95% CI = 0.82–2.25). The OR for those actually having the PPI dispensed during the hazard period was 1.26 (95% CI = 0.92–1.72). For those without a previous MI in the last 5 years, the OR for patients having a PPI prescription written within the hazard period was 1.66 (95% CI = 1–2.76) which was higher than that seen during the control periods suggesting that an MI may not have been considered in those presenting with mild symptoms with no previous cardiac history. While the number of prescriptions increased during the hazard period, when looking at actual dispense dates, that increase attenuated suggesting early MI symptoms may have been mistaken for dyspepsia and a subsequent prescription for a PPI was written as opposed to the PPIs actually causing the MI.

℞

Case report

- A 54-year-old male hospitalized with lightheadedness and syncope was found to have second-degree Mobitz type 1 AV block with 5:4 AV conduction [6A]. Aortic valve sclerosis was found on transthoracic echocardiogram. His history was significant for dyslipidemia, coronary artery disease, and anxiety and he was a former smoker. His home medications included trazodone 50 mg at bedtime, omeprazole 20 mg and simvastatin 20 mg at bedtime. He had doubled his trazodone dose to 100 mg the night before to calm anxiety. Trazodone and omeprazole were discontinued and all symptoms resolved by Day 3. Inhibition of CYP3A4 by omeprazole was thought to contribute to trazodone accumulation and toxicity.

  Use trazodone with caution in patients with underlying cardiovascular disease due to proarrhythmic potential, especially if patient is also on omeprazole.

Nervous System

A population-based case-crossover study evaluated PPI use within 7, 14 and 28 days of first diagnosis of any headache documented within the patient's medical record [7MC]. Data were obtained from 314 201 patients (>18 years old) from the Taiwan National Health Insurance Research Database. The adjusted OR for headache occurring within 7 days of PPI use was 1.41 (95% CI 1.14–1.74; $p < 0.002$); within 14 days of PPI use, the adjusted OR was 1.36 (95% CI 1.16–1.59; $p < 0.001$) and within 28 days of PPI use, the adjusted OR was 1.20 (95% CI 1.07–1.35; $p = 0.002$). Patients <45 years old and females were more likely to get headaches [adjusted OR = 1.68 (95% CI 1.22–2.31; $p = 0.002$) and 1.76 (95% CI 1.31–2.38; $p < 0.001$), respectively]. Esomeprazole and lansoprazole were most associated with headaches [adjusted OR = 1.78 (95% CI 1.01–3.12; $p = 0.046$) and 1.72 (95% CI 1.21–2.47; $p = 0.002$), respectively]. Most patients reported "nonspecific" headache versus tension headache or migraine headache.

If patient develops headache with one PPI, an alternative PPI may be tried. Lansoprazole and esomeprazole were most associated with headache in the study described above.

Endocrine

Case report

- A 32-year-old female with a 6-month GERD history was diagnosed with erosive esophagitis and started on esomeprazole 40 mg daily [8A]. She presented after 7 days of esomeprazole with galactorrhea. Fasting prolactin level was 275 ng/mL and estradiol level on day 6 of her menstrual cycle was 656 pg/mL (reference range 20–145 pg/mL for follicular phase). Symptoms resolved 3 days after discontinuing esomeprazole and prolactin and estradiol levels returned to normal. Prolactin level after 7 days decreased to 23 ng/mL and her estradiol level was 390 pg/mL on day 16 of menstrual cycle (reference range 112–443 pg/mL for periovulatory phase). After 1 month, the patient restarted her esomeprazole on her own and again experienced galactorrhea. Mild CYP3A4 inhibition by esomeprazole may decrease estrogen metabolism. Estrogen was postulated to stimulate prolactin release leading to potential galactorrhea.

Electrolyte Balance

A prospective, population-based cohort study evaluated the association between acid suppressive therapy (PPI or H2RA) and hypomagnesemia in the general population [9MC]. A total of 9818 individuals were stratified according to PPI use, H2RA use or no acid suppressive therapy. Adjustments were made for age, sex, body mass index, kidney function, comorbid conditions, alcohol use, and diuretic use. Patients on PPIs were two times more likely to develop hypomagnesemia (95% CI 1.36–2.93). The odds of hypomagnesemia increased to 7.22 in those on PPIs and loop diuretics (95% CI 1.69–30.83). The risk of hypomagnesemia with PPIs was only seen with prolonged use (182–2618 days; OR = 2.99; 95% CI

1.73–5.15). The odds of hypomagnesemia in those on H2RAs also increased twofold; however, there was no interaction noted with loop diuretics as seen with PPIs (95% CI 1.08–3.72).

A prospective study evaluated the prevalence of hypomagnesemia in hospitalized elderly patients and the effect of PPI duration on developing hypomagnesemia [10r]. There were 260 patients, all ≥ 65 years old, included. Hypomagnesemia occurred in 16.5% (95% CI = 12.2–21.6%). Although not statistically significant, patients on PPI for >6 months had an increased prevalence of hypomagnesemia (19.9%); $p = 0.10$. Magnesium levels were not correlated with age, gender, potassium levels, diuretic use, serum creatinine, or other comorbid conditions.

Patients expected to be on long-term PPI therapy (e.g., >1 year) should have baseline magnesium concentration measured then monitored periodically. If hypomagnesemia is found, magnesium replacement should be considered.

Hematologic

Case report

- A 50-year-old male hospitalized with ischemic cardiomyopathy and GERD developed thrombocytopenia within 6 days of switching from omeprazole to pantoprazole [11A]. Platelet counts dropped from 177×10^3 to 47×10^3 per mm^3. Pantoprazole was the only new medication started in hospital except for heparin which was discontinued on Day 3 when platelets were 94×10^3 per mm^3. The heparin-induced thrombocytopenia panel was negative and platelets continued to decline until pantoprazole was discontinued on Day 6. Upon discharge, he was changed to famotidine and platelets were 283×10^3 per mm^3 1 week later. A previous admission 5 months prior noted a similar effect after switching from omeprazole to pantoprazole where platelets declined from 183×10^3 to 57×10^3 per mm^3 by Day 3.

Gastrointestinal

A prospective cohort study evaluated the incidence of small bowel bacterial overgrowth (SBBO) in 40 children (3–18 years old) before and after treatment with 3 months of PPI therapy [12c]. Symptoms including abdominal pain, nausea, vomiting, diarrhea, constipation, heartburn, bloating, flatulence, and eructation within the previous 4 weeks were also assessed via questionnaire. A total of 22.5% of children were diagnosed with SBBO ($p = 0.011$). Those diagnosed with SBBO experienced more abdominal symptoms than those without SBBO. Conclusions highlighted the need to consider SBBO in children on PPIs who have continued symptoms after a course of therapy. A glucose breath hydrogen test is helpful to assess for

SBBO prior to empirically prolonging PPIs which are linked to causing proliferation of nonpathogenic bacteria in the upper small intestines due to increased gastric pH.

Case report

- A 12-year-old female with ulcerative colitis presented with abdominal pain, arthralgia, vomiting and bloody diarrhea [13A]. She was on infliximab 5 mg/kg IV every 8 weeks for ulcerative colitis and esomeprazole 20 mg daily for 2 years for gastritis. Due to antibody formation, infliximab was changed to adalimumab. During this evaluation, she was diagnosed with Menetrier disease so her esomeprazole was increased to 40 mg daily. After 4 months, she developed an allergy to adalimumab and colectomy was scheduled. Endoscopic findings and biopsy prior to colectomy showed a hyperplastic polyp with proton pump inhibitor effect. Esomeprazole was discontinued and repeat endoscopy 1 year later showed improvement of the gastric polyp.

Liver

An observational study prospectively followed 272 cirrhotic patients to determine if PPIs affected overall survival [14C]. Patients (18–84 years old) were followed from the time of enrollment until death, liver transplantation, or lost to follow-up. There were 213 (78.3%) patients on PPIs. Patients were followed for a median of 2676 days. There were 31.6% of patients who died and 14% who had a liver transplant during the study. Proton pump inhibitors were an independent risk factor for increased mortality (HR = 2.33; 95% CI 1.264–4.296; $p = 0.007$).

A population-based, nested case–control study examined the association between PPIs and cryptogenic liver abscess [15C]. Proton pump inhibitors increase gastric pH which may ultimately lead to overgrowth of virulent *Klebsiella pneumoniae* in the intestines which may be translocated to the liver via the portal circulation. This predisposes the patient to the developing a liver abscess. The study included 958 patients >20 years old with liver abscess and 3832 matched controls for sex and age hospitalized with a primary diagnosis of pyogenic liver abscess. Data were obtained retrospectively from the Taiwan National Health Insurance Research Database. Patients with a cryptogenic liver abscess were 4.7 times more likely to have a PPI prescription within the previous 30 days versus controls; adjusted OR = 4.7 (95% CI = 2.9–7.8). The adjusted OR increased to 6.5 (95% CI = 2.8–14.9) when considering cumulative defined daily dose (DDD) of PPIs within 90 days.

Skin

Case report

- An 86-year-old Hispanic female presented with a 2-month history of nausea, dyspepsia, postprandial bloating, and loss of appetite [16A]. Her history was significant for breast cancer diagnosed a year ago. At 9 months after her breast cancer diagnosis, up until the current presentation, she was cancer free. Omeprazole 20 mg daily was started for GERD. On Day 6 of omeprazole, she developed severe neck pain and on Day 8 had blisters in the palm of her hands. On Day 8, she presented to the Emergency Department where the omeprazole was stopped and she received supportive care. After a 5-day course of prednisone, the neck pain and blisters on her hands improved, but she still had GERD symptoms; therefore, esomeprazole 20 mg daily was started. Six hours after first dose, the blisters on her hands and the neck pain returned. The infiltrates on her hands revealed mostly of neutrophils. She was diagnosed with Sweet's syndrome, an acute febrile neutrophilic dermatosis. Her cancer had returned and she had metastases to her stomach. While Sweet's syndrome has also been associated with cancer, the symptoms in this patient resolved when the PPIs were discontinued despite the return of her cancer, providing evidence that the development of Sweet's syndrome was probably secondary to PPI use.

Musculoskeletal

A prospective, open-label comparative parallel study evaluated the association between PPIs and change in bone mineral density (BMD) of the lumbar spine, femur neck, and total hip after 1 year [17C]. Incidence of new-onset osteoporosis was also assessed. A total of 209 patients, 18–65 years old, who were newly started on PPI maintenance therapy were included. Patients were stratified into four groups—placebo, esomeprazole 20 mg, lansoprazole 30 mg, omeprazole 20 mg, or pantoprazole 40 mg and matched for age, gender, body mass index, and baseline bone mineral density values. Overall, PPIs showed a significant decrease in femur neck and total hip T scores ($p = 0.001$). Variation in total lumbar spine T score, femur neck T score, and total hip score that can be accounted for by PPI use was 2.8%, 2.6%, and 2.1%, respectively. Esomeprazole was the only PPI independently associated with bone mineral density reductions. While not statistically significant, there were 22.2% new cases of osteoporosis diagnosed in the PPI group versus 11.9% in the control group ($p = 0.138$).

Infection Risk

A population-based retrospective, cohort study evaluated the association between acid suppressive therapy (PPI or H2RA) and stroke-associated pneumonia [18MC]. Patients with new-onset stroke were identified from the Taiwan National Health Insurance Research Database. Patients followed for about a year to determine if pneumonia occurred. Patients were matched 1:2 for age, sex, monthly income, and urbanization. A total of 7965 patients with new-onset stroke were identified

and 6.9% developed pneumonia. Approximately 40% developed pneumonia within 3 months after stroke. Acid suppressive therapy was an independent risk factor for developing acute stroke-associated pneumonia (adjusted HR = 1.44; 95% CI 1.18–1.75; $p < 0.01$). The risk of chronic stroke-associated pneumonia (occurring after 1 month of stroke) was increased only with PPIs (adjusted HR = 1.46; 95% CI 1.04–2.05).

A population-based retrospective cohort study evaluated the association between PPIs and pneumonia risk in patients with chronic kidney disease (CKD) [19C]. A total of 8076 patients were identified from the Taiwan Health Insurance Research Database. Those with CKD receiving a PPI were followed for 5 years or until the occurrence of pneumonia ($n = 277$). A total of 19.1% (53/277) of patients with CKD on a PPI developed pneumonia (adjusted HR = 2.21; 95% CI 1.59–3.07; $p < 0.001$). Of the remaining 7799 patients who were not on a PPI, only 7.3% developed pneumonia. This study was unique because it specifically looked at pneumonia risk in patients with CKD.

A prospective trial evaluated the effect of certain chronic medications on infection rates in 400 cirrhotic patients [20C]. Proton pump inhibitors were the most frequent chronic therapy used (67%) and was an independent risk factor for developing an infection (OR = 2; 95% CI 1.2–3.2; $p = 0.001$). Infections were seen in 39% of patients on PPIs versus only 26% with controls ($p = 0.008$). No differences were noted in the type of infections PPIs versus other therapies.

A retrospective cohort study evaluated the association between PPIs and risk of initial *Clostridium difficile* infection recurrence within 90 days of initial infection [21C]. A total of 754 patients with health-care associated *Clostridium difficile* infections were included. Recurrent infection occurred in 28.8% of patients on a PPI versus 20.6% in those not on a PPI ($p = 0.007$). Mortality rate within 15–90 days after initial *Clostridium difficile* infection was 10.3% in patients on a PPI versus 4.7% in those not on a PPI ($p = 0.007$). Proton pump inhibitors were an independent risk factor associated with *Clostridium difficile* infection recurrence.

In order to decrease risk of infection, clinicians should evaluate the indication for PPIs and make sure that there is a clear indication supported by the literature. Use PPIs for the shortest duration possible.

Drug–Drug Interaction, Clopidogrel

Important drug interactions with clopidogrel were assessed in one review that included 58 articles [22R]. The review highlighted omeprazole and esomeprazole as the PPIs most likely to decrease exposure to clopidogrel's active metabolite due to CYP2C19 inhibition. Separating clopidogrel and omeprazole by up to 12 hours was not beneficial in preventing this drug interaction. Pantoprazole and rabeprazole did not affect the conversion of clopidogrel. Interestingly, when higher doses of clopidogrel were used acutely (300–600 mg), platelet reactivity changes were not seen indicating that higher doses may be able to overcome the interaction between clopidogrel and omeprazole. Histamine-2 receptor antagonists did affect conversion of clopidogrel to its active metabolite. Prasugrel did not interact with omeprazole or esomeprazole.

A meta-analysis including 39 studies evaluated cardiovascular outcomes associated with clopidogrel and PPIs used concomitantly [23M]. Gastrointestinal bleeding rates were also assessed. While the incidence all-cause mortality, myocardial infarction, stent thrombosis, and cerebrovascular accidents were higher in patients receiving both medications, the majority of the studies were non-randomized, observational trials. The authors performed a pre-specified subgroup analysis including only the eight randomized-controlled studies or propensity score matched populations which represented 23 552 patients. Factors that were assessed included incidence of (1) dual antiplatelet therapy; (2) percutaneous coronary intervention; (3) acute coronary syndrome; (4) stratification by risk based on CYP2C19 inhibition (omeprazole, esomeprazole and lansoprazole have the highest risk for CYP2C19 interactions). There were no differences in mortality or ischemic events in those on clopidogrel +/− a PPI. Those on lower risk PPIs (pantoprazole or rabeprazole) demonstrated an association with adverse cardiovascular outcomes suggesting that PPI use may be more of a marker of patients who have an increased underlying cardiovascular risk more so than actually causing the adverse outcome. Beneficially, there was a 60% decrease in gastrointestinal bleeding in patients on a PPIs. Comorbid risks that were not equally randomized among the groups may have accounted for the increased adverse outcomes seen in the pooled analysis.

A retrospective propensity score-adjusted cohort trial assessed the incidence of ischemic stroke in outpatients recently started on clopidogrel who were also receiving a PPI [24C]. Pantoprazole served as the reference PPI due to low CYP2C19 inhibitory activity. The primary endpoint was hospitalization for acute ischemic stroke within 180 days of starting concomitant therapy with clopidogrel and a PPI. Ischemic stroke occurred in 2.4% of patients receiving clopidogrel and a PPI (95% CI 2.3–2.5). The rate of stroke was not found to be different in those receiving clopidogrel-pantoprazole versus any other PPI with clopidogrel.

A systematic review of 35 studies evaluated the cardiovascular efficacy and safety of dual antiplatelet therapy (DAPT) used concomitantly with a PPI [25M]. Five of these studies (4 randomized-controlled studies and 1 observational study) evaluated omeprazole with DAPT versus placebo with DAPT. The other 30 observational studies evaluated the PPIs as a class versus no PPI use. The clinical outcomes measured at 1 year included composite ischemic endpoints, death from all cause, nonfatal myocardial infarction, stroke, revascularization and stent thrombosis. Proton pump inhibitors were associated with more cardiovascular events versus controls. However, this was not seen from the randomized trials looking specifically at omeprazole versus placebo, where no difference in ischemic events was seen. There was a decrease in upper gastrointestinal bleeding in patients receiving PPIs. Poor cardiovascular outcomes in patients on DAPT plus a PPI seen in the observational studies conflicted with results seen when only the randomized-controlled trials were considered.

A systematic review assessed the associated risk of individual PPIs on cardiovascular events in patients taking DAPT [26M]. This was part of a larger systematic review described above [25M]. Only studies that evaluated individual PPIs and reported on cardiovascular outcomes at 1 year were included. A total of 6 observational trials were identified. Omeprazole was the least likely to be associated with adverse cardiovascular events with a HR of 1.16 (95% CI 0.93–1.44). Pantoprazole was the most likely associated with increased cardiovascular events (HR = 1.38; 95% CI 1.12–1.7) followed by lansoprazole (HR = 1.29; 95% CI 1.09–1.52) then esomeprazole (HR = 1.27; 95% CI 1.02–1.58).

A retrospective analysis of hemorrhagic and thromboembolic events reported to the Food and Drug Administration Adverse Event Reporting System was performed in patients on DAPT plus a PPI [27C]. A total of 2 257 902 reports were analyzed using a reporting odds ratio (ROR) and logistic regression. The adjusted ROR for hemorrhagic events occurring in those just on DAPT was 4.4 (95% CI 4.02–4.81) and it was 3.4 (95% CI 2.84–4.06) for those on DAPT plus a PPI. The adjusted ROR for thromboembolic events occurring in those just on DAPT was 2.37 (9%% CI 2.16–2.59) and it was 2.38 (95% CI 2–2.84) for those on DAPT plus a PPI.

A prospective, international, multicenter trial evaluated the relationship of platelet reactivity and cardiovascular outcomes in patients on clopidogrel after drug-eluting stent implantation who also received a PPI [28MC]. A total of 8582 patients were followed for 2 years. At time of stent placement, 31.4% were on a PPI. The use of PPIs was an independent risk factor associated with high platelet reactivity (OR = 1.38; 95% CI 1.25–1.52; $p = 0.001$). After propensity-adjusted multivariable analysis, patients discharged on a PPI was also an independent risk factor associated with negative cardiac outcomes (e.g., cardiac death, myocardial infarction, revascularization) 2 years post-discharge; HR = 1.21 (95% CI 1.04–1.42; $p = 0.02$).

Much of the data on the PPIs and clopidogrel drug interaction is from observational studies. In reality, omeprazole is the most likely to interact with clopidogrel. Esomeprazole carries a warning also since it is the isomer of omeprazole. In patients on clopidogrel and alternative PPI (other than omeprazole, and possibly esomeprazole) should be chosen.

Drug–Drug Interaction, Erlotinib

The solubility of erlotinib is pH-dependent and therefore, concomitant PPI use should be avoided due to decreased absorption. A population-based, retrospective cohort study in 507 patients (average age = 64 years old) with advanced NSCLC receiving erlotinib evaluated how many were also receiving concurrent acid suppressive therapy (PPI or H2RA) and what effect it had on clinically important outcomes [29C]. Progression-free and overall survival rates were the primary endpoints. There were 124 patients on concurrent erlotinib and acid suppressive therapy, of which 93% were on a PPI. Pantoprazole accounted for 43% of PPI use, followed by omeprazole (29%), lansoprazole (16%), and rabeprazole (5%). Median progression-free survival was 1.4 months for those on acid suppressive therapy versus 2.3 months for controls (HR = 1.7; $p < 0.001$). Median overall survival was 12.9 months for those on acid suppressive therapy versus 16.8 months for controls (HR = 1.38; $p = 0.003$). This study was unique because it was done in patients with NSCLC where decreased efficacy due to drug interactions could affect not only disease progression, but also overall survival. Previous studies were in healthy volunteers.

It is recommended to avoid using PPIs concomitantly with erlotinib if possible. If using a histamine-2 receptor antagonist (H2RA) in place of a PPI, erlotinib should be administered 2 hours before the H2RA or 10 hours after the H2RA.

Drug–Drug Interaction, HIV

The prevalence of clinically significant drug interactions in 268 HIV-positive patients was assessed in a cross-sectional study [30c]. Patients were 18–81 years old who had at least one active prescription for an antiretroviral medication and was on the interacting medication for at least 1 week. There were 102 (34.9%) clinically significant drug interactions identified. Of those, PPIs were one of seven classes that made up 75% of those clinically significant drug interactions. Clinically significant drug interactions were reported with PPIs used concomitantly with atazanavir due to decreased atazanavir AUC.

Concurrent administration of a PPI is not recommended in antiretroviral-experienced patients. In those who are antiretroviral-naïve—it is recommended to give atazanavir 12 hours after the PPI. The PPI dose should not exceed the equivalent of omeprazole 20 mg/day.

Drug–Drug Interaction, Serotonin Receptor Reuptake Inhibitors (Citalopram, Escitalopram, Sertraline)

A retrospective study evaluated PPI effects on citalopram, escitalopram, and sertraline concentrations, all metabolized via CYP2C19 [31C]. There were 831 patients receiving either citalopram, escitalopram or sertraline with concomitant PPI use. Concentrations for all three serotonin receptor reuptake inhibitors (SSRIs) were significantly increased versus controls. The PPIs affected the SSRI concentrations at varying levels. Citalopram concentrations were 35.3% higher with omeprazole, 32.8% with esomeprazole and 14.7% with lansoprazole ($p < 0.001$, $p < 0.001$ and $p < 0.043$, respectively). Escitalopram concentrations were most affected by PPIs with a 93.9% increase with omeprazole, 81.8% increase with esomeprazole, 20.1% with lansoprazole, and 21.6% with pantoprazole ($p < 0.001$, $p < 0.001$, $p = 0.008$, and $p = 0.002$, respectively). Sertraline concentrations were significantly increased only by esomeprazole (38.5%; $p = 0.0014$).

Because omeprazole and esomeprazole are moderate inhibitors of CYP2C19, they may increase the serum concentration of citalopram and escitalopram. Dose of citalopram should be limited to a maximum of 20 mg/day. May consider lower doses of escitalopram.

Drug–Drug Interaction, Voriconazole

A retrospective study evaluated the magnitude of effect of CYP inhibitors and/or CYP inhibitors plus CYP inducers on voriconazole trough concentrations in 83 hematological patients (41–62 years old) [32c]. Thirty-five patients received omeprazole or pantoprazole (CYP inhibitors) and 21 patients received (omeprazole or pantoprazole) plus a CYP inducer (methylprednisolone, dexamethasone, phenobarbital, rifampin, or carbamazepine). Voriconazole troughs were most affected by co-administration with a CYP inhibitor alone. A twofold increase in dose-normalized voriconazole troughs was seen in those on omeprazole or pantoprazole. The odds of the voriconazole trough being supratherapeutic (>5.5 mg/L) was 23.22 higher when co-administered with omeprazole or pantoprazole (95% CI 3.01–179.09; $p = 0.003$). The odds of a supratherapeutic voriconazole trough decreased to 3.53 when both a CYP inhibitor (omeprazole or pantoprazole) and a CYP inducer were administered (95% CI 0.36–34.95; $p = 0.28$). Co-administration of a CYP inducer alone resulted in a mean decrease in the dose-normalized voriconazole trough (range 1.65–4.19 mg/dL).

In patients receiving omeprazole doses of 40 mg/day, consider decreasing the dose by half when initiating voriconazole therapy.

Drug–Drug Interaction, Warfarin

The effect of CYP2C19 genotypes on the interaction between warfarin and PPIs was assessed in a prospective observational study of 82 post-surgical Japanese patients (mean age = 67.9 years old) whose CYP2C19 genotypes had been analyzed in advance [33c]. Patients were randomized to either lansoprazole or rabeprazole used concurrently with warfarin. The INR was monitored at Day 4, 8, 14, 1 month and 2 months after surgery. Patients on lansoprazole who were intermediate-metabolizers of CYP2C19 had maximum INR values (3.36 + 0.98). These were higher than with rabeprazole (2.29 ±0.55); $p < 0.0001$. The INR was > 3.5 in 15 patients receiving lansoprazole but only in 2 patients receiving rabeprazole; $p = 0001$. In addition, there were ten bleeding events with lansoprazole versus no bleeding with rabeprazole; $p = 0.015$. Lansoprazole combined with CYP2C19 intermediate-metabolizer genotype were independent predictors of bleeding complications after surgery (OR = 2.39; 95% CI = 1.1–29.4; $p = 0009$).

ANTICONSTIPATION AND PROKINETIC

Domperidone [SED-15, 1178; SEDA-35, 633; SEDA-36, 541, SEDA-37, 445]

Drug–Drug Interactions, Erythromycin, Pioglitazone, Ketoconazole

A review summarized the drug interactions with domperidone which is primarily metabolized by CYP3A4, and to a lesser extent CYP1A2, CYP2D6, and CYP2C8 [34R]

- Erythromycin and pioglitazone (CYP3A4 inhibitors) have been shown *in vivo* to increase domperidone systemic exposure by 2.5- and 2-fold, respectively.
- Ketoconazole increased domperidone systemic exposure threefold in a randomized placebo-controlled, double-blind, crossover study in healthy volunteers leading to a significantly higher QTc in males, 15.9 ms higher ($p < 0.001$). The difference was not significantly different in females.

Concurrent use of domperidone with moderate and strong CYP3A4 inhibitors is not recommended.

Erythromycin [SED-15, 1237]

Case report

- A 28-year-old male treated for 2 years with olanzapine (20 mg/day) and trihexyphenidyl (2 mg/day) for schizophrenia developed pityriasis rosea [35A]. He was treated with erythromycin 250 mg four times daily and cetirizine 10 mg daily for 5 days. On Day 4, he began feeling restless and was diagnosed with akathisia which resolved 3 days after erythromycin discontinuation.

Caution may be needed when combining erythromycin, which is known to cause akathisia, with other agents known to cause akathisia, such as second-generation antipsychotics. Educate patient to report signs of akathisia.

Metoclopramide [SED-15, 2317; SEDA-35, 634, SEDA-36, 542, SEDA-37, 446]

Neuromuscular Function

A meta-analysis comprising 11 randomized-controlled crossover and double-blind trials, in patients 18–80 years old, compared metoclopramide continuous infusion ($n = 608$) and metoclopramide intravenous bolus administration ($n = 595$) to determine rates of extrapyramidal symptoms (EPS) [36M]. Continuous infusion produced 8% less EPS (95% CI 5–11%; $I2 = 65\%$). Nine studies showed a trend towards decreased EPS, with three having a significant difference. Studies scoring ≥ 3 on the Jadad scale showed a larger difference in EPS effects between the two groups, favoring continuous infusion. Limitations were that studies included concomitant medications that could modify the effects of metoclopramide and varying doses that were used.

Patients at increased risk of EPS may benefit from continuous infusion instead of bolus therapy for metoclopramide if therapy is indicated.

Drug–Drug Interaction, Fluoxetine, Digoxin, Levadopa, Sertraline, and Venlafaxine

A review summarized the drug interactions with metoclopramide, an inhibitor of CYP2D6 [34R]. Fluoxetine increased the area under the curve (AUC) of metoclopramide by twofold, while decreasing clearance 1.5-fold in healthy subjects. An AUC decrease was reported with digoxin in healthy male subjects. Levodopa reached higher peak concentrations faster in healthy subjects. Of note, the most clinically significant drug interaction occurred when metoclopramide was given in with sertraline or venlafaxine.

Case reports

- A 21-year-old female experienced forced extension of the neck, lateral deviation of the eyes, and non-rigid opening of the jaw 24 hours after receiving metoclopramide 10 mg twice daily for 2 days for postoperative nausea [37A]. Similar reactions are generally seen with doses >30 mg per day.
- Acute dyslalia, dysphonia, dysphagia and facial rhythmic jerks were observed in a 61-year-old female 8 hours after taking metoclopramide 20 mg orally [38A]. She had myoclonus in the orbicularis oculi, orbicularis oris and palatopharyngeal.
- Asystolic cardiac arrest was observed after administration of metoclopramide 10 mg intravenously over 5 seconds to a 28-year-old male with newly diagnosed hypertension and hyperlipidemia [39A]. Myocardial infarction was ruled out. Serum potassium was 3.1 mEq/L, and in combination with rapid intravenous administration, could have contributed to the patient's cardiac arrest immediately following metoclopramide.

Patients should be monitored for serotonin syndrome and extrapyramidal symptoms if concurrent use of serotonin modulating agents or dopaminergic agents and metoclopramide is needed.

Mineral Oil

Case report

- A 40-year-old male was admitted on three instances with progressive respiratory distress over a few weeks [40A]. He first presented with a sternum fracture, secondly with fever, cough, elevated C-reactive protein and leukocytosis diagnosed as pneumonia. On his third admission, he was in acute hypoxic respiratory failure with oxygen saturations 83% on room air and 91% with 15 L/minute oxygen. Chest X-ray revealed interstitial infiltrates due to pulmonary edema and atelectasis. He had been injecting mineral oil with anabolic steroids in biceps and observed blood upon aspiration of the needle and experienced hemoptysis consistent with intravascular administration. He was diagnosed with subacute fat-embolism like syndrome.

Polyethylene glycol [SEDA-35, 646; SEDA-36, 553; SEDA-37, 447]

Case reports

- A 39-year-old male ingested polyethylene glycol (PEG) for routine bowel cleansing prior to colonoscopy [41A]. Five minutes later, he developed a rash, swelling, itching, tingling in arms, dizziness, dysphagia, and dyspnea. He presented to the emergency department within 30 minutes in a state of shock with a blood pressure of 41/31 mmHg, HR 102 beats/minute, RR of 28 breaths/minute and temperature of 36 °C. He had no chronic medical conditions and no known allergies. Twenty hours after presentation and treatment all symptoms resolved.
- A 30-year-old female with chronic diarrhea was scheduled to undergo endoscopy and small bowel series [42A]. She was given PEG 3350 bowel preparation, taken previously without adverse effects. Her throat became itchy and she experienced generalized pruritus and chest pressure within a few minutes. Symmetric erythema on forearms and hives on her chest developed. Symptoms were alleviated with an antihistamine and corticosteroids. Biopsy confirmed a diagnosis of nodular lymphoid hyperplasia (NLH). Mucosal breaks due to NLH and impaired mucosal barrier due to diarrhea could have increased the systemic absorption of PEG 3350.

  Allergic reactions to PEG are uncommon, however should not be ruled out, even with previous exposure with no reaction. PEG should be avoided in patients with prior history of allergic reaction.

ANTIDIARRHEAL AND ANTISPASMODIC AGENTS

Trauma, Injury

A retrospective case–control study evaluated risk of injury associated with antispasmodic and anticholinergic agents in patients ≥65 years old [43C]. Medications were belladonna alkaloids with phenobarbital, diphenoxylate w/atropine, clidinium w/chlordiazepoxide, propantheline, dicyclomine, and hyoscamine. There were 302 cases out of 54 152 (0.6%) who had exposure to one of the identified medications; with dicyclomine being the most commonly used. Current users had a 1.16-fold increased risk of injury (95% CI = 1.01–1.34; $p = 0.03$). Patients using the medication for a shorter duration (≤60 days) had an increased risk of injury (OR = 1.31; 95% CI 1.01–1.70; $p = 0.04$). Long-term use was not associated with a significant difference, however did show a greater risk.

Eluxadoline

Drug–Drug Interactions, Cyclosporine, Probenecid

A prospective, crossover study was conducted in 30 healthy volunteers to determine the pharmacokinetic effects of cyclosporine, an organic anion transporting polypeptide 1B1 (OATP1B1) and multi-drug resistance-associated protein 2 (MRP2) inhibitor; and probenecid, an organic anion transporter 3(OAT3) and MRP2 inhibitor, on single doses of eluxadoline [44c]. Blood and urine samples were used to assess eluxadoline concentrations after administration alone or in combination with either cyclosporine or probenecid. Cyclosporine-mediated inhibition, primarily through OATP1B1, had larger effects on eluxadoline versus probenecid. The half-life in combination with cyclosporine was 7.4 hours, 5.1 hours in combination with probenecid and 3.7 hours alone. The OATP1B1 inhibition showed increased oral bioavailability and decreased biliary clearance, likely leading to a major systemic drug interaction.

Eluxadoline dose should be reduced if combined with OATP1B1 inhibitors and patient should be monitored for eluxadoline toxicities including constipation, abdominal pain, and mental alertness.

Loperamide [SED-15, 2159; SEDA-37, 450]

Case reports

- A 54-year-old female presented with two previous episodes of syncope and was found to have sinus arrest, slow junctional escape rhythm and recurrent premature ventricular contractions on electrocardiogram (ECG) [45A]. An EKG, coronary angiogram and right heart catheterization were normal. She was treated with amiodarone, lidocaine and a pacemaker was inserted in an attempt to control the ventricular arrhythmias. Cardiopulmonary resuscitation including electrical cardioversion and intubation/mechanical ventilation was used following an episode of polymorphic ventricular tachycardia. Due to diarrhea associated with a cholecystectomy 8 years prior, the patient had been self-treating with loperamide, increasing the dose over time. For 2 years, she was taking nine times the recommended daily dose. An implantable cardioverter defibrillator was implanted for secondary prevention of arrhythmic cardiac death. Two months post-discharge and loperamide discontinuation, no ventricular tachycardia or bradycardia episodes were reported.

- A 25-year-old female, with no significant medical history, presented with a 2-week history of persistent abdominal discomfort [46A]. An ECG showed QTc and corrected QTc interval of 492 and 527 ms, respectively. Two weeks after being treated symptomatically, she returned and her ECG showed QTc and corrected QTc interval of 480 and 490 ms, respectively, as well as an intraventricular conduction defect with QRS interval of 140 ms and nonspecific T wave abnormalities. Long QTc syndrome was diagnosed. A dual-chamber implantable cardioverter defibrillator was implanted. Six weeks later, she developed multiple episodes of non-sustained ventricular tachycardia with wide QRS duration, and frequent polymorphic ventricular tachycardic runs. Multiple bottles of loperamide were found in her apartment and her loperamide concentration was elevated at 32 ng/mL. Two months after discharge with continued loperamide abuse, she died due to cardiopulmonary arrest.
- A 30-year-old male took 25 times the recommended dose of loperamide at 400 mg/day for 1 week, presenting with syncope [47r]. An ECG showed QTc of 704 ms and QRS of 192 ms. Twenty hours after his last 400 mg dose, his loperamide concentration was 120 ng/mL. After 70.5 hours, loperamide concentration was 20 ng/mL. After 13 days, he was discharged with a QRS of 94 ms and QTc/corrected QTc of 406 and 483 ms, respectively.
- A 43-year-old female reported taking 288 mg loperamide. Her QTc was 684 ms and frequent premature ventricular contractions and multiple episodes of torsades de pointe occurred [48A].
- A 28-year-old male taking 792 mg of loperamide daily displayed syncope and ventricular tachycardia. Loperamide concentration was 130 ng/mL (therapeutic range 0.24–1.2 ng/mL) and QTc was 647 ms [48A].

- A 33-year-old male ingested 120–200 mg loperamide in a six hour period, resulting in a concentration of 77 ng/mL and a QTc interval of 636 ms [48A].
- A 33-year-old male ingested 280 mg of loperamide in a 7-hour period and presented with a QTc interval of 490 ms and loperamide concentration of 33 ng/mL [48A].

Loperamide, especially at significantly higher doses than the maximum daily recommended dose (16 mg/day), should be avoided in patients with QTc prolongation. QTc monitoring should be considered in patients with a prolonged QTc at approved doses.

Octreotide

Case reports

- Within the first 20 minutes of life, after urgent caesarean section due to fetal distress, a baby boy developed a seizure and blood glucose was 10 mg/dL [49A]. Continuous intravenous glucose infusion up to 30 mg/kg/minute was given and the patient had high insulin levels (22.9 MU/L). Liver enzymes were elevated at birth. He was diagnosed with congenital hyperinsulinism at 5 days and started on diazoxide, hydrocholorthiazide and continuous intravenous octreotide. By 3 weeks, his liver enzymes normalized, however, by 4 weeks aspartate aminotransferase (AST), alanine aminotransferase (ALT) and serum bilirubin were elevated again. At 45 days of age, AST (643 IU/L), ALT (538 IU/L), direct bilirubin (17 mg/dL) and bilirubin (20.1 mg/dL) were elevated. All reasonable causes of liver injury were excluded and octreotide-induced liver injury was the most likely cause. Treatment was stopped, resulting in decreased bilirubin within 2 days and aminotransferases lowering. All hepatic enzymes had normalized at 3 months.
- A 77-year-old male with inoperable metastatic pancreatic neuroendocrine tumor secreting insulin and gastrin experienced multiple episodes of hypoglycemia [50A].

Insulin levels were elevated (58 mU/L) with plasma glucose levels approximately 2.3 mmol/L. Diazoxide, dexamethasone and subcutaneous octreotide were initiated. Long-acting octreotide (LAR) was started at 20 mg monthly, then 30 mg monthly after frequent episodes of hypoglycemia. One week after dose escalation, the patient experienced unconscious hypoglycemic collapse with plasma glucose levels <1.5 mmol/L. Octreotide LAR was stopped but he continued to have episodes of hypoglycemia warranting 20% dextrose infusions. Blood glucose levels stabilized after two cycles of peptide receptor radionuclide therapy (PRRT). No symptoms of hypoglycemia were reported at 24-month follow-up.

Because octreotide-induced liver injury and hypoglycemia are rare, routine monitoring of AST/ALT and blood glucose would not be recommended.

ANTIEMETIC AGENTS

Netupitant [SEDA-37, 452]

Drug–Drug Interaction, Dexamethasone, Ketoconazole, Rifampin

A randomized, open-label, three-period crossover study assigned patients to oral dexamethasone (20 mg on Day 1; and 8 mg twice daily on Days 2–4) +/− netupitant (100, 300, and 450 mg) on Day 1 [51R]. Netupitant increased dexamethasone exposure in a dose-dependent fashion. The AUC was increased by 48%, 72%, and 75% on Day 1; and by 75%, 140%, and 170% on Day 4 with 100, 300, and 450 mg, respectively. Netupitant exposure was significantly increased (AUC increased 140%) after administration with ketoconazole, a CYP3A4 inhibitor, and significantly decreased (AUC decreased by 83%) after administration with rifampin, a CYP3A4 inducer.

Netupitant dose adjustment may be required with concomitant use of CYP3A4 inhibitors and CYP3A4 inducers. Individual drug combinations should be assessed for concurrent use. Dexamethasone should be reduced by 50% when given with netupitant.

Ondansetron [SED-15, 1365; SEDA-35, 635; SEDA-36, 544; SEDA-37, 453]

Gastrointestinal

A 21-week pregnant 29-year-old female experienced severe nausea and vomiting [52r]. She had been treated for 3 months with varying doses (4–8 mg/day) of ondansetron resulting in intestinal obstruction.

Immunologic

Two episodes of hypersensitivity were observed in a 29-year-old female receiving 8 mg intravenous ondansetron prior to chemotherapy [53A]. The first episode occurred 15 minutes after administration, displaying as vulvovaginal pruritus. The second episode appeared 10 minutes later where she experienced odynophagia with dyspnea and generalized pruritus. Skin testing revealed tolerance to granisetron with cross-reactivity between ondansetron, palonsetron, and tropisetron.

Intestinal obstruction and hypersensitivity reactions are extremely rare with ondansetron, but should not be ruled out if symptoms are consistent with above case reports.

Prochlorperazine [SED-15, 2930]

Case report

• A 10-week pregnant 32-year-old female presented to the emergency department with stroke- like symptoms including sudden-onset slurred speech, left chest, shoulder and neck pain, left arm and leg weakness, and paresthesias [54A]. One day earlier she took oral prochlorperazine, consuming four 10 mg doses, with the last dose one hour prior to symptom onset. Tongue protrusion and rolling consistent with extrapyramidal symptoms. Two episodes occurred responding to intravenous diphenhydramine, suggesting hemidystonia mimicking acute stroke.

Extrapyramidal symptoms (EPS) are more common with increased doses, use with other agents that are likely to cause EPS and younger patients. Patients should be educated on the risk and seek medical attention if symptoms occur.

Promethazine [SED-15, 2938]

Case report

• A 19-year-old male received intramuscular promethazine in his gluteal region for a 5-day history of vomiting, headache, fever and diarrhea [55A]. Five days later, he complained of pain in the area of injection with a new pruritic rash. MRI revealed gluteal soft tissue abscess and was found to have methicillin-sensitive *Staphylococcus aureus* bacteremia.

Treatment of soft tissue abscess caused by promethazine should be treated in the same manner as other skin and soft tissue infections.

Rolapitant

General

Two randomized, placebo-controlled trials with 1087 patients (rolapitant = 544; control = 543) reported the safety of rolapitant 180 mg for prevention of chemotherapy-induced nausea and vomiting in patients receiving moderately or highly emetogenic chemotherapy [56R]. All received granisetron and dexamethasone. A pooled analysis of both trials showed the most common adverse effects were dyspepsia, headache, constipation, and hiccups (<2%). Treatment-emergent adverse effects of grade 3–5 were present and similar in 16% of both groups.

Patients should be educated on most common adverse effects that will resolve upon discontinuation of the drug if bothersome.

ANTIINFLAMMATORY AGENTS

6-Mercaptopurine [SED-15, 377; SEDA-37, 455]

Endocrine, Pancreatitis

A review on thiopurine-induced pancreatitis (TIP) showed an incidence of 3.25% in 400 patients treated for inflammatory bowel disease (IBD) [57r]. Onset of symptoms ranged from 8 to 32 days with elevated serum amylase levels. Hospitalization was required in 57%. Similar findings were found in Spain, with 3.1% of a cohort from nine hospitals showing TIP with symptom onset within 35 days. Female gender was a risk factor for developing TIP (OR 3.4, 95% CI 1.3–9.3).

Aminosalicylates [SED-15, 138; SEDA-35, 647; SEDA-36, 555; SEDA-37, 454]

A meta-analysis examined the risk of lymphoma in patients with IBD who were treated with azathioprine and 6-mercaptopurine [58M]. A prior meta-analysis was updated to include an additional seven population-based studies, five referral center studies and an update on one population-based study. Studies included those specifically evaluating cancer as an adverse outcome in IBD patients who had received azathioprine or 6-mercaptopurine. Ten referral center studies and eight population-based studies were included. There were 93 cases of lymphoma with a standardized incidence ratio (SIR) of 4.92 (95% CI, 3.10–7.78). Current users were at an increased risk (SIR = 5.71). Patients aged 0–29 had the highest risk (SIR = 6.99). Onset of lymphoma was highest in those with 1–2 years of exposure (SIR 4.31, 95% CI, 1.85–10.1) and >3 years exposure (SIR 4.84, 95% CI, 2.88–8.11).

Case report

• A 23-year-old male with ulcerative colitis was initiated on 5-aminosalicylate (5-ASA) 3000 mg/day [59A]. Due to flares of his bowel disease, the dose was increased to 4500 mg/day. Routine lab work revealed a twofold serum creatinine increase from baseline (2 mg/dL), but was attributed to diarrhea, dehydration and inflammatory bowel disease. His serum creatinine rose to 4 mg/dL 7 months later when he was in clinical remission. Urinary output was normal and he reported no other symptoms. Kidney biopsy revealed chronic tubulointerstitial nephritis. He was treated and 5-ASA was stopped. Two years later his renal function was stable.

Azathioprine [SED-15, 377; SEDA-36, 555]

Endocrine, Pancreatitis

A prospective cohort study of first prescription data was conducted to determine the incidence of azathioprine-induced acute pancreatitis [60C]. There were 510 patients analyzed, with 7.25% experiencing azathioprine-induced acute pancreatitis ($p < 0.00001$). Median duration of exposure was 21 days. Only 43% of patients required hospitalization. No statistical difference was seen in the incidence experienced in patients with Crohn's disease (8.6%) versus ulcerative colitis (3.2%) ($p = 0.055$). Smoking was a significant risk factor (OR = 3.24; 95% CI = 1.74–6.02; $p = 0.0002$) and incidence was shown to be increased by 2.8 times for those who smoked >3 packs/week ($p = 0.021$). Nausea was the most frequently reported adverse effect (12.2%) leading to medication discontinuation.

Adverse effects from azathioprine in pediatric patients ($n = 82$) treated for atopic dermatitis were reviewed [61c]. Clinical adverse events were seen in 20% of patients. Most common adverse effects were cutaneous viral infections (12%). Laboratory abnormalities were also observed, with 40% of patients having adverse effects on blood indices (hepatic transaminases >50 U/L, leukocyte count $<4.0 \times 10^9$/L, lymphocytes $<1.0 \times 10^9$/L, and neutrophils $<1.0 \times 10^9$/L), including 29% involving CBC, 13% involving liver transaminases and 2.5% involving both. Therapy discontinuation occurred in 6% of patients. Timing of adverse effects was towards the beginning of treatment or after dosage increases.

Case reports

• A 57-year-old male on azathioprine 100 mg daily for 80 days for Crohn's disease was increased to 450 mg daily 1 day prior to presenting with fevers, chills and myalgia [62A]. Elevated WBC count and chest X-ray were concerning for infectious etiology. Post-discharge, he resumed azathioprine and five hours later reported the same symptoms with the addition of arthralgia in both ankles and knees. Due to elevated WBC count and fever, it was determined to be infectious. The day after the second admission and within 5 hours of resuming azathioprine, he experienced the same symptoms plus erythematous papular rash on the back and knees. After three admissions in a 9-day period, symptoms were attributed to azathioprine hypersensitivity.

• A 42-year-old female with a 5-year history of rheumatoid arthritis received treatment with rituximab and azathioprine achieving a complete response [63A]. Three months after initiating azathioprine, she developed a cough and subcutaneous nodules on her right leg. Biopsy confirmed subcutaneous rheumatoid nodules which disappeared 2 months after discontinuation of azathioprine.

Mesalamine

Case report

- A 31-year-old healthy male developed progressive and severe cardiomyopathy leading to cardiogenic shock 3 days after initiation of mesalamine 2.4 g twice daily [64A]. He presented with chest pain, elevated troponin and increased inflammatory markers. He suffered a cerebrovascular event exhibiting signs of acute right hemiplegia, right facial droop and dysarthria. Multiple acute and deep white matter infarcts were seen. Rapid improvement seen with discontinuation of mesalamine led to a diagnosis of mesalamine-induced cardiomyopathy, even though rapid onset is not typical.

Sulfasalazine

Case reports

- A 28-year-old male was initiated on sulfasalazine (500 mg three times daily) for ankle joint arthritis 13 days prior to presenting to the emergency department with fever, facial and neck edema, erythematous rash, cervical lymphadenopathy, shortness of breath and malaise [65A]. Since childhood, he had episodes of periodic fever syndrome where he experienced fever and lymphadenopathy. The patient progressed to cardiogenic shock and died eight hours later. Autopsy revealed cause of death to be acute heart failure due to eosinophilic myocarditis secondary to sulfasalazine.
- A 25-year-old male taking sulfasalazine (4 g daily) for ulcerative colitis developed DRESS (drug reaction with eosinophilia and systemic symptoms) and agranulocytosis within 8 weeks of initiation [66A]. He discontinued sulfasalazine after development of eruptions and facial edema. One week later, he presented with a temperature of 40 °C and diffuse skin desquamation on face and trunk. Upon hospitalization, his white blood cell count was 1×10^9/L and dropped to 0.1×10^9/L 48 hours later. Colony stimulating factor was initiated and continued for 3 days until his neutrophil count increased to 2.2×10^9/L.

Thiopurines [SEDA-37, 455]

A retrospective chart review including 351 patients with current or previous azathioprine or 6-mercaptopurine use was analyzed over a median follow-up duration of 5.8 years to determine the first adverse effect that led to the discontinuation [67C]. Hypersensitivity (7.1%) and pancreatitis (6.2%) were the most common adverse effects with a median time to discontinuation of 31 and 29 days, respectively, followed by gastrointestinal toxicity (5.4%), leukopenia (3.7%), hepatotoxicity (3.4%) and infection (1.1%). Age and sex were predictive factors of adverse effects with patients over 40 years old at time of initiation more likely to discontinue the medication ($p = 0.007$). Patients over 40 years old and female had a 2.8-fold increased risk of discontinuing due to an adverse effect (95% CI 1.4–5.6).

Benefits of antiinflammatory agents generally outweigh the potential risks. In patients experiencing pancreatitis, it is generally mild and the use of another thiopurine can be considered. The absolute risk of lymphoma is relatively low, but should be strongly cautioned in patients with a history of lymphoma. For patients experiencing hypersensitivity reactions, the offending agent should be immediately withdrawn and not resumed.

ANTICHOLINERGIC AGENTS

Glycopyrrolate

Case report

- A 22-year-old female scheduled to undergo laparotomy for ovarian cyst removal was premedicated with ondansetron 4 mg IV and glycopyrrolate 0.2 mg IV [68A]. The patient's SpO2 began to decline, followed by shallow breathing within the first minute of administration. She went into respiratory arrest, requiring 100% oxygen. Heart rate increased to 110 beats/minute, blood pressure was 140/90 mmHg and developed sinus tachycardia. Intubation occurred after 5 minutes of receiving mask ventilation. Her respiratory arrest was most likely attributable to glycopyrrolate due to an increase in heart rate, as opposed to bradycardia which is generally seen with respiratory arrest due to ondansetron.

  Caution should be used when administering glycopyrrolate IV for respiratory arrest. No specific recommendations are noted.

Scopolamine

Case report

- A 62-year-old female developed scopolamine withdrawal syndrome on multiple occasions after transdermal scopolamine use for prevention of motion sickness [69A]. When worn less than 2 days behind the ear and removed, she experienced no adverse effects.

On two occasions, she experienced dizziness, drowsiness, sweating, fatigue and nausea after wearing the patch for greater than 2 days, up to 7 days. Symptoms began 24–36 hours after removal. One month later, she wore the scopolamine patch for 7 days and 24 hours after removal experienced pronounced drowsiness and malaise, severe asthenia, inability to stand, and hypotension (systolic blood pressure <100 mmHg) requiring midodrine. Her symptoms dissipated after several days. In rat models, chronic use of scopolamine leads to increased density and sensitivity of muscarinic receptors, and is one possible mechanism of her withdrawal symptoms.

Transdermal scopolamine patch is extensively used and reports of withdrawal are not reported. Patients with chronic use of scopolamine may be at an increased risk.

MISCELLANEOUS AGENTS

Misoprostol [SED-15, 2357]

Cardiovascular

There have been 63 reported cardiovascular and neurologic events in patients treated with misoprostol (22 cases of myocardial infarction, 19 cases of angina, 14 cases of stroke and 3 cases of TIA) [70r]. Patients potentially at increased risk include those who are administered misoprostol vaginally due to the increased bioavailability, as well as risk factors for cardiovascular disease. Of the six myocardial infarction cases, four occurred in smokers using 800 mcg intravaginally.

A prospective, randomized trial comparing oral, sublingual and vaginal misoprostol in first and second trimester abortions in 150 women showed similar adverse effect profiles except for fever and diarrhea [71C]. Females who received sublingual, vaginal, and oral misoprostol experienced fever at rates of 24%, 36% and 12%, respectively ($p = 0.019$). Significant difference was shown between vaginal and oral administration, with vaginal administration being significantly higher ($p = 0.005$). Vaginal administration had the lowest rate (6%) of diarrhea compared to sublingual (22%) and oral (28%); $p = 0.014$.

Misoprostol should be used with caution in patients with cardiovascular disease, especially those who are current smokers.

Orlistat

Case report

- A 54-year-old male with a body mass index of 31 on orlistat for 7 days presented to the emergency department with abdominal pain, nausea and vomiting that had lasted for 24 hours [72A].

Abdominal CT showed peripancreatic fat tissue edema and heterogenous pancreatic appearance. Serum amylase was significantly elevated (2409 U/L), C-reactive protein = 136 mg/L, and lactate dehydrogenase = 835 U/L. The patient was determined to be in the initial stages of edematous pancreatitis. Unlike a previous case of orlistat-induced pancreatitis in which serum amylase levels were not elevated, they were markedly increased in this patient.

Development of severe abdominal pain with use of orlistat should lead to a consideration of pancreatitis, prompting appropriate imaging and laboratory studies. Risk may be increased in patients with other risk factors for acute pancreatitis including alcohol use and high triglyceride levels.

BIOLOGICS

See Chapter 36 for further information.

STEROIDS

See Chapter 38 for further information.

References

[1] Cohen S, Bueno de Mesquita M, Mimouni FB. Adverse effects reported in the use of gastroesophageal reflux disease treatments in children: a 10 years literature review. Br J Clin Pharmacol. 2015;80(2):200–8 [M].

[2] Banihani SA. Histamine-2 receptor antagonists and semen quality. Basic Clin Pharmacol Toxicol. 2016;118(1):9–13 [R].

[3] Poudel RR, Kafle NK. Tizanidine-induced acute severe cystitis in a female taking famotidine. Clin Pharmacol. 2015;7:83–5 [A].

[4] Shah NH, LePendu P, Aauer-Mehren A, et al. Proton pump inhibitor usage and the risk of myocardial infarction in the general population. PLoS One. 2015;10(6):e0124653. http://dx.doi.org/10.1371/journal [MC].

[5] Turkiewicz A, Vicente RP, Ohlsson H, et al. Revising the link between proton-pump inhibitors and risk of acute myocardial infarction—a case-crossover analysis. Eur J Clin Pharmacol. 2015;71:125–9 [MC].

[6] Akinseye OA, Alfishawy M, Radparvar F, et al. Trazodone and omeprazole interaction causing frequent second-degree Mobitz type 1 atrioventricular (AV) block (Wenckebach Phenomenon) and syncope: a case report and literature review. Am J Case Rep. 2015;16:319–21 [A].

[7] Liang JF, Chen YT, Fuh JL, et al. Proton pump inhibitor-related headaches: a nationwide population-based case-crossover study in Taiwan. Cephalalgia. 2015;35(3):203–10 [MC].

[8] Pipaliya N, Solanke D, Rathi C, et al. Esomeprazole induced galactorrhea: a novel side effect. Clin J Gastroenterol. 2016;9(1):13–6 [A].

[9] Kieboom BCT, Kiefte-de Jong JC, Eijgelsheim M, et al. Proton pump inhibitors and hypomagnesemia in the general population: a population-based cohort study. Am J Kidney Dis. 2015;66(5):775–82 [MC].

[10] Pastorino A, Greppi F, Bergamo D, et al. Proton pump inhibitors and hypomagnesemia in polymorbid elderly adults. J Am Geriatr Soc. 2015;63(1):179–80 [r].

[11] Kallam A, Singla A, Silberstein P. Proton pump induced thrombocytopenia: a case report and review of the literature. Platelets. 2015;26(6):598–601 [A].

[12] Sieczkowska A, Landowski P, Zagozdzon P, et al. Small bowel overgrowth associated with persistence of abdominal symptoms in children treated with a proton pump inhibitor. J Pediatr. 2015;166(5):1310–2 [c].

[13] Parks T, Ragland KL, Subramony C, et al. Menetrier Mimicker complicating ulcerative colitis: proton-pump inhibitor-induced hyperplastic polyps. J Pediatr. 2015;167:776 [A].

[14] Dultz G, Piiper A, Zeuzem B, et al. Proton pump inhibitor treatment associated with the severity of liver disease and increased mortality in patients with cirrhosis. Aliment Pharmacol Ther. 2015;41:459–66 [C].

[15] Wang YP, Liu CJ, Chen TH, et al. Proton pump use significantly increases the risk of cryptogenic liver abscess: a population-based study. Aliment Pharmacol Ther. 2015;41:1175–81 [C].

[16] Cohen PR. Proton pump inhibitor-induced Sweet's syndrome: report of acute febrile neutrophilic dermatosis in a woman with recurrent breast cancer. Dermatol Pract Concept. 2015;5(2):113–9. 23. [A].

[17] Bahtiri E, Islami H, Hoxha R, et al. Esomeprazole use is independently associated with significant reduction of BMD: 1-year prospective comparative safety study of four proton pump inhibitors. J Bone Miner Metabol. 2016;34(5):571–9. http://dx.doi.org/10.1007/s00774-015-0699-6 [C].

[18] Ho SW, Yang SF, Yeh YT, et al. Risk of stroke-associated pneumonia with acid-suppressive drugs: a population-based cohort study. Medicine. 2015;94(29):e1227 [MC].

[19] Chen CH, Lin HC, Lin HL, et al. Proton pump inhibitor usage and the associated risk of pneumonia in patients with chronic kidney disease. J Microbiol Immunol Infect. 2015;48:390–6 [C].

[20] Merli M, Lucidi C, Di Gregorio V, et al. The chronic use of beta-blockers and proton pump inhibitors may affect the rate of bacterial infections in cirrhosis. Liver Int. 2015;35:362–9 [C].

[21] McDonald EG, Milligan J, Frenette C, et al. Continuous proton pump inhibitor therapy and the associated risk of recurrent Clostridium difficile infection. JAMA Intern Med. 2015;175(5):784–91 [C].

[22] Wang JY, Chen M, Zhu LL, et al. Pharmacokinetic drug interactions with clopidogrel: updated review and risk management in combination therapy. Ther Clin Risk Manag. 2015;11:449–67 [R].

[23] Cardoso RN, Benjo AM, DiNicolantonio JJ, et al. Incidence of cardiovascular events and gastrointestinal bleeding in patients receiving clopidogrel with and without proton pump inhibitors: an updated meta-analysis. Open Heart. 2015;2:e000248. http://dx.doi.org/10.1136/openht-2015-000248 [M].

[24] Leonard CE, Bilker WB, Brensinger CM, et al. Comparative risk of ischemic stroke among users of clopidogrel together with individual proton pump inhibitors. Stroke. 2015;46:722–31 [C].

[25] Melloni C, Washam JB, Jones WS, et al. Conflicting results between randomized trials and observational studies on the impact of proton pump inhibitors on cardiovascular events when coadministered with dual antiplatelet therapy: systematic review. Circ Cardiovasc Qual Outcomes. 2015;8:47–55 [M].

[26] Sherwood MW, Melloni C, Jones WS. Individual proton pump inhibitors and outcomes in patients with coronary artery disease on dual antiplatelet therapy: a systematic review. J Am Heart Assoc. 2015;4:e002245. http://dx.doi.org/10.1161/JAHA.115.002245 [M].

[27] Suzuki Y, Suzuki H, Umetsu R, et al. Analysis of the interaction between clopidogrel, aspirin, and proton pump inhibitors using the FDA Adverse Event Reporting System Database. Biol Pharm Bull. 2015;38:680–6 [C].

[28] Weisz G, Smilowitz NR, Kirtane AJ. Proton pump inhibitors, platelet reactivity, and cardiovascular outcomes after drug-eluting stents in clopidogrel-treated patients—the ADAPT-DES study. Circ Cardiovasc Interv. 2015;8:e001952. http://dx.doi.org/10.1161/CIRCINTERVENTIONS.114.001952 [MC].

[29] Chu MP, Ghosh S, Chambers CR, et al. Gastric acid suppression is associated with decreased erlotinib efficacy in non-small cell lung cancer. Clin Lung Cancer. 2015;16(1):33–9 [C].

[30] Iniesta-Navalon C, Franco-Miguel JJ, Gascon-Canovas JJ, et al. Identification of potential clinically significant drug interactions in HIV-infected patients: a comprehensive therapeutic approach. HIV Med. 2015;16:273–9 [c].

[31] Gjestad C, Westin AA, Skogvoll E, et al. Effect of proton pump inhibitors on the serum concentrations of the selective serotonin reuptake inhibitors citalopram, escitalopram, and sertraline. Ther Drug Monit. 2015;37:90–7 [C].

[32] Cojutti P, Candoni A, Forghieri F, et al. Variability of voriconazole trough levels in haematological patients: influence of comedications with cytochrome P450 (CYP) inhibitors and/or with CYP inhibitors plus CYP inducers. Basic Clin Pharmacol Toxicol. 2016;118(6):474–9. http://dx.doi.org/10.1111/bcpt.12530 [c].

[33] Hata M, Shiono M, Akiyama K, et al. Incidence of drug interaction when using proton pump inhibitor and warfarin according to cytochrome P450 2C19 (CYP2C19) genotype in Japanese. Thorac Cardiovasc Surg. 2015;63:45–50 [c].

[34] Youssef AS, Parkman HP, Nagar S. Drug-drug interactions in pharmacologic management of gastroparesis. Neurogastroenterol Motil. 2015;27:1528–41 [R].

[35] Sachdeva A, Rathee R. Akathisia with erythromycin: induced or precipitated? Saudi Pharm J. 2015;23:541–3 [A].

[36] Cavero-Redondo I, Alvarez-Bueno C, Pozuelo-Carrascosa DP, et al. Risk of extrapyramidal side effects comparing continuous vs bolus intravenous metoclopramide administration: a systematic review and meta-analysis of randomized controlled trials. J Clin Nurs. 2015;24:3638–46 [M].

[37] Leus M, van de Ven A. An acute dystonic reaction after treatment with metoclopramide. N Engl J Med. 2015;373(14):e16 [A].

[38] Immovilli P, Rota E, Morelli N, et al. Metoclopramide-induced facial and platopharyngeal myoclonus. Neurology. 2015;84:1284 [A].

[39] Al-Shaer MH, Mustafa MS, Scalese MJ. Metoclopramide-induced asystolic cardiac arrest. Ann Pharmacother. 2015;49(5):610–1 [A].

[40] Hjort M, Groth-Heoberg LC, Almind M, et al. Subacute fat-embolism-like syndrome following high-volume intramuscular and accidental intravascular injection of mineral oil. Clin Toxicol. 2015;53(4):230–2 [A].

[41] Lee SH, Cha JM, Lee J, et al. Anaphylactic shock caused by ingestion of polyethylene glycol. Intest Res. 2015;13(1):90–4 [A].

[42] Zhang H, Henry WA, Chen LA, et al. Urticaria due to polyethylene glycol-3350 and electrolytes for oral solution in a patient with jejunal nodular lymphoid hyperplasia. Ann Gastroenterol. 2015;28:148–50 [A].

[43] Spence MM, Karim FA, Lee EA, et al. Risk of injury in older adults using gastrointestinal antispasmodic and anticholinergic medications. J Am Geriatr Soc. 2015;63:1197–202 [C].

[44] Davenport JM, Convington P, Bonifacio L, et al. Effect of uptake transporters OAT3 and OATP1B1 and efflux transporter MRP2 on the pharmacokinetics of eluxadoline. J Clin Pharmacol. 2015;S5(5):S34–42 [c].

[45] Spinner HL, Lonardo NW, Mulamalla R, et al. Ventricular tachycardia associated with high-dose chronic loperamide use. Pharmacotherapy. 2015;35(2):234–8 [A].

[46] Enakpene EO, Riaz I, Shirazi FM, et al. The long QT teaser: loperamide abuse. Am J Med. 2015;128(10):1083–6 [A].

[47] Eggleston W, Nacca N, Marraffa JM. Loperamide toxicokinetics: serum concentrations in the overdose setting. Clin Toxicol. 2015;53:495–6 [r].

[48] Mancano MA. ISMP adverse drug reactions. Hosp Pharm. 2015;50(5):351–5 [A].

[49] Levy-Khademi F, Irna S, Avnon-Ziv C, et al. Octreotide-associated cholestasis and hepatitis in an infant with congenital hyperinsulinism. J Pediatr Endocrinol Metab. 2015;28(3-4): 449–51 [A].

[50] Abell SK, Teng J, Dowling A, et al. Prolonged life-threatening hypoglycaemia following dose escalation of octreotide LAR in a patient with malignant polysecreting pancreatic neuroendocrine tumour. Endocrinol Diabetes Metab Case Rep. 2015;140097. http://dx.doi.org/10.1530/EDM-14-0097 [A].

[51] Natale JJ, Spinelli T, Calcagnile S, et al. Drug-drug interaction profile of components of a fixed combination of netupitant and palonosetron: review of clinical data. J Oncol Pharm Pract. 2015;22(3):485–95 [R].

[52] Fejzo MS, MacGibbon K, Mullen P. Intestinal obstruction is a rare complication of ondansetron exposure in hyperemesis gravidarum. Reprod Toxicol. 2015;57:207 [r].

[53] Nunez G, Mamol A, Ariza R. Ondansetron hypersensitivity: a clinical diagnosis protocol and cross-reactivity study. J Investig Allergol Clin Immunol. 2015;25(3):214–36 [A].

[54] Coralic Z, Kim AS, Vinson DR. Prochlorperazine-induced hemidystonia mimicking acute stroke. West J Emerg Med. 2015;16(4):572–4 [A].

[55] Snyder LTS, Letizia A, Hartzell J. Gluteal abscess and bacteremia following promethazine injection in a Marine. Mil Med. 2015;180(6):e732–4 [A].

[56] Rapoport BL, Chasen MR, Gridelli C, et al. Safety and efficacy of rolapitant for prevention of chemotherapy-induced nausea and vomiting after administration of cisplatin-based highly emetogenic chemotherapy in patients with cancer: two randomized, active-controlled, double-blind, phase 3 trials. Lancet. 2015;16:1079–89 [R].

[57] Ledder O, Lemberg DA, Day AS. Thiopurine-induced pancreatitis in inflammatory bowel diseases. Expert Rev Gastroenterol Hepatol. 2015;9(4):399–403 [r].

[58] Kotylar DS, Lewis JD, Beaugerie L, et al. Risk of lymphoma in patients with inflammatory bowel disease treated with azathioprine and 6-mercaptopurine: a meta-analysis. Clin Gastroenterol Hepatol. 2015;13:847–58 [M].

[59] Magalhaes-Costa P, Matos L, Chagas C. Chronic tubulointerstitial nephritis induced by 5-aminosalicylate in an ulcerative colitis

patient: a rare but serious adverse event. BMJ Case Rep. 2015; http://dx.doi.org/10.1136/bcr-2014-207928 [A].

[60] Teich N, Mohl W, Bokemeyer B, et al. Azathioprine-induced acute pancreatitis in patients with inflammatory bowel disease-a prospective study on incidence and severity. J Crohn's Colitis. 2015;10(1):61–8 [C].

[61] Fuggle NR, Bragoli W, Mech B, et al. The adverse effect profile of oral azathioprine in pediatric atopic dermatitis, and recommendations for monitoring. J Am Acad Dermatol. 2015;72(1):108–14 [c].

[62] Mookherjee S, Narayanan M, Uchiyama T, et al. Three hospital admissions in 9 days to diagnose azathioprine hypersensitivity in a patient with Crohn's disease. Am J Ther. 2015;22:e28–32 [A].

[63] Vera Kellet C, Gonzalez Bombardieri S, Andino Navarrete R, et al. Azathioprine-induced accelerated cutaneous and pulmonary nodulosis in a patient with rheumatoid arthritis. An Bras Dermatol. 2015;90(3 Suppl 1):S162–4 [A].

[64] Fleming K, Ashcroft A, Alexakis C, et al. Proposed case of mesalazine-induced cardiomyopathy in severe ulcerative colitis. World J Gastroenterol. 2015;21(11):3376–9 [A].

[65] Jeremic I, Vujasinovic-Stupar N, Terzic T, et al. Fatal sulfasalazine-induced eosinophilic myocarditis in a patient with periodic fever syndrome. Med Princ Pract. 2015;24:195–7 [A].

[66] Fathallah N, Slim R, Rached S, et al. Sulfasalazine-induced DRESS and severe agranulocytosis successfully treated by granulocyte colony-stimulating factor. Int J Clin Pharm. 2015;37:563–5 [A].

[67] Moran GW, Dubeau MF, Kaplan GG, et al. Clinical predictors of thiopurine-related adverse events in Crohn's disease. World J Gastroenterol. 2015;21(25):7795–804 [C].

[68] D'souza S, Gowler V. Glycopyrrolate-induced respiratory arrest: an unusual side effect. Acta Anaesthesiol Scand. 2015;29:406–7 [A].

[69] Manno M, Di Renzo G, Bianco P, et al. Unique scopolamine withdrawal syndrome after standard transdermal use. Clin Neuropharmacol. 2015;38(5):204–5 [A].

[70] Anonymous. Misoprostol: serious cardiovascular events, even after a single dose. Rev Prescrire. 2015;35(376):108–10 [r].

[71] Deepika N, Krishna M, Inderjeet P, et al. Comparative study of misoprostol in first and second trimester abortions by oral, sublingual, and vaginal routes. J Obstet Gynecol India. 2015;65(4):246–50 [C].

[72] Kose M, Emet S, Akpinar TS, et al. An unexpected result of obesity treatment: orlistat-related acute pancreatitis. Case Rep Gatroenterol. 2015;9:152–5 [A].

35

Drugs That Act on the Immune System: Cytokines and Monoclonal Antibodies

Tristan Lindfelt[1]

Department of Clinical Sciences, Touro University California College of Pharmacy, Vallejo, CA, USA
[1]Corresponding author: tristan.lindfelt@tu.edu

CYTOKINES

Bone Morphogenetic Proteins [SEDA-35, 659; SEDA-36, 561; SEDA-37, 461]

RESPIRATORY AND MUSCULOSKELETAL

In a retrospective chart review of 37 patients who underwent a 3-level anterior cervical discectomy and fusion, rh-BMP2 at low doses (0.26–0.35 mg/level) did not cause complications due to airway or cervical swelling or hematoma formation [1c].

Colony-Stimulating Factors [SEDA-35, 659; SEDA-36, 563; SEDA-37, 461]

Filgrastim-sndz

Filgrastim-sndz is the first biosimilar approved by the United States Food and Drug Administration. It was approved in March 2015. It has already been in use in Europe for several years.

OBSERVATIONAL STUDY

A multi-center, international, prospective, observational, open-label study of the use of filgrastim-sndz was conducted to determine the safety and efficacy of this biosimilar. A total of 1496 patients enrolled in this trial with various cancer diagnoses although a majority (77.2%) had a solid tumor. All patients were treated with myelosuppressive chemotherapy. The adverse effect profile was similar to what has been seen with filgrastim in the past. Bone pain was the most common adverse effect and was reported by 24.7% of patients. Four serious adverse events occurred during the course of the study and included bone pain, drug hypersensitivity, vulval abscesses and loss of consciousness. None of the 61 deaths occurring during the study period were attributed to filgrastim-sndz or neutropenia [2c].

Thrombopoietin Agonists [SEDA-36, 568]

Eltrombopag

OBSERVATIONAL STUDY

In a study designed to determine the safety and efficacy of eltrombopag in children with chronic immune thrombocytopenia, 92 subjects were randomized in a 2:1 ratio to receive eltrombopag or placebo. Eltrombopag doses were weight-based. Five patients in the eltrombopag-treated group experienced serious adverse events including gingivitis ($n=1$), influenza ($n=1$), aseptic meningitis ($n=1$), pneumonia ($n=1$) and fungal pneumonia ($n=1$) [3c].

CARDIOVASCULAR

Two cases of myocardial infarctions (MI) in a patient receiving eltrombopag for HIV-associated immune thrombocytopenic purpura (ITP) were reported. The first patient was a 43-year-old African American female with chronic heart failure, coronary artery disease and morbid obesity in addition to HIV. She developed an ST-elevation MI after taking eltrombopag 50 mg daily for 12 months. Following angioplasty and stent replacement, she was re-started on eltrombopag and 5 months later died from complications due to a second MI [4A]. In other case report, a 53-year-old male with ITP for the past 30 years presented with an ST-elevation MI. He had started eltrombopag 50 mg per day 2 months prior to the MI and had no other risk factors for coronary artery disease [5A].

Romiplostim

CARDIOVASCULAR

A case of presumed pulmonary embolism (PE) was reported in a 32-year-old Caucasian male patient with HIV-associated ITP. The patient used romiplostim 2–3 mcg/kg weekly prior to lumbar surgery. The patient died one day post-procedure. The PE was not confirmed by autopsy [4A].

Interferons [SEDA-35, 660; SEDA-36, 564; SEDA-37, 461]

Interferon Alpha [SEDA-35, 660; SEDA-36, 564; SEDA-37, 461]

IMMUNOLOGIC

A case of protracted anaphylaxis was reported in a 61-year-old Japanese male receiving pegylated interferon alpha for the treatment of chronic hepatitis C. Patient had a past medical history of hypertension and diabetes mellitus. A skin prick test with undiluted pegylated interferon alfa-2a was given and tolerated well. The patient was then given an injection of 180 mcg in their upper arm. One hour and 20 minutes later, the patient developed itching, fever, hypotension and loss of consciousness. His blood pressure decreased to 66/48 mm Hg and his oxygen saturation on room air fell to 88%. He was given intramuscular epinephrine 0.5 mg, intravenous chlorpheniramine 5 mg and intravenous hydrocortisone 200 mg and recovered. Three hours after the pegylated interferon alfa-2a dose, the symptoms returned and the patient was given additional doses of epinephrine and hydrocortisone and oxygen 10 L/minute was initiated. Patient had edematous changes in the small intestine mucosa and mild swelling of the larynx. Five hours following the pegylated interferon alfa-2a administration, patients' symptoms of anaphylaxis returned again. Patient was given a third dose of epinephrine and intravenous methylprednisolone. He remained on oxygen for 15 hours and signs of erythema resolved at 24 hours post-pegylated interferon alfa-2a. Pegylated interferon alfa-2a was discontinued. Previous reported cases of anaphylaxis due to interferon alfa-2a were monophasic and not protracted as in this case [6A].

Interferon Beta [SEDA-35, 664; SEDA-36, 566; SEDA-37, 462]

IMMUNOLOGIC

A 45-year-old female with a history of multiple sclerosis presented with acute febrile neutrophilic dermatosis, Sweet's syndrome, one day following an interferon beta-1b subcutaneous injection. She presented with widespread, painful erythematous papules and pustules and fever. The interferon was discontinued and patient received oral methylprednisolone. The symptoms resolved [7A].

SENSORY SYSTEMS—EYES

A 49-year-old female with a history of multiple sclerosis received interferon beta-1a 44 mcg subcutaneously three times weekly for 4 years. An ocular exam showed intraretinal hemorrhages in the periphery of both eyes. The patient was asymptomatic [8A].

INTERLEUKINS [SEDA-35, 665; SEDA-36, 567; SEDA-37, 462]

Interleukin-2 (Aldesleukin) [SEDA-35, 665; SEDA-36, 567]

GASTROINTESTINAL

A 1½-year-old experienced enterocolitis following treatment with interleukin-2, dinutuximab and isotretinoin. The patient was initially admitted for treatment of localized stage 3 N Myc-amplified neuroblastoma. The patient received chemotherapy followed by a hematopoietic stem cell transplant. Eighty days post-transplant, the patient received radiation and began therapy with interleukin-2, dinutuximab and isotretinoin. The patient developed abdominal distension, fever, and diarrhea followed by hypotensive shock and disseminated intravascular coagulation on the third day of this treatment regimen. On CT scan, enterocolitis was diagnosed. Interleukin-2 and dinutuximab were discontinued and isotretinoin was maintained. The patient underwent colonic resection 2 months later. Authors report this adverse effect was likely due to interleukin-2 or dinutuximab [9A].

Anakinra (Interleukin-1 Receptor Antagonist) [SEDA-35, 665; SEDA-37, 462]

INFECTION RISK

A case of tuberculosis pyomyositis was reported in an 85-year-old Caucasian male receiving therapy with anakinra and steroids for rheumatoid arthritis. The patient presented with a fever, redness, swelling and induration on lateral side of hip and thigh. Tuberculosis pyomyositis was confirmed by culture. The patient initiated therapy for tuberculosis. The patient was not tested for tuberculosis prior to starting therapy with anakinra and steroids [10A].

TUMOR NECROSIS FACTOR ALFA (TNF-α) ANTAGONISTS [SEDA-35, 666; SEDA-36, 568; SEDA-37, 462]

SKIN

Three patients developed amicrobial pustulosis after receiving treatment with tumor necrosis factor alfa antagonists for inflammatory bowel disease. One patient developed this after 6 months of therapy with adalimumab and two patients after 9 months of treatment with infliximab. Epidermal spongiform pustules with dermal neutrophilic and lymphocytic infiltrate were found in the patients' skin folds, genital regions and scalp. The tumor necrosis factor alfa antagonists were discontinued and all patients experienced resolution following treatment with steroids [11A].

Adalimumab [SEDA-35, 669; SEDA-36, 568; SEDA-37, 462]

SENSORY SYSTEMS—EYES

Peripheral corneal infiltrates with features of immune infiltrates developed in a 34-year-old Caucasian woman with Crohn's disease after 4 years of adalimumab treatment. She developed red eyes 36 hours following a dose of adalimumab. She was treated with topical dexamethasone and the infiltrates resolved. Upon re-challenge with adalimumab, the corneal infiltrates returned [12A].

SKIN

A 75-year-old African American woman with grey-white hair experienced hair re-pigmentation after 4 months of therapy with adalimumab for rheumatoid arthritis. Dark brown-black hairs were observed on the posterior occipital, lateral, parietal and frontal scalp regions. She denied use of any cosmetic or topical products that could have led to re-pigmentation. Therapy with adalimumab was not discontinued but the patient later changed to golimumab due to decreased efficacy [13A].

INFECTION RISK

A case of Majocchi's granuloma, a dermatophyte infection, was reported in a 43-year-old Taiwanese male with a history of plaque psoriasis. The patient developed numerous tender nodules 1 month after beginning standard-dose adalimumab. He was initially treated for bacterial folliculitis with no success. Skin biopsies and fungal culture were performed and confirmed the diagnosis of Majocchi's granuloma. The patient underwent treatment with terbinafine for 12 weeks and the lesions improved [14A].

A 46-year-old female with a 20-year history of rheumatoid arthritis developed scabies 5 days after receiving her second dose of adalimumab. Adalimumab was discontinued and a skin hypersensitivity reaction was suspected. However, the skin lesions did not heal after more than 2 months despite the discontinuation of adalimumab and treatment with steroids and an antihistamine. Scabies was diagnosed and resolved after several treatments with 10% crotamiton. Adalimumab was re-started without issue [15A].

SEXUAL FUNCTION

A case of prolonged priapism was reported in a 58-year-old Hispanic male after receiving his first dose of adalimumab for sero-positive erosive rheumatoid arthritis. The erection lasted for 17 days despite urologic interventions [16A].

Etanercept [SEDA-35, 669; SEDA-37, 463]

HEMATOLOGIC

A 47-year-old female with a 20-year history of rheumatoid arthritis developed small bruises and a hematoma after 11 months of therapy with etanercept 50 mg weekly. Her aPTT was 2.48 and an anti-factor VIII antibody was detected. She was diagnosed with acquired hemophilia [17A].

Infliximab [SEDA-35, 672; SEDA-36, 575; SEDA-37, 464]

NERVOUS SYSTEM

A 43-year-old woman with a 12-year history of ulcerative colitis presented for care complaining of a 3-day history of diplopia and a mild headache. Her ulcerative colitis had been treated with azathioprine and then methotrexate in the past but she had initiated infliximab 9 weeks prior to presenting with the ocular symptoms. Her past medical history was significant for mesenteric ischemia likely due to factor V leiden deficiency for which she was receiving chronic anticoagulation with warfarin. On presentation, the patient had mild ophthalmoparesis, pupillary unresponsiveness, lid twitches and lid hops. She had a high anti-Gq1b antibody titer of 6400. Her tendon reflexes were normal and ataxia was not noted. No treatment was given and symptoms revolved after 10 weeks. The anti-Gq1b titer decreased to 200 [18A].

INFECTION RISK

A case of Blastomyces dermatitidis was reported in a 9-year-old male receiving infliximab and methotrexate for the treatment of juvenile idiopathic rheumatoid arthritis. The patient presented with an indurated plaque and crusting on his ear. He was given topical and oral antibiotics with no improvement. Biopsy and tissue culture confirmed the diagnosis of the fungal infection and he was given oral fluconazole in addition to discontinuing infliximab [19A].

URINARY TRACT

Nephrotic syndrome was reported in a 61-year-old male with an extensive history of ulcerative colitis and hypertension. He developed symptoms following his fifth infusion of infliximab. These symptoms included severe edema, hypertension and acute renal failure. He was treated with dialysis, albumin, anticoagulants and methylprednisolone. The nephrotic syndrome persisted despite discontinuation of infliximab and treatment with steroids and mycophenolate was initiated. The patient experienced another episode of severe nephrotic syndrome the following year. An underlying kidney process or past exposure to etidronate for osteoporosis cannot be ruled out as contributors to the nephrotic syndrome [20A].

MONOCLONAL ANTIBODIES [SEDA-35, 672; SEDA-36, 568; SEDA-37, 465]

Ado-Trastuzumab Emtansine

SKIN

A 45-year-old female with metastatic breast cancer developed mucositis, desquamation on the palms of her hands (plus orange discoloration) and soles of her feet following five cycles of treatment with ado-trastuzumab (dosed at 3.6 mg per kilogram intravenously every 3 weeks). Laboratory values were within normal limits and the signs and symptoms were characteristic of hand foot syndrome and carotenoderma. Ado-trastuzumab was discontinued due to progressive disease and the dermatologic symptoms resolved within 2 weeks [21A].

Alemtuzumab [SEDA-35, 672; SEDA-36, 569; SEDA-37, 465]

RESPIRATORY

Diffuse alveolar hemorrhage developed in an 18-year-old male who received one dose of alemtuzumab 30 mg subcutaneously with renal transplantation from a deceased donor. The patient developed acute onset shortness of breath, hemoptysis and fever 3 days after transplant and required ventilator support 2 days later. There was no evidence of an infection and pulmonary angiogram showed bilateral upper and lower lobe opacities with pleural effusion. Plasma electrophoresis, tacrolimus and steroids were given but the patient expired 31 days post-transplant due to worsening respiratory function and graft failure [22A].

Bevacizumab [SEDA-36, 570; SEDA-37, 465]

CARDIOVASCULAR

Hypotension developed in a neonate treated with intravitreal bevacizumab for retinopathy of prematurity. Twin A (a girl) and Twin B (a boy) were born at 26 weeks of gestation and weighed 775 grams and 800 grams, respectively. Although both received 0.625 mg of bevacizumab intravitreally along with 0.3 mg intravenous ketamine and local 0.25% atropine, only Twin B developed hypotension at 22 hours following bevacizumab. Twin B's blood pressure decreased to 42/24 and he also experienced feeding intolerance and oxygen desaturation. On the second day, his blood pressure remained low and he experienced more severe desaturation leading to intubation with mechanical ventilation. Dopamine and intravenous antibiotics were started. On day three, Twin B's blood pressure improved. On day six, the antibiotics and dopamine were discontinued and he was extubated on the following day. Authors attribute the hypotension to bevacizumab rather than ketamine due to the time of onset at 22 hours which is more fitting with bevacizumab's prolonged half-life of 11–50 days (as opposed to 2–3 hours with ketamine) [23A].

URINARY TRACT

Gross hematuria was reported in an 81-year-old woman with neovascular age related macular degeneration receiving intravitreal bevacizumab injections. She reported two episodes of gross hematuria following repeated bevacizumab injections. A urological exam was normal and the hematuria resolved upon discontinuing the bevacizumab. One year later, she received three additional bevacizumab injections and again, reported gross hematuria. At this time, a urological exam revealed a high grade urothelial carcinoma in the right ureter which was surgically removed. Bevacizumab was re-initiated and no further episodes of gross hematuria were reported [24A].

SKIN

A 68-year-old female with metastatic colon cancer and hypertension developed drug-induced lupus erythematosus after receiving chemotherapy with capecitabine (2000 mg/m2/day on days 1–14), oxaliplatin (130 mg/m2 intravenously on day 1) and bevacizumab (7.5 mg/kg intravenously on day 1) for two cycles. She presented with arthralgia, myalgia and prolonged thrombocytopenia. Chemotherapy was discontinued and hydroxychloroquine and methylprednisolone were initiated. Platelets increased and joint pain resolved [25A].

Brentuximab [SEDA-36, 573]

IMMUNOLOGIC

Cytokine release syndrome was reported in a 64-year-old male Caucasian with relapsed systemic anaplastic large cell lymphoma following his first dose of brentuximab. The patient experienced fever, chills, dyspnea and catecholamine-dependent shock [26A].

Catumaxomab

Catumaxomab is a monoclonal antibody which targets the epithelial cell adhesion molecule (EpCAM) and CD3 antigen on T cells. It is used intraperitoneally in the European Union for the treatment of malignancy-related ascites in EpCAM-positive epithelial carcinomas.

OBSERVATIONAL STUDY

A phase I study was conducted to determine the maximum tolerated dose of intravenous catumaxomab. Sixteen patients with epithelial cancers expressing EpCAM were enrolled and given 2, 4, 7 or 10 mcg doses weekly for 4 weeks. The maximum tolerated dose was found to be 7 mcg. One patient received the 10 mcg dose and died due to hepatic failure. The most common adverse effects were symptoms of cytokine release and hepatotoxicity [27c].

Daclizumab [SEDA-35, 675; SEDA-36, 574; SEDA-37, 467]

OBSERVATIONAL STUDY

Daclizumab high power yield (HYP) was compared with interferon beta-1a for the treatment of relapsing multiple sclerosis in a phase III study of 1841 patients. The study was randomized and double-blinded. Patients received daclizumab 150 mg subcutaneously every 4 weeks or interferon beta-1a 30 mcg intramuscularly once weekly for up to 144 weeks. Annualized relapse rate was the primary endpoint and was 45% lower in the daclizumab group. Disability progression at 12 weeks was not different between the two treatment groups. Serious adverse events were reported in 15% of the patients in the daclizumab HYP group as compared to 10% of the interferon beta-1a group. Several types of adverse effects were more common in the daclizumab group as compared with the interferon beta-1a group including infections (65% vs. 57%), serious infections (4% vs. 2%), cutaneous events (37% vs. 19%), and elevations in liver function tests greater than five times the upper limit of normal (6% vs. 3%) [28C].

Daratumumab

Daratumumab is a novel monoclonal antibody approved by the United States Food and Drug Administration in November 2015 for patients with previously treated multiple myeloma. Patients must have at least three prior treatments. It has breakthrough designation and approval was accelerated. Daratumumab is directed against CD38 which is expressed on multiple myeloma cells.

OBSERVATIONAL STUDY

The safety, efficacy and pharmacokinetics of daratumumab in relapsed multiple myeloma were investigated in a multi-center, open-label phase I–II trial. All patients enrolled had relapsed multiple myeloma or relapsed multiple myeloma refractory to two or more previous therapies. The first part of the study involved dose-escalation up to 24 mg per kilogram of body weight in 32 patients. No maximum tolerated dose was identified.

In the second part of the study, 72 patients were given 8 mg per kilogram (21 patients) or 16 mg per kilogram (51 patients) doses administered once weekly, twice monthly or monthly for up to a 2-year period of time. Pneumonia (5 patients) and thrombocytopenia (4 patients) were the most common grade 3 or 4 adverse events. Other grade 3 or 4 toxicities included neutropenia (2 patients), leukopenia (2 patients), anemia (2 patients) and hyperglycemia (2 patients). A majority of patients (71%) experienced grade 1 or 2 infusion reactions with only one patient having a grade 3 infusion reaction. The rate of infusion reactions decreased after the first dose with only 9% of the 8 mg per kilogram group and 7% of the 16 mg per kilogram group experiencing infusion reactions with more than one dose. Adverse events that occurred in at least 25% of patients included fever, allergic rhinitis and fatigue. Cough occurred in 21% of patients and nasopharyngitis in 24% of patients. Neutropenia occurred in 5 patients who received the 16 mg per kilogram dose.

In terms of efficacy, 36% of patients in the 16 mg per kilogram arm and 10% of patients in the 8 mg per kilogram arm had an overall response to daratumumab. Two patients experienced a complete response in the 16 mg per kilogram arm. Median progression free survival was 5.6 months in the 16 mg per kilogram group. Approximately 65% of patients who had a response to daratumumab remained disease free at 12 months [29c].

Dinutuximab

Dinutuximab is an anti-GD2 monoclonal antibody that was FDA approved in March 2015 for the treatment of high risk neuroblastoma in pediatric patients who achieved at least a partial response to prior therapy. It is approved for use in combination with a GCSF, aldesleukin and isotretinoin.

Refer to Section "Aldesleukin".

Elotuzumab

Elotuzumab is a new monoclonal antibody directed against the Signaling Lymphocyte Activation Molecule Family 7 or SLAMF7. It was FDA approved in November 2015 for the treatment of multiple myeloma in patients with one to three prior therapies. It should be used in combination with lenalidomide and dexamethasone.

OBSERVATIONAL STUDY

In a phase II, multi-center study in the United States, Canada, France and Germany, the efficacy of elotuzumab in patients with relapsed multiple myeloma was investigated. Seventy-three adult patients with a good performance status were enrolled. Patients had between one and three prior therapies but none contained lenalidomide. They were randomized in a 1:1 fashion to receive elotuzumab 10 mg per kilogram (36 patients) or 20 mg per kilogram (37 patients). Elotuzumab was given in combination with lenalidomide and dexamethasone. Cycles were 28 days in length. Patients received treatment until disease progression or intolerable toxicities developed. The primary endpoint was objective response. An objective response was achieved by 84% of patients, 33 (92%) in the 10 mg per kilogram dosing group and 28 (76%) in the 20 mg per kilogram group. There were no deaths attributed to elotuzumab. The most common treatment-related adverse effects were diarrhea (48 patients, 66%), muscle spasms (45 patients, 62%), and fatigue (41 patients, 56%). Grade 3 or 4 toxicities developed in 57 patients (78%) and the most common were lymphopenia (15 patients, 21%) and neutropenia (14 patients, 19%) [30c].

A randomized, phase III study compared elotuzumab plus lenalidomide and dexamethasone to a control group of lenalidomide and dexamethasone in 646 patients. Median progression free survival was 19.4 months compared with 14.9 months in the control group. Similar to the above study, lymphocytopenia and neutropenia were the commonly reported grade 3 or 4 adverse events. Other common grade 3 or 4 adverse events included fatigue and pneumonia. Infusion reactions (pyrexia, chills and hypertension) developed in 33 patients and were considered to be grade 1 or 2 in 29 of these patients. A majority (70%) occurred with the first dose. Infections developed in 81% of the treatment group compared with 74% of the control group [31C].

Evolocumab

Evolocumab is a PCSK9 inhibitor used as an adjunct to statin therapy for adults with heterozygous or homozygous familial hypercholesterolemia or atherosclerotic cardiovascular disease who need further lowering of low density lipoprotein (LDL) cholesterol. For patients with homozygous familial hypercholesterolemia it can also be used as adjunct therapy to ezetimibe and apheresis. Evolocumab is the second drug approved in this therapeutic class (alirocumab is also a PCSK9 inhibitor). Endogenously, PCSK9 works to decrease the number of LDL-removing receptors on the liver. With evolocumab, more LDL can be removed from the bloodstream.

OBSERVATIONAL STUDY

The efficacy and safety of evolocumab for lipid reduction and cardiovascular events were examined in two open-label, randomized trials of 4465 patients. Patients were randomized in a 2:1 ratio to receive evolocumab plus standard therapy or standard therapy alone. Use of evolocumab resulted in a 61% decrease in LDL compared with standard therapy. Evolocumab also reduced the rates of cardiovascular events at 1 year compared with the standard therapy group. A similar overall rate of adverse events (including serious adverse events) was reported between groups. Neurocognitive events

(delirium, confusion, cognitive and attention disorders, dementia, amnesic disturbances, issues with thinking and perception and mental impairment disorders) were reported more frequently in the evolocumab group (27 patients, 0.9%) compared with standard therapy (4 patients, 0.3%). Injection site reactions, arthralgia, headache, limb pain and fatigue were also more common in evolocumab-treated patients [32C].

In another trial, evolocumab was compared with placebo in patients with heterozygous familial hypercholesterolemia. This was a multi-center, randomized, placebo-controlled trial with 331 patients. Patients were randomized in a 2:1 fashion to receive evolocumab or placebo. In evolocumab-treated patients, nasopharyngitis (9% versus 5% in placebo group) and muscle-related adverse events (5% vs. 1%) occurred more frequently [33C].

Idarucizumab

Idarucizumab in a monoclonal antibody that serves as an antidote for dabigatran and aids in reversal of dabigatran's anticoagulant effects.

OBSERVATIONAL STUDY

A prospective cohort study was conducted to examine the safety of a 5-gram idarucizumab dose in reversing the anticoagulant effects of dabigatran. The study enrolled 90 patients with 51 patients having an episode of serious bleeding and 39 patients requiring an urgent procedure. There were 18 deaths in the study, nine in each group. No deaths were attributed to idarucizumab. Thrombotic events were classified as being early (within 72 hours of idarucizumab administration) or late (greater than 72 hours post-administration) and occurred in 5 patients. A deep vein thrombosis (DVT) and pulmonary embolism (PE) developed in one patient in the early period. In the late period, one patient developed DVT, PE and left atrial thrombus, one patient had DVT alone, one patient had a non ST elevation myocardial infarction and one patient suffered an ischemic stroke. No patients were receiving antithrombotic therapy at the time of the thrombotic events. Including the deaths and thrombotic events, 21 serious adverse drug events were reported. Two patients experienced a gastrointestinal hemorrhage and one patient each experienced post-operative wound infection, delirium, pulmonary edema and right ventricular failure [34c].

Ipilimumab [SEDA-36, 576]
HEMATOLOGIC

Febrile neutropenia was reported in a 35-year-old male 14 days after his third dose of ipilimumab (3 mg per kilogram, administered every 3 weeks). The patient was not on any other medications. A blood culture and urine culture were negative and a bone marrow biopsy showed no evidence of melanoma. After a complicated clinical course, the patient succumbed to melanoma [35A].

SENSORY SYSTEM—EYES

A 46-year-old male developed retinopathy following his third dose of ipilimumab (3 mg per kilogram) for the treatment of melanoma. He complained of blurred vision and photophobia and was initially diagnosed with Vogt–Koyanagi–Harada (VKH) syndrome. He was treated with dexamethasone 10 mg four times a day for 3 days with no improvement. Further evaluation showed bilateral serous retinal detachments in the macula that were not consistent with VKH. The fourth dose of ipilimumab was held due to increased liver function tests. At 1 week, improvement was noticed in the extent of the detachment and visual acuity. At 2 weeks, the detachment had resolved in the right eye and the left eye continued to improve [36A].

Bilateral retinal detachments and thickening of the choroid were reported in a woman in her early 70s. She received three doses of ipilimumab and then underwent surgery due to melanoma. After recovery, maintenance ipilimumab was initiated and 4 weeks after the first dose, the patient noted decreased vision, photophobia, and ocular tenderness on palpation, nausea, itchiness and weight loss. Additional testing revealed decreased visual acuity, the retinal detachments and thickening of the choroid. Ipilimumab was permanently discontinued. The patient was treated with topic and then systemic corticosteroids. Symptoms resolved after 6 months [37A].

Mepolizumab

Mepolizumab is a new monoclonal antibody which acts as an antagonist for the interleukin-5 receptor and inhibits the action of eosinophils, a culprit in airway inflammation. It is used in severe asthma as an addition to maintenance therapy.

A recent meta-analysis examined the effects of mepolizumab compared to placebo on asthma exacerbations and health related quality of life in adults and children with asthma. Randomized controlled trials were included in the analysis. Authors stated that the quality of evidence for adverse effects was low and they were unable to combine the results for analysis. Of the eight studies included in the meta-analysis, five reported serious adverse events but none were attributed to mepolizumab. Other adverse effects were reported in six of the studies and included the following: upper respiratory tract infections, asthma, headache, rhinitis, bronchitis, sinusitis, viral infection, injury, back pain, nausea, pharyngitis, rash, infusion and injection-related reactions [38M].

Necitumumab

Necitumumab is a novel monoclonal antibody recently developed which targets the epidermal growth factor receptor (EGFR) and is efficacious in treating metastatic squamous non-small cell lung cancer (NSCLC).

OBSERVATIONAL STUDY

A multi-center, open-label phase III study was conducted in patients with stage IV squamous NSCLC with good performance status and no prior chemotherapy. There were 1093 patients enrolled in the study and they were randomized 1:1 to receive therapy with gemcitabine, cisplatin and necitumumab or gemcitabine and cisplatin alone. Overall survival was the primary endpoint and was found to be longer in the group treated with necitumumab. In terms of adverse events, 72% of the necitumumab group experienced at least one grade 3 or worse adverse effect compared to 62% in the other group. More patients (48% versus 38%) in the necitumumab group experienced severe adverse effects. The grade 3 and grade 4 toxicities which were more common in necitumumab-treated patients included hypomagnesemia and rash. In the necitumumab group, 3% of the deaths were attributed to the medications compared with 2% in the control group [39C].

Another randomized, open-label phase III study examined the role of necitumumab combined with cisplatin and pemetrexed compared with cisplatin and pemetrexed alone in patients with stage IV nonsquamous NSCLC. No difference in overall survival was noted and trial enrollment was halted. The adverse effects due to necitumumab are similar to those noted previously with the addition of more grade 3 or higher venous thromboembolic events in patients treated with necitumumab (8% compared to 4% in the cisplatin plus pemetrexed group) [40C].

Nivolumab

Nivolumab is a monoclonal antibody directed against the programmed death immune checkpoint inhibitor (PD-1 receptor). It first gained approval in the United States for use in metastatic melanoma and more recently had earned FDA approval for use in metastatic non-small cell lung cancer with progression following platinum-based chemotherapy. It is also used for clear cell renal cell carcinoma.

OBSERVATIONAL STUDY

A randomized trial investigated nivolumab compared with docetaxel in the treatment of advanced non-squamous NSCLC. Overall survival was the primary endpoint and was significantly longer in the nivolumab-treated group. The frequency of adverse events was similar between the two groups although there were fewer grade 3 and 4 adverse events in the nivolumab group. The most common adverse effects of any grade in the nivolumab included fatigue (16%), nausea (12%), decreased appetite (10%), and asthenia (10%). Other adverse effects in the nivolumab group included rash, pruritus, diarrhea, hypothyroidism, increases in alanine aminotransferase, infusion related reactions, peripheral edema, myalgia, anemia and pneumonitis. No patients developed febrile neutropenia or leukopenia in the nivolumab group. One patient in the nivolumab group died due to encephalitis [41C].

In another randomized, open-label phase III trial in patients with advanced renal cell carcinoma, nivolumab was compared with everolimus. The adverse effects in the nivolumab group were similar to the previously mentioned study but also included cough, dyspnea, mucosal inflammation, dysgeusia, hyperglycemia, stomatitis, hypertriglyceridemia and epistaxis [42C].

SKIN

Skin eruptions resembling psoriasis developed in an 80-year-old man following his fourth dose of nivolumab for primary oral mucosa melanoma. Symptoms resolved with systemic steroids. At the 3-month follow-up, no melanoma cells were found on biopsy [43A].

ENDOCRINE

Four patients (two males and two females, aged 55–83 years old) developed insulin-dependent diabetes mellitus following treatment with nivolumab for different indications. They were treated with insulin and remained on insulin for treatment of their diabetes [44A].

Nimotuzumab [SEDA-36, 579]

OBSERVATIONAL STUDY

A phase II trial in 21 patients investigated nimotuzumab in combination with capecitabine and concurrent radiotherapy. All patients had locally advanced rectal cancer and a vast majority was nodal positive. Grade 3 diarrhea and leukopenia were experienced by 9.5% and 4.8% of patients, respectively. The most common Grade 1 and Grade 2 toxicities were radiation dermatitis, nausea and vomiting, leukocytopenia, diarrhea and proctitis [45c].

Obinutuzumab [SEDA-36, 578]

INFECTION RISK

Although infections with obinutuzumab use have been reported, new information has been added to the literature. In a case series, two patients developed invasive fungal infections following their third dose of obinutuzumab for refractory chronic lymphocytic leukemia. Both patients had received cytotoxic chemotherapy for several years prior to obinutuzumab but had not developed invasive fungal infections despite neutropenia. One of these patients, a 40-year-old male, received prophylaxis with itraconazole and cotrimoxazole yet developed an infection with Pneumocystis jirovecii and Candida kruseii.

This patient died from multiorgan failure. The second patient, a 38-year-old male, received pentamidine for prophylaxis against Pneumocystis jirovecii yet likely developed pneumonia due to this organism as well as evidence of Penicillium marneffei in his bone marrow. This patient went on to receive additional doses of obinutuzumab with cotrimoxazole and itraconazole for prophylaxis [46A].

Panitumumab [SEDA-35, 678]

SKIN

A 76-year-old woman presented with a 2-month history of painful scalp lesions which were interfering with her sleep. These lesions were confirmed to be severe folliculitis with secondary impetiginization. She initiated monotherapy for metastatic bowel cancer 6 months prior to presentation. Due to the lesions, panitumumab was discontinued [47A].

Pembrolizumab

SKIN

Bullous pemphigoid was diagnosed in a 75-year-old man 30 days after the completion of cycle six of pembrolizumab. Pembrolizumab had been stopped due to disease progression of the patient's metastatic melanoma. The patient had also developed spongiotic dermatitis after cycle 3 which was treated with topical steroids. The bullous pemphigoid was responsive to oral prednisone and then dexamethasone [48A].

MUSCULOSKELETAL

Two patients developed acute onset polyarticular inflammatory arthritis following 11 and 14 months of treatment with pembrolizumab. Both patients were treated with bisphosphonates and salazopyrin [49A].

Ramucirumab

Ramucirumab is a monoclonal antibody which targets the vascular endothelial growth factor receptor 2 (VEGFR2). This leads to decreased angiogenesis within tumors. It is used in the treatment of advanced or metastatic gastric, colorectal and non-small cell lung cancer.

CARDIOVASCULAR

A male patient with stage IV KRAS wild-type rectal adenocarcinoma with liver and pulmonary metastases developed a sporadic angioma on his lower right leg following two cycles of chemotherapy with ramucirumab, cetuximab and irinotecan. No pain or pruritus accompanied the lesion. The p.T771R KDR mutation was found within the angioma. Chemotherapy was continued with no change to the vascular lesion [50A].

Rituximab [SEDA-35, 678; SEDA-36, 581; SEDA-37, 467]

CARDIOVASCULAR

A 61-year-old woman developed coronary artery vasospasm 15 minutes after initiation of a rituximab infusion. She reported chest pain, experienced diaphoresis and vomited twice. It was her sixth cycle of gemcitabine, cisplatin, dexamethasone and rituximab. Additionally, the patient had received other rituximab-containing regimens in the past with no episodes of vasospasm. Her past medical history was not significant for any history of cardiovascular disease. Electrocardiogram showed ST segment elevations. Angiogram showed posterior descending artery vasospasm and mild coronary artery disease [51A].

INFECTION RISK

A brain abscess was reported in a 52-year-old Saudi American woman with pemphigus vulgaris and diabetes shortly after rituximab was added to her treatment regimen of azathioprine and a corticosteroid. Patient presented with low-grade fever, headache and one-sided weakness 2 weeks after her second dose of rituximab. The patient also had a blood culture positive for Listeria monocytogenes. The patient recovered after 6 weeks of therapy with ampicillin and gentamicin [52A].

Secukinumab

Secukinumab is a novel monoclonal antibody which targets and inhibits interleukin-17A. It is used in the treatment of ankylosing spondylitis, plaque psoriasis, and psoriatic arthritis.

OBSERVATIONAL STUDY

Two randomized, placebo-controlled phase III trials (containing 371 and 219 patients) were conducted to investigate the efficacy of secukinumab in ankylosing spondylitis. The primary endpoint was improvement in Assessment of Ankylosing Spondyloarthritis International Society response criteria. Use of secukinumab was associated with significant improvements in ankylosing spondylitis. Infections occurred at a higher rate in secukinumab-treated patients when compared with placebo. Candidiasis and neutropenia were also reported. Four patients in the first trial and one patient in the second trial developed cancer during the study period and secukinumab was discontinued. Other adverse events included cardiac issues, Crohn's disease and uveitis [53C].

The efficacy of secukinumab was also examined in 606 psoriatic arthritis patients in a double-blind, placebo-controlled, randomized, phase III trial. The adverse events reported were similar to the previously reported trial with the addition that six secukinumab-treated patients suffered a stroke (0.6 per 100 patient years) [54C].

Trastuzumab [SEDA-35, 680; SEDA-36, 582; SEDA-37, 468]

CARDIOVASCULAR

A right middle cerebral artery embolism was reported in a 67-year-old male with stage IV HER2-positive gastric cancer receiving chemotherapy with cisplatin, fluorouracil and trastuzumab. The patient presented with left hemiplegia and an MRI showed a middle cerebral artery occlusion 4 days after chemotherapy initiation. No additional chemotherapy was given due to the poor performance status of the patient. Brain metastases were not apparent for the patient but tumor microemboli and his status as a current smoker may have contributed to the embolism [55A].

Ustekinumab [SEDA-36, 583]

HEMATOLOGIC

A case of thrombotic thrombocytopenic purpura (TTP) was reported in a 36-year-old male patient treated with ustekinumab and methotrexate for psoriasis. The patient had received treatment with ustekinumab for approximately 1 year prior to developing TTP. The patient died 14 days after admission despite supportive care measures. Authors cannot exclude an idiopathic cause for the TTP [56A].

References

[1] Pourtaheri S, Hwang K, Faloon M, et al. Ultra-low-dose recombinant human bone morphogenetic protein-2 for 3-level anterior cervical diskectomy and fusion. Orthopedics. 2015;38(4):241–5 [c].

[2] Gascon P, Aapro M, Ludwig H, et al. Treatment patterns and outcomes in the prophylaxis of chemotherapy-induced (febrile) neutropenia with biosimilar filgrastim (the MONITOR-GCSF study). Support Care Cancer. 2016;24:911–25 [c].

[3] Grainger JD, Locatelli F, Chotsampancharoen T, et al. Eltrombopag for children with chronic immune thrombocytopenia (PETIT2): a randomised, mulicentre, placebo-controlled trial. Lancet. 2015;386:1649–58 [c].

[4] Kowalczyk M, Rubinstein PF, Aboulafia DM. Initial experience with the use of thrombopoetin receptor agonists in patients with refractory HIV-associated immune thrombocytopenic purpura: a case series. J Int Assoc Provid AIDS Care. 2015;14(3):211–6 [A].

[5] Gunes H, Kivrak T. Eltrombopag induced thrombosis: a case with acute myocardial infarction. Curr Drug Saf. 2016;11:174–6 [A].

[6] Sakatani A, Doi Y, Matsuda T, et al. Protracted anaphylaxis developed after peginterferon alfa-2a administration for chronic hepatitis C. World J Gastroenterol. 2015;21(9):2826–9 [A].

[7] Kim YJ, Lee HY, Lee JY, et al. Interferon beta-1b-induced Sweet's syndrome in a patient with multiple sclerosis. Int J Dermatol. 2015;54(4):456–8 [A].

[8] Bakri S, Swanson J. Asymptomatic peripheral retinal hemorrhages as a manifestation of interferon beta-1a retinopathy. Semin Ophthalmol. 2015;30(1):56–7 [A].

[9] Levy G, Bonnevalle M, Rocourt N, et al. Necrotizing enterocolitis as an adverse effect of recombinant interleukin-2 and ch14.18 in maintenance therapy for high-risk neuroblastoma. J Pediatr Hematol Oncol. 2015;37(4):250–2 [A].

[10] Migkos M, Somarakis G, Markatseli T, et al. Tuberculosis pyomyositis in a rheumatoid arthritis patient treated with anakinra. Clin Exp Rheumatol. 2015;33(5):734–6 [A].

[11] Marzano A, Tavecchio S, Berti E, et al. Paradoxical autoinflammatory skin reaction to tumor necrosis factor alpha blockers manifesting as amicrobial pustulosis of the folds in patients with inflammatory bowel diseases. Medicine (Baltimore). 2015;94(45):e1818 [A].

[12] Matet A, Daruich A, Beydoun T, et al. Systemic adalimumab induces peripheral corneal infiltrates: a case report. BMC Ophthalmol. 2015;15:57 [A].

[13] Tintle S, Dabade T, Kalish R, et al. Repigmentation of hair following adalimumab therapy. Dermatol Online J. 2015;21(6), pii:13030/qt6fn0t1xz, [A].

[14] Chou W, Hsu C. A case report of Majocchi's granuloma associated with combined therapy of topical steroids and adalimumab. Medicine (Baltimore). 2016;95(2):e2245 [A].

[15] Markovic I, Puksic S, Gudelj G, et al. Scabies in a patient with rheumatoid arthritis treated with adalimumab—a case report. Acta Dermatovenerol Croat. 2015;23(3):195–8 [A].

[16] Kreitenberg A, Ortiz E, Arkfeld D. Priapism after tumor necrosis factor alpha inhibitor use. Clin Rheumatol. 2015;34(4): 801–2 [A].

[17] Banse C, Benhamou Y, Lequerre T, et al. Acquired hemophilia possibly induced by entanercept in a patient with rheumatoid arthritis. Joint Bone Spine. 2015;82(3):200–2 [A].

[18] Ratnarajan G, Thompson A, Dodridge C, et al. Novel variant of Miller Fisher syndrome occurring with tumor necrosis factor alfa antagonist therapy. JAMA Neurol. 2015;72(11):1377–8 [A].

[19] Smith R, Boos M, Burnham J, et al. Atypical cutaneous blastomycosis in a child with juvenile idiopathic rheumatoid arthritis on infliximab. Pediatrics. 2015;136(5):e1386–9 [A].

[20] Dumitrescu G, Dahan K, Treton X, et al. Nephrotic syndrome after infliximab treatment in a patient with ulcerative colitis. J Gastrointestin Liver Dis. 2015;24(2):249–51 [A].

[21] Dholaria B, Srinivasan S. T-DM1-related carotenoderma and hand-foot syndrome. Lancet. 2015;385(9977):1509–10 [A].

[22] Tahir W, Hakeem A, Baker R, et al. Diffuse alveolar hemorrhage: a fatal complication after alemtuzumab induction therapy in renal transplantation. Transplant Proc. 2015;47(1):151–4 [A].

[23] Wu L, Yang Y, Lin C, et al. Hypotension associated with intravitreal bevacizumab therapy for retinopathy of prematurity. Pediatrics. 2016;137(2):1–4 [A].

[24] Lemor D, Lazar D, Mazzulla D. Recurrent hematuria in patient with a previously undiagnosed transitional cell carcinoma of the right ureter after intravitreal bevacizumab (Avastin) injection: a case report. Retin Cases Brief Rep. 2015;9(1):45–6 [A].

[25] Ozaslan E, Eroglu E, Gok K, et al. Drug induced lupus erythematosus due to capecitabine and bevacizumab treatment presenting with prolonged thrombocytopenia. Rom J Intern Med. 2015;53(3):282–5 [A].

[26] Alig S, Dreyling M, Seppi B, et al. Severe cytokine release syndrome after the first dose of brentuximab vedotin in a patient with relapsed systemic anaplastic large cell lymphoma (sALCL): a case report and review of the literature. Eur J Haematol. 2015;94(6):554–7 [A].

[27] Mau-Sorensen M, Dittrich C, Dienstmann R, et al. A phase I trial of intravenous catumaxomab: a bispecific monoclonal antibody targeting EpCAM and the T cell coreceptor CD3. Cancer Chemother Pharmacol. 2015;75(5):1065–73 [c].

[28] Kappos L, Wiendl H, Selmaj K, et al. Daclizumab HYP versus interferon beta-1a in relapsing multiple sclerosis. N Engl J Med. 2015;373(15):1418–28 [C].

[29] Lokhorst H, Plesner T, Laubach J, et al. Targeting CD38 with daratumumab monotherapy in multiple myeloma. N Engl J Med. 2015;373(13):1207–19 [c].

[30] Richardson P, Jagannath S, Moreau P, et al. Elotuzumab in combination with lenalidomide and dexamethasone in patients with relapsed multiple myeloma: final phase 2 results from randomised, open-label, phase 1b-2 dose-escalation study. Lancet Haematol. 2015;2(12):e516–27 [c].

[31] Lonial S, Dimopoulos M, Palumbo A, et al. Elotuzumab therapy for relapsed or refractory multiple myeloma. N Engl J Med. 2015;373(7):621–31 [C].

[32] Sabatine M, Giugliano R, Wiviott S, et al. Efficacy and safety of evolocumab in reducing lipids and cardiovascular events. N Engl J Med. 2015;372(16):1500–9 [C].

[33] Raal F, Stein E, Dufour R, et al. PCSK9 inhibition with evolocumab (AMG 145) in heterozygous familial hypercholesterolemia (RUTHERFORD-2): a randomised, double-blind, placebo-controlled trial. Lancet. 2015;385:331–40 [C].

[34] Pollack C, Reilly P, Eikelboom J, et al. Idarucizumab for dabigatran reversal. N Engl J Med. 2015;373:511–20 [c].

[35] Wozniak S, Mackiewicz-Wysocka M, Krokowicz L, et al. Febrile neutropenia in a metastatic melanoma patient treated with ipilimumab—a case report. Oncol Res Treat. 2015;38(3):105–8.

[36] Crews J, Agarwal A, Jack L, et al. Ipilimumab-associated retinopathy. Ophthalmic Surg Lasers Imaging Retina. 2015;46(6):658–60 [A].

[37] Mantopoulos D, Kendra K, Letson A, et al. Bilateral choroidopathy and serous retinal detachments during ipilimumab treatment for cutaneous melanoma. JAMA Ophthalmol. 2015;133(8):965–7 [A].

[38] Powell C, Millan S, Dwan K, et al. Mepolizumab versus placebo for asthma. Cochrane Database Syst Rev. 2015;27(7):CD010834 [M].

[39] Thatcher N, Hirsch F, Luft A, et al. Necitumumab plus gemcitabine and cisplatin versus gemcitabine and cisplatin alone as first-line therapy in patients with stage IV squamous non-small-cell lung cancer (SQUIRE): an open-label, randomised, controlled phase 3 trial. Lancet Oncol. 2015;16(7):763–74 [C].

[40] Paz-Ares L, Mezger J, Ciuleanu T, et al. Necitumumab plus pemetrexed and cisplatin as first-line therapy in patients with stage IV non-squamous non-small cell lung cancer (INSPIRE): an open-label, randomised, controlled phase III trial. Lancet Oncol. 2015;6(3):328–37 [C].

[41] Borghaei H, Paz-Ares L, Horn L, et al. Nivolumab versus docetaxel in advanced non-squamous non-small cell lung cancer. N Engl J Med. 2015;373(17):1627–39 [C].

[42] Motzer R, Escudier B, McDermott D, et al. Nivolumab versus everolimus in advanced renal cell carcinoma. N Engl J Med. 2015;373(19):1803–13 [C].

[43] Ohtsuka M, Miura T, Mori T, et al. Occurrence of psoriaform eruption during nivolumab for primary oral mucosa melanoma. JAMA Dermatol. 2015;151(7):797–9 [A].

[44] Hughes J, Vudattu N, Sznol M, et al. Precipitation of autoimmune diabetes with anti-PD-1 immunotherapy. Diabetes Care. 2015;38(4):e55–7 [A].

[45] Jin T, Zhu Y, Luo J, et al. Prospective phase II trial of nimotuzumab in combination with radiotherapy and concurrent capecitabine in locally advanced rectal cancer. Int J Colorectal Dis. 2015;30(3):337–45 [c].

[46] Tse E, Leung R, Kwong YL. Invasive fungal infections after obinutuzumab monotherapy for refractory chronic lymphocytic leukemia. Ann Hematol. 2015;94:165–7 [A].

[47] Rodriguez-Bandera A, Gomez-Fernandez C, Vorlicka K, et al. Severe folliculitis with secondary impetiginization in the scalp of a woman treated with panitumumab. Int J Dermatol. 2015;54(6): e226–9 [A].

[48] Carlos G, Anforth R, Chou S, et al. A case of bullous pemphigoid in a patient with metastatic melanoma treated with pembrolizumab. Melanoma Res. 2015;25(3):265–8 [A].

[49] Chan M, Kefford R, Carlino M, et al. Arthritis and tenosynovitis associated with anti-PD1 antibody pembrolizumab in metastatic melanoma. J Immunother. 2015;38(1):37–9 [A].

[50] Young H, Lim B, Odell I, et al. Somatic p.T771R KDR (VEGFR2) mutation arising in sporadic angioma during ramucirumab treatment. JAMA Dermatol. 2015;151(11):1240–3 [A].

[51] Ke C, Khosla A, Davis M, et al. A care of coronary vasopasm after repeat rituximab infusion. Case Rep Cardiol. 2015;2015:523149. http://dx.doi.org/10.1155/2015/523149 [A].

[52] Al-Harbi T, Al-Muammar S, Ellis R. Brain abscess following rituximab infusion in a patient with pemphigus vulgaris. Am J Case Rep. 2015;16:65–8 [A].

[53] Baeten D, Sieper J, Braun J, et al. Secukinumab, an interleukin-17a inhibitors, in ankylosing spondylitis. N Engl J Med. 2015;373(26):2534–48 [C].

[54] Mease P, McInnes I, Kirkham B, et al. Secukinumab inhibition of interleukin-17a in patients with psoriatic arthritis. N Engl J Med. 2015;373(14):1329–39 [C].

[55] Takahama T, Takeda M, Nishina S, et al. A case of severe cerebral embolism after chemotherapy for HER2-positive gastric cancer. BMC Res Notes. 2015;26(8):100 [A].

[56] Philippe L, Badie J, Faller J, et al. Fatal thrombotic thrombocytopenic purpura in a psoriasis patient treated with ustekinumab and methotrexate. Acta Derm Venereol. 2015;95(4):495–6 [A].

36

Drugs That Act on the Immune System: Immunosuppressive and Immunostimulatory Drugs

Calvin J. Meaney[1], Spinel Karas

Department of Pharmacy Practice, School of Pharmacy and Pharmaceutical Sciences, State University of New York at Buffalo, Buffalo, NY, USA

[1]Corresponding author: cjmeaney@buffalo.edu

IMMUNOSUPPRESSIVE DRUGS

Belatacept [SEDA-34, 609]

Comparative Studies

The novel combination of belatacept and a mammalian target of rapamycin (mTOR) inhibitor post-renal transplant was reviewed [1R]. Compared to tacrolimus and mycophenolate mofetil, belatacept and sirolimus had better renal function (GFR 54 mL/min vs. 62 mL/min, respectively), lower incidence of serious infections (13% vs. 8%, respectively) but higher incidence of malignancy (0% vs. 4%, respectively).

Systematic Reviews

A systematic review and meta-analysis included six randomized controlled trials comparing belatacept to calcineurin inhibitor based immunosuppression post-renal transplant [2M]. Renal function, blood pressure, and triglycerides were better in belatacept compared to calcineurin inhibitor treatment: mean differences at 12 months were +11.7 mL/min/1.73 m² in calculated glomerular filtration rate (GFR), −7.2 mmHg in systolic blood pressure, and −32.9 mg/dL in triglycerides. There was a lower risk of new-onset diabetes after transplantation with belatacept compared to calcineurin inhibitor regimens (OR 0.43, 95% CI 0.24–0.78). Rates of post-transplant lymphoproliferative disorder, skin cancer, and other malignancies were not different between groups.

CYCLOPHOSPHAMIDE [SED-15, 1025; SEDA-34, 612; SEDA-35, 700; SEDA-36, 592]

Infection, malignancy, infertility, and genetic predisposition to adverse effects were highlighted in a review of cyclophosphamide when used in the treatment of anti-neutrophil cytoplasm antibody-associated systemic vasculitis [3R].

Observational Studies

A 10-year follow-up to a prospective, open-label study of cyclophosphamide and steroids in 58 adults with idiopathic membranous nephropathy provided insight into adverse effects in this population [4c]. Gastrointestinal intolerance (1), pancreatitis (1), herpes zoster (2), myelosuppression (2), tuberculosis (9), and unspecific drug reactions (3) occurred during the follow-up period, during which 43.1% of patients experienced a serious complication of therapy.

Adverse effects of cyclophosphamide in Chinese patients were investigated in 419 patients with autoimmune diseases [5C]. The side effect profile was not different than other populations. Risk factors for gastrointestinal effects were noted to be female gender, length of therapy, and use of intravenous route of administration. Females were also at higher risk of myelosuppression and alopecia. Hemorrhagic cystitis did not occur in any patient.

A prospective observational study of 100 patients compared the toxicity profiles of 5-fluorouracil, doxorubicin (Adriamycin®), and cyclophosphamide (FAC) to Adriamycin® and paclitaxel (AT) regimens in breast cancer [6C]. Distinct toxicity profiles were observed; the FAC regimen had more anemia, leukopenia, stomatitis, peripheral neuropathy, hyperpigmentation, and photosensitivity than the AT regimen.

Analysis of vincristine, doxorubicin, and cyclophosphamide compared to vincristine, doxorubicin, and ifosfamide for Ewing sarcoma revealed more frequent severe toxicity in females in the 856 patients studied [7C]. Toxicities more severe in females included anemia, leukopenia, thrombocytopenia, infection, diarrhea, renal toxicity, hyperbilirubinemia, and peripheral neuropathy. There were minimal toxicity differences between treatment regimens.

Cardiovascular

Cardiotoxicity of chemotherapy was analyzed from the United States Food and Drug Administration Adverse Event Reporting System database (2004–2012) [8C]. Anthracyclines, in particular trastuzumab, were most often associated with cardiotoxicity. Combination of trastuzumab and cyclophosphamide was also associated with a significant increase in cardiotoxicity (reported OR 16.8, 95% CI 13.3–21.3).

Pulmonary

Cyclophosphamide was the suspected culprit agent in 43.2% of pulmonary veno-occlusive disease cases in a recent review [9R]. This was confirmed with animal studies wherein cyclophosphamide induced pulmonary hypertension changes.

Urinary Tract

Hemorrhagic cystitis is a well-known toxicity of cyclophosphamide. A retrospective study of 1018 patients receiving cyclophosphamide for rheumatic diseases investigated risks for development of this complication [10C]. Use of mesna, an agent that has been shown to reduce the risk of hemorrhagic cystitis in cancer patients, was not associated with a lower risk in this population. Cumulative cyclophosphamide dose was the only variable to be associated with a higher risk (HR for each 10 g dose increment: 1.24, $P < 0.001$). Results should be interpreted cautiously given the retrospective design, especially as they pertain to the use of mesna which is well accepted to reduce hemorrhagic cystitis risk.

Skin

A female with rheumatoid vasculitis developed toxic epidermal necrolysis while receiving cyclophosphamide and mesna [11A]. The reaction resolved after discontinuation of cyclophosphamide and administration of intravenous immunoglobulin.

Musculoskeletal

A rat model of breast cancer treated with cyclophosphamide, epirubicin, and 5-fluorouracil revealed mechanisms of bone disease associated with this regimen [12E]. Lower trabecular bone volume, increased osteoclast density and size, and less bone marrow cellularity were observed after 6 cycles of treatment.

Genetic Factors

Adverse effect associations with three alleles in CYP2B6 (CYP2B6*4 [rs2279343], CYP2B6*5 [rs3211371] and CYP2B6*9 [rs3745274]) were evaluated in 145 female breast cancer patients receiving cyclophosphamide-based therapy [13C]. There were no associations with the three CYP2B6 polymorphisms or the haplotypes with hematologic toxicities. Limitations include the small number of patients and low variant allele frequencies (0.07–0.29) coupled with toxicities determined by chart review.

Cyclophosphamide toxicities in 256 cancer patients were evaluated for their association to GSTP1 (rs1695) and *ABCC4* (rs9561778) polymorphisms [14C]. The *ABCC4* genotypes of GT and TT were associated with anemia (OR 2.10, 95% CI 1.18–3.74), neutropenia (OR 2.44, 95% CI 1.35–4.40), leukopenia (OR 2.28, 95% CI 1.23–4.22), and gastrointestinal toxicities (OR 2.62, 95% CI 1.22–5.59) compared to the GG wild-type. No associations were observed for the GSTP1 polymorphism and toxicities.

Rituximab, cyclophosphamide, doxorubicin, vincristine, and prednisone comprise the common "R-CHOP" chemotherapeutic regimen. The rs2229109 polymorphism in *ABCB1* was associated with more vomiting ($P = 0.003$) and diarrhea ($P = 0.007$) in 760 patients with non-Hodgkin lymphoma receiving R-CHOP compared to wild type [15C]. The rs20572 and rs9024 polymorphisms in *CBR1* were associated with worse anemia, thrombocytopenia, and diarrhea in the same patients compared to wild type ($P < 0.05$ for all). A major concern with these data are the large number of associations made between groups and different toxicities without statistical adjustment for multiple comparisons.

Genetic associations to adverse effects of cyclophosphamide were investigated in 189 Chinese patients with systemic lupus erythematosus (SLE) [16C]. *CYP2B6* −750TT genotype was associated with less gastrointestinal toxicity (OR 0.2348, 95% CI 0.107–0.523). *CYP2C19*2* polymorphism, *1/*1 allele was associated with less gastrointestinal toxicity (OR 0.157, 95% CI 0.057–0.430), infection (OR 0.260, 95% CI 0.119–0.568) and leukopenia (OR 0.194, 95% CI 0.092–0.409). Extensive, intermediate, and poor were identified with *CYP2B6* −750T > C and *CYP2C19*2* polymorphisms. Extensive metabolizers had higher rates of gastrointestinal toxicity (OR 7.58, 95% CI 2.93–19.58, *P* < 0.0001) and leukopenia (OR 7.54, 95% CI 2.95–19.26, *P* < 0.0001) compared to intermediate metabolizers. Increased 4-OH-cyclophosphamide concentrations were postulated to cause this worse adverse effect profile.

CYCLOSPORINE (CICLOSPORIN) *[SED-15, 743; SEDA-34, 609; SEDA-35, 699; SEDA-36, 591]*

Observational Studies

A retrospective study examined adverse effects of 267 atopic dermatitis patients receiving cyclosporine [17C]. Twenty-four percent (57/234) of patients discontinued therapy due to adverse effects including increase in serum creatinine (10%), hypertension (7%), neurological symptoms (6%), fatigue (4%), and GI symptoms (4%).

Another retrospective study showed that adverse effects could often occur even at low cyclosporine doses [18c]. When adult patients (*n* = 88) who had undergone penetrating keratoplasty were given cyclosporine (a loading dose of 5 mg/kg/day followed by 2.5–3.5 mg/kg/day) to achieve target trough concentration of 120–150 ng/mL, 82% of patients experienced adverse effects. The most commonly reported adverse effects include herpes keratitis (31.8%), hypertension (14.8%), and hepatotoxicity (6.8%). Herpes keratitis was more likely to occur in patients treated with cyclosporine compared to those not treated with cyclosporine (31.8% vs. 16.8%; *P* = 0.005).

Adverse effects of immunosuppressive therapy consisting of steroids, mycophenolate mofetil, and cyclosporine (51%) or tacrolimus (49%) were described in a retrospective study of 55 pediatric renal transplant patients [19c]. The most commonly reported adverse effects of cyclosporine included hypertension (69%), hypercholesterolemia (38%), hyperglycemia (16.3%), and hypertrichosis (14.5%). Adverse effects of cyclosporine in pediatric population were generally similar to those seen in adults.

Comparative Studies

In a prospective, cross-sectional study, a regimen of cyclosporine and mycophenolate mofetil (MMF; *n* = 82) was compared to tacrolimus and enteric-coated mycophenolate sodium (EC-MPS; *n* = 67) to assess adverse

effects in renal transplant recipients [20C]. Gingival hyperplasia (OR 28.1, 95% CI 9.2–82.7; *P* < 0.001), hirsutism (OR 11.6, 95% CI 3.9–34.2; *P* < 0.001), skin changes (OR 4.10, 95% CI 1.6–10.7; *P* = 0.004), and tremor (OR 2.22, 95% CI 1.1–4.6; *P* = 0.031) were more frequent with cyclosporine [20C]. Insomnia (OR 2.34, 95% CI 1.10–5.00), diarrhea (OR 4.17, 95% CI 1.69–10.2) and dyspepsia (OR 2.93, 95% CI 1.41–6.10) were more frequent with tacrolimus. Additionally, total cholesterol, low-density lipoprotein (LDL) and triglycerides (TG) were higher in patients receiving cyclosporine compared to tacrolimus, although more patients on cyclosporine received concomitant prednisone. Gastrointestinal, neurologic, and aesthetic adverse effect domains were more severe in female patients compared to males (*P* = 0.022, *P* = 0.022, and *P* < 0.001, respectively). Associations to polymorphisms in *ABCB1* revealed a 2.6-fold higher gastrointestinal adverse effect score with the CTT (1236C-2677T-3435T) haplotype compared to wild-type CGC (*P* = 0.018) and a 3.2-fold higher aesthetic adverse effect score with the TTC haplotype compare to wild type (*P* = 0.005). The open-label, observational nature of this study makes interpretation difficult, but it is one of the first to use a systematic, standardized, and validated approach to adverse effect assessment in this patient population.

Cardiovascular

Hypertension with electrolyte imbalance (hypokalemia, hypophosphatemia, and hypocalcemia) was reported in a 12-year-old female with Fanconi anemia who received cyclosporine for graft-versus-host disease (GvHD) prophylaxis after hematopoietic stem cell transplantation [21A].

In a single-center, retrospective study, renal transplant recipients (*n* = 386) were assessed for risk factors of lipid abnormalities [22C]. Thirty-six percent (140/386) of patients received cyclosporine with mean trough concentration of 70.0 ng/mL. The authors reported that among total population, 43% of patients received statin therapy, but the total number of patients who received both cyclosporine and statin was not indicated. In contrast to previous study results, cyclosporine did not significantly increase the risk of lipid abnormalities (OR 1.72, 95% CI: 0.57–5.15). This is potentially due to administration of relatively low dose of cyclosporine (mean trough concentration 70.0 ng/mL) as the cyclosporine dose decreased over time post-transplantation (mean post-plantation period 8.4 years).

Eyes

A case of diplopia was reported in a 42-year-old female with idiopathic membranous nephropathy who received prednisone and tacrolimus (trough concentration

6–8 ng/mL) [23A]. Tacrolimus was switched to low dose cyclosporine (trough concentration 44–59 ng/mL) after she developed diplopia at 3 months of tacrolimus therapy, but the symptom did not resolve. Complete recovery occurred after 6 days of discontinuation of cyclosporine. The authors concluded that diplopia could occur in recommended therapeutic doses of calcineurin inhibitors (i.e. tacrolimus, cyclosporine).

Endocrine

A review by Montero and Pascual discussed mechanisms of cyclosporine-induced post-transplant diabetes mellitus [24R]. Cyclosporine appears to have a direct toxic effect on the pancreatic β cells, which lead to decrease in insulin synthesis and secretion.

Fertility

Georgiou et al. reviewed the effect of cyclosporine on fertility of male post-renal transplant patients [25R]. The analysis is based on small studies making it difficult to draw a firm conclusion. Nonetheless, several studies included in the analysis have shown that cyclosporine can adversely affect male fertility. Cyclosporine has been found to decrease several fertility-associated parameters (i.e. testosterone, sperm motility, sperm counts, testicular volume) as compared to healthy controls.

Drug–Drug Interactions

Statin-induced myopathy with elevated serum creatine kinase levels was reported in an 88-year-old Chinese male patient receiving atorvastatin (20 mg once daily) with cyclosporine (150 mg twice daily) for 8 months [26A]. Investigators suggested that cytochrome CYP3A4 inhibition by cyclosporine might have resulted in increased plasma atorvastatin concentrations and myopathy.

EVEROLIMUS [SED-15, 1306; SEDA-34, 614; SEDA-35, 701; SEDA-36, 592]

Observational Studies

Everolimus and low-dose cyclosporine were compared to MMF and standard-dose calcineurin inhibitor in 105 pediatric renal transplant patients [27C]. While renal function was similar between the two regimens at 4 years post-transplant, the everolimus group had less BK polyomavirus replication (3% vs. 17%, $P=0.04$) but more hypertension (91% vs. 69%, $P=0.049$) and hyperlipidemia (total cholesterol: 222 ± 56 mg/dL vs. 165 ± 36 mg/dL, $P<0.001$) compared to the MMF regimen.

Grade 3 or higher toxicities of everolimus were stomatitis, dyspnea, vomiting, and thrombocytopenia among 22 Chinese patients with non-small cell-lung cancer [28c].

The adverse effect profile of mTOR inhibitors, including everolimus, for tuberous sclerosis complex was reviewed [29R]. The authors conclude that while adverse effects such as infection, metabolic and hematologic derangements, and renal dysfunction occur in this population, the overall safety profile of everolimus is better in tuberous sclerosis complex compared to the renal transplant population.

Comparative Studies

A multi-center, randomized, open-label phase 3 trial compared nivolumab to everolimus for renal cell carcinoma in 821 patients [30C]. Any side effect occurred in 79% of nivolumab compared to 88% of everolimus patients. The everolimus group had more grade 3 or 4 adverse events and a lower quality of life compared to nivolumab.

A multi-center, retrospective study compared the adverse effects of everolimus and temsirolimus in 196 Japanese patients with renal cell carcinoma [31C]. Rates of adverse effects for everolimus compared to temsirolimus were: stomatitis 56% vs. 30% ($P<0.001$), pneumonitis 38% vs. 22% ($P=0.018$), asthenia 11% vs. 23% ($P=0.027$), rash 20% vs. 36% ($P=0.018$), and fatigue 33% vs. 48% ($P=0.032$), respectively. Risks for pneumonitis were male gender (OR 3.65, 95% CI 1.44–9.26) and everolimus treatment (OR 2.00, 95% CI 1.01–3.96).

Systematic Reviews

Ten clinical trials were included in a meta-analysis of everolimus toxicities in solid tumors [32M]. The relative risks (RR) were 1.31 ($P<0.002$) for fatigue, 2.54 ($P=0.0001$) for hyperlipidemia, 3.06 ($P<0.0001$) for hyperglycemia, and 2.96 ($P<0.003$) for elevated alanine aminotransferase.

A meta-analysis of 56 prospective trials ($n=9760$) compared treatment-related fatigue of everolimus to temsirolimus [33M]. All-grade fatigue was higher with everolimus (RR 1.85, 95% CI 1.71–2.01); however, no differences were observed for severe fatigue.

Cardiovascular

Holdaas et al. reviewed dyslipidemia associated with mTOR inhibitors in transplant patients [34R]. They concluded that the lipid panel should be routinely monitored, but dyslipidemia is not an absolute barrier to use mTOR inhibitors.

The effect of conversion from cyclosporine to everolimus on cardiac function was evaluated in 39 renal transplant patients [35c]. At 3 years of follow-up, no differences in cardiac function (left ventricle diastolic and systolic function, left ventricle mass and morphology) were observed.

Pulmonary

A phase 2 trial investigated the combination of letrozole and everolimus for advanced non-small-cell lung cancer [36c]. The study was stopped after enrolling 5 patients as 3 patients developed severe pulmonary toxicity.

Non-infectious pneumonitis was reported in a 72-year-old male on everolimus for metastatic renal cell carcinoma [37A].

Everolimus-induced pneumonitis occurred in 58% (23/40) of patients with Waldenstrom macroglobulinemia [38c]. Radiographic features of the pneumonitis were described in detail through computed tomography assessment.

Interstitial lung disease caused by mTOR inhibitors used in oncology was reviewed [39R]. The authors proposed a new diagnostic system and clinical management algorithm.

Mouth and Teeth

A case series of three patients with stomatitis (2 on everolimus, 1 on sirolimus) highlighted the difficulty in diagnosis and management of this well-known side effect [40A]. Stomatitis was dose dependent, and corticosteroids appeared to have a beneficial effect in treatment and prevention.

Urinary Tract

A 47-year-old male renal transplant recipient experienced two episodes of acute renal dysfunction after conversion from tacrolimus to everolimus [41A]. The first was associated with lymphopenia and, the second occurred when the patient began consuming 2–3 glasses of grapefruit juice per day (a known p-glycoprotein inhibitor). The nephrotoxic potential of everolimus was reviewed from the literature. Possible mechanisms included renal epithelial cell damage, interstitial fibrosis and tubular atrophy, proteinuria, and alteration of intracellular everolimus concentration through transmembrane efflux pump activity (p-glycoprotein).

Skin

Macdonald et al. reviewed cutaneous side effects of mTOR inhibitors including everolimus [42R]. Stomatitis and rash were most common with mTOR inhibitors for which local treatments are most often sufficient. Less common cutaneous side effects included inflammatory eruptions, nail toxicity, alopecia, and hypertrichosis.

A 38-year-old female renal transplant recipient developed severe oral and perianal ulcers while on everolimus [43A]. Trough concentration of everolimus was 11.7 ng/mL, above the target range of 3–8 ng/mL, at presentation. The ulcers healed after everolimus discontinuation; however, aesthetic and functional impairment of the upper lip resulted in permanent deformity.

A meta-analysis of 11 trials ($n = 4752$) described the incidence of stomatitis associated with everolimus and temsirolimus in cancer patients [44M]. Use of mTOR inhibitors increased the risk of all-grade stomatitis (RR 4.04, 95% CI 3.13–5.22) and severe stomatitis (RR 8.84, 95% CI 4.07–19.22). Risks of high-grade stomatitis with individual agents were higher with everolimus (RR 9.67, 95% CI 4.05–23.1) compared to temsirolimus (RR 6.22, 95% CI 1.11–34.8), but the comparison was not statistically significant ($P = 0.65$).

Drug–Drug Interactions

Lempers et al. reviewed drug interactions of azole antifungals with immunosuppressants, including everolimus [45R]. The authors provided a stepwise approach to management of these interactions and advocated for frequent therapeutic drug monitoring of the immunosuppressive agent.

A case report described a decline in everolimus trough concentration from 10.1 to 4.2 ng/mL after initiation of fenofibrate 160 mg per day [46A]. After withdrawal of fenofibrate, everolimus concentration increased to 11.5 ng/mL. This interaction was likely to result of fenofibrate-mediated CYP3A4 induction.

FINGOLIMOD [SEDA-34, 616; SEDA-35, 703; SEDA-36, 593]

The safety of fingolimod in the treatment of multiple sclerosis was reviewed [47R]. Infections, arrhythmias, sudden death, progressive multifocal leukoencephalopathy, macular edema, and pregnancy outcomes were discussed.

Comparative Studies

A multi-center, double-blind, placebo-controlled trial of 142 multiple sclerosis patients evaluated 3 conversion regimens from natalizumab to fingolimod [48C]. Mild or moderate adverse effects occurred in 58.5% of patients during fingolimod treatment and were mostly headache (8.5%), dizziness (2.8%), nasopharyngitis (6.3%), and urinary tract infection (2.8%). Ten serious adverse events occurred but no opportunistic infections were observed in this short (24 weeks) trial.

Observational Studies

A registry study compared safety and drug discontinuation rates of natalizumab to fingolimod in 1516 multiple sclerosis patients [49C]. Discontinuation rates at 1 year were 20.3% for fingolimod and 13.4% for natalizumab treatment. Adverse effects leading to discontinuation were 10.5% for fingolimod and 3.4% for natalizumab.

Systematic Reviews

A Cochrane meta-analysis reviewed 39 trials ($n = 25\,113$) of immunosuppressants used to treat multiple sclerosis [50M]. Fingolimod was associated with a higher risk of discontinuation due to adverse effects over 24 months compared to placebo (RR 1.69, 95% CI 1.32–2.17).

Cardiovascular

The effect of fingolimod on cardiac function was compared to natalizumab in 78 patients over a 12-month period [51c]. At 6 months, left ventricular ejection fraction (LVEF) decreased from 63% to 59% ($P = 0.0001$) and end-systolic volume increased (data not provided, $P = 0.01$) in the fingolimod group compared to no changes in the natalizumab group. A 10% decline in LVEF occurred in 30% of fingolimod patients. While statistically significant, these results do not hold significant clinical relevance. Additionally, the LVEF rebounded at month 12 in fingolimod-treated patients to near baseline values.

Nervous System

A 38-year-old female with multiple sclerosis developed posterior reversible encephalopathy syndrome at month 21 of fingolimod treatment [52A]. For unknown reasons, fingolimod was continued for 16 days after initial presentation. Upon discontinuation, she made a partial recovery.

Sensory Systems

Two cases of fingolimod-associated macular edema were successfully treated with intravitreal triamcinolone which allowed for continuation of fingolimod therapy [53A].

A 31-year-old male on fingolimod for 1 month developed macular edema and retinal hemorrhage which completely resolved 24 months after discontinuation [54A].

Hematologic

The effect of fingolimod on platelet count was investigated in 80 multiple sclerosis patients [55c]. Platelet count was 256.5 ± 66.3 $(\times 10^6)$ prior to treatment and 230.0 ± 49.7 $(\times 10^6)$ 1 month into therapy ($P < 0.01$). While this drop was deemed statistically significant, the clinical relevance is minimal.

Infection Risk

A 37-year-old female receiving fingolimod for multiple sclerosis developed visceral leishmaniasis [56A]. She made a full recovery after amphotericin B treatment.

GLATIRAMER [SEDA-34, 617; SEDA-35, 703; SEDA-36]

Observational Studies

A German registry analysis from 1998 to 2012 identified glatiramer as a top 10 prescription drug to cause anaphylactic reactions [57C].

Systematic Reviews

A Cochrane meta-analysis reviewed 39 trials ($n = 25\,113$) of immunosuppressants used to treat multiple sclerosis [50M]. Glatiramer was not associated with a higher risk of discontinuation due to adverse effects over 24 months compared to placebo (RR 1.19, 95% CI 0.84–1.70).

Skin

A 51-year-old female patient developed glatiramer-induced urticaria [58A]. Desensitization over 3 hours (20 ng–20 mg) resulted in no adverse events, and the patient was able to tolerate therapy through 3 months of follow-up.

Panniculitis, skin necrosis, and lipoatrophy occurred in a 36-year-old female following glatiramer injections [59A]. The necrotic lesion healed in 2 months after discontinuation of glatiramer.

LEFLUNOMIDE [SED-15, 2015; SEDA-34, 618; SEDA-35, 703; SEDA-36, 594]

Systematic Reviews

A meta-analysis of 11 trials ($n = 254$) evaluated the safety of leflunomide for lupus nephritis in Chinese patients [60M]. Compared to cyclophosphamide, leflunomide had less liver damage (RR 0.53, 95% CI 0.33–0.87), alopecia (RR 0.38, 95% CI 0.17–0.85), leukopenia (RR 0.25, 95% CI 0.08–0.77) and infection (RR 0.54, 95% CI 0.32–0.92). Gastrointestinal adverse effects, rash, and herpes zoster infections were similar between leflunomide and cyclophosphamide.

Liver

Hepatotoxicity is a well-known side effect of leflunomide. Total glucosides of paeony (TGP) are an extract of a Chinese traditional herbal medicine. TGP was studied for hepatoprotective effects in 268 rheumatoid arthritis patients receiving leflunomide with methotrexate in an open-label, randomized study [61C]. Abnormal liver function tests occurred in 11.4% of the TGP group compared to 23.3% of the no TGP group ($P = 0.013$). Elevation of ALT or AST greater than three times the upper limit of normal occurred in 1.6% of the TGP group compared to 7.8% of the no TGP group ($P = 0.022$).

Skin

A case series described 17 patients with drug reaction with eosinophilia and systemic symptoms (DRESS) [62c]. One of the culprit drugs was leflunomide. The outcome for the patient on leflunomide was not specifically stated, but 76.5% of the patients had complete recovery following culprit drug discontinuation and system corticosteroids.

Infection Risk

A population-based nested case–control study in Ontario characterized the risk of tuberculosis and non-tuberculosis mycobacterium infections in rheumatoid arthritis patients [63C]. Leflunomide was associated with an increased risk of both tuberculosis (adjusted OR 4.02, 95% CI 1.08–15.0) and non-tuberculosis mycobacterium infections (adjusted OR 2.74, 95% CI 1.59–4.70).

Genetic Factors

Discontinuation of leflunomide was higher among rheumatoid arthritis patients ($n = 105$) with the *CYP1A2* rs762551 C allele (HR 2.29, 95% CI 2.24–2.34) [64C]. However, exposure to teriflunomide, the active metabolite of leflunomide, was not associated with discontinuation. Analysis of *CYP2C19* phenotype, *ABCG2* rs2231142 polymorphism, *DHODH* rs3213422 polymorphism, and *DHODH* haplotype II did not reveal any association with leflunomide discontinuation.

MYCOPHENOLIC ACID [SED-15, 2402; SEDA-34, 622; SEDA-35, 704; SEDA-36, 594]

Systematic Reviews

A systematic review compared mycophenolate mofetil (MMF) to azathioprine in 3301 patients [65M]. There were no significant differences in cytomegalovirus (CMV) infection between azathioprine and MMF (RR 1.06, 95% CI: 0.85–1.32); however, MMF therapy had a higher incidence of tissue-invasive CMV disease (RR 1.70, 95% CI 1.10–2.61). Gastrointestinal-associated adverse effects were more common in MMF-treated patients, whereas thrombocytopenia and elevated liver enzymes were more common in azathioprine-treated patients.

Strathie Page and Tait reviewed adverse effects of MMF in dermatologic uses [66R].

Observational Studies

A retrospective study examined adverse effects of 104 patients with atopic dermatitis receiving MMF or enteric-coated mycophenolate sodium (EC-MPS). Twenty-two percent (18/82) of patients discontinued therapy due to adverse effects including neurological symptoms (10%), gastrointestinal symptoms (6%), flu-like symptoms (4%), and shortness of breath (4%) [17C].

Twenty liver transplant recipients were assessed for adverse effects of MMF combined with everolimus [67c]. Note that a calcineurin inhibitor (tacrolimus or cyclosporine) was not given to prevent nephrotoxicity and neurotoxicity. The most commonly reported adverse effects included dyslipidemia in 25%, CMV infection in 25%, and myelotoxicity in 25%. Proteinuria (>1 g/day) was reported in 1 patient (5%). Although the combination of everolimus and MMF without a calcineurin inhibitor could prevent nephrotoxicity and neurotoxicity, caution is warranted due to high rejection rate observed in this study (35%).

Comparative Studies

In a single-center, prospective, randomized clinical trial, the risk of infection and gastrointestinal adverse effects was compared between EC-MPS and MMF among 101 Asian renal transplant recipients ($n = 101$) [68C]. Concomitant immunosuppression was tacrolimus and methylprednisolone. There was no significant difference in infection rate between EC-MPS and MMF (40% vs. 49%, $P=0.362$). However, the incidence of serious infection (i.e. septic shock, multiple organ dysfunction syndrome) was significantly higher with MMF compared to EC-MPS (11.8% vs. 0%, respectively; $P=0.056$). No differences were observed for gastrointestinal adverse effects (41.2% MMF vs. 24% EC-MPS, $P=0.066$), but serious diarrhea (9.8%) was only reported in patients receiving MMF.

In a single-center, prospective, semi-randomized clinical trial, the risk of adverse effects associated with EC-MPS was compared to MMF among Chinese liver transplant recipients ($n=92$) [69c]. There was no significant difference in the incidence rates of adverse events between EC-MPS and MMF (48.8% vs. 47.8%, P-value not provided). The most common adverse effects were infection and gastrointestinal complaints (i.e. abdominal pain, constipation, and diarrhea).

Cardiovascular

A 12-year-old female developed hypertension associated with hyperaldosteronism while receiving MMF [21A]. She had developed hypertension from cyclosporine and was converted to MMF for prevention of GvHD but the hypertension persisted while on MMF. Both hypertension and hyperaldosteronism resolved after MMF dose reduction.

In a cohort study, 126 renal transplant recipients receiving MMF, tacrolimus, and steroid were evaluated to determine clinical and genetic characteristics associated with dyslipidemia [70C]. Dyslipidemia was observed in 35% of patients 1 year after transplantation. Significant risk factors associated with dyslipidemia were: female gender ($P=0.021$), use of high, body-weight based, dose of MMF ($P=0.012$), and use of high, body-weight based, dose of prednisolone ($P=0.023$). The glucocorticoid receptor (NR3C1) *Bcl1* G allele was associated with a higher incidence of dyslipidemia (OR 2.6, 95% CI 1.8–12.2).

Gastrointestinal

Death secondary to MMF-associated gastrointestinal toxicity occurred in a 56-year-old male liver transplant recipient [71A]. Severe diarrhea (>10 times/day) associated with nausea and vomiting led to volume depletion and eventual death.

In a phase III, open-label, single-arm study, adverse effects were assessed for 111 autoimmune disease patients who switched from MMF to EC-MPS [72C]. The mean change in gastrointestinal symptom rating scale (GSRS) at the 6- to 8-week follow-up visit was -0.28 ± 0.92 ($P=0.002$). At follow-up, 39.6% of patients experienced

gastrointestinal-associated symptoms including diarrhea (14.4%), nausea (11.7%), dyspepsia (7.2%), and abdominal pain (4.5%). The clinical significance of this study is unclear since not all patients had gastrointestinal adverse effects prior to conversion and the small observed change in GSRS is not likely clinically relevant.

Urinary Tract

Huang et al. used quantitative assays to assess the risk factors for BK virus-associated nephropathy in renal transplant recipients ($n=615$) [73C]. The authors concluded that concurrent use of tacrolimus with mycophenolic acid (OR$=12.4$, $P=0.001$) and pneumonia (OR$=3.7$, $P=0.001$) after kidney transplantation may increase the risk of BK virus nephropathy.

Infection Risk

A meta-analysis of 5 randomized controlled trials in renal transplant recipients indicated a significantly lower incidence of pneumonia with EC-MPS compared to with MMF (RR 0.32, 95% CI 0.13–0.79) [74M].

In a retrospective study, 268 patients who received hematopoietic cell transplantation were assessed for the effect of MMF dose (2 g/day vs. 3 g/day) on risk of infection [75C]. Investigators concluded that the increased MMF dose had no significant effect on bacterial infections, measured by infection density function per 1000 patients days, on either early (days 0–45; 13.65 vs 18.40, $P=0.05$) or late (days 181–365; 0.74 vs. 1.49, $P=0.03$) post-transplantation time period. Note that P-values of less than 0.01 were considered statistically significant due to multiple comparisons.

Response to influenza vaccination was diminished among transplant patients receiving MMF (RR 0.72, 95% CI 0.60–0.88) compared to other immunosuppressive drugs [76M].

Drug–Drug Interactions

A single-center, open-label, randomized study investigated the pharmacokinetic drug–drug interaction of proton pump inhibitors and mycophenolic acid formulations [77c]. In contrast to previously reported literature, co-administration of either MMF (500–1000 mg twice daily) or EC-MPS (360–720 mg twice daily) with pantoprazole (40 mg daily) had no clinically relevant effect on the pharmacokinetics of mycophenolic acid in renal transplant recipients ($n=20$).

In a rat pharmacokinetic study, concomitant use of glycyrrhizin (an active component of liquorice root) and EC-MPS for 14 days resulted in increased exposure of total and free mycophenolic acid by 28% and 44%, respectively ($P<0.001$) [78E].

SIROLIMUS (RAPAMYCIN) [SED-15, 3148; SEDA-34, 626; SEDA-35, 705; SEDA-36, 594]

Systematic Reviews

The use of mTOR inhibitors for vascular anomalies was reviewed in a systematic review (n = 84) [79M]. The safety profile was mild, and the most frequent side effect was stomatitis.

Sirolimus for the prevention of GvHD was reviewed in a meta-analysis of 5 trials [80M]. Adverse effects included sinusoidal obstructive syndrome (RR 2.24, 95% CI 1.26–4.01) and thrombotic microangiopathy (RR 2.48, 95% CI 0.87–7.06). CMV reactivation was no different with sirolimus treatment (RR 0.64, 95% CI 0.35–1.18).

Cardiovascular

A retrospective study over 11 years evaluated the risk of cardiovascular disease while on sirolimus therapy post-liver transplant (n = 803) [81C]. Six percent of sirolimus-treated patients developed coronary artery disease or cerebrovascular accidents compared to 7% of non-sirolimus-treated patients. There was no difference in the risk of cardiovascular outcomes with sirolimus on multivariate analysis.

Pulmonary

Non-infectious pneumonitis was associated with sirolimus in a stem cell transplant patient [82A]. Discontinuation of sirolimus and steroid treatment led to resolution of symptoms.

An 8-year-old male stem cell transplant recipient developed interstitial lung disease associated with sirolimus [83A]. His symptoms improved after sirolimus discontinuation.

Sirolimus was associated with acute respiratory distress in 2 solid organ transplant recipients [84A]. After sirolimus discontinuation and systemic steroids, the symptoms quickly resolved.

Hematology

A 71-year-old male developed bilateral lymphedema while on sirolimus post-renal transplant [85A]. It resolved after conversion to tacrolimus.

Liver

Sirolimus toxicity with hepatic dysfunction occurred in a 51-year-old male stem cell transplant recipient [86A]. Automated red cell exchange decreased the sirolimus concentration from 22.6 to 10.3 ng/mL and also decreased the liver enzymes. The large volume of distribution necessitated repeated red cell exchanges for continued sirolimus removal.

Skin

A 71-year-old male on sirolimus developed severe radiation toxicity (grade 4 mucositis and esophagitis), disproportionate to the dose of radiation delivered [87A].

Drug–Drug Interactions

A 65-year-old male allogeneic hematopoietic cell transplant patient developed supratherapeutic sirolimus and tacrolimus concentrations after initiation of clotrimazole troches for oral candidiasis [88A]. Sirolimus trough concentration increased from 13.1 to >30.0 ng/mL within 3 days of clotrimazole initiation. Elevated concentrations were likely the result of CYP3A4 inhibition mediated by clotrimazole. After holding the medications and administering phenytoin to induce metabolism, the immunosuppressive drug concentrations declined.

A dosing algorithm for sirolimus and tacrolimus in combination with azole antifungals was developed from a retrospective study of 28 allogeneic hematopoietic stem cell transplant patients [89c]. A 50–75% dose reduction was recommended for tacrolimus and sirolimus when combined with therapeutic doses of azole antifungals to maintain therapeutic trough concentrations. Frequent therapeutic drug monitoring is advised because of the pharmacokinetic variability in tacrolimus and sirolimus along with the differential effects of the various azole antifungals on CYP3A4 and p-glycoprotein.

TACROLIMUS [SED-15, 3279; SEDA-34, 629; SEDA-35, 705; SEDA-36, 596]

Systemic Reviews

A systematic review of non-randomized trials in patients with refractory dermatomyositis/polymyositis (n = 134) who received tacrolimus treatment revealed that nephrotoxicity (11.6%), hypomagnesemia (9.7%), tremors (8.7%), and hypertension (8.7%) was the most common adverse effects [90M].

Observational Studies

A prospective study investigated adverse effects in renal transplant recipients (n = 123) who underwent 1 mg:1 mg conversion of tacrolimus from extended-release regimen (Advagraf®) to immediate-release regimen (Prograf®) [91C]. Nine percent of patients reported adverse effects, mainly including tremor and alopecia, which were potentially due to increased tacrolimus trough concentration ($P=0.000$).

In a multicenter, prospective study, patients with ulcerative colitis ($n=49$) were assessed for adverse effects of oral tacrolimus as a rapid induction therapy [92c]. Tacrolimus was titrated from an initial dose of 0.1 mg/day, to achieve a trough blood concentration of 10–15 ng/mL within the first 7 days. The most commonly reported adverse effects include hypomanesemia (<1.7 mg/dL; 74.1%), elevated blood glucose (>120 mg/dL; 48.6%), tremor (35.7%), headache (9.5%), nausea (7.1%), and elevated serum creatinine (>1.2 mg/dL; 5.4%).

In a single-center, prospective study, patients with SLE ($n=57$) were assessed for adverse effects of maintenance therapy consisting of tacrolimus plus prednisolone (≤20 mg/day) [93c]. Tacrolimus target trough concentration was 5–10 ng/mL. After 1 year, 5/57 patients reported adverse effects. Of the 30 patients with renal complications of SLE, 1 developed an adverse effect (pruritis) compared to 4/27 patients without renal complications (rhabdomyolysis, muscle cramp, alopecia, and diarrhea).

A post-marking surveillance study described adverse effects of tacrolimus when added to biological disease-modifying anti-rheumatic drugs (DMARDs) [94C]. Adverse effects occurred in 10.5% (18/172) of patients. Serious adverse effects (herpes zoster, myocardial infarction) were observed in two patients.

Comparative Studies

There are several reviews that compare adverse effects of tacrolimus between extended-release and immediate-release formulations [95R,96R]. A review by Singh et al. revealed that there is no significant difference in the rate of adverse effects (i.e. diabetes mellitus, hypertension, hyperlipidemia) between extended-release tacrolimus (Advagraf®, Astagraf XL™) and immediate-release tacrolimus (Prograf®) in solid organ transplant recipients [95R]. Consistently, Coilly et al. concluded that there was no difference in adverse event rates between extended-release (Advagraf®) and immediate-release (Prograf®) regimen in de novo liver transplant recipients (89.9% vs. 93.2%, P-value not provided) [96R]. The most commonly reported adverse events for both once-a-day and twice-a-day regimens were: metabolism and nutrition disorders including diabetes (39.7% vs. 46.6%), infections (39.2% vs. 33.3%), nervous system disorders (27.0% vs. 31.6%), hypertension (20.7% vs. 21.8%), renal insufficiency (21.9% vs. 20.5%), psychiatric disorders (17.3% vs. 15.8%), blood and lymphatic disorders (16.5% vs. 15.0%), gastrointestinal disorders (15.6% vs. 15.0%), and CMV infection (9.3% vs. 4.7%). These results were consistent with a recent single-center, randomized, open-labeled study that compared Advagraf® ($n=49$) to

Prograf® ($n=50$) in stable renal transplant recipients ($n=99$) [97c]. There was no difference in adverse event rates between Advagraf® and Prograf® ($P>0.05$). The most common adverse reactions associated with both Prograf® and Advagraf® were increased serum creatinine (12.0% vs 14.3%), nasopharyngitis (20.0% vs 10.2%), urinary tract infection (10.0% vs 8.2%), and rhinorrhea or rhinitis (4.0% vs 4.1%).

In a prospective, randomized, open-labeled trial, standard-dose tacrolimus was compared with everolimus plus reduced-dose tacrolimus regimen in de novo liver transplant recipients ($n=719$) [98C]. During 24–36 months of treatment, 76.8% of patients receiving standard-dose tacrolimus (target trough concentration 6–10 ng/mL) and 82.1% of patients receiving everolimus (target trough concentration 3–8 ng/mL) and reduced-dose tacrolimus (target trough concentration 3–5 ng/mL) regimen reported one or more adverse events ($P=0.335$). There was no difference in serious adverse event rates between standard-dose tacrolimus and everolimus plus reduced-dose tacrolimus regimens during that period (30.2% vs. 22.4%, $P=0.228$). The most commonly reported serious adverse events for both standard-dose tacrolimus and everolimus plus reduced-dose tacrolimus regimens were: diarrhea (1.6% vs. 2.8%), pyrexia (1.6% vs. 2.8%), and pneumonia (2.4% vs. 1.9%).

In a prospective, open-labeled trial, tacrolimus and MMF combination was compared to tacrolimus and sirolimus combination in renal transplant recipients at high immunologic risk [99c]. At 12 months of follow-up, BK virus infection ($P=0.031$), dyslipidemia ($P=0.004$), and lymphocele ($P=0.02$) were significantly more frequent in patients receiving tacrolimus and sirolimus ($n=28$) compared to those receiving tacrolimus and MMF ($n=69$).

Cardiovascular

A case of tacrolimus-induced cardiomyopathy was reported in a 62-year-old female renal transplant recipient [100A]. Tacrolimus target trough concentration was 3–10 ng/mL. After 6 months post-transplantation, she was admitted to hospital three times with heart failure and acute renal allograft dysfunction. Carvedilol, isosorbide mononitrate, hydralazine, and torsemide were initiated after the first hospital admission, but the symptoms did not resolve. Left ventricular ejection fraction (LVEF) was reduced from 63% to 40% at the third hospital admission. LVEF normalized to 56% 3 months after tacrolimus discontinuation. Both heart failure exacerbation and acute renal allograft dysfunction were not observed over the 3-year follow-up period.

Pregnancy

Tacrolimus adverse effect profile was reviewed for pregnant female solid organ transplant recipients [101R]. Tacrolimus (pregnancy category C) is not associated with an increased risk of congenital malformation, but it has been associated with neonatal hyperkalemia and renal impairment.

Drug–Drug Interaction

A review discussed drugs that affect tacrolimus blood concentration in *de novo* heart and lung transplant recipients [102R]. Drugs that increase tacrolimus concentration include: glucocorticoids, macrolides (i.e. erythromycin, clarithromycin), azoles, levofloxacin, basiliximab, calcium antagonists (i.e. verapamil, diltiazem, nifedipine, amlodipine, etc.), omeprazole, HIV protease inhibitors (i.e. nelfinavir, ritonavir), amiodarone, and theophylline, among others. Drugs that decrease tacrolimus concentration include: glucocorticoids, carbamazepine, phenytoin, phenobarbital, and rifampin, among others.

A 30-year-old female lung transplant recipient with a mediastinal *Aspergillus fumigatus* infection experienced an increase in tacrolimus concentration after the addition of isavuconazole [103A]. Tacrolimus trough concentration was increased despite an empiric dose reduction of tacrolimus from 3.5 mg twice-a-day to 2 mg twice-a-day following isavuconazole initiation. Tacrolimus dosage reduction to 72% resulted in attainment of target trough concentration (6–8 ng/mL).

TEMSIROLIMUS [SEDA-34, 632; SEDA-35, 707; SEDA-36, 597]

Observational Studies

The association of baseline chronic kidney disease with toxicity was assessed in a retrospective study of renal cell carcinoma patients ($n = 102$; 11/102 on temsirolimus) [104C]. Baseline GFR of less than 60 mL/min/1.73 m^2 was associated with higher odds of severe toxicity (OR 4.74, 95% CI 1.67–13.4).

A retrospective analysis was completed in 38 patients receiving temsirolimus for renal cancer [105c]. Adverse effects were similar to prior reports of temsirolimus and included 12 (31.6%) grade 3 or 4 toxicities. Anemia, thrombocytopenia, rash, mucositis, fatigue, and increased serum creatinine were the most commonly reported (>20%) adverse effects.

Grade 3 or 4 toxicities were reported in 15 patients with follicular lymphoma treated with temsirolimus, bendamustine, and rituximab [106c]. These included neutropenia (27%), leukopenia (40%), and thrombocytopenia (13%).

A phase I/II trial investigated the combination of temsirolimus and bevacizumab for previously treated renal cell carcinoma [107c]. Anemia (71%), neutropenia (15%), thrombocytopenia (40%), hypercholesterolemia (63%), hypertriglyceridemia (63%), proteinuria (48%), fatigue (65%), mucositis (67%) and rash (42%) were the most commonly experienced side effects. Temsirolimus dose reduction due to toxicity was required in 59.6% of the evaluated patients.

THIOPURINES [SED-15, 377; SEDA-34, 633; SEDA-35, 709; SEDA-36, 598]

Observational Studies

Among 67 patients on azathioprine for SLE, discontinuation occurred in 30 (45%) of the patients [108c]. However, toxicity was the reason for discontinuation in only 3 of those patients indicating a generally well-tolerated treatment.

Safety of azathioprine was assessed in 82 pediatric atopic dermatitis patients [109c]. Hematologic adverse effects occurred in 41% of patients with 2 patients discontinuing therapy. Clinic adverse effects (hepatotoxicity, infection, gastrointestinal upset, headache, lethargy, and nausea) occurred in 20% of patients with 2 patients discontinuing therapy. Most adverse effects were observed within 9 months of starting azathioprine. Factors including age, sex, TMPT activity, or drug dose were not predictors of adverse effect manifestations.

A retrospective study of 351 Crohn's disease patients aimed to describe the incidence and predictors of thiopurine adverse effects [110C]. Thirty-one percent of patients discontinued thiopurine due to adverse effects: hypersensitivity reactions, pancreatitis, gastrointestinal toxicity, leukopenia, hepatotoxicity, and infection. Females over the age of 40 were most likely to discontinue due to an adverse effect.

Systematic Reviews

Amin et al. reviewed the metabolic pathways of azathioprine and 6-mercaptopurine with a focus on dosing strategies to minimize adverse effects [111R]. Goel et al. and Goldberg et al. also reviewed thiopurines used for inflammatory bowel disease (IBD) with discussion of strategies to avoid toxicity [112R,113R].

Cardiovascular

A 55-year-old female developed paroxysmal atrial fibrillation 2 hours after receiving azathioprine 50 mg

[114A]. The arrhythmia resolved after discontinuation of azathioprine, indicating a moderate probability of causation.

Endocrine

Azathioprine-induced acute pancreatitis is reported in several studies [115A,116C]. Gallego-Gutierrez et al. described 2 pediatric male Crohn's disease patients with azathioprine-induced acute pancreatitis [115A]. After azathioprine withdrawal, both patients were able to tolerate 6-mercaptopurine treatment without further adverse events. In another prospective registry trial, azathioprine-induced pancreatitis occurred in 7.3% of 510 IBD patients [116C]. Smoking was identified as a risk factor for this adverse event (OR 3.24, 95% CI 1.74–6.02) with a dose-dependent effect. The course of pancreatitis was generally mild and resolved in all patients within significant sequelae.

Pancreatitis induced by thiopurines was reviewed with a discussion on genetic predisposition [117R].

Hematologic

To predict post-high-dose methotrexate myelotoxicity, two major active 6-mercaptopurine (6-MP) metabolites, methylated 6-MP metabolites and 6-thioguanine nucleotides (6-TGN), were investigated in 17 pediatric acute lymphoblastic leukemia (ALL) patients under methotrexate/6-MP maintenance therapy [118c]. Based on multiple linear regression analyses at 48 hours after high-dose methotrexate administration, erythrocyte concentrations of methylated 6-MP metabolites and 6-TGN were significant predictors of neutrophil nadir ($P < 0.0001$ for both); erythrocyte concentration of methylated 6-MP metabolites was a significant predictor of thrombocyte nadir ($P < 0.0001$) after high-dose methotrexate administration.

Liver

Drug-induced liver injury was reviewed with identification of azathioprine as a top offending agent [119R].

Skin

Sweet's syndrome was reported in a 50-year-old patient on azathioprine [120A].

Hair

Hair loss occurred in two female patients receiving azathioprine determined to be anagen effluvium (abrupt shedding of hair while in growth phase) [121A]. Hair regrowth occurred after azathioprine discontinuation in both cases.

Immunologic

Azathioprine hypersensitivity reaction was reported in a 57-year-old male with Crohn's disease [122A]. His symptoms completely resolved after azathioprine discontinuation.

Infection Risk

CMV infection was more common with azathioprine (77%) and MMF (72%) compared to everolimus (35%; $P < 0.0001$) in a cohort of heart transplant recipients [123C].

Mutagenicity

A high cumulative dose of azathioprine was associated with an increased risk of cervical cancer in a population-based cohort study of autoimmune disease patients (HR 2.2, 95% CI 1.2–3.9) [124C].

Pregnancy

The impact of thiopurines on pregnancy outcomes of patients with IBD was investigated in a meta-analysis of 312 pregnant females treated with thiopurines compared to 1149 pregnant controls [125C]. There was a higher risk of congenital abnormalities in the thiopurine group (OR 2.95, 95% CI 1.03–8.43). However, other pregnancy outcomes including low birth weight, premature delivery, spontaneous abortion, and neonatal adverse outcomes were no different between thiopurine and control groups.

SPECIAL REVIEW

Association of Genetic Factors and Adverse Effects of Thiopurines

Inosine triphosphate pyrophosphohydrolase (ITPA) metabolizes inosine triphosphate, a toxic metabolite of 6-mercaptopurine, to the non-toxic inosine monophosphate. Polymorphisms in ITPA were investigated in 70 pediatric patients with ALL for association to toxicities of 6-mercaptopurine [126c]. The ITPA 94C > A, 138G > A, IVS2 + 21A > C, and IVS3 + 101G > A polymorphisms were studied. Compound mutant alleles in all four positions were associated with leukopenia (OR 9.2, 95% CI 0.97–70.0, P = 0.05), neutropenia (OR 8.8, 95% CI 1.04–74.9, P = 0.04), and hepatotoxicity defined by ALT elevation (OR 15.4, 95% CI 3.0–75.9, P = 0.001) and AST elevation (OR 9.6, 95% CI 2.0–44.6, P = 0.004). Thus, these polymorphisms are likely associated with poor activity of ITPA, elevation in inosine triphosphate concentrations, and subsequent toxic effects.

Thiopurine S-methyltransferase (TMPT) activity has been used to optimize thiopurine therapy for years. In a prospective, multicenter, controlled trial, adverse effects were assessed between standard treatment and thiopurine dose adjustment based on TMPT activity (determined by genotyping) [127C]. There was no difference in hematologic side effects (RR 0.93, 95% CI 0.57–1.52) at 20 weeks. Of the patients with TMPT variants who require lower thiopurine doses, 2.6% developed hematologic side effects in the dose-adjusted group compared to 22.9% in the standard-dose group (RR 0.11, 95% CI 0.01–0.85).

TMPT activity was measured in 101 Behcet's disease patients and compared to healthy controls, SLE, and vasculitis patients [128C]. TMPT levels were similar across the patient groups, including health controls. Azathioprine-associated adverse effects were rare, but those patients with adverse effects had lower TMPT levels (14.08 ± 9.49 ng/mL) compared to those without adverse effects (25.62 ± 12.68 ng/mL; P = 0.013).

Association of hematologic toxicity and genetic polymorphisms in genes involved in 6-mercaptopurine metabolism was determined in 70 patients with ALL [129c]. Leukopenia was associated with polymorphisms: ITPA rs1127354 (CC vs. CA genotypes: HR 2.32, 95% CI 1.34–4.01), ITPA rs7270101 (CC vs. AA genotypes: HR 2.03, 95% CI 1.31–3.17), IMPDH1 rs2278293 (TT vs. CC genotypes: HR 0.59, 95% CI 0.40–0.89), SLC28A2 rs2431775 (AA vs. TT genotypes: HR 2.02, 95% CI 1.45–2.82), SLC29A1 rs747199 (CC vs. GG/CG genotypes: HR 0.69, 95% CI 0.52–0.92), SLC28A3 rs10868138 (AG/GG vs. AA genotypes: HR 1.56, 95% CI 1.16–2.11), and ABCC4 rs2274407 (CC vs. AA/CA genotypes: HR 1.90, 95% CI 1.39–2.60). Male sex was associated with a lower risk of leukopenia (HR 0.56, 95% CI 0.44–0.71).

A retrospective study of 132 pediatric IBD patients investigated numerous genetic polymorphisms with thiopurine toxicities [130C]. Neutropenia was associated with ADK rs10824095 (OR 6.22, P = 0.004), SLC29A1 rs747199 (OR 5.68, P = 0.016), and TYMS rs34743033 (OR 3.85, P = 0.045). Lymphopenia was associated with ABCC1 rs2074087 (OR 3.41, P = 0.022), IMPDH1 rs2278294 (OR 0.28, P = 0.027), and IMPDH2 rs11706052 (OR 3.64, P = 0.034). However, multiple testing of 70 polymorphisms may have resulted in false-positive associations.

The effect of TMPT activity on hematologic and liver toxicity of 6-mercaptopurine was investigated in 411 children with ALL given high-dose methotrexate [131C]. The decline in leukocytes or neutrophils did not differ between TMPT intermediate activity and high activity. Rather, the dose of 6-mercaptopurine was significantly related to leukopenia, neutropenia, thrombocytopenia, and rise in aminotransferases (P < 0.0001 for all).

A meta-analysis of 14 trials of IBD patients (n = 2206) found that TMPT polymorphisms (lower TMPT activity) were associated with cumulative adverse effects (OR 3.36, 95% CI 1.81–6.19) and hematologic toxicity (OR 6.67, 95% CI 3.88–11.47) of thiopurines [132M]. No associations between TMPT polymorphisms and hepatotoxicity, pancreatitis, or gastrointestinal adverse effects were observed. A similar meta-analysis in autoimmune diseases (11 trials, n = 651) found associations with TMPT polymorphisms and cumulative adverse effects (OR 3.12, 95% CI 1.48–6.56), hematologic toxicity (OR 3.76, 95% CI 1.97–7.17) and gastrointestinal adverse effects (OR 6.43, 95% CI 2.04–20.25) [133M]. No association was observed for hepatotoxicity.

Pharmacogenetic associations with toxicity of 6-mercaptopurine were included in a review of ALL treatments [134R]. The influence of genetic variability on response to thiopurines was also reviewed [135R].

The associations between TMPT and ITPA polymorphisms and azathioprine toxicities were investigated in 48 IBD patients [136c]. All patients were wild type for TMPT, so no associations were investigated after genotyping. The ITPA 94C > A polymorphism was more prevalent in the group of patients with leukopenia (70.0%) compared to those without leukopenia (31.6%; P < 0.05). Concentrations of the myelotoxic 6-thioguanine nucleotide (6-TGN) metabolite were not different among leukopenic versus non-leukopenic patients.

TMPT and ITPA polymorphisms were also investigated in 551 Lithuanian IBD patients for their association to azathioprine side effects [137C]. Leukopenia and myelotoxicity were associated with mutant alleles (all combined) of TMPT compared to wild type (P = 0.01 and P = 0.001, respectively). No associations were observed for ITPA polymorphisms and azathioprine adverse effects.

Polymorphisms in ITPA, MRP4, MTHFR, RFC1, and SLCO1B1 were not associated with leukocyte or ALT values in 53 pediatric leukemia patients [138c].

The NUDT15 rs116855232 polymorphism was investigated in 92 Japanese pediatric ALL patients for association to 6-mercaptopurine toxicity [139c]. The T allele was associated with leukopenia (OR 7.20, 95% CI 2.49–20.8) and 6-mercaptopurine dose reduction. Hepatotoxicity occurred in 10 patients, all with the CC genotype.

Drug Formulations

A novel 6-mercaptopurine formulation was developed for Crohn's disease that has a delayed-release and minimal systemic absorption. This was compared to conventional 6-mercaptopurine in 70 patients over a 12-week double-blinded study [140c]. Side effects occurred in 67.5% of patients on the novel delayed-release formulation compared to 95.8% on the conventional formulation (P = 0.0079). Leukocytes were within the normal range in 87.0% of patients on the novel delayed-release formulation compared to 69.2% on the conventional formulation (P-value not provided). Hepatotoxicity was also less with the novel formulation (2.5%) compared to the conventional formulation (8.3%; P-value not provided).

A novel oral liquid formulation of 6-mercaptopurine was designed for pediatric leukemia patients. The palatability of this novel liquid formulation was subjectively improved compared to the conventional tablet formulation in 15 patients [141c]. However, significant differences in the pharmacokinetics were noted in this study, necessitating future investigation to determine appropriate dose conversions.

IMMUNOENHANCING DRUGS

Levamisole [SED-15, 2028; SEDA-34, 638; SEDA-35, 710; SEDA-36, 460]

Nervous System

A 22-year-old male with chronic abuse of cocaine adulterated with levamisole-induced leukoencephalopathy mimicking Susac's syndrome [142A]. While a definitive diagnosis was not made, the authors suspected levamisole and/or cocaine as the culprit agent(s). The patient died of infectious complications from intensive immunosuppression.

Multifocal leukoencephalopathy was described in two patients with a history of levamisole-adulterated cocaine abuse [143A]. Causality to cocaine and/or levamisole was unable to be determined, but an immune-mediated mechanism of levamisole-induced leukoencephalopathy was proposed. Both patients clinically improved following steroids and plasma exchange.

References

[1] Diekmann F. Immunosuppressive minimization with mTOR inhibitors and belatacept. Transpl Int. 2015;28(8):921–7 [R].

[2] Talawila N, Pengel LH. Does belatacept improve outcomes for kidney transplant recipients? A systematic review. Transpl Int. 2015;28(11):1251–64 [M].

[3] Wong L, Harper L, Little MA. Getting the balance right: adverse events of therapy in anti-neutrophil cytoplasm antibody vasculitis. Nephrol Dial Transplant. 2015;30(Suppl 1):i164–70 [R].

[4] Ram R, Guditi S, Kaligotla Venkata D. A 10-year follow-up of idiopathic membranous nephropathy patients on steroids and cyclophosphamide: a case series. Ren Fail. 2015;37(3):452–5 [c].

[5] Li J, Dai G, Zhang Z. General adverse response to cyclophosphamide in Chinese patients with systemic autoimmune diseases in recent decade-a single-center retrospective study. Clin Rheumatol. 2015;34(2):273–8 [C].

[6] Shajahan J, Pillai PS, Jayakumar KN. A prospective comparative study of the toxicity profile of 5-flurouracil, adriamycin, cyclophosphamide regime vs adriamycin, paclitaxel regime in patients with locally advanced breast carcinoma. J Clin Diagn Res. 2015;9(12):FC01–6 [C].

[7] van den Berg H, Paulussen M, Le Teuff G, et al. Impact of gender on efficacy and acute toxicity of alkylating agent-based chemotherapy in Ewing sarcoma: secondary analysis of the Euro-Ewing99-R1 trial. Eur J Cancer. 2015;51(16):2453–64 [C].

[8] Wittayanukorn S, Qian J, Johnson BS, et al. Cardiotoxicity in targeted therapy for breast cancer: a study of the FDA adverse event reporting system (FAERS). J Oncol Pharm Pract. 2015; doi: 1078155215621150 [Epub ahead of print] [C].

[9] Ranchoux B, Gunther S, Quarck R, et al. Chemotherapy-induced pulmonary hypertension: role of alkylating agents. Am J Pathol. 2015;185(2):356–71 [R].

[10] Yilmaz N, Emmungil H, Gucenmez S, et al. Incidence of cyclophosphamide-induced urotoxicity and protective effect of mesna in rheumatic diseases. J Rheumatol. 2015;42(9):1661–6 [C].

[11] Chowdhury AC, Misra DP, Patro PS, et al. Toxic epidermal necrolysis due to therapy with cyclophosphamide and mesna: a case report of a patient with seronegative rheumatoid arthritis and rheumatoid vasculitis. Z Rheumatol. 2016;75:200–2 [A].

[12] Fan C, Georgiou KR, McKinnon RA, et al. Combination chemotherapy with cyclophosphamide, epirubicin and 5-fluorouracil causes trabecular bone loss, bone marrow cell depletion and marrow adiposity in female rats. J Bone Miner Metab. 2016;34:277–90 [E].

[13] Haroun F, Al-Shaar L, Habib RH, et al. Effects of CYP2B6 genetic polymorphisms in patients receiving cyclophosphamide combination chemotherapy for breast cancer. Cancer Chemother Pharmacol. 2015;75(1):207–14 [C].

[14] Islam MS, Islam MS, Parvin S, et al. Effect of GSTP1 and ABCC4 gene polymorphisms on response and toxicity of cyclophosphamide-epirubicin-5-fluorouracil-based chemotherapy in Bangladeshi breast cancer patients. Tumour Biol. 2015;36(7):5451–7 [C].

[15] Jordheim LP, Ribrag V, Ghesquieres H, et al. Single nucleotide polymorphisms in ABCB1 and CBR1 can predict toxicity to R-CHOP type regimens in patients with diffuse non-Hodgkin lymphoma. Haematologica. 2015;100(5):e204–6 [C].

[16] Shu W, Guan S, Yang X, et al. Genetic markers in CYP2C19 and CYP2B6 for prediction of cyclophosphamide's 4-hydroxylation, efficacy and side effects in Chinese patients with systemic lupus erythematosus. Br J Clin Pharmacol. 2016;81(2):327–40 [C].

[17] Garritsen FM, Roekevisch E, van der Schaft J, et al. Ten years experience with oral immunosuppressive treatment in adult patients with atopic dermatitis in two academic centres. J Eur Acad Dermatol Venereol. 2015;29(10):1905–12 [C].

[18] Lee JJ, Kim MK, Wee WR. Adverse effects of low-dose systemic cyclosporine therapy in high-risk penetrating keratoplasty. Graefes Arch Clin Exp Ophthalmol. 2015;253(7):1111–9 [c].

[19] Yilmaz A, Yuruk Yildirim Z, Pehlivanoglu C, et al. Side effects of immunosupression in pediatric renal transplantation. Pediatr Transplant. 2015;19:104 [c].

[20] Venuto RC, Meaney CJ, Chang S, et al. Association of extrarenal adverse effects of posttransplant immunosuppression with sex and ABCB1 haplotypes. Medicine. 2015;94(37):e1315 [C].

[21] Rabah F, Beshlawi I, El-Naggari M, et al. Determining the etiology of pediatric hypertension; a hard nut to crack. Pediatr Nephrol. 2015;30(9):1622–3 [A].

[22] Ichimaru N, Yamanaka K, Kato T, et al. Risk factors and incidence for lipid abnormalities in kidney transplant patients. Transplant Proc. 2015;47(3):672–4 [C].

[23] Bahri NS, Adam-Eldien R, Gupta A. Isolated diplopia caused by calcineurin inhibitor therapy in a patient with idiopathic calcineurin membranous nephropathy. J Investig Med. 2015;63(2):326–7 [A].

[24] Montero N, Pascual J. Immunosuppression and post-transplant hyperglycemia. Curr Diabetes Rev. 2015;11(3):144–54 [R].

[25] Georgiou GK, Dounousi E, Harissis HV. Calcineurin inhibitors and male fertility after renal transplantation—a review. Andrologia. 2016;48:483–90 [R].

[26] Mo L, He J, Yue Q, et al. Increased dosage of cyclosporine induces myopathy with increased seru creatine kinase in an

elderly patient on chronic statin therapy. J Clin Pharm Ther. 2015;40(2):245–8 [A].

[27] Brunkhorst LC, Fichtner A, Hocker B, et al. Efficacy and safety of an everolimus- vs. a mycophenolate mofetil-based regimen in pediatric renal transplant recipients. PLoS One. 2015;10(9): e0135439 [C].

[28] Ju Y, Hu Y, Sun S, et al. Toxicity and adverse effects of everolimus in the treatment of advanced nonsmall cell lung cancer pretreated with chemotherapy—Chinese experiences. Indian J Cancer. 2015;52(Suppl 1):e32–6 [c].

[29] Somers MJ, Paul E. Safety considerations of mammalian target of rapamycin inhibitors in tuberous sclerosis complex and renal transplantation. J Clin Pharmacol. 2015;55(4):368–76 [R].

[30] Motzer RJ, Escudier B, McDermott DF, et al. Nivolumab versus everolimus in advanced renal-cell carcinoma. N Engl J Med. 2015;373(19):1803–13 [C].

[31] Nozawa M, Ohzeki T, Tamada S, et al. Differences in adverse event profiles between everolimus and temsirolimus and the risk factors for non-infectious pneumonitis in advanced renal cell carcinoma. Int J Clin Oncol. 2015;20(4):790–5 [C].

[32] Abdel-Rahman O, Fouad M. Risk of fatigue and hepatic and metabolic toxicities in patients with solid tumors treated with everolimus: a meta-analysis. Future Oncol. 2015;11(1):79–90 [M].

[33] Peng L, Zhou Y, Ye X, et al. Treatment-related fatigue with everolimus and temsirolimus in patients with cancer—a meta-analysis of clinical trials. Tumour Biol. 2015;36(2):643–54 [M].

[34] Holdaas H, Potena L, Saliba F. mTOR inhibitors and dyslipidemia in transplant recipients: a cause for concern? Transplant Rev (Orlando). 2015;29(2):93–102 [R].

[35] Murbraech K, Massey R, Undset LH, et al. Cardiac response to early conversion from calcineurin inhibitor to everolimus in renal transplant recipients—a three-yr serial echocardiographic substudy of the randomized controlled CENTRAL trial. Clin Transplant. 2015;29(8):678–84 [c].

[36] Singhal N, Vatandoust S, Brown MP. Phase II study evaluating efficacy and safety of everolimus with letrozole for management of advanced (unresectable or metastatic) non-small cell lung cancer after failure of platinum-based treatment: a preliminary analysis of toxicity. Cancer Chemother Pharmacol. 2015;75(2):325–31 [c].

[37] Badar Q, Masood N, Abbasi AN. Everolimus induced pneumonitis. Gulf J Oncolog. 2015;1(18):18–24 [A].

[38] Nishino M, Boswell EN, Hatabu H, et al. Drug-related pneumonitis during mammalian target of rapamycin inhibitor therapy: radiographic pattern-based approach in Waldenstrom macroglobulinemia as a paradigm. Oncologist. 2015;20(9):1077–83 [c].

[39] Willemsen AE, Grutters JC, Gerritsen WR, et al. mTOR inhibitor-induced interstitial lung disease in cancer patients: comprehensive review and a practical management algorithm. Int J Cancer. 2016;138:2312–21 [R].

[40] Meiller TF, Varlotta S, Weikel D. Recognition and management of oral mucosal injury caused by mammalian target of rapamycin inhibitors: a case series. Case Rep Oncol. 2015;8(2):369–77 [A].

[41] Barbari A, Maawad M, Kfoury Kassouf H, et al. Mammalian target of rapamycin inhibitors and nephrotoxicity: fact or fiction. Exp Clin Transplant. 2015;13(5):377–86 [A].

[42] Macdonald JB, Macdonald B, Golitz LE, et al. Cutaneous adverse effects of targeted therapies: part II: inhibitors of intracellular molecular signaling pathways. J Am Acad Dermatol. 2015;72(2):221–36 [R].

[43] Pasin VP, Pereira AR, Carvalho KA, et al. New drugs, new challenges for dermatologists: mucocutaneous ulcers secondary to everolimus. An Bras Dermatol. 2015;90(3 Suppl 1):165–7 [A].

[44] Shameem R, Lacouture M, Wu S. Incidence and risk of high-grade stomatitis with mTOR inhibitors in cancer patients. Cancer Invest. 2015;33(3):70–7 [M].

[45] Lempers VJ, Martial LC, Schreuder MF, et al. Drug-interactions of azole antifungals with selected immunosuppressants in transplant patients: strategies for optimal management in clinical practice. Curr Opin Pharmacol. 2015;24:38–44 [R].

[46] Mir O, Poinsignon V, Arnedos M, et al. Pharmacokinetic interaction involving fenofibrate and everolimus. Ann Oncol. 2015;26(1):248–9 [A].

[47] Gajofatto A, Turatti M, Monaco S, et al. Clinical efficacy, safety, and tolerability of fingolimod for the treatment of relapsing-remitting multiple sclerosis. Drug Healthc Patient Saf. 2015;7:157–67 [R].

[48] Kappos L, Radue EW, Comi G, et al. Switching from natalizumab to fingolimod: a randomized, placebo-controlled study in RRMS. Neurology. 2015;85(1):29–39 [C].

[49] Frisell T, Forsberg L, Nordin N, et al. Comparative analysis of first-year fingolimod and natalizumab drug discontinuation among Swedish patients with multiple sclerosis. Mult Scler. 2016;22(1):85–93 [C].

[50] Tramacere I, Del Giovane C, Salanti G, et al. Immunomodulators and immunosuppressants for relapsing-remitting multiple sclerosis: a network meta-analysis. Cochrane Database Syst Rev. 2015;9:CD011381 [M].

[51] Racca V, Di Rienzo M, Cavarretta R, et al. Fingolimod effects on left ventricular function in multiple sclerosis. Mult Scler. 2016;22(2):201–11 [c].

[52] Linda H, von Heijne A. A case of posterior reversible encephalopathy syndrome associated with gilenya((R)) (fingolimod) treatment for multiple sclerosis. Front Neurol. 2015;6:39 [A].

[53] Thoo S, Cugati S, Lee A, et al. Successful treatment of fingolimod-associated macular edema with intravitreal triamcinolone with continued fingolimod use. Mult Scler. 2015;21(2):249–51 [A].

[54] Ueda N, Saida K. Retinal hemorrhages following fingolimod treatment for multiple sclerosis; a case report. BMC Ophthalmol. 2015;15:135 [A].

[55] Farrokhi M, Beni AA, Etemadifar M, et al. Effect of fingolimod on platelet count among multiple sclerosis patients. Int J Prev Med. 2015;6:125 [c].

[56] Artemiadis AK, Nikolaou G, Kolokythopoulos D, et al. Visceral leishmaniasis infection in a fingolimod-treated multiple sclerosis patient. Mult Scler. 2015;21(6):795–6 [A].

[57] Sachs B, Fischer-Barth W, Merk HF. Reporting rates for severe hypersensitivity reactions associated with prescription-only drugs in outpatient treatment in Germany. Pharmacoepidemiol Drug Saf. 2015;24(10):1076–84 [C].

[58] Syrigou E, Psarros P, Grapsa D, et al. Successful rapid desensitization to glatiramer acetate in a patient with multiple sclerosis. J Investig Allergol Clin Immunol. 2015;25(3):214–5 [A].

[59] Watkins CE, Litchfield J, Youngberg G, et al. Glatiramer acetate-induced lobular panniculitis and skin necrosis. Cutis. 2015;95(5):E26–30 [A].

[60] Cao H, Rao Y, Liu L, et al. The efficacy and safety of leflunomide for the treatment of lupus nephritis in Chinese patients: systematic review and meta-analysis. PLoS One. 2015;10(12):e0144548 [M].

[61] Xiang N, Li XM, Zhang MJ, et al. Total glucosides of paeony can reduce the hepatotoxicity caused by methotrexate and leflunomide combination treatment of active rheumatoid arthritis. Int Immunopharmacol. 2015;28(1):802–7 [C].

[62] Sultan SJ, Sameem F, Ashraf M. Drug reaction with eosinophilia and systemic symptoms: manifestations, treatment, and outcome in 17 patients. Int J Dermatol. 2015;54(5):537–42 [c].

[63] Brode SK, Jamieson FB, Ng R, et al. Increased risk of mycobacterial infections associated with anti-rheumatic medications. Thorax. 2015;70(7):677–82 [C].

[64] Hopkins AM, Wiese MD, Proudman SM, et al. Genetic polymorphism of CYP1A2 but not total or free teriflunomide concentrations is associated with leflunomide cessation in rheumatoid arthritis. Br J Clin Pharmacol. 2016;81(1):113–23 [C].

[65] Wagner M, Earley AK, Webster AC, et al. Mycophenolic acid versus azathioprine as primary immunosuppression for kidney transplant recipients. Cochrane Database Syst Rev. 2015;(12): Cd007746 [M].

[66] Strathie Page SJ, Tait CP. Mycophenolic acid in dermatology a century after its discovery. Australas J Dermatol. 2015;56(1):77–83 [R].

[67] Jimenez-Perez M, Gonzalez Grande R, Rando Munoz FJ, et al. Everolimus plus mycophenolate mofetil as initial immunosuppression in liver transplantation. Transplant Proc. 2015;47(1):90–2 [c].

[68] Feng JJ, Zhang LW, Zhao P, et al. Enteric-coated mycophenolate sodium given in combination with tacrolimus has a lower incidence of serious infections in Asian renal-transplant recipients compared with mycophenolate mofetil. Int J Clin Pract. 2015;69(S183):1–7 [C].

[69] Wang Z, He JJ, Liu XY, et al. The evaluation of enteric-coated mycophenolate sodium in cardiac deceased donor liver transplant patients in China. Immunopharmacol Immunotoxicol. 2015;37(6):508–12 [c].

[70] Numakura K, Kagaya H, Yamamoto R, et al. Characterization of clinical and genetic risk factors associated with dyslipidemia after kidney transplantation. Dis Markers. 2015;2015:179434 [C].

[71] Deutsch J, Rodriguez S, Pyrsopoulos N. Severe mycophenolate mofetil related diarrhea in a post-transplant patient. Am J Gastroenterol. 2015;110:S473 [A].

[72] Manger B, Hiepe F, Schneider M, et al. Impact of switching from mycophenolate mofetil to enteric-coated mycophenolate sodium on gastrointestinal side effects in patients with autoimmune disease: a phase III, open-label, single-arm, multicenter study. Clin Exp Gastroenterol. 2015;8:205–13 [C].

[73] Huang G, Wang C, Luo X, et al. Analysis on BK virus associated nephropathy related risk factors in renal transplant recipients. Zhonghua Yi Xue Za Zhi. 2015;95(38):3124–7 [C].

[74] Lu KP, Zhang J, Lin LM, et al. Efficacy and safety of enteric-coated mycophenolate sodium versus mycophenolate mofetil in renal transplant recipients: a meta-analysis. CJEBM. 2015;15(6):681–6 [M].

[75] Bejanyan N, Rogosheske J, DeFor T, et al. Higher dose of mycophenolate mofetil reduces acute graft-versus-host disease in reduced-intensity conditioning double umbilical cord blood transplantation. Biol Blood Marrow Transplant. 2015;21(5):926–33 [C].

[76] Karbasi-Afshar R, Izadi M, Fazel M, et al. Response of transplant recipients to influenza vaccination based on type of immunosuppression: a meta-analysis. Saudi J Kidney Dis Transpl. 2015;26(5):877–83 [M].

[77] Rissling O, Glander P, Hambach P, et al. No relevant pharmacokinetic interaction between pantoprazole and mycophenolate in renal transplant patients: a randomized crossover study. Br J Clin Pharmacol. 2015;80(5):1086–96 [c].

[78] Liu Q, Jiao Z, Zhong M, et al. Effect of long-term coadministration of compound glycyrrhizin tablets on the pharmacokinetics of mycophenolic acid in rats. Xenobiotica. 2016;46(7):627–33 [E].

[79] Nadal M, Giraudeau B, Tavernier E, et al. Efficacy and safety of mammalian target of rapamycin inhibitors in vascular anomalies: a systematic review. Acta Derm Venereol. 2016;96:448–52 [M].

[80] Wang L, Gu Z, Zhai R, et al. The efficacy and safety of sirolimus-based graft-versus-host disease prophylaxis in patients undergoing allogeneic hematopoietic stem cell transplantation: a meta-analysis of randomized controlled trials. Transfusion. 2015;55(9):2134–41 [M].

[81] Weick A, Chacra W, Kuchipudi A, et al. Incidence of cardiovascular and cerebrovascular events associated with sirolimus use after liver transplantation. Transplant Proc. 2015;47(2):460–4 [C].

[82] Garcia E, Buenasmananas D, Martin C, et al. Sirolimus associated pneumonitis in a hematopoietic stem cell transplant patient. Med Clin (Barc). 2015;145(1):21–3 [A].

[83] Garrod AS, Goyal RK, Weiner DJ. Sirolimus-induced interstitial lung disease following pediatric stem cell transplantation. Pediatr Transplant. 2015;19(3):E75–7 [A].

[84] Wang WL, Yu LX. Acute respiratory distress attributed to sirolimus in solid organ transplant recipients. Am J Emerg Med. 2015;33(1):124.e1–4 [A].

[85] Al Gain M, Crickx B, Bejar C, et al. Sirolimus-induced lymphedema in a kidney-transplant recipient: partial recovery after changeover to tacrolimus. Ann Dermatol Venereol. 2015;142(5):350–5 [A].

[86] Galera P, Martin HC, Welch L, et al. Automated red blood cell exchange for acute drug removal in a patient with sirolimus toxicity. J Clin Apher. 2015;30(6):367–70 [A].

[87] Manyam BV, Nwizu TI, Rahe ML, et al. Early and severe radiation toxicity associated with concurrent sirolimus in an organ transplant recipient with head and neck cutaneous squamous cell carcinoma: a case report. Anticancer Res. 2015;35(10):5511–4 [A].

[88] El-Asmar J, Gonzalez R, Bookout R, et al. Clotrimazole troches induce supratherapeutic blood levels of sirolimus and tacrolimus in an allogeneic hematopoietic cell-transplant recipient resulting in acute kidney injury. Hematol Oncol Stem Cell Ther. 2015; http://dx.doi.org/10.1016/j.hemonc.2015.11.001 [Epub ahead of print] [A].

[89] Peksa GD, Schultz K, Fung HC. Dosing algorithm for concomitant administration of sirolimus, tacrolimus, and an azole after allogeneic hematopoietic stem cell transplantation. J Oncol Pharm Pract. 2015;21(6):409–15 [c].

[90] Ge Y, Zhou H, Shi J, et al. The efficacy of tacrolimus in patients with refractory dermatomyositis/polymyositis: a systematic review. Clin Rheumatol. 2015;34(12):2097–103 [M].

[91] Melo MJ, Goncalves J, Guerra JO, et al. Impact of conversion from Advagraf to twice-daily generic tacrolimus in kidney transplant recipients: a single-center study. Transplant Proc. 2015;47(4):911–3 [C].

[92] Kawakami K, Inoue T, Murano M, et al. Effects of oral tacrolimus as a rapid induction therapy in ulcerative colitis. World J Gastroenterol. 2015;21(6):1880–6 [c].

[93] Ishii S, Miwa Y, Otsuka K, et al. Influence of renal complications on the efficacy and adverse events of tacrolimus combination therapy in patients with systemic lupus erythematosus (SLE) during a maintenance phase: a single-centre, prospective study. Lupus Sci Med. 2015;2(1):e000091 [c].

[94] Ishida K, Shiraki K, Yoshiyasu T. Evaluation of the safety and effectiveness of add-on Tacrolimus in patients with rheumatoid arthritis who failed to show an adequate response to biological DMARDs: the interim results of a specific drug use-results survey of tacrolimus. Drugs R&D. 2015;15(4):307–17 [C].

[95] Singh N, Von Visger J, Zachariah M. Extended release once a day tacrolimus. Curr Opin Organ Transplant. 2015;20(6):657–62 [R].

[96] Coilly A, Calmus Y, Chermak F, et al. Once-daily prolonged release tacrolimus in liver transplantation: experts' literature review and recommendations. Liver Transpl. 2015;21(10):1312–21 [R].

[97] Yang SS, Choi JY, Cho WT, et al. A single center, open-label, randomized pilot study to evaluate the safety and efficacy of tacrolimus modified release, Advagraf, versus tacrolimus twice daily, Prograf, in stable renal recipients (single). Transplant Proc. 2015;47(3):617–21 [c].

[98] Fischer L, Saliba F, Kaiser GM, et al. Three-year outcomes in de novo liver transplant patients receiving everolimus with reduced tacrolimus: follow-up results from a randomized, multicenter study. Transplantation. 2015;99(7):1455–62 [C].

[99] Lee J, Lee JJ, Kim BS, et al. A 12-month single arm pilot study to evaluate the efficacy and safety of sirolimus in combination with tacrolimus in kidney transplant recipients at high immunologic risk. J Korean Med Sci. 2015;30(6):682–7 [c].

[100] Bowman LJ, Brennan DC, Delos-Santos R, et al. Tacrolimus-induced cardiomyopathy in an adult renal transplant recipient. Pharmacotherapy. 2015;35(12):1109–16 [A].

[101] Durst JK, Rampersad RM. Pregnancy in women with solid-organ transplants: a review. Obstet Gynecol Surv. 2015;70(6):408–18 [R].

[102] Sikma MA, van Maarseveen EM, van de Graaf EA, et al. Pharmacokinetics and toxicity of tacrolimus early after heart and lung transplantation. Am J Transplant. 2015;15(9):2301–13 [R].

[103] Kim T, Jancel T, Kumar P, et al. Drug-drug interaction between isavuconazole and tacrolimus: a case report indicating the need for tacrolimus drug-level monitoring. J Clin Pharm Ther. 2015;40:609–11 [A].

[104] Nouhaud FX, Pfister C, Defortescu G, et al. Baseline chronic kidney disease is associated with toxicity and survival in patients treated with targeted therapies for metastatic renal cell carcinoma. Anticancer Drugs. 2015;26(8):866–71 [C].

[105] Afshar M, Pascoe J, Whitmarsh S, et al. Temsirolimus for patients with metastatic renal cell carcinoma: outcomes in patients receiving temsirolimus within a compassionate use program in a tertiary referral center. Drug Des Devel Ther. 2015;9:13–9 [c].

[106] Hess G, Keller U, Scholz CW, et al. Safety and efficacy of temsirolimus in combination with bendamustine and rituximab in relapsed mantle cell and follicular lymphoma. Leukemia. 2015;29(8):1695–701 [c].

[107] Merchan JR, Qin R, Pitot H, et al. Safety and activity of temsirolimus and bevacizumab in patients with advanced renal cell carcinoma previously treated with tyrosine kinase inhibitors: a phase 2 consortium study. Cancer Chemother Pharmacol. 2015;75(3):485–93 [c].

[108] Croyle L, Hoi A, Morand EF. Characteristics of azathioprine use and cessation in a longitudinal lupus cohort. Lupus Sci Med. 2015;2(1):e000105 [c].

[109] Fuggle NR, Bragoli W, Mahto A, et al. The adverse effect profile of oral azathioprine in pediatric atopic dermatitis, and recommendations for monitoring. J Am Acad Dermatol. 2015;72(1):108–14 [c].

[110] Moran GW, Dubeau MF, Kaplan GG, et al. Clinical predictors of thiopurine-related adverse events in Crohn's disease. World J Gastroenterol. 2015;21(25):7795–804 [C].

[111] Amin J, Huang B, Yoon J, et al. Update 2014: advances to optimize 6-mercaptopurine and azathioprine to reduce toxicity and improve efficacy in the management of IBD. Inflamm Bowel Dis. 2015;21(2):445–52 [R].

[112] Goel RM, Blaker P, Mentzer A, et al. Optimizing the use of thiopurines in inflammatory bowel disease. Ther Adv Chronic Dis. 2015;6(3):138–46 [R].

[113] Goldberg R, Irving PM. Toxicity and response to thiopurines in patients with inflammatory bowel disease. Expert Rev Gastroenterol Hepatol. 2015;9(7):891–900 [R].

[114] Dogan P, Grbovic E, Inci S, et al. Azathioprine-induced atrial fibrillation. Intractable Rare Dis Res. 2015;4(4):207–9 [A].

[115] Gallego-Gutierrez S, Navas-Lopez VM, Kolorz M, et al. Successful mercaptopurine usage despite azathioprine-induced pancreatitis in paediatric Crohn's disease. J Crohns Colitis. 2015;9(8):676–9 [A].

[116] Teich N, Mohl W, Bokemeyer B, et al. Azathioprine-induced acute pancreatitis in patients with inflammatory bowel diseases—a prospective study on incidence and severity. J Crohns Colitis. 2016;10(1):61–8 [C].

[117] Ledder O, Lemberg DA, Day AS. Thiopurine-induced pancreatitis in inflammatory bowel diseases. Expert Rev Gastroenterol Hepatol. 2015;9(4):399–403 [R].

[118] Vang SI, Schmiegelow K, Frandsen T, et al. Mercaptopurine metabolite levels are predictors of bone marrow toxicity following high-dose methotrexate therapy of childhood acute lymphoblastic leukaemia. Cancer Chemother Pharmacol. 2015;75(5):1089–93 [c].

[119] Bjornsson ES. Drug-induced liver injury: an overview over the most critical compounds. Arch Toxicol. 2015;89(3):327–34 [R].

[120] Imhof L, Meier B, Frei P, et al. Severe sweet's syndrome with elevated cutaneous interleukin-1beta after azathioprine exposure: case report and review of the literature. Dermatology. 2015;230(4):293–8 [A].

[121] Gupta P, Shaffrali F. An unusual side effect of azathioprine. Clin Exp Dermatol. 2015;40(8):929–30 [A].

[122] Mookherjee S, Narayanan M, Uchiyama T, et al. Three hospital admissions in 9 days to diagnose azathioprine hypersensitivity in a patient with Crohn's disease. Am J Ther. 2015;22(2):e28–32 [A].

[123] Durante-Mangoni E, Andini R, Pinto D, et al. Effect of the immunosuppressive regimen on the incidence of cytomegalovirus infection in 378 heart transplant recipients: a single centre, prospective cohort study. J Clin Virol. 2015;68:37–42 [C].

[124] Dugue PA, Rebolj M, Hallas J, et al. Risk of cervical cancer in women with autoimmune diseases, in relation with their use of immunosuppressants and screening: population-based cohort study. Int J Cancer. 2015;136(6):E711–9 [C].

[125] Mozaffari S, Abdolghaffari AH, Nikfar S, et al. Pregnancy outcomes in women with inflammatory bowel disease following exposure to thiopurines and antitumor necrosis factor drugs: a systematic review with meta-analysis. Hum Exp Toxicol. 2015;34(5):445–59 [C].

[126] Azimi F, Mortazavi Y, Alavi S, et al. Frequency of ITPA gene polymorphisms in Iranian patients with acute lymphoblastic leukemia and prediction of its myelosuppressive effects. Leuk Res. 2015;39(10):1048–54 [c].

[127] Coenen MJ, de Jong DJ, van Marrewijk CJ, et al. Identification of patients with variants in TPMT and dose reduction reduces hematologic events during thiopurine treatment of inflammatory bowel disease. Gastroenterology. 2015;149(4):907–917.e7 [C].

[128] Emmungil H, Durusoy R, Kalfa M, et al. Plasma thiopurine S-methyltransferase levels and azathioprine-related adverse events in patients with Behcet's disease. Clin Exp Rheumatol. 2015;33(6 Suppl 94):S40–5 [C].

[129] Hareedy MS, El Desoky ES, Woillard JB, et al. Genetic variants in 6-mercaptopurine pathway as potential factors of hematological toxicity in acute lymphoblastic leukemia patients. Pharmacogenomics. 2015;16(10):1119–34 [c].

[130] Lee MN, Kang B, Choi SY, et al. Impact of genetic polymorphisms on 6-thioguanine nucleotide levels and toxicity in pediatric patients with IBD treated with azathioprine. Inflamm Bowel Dis. 2015;21(12):2897–908 [C].

[131] Levinsen M, Rosthoj S, Nygaard U, et al. Myelotoxicity after high-dose methotrexate in childhood acute leukemia is influenced by 6-mercaptopurine dosing but not by intermediate thiopurine methyltransferase activity. Cancer Chemother Pharmacol. 2015;75(1):59–66 [C].

[132] Liu YP, Wu HY, Yang X, et al. Association between thiopurine S-methyltransferase polymorphisms and thiopurine-induced adverse drug reactions in patients with inflammatory bowel disease: a meta-analysis. PLoS One. 2015;10(3):e0121745 [M].

[133] Liu YP, Xu HQ, Li M, et al. Association between thiopurine S-methyltransferase polymorphisms and azathioprine-induced

adverse drug reactions in patients with autoimmune diseases: a meta-analysis. PLoS One. 2015;10(12):e0144234 [M].

[134] Mei L, Ontiveros EP, Griffiths EA, et al. Pharmacogenetics predictive of response and toxicity in acute lymphoblastic leukemia therapy. Blood Rev. 2015;29(4):243–9 [R].

[135] Roberts RL, Barclay ML. Update on thiopurine pharmacogenetics in inflammatory bowel disease. Pharmacogenomics. 2015;16(8):891–903 [R].

[136] Odahara S, Uchiyama K, Kubota T, et al. A prospective study evaluating metabolic capacity of thiopurine and associated adverse reactions in Japanese patients with inflammatory bowel disease (IBD). PLoS One. 2015;10(9):e0137798 [c].

[137] Steponaitiene R, Kupcinskas J, Survilaite S, et al. TPMT and ITPA genetic variants in Lithuanian inflammatory bowel disease patients: prevalence and azathioprine-related side effects. Adv Med Sci. 2015;61(1):135–40 [C].

[138] Suzuki R, Fukushima H, Noguchi E, et al. Influence of SLCO1B1 polymorphism on maintenance therapy for childhood leukemia. Pediatr Int. 2015;57(4):572–7 [c].

[139] Tanaka Y, Kato M, Hasegawa D, et al. Susceptibility to 6-MP toxicity conferred by a NUDT15 variant in Japanese children with acute lymphoblastic leukaemia. Br J Haematol. 2015;171(1): 109–15 [c].

[140] Israeli E, Goldin E, Fishman S, et al. Oral administration of non-absorbable delayed release 6-mercaptopurine is locally active in the gut, exerts a systemic immune effect and alleviates Crohn's disease with low rate of side effects: results of double blind Phase II clinical trial. Clin Exp Immunol. 2015;181(2):362–72 [c].

[141] Tiphaine Ade B, Hjalgrim LL, Nersting J, et al. Evaluation of a pediatric liquid formulation to improve 6-mercaptopurine therapy in children. Eur J Pharm Sci. 2016;83:1–7 [c].

[142] Hantson P, Di Fazio V, Del Mar Ramirez Fernandez M, et al. Susac-like syndrome in a chronic cocaine abuser: could levamisole play a role? J Med Toxicol. 2015;11(1):124–8 [A].

[143] Vosoughi R, Schmidt BJ. Multifocal leukoencephalopathy in cocaine users: a report of two cases and review of the literature. BMC Neurol. 2015;15:208 [A].

37

Corticotrophins, Corticosteroids, and Prostaglandins

Alison Brophy*,†,1, *Sidhartha D. Ray*‡

*Ernest Mario School of Pharmacy, Rutgers, The State University of New Jersey, Piscataway, NJ, USA
†Saint Barnabas Medical Center, Livingston, NJ, USA
‡Department of Pharmaceutical Sciences, Manchester University College of Pharmacy, Natural and Health Sciences, Fort Wayne, IN, USA
1Corresponding author: aabrophy@pharmacy.rutgers.edu

EDITOR'S NOTES

In this chapter adverse effects and reactions that arise from the oral or parenteral administration of corticosteroids (glucocorticoids and mineralocorticoids) are covered. Other routes of administration are dealt with in the sections after that; inhalation and nasal administration are dealt with in Chapter 15 topical administration to the skin in Chapter 13, and ocular administration in Chapter 46.

All the uses of prostaglandins are covered in this chapter, apart from topical administration to the eyes, which is covered in Chapter 46.

CORTICOTROPHINS [SED-15, 906; SEDA-33, 841; SEDA-34, 653; SEDA-35, 719; SEDA-36, 603; SEDA-37, 491]

Adrenocorticotropic hormone (ACTH) is most commonly used for infantile spasm; corticosteroids are the alternative therapy for this condition. A major review by Cochrane libraries sought to compare ACTH to corticosteroids but identified only 1 randomized controlled cross-over study with 5 children and described no adverse reactions [1M].

Cardiovascular

A retrospective evaluation of ACTH versus prednisone for infantile spasms that failed to respond to vigabatrin identified hypertension as the primary adverse event reported in 5 of 19 patients treated. Additional side effects included hyponatremia, hypokalaemia, or infection with H1N1 virus [2c].

Hematologic

In a 6-year-old boy treated with ACTH 0.01 mg/kg/day daily for 13 days fibrinogen decreased from 235.5 to 66.6 mg/dL. The medication was discontinued and on day-17 fibrinogen was 233 mg/dL. Authors did not propose a mechanism but cautioned about the bleeding risk from ACTH and need for supplementation if clinical bleeding occurs [3A].

Drug Tolerance

Two cases of long-term use of ACTH refractory epilepsy are described. Patients were treated for at least 1 year and followed for 1 year following treatment. A 5-year-old male and 3-year-old female demonstrated no significant side effects. Both patients saw resolution of epileptic activity during treatment and demonstrated developmental gains during and following treatment [4A].

SYSTEMIC GLUCOCORTICOIDS [SED-15, 906; SEDA-33, 841; SEDA-34, 653; SEDA-35, 719; SEDA-36, 604; SEDA-37, 492]

Glucocorticoids are noted to be associated with significant long- and short-term side effects. A recent review of corticosteroid use in rheumatoid arthritis highlighted that with recent advancements side effects can be management; for example bisphosphonates for prevention of bone loss. However, significant risks for infection persist [5R]. Novel glucocorticoids and preparations in development work to improve target receptor selectivity, extend duration of action, and allow liposomal delivery. All novel approaches to therapy offer the potential of minimizing corticosteroid study effects [6R,7c]. Patients and practitioners survived regarding inhaled and systemic corticosteroid use in asthma reported concerns over side effects. More than one oral steroid-associated side effect was reported by 88% of the 205 patients surveyed. This was associated with decreased adherence to therapy. Statistically significant differences were found between the patient reported rate of adverse effects and the clinician predicted rate in the survey of 244 clinicians. This highlights the potential to underestimate the rate of side effects and implications on patients [8]. Recent reports of study results, reviews of existing data, and adverse reactions for currently available glucocorticoids are presented below.

Systematic Review

The Cochrane library published several meta-analyses with new data related to corticosteroids. The use of prednisone in cystic fibrosis evaluation identified 3 studies with more than 300 patients demonstrating delayed progression of disease with treatment. However, risk of growth retardation in children was identified to be dose related [9M]. Use of adjunctive steroids for the treatment of *Pneumocystis jiroveci* pneumonia in HIV infection patients identified benefit in patient with severe hypoxemia in 6 studies with 242 patients [10M]. In two trials with 132 neonatal patients with bacterial meningitis use of adjunctive corticosteroids was associated with reduced risk of death and hearing loss [11M]. Authors were unable to complete a meta-analysis of steroid use for the common cold due to low quality of available evidence but concluded corticosteroids are of limited benefit [12M]. Oral budesonide for ulcerative colitis was evaluated in comparison to placebo, prednisone, and mesalamine in six studies with 1088 participants. Moderate evidence supported budesonide for induction of remission in active ulcerative colitis. Reported adverse events included worsening ulcerative colitis, headache, pyrexia, insomnia, back pain, nausea, abdominal pain, diarrhoea, flatulence and nasopharyngitis [13M]. Ten studies with 5700 infants determined there was short-term benefit to repeated courses of steroids for prenatal steroids in preterm birth to prevent respiratory distress syndrome and serious infant outcomes. However, there was association with low mean birth weight [14]. The use of corticosteroids for acute optic neuritis either intravenous or oral was not associated with improved outcomes at 6 months after treatment [15M]. After reviewing 15 studies with 1926 patients, authors determined there was varied evidence for efficacy of

opioids in cancer patients. Corticosteroids, mostly dexamethasone, did decrease acute pain, but little documentation of adverse effects was available [16M]. The final significant meta-analysis was published in the *Annuals of Internal Medicine* and explored the controversy surrounding the use of corticosteroids in patients hospitalized with community acquired pneumonia. A total of 13 randomized controlled trials with nearly 2000 patients demonstrated no statistically significant decrease in mortality, RR, 0.67 [95% CI, 0.45–1.01]; I2 = 6%. There was a significant increase in the rate of hyperglycemia requiring treatment, RR, 1.49 [CI, 1.01–2.19]; I2 = 6% [17M].

Nervous System

A commentary published by an FDA scientist reviewed the decision to continue to label epidural corticosteroids for the risk of serious neurologic events. Despite the low risk the advisory committee for the FDA felt it remained important to remind clinicians. A total of 90 serious events from 1997 to 2014 are reported including paraplegia quadriplegia. Spinal cord infarction, stroke, and infection were also reported [18r].

Psychiatric

A prospective observational cohort study evaluated 1112 intensive care unit (ICU) patients and found no difference between those treated with corticosteroids and not treated for risk of transition to ICU delirium adjusted OR, 1.08; 95% CI, 0.89–1.32. There was also no difference found with increasing corticosteroid dose, adjusted OR, 1.00; 95% CI, 0.99–1.01 per 10 mg increase in prednisone equivalent [19C]. A case report of a 58-year-old man with idiopathic thrombocytopenic purpura describes development of prolonged acute psychosis. This patient had been treated with multiple previous courses of high dose corticosteroids, including 100 mg prednisone daily, with no mental health issues. The patient was initiated on his third cycle of treatment with 4 days of 40 mg dexamethasone. He developed unusual behaviour and inability to care for himself with delusional thinking. Treatment with quetiapine titrated up to 800 mg per day and aripiprazole was trialled as well. The patient was found naked at times, speaking in religious tongues. The patient required treatment for 6 months including trials of electroconvulsion therapy before gradual resolution of symptoms occurred. Author's highlighted the dose-dependent risk of psychosis and varying duration of symptoms [20A].

Sleep

Continuous subcutaneous administration of hydrocortisone was compared to three times a day oral administration in patients with Addison's disease. Improved circadian rhythm control was found with the subcutaneous administration and no difference in insulin sensitivity [21c].

Endocrine

The REDUCE trial evaluated 5 versus 14 days of prednisone therapy for chronic obstructive pulmonary disease (COPD) exacerbation. Cortisol levels were measured in patients on day 6, at hospital discharge and up to 180 days follow-up. Pathologic tests were found initially in 63% of patients which decreased to 2%. There was no difference between prednisone treatment groups and abrupt termination of treatment appeared safe [22C].

A matched study of 168 pregnant women with inflammatory bowel disease (IBD) compared to 381 pregnant women without IBD to assess the risk of intrapartum corticosteroid use. Gestational diabetes occurred in 6.9% versus 1.8% ($p = 0.003$) of women with IBS compared to those without [23C]. A meta-analysis assessing the risk of developing adrenal insufficiency after corticosteroid use found prevalence of the side effect ranging from 2.4% for low dose to 21.5% for high dose. For short-term therapy the risk of 1.4% comparted to long-term therapy with 27.4% rate. The analysis included 74 studies and 3753 patients [24M].

Hematologic

A double-blind, randomized, placebo controlled trial of 65 patients with rhinosinusitis with nasal polyps evaluated 1 mg/kg of prednisolone in endoscopic sinus surgery. There was no difference between groups for intraoperative bleeding [25c].

Gastrointestinal

A 12-year-old boy with pseuodohypoaldosteronism, chronic lung disease, and gastrostomy presented with abdominal pain and was found to have diffuse pneumatosis intestinalis along the ascending, descending, and transverse colon. He was admitted to surgical service monitored with serial exams and antibiotics. He was discharged after 4 days. Chronic steroid use can cause atrophy of gastrointestinal lymphoid tissue decreasing submucosal integrity and increasing the risk for translocation of air [26A]. A double-blinded placebo controlled cross-over study of 10 days of prednisone in patient with asthma demonstrated no changes in dietary intake, appetite, or body weight during treatment. However, patients reported sleep disturbances and gastrointestinal disturbances during prednisone treatment [27c].

Liver

A 35-year-old women treated with 1 g pulse dose methylprednisolone for multiple sclerosis and optic neuritis developed acute hepatitis on two separate occasions, 4 years apart, within days of treatment. During the second episode her labs included; AST 972 mU/mL, ALT1419 mU/mL, INR 1.6. One month later, a wedge biopsy showed liver parenchyma septation. Following 9 months of methylprednisolone withdrawal a core liver needle biopsy was repeated and changes had resolved [28A].

Musculoskeletal

A review article of the effects of corticosteroids on osteoclast activity identified that initially treatment with bisphosphonates will improve bone integrity. However, after 2 years of corticosteroids and bisphosphonates there are increased fracture risks due to dampened bone remodelling [29r].

Neuromuscular Function

A retrospective evaluation of 527 patients with Guillain–Barre syndrome found greater improvement in functional scores for mechanically ventilated patients treated with IVIG alone compared to IVIG plus corticosteroids. Corticosteroids were detrimental for short-term prognosis, $p < 0.05$ [30r].

Immunologic

A 35-year-old women received intralesional injection of triamcinolone for alopecia areata. She had previously been treated with the same strategy four times over a period of 14 years. Three days after this course was initiated she developed tender itchy scaly nodules. They were treated and resolved with topical clobetasone over 7 days. Patch testing was performed and was negative for triamcinolone. Finally intradermal testing was positive with a 15-mm wheal reaction, edema, erythema, and itching [31A]. Similarly, a retrospective review of 23 cases of skin testing for corticosteroid allergy noted the difference in response for skin prick testing and intradermal testing. There was both false-positive and false-negative reactions and cross-reactivity between agents [32r].

Infection Risk

A retrospective case series of 23 cases of pulmonary nocardiosis over 22 years at an Asian hospital noted that all but one case was receiving immunosuppressants including corticosteroids. Cytotoxic agents and corticosteroid doses were decreased or discontinued during treatment [33r].

Death

A meta-analysis of corticosteroid use in influenza patients included 3059 patients from 16 observational studies. Corticosteroids were associated with increased risk of death, OR, 2.12; 95% CI, 1.36–3.29 [34M]. Conversely, in a meta-analysis of corticosteroids in acute respiratory distress syndrome no effect on mortality could be determined. The analysis included 11 studies with 949 patients. Odd ratio for corticosteroids and mortality was 0.77: 95% CI, 0.58–1.03 [35M].

Drug Resistance

A prospective study of 54 wrists in 49 patients determined 79% of wrists responded to 1 initial injection of dexamethasone or triamcinolone for carpal tunnel syndrome. The only risk factor for non-response identified was diabetes [36c].

Pregnancy

A systematic review of corticosteroid use in pregnancy identified that the use of corticosteroids during pregnancy has risen from 1999–2000 to 2008–2009. In addition no association with systemic oral steroids and miscarriage or congenital malformation was highlighted; however, confidence intervals were very large. Conversely with inhaled steroids an increased risk of miscarriage was noted [37M].

Pharmacogenetics

Analysis of the genomes of 489 white children in the Children Asthma Management program identified 2 single nucleotide polymorphisms (SNP) associated with decreased bone mineral accretion (BMA). The children had been treated with short pulse steroids. The SNP's, rs9896933 and rs2074439, are related to the tubulin pathway. The BMA worsen as prednisone dose increased and number of mutant alleles of the 2 SNP's increased [38R]. Also in adult asthmatic patients glucocorticoid non-responsiveness was linked to decrease receptor expression with impaired nuclear translocation [39r]. In children treated with corticosteroids for acute lymphoblastic leukemia osteonecrosis of the jaw is a major adverse effect. The effect was found to be associated with a SNP rs10989682 near the glutamate receptor locus. Other vascular phenotypes were associated with the glutamate receptor locus including cerebral ischemia, arterial embolism and thrombosis [40R].

PROSTAGLANDINS AND ANALOGUES
[SED-15, 2955; SEDA-33, 846; SEDA-34, 660; SEDA-35, 725; SEDA-36, 604; SEDA-37, 494]

See also Chapter 46.

Epoprostenol (PGI2)

A review of epoprostenol for pulmonary arterial hypertension (PAH) highlighted a number of common adverse effects in dose initiation were flushing, headache, nausea, vomiting, hypotension, anxiety and chest pain. The most common adverse effects in chronic administration included those above and jaw pain, myalgia, diarrhea, musculoskeletal pain, tachycardia, chills, fever, flu-like symptoms, and hypesthesia. These all occurred in more than 10% of patients. Authors also discuss the risk of bleeding in patients with idiopathic pulmonary hypertension due to use of anticoagulation and the antiplatelet activity of epoprostenol [41R].

Cerebrovascular

A randomized placebo controlled trial of epoprostenol for patients with subarachnoid haemorrhage for day 5 to day 10 post bleed. No statistically significant difference in cerebral blood flow was found. A non-significant decrease in delayed ischemic neurologic deficits and angiography confirmed vasospasm was noted [42c].

Iloprost (PGI2 Analogue) [SED-15, 1716; SEDA-33, 847; SEDA-34, 660; SEDA-35, 726; SEDA-36, 604; SEDA-37, 495]

Respiratory

A review of inhaled prostacyclin therapy highlighted the approval of iloprost for inhaled administration. Side effects highlighted include cough and wheeze [43R].

Hematologic

A Greek study of 110 patients with heparin-induced thrombocytopenia undergoing cardiac surgery determines that addition of intravenous iloprost at 10 ng/kg/min to heparin was safe. Dose titration was completed based on intraoperative measurement of platelet activity due to HIT antibodies, and antiplatelet activity of iloprost was able to prevent thrombosis [44c].

Skin

A 65-year-old man admitted for iloprost initiation developed a linear erythema reaction twice when the infusion was initiated in peripheral intravenous catheters. The reaction resolved after 2 hours. A peripherally inserted central catheter was placed the next day allowing for treatment without incident. The proposed mechanism was due to cutaneous vasodilation [45A].

Treprostinil

Treprostinil is administered as a subcutaneous infusion or orally tablet. Administration through the subcutaneous route puts patients at risk for injection site reactions. The controlled release tablets are administered twice daily. Reported adverse events include nausea, vomiting, diarrhoea, jaw pain, flushing, abdominal pain, flushing, headache, and pain in extremities, and dyspnea [46R,47R].

Pregnancy

Administration of intravenous treprostinil to 30-year-old women was successful during pregnancy from 23 to 33 weeks gestation. The infant was born via elective caesarean section with favourable outcome. The patient was also administered enoxaparin and oxygen therapy [48A].

Latanoprost (PGF2α Analogue) [SED-15, 2002; SEDA-33, 847; SEDA-34, 660; SEDA-35, 726; SEDA-36, 604; SEDA-37, 496]

Dermatologic

A systematic review of alternative uses for latanoprost identified potential indications for androgenic alopecia, chemotherapy-induced alopecia, and alopecia areata. These disorders with hypopigmentation respond to PGF2α analogs [49R]. Latanoprost administered in combination with laser therapy was used with limited side effects for 22 patients with bilateral stable vitiligo lesions. Significant improvement in pigmentation of lesions was found after treatment with latanoprost [50c]. A 61-year-old women with androgenetic alopecia was treated with topical latanoprost 0.1% solution. She developed pustules, erosions, scales of scalp. Clinical and histologic diagnosis was erosive pustular dermatosis of the scale. Latanoprost was stopped and the patient was treated with oral methylprednisolone, topical clobetasol, and oral zinc sulphate. At 6 weeks resolution was observed [51A].

Bimatoprost (PGF2α Analogue)

Eyes

In a randomized placebo controlled study of brimatoprost for treatment of chemotherapy-induced eyelash hypotrichosis, the most common reported adverse effects were conjunctival hyperemia (16.7%) and punctate keratitis (9.4%) [52]. A review article of use of bimatoprost for hypotrichosis of the eyelash highlighted the following adverse effects: eye pruritus, conjunctival hyperemia, skin hyperpigmentation, ocular irritation, dry eye symptoms, and erythema of the eyelid [53r].

Misoprostol (PGE1 Analogue) [SED-15, 2357; SEDA-33, 847; SEDA-34, 660; SEDA-35, 726; SEDA-36, 612; SEDA-36, 496]

Misoprostol is used for a variety of indications in women including induction of labor, cervical ripening, incomplete miscarriage, postpartum haemorrhage, placement of intra uterine devices, and before hysteroscopy [54R]. A review of misoprostol for labor induction highlighted side effects of fever, chills, tachysystole, vomiting, and diarrhea [55R].

Cardiovascular

The French Pharmacovigilance committee identified 63 reports of cardiovascular and neurovascular events up to 2012 in patients treated with misoprostol. Events included myocardial infarction, stroke, angina, and transient ischemic attacks. Risk factors include obesity, smoking, age greater than 35, and vaginal administration or dose [56r].

Respiratory

A prospective analysis of administration of misoprostol to 234 women with asthma did not identify any patients experiencing asthma exacerbation during hospitalization [57C].

Nervous System

In a prospective study of misoprostol vaginally versus intramuscular oxytocin, shivering was the most common and significant side effect noted for women in the third stage of labor [58C].

Musculoskeletal

A 30-year-old women with previous history of caesarean section was administered 400 mcg of misoprostol for surgical termination of pregnancy due to fetal malformation. One hour after administration she developed heavy vaginal bleeding and was taken emergently to the operating room for evacuation of the fetus and attempts to control haemorrhage. Six units of red blood cells, 4 units of frozen plasma and 1 unit of platelets were administered and a Foley balloon was inserted. A ultrasound image showed complete disruption of the myometrium with large hematoma consistent with dehiscence of the uterine scar from previous caesarean section [59A]. In a study of 188 women, comparing sublingual misoprostol to intracervical dinoprostone gel for cervical ripening after 34 weeks gestation more maternal side effects were reported with misoprostol $p = 0.026$. The side effect reported was uterine tachysystole [60C].

Drug Formulations

Administration of intravaginal misoprostol is currently completed using partial or full oral tablet fragments. This is challenging due to measurements and in ability to remove the drug after administration if adverse effects occur. A novel vaginal insert of 200 mcg releases 7 mcg per hour through a polymer matrix. In studies there were high rates of uterine tachysystole versus comparator interventions [61R].

Selexipag (Prostacyclin IP Receptor Agonist)

The beneficial effects of prostaglandins in PAH are well established. As discussed previously short half-life and limited oral products, pose challenges to use. Selexipag is a novel orally active selective IP (prostacyclin) receptor agonist. It is a prodrug which is rapidly hydrolysed to its active metabolite. It exhibits high selectivity for the human IP receptor over other receptors with a longer half life of 7.9 hours. During a phase 1 study in healthy male subjects reported side effects included nausea, headache, and dizziness [62]. In the phase II trial of 1156 patients, 41.6% of patients treated with selexipag and 27% of patients treated with placebo experienced the composite primary endpoint of death or complication related to PAH; HR 0.60; 99% CI, 0.46–0.78; $p < 0.001$. Adverse events reported in the selexipag group included headache, diarrhea, nausea, and jaw pain [63C].

Cardiovascular

A prospective study of selexipag compared to placebo or moxifloxacin in 91 and 68 patients respectively analysed QTc interval in a nested cross-over design. No significant QTc prolongation was identified with selexipag [64C].

References

[1] Mehta V, Ferrie CD, Cross JH, et al. Corticosteroids including ACTH for childhood epilepsy other than epileptic spasms. Cochrane Database Syst Rev. 2015;(6). Art. No.: CD005222. [M].

[2] Jones K, Snead OC, Boyd J, et al. Adrenocorticotropic hormone versus prednisolone in the treatment of infantile spasms post vigabatrin failure. J Child Neurol. 2015;30(5):595–600 [c].

[3] Kamei A, Araya N, Akasaka M, et al. Hypofibrinogenemia caused by adrenocorticotropic hormone for infantile spasms: a case report. Brain Dev. 2015;37(1):137–9 [A].

[4] Inui T, Kobayashi T, Kobayashi S, et al. Efficacy of long term weekly ACTH therapy for intractable epilepsy. Brain Dev. 2015;37(4):449–54 [A].

[5] Bijlsma JWJ, Jacobs JWG, Buttgereit F. Glucocorticoids in the treatment of rheumatoid arthritis. Clin Exp Rheumatol. 2015;33(Suppl 92):S34–6 [R].

[6] Buttgereit F, Spies CM, Bijlsma JWJ. Novel glucocorticoids: where are we now and where do we want to go? Clin Exp Rheumatol. 2015;33(Suppl 92):S29–33 [R].

[7] Dolle S, Hielshcer N, Bareille PJ, et al. Clinical efficacy and tolerability of a novel selective corticosteroid in atopic dermatitis—two randomized controlled trials. Skin Pharmacol Physiol. 2015;28:159–66 [c].

[8] Cooper V, Metcalf L, Versnel J, et al. Patient-reported side effects, concerns and adherence to corticosteroid treatment for asthma, and comparison with physician estimates of side-effect prevalence: a UK-wide, cross-sectional study. NPJ Prim Care Respir Med. 2015;25:15026 [c].

[9] Cheng K, Ashby D, Smyth RL. Oral steroids for long-term use in cystic fibrosis. Cochrane Database Syst Rev. 2015;(12). Art. No.: CD000407. [M].

[10] Ewald H, Raatz H, Boscacci R, et al. Adjunctive corticosteroids for Pneumocystis jiroveci pneumonia in patients with HIV infection. Cochrane Database Syst Rev. 2015;(4). Art. No.: CD006150. [M].

[11] Ogunlesi TA, Odigwe CC, Oladapo OT. Adjuvant corticosteroids for reducing death in neonatal bacterial meningitis. Cochrane Database Syst Rev. 2015;(11). Art. No.: CD010435. [M].

[12] Hayward G, Thompson MJ, Perera R, et al. Corticosteroids for the common cold. Cochrane Database Syst Rev. 2015;(10). Art. No.: CD008116. [M].

[13] Sherlock ME, MacDonald JK, Griffiths AM, et al. Oral budesonide for induction of remission in ulcerative colitis. Cochrane Database Syst Rev. 2015;(10). Art. No.: CD007698. [M].

[14] Crowther CA, McKinlay CJD, Middleton P, et al. Repeat doses of prenatal corticosteroids for women at risk of preterm birth for improving neonatal health outcomes. Cochrane Database Syst Rev. 2015;(7). Art. No.: CD003935. [M].

[15] Gal RL, Vedula SS, Beck R. Corticosteroids for treating optic neuritis. Cochrane Database Syst Rev. 2015;(8). Art. No.: CD001430. [M].

[16] Haywood A, Good P, Khan S, et al. Corticosteroids for the management of cancer-related pain in adults. Cochrane Database Syst Rev. 2015;(4). Art. No.: CD010756. [M].

[17] Siemieniuk RAC, Meade MO, Alonso-Coello P, et al. Corticosteroid therapy for patients hospitalized with community-acquired Pneumonia. Ann Intern Med. 2015;163:519–28 [M].

[18] Racoosin JA, Seymour SM. Cascio et al. serious neurologic events after the epidural glucocorticoid injection—the FDA's risk assessment. N Engl J Med. 2015;373(24):2299–301 [r].

[19] Wolters AE, Veldhuijzen DS, Zaal IJ, et al. Systemic corticosteroids and transition to delirium in critically ill patients. Crit Care Med. 2015;43:e585–8 [C].

[20] Gable M, Depry D. Sustained corticosteroid-induced mania and psychosis despite cessation: a case study and brief literature review. Int J Psychiatry Med. 2015;50(4):398–404 [A].

[21] Bjornsdottir S, Oksnes M, Isaksson M, et al. Circadian hormone profiles and insulin sensitivity in patients with Addison's disease: a comparison of continuous subcutaneous hydrocortisone infusion with conventional glucocorticoid replacement therapy. Clin Endocrinol. 2015;83(1):28–35 [c].

[22] Schuetz P, Leuppi JD, Bingisser R, et al. Prospective analysis of adrenal function in patients with acute exacerbations of COPD: the reduction in the use of corticosteroids in exacerbated COPD (REDUCE) trial. Eur J Endocrinol. 2015;173(1):19–27 [C].

[23] Leung YPY, Kaplan GG, Coward S, et al. Intrapartum corticosteroid use significantly increases the risk of gestational diabetes in women with inflammatory bowel disease. J Crohns Colitis. 2015;9(3):223–30 [C].

[24] Broersen LHA, Pereira AM, Jorgensen JOL, et al. Adrenal insufficiency in corticosteroids use: systematic review and meta-analysis. J Clin Endocrinol Metab. 2015;100(6):2171–80 [M].

[25] Gunel C, Basak HS, Bleier BS. Oral steroids and intraoperative bleeding during endoscopic sinus surgery. B-ENT. 2015;11(2):123–8 [c].

[26] Cruz AT, Naik-Mathuria BJ, Bisset GS. Pneumatosis intestinalis in a corticosteroid-dependent child. J Emerg Med. 2015;48(5):607–8 [A].

[27] Berthon BS, Gibson PG, McElduff P, et al. Effects of short-term oral corticosteroid intake on dietary intake, body weight and body composition in adults with asthma—a randomized controlled trial. Clin Exp Allergy. 2015;45(5):908–19 [c].

[28] Grilli E, Galati V, Petrosillo N, et al. Incomplete septal cirrhosis after high-dose methylprednisolone therapy and regression of liver injury. Liver Int. 2015;35:674–6 [A].

[29] Teitelbaum SL. Glucocorticoids and the osteoclast. Clin Exp Rheumatol. 2015;33(Suppl 92):S37–9 [r].

[30] Wu X, Zhang B, Li C, et al. Short-term prognosis of mechanically ventilated patients with Guillain–Barre syndrome is worsened by corticosteroids as an add-on therapy. Medicine. 2015;94(43): e1898 [r].

[31] Kreeshan FC, Hampton P. Delayed hypersensitivity reaction to intralesional triamcinolone acetonide following treatment for

alopecia areata. Intradermal testing. J Dermatol Case Rep. 2015;9(4):107–9 [A].

[32] B aker A, Empson M, The R, et al. Skin testing for immediate hypersensitivity to corticosteroids: a case series and literature review. Clin Exp Allergy. 2015;45:669–76 [r].

[33] Li S, Song XY, Zhao YY, et al. Clinical analysis of pulmonary nocardiosis in patients with autoimmune disease. Medicine. 2015;94(39):e1561 [r].

[34] Rodrigo C, Leonardi-Bee J, Nguyen-Van-Tam JS, et al. Effect of corticosteroid therapy on influenza-related mortality: a systematic review and meta-analysis. J Infect Dis. 2015;212(2):183–94 [M].

[35] Horita N, Hasshimoto S, Miyazawa N, et al. Impact of corticosteroids on mortality in patients with acute respiratory distress syndrome: a systematic review and meta-analysis. Intern Med. 2015;54:1473–9 [M].

[36] Blazar PE, Floyd IV WE, Han CH, et al. Prognostic indicators for recurrent symptoms after a single corticosteroid injection for carpal tunnel syndrome. J Bone Joint Surg Am. 2015;97:1563–70 [c].

[37] Bjorn AMB, Ehrenstein V, Nohr EA, et al. Use of inhaled and oral corticosteroids in pregnancy and the risk of malformations or miscarriage. Basic Clin Pharmacol Toxicol. 2015;116(4):308–14 [M].

[38] Park HW, Ge B, Tse S, et al. Genetic risk factors for decreased bone mineral accretion in children with asthma receiving multiple oral corticosteroid bursts. J Allergy Clin Immunol. 2015;136(5):1240–6 [R].

[39] Chang PJ, Michaeloudes C, Zhu J, et al. Impaired nuclear translocation of the glucocorticoid receptor in corticosteroid-insensitive airway smooth muscle in severe asthma. Am J Respir Crit Care Med. 2015;191(1):54–62 [r].

[40] Karol SE, Yang W, Van Driest SL, et al. Genetics of glucocorticoid-associated osteonecrosis in children with acute lymphoblastic leukemia. Blood. 2015;126(15):1770–6 [R].

[41] Saito Y, Nakamura K, Akagi S, et al. Epoprostenol sodium for treatment of pulmonary arterial hypertension. Vasc Health Risk Manag. 2015;11:265–70 [R].

[42] Rasmussen R, Wettersley J, Stavngaard T, et al. Effects of prostacyclin on cerebral blood flow and vasospasm after subarachnoid hemorrhage. Stroke. 2015;46:37–41 [c].

[43] Hill NS, Preston IR, Roberts KE. Inhaled therapies for pulmonary hypertension. Respir Care. 2015;60(6):794–802 [R].

[44] Palatianos G, Michanlis A, Alivizatos P. Perioperative use of iloprost in cardiac surgery patients diagnosed with heparin-induced thrombocytopenia-reactive antibodies or with true HIT (HIT-reactive antibodies plus thrombocytopenia): an 11-year experience. Am J Hematol. 2015;90(7):608–17 [c].

[45] Parham G, Reed M. Linear erythematous cutaneous adverse reaction during intravenous iloprost administration. Intern Med J. 2015;45(11):1197–8 [A].

[46] Patel BB, Feng Y, Cheng-Lai A. Pulmonary arterial hypertension: a review in pharmacotherapy. Cardiol Rev. 2015;23(1):33–51 [R].

[47] Feldman J, Im Y, Gill K. Oral treprostinil diethanolamine for pulmonary arterial hypertension. Expert Rev Clin Pharmacol. 2015;8(1):55–60 [R].

[48] Rosengarten D, Kramer R. Pregnancy in a woman with pulmonary hypertension: favorable outcome with intravenous treprostinil. Clin Exp Obstet Gynecol. 2015;42(3):390–1 [A].

[49] Choi YM, Diehl J, Levins PC. Promising alternative clinical use of prostaglandin F2α analogs: beyond the eyelashes. J Am Acad Dermatol. 2015;72:712–6 [R].

[50] Anbar TS, El-Ammawi TS, Abdel-Rahman AT, et al. The effect of latanoprost on vitiligo: a preliminary comparative study. Int J Dermatol. 2015;54(5):587–93 [c].

[51] Vaccaro M, Barbuzza O, Borgia F, et al. Erosive pustular dermatosis of the scalp following topical latanoprost for androgenetic alopecia. Dermatol Ther. 2015;28(2):65–7 [A].

[52] Wirta D, Baumann L, Bruce S, et al. Safety and efficacy of bimatoprost for eyelash growth in postchemotherapy subjects. J Clin Aesthet Dermatol. 2015;8(4):11–20 [R].

[53] Fagien S. Management of hypotrichosis of the eyelashes: focus on bimatoprost. Plast Surg Nurs. 2015;35(2):82–91 [r].

[54] Marret H, Simon E, Beucher G, et al. Overview and expert assessment of off-label use of misoprostol in obstetrics and gynecology: review and report by the college national des gynecologues obstetriciens francais. Eur J Obstet Gynecol Reprod Biol. 2015;187:80–4 [R].

[55] Wing DA, Sheibani L. Pharmacotherapy options for labor induction. Expert Opin Pharmacother. 2015;16(11):1657–68 [R].

[56] [No authors listed in pubmed]. Misoprostol: serious cardiovascular events, even after a single dose. Prescrire Int. 2015;24(162):183–4 [r].

[57] Thompson MR, Towers CV, Howard BVC, et al. The use of prostaglandin E1 in peripartum patients with asthma. Am J Obstet Gynecol. 2015;212(392):e1–3 [C].

[58] Priya GP, Veena P, Chaturvedula L, et al. A randomized controlled trial of sublingual misoprostol and intramuscular oxytocin for the prevention of postpartum haemorrhage. Arch Gynecol Obstet. 2015;292:1231–7 [C].

[59] Stitely ML, Craw S, Africano E, et al. Uterine scar dehiscence associated with misoprostol cervical priming for surgical abortion: a case report. J Reprod Med. 2015;60(9–10):445–8 [A].

[60] Jha N, Sagili H, Jayalakshmi D, et al. Comparison of the efficacy and safety of sublingual misoprostol with intracervical dinoprostone gel for cervical ripening in prelabour rupture of membranes after 34 weeks gestation. Arch Gynecol Obstet. 2015;291:39–44 [C].

[61] Stephenson ML, Wing DA. A novel misoprostol delivery system for induction of labor: clinical utility and patient considerations. Drug Des Devel Ther. 2015;9:2321–7 [R].

[62] Kaufmann P, Okubo K, Bruderer S, et al. Pharmacokinetics and tolerability of the novel oral prostacyclin IP receptor agonist selexipag. Am J Cardiovasc Drugs. 2015;15:195–203 [c].

[63] Sitbon O, Channick R, Chin KM, et al. Selexipag for the treatment of pulmonary arterial hypertension. N Engl J Med. 2015;373:2522–33 [C].

[64] Hoch M, Darpo B, Remenova T, et al. A thorough QT study in the context of an uptitration regimen with selexipag, a selective oral prostacyclin receptor agonist. Drug Des Devel Ther. 2014;9:175–85 [C].

38

Sex Hormones and Related Compounds, Including Hormonal Contraceptives

Sandra L. Hrometz[1]

Department of Pharmaceutical Sciences, Manchester University College of Pharmacy, Natural and Health Sciences, Fort Wayne, IN, USA

[1]Corresponding author: slhrometz@manchester.edu

ESTROGENS: [SED-15, 1253; SEDA-35, 731; SEDA-36, 615; SEDA-37, 499]

Diethylstilbestrol (DES)

DES is a nonsteroidal estrogen that was prescribed for decades to pregnant women in order to prevent miscarriage and premature delivery. It was banned in the United States in 1972 and in France in 1977. *In utero* exposure of females to DES is associated with clear cell adenocarcinoma of the cervix, genital tract malformation, subfertility and breast cancer later in life. Male offspring also have genital tract malformation, most commonly hypospadias [1R].

Reproductive System Effects

DES was administered orally at a dose of 0.05 mcg/kg/day to pregnant mice from gestational day 11 to birth. These original mice were designated F_0. The offspring of F_0 were F_1, the offspring of F_1 were F_2 and the offspring of F_2 were F_3 to study the *in utero* effects of DES over three generations. Reproductive system function was studied as the mice aged (time points at 3, 6 and 9 months of age). Compared to control mice (receive vehicle only), the age of first estrus was significantly earlier in the F_1 generation ($p \leq 0.05$) and significantly delayed in the F_3 generation ($p \leq 0.05$). When looking at pregnancy success, there was no change in the number of pups per litter in mothers aged 3, 6 and 9 months in the F_2 and F_3 generations (data not reported for the F_1 generation). With respect to the number of dead pups per litter, there was a significantly lower incidence for mothers aged 6 months in the F_3 generation ($p \leq 0.05$) only. There were no statistically significant changes in the weights of the female mice, the age of vaginal opening, the fertility rate, or the pregnancy rate in any of the generations at 3, 6 or 9 months [2E].

Non-Reproductive System Effects

A fascinating animal study reported on the effects of DES on both maternal and offspring behavior. The authors reported two major findings: (1) aberrant maternal behavior from mothers receiving DES influenced the behavior of the offspring and (2) the influence of gestational DES on offspring behavior differed between the sexes. Pregnant mice were administered DES (DES-m) or an oil control (OIL-m), and their maternal behaviors were monitored postpartum. Overall there was a significant decrease in arched-back posturing over the pups ($p < 0.01$) and an increased amount of time lying motionless outside of the nest (no pups suckling) in the DES-treated mothers compared to the oil controls ($p < 0.05$). All other behaviors (licking, nest building, self-grooming, etc.) were similar between the two groups. The indirect effects of aberrant maternal behavior were also measured in offspring. The drug- and control-treated mothers (DES-m and OIL-m, respectively) were given foster-pups with and without gestational DES exposure (DES-p and OIL-p, respectively). The behavior of the foster-pups was monitored for their level of ambulation in an open-field, anxiety and passive avoidance.

Female mice (OIL-p) reared by DES foster-mothers (DES-m) showed significantly less open-field ambulation and higher levels of anxiety and passive avoidance than those reared by the control foster-mothers (OIL-m) ($p < 0.05$). Additionally, female mice who were exposed to DES *in utero* (DES-p) and reared by DES foster-mothers (DES-m) showed significantly less open-field ambulation and higher levels of anxiety and passive avoidance than those who did not receive DES *in utero* (OIL-p) (*p* < 0.05). Alternatively, male mice (OIL-p) reared by DES foster-mothers (DES-m) exhibited more hyperactivity in the open-field test than those reared by oil-exposed foster-mothers (OIL-m). Additionally, male pups reared by a control foster-mother (OIL-m) were significantly more active in the open-field test if exposed to DES *in utero* (DES-p) compared to those who did not receive DES *in utero* (OIL-p) (*p* < 0.01) [3E].

A recent case report of a DES-exposed (in utero) patient described the recurrence of liver metastases 24 years after initial treatment for clear cell adenocarcinoma of the cervix. The cervical cancer was successfully treated with brachytherapy and surgery. Fourteen years later, she underwent radical hysterectomy and right annexectomy for an abnormal uterine mass and a leiomyoma. Ten years after the hysterectomy, she was diagnosed with multiple hepatic masses and peritoneal cancinomatosis. The liver tumors were considered a metastatic diffusion of the previously treated clear cell adenoma. This appears to be the first published case of liver metastases from clear cell cervical adenocarcinoma brought about by DES exposure in utero [4A].

Hormone Replacement Therapy (HRT): [SEDA-15, 1684, 1686, 1692; SEDA-35, 732; SEDA-36, 616; SEDA-37, 500–503]

Abbreviations: EPT, estrogen and progestin therapy; ET, estrogen therapy; HRT, hormone replacement therapy; LNG, levonorgestrel; MHT, menopausal hormone therapy; NIH-AARP, National Institute of Health—American Association of Retired People; PAI-1, plasminogen activator inhibitor-1; WHI, Women's Health Initiative.

The Endocrine Society appointed a task force to create evidence-based recommendations for clinical practice guidelines for treatment of menopausal symptoms. The updated guidelines were published in November 2015. Updates and analysis of HRT for menopause have been rampant since the 2002 WHI MHT report that HRT increased the risk of cardiovascular disease, deep vein thrombosis, stroke, breast cancer and all-cause mortality. Sub-group analysis revealed that the women who experienced these adverse effects tended to be older (>60 years) were beyond 10 years out for the onset of menopause symptoms and had specific cardiovascular and breast cancer risk factors. Repeated analysis of WHI data and spin-off studies has given repeated reports that the benefits of HRT can outweigh risks in most women who are within 10 years of the initiation of menopausal symptoms, less than 60 years of age and are not in possession of cardiovascular and breast cancer risk factors. The 2015 guidelines emphasize that HRT should be individualized based upon clinical factors and patient preference. Additionally, they recommend that women should be screened for cardiovascular and breast cancer risk before initiation of HRT as a way of choosing the most appropriate therapy that will yield the best risk-to-benefit ratio. It is also important to note that newest guidelines recommend HRT be limited to the treatment to vasomotor and urogenital symptoms of climacteric [5S].

In women who have had their uterus removed, hormone therapy can be limited to replacement with estrogen alone, while women with a uterus must receive combination EPT. Use of unopposed estrogen in a woman with a uterus increases the risk of endometrial cancer.

Cardiovascular Risk

Due to the increased risk of clot formation, studies have looked at hormone-induced alterations in the expression of inflammatory and hemostatic markers.

Platelet hemostasis was measured in women receiving HRT in the form of patches containing 50 mcg 17-beta estradiol and 170 mcg norethisterone acetate/day without (group 1) and with (group 2) a low dose acetylsalicylic acid (ASA). All of the 92 postmenopausal women in the study (treatment groups and control) had at least two risk factors for arterial thrombosis (smoking, hypertension, visceral obesity, elevated blood lipids, elevated PAI-1, increased fibrinogen, increased clotting factor VII activity). Platelet count and the expression of platelet fibrinogen receptor GP IIb/IIIa were measured at baseline and after 3 months of hormone use. After 3 months, group 1 (hormone without ASA) had a statistically significant decrease in platelet count (*p* = 0.004) and GP IIb/IIIa (*p* = 0.022). Although there was a decrease in the platelet count and GP IIb/IIIa from baseline to 3 months for group 2 (hormone with ASA), it was not statistically significant [6c].

Cancer Risk

COLORECTAL CANCER (CRC)

There is a well-established association between use of post-menopausal hormones and lower CRC risk. A retrospective observational study looked at 2053 post-menopausal women who were diagnosed with CRC in the NIH-AARP Diet and Health Study. These women were followed for a median of 7.7 years. During this time, there were 759 deaths. The group looked at a number of reproductive and hormonal factors in search of correlations to CRC survival time. No associations with CRC mortality were found in those with a history of oral contraceptive use (user versus never used). There was also no association with CRC-specific (HR=0.98, 95% CI 0.68–1.43) or all-cause death (HR=1.13, 95% CI 0.89–1.43) in women who reported being previous HRT users (for either <5 years or more than 5 years) compared to those reporting that they never used menopausal HRT. However, in women who reported current HRT at baseline, there was a 21% lower risk of all-cause death (HR=0.79, 95% CI 0.66–0.94) and a 24% lower risk of CRC death (HR=0.76, 95% CI 0.59–0.99). There were not enough subjects to look at the types of HRT used; however, the participants reported estrogen only, sequential EPT, continuous EPT and unknown types of preparations [7MC].

REPRODUCTIVE CANCER

The Collaborative Group on Epidemiological Studies of Ovarian Cancer published a meta-analysis of 52 studies concerning risk of ovarian cancer in post-menopausal women with the use of MHT. The analysis (17 prospective and 35 retrospective studies) included 21 488 ovarian cancer cases in post-menopausal women. Subjects were categorized as current users, previous users and those who never used MHT. The current users were divided into those who have been using MHT for less than or greater than 5 years. Previous users were categorized as having stopped MHT less than or greater than 5 years ago.

They reported that the relative risk of ovarian cancer is significantly increased in current users of MHT compared to those who never used MHT. The increased risk in current users of MHT included those using less than and also more than 5 years ($p < 0.00001$). They also reported a significant increase in risk in women who were past users. Specifically, in women who stopped using MHT for less than 5 years, the increased risk of ovarian cancer only occurred in those who had used MHT for 5 or more years ($p = 0.00002$). In women who stopped using MHT for more 5 years, the increased risk of ovarian cancer only occurred in those who had used MHT for five or more years ($p = 0.008$). This is just a summary of overall findings. Based upon additional parameters, the author's concluded that there is an "increased risk, and it may be largely or wholly causal" [8MC].

Shapiro and colleagues published an article evaluating the meta-analysis of the original study [8MC], and reported that the meta-analysis did not establish whether current or recent use of MHT caused ovarian cancer and that it is a stronger likelihood that women with early symptoms of undiagnosed ovarian cancer (such as dyspareunia, lower abdominal pain or discomfort, recurrent bladder infections) were mistakenly treated as perimenopausal with MHT. They conclude that rather than MHT actually causing ovarian cancer, it may be that undiagnosed ovarian cancer caused MHT use [9MC].

Risk of primary fallopian tube cancer (PFTC) with use of MHT was studied using the Finnish National Population Register and Prescription Register data from 1995 to 2007. The participants were women aged 50–85 that either had PFTC ($n = 360$) or were age- and location-matched controls ($n = 3442$). The increased risk of cancer seemed to be related to the type of therapy and duration of use. Specifically, there was an increased risk of PFTC in women who used a combination estradiol and LNG-releasing intrauterine system for more than 5 years compared to matched controls ($p = 0.032$). Additionally, compared to matched controls, there was a significant risk in women using sequential EPT, meaning a progestin is added to estradiol for 10–14 days every 1–3 months ($p < 0.0001$) [10MC].

CENTRAL NERVOUS SYSTEM (CNS) CANCER

A large prospective study was published at the end of 2014 and not included in SEDA-37. This study utilized the UK General Practice Research Database (GPRD), which contains about 10 million patient records since 1987. Researchers collected information on MHT prescriptions in women between the ages of 50 and 79 with CNS tumors between 1987 and 2011 ($n = 3500$). Each case of a primary malignant or benign CNS tumor was matched with 13 997 age-matched controls from the same database. The tumors identified and characterized as "all CNS tumors" ($n = 3500$), gliomas ($n = 689$), meningiomas ($n = 1197$), acoustic neuromas ($n = 439$) and pituitary tumors ($n = 273$). Overall 30% of cases and 27% of controls had at least one HT prescription during the observation period. Compared to non-users, women with ≥ 1 prescription for HT were at significantly increased risk of having a CNS tumor ($p < 0.0001$). A significant increase in risk was specifically noted for meningiomas ($p = 0.001$) and acoustic neuromas ($p = 0.01$). The increased risk for gliomas and pituitary tumors was not statistically significant.

The group also performed a meta-analysis of their UK GPRD findings plus eight published studies. A significantly increased risk was noted for "all CNS tumors" and specifically meningiomas when comparing women using some type of MHT compared to those never using MHT. When examining women taking ET only, there was a significant increase in risk for "all" CNS tumors, gliomas and meningiomas compared to those who never used MHT. When examining women with exposure to EPT versus non-users of MHT, there was not a significant increase in relative risk. When comparing the two HRT regimens, the ET only women had a significantly greater risk of CNS tumors than the EPT women ($p < 0.005$ for each tumor type) [11MC].

Hormonal Contraceptives and Emergency Contraceptives [SEDA-15, 1642, 1645, 2225; SEDA-35, 733–734, 736–737; SEDA-36, 618, 622–623; SEDA-37, 501–504, 506]

Abbreviations: aPTT, activated partial thromboplastin time; BMC, bone mineral content; BMD, bone mineral density; CHC, combination hormonal contraceptive; COC, combined oral contraceptive; CRP, C reactive protein; CVC, combination vaginal contraceptive; DRSP, drospirenone; EC, emergency contraception; EE, ethinyl estradiol; HC, hormonal contraceptive; IUD, intrauterine device; LNG, levonorgestrel; MPA, medroxyprogesterone; OR, odds ratio; PAI-1, plasminogen activator inhibitor-1; sCD40L, soluble CD40 ligand.

Thromboembolism

Due to the increased risk of clot formation, multiple studies have looked at hormone-induced alterations in the expression of inflammatory and hemostatic markers. Recent publications have suggested that the increased risk of thrombosis with the third-generation progestins (DSRP, desogestrel, etonogestrel, norgestimate) is because they have less anti-estrogen activity compared to first-generation (norethindrone) and second-generation (LNG) products. The possible end result is that they are less potent to counterbalance the prothrombic effects of the estrogen.

Venothromboembolism (VTE)

A 2015 systematic review and meta-analysis reported on the use of COC and the risk of developing cerebral venous sinus thrombosis. In women aged 15–50 taking an oral HC, the pooled odds of developing cerebral venous thrombosis is 7.59 times higher than non-users (OR 7.59; 95% CI 3.82–15.09). In their review and analysis of the literature, the authors were not able to find enough specific information to offer conclusions concerning non-oral forms of CHC, specific types of hormones used in contraceptives or the duration of use that puts an individual at higher risk for cerebral venous sinus thrombosis. However, their final recommendation is to use non-hormonal contraceptives in women with pre-existing thrombosis risk factors (smoking, immobility, history of thrombosis or thrombophilia, or a past history of cerebral venous sinus thrombosis) [12M].

The VTE risk among the different types of progestins used in CHC was examined in a large observational study that utilized the CPRD (Clinical Practice Research Datalink) and QResearch databases in the UK. The subjects were women aged 15–49 with a first diagnosis of VTE between 2001 and 2013. Analysis was performed on 5062 cases of VTE from CPRD (matched to 19 683 non-VTE controls) and 5500 cases of VTE from QResearch (matched to 22 396 non-VTE controls). Overall findings were that current exposure to any CHC was associated with an increased risk of VTE compared to no exposure in the previous year. Preparations containing gestodene, desogestrel, DRSP and cyproterone were associated with significantly higher risks of VTE than those containing either LNG or norgestimate. The number of extra VTE cases per year per 10 000 treated women was highest for desogestrel and cyproterone [13MC].

Hemostatic and Inflammatory Markers

The effect of CHC to change clotting factors as early during the first month of use was studied in a single-arm, open-label pilot study in 17 females aged 18–35. To examine the clotting factor changes during the first cycle of CHC use, repeated blood samples were collected throughout the duration of a 21-day cycle of CHC containing 30 mcg EE and 150 mcg LNG. Levels of D-dimer more than doubled after 6 days of using the CHC and remained elevated at day 21 ($p = 0.012$) compared to baseline. A significant increase in Factor VIII activity was seen after 2 days of using the CHC, but declined to levels that were not significantly increased by day 21. There was not a significant increase in Protein C with the first cycle of use of the CHC [14c].

Plasma expression of hemostatic factors was measured in a small study of 70 healthy women aged 18–30, divided into groups receiving no CHC, 3 mg DRSP with 20 mcg EE (DRSP/20EE), 3 mg DRSP with 30 mcg EE (DRSP/30EE) or 0.15 mg LNG with 30 mcg EE (LNG/30EE). Compared to control, the highest number of significant alterations in markers favoring hypercoagulability occurred with the product containing the lowest estrogen content, DRSP/20EE. All three products resulted in a significant decrease in prothrombin time compared to control ($p < 0.01$ for all three). Although there were similar trends (increases/decreases) among the three products, only DRSP/20EE showed significant changes in aPTT (decreased), fibrinogen (increased) and D-dimer (increased) compared to control ($p = 0.02$, $p = 0.02$, $p < 0.01$, respectively). D-dimer is a product of fibrin degradation and is dependent on fibrin formation and fibrinolysis. The concentration of Protein S significantly decreased in both DRSP products compared to control ($p < 0.01$), while the amount of Protein C significantly decreased only for the LNG containing product ($p < 0.01$). Protein S and Protein C are mediators of endogenous anticoagulation processes. Lastly, DRSP/30EE had a significant decrease in the activity of the antifibrinolytic variable, PAI-1 ($p < 0.01$). The authors suggest that significant changes in hemostatic variables seen with the lower doses of EE in COC products (20 mcg compared to 30 mcg) provide evidence against estrogen being the sole contributor to thrombosis. They also stated that these findings, although statistically significant, were not verified to have clinical significance [15c].

In a small clinical trial of 79 females aged 19–30, differences in expression of inflammation markers were examined in those using oral and vaginal contraceptive products. According to the authors, circulating levels of CRP are considered a marker of a hepatic protein response to acute inflammation. CRP is also used as an inflammatory marker to assess the risk for cardiovascular disease and stroke. Levels of sCD40L were measured, since an elevated concentration suggests *in vivo* platelet activation. There were 29 subjects in the COC group, 20 in the CVC group and 30 nonusers. Subjects in the CHC groups must have used the contraceptive for a minimum of 6 months, while the non-users could not have used a CHC for at least 6 months. Information on medical history, physical activities, dietary and sleeping habits was collected. Both oral and vaginal contraceptive users had higher levels of CRP ($p < 0.0001$ and $p < 0.001$, respectively) compared to nonusers. Only COC users exhibited elevated sCD40L. Levels of sCD40L were significantly higher for COC compared to CVC ($p < 0.01$) and non-users ($p < 0.01$). There was not a significant difference in sCD40L between the CVC and non-users ($p = 0.89$). The authors did not report the specific types of progestin in the COC products, but NuvaRing contains etonogestrel, which is a third-generation progestin (the active metabolite of desogestrel) [16c].

Multiple blood biomarkers for coagulation and inflammation were compared in women taking either a COC or CVC (NuvaRing), for a minimum of 6 months. The study included 159 healthy women between 19 and 30 years of age. Due to small sample size, the COC group (51 participants) was not divided into the specific type or dose of hormone. The control group (64 participants) had to be hormone free for a minimum of 6 months prior to the study. Both groups of contraceptive users had elevated levels of factor VII ($p < 0.0001$). With respect to markers of inflammation, CHC users had significantly higher levels of CRP compared to controls ($p < 0.0001$). Additionally, levels of E-selectin (an endothelial activation molecule) ($p = 0.0009$ for COC and $p = 0.0023$ for CVC) and P-selectin (a platelet activation molecule) ($p < 0.0001$ for COC and $p = 0.0067$ for CVC) were significantly lower in those taking CHC, which the authors stated to be an indication that a non-endothelial activation pathway was responsible for the increase in CRP levels. CD40 ligand (a marker of platelet activation) was significantly higher in users of COC compared to control and CVC ($p < 0.0001$). There was not a significant difference in CD40 ligand levels between control and CVC users ($p = 0.167$). For markers of coagulation, CHC users had significantly lower levels of tissue factor pathway inhibitor, which is indicative of a hypercoagulable state ($p = 0.0117$ for COC and $p = 0.0206$ for CVC). Other coagulation markers that were modified in CHC users included PAI-1, tissue factor, thrombin/antithrombin and soluble thrombomodulin. The breakdown

for specific progestins in the COC users is the following: 19.6% norethindrone (first generation), 13.7% LNG (second generation) and 66.7% used DRSP, desogestrel or norgestimate (third generation). The CVC, NuvaRing, also contains the third-generation progestin, etonogestrel [17C].

Skeletal Effects

The effects of COC on bone were investigated in a non-randomized parallel-control study of females aged 12–19. Participants in the treatment group ($n = 35$) received a low dose COC containing 20 mcg EE and 150 mcg desogestrel, while the control group ($n = 26$) did not receive a COC. Use of hormonal contraceptives will shut down the hypothalamic–pituitary–gonadal axis and thus the endogenous production of ovarian hormones. If the individual is not being supplied with an adequate amount of exogenous estrogen (via the COC), a state of hypogonadism (and decreased bone development) can result. This is a proposed mechanism for the decreased BMD occurring with the use of depot MPA, which is a progestin only product. Previous studies using higher doses of COC do not show a negative effect on BMD, possibly because enough exogenous estrogen is being provided to maintain normal bone development and growth. The researchers set out to specifically investigate the effect of a COC with a low estrogen content on bone mass acquisition in an adolescent population over a 1-year period. Labs and DEXA (dual energy X-ray absorptiometry) scans were measured at baseline and after 1 year of the COC use. Overall, the increase in lumbar, subtotal and whole body BMC was significantly lower in those taking the COC ($p < 0.05$ for all 3 parameters). Although there was also a substantial decrease in BMD, it was not statistically significant [18c].

Ectopic Pregnancy

An ectopic pregnancy is defined as implantation of a fertilized egg outside of the uterus. As the fetus enlarges, it requires a greater blood supply and physical space. The uterus is the only organ that possesses the required blood supply and capability to expand in order to accommodate the fetus for a successful pregnancy. If the organ in which the ectopic pregnancy is attached ruptures, this can lead to massive hemorrhage, infertility or death to the mother. In general, the estimated ectopic pregnancy rate in women not using contraceptives is 2.1 per 1000 women-years and 9.24 per 1000 women-years in women who are trying to become pregnant. Since this is such a dramatic and dangerous occurrence, determining a cause or factor that increases the risk of ectopic pregnancy is very important.

A large review investigated the incidence of ectopic pregnancy in women using progestin contraceptive implants (53 studies) and injectable progestin contraceptives (28 studies). With respect to the implants, there were a total of 28 studies for Norplant (LNG-containing implant), and the incidence of ectopic pregnancy was 0.1–2.9 per 1000 women-years. There were a total of 11 studies for other marketed LNG-containing implants (Jadelle, Sino-implant, Sino-implant II) which reported the range of ectopic pregnancy to be from 0.2 to 0.8 per 1000 women-years. There were only two studies reporting on pregnancy occurrence with etonogestrel-containing implants (Implanon, Nexplanon). One of those studies with the etonogestrel product had no pregnancies, and the other reported 5 ectopic pregnancies, but it was not clear if those pregnancies were due to a method or a product failure. For contraceptive injections, the cases of ectopic pregnancy in the literature for depot MPA and nor-ethisterone were too scarce to report. In general the pregnancy rates for the injectable products were low and details on the location of pregnancy (intrauterine versus ectopic) was not complete. The authors pointed out that only six reports of ectopic pregnancy in three studies exist in nearly 50 years of published literature [19R].

A retrospective, case-controlled study at 5 hospitals in China examined the risk of ectopic pregnancy with previous or current use of LNG-EC pills. Women with ectopic pregnancy were identified ($n = 2411$) using diagnostic criteria from the American Congress of Obstetricians and Gynecologists. The study group was compared to 2416 matched women with intrauterine pregnancies and 2419 match non-pregnant women as controls. Compared to non-users of contraceptives, users of LNG-EC had a reduced risk of pregnancy in general (ectopic or intrauterine). Multivariate analysis revealed that previous use of LNG-EC (even repeated use) did not correlate with an increased risk of ectopic pregnancy. Additionally, there was no significant association between the numbers of LNG-EC used within the last year to the risk of ectopic pregnancy in the current cycle.

The study also looked at a subset of women who took EC and then engaged in further acts of intercourse during the same cycle. Compared to women who did not have further intercourse in the same cycle after using the EC, those who did engage in further acts of unprotected intercourse were at higher risk of ectopic pregnancy following EC failure. Women who had further acts of intercourse and used repeated doses of LNG-EC in the same cycle were also at an increased risk of ectopic pregnancy compared to those not engaging in further acts of intercourse after the first EC use. The authors speculated that the reason behind this was the effect of progestin to decrease fallopian tube motility which could cause implantation of a fertilized egg in the fallopian tube [20MC].

Adverse Effects with Transdermal CHC

Benefits of a transdermal patch CHC include increased compliance and more consistent blood levels of hormones. The transdermal CHC, Ortho Evra (ethinyl estradiol and norelgestromin) recently (2014) made a change to the packet-insert to disclose that the area under the curve concentration of estrogen is 60% higher than a COC containing 35 mcg of ethinyl estradiol. Additionally, this increased exposure to estrogen may increase the risk of adverse reactions, including thromboembolism.

A new transdermal product containing EE and LNG is currently undergoing Phase 3 studies. The new transdermal product, Twirla, has been shown to maintain serum estrogen levels equivalent to a COC containing 30 mcg of EE. The safety and tolerability were summarized using data from two open-label, randomized, multicenter, parallel-group clinical studies. Twirla was compared to two COC products: a 20 mcg EE with 100 mcg of LNG (COC20) and a 30 mcg EE with 150 mcg LNG (COC30). With the exception of application sites reactions (which occurred in 4.9% of participants), the severity and incidence of adverse events with the new transdermal CHC were similar to those of COC20 and COC30. The studies lacked the statistical power to report clot risk in any of the products [21R].

Adverse Effects with the Intrauterine Device (IUD)

The 3-year efficacy and safety of a 52 mg LNG-releasing IUD system designed for up to 7 years of use were recently published. The study included 1600 women aged 16–35 and 151 women aged 36–45. The most common adverse effect was expulsion of the implanted device. The incidence of complete and partial expulsion was 3.5%. Most expulsions (80.6%) occurred in the first year of device implantation, with 10 occurring within the first 30 days, 17 occurring within the first 3 months, 30 occurring within the first 6 months, and 50 occurring within the first 12 months. Nulliparous women had a significantly lower expulsion frequency than parous women (2.0% compared to 5.6%, respectively; $p < 0.0001$).

At least one adverse event was noted in 83.3% of 16–35 year olds and 86.8% of 36–45 year olds. The most common adverse reactions reported were vaginal infection (26.3%), acne (12.3%), headache/migraine (9.8%), nausea or vomiting (7.9%), dyspareunia (7%), abdominal discomfort or pain (6.8%), breast tenderness or pain (6.7%), pelvic discomfort or pain (6.1%), depression or depressed mood (5.4%) and mood changes (5.2%). Overall, 12.3% of participants discontinued product use due to an adverse event. The most common adverse events leading to product discontinuation were expulsion (3.5%), bleeding complaints (1.5%), acne (1.3%) and mood swings (1.3%). Discontinuation for all bleeding-related complaints combined occurred in 26 (1.5%) LNG20 users. Over the course of the 3-year study, there were six recorded pregnancies, four of which were ectopic. None of the pregnancies occurred in the 36–45-year-old age group [22MC].

A delayed-type hypersensitivity reaction was reported in a 37-year-old multiparous women using the Nexplanon® (etonogestrel) implant. She had no history of hypersensitivity reactions (including seasonal allergies). Three months after insertion of the implant, she complained of mild itching at the insertion site. A few months later, she developed nonpainful small cutaneous maculopapular lesions of the skin surrounding the implant. Symptoms worsened and 1 year after insertion of the implant, she presented with skin redness and moderate arm edema, without fever, leukocytosis or eosinophilia. The implant was removed. There was some fibrosis surrounding the implant. When the device was surgically removed, it appeared fractured in several segments. Histological exam showed active macrophagic and mastocytic reactions of the tissue surrounding the implant. One week after device removal, there was total regression of symptoms and a 6-month follow-up revealed no late complications [23A].

Abortifacients [SEDA-15, 2344; SEDA-35, 738; SEDA-36, 625; SEDA-37, 506–507]

A retrospective observational cohort study to estimate the complication rate within 6 weeks of different types of abortions was performed using 2009–2010 abortion data from Medicaid records in the state of California. The types of abortions were classified as a medical abortion (mifepristone and misoprostol), first-trimester aspiration abortion and second-trimester or later procedures. Complications were categorized as minor and major. A major complication was defined as a serious unexpected adverse event requiring hospital admission, surgery or a blood transfusion. Major complications included incomplete abortion, failed abortion, hemorrhage, infection, uterine perforation and other/undetermined. A minor complication was defined as all other expected adverse effects but also included incomplete abortion, failed abortion, hemorrhage, infection, anesthesia-related, uterine perforation and other/undetermined.

For the 11 319 medication abortions performed, there were a total of 588 complications (rate of 5.19/100; 95% CI 4.79–5.60). Out of these, 35 were major complications (rate of 0.31/100; 95% CI, 0.21–0.41) and 553 were minor complications (rate of 4.88/10; 95% CI, 4.49–5.28). The most common complication of medical abortion was incomplete abortion, followed by infection, hemorrhage and failed abortion. Compared to first-trimester aspiration abortion, the medical abortion had a significantly higher number of total complications (5.19% compared to 1.26%, $p < 0.001$) [24MC].

Selective Estrogen Receptor Modulators (SERMs): Tamoxifen [SED-15, 3296; SEDA-35, 735; SEDA-36, 619; SEDA-37, 504]

A small study looked at the effect of long-term tamoxifen treatment on cognitive function in postmenopausal women with breast cancer. There were 107 participants in the study; 20 women who underwent surgical

operation with or without radiotherapy plus adjuvant tamoxifen (tamoxifen group), 43 women who underwent surgical operation with or without radiotherapy (surgical group) and 44 healthy controls matched to both the tamoxifen and surgical groups for age and education level (control). The range for the mean age of the participants was 61–62 years, and their age at menopause was 47–48 years of age. The only demographic that was significantly different between groups was marital status. Women in the tamoxifen group were current tamoxifen users and had been using for at least 12 months. A battery of tests was performed, including those for cognitive function, memory (verbal, visual, working), executive functioning and processing speed, physical function, symptoms of treatment and health-related quality of life (anxiety, fatigue, depression, menopausal symptoms). Overall, the tamoxifen group scored significantly lower in the cognitive functioning scale compared to the surgical ($p < 0.05$) and control ($p < 0.05$) groups. Specifically, verbal memory was significantly lower compared to both the surgical ($p < 0.05$) and control ($p < 0.05$) groups, while language fluency performance was significantly lower than the control group ($p < 0.05$), but not the surgical group. When looking at health related quality of life, the three groups did not differ on reported levels of fatigue, pain, anxiety and depression ($p > 0.05$). With respect to symptoms of treatment, those in the tamoxifen group had significantly more constipation compared to the others ($p < 0.05$) [25C].

Anabolics, Androgens and Related Compounds [SEDA-35, 739; SEDA-36, 628; SEDA-37; SEDA-37, 507–508]

Abbreviations: AAS, anabolic androgenic steroid; DVT, deep venous thrombosis; HR, hazard ratios; MI, myocardial infarction; PE, pulmonary embolism; RR, relative risk; VTE, venothromboembolism.

The use of high doses of AAS is well known to lead to a number of medical complications such as hypertension, atherosclerosis, myocardial hypertrophy and infarct, abnormal blood clotting, hepatotoxicity and hepatic tumors, tendon damage, reduced libido and psychiatric/behavioral symptoms [26R].

Cardiovascular

The risk of MI with testosterone replacement therapy use was investigated in a case-controlled study using the IMS LifeLink health plan claims database. For data between 2001 and 2011, 30 066 MI cases in men aged 45–80 and 120 264 corresponding controls were identified. The primary outcome was a new-onset acute MI. A total of 515 men in the MI group and 1954 in the control group were testosterone therapy users, which was defined as having at least one prescription for testosterone filled within the last year. The formulation (gel, patch, injection) and timing of use (current, previous, first-time user) were characterized for each group. The mean age of the men at index date was 70.4 years, and the mean duration of follow-up was 2.8 years. The authors found that current use of testosterone (a prescription was received within the last 90 days) was not associated with a significant increased risk of MI, unless the man was a first time user (received their first testosterone prescription within the last 90 days) (RR 1.04; 95% CI 1.06–1.87). Among the different testosterone formations in the first time users, only the topical gels reached statistical significance since it accounted for more 55% of testosterone therapy (RR 1.49; 95% CI 1.02–2.18). The authors stated that the other formulations did not reach statistical significant, possibly due to insufficient power. There was no association between MI and past testosterone users and no differences among the different formulations. The authors concluded that there was a statistically significant association between first-time testosterone therapy exposure and MI, but the absolute risk was low [27C].

The effect of long-term testosterone administration on subclinical atherosclerosis progression was examined in older men with low or low–normal testosterone levels. This was a placebo-controlled, double-blind, parallel-group randomized clinical trial employing 156 men to use 7.5 g of 1% testosterone gel and 152 to use a placebo gel packet every day for 3 years. The dose was adjusted to achieve testosterone levels between 500 and 900 ng/dL. Baseline free and total testosterone levels were similar between the two groups. The free and total testosterone did not significantly change in the placebo group (51 and 330 ng/dL, respectively); however, the levels increased to 104 ng/dL in testosterone free and 565 ng/dL in total testosterone in the treatment group. The primary outcomes were common carotid artery intima-media thickness and coronary artery calcium. Secondary outcomes included sexual dysfunction and health-related quality of life. The mean age of the men was 67.6 years and comorbidities included hypertension (42%), diabetes (15%), cardiovascular disease (15%) and obesity (27%). There was not a significant difference in the rate of change in intima-media thickness between the two groups (0.010 mm/year for placebo and 0.012 mm/year for treatment). The rate of change in the coronary artery calcium score was also not significant between the groups ($p = 0.54$). Lastly, 3 years of testosterone administration did not improve overall sexual function or health-related quality of life in the older men [28C].

The prevalence of thrombotic events in elderly men (>65 years of age) taking testosterone replacement therapy for hypogonadism was investigated in a retrospective study. The subjects included 217 hypogonadal men taking testosterone ($n = 153$) and controls who also

had hypogonadism but were not taking testosterone ($n = 64$). Total testosterone (ng/dL) and estradiol (ng/dL) levels were both significantly higher in men receiving testosterone ($p < 0.001$ for both). All-cause mortality and the occurrence of MI, transient ischemic attack, cerebrovascular accident and DVT/PE were evaluated. Mean follow-up was 3.8 ± 2.7 years in those receiving testosterone and 3.4 ± 2.8 years for control. Although none of the men receiving testosterone therapy died, five of the control hypogonadal men died ($p = 0.007$) of metastatic prostate cancer, metastatic lung cancer and chronic obstructive pulmonary disease. There were four thrombotic events (a MI, a PE and two cerebrovascular accidents) in the testosterone group and one cerebrovascular event in the control group, although these differences were not statistically significant ($p = 0.8$). There was also not a significantly increased risk of all-cause mortality between the two groups [29C].

A retrospective cohort study utilized databases from the United States and United Kingdom to identify 544 115 men ≥18 years of age using different testosterone formulations (transdermal patches, intramuscular injections and topical gels). The subjects were newly initiated users of testosterone, meaning they had no history of previous testosterone use or had a minimum of 180-day washout period free of documented testosterone use. The study compared the cardiovascular safety between the different dosage forms. In the study, 37.4% used injection, 6.9% used the patch and 55.8% use a gel formulation. The results showed that testosterone injection users had higher hazards of cardiovascular events (MI, unstable angina and stroke (HR 1.26; 95% CI 1.18–1.35), hospitalization (HR 1.16; 95% CI 1.13–1.19) and death (HR 1.34; 95% CI 1.15–1.56)), but not VTE compared to gel formulations. Additionally, transdermal patches did not have increased hazards of cardiovascular events, hospitalization, death or VTE compared to gel preparations. The authors reported that the injectable form of testosterone were associated with a greater risk of cardiovascular events, hospitalizations and death compared to topical gels. Additionally, the patches and gels had similar risk profiles. The author's conclusions are that their analysis "suggests" that the testosterone injections "may" have increased risks does not communicate a definitive recommendation of using one formulation over others [30C].

Anabolic Steroids

Anabolic androgens consist of testosterone and synthetic derivatives that have been modified to enhance anabolic effects over androgenic effects. Coveted anabolic effects include muscle growth, erythropoiesis, reduced body fat, faster recovery from muscle strain/injury and increased intensity in the ability to physically train longer and harder.

Cardiovascular

Prolonged misuse of AAS can have fatal effects, especially on the cardiovascular system since there is an increase of sudden cardiac death, MI, altered serum lipoproteins, clot formation and cardiac hypertrophy. Histological, toxicology and autopsy findings in 19 deaths related to AAS abuse between 1990 and 2012 revealed that cardiac causes were responsible for death in 18 cases, and one death was due to a DVT that resulted in bilateral PE [31R].

Psychological

A thorough review by Piacentino and colleagues reviewed the psychological factors involved with abuse of AAS in athletes. Athletes using AAS are shown to present with psychiatric symptoms such as somatoform (dysmorphia), eating, mood and schizophrenia-related disorders. As some psychiatric disorders are typical of athletes, there is question as whether the preexistence of psychopathology promotes use of AAS or is the psychopathology is caused by abuse of AAS. The authors conclude that the bulk of available data, combined with data from animal studies suggest the development of specific psychopathology, increased aggressiveness, mood destabilization (depression with long-term use, anxiety and withdrawal and hypomania with short-term use, suicide), eating disorders, behavior abnormalities and psychosis after AAS abuse/dependence [26R].

References

[1] Fenichel P, Brucker-Davis F, Chevalier N. The history of Distilbene (Diethylstilbestrol) told to grandchildren—the transgenerational effect. Ann Endocrinol. 2015;76:253–9 [R].

[2] Ziv-Gal A, Wang W, Zhou C, et al. The effects of in utero bisphenol A exposure on reproductive capacity in several generations of mice. Toxicol Appl Pharmacol. 2015;284:354–62 [E].

[3] Tomihara K, Zoshiki T, Kukita SY, et al. Effects of diethylstilbestrol exposure during gestation on both maternal and offspring behavior. Front Neurosci. 2015;9:1–8 [E].

[4] Adani-lfe A, Goldschmidt E, Innominato P, et al. Very late recurrence of diethylstilbestrol-related clear cell carcinoma of the cervix: case report. Gynecol Oncol Res Pract. 2015;2:3 [A].

[5] Stuenkel CA, Davis SR, Gompel A, et al. Treatment of symptoms of the menopause: an Endocrine Society clinical practice guideline. J Clin Endocrinol Metab. 2015;100(11):3975–4011 [S].

[6] Stachowiak G, Pertyński T, Pertyńska-Marczewska M. Effect of transdermal hormone therapy on platelet haemostasis in menopausal women. Ann Agric Environ Med. 2015;22(1):167–71 [c].

[7] Arem KH, Park Y, Felix AS, et al. Reproductive and hormonal factors and mortality among women with colorectal cancer in the NIH-AARP diet and health study. Br J Cancer. 2015;113:562–8 [MC].

[8] Beral V, Gaitskell K, Herman C, et al. Menopausal hormone use and ovarian cancer risk: individual participant meta-analysis of 52 epidemiological studies. Lancet. 2015;385:1835–42 [MC].

[9] Shapiro S, Stevenson JC, Mueck AO, et al. Misrepresentation of the risk of ovarian cancer among women using menopausal hormones. Spurious findings in a meta-analysis. Maturitas. 2015;81:323–6 [MC].

[10] Koskela-Niska V, Pukkala E, Lyytinen H, et al. Postmenopausal hormone therapy-also use of estradiol plus levonorgestrel-intrauterine system is associated with an increased risk of primary fallopian tube carcinoma. Int J Cancer. 2015;137:1947–52 [MC].

[11] Benson VS, Kirichek O, Beral V, et al. Menopausal hormone therapy and central nervous system tumor risk: large UK prospective study and meta-analysis. Int J Cancer. 2015;136:2369–77 [MC].

[12] Amoozegar F, Ronksley PE, Sauve R, et al. Hormonal contraceptives and cerebral venous thrombosis risk: a systematic review and meta-analysis. Front Neurol. 2015;6:7. http://dx.doi.org/10.3389/fneur.2015.00007 [M].

[13] Vinogradova Y, Coupland C, Hippisley-Cox J. Use of combined oral contraceptives and risk of venous thromboembolism: nested case-control studies using the QResearch and CPRD databases. BMJ. 2015;350:h2135 [MC].

[14] Westhoff CL, Eisenberger A, Tang R, et al. Clotting factor changes during the first cycle of oral contraceptive use. Contraception. 2016;93:70–6 [c].

[15] Stocco B, Fumagalli HF, Franceschini SA, et al. Comparative study of the effects of combined oral contraceptives in hemostatic variables: an observational preliminary study. Medicine. 2015;94(4):e385. http://dx.doi.org/10.1097/MD.0000000000000385 [c].

[16] Divani AA, Luo X, Datta YH, et al. Effect of oral and vaginal hormonal contraceptives on inflammatory blood biomarkers. Mediators Inflamm. 2015;2015:379501. http://dx.doi.org/10.1155/2015/379501 [c].

[17] Divani AA, Luo X, Brandy KR, et al. Oral versus vaginal combined hormonal contraceptives' effect on coagulation and inflammatory biomarkers among young adult women. Clin Appl Thromb Hemost. 2015;18(5):487–94 [C].

[18] Biason TP, Goldberg TBL, Kurokawa CS, et al. Low-dose combined oral contraceptive use is associated with lower bone mineral content variation in adolescents over a 1-year period. BMC Endocr Disord. 2015;15:15. http://dx.doi.org/10.1186/s12902-015-0012-7 [c].

[19] Callahan R, Yacobson I, Halpern V, et al. Ectopic pregnancy with use of progestin-only injectables and contraceptive implants: a systematic review. Contraception. 2015;92(6):514–22 [R].

[20] Zhang J, Li C, Zhao W, et al. Association between levonorgestrel emergency contraception and the risk of ectopic pregnancy: a multicenter case-control study. Sci Rep. 2015;5:8487. http://dx.doi.org/10.1038/srep08487 [MC].

[21] Kaunitz AM, Archer DF, Mishell DR, et al. Safety and tolerability of a new low-dose contraceptive patch in obese and nonobese women. Am J Obstet Gynecol. 2015;212:318.e1–8 [R].

[22] Eisenberg DL, Schreiber CA, Turok DK, et al. Three-year efficacy and safety of a new 52-mg levonorgestrel-releasing intrauterine system. Contraception. 2015;92:10–6 [MC].

[23] Serati M, Bogani G, Kumar S, et al. Delayed-type hypersensitivity reaction against Nexplanon®. Contraception. 2015;91:91–2 [A].

[24] Upadhyay UD, Desai S, Zlidar V, et al. Incidence of emergency department visits and complications after abortion. Obstet Gynecol. 2015;125(1):175–83 [MC].

[25] Boele FW, Schilder CMT, de Roode M. Cognitive functioning during long-term tamoxifen treatment in postmenopausal women with breast cancer. Menopause. 2015;22(1):17–25 [C].

[26] Piacentino D, Kotzalidis GD, del Casale A, et al. Anabolic-androgenic steroid use and psychopathology in athletes. A systematic review. Curr Neuropharmacol. 2015;13:101–21 [R].

[27] Etminan M, Skeldon SC, Goldenberg SL, et al. Testosterone therapy and risk of myocardial infarction: a pharmacoepidemiologic study. Pharmacotherapy. 2015;35(1):72–8 [C].

[28] Basaria S, Harman SM, Travison TG, et al. Effects of testosterone administration for 3 years on subclinical atherosclerosis progression in older men with low or low-normal testosterone levels. JAMA. 2015;314(6):570–81 [C].

[29] Ramasamy R, Scovell J, Mederos M, et al. Association between testosterone supplementation therapy and thrombotic events in elderly men. Urology. 2015;86:283–5 [C].

[30] Layton JB, Meier CR, Sharpless JL, et al. Comparative safety of testosterone dosage forms. JAMA Intern Med. 2015;175(7):1187–96 [C].

[31] Frati P, Busardo FP, Cipolloni L, et al. Anabolic androgenic steroid (AAS) related deaths: autoptic, histopathological and toxicological findings. Curr Neuropharmacol. 2015;13:146–59 [R].

39

Thyroid hormones, Iodine and Iodides, and Antithyroid Drugs

Rahul Deshmukh*, Ajay N Singh†, Mark Martinez‡, Nidhi Gandhi‡, Karyn I. Cotta†, Harish Parihar‡, Vicky V. Mody§,1

*Department of Pharmaceutical Sciences, College of Pharmacy, Rosalind Franklin University of Medicine and Science, North Chicago, Il, USA

†Department of Pharmaceutical Sciences, South University School of Pharmacy, Savannah, GA, USA

‡Department of Pharmacy Practice, PCOM School of Pharmacy, Suwanee, GA, USA

§Department of Pharmaceutical Sciences, PCOM School of Pharmacy, Suwanee, GA, USA

1Corresponding author: vickymo@pcom.edu

THYROID HORMONES [SED-15, 3409; SEDA-31, 687; SEDA-32, 763; SEDA-33, 881; SEDA-34, 679; SEDA-35, 747; SEDA-36, 635; SEDA-37, 513]

Thyroid hormones mimicking agents such as eprotirome, levothyroxine (T4), and triiodothyronine (liothyronine, T3) are used in the treatment of both overt and subclinical hypothyroidism. Both conditions are presented with elevated TSH levels; however, overt clinical hypothyroidism is further defined by low levels of free triiodothyronine (fT3) and free levothyroxine (fT4). Patients presenting with overt or subclinical hypothyroidism are at increased risk of developing cardiovascular disease; hence, care has to be sought as soon as discovered.

Eprotirome

Eprotirome, selectively acts on the hepatic β receptor. The use of eprotirome has been shown to lower serum low-density lipoprotein (LDL) cholesterol concentrations in patients with dyslipidemia. Abnormal lipid levels put patients at risk for cardiovascular disease, which sometimes becomes difficult to reverse with stand-alone statin therapy [1R]. The use of thyroid hormone mimetics in these patients can help lower levels of LDL cholesterol.

Increase in Liver Enzymes

Angelin B and coworkers conducted a multicentre, randomized, placebo-controlled, double-blind study to evaluate the efficacy and safety of eprotirome, in 98 patients with primary hypercholesterolaemia [2C]. These 98 patients were divided into 3 subgroups of 20 patients in group 1, 38 patients in group 2, and 40 patients in group 3. The patients in group 1 received a placebo, whereas, both patients in group 2 and 3 received 100 and 200 μg of eprotirome, respectively. While eprotirome was able to reduced serum LDL cholesterol levels by $23 \pm 5\%$ and $31 \pm 4\%$, in group 2 and 3, respectively, as compared with $2 \pm 6\%$ for placebo ($p < 0.0001$), an increase in liver enzymes was observed in all patients. In fact 7 patients withdrew from the study as their serum ALT levels exceeded the predefined limit [2C].

Levothyroxine

Levothyroxine remains the mainstay of current treatment for hypothyroidism, and the mean dosage prescribed for levothyroxine therapy is 1.6 μg/kg/day. Intestinal absorption of levothyroxine varies from patient to patient and is usually in the range of 60–80% of the dose administered.

Quality of Life

Primary hypothyroidism can affect the quality of life (QOL). Kelderman-Bolk and coworkers studied the relation between QOL and various parameters in hypothyroid patients who were taking levothyroxine [3R]. They evaluated the QOL in 90 patients (20 males and 70 females) who were treated for primary hypothyroidism using Short-Form 36, Hospital Anxiety and Depression Scale and MFI20. The Post hoc analysis was performed on the relation of QOL at baseline, BMI, thyroid hormones, and other serum values. It was found that there exists an inverse relationship between QOL and BMI, and a decreased QOL was observed in hypothyroid patients on thyroxine treatment. This was mainly due to their higher body weight (BMI) and hence the authors concluded that weight gain should be one of the focus while treating hypothyroid patients as it can decrease their QOL.

Rheumatoid Arthritis (RA)

Levothyroxine has been shown to increase the risk of developing rheumatoid arthritis for patients with autoimmune disorders [4R]. In this study authors compared 1998 patients using levothyroxine along with 2252 controls for incident RA cases. They found that patients on levothyroxine were at twofold risk for RA [4R].

Vitamin D Deficiency

The use of levothyroxine has also been implicated for vitamin D deficiency. Authors compared 25-hydroxy-vitamin D and parathyroid hormone (PTH) levels between four groups of non-lactating women [5C]. Group A consisted of 14 hypothyroid women with post-partum thyroiditis, Group B included 14 euthyroid females with post-partum thyroiditis, Group C included 16 female with non-autoimmune hypothyroidism, and group D was a control which included 15 healthy euthyroid females. The patients in both groups A and C were treated with L-thyroxine for 6 months. After 6 months, it was found that the serum levels of 25-hydroxyvitamin D were lowered in group A than in group B, as well as in group C in comparison with group D. Hence, the authors concluded that there is an association of vitamin D status with post-partum thyroiditis and levothyroxine treatment.

Multiple Subungual Pyogenic Granulomas

A 54-year-old woman who was taking levothyroxine for hypothyroidism for 3 months presented with rapidly growing lesions in her nail beds [6R]. Examination revealed red nodules that had invaded beneath the nail plates. The patient also took venlafaxine 75 mg use once a day for depression for 10 years and intermittent ibuprofen use (which was stopped a year ago) for osteoarthritis. A wide excision was performed but the symptoms relapsed as noted during the 3-month follow-up period. Levothyroxine treatment was stopped and the symptoms did not recur [6R].

Bone Loss

Effects of levothyroxine (LT4) on bone and bone metabolism are controversial [7C]. To address this author examined mean bone losses in 93 patients with well-differentiated carcinoma over 12 months after initiating levothyroxine therapy. It was found that there was a mean bone losses in the lumbar spine, femoral neck, and total hip; however, the loss was more prominent in postmenopausal women. Authors also observed that the loss was higher in postmenopausal women who received no supplementation of calcium/vitamin D. Hence, the authors concluded that TSH-suppressive levothyroxine therapy can accelerate bone loss predominantly in postmenopausal women and mainly during the early post-thyroidectomy period but the loss can be reduced by adding calcium/vitamin D to the therapy.

On the similar lines Nyandege and coworkers have suggested that the concomitant use of bisphosphonates and other medications, which can stimulates bone metabolism such as acid-suppressive therapy, levothyroxine, thiazolidinediones (TZDs), and selective serotonin reuptake inhibitors (SSRIs), can increase the risk of fracture [8R]. Authors found that the concomitant use of acid suppressive agents with bisphosphonate can increase the risk of fracture. However, they suggested that TZDs, SSRIs, and levothyroxine can have similar implications based on their pharmacological action. Hence, precaution should to be taken while using bisphosphonates along with these other medications.

CARDIOVASCULAR DISORDERS

A prospective, controlled, single-blind study was conducted by Bakiner et al. to determine plasma Fetuin A levels in hypothyroid patients ($n=39$) before and after levothyroxine treatment. Additionally, authors wanted to figure out if there is any association between Fetuin A levels and cardiovascular risk in those patients [9C]. Authors found that there was no correlation between Fetuin A levels and cardiovascular risk factors; however, the mean HDL cholesterol levels decreased in those patients from 49.3 (23–83.9) to 44 (28.3–69.0) [9C].

Drug Overdose

The pharmacological effects of levothyroxine on cardiac cells are well know where in high doses of levothyroxine can cause severe toxic effects in the patient [10A]. Stuijver et al. reported a case of 23-year-old woman who attempted suicide by ingesting 25 mg of levothyroxine [10A]. The patient experienced hypercoagulation and a hypofibrinolytic effect, reflecting an increased risk of venous thrombosis [10A]. Similarly, a 61-year-old patient who accidentally ingested 1000 times excess of levothyroxine rather than the actual dose of 50 mg exhibited altered mental consciousness, acute respiratory failure, and atrial fibrillation [11A].

Drug–Drug Interaction

Levothyroxine can interact with various other drugs. In an observational study carried out by Irving and coworkers, the authors wanted to evaluate the effect of drugs co-administered on thyroxine [12C]. This study evaluated 10 999 patients (mean age 58 years, 82% female) who were prescribed levothyroxine on at least three occasions within a 6-month period, prior to the start of a study. They found that both iron and calcium supplements, proton pump inhibitors, and oestrogen were responsible for the increase in serum TSH concentration (7.5%, 4.4%, 5.6% and 4.3%), respectively. However, there was a decrease in the TSH concentration (0.17 mU/L) for those patients on statins. Hence, the authors concluded that there is a significant interaction between levothyroxine and iron, calcium, proton pump inhibitors, statins and oestrogens. Co-administration of these drugs with levothyroxine may reduce the effectiveness of levothyroxine therapy, and hence the TSH concentrations in those patients should be carefully monitored.

The amount of levothyroxine absorbed can also be affected by the co-administration of other drugs such as ciprofloxacin or rifampin [13A]. In a randomized, double-blind, placebo-controlled study on 8 healthy volunteers who received either 1000 µg of levothyroxine and placebo, or 1000 µg of levothyroxine and 750 mg ciprofloxacin, or 1000 µg of levothyroxine and 600 mg rifampin authors found that the co-administration of ciprofloxacin significantly decreased the area T4 levels by ~39% ($p = 0.035$), whereas, rifampin co-administration significantly increased T4 by 25% ($p = 0.003$).

Octreotide

The use of preoperative administration of octreotide in cohort of patients with TSH secreting pituitary adenomas (TSHoma) was evaluated by Fukuhara et al. [14C]. Authors discovered that of 81 patients who underwent surgery for TSHoma at Toranomon Hospital between January 2001 and May 2013, 44 received preoperative short-term octreotide. Further, among these 44 patients 19 received octreotide as a subcutaneous injection, and 24 patients received octreotide as a long-acting release (LAR) injection, and one of them was excluded due to side effects. It was found that the use of short-term preoperative octreotide administration was highly effective in suppressing TSHoma shrinkage. Some common side effects such as mild diarrhea (5 patients), constipation (1 patient), nausea and elevation of bilirubin (1 patient) were observed. Hence, the authors concluded that

preoperative octreotide are effective in suppressing TSHoma and should be recommended to patients to avoid problems with hyperthyroidism.

IODINE AND IODIDES [SED-15, 1896; SEDA-32, 764; SEDA-33, 883; SEDA-34, 680; SEDA-35, 752; SEDA-36; SEDA-37, 514]

Dietary Iodine

Iodine is an essential component of thyroid hormones, and Iodine deficiency can have serious adverse effects on one's growth and development. The deficiency of iodine in pregnant women can result in spontaneous abortion, stillbirth, and cretinism. The World Health Organization (WHO) recommends the use of iodinated salt to compensate for any iodine deficiency. Moreover, WHO also reports the most common side effects reported for iodine deficiency [12C].

Excessive iodine intake can severely effect TSH levels. In one study, infants (aged 6–24 months), who were exposed to excessive iodine, were found to have subclinical hypothyroidism [15C]. Water was assumed to be the source of excessive intake of iodine in lactating mother of those infants [16C].

Higher dietary iodine in iodine-deficient areas can also be correlated to thyroid cancer. In fact, it was observed that patients who lived in iodine-deficient areas had a higher risk of thyroid cancer if they had a diet high in iodine than those compared with the ones living in non deficient areas [17M]. Similar correlation was found in cruciferous vegetables [17M]. Thus the authors implied that dietary roles play an important part in thyroid cancer [17M].

In another case a 4-year-old boy who had severe allergy and was on highly restrictive iodine-deficient diet developed goitre and significant thyroid dysfunction [18A]. His diet was restricted to "cow's milk protein, soya (33.7 kUA/L), wheat and egg (>100 kUA/L), fish cod (65.2 kUA/L), shellfish and peanuts (>100 kUA/L) and tree nuts (1.4–6.8 kUA/L) (normal reference range <0.35 kUA/L)". He was on Flixotide, salbutamol, cetirizine hydrochloride, and fluticasone propionate nasal spray and steroid creams for his atopic disorders [18A]. His TSH levels were slightly raised, whereas, his T4 levels were low, suggesting secondary hypothyroidism. Later a soft and smooth goiter was found during following assessments which was correlated to the severe deficiency in dietary iodine [18A].

Iodine-125 Brachytherapy

Iodine-125 has a relatively long half-life (59.4 days) and emits low-energy photons (35 keV), making it a preferred isotope for radiation therapy (brachytherapy, BT) to treat prostate cancer and brain tumors.

Ophthalmic Side Effect

Application of I-125 brachytherapy in the treatment of intraocular tumor has been associated with radiation-induced ophthalmic side effects. The radiation affects the organs around the ocular cavity, eyelids, eyelashes, conjunctiva, tear production, corneal surface, sclera, and ocular muscles. Within the eye, radiation can cause iritis, uveitis, synechiae, neovascular glaucoma, cataract, posterior neovascularization, hemorrhage, retinal detachment, retinopathy, and optic neuropathy [19S]. Radiation side effects from I-125 brachytherapy can result in loss of vision and quality of life.

Tsui and coworkers reported a decrease in visual acuity, contrast sensitivity, and color vision in patients with choroidal and ciliary body melanoma (CCM) [20C]. Authors measured visual acuity, contrast sensitivity and color vision in 37 patients, 1, 2, and 3 years after I-125 brachytherapy. These 37 patients were grouped into 4 groups. Prior to (group 1), 1 year after (group 2), 2 years after (group 3), and 3 years (group 4). It was found that after brachytherapy, group 1, 2, 3, and 4 had mean best-corrected visual acuity of 77 letters (20/32), 65 letters (20/50), 56 letters (20/80) and 47 letters (20/125), respectively, and a contrast sensitivity of 30, 26, 22 and 19 letters; color vision of 26, 20, 17 and 14 test figures, respectively. Radiation-induced mid-choroid, macula melanoma, radiation maculopathy and radiation optic neuropathy were also reported for these patients [20C].

In a study, comparing the transscleral resection without hypotensive anesthesia vs I-125 brachytherapy, for the treatment of choroidal melanoma, radiation induce side effects were reported. The most common side effects for I-125 brachytherapy in 53 patients were radiation-induced retinopathy (45.3%), neovascular glaucoma (28.3%), and macular oedema (24.5%) [21R].

A 69-year-old female who underwent I-125 brachytherapy in scleral buckle was diagnosed with decreased vision and occasional floaters in the left eye [22A].

Lower Abdominal Side Effects

Iodine-125 brachytherapy in the treatment of localized prostate cancer is associated with radiation-induced bowel symptoms, decrease erectile function, and lower urinary tract symptoms. Among these symptoms, lower urinary tract symptoms are the most manifested.

In a single-center longitudinal study (1994–2007) conducted by Wilson and coworkers, 207 patients with localized prostate cancer were monitored for the biochemical disease-free survival and side effects of I-125 brachytherapy. The peak incidences of late grade 3 or higher urinary and rectal toxicities were 10.7% and 1.1%, respectively [23R].

In a nationwide multi-institutional study aimed at comparing the use of I-125 brachytherapy for permanent seed implant (PI) and combination therapy with PI and external beam radiation therapy (EBRT), Ohashi and coworkers reported urinary and rectal toxicity profiles as the major side effects [24R]. Grade 2+ acute urinary toxicities developed in 7.36% (172 of 2337) of patients and grade 2+ acute rectal toxicities developed in 1.03% (24 of 2336) of the patients. Grade 2+ late urinary and rectal toxicities developed in 5.75% (133 of 2312) and 1.86% (43 of 2312) of the patients, respectively. A higher incidence of grade 2+ acute urinary toxicity occurred in the PI group than in the EBRT group (8.49% vs 3.66%; $p < 0.01$). Acute rectal toxicity outcomes were similar between the treatment groups.

Keyes and coworkers evaluated the long-term effect of I-125 brachytherapy on erectile function (EF) of prostate cancer patients [25R]. In this study ($n = 2929$), EF was significantly reduced 6 weeks after brachytherapy, with gradual decline thereafter. EF preservation at 5 years for age younger than 55, 56–59, 60–64, 65–69, and 70 years and older was 82%, 73%, 58%, 39%, and 23%, respectively. Comparisons of the 5-year age-related and treatment-related EF decline show that 50% of the long-term EF decline is related to aging.

Eriguchi and coworkers reported neoadjuvant androgen deprivation therapy (NADT) as a key factors associated with urinary toxicities in localizes prostate cancer treated with I-125 brachytherapy [26R]. In this study authors evaluated 1313 patients, between 2003 and 2009 to examine the role of base line international prostate symptom score, biologically effective dose (BED), age, and NADT. Urinary symptom flare and urinary Grade 2 or higher (G2+) toxicity occurred in 51%, 58%, and 67% ($p = 0.025$) and 16%, 22%, and 20% ($p = 0.497$) of the <180, 180–220, and >220 Gy BED groups, respectively. When patients were divided into four groups according to prostate volume (<30 or ≥30 cc) and NADT use, urinary G2+ toxicity was most commonly observed in those patients with larger prostates who received NADT, and least in the patients with smaller prostates and no NADT.

Strom and coworkers reported a comparative study on prostate cancer patients who were treated with either high-dose-rate (HDR) brachytherapy, low-dose-rate (LDR) brachytherapy, intensity-modulated radiation therapy (IMRT), and monotherapy to investigate the effect on their urinary, bowel, and sexual health-related quality-of-life (HRQOL) [27R]. Study was conducted between years 2002 and 2013 with median follow-up of 32 months. The authors observed that patients on both HDR brachytherapy ($n = 85$, 2700–2800 cGy in two fraction) and IMRT ($n = 79$, monotherapy to 7400–8100 cGy in 37–45 fractions) had significantly less deterioration in their urinary incontinence and HRQOL than those on LDR ($n = 249$, monotherapy to 14 500 cGy in one fraction) brachytherapy patients as seen 1 and 3 months after irradiation. Additionally, HDR brachytherapy patients had worse sexual HRQOL than both LDR brachytherapy and IMRT patients after treatment.

Lower urinary tract symptoms and bowl symptoms were also reported for the rectal cancer patients. In a study of 17 rectal patients, I-125 brachytherapy was found as independent risk factor for urinary dysfunction [28C]. Peters and coworkers reported the dose-dependent GI toxicity associated with I-125 brachytherapy in rectal cancer patients. Total salvage (TS) patients with severe GI toxicity (41%, $n = 11$) showed significantly higher rectal doses than TS patients without GI toxicity (59%, $n = 16$) [29C].

Iodine-131

Iodine-131 (^{131}I) is the most commonly used iodine radioisotope, and it decays mostly by beta-emission (606 keV; 90%). It is notable for causing death in cells that it penetrates and other cells up to several millimeters away. For this reason, ^{131}I is used for the treatment of thyrotoxicosis (hyperthyroidism) and some types of thyroid cancer that absorb iodine. The ^{131}I isotope is also used as a radioactive label for certain radiopharmaceutical therapies, e.g. ^{131}I-metaiodobenzylguanidine (^{131}I-MIBG) for treating pheochromocytoma and neuroblastoma. Iodine-131 also emits high-energy gamma radiation (364 keV, 10%) that can be used for imaging [30C]. Adverse reactions with the use of ^{131}I include myelotoxicity, swelling and tenderness of salivary glands, nausea, vomiting, dry mouth, and hypothyroidism [31C].

Hematological Toxicity

Safety and efficacy of radio immunotherapy (RTI) using I-131 tositumomab in treatment of non-Hodgkin's lymphoma were reported by Hadid and coworkers [32C]. This institutional study of 48 patients report manageable but predominantly hematological toxicity.

Hypothyroidism

The incidence of hypothyroidism following the I-131 treatment in Grave's disease was reported by Husseni [33C]. The retrospective analysis was performed on 272 patients who were treated with low activity dose (370 MBq, 125 patients) vs those treated with high activity dose (555 MBq, 147 patients). The incidence of hypothyroidism following the first low activity was 24.8% with a high treatment failure rate of 58.4%, compared with 48.3% and 32% following high activity.

Radio Necrosis

Reulen and coworkers reported radio necrosis in six patients ($n = 55$) who were treated with I-131 or Y-90 labeled anti-tenascin monoclonal antibody in WHO grade III and IV gliomas [34R].

ANTITHYROID DRUGS [SEDA-32,765; SEDA-33, 884; SEDA-34, 681; SEDA-35, 754; SEDA-36, 638; SEDA-37, 518]

Thionamides, a class of antithyroid drugs (ATDs), are compounds that are known to inhibit thyroid hormone synthesis. Iodine is incorporated into thyroglobulin for the production of thyroid hormone, which is achieved after the oxidation of iodide by peroxide. Thionamides inhibit organification of iodine to tyrosine residues in thyroglobulin and the subsequent coupling of iodotyrosines [35R]. The commonly available thionamides are propylthiouracil (PTU) and methimazole (MMI). MMI has some intrinsic pharmacokinetic advantages over propylthiouracil in terms of longer half-life, resulting in once daily dosing and higher patient compliance. MMI is also known to exhibit less hepatotoxicity compared to PTU. Carbimazole (CBZ), which is a prodrug of methimazole, is currently not available in the Unites States.

COMMON SIDE EFFECTS

Some of the common side effects associated with PTU and MMI include pruritus, rash, urticaria, arthralgias, arthritis, fever, abnormal taste sensation, nausea, and vomiting. These adverse effects were observed in 13% of patients ($n = 389$) taking thionamide drugs in one study [36C].

AGRANULOCYTOSIS

Agranulocytosis, although not common, is a serious complication of thionamide therapy. A prevalence of as high as 0.5% has been observed within the first 2 months of treatment with thionamide drugs [37R,38R]. The risk of agranulocytosis is higher for ATDs when compared to 20 other classes of drugs associated with this rare complication [39R]. A 41-year-old woman receiving MMI for Grave's disease was reported to outpatient care with high fever, lymphadenopathy and other symptoms. A diagnosis of neutropenia was made and granulocyte colony-stimulating factor was administered leading to recovery [40A]. A Chinese study reports a 51-year-old Chinese male diagnosed as hyperthyroidism. After 4 weeks' treatment with MMI 20 mg/day, the patient developed agranulocytosis and severe cholestatic hepatotoxicity. The patient's symptoms and laboratory abnormalities disappeared after the withdrawal of MMI. The authors report this as one of the rare cases of synchronous ATD-induced agranulocytosis and severe hepatotoxicity in patients with hyperthyroidism [41A]. In a unique case of a patient with agranulocytosis that was caused by MMI and suffering from invasive pulmonary aspergillosis (IPA), the patient exhibited unusual maxillofacial soft tissue swelling that required treatment with voriconazole to normalize the tissue swelling and maxillofacial ulcer [42A]. For the first time, a Korean study reported that a patient with Graves' disease developed post-infectious Guillain–Barre syndrome (GBS) during a course of MMI-induced agranulocytosis [43A]. MMI-induced neutropenia and ecthyma was also reported in a pregnant patient with hyperthyroidism. The patient subsequently had to undergo a thyroidectomy [44A]. A 37-year-old female who was started on MMI for hyperthyroidism was presented to medical facility for evaluation of suspected thyroid storm. The patient was diagnosed with sepsis mimicking thyroid storm as a result of MMI-induced agranulocytosis [45A]. In a Korean study, researchers identified a susceptibility locus of antithyroid drug (ATD)-induced agranulocytosis. A single-nucleotide polymorphism (SNP), rs185386680, showed the strongest association with ATD-induced agranulocytosis. HLA-B*38:02:01 was associated with carbimazole (CMZ)/methimazole (MMI)-induced agranulocytosis. The authors concluded that screening for the risk allele may help prevent agranulocytosis in populations in which the frequency of the risk allele is high [46C].

The EIDOS and DoTS descriptions of thionamide-induced agranulocytosis are shown in Figure 1.

ANCA-POSITIVE VASCULITIS

Propylthiouracil (PTU)-associated vasculitis is normally associated with tetrad of fever, sore throat, arthralgia, and skin lesions but may also involve multiple systems. Recently a perinuclear antineutrophil cytoplasmic antibody-associated vasculitis developed during treatment with PTU for Grave's disease was reported [47R]. A case of a 55-year-old man with toxic multinodular goiter on MMI treatment for 6 months developed ANCA-positive leukocytoclastic vasculitis with hemorrhagic

and necrotic bullous lesions of lower extremities. The vasculitis resolved after termination of MMI therapy. The case highlights the importance of monitoring for variable manifestations of vasculitis in patients treated with MMI [48A]. A case of a young girl with Graves' disease with symptoms of fatigue, fever, episcleritis, and arthritis was investigated. A multidisciplinary diagnostic work-up was used to diagnose a case of PTU-induced ANCA-positive vasculitis. PTU-withdrawal, along with high-dose corticosteroids treatment resulted in a favorable clinical outcome [49A]. A 42-year-old woman, on PTU for management of Graves' disease, was being evaluated for acute renal and hepatic failure. Renal and hepatic failures were attributed to PTU-induced c-ANCA production. Despite multiple clinical interventions, the patients' condition deteriorated and eventually leads to a fatal outcome after 20 days of intervention. The medical team report that PTU can cause ANCA-associated vasculitis resulting in multi-organ failure [50R]. In another case study, a 27-year-old woman presenting with refractory hypoxaemic respiratory failure, haemoptysis, and thyrotoxicosis was attributed by the authors as a rare manifestation of propylthiouracil therapy resulting from the development of c-ANCA [51A]. A 34-year-old female was being treated for autoimmune hyperthyroidism, 6 weeks later she exhibited purpuric plaques with central necrosis on the gluteal areas [52A]. Laboratory results showed the presence of cryoglobulin, cryofibrinogen, and c-ANCA. PTU is considered to be the most common inducer of ANCA-associated microscopic polyangiitis [53R]. When PTU was stopped and replacing it with MMI, the skin lesions improved within a week, but the cryoglobulins, cryofibrinogens, c-ANCA and anti-SSA remained positive even after 5 months.

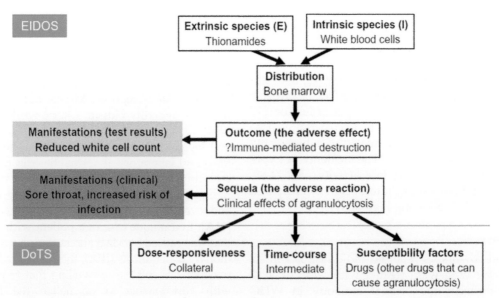

FIG. 1   EIDOS and DoTS description of thionamide-induce agranulocytosis.

HEPATOTOXICITY

Hepatotoxicity is a rare complication of drug-induced liver injury (DILI). DILI is a major problem for pharmaceutical industry and drug development. Although MMI has been associated with liver disease, it is typically due to cholestatic dysfunction, not hepatocellular inflammation [54R]. Due to the idiosyncratic nature of the injury, the understanding of the mechanism of these toxicities is limited. It appears that reactive metabolite formation and immune-mediated toxicity may play a role in antithyroids liver toxicity, especially those caused by MMI, though other mechanism including reactive metabolites formation, oxidative stress induction, intracellular targets dysfunction may be possible [55H]. In a retrospectively study analyzing 77 patients presenting with newly diagnosed overt hyperthyroidism, the authors evaluated the liver function tests (LTF). The researchers found that MMI treatment can induce insignificant LFT elevation. They concluded that MMI can be safely administered in hyperthyroid patients with abnormal LFT [56R]. In another retrospective study, authors examined the prevalence of thyrotoxicosis and gestational ATD use in women who delivered from 1996 to 2010. The authors report that gestational ATD exposure occurred in 1.29 per 1000 mother–infant pairs but a much larger maternal population had thyrotoxicosis but no drug exposure. Infants of mothers with gestational ATD use or diagnosed thyrotoxicosis were more likely to be preterm and admitted to the neonatal intensive care unit. Furthermore, rates of congenital malformation in babies had not association with drug exposure [57R].

PANCREATITIS

Pancreatitis has very rarely been reported in association with MMI treatment [58A]. A population-based case–control study analyzing the database of the Taiwan National Health Insurance Program involving 5764 individuals aged 20–84 years with a first attack of acute pancreatitis from 1998 to 2011 was evaluated to estimate the relative risk of acute pancreatitis associated with the use of MMI. The study did not detect a substantial association between the use of MMI and risk of acute pancreatitis [59C]. Recently, a sixth case of MMI-induced pancreatitis (according to the authors), in a patient with toxic multinodular goiter was reported. The authors suggest to explore the possibility of pancreatitis in subjects treated with MMI in the presence of suggestive symptoms. Discontinuation of the drug is recommended if the diagnosis is confirmed by elevated pancreatic enzymes [60A].

TERATOGENICITY AND BIRTH DEFECTS

MMI has been associated with a rare fetal scalp defect, an aplasia cutis [61R]. More serious congenital malformations such as choanal atresia and tracheoesophageal fistulas, also called MMI embryopathy, have also been associated with MMI use. A recent review article analyzed 92 papers discussing use of MMI and birth defects. The review concludes that MMI use in early pregnancy may lead to birth defects in 2–3% of the exposed children and that the defects are often severe. Proposals are given on how to minimize the risk of birth defects in fertile women treated for hyperthyroidism with ATDs [62R]. In a recent study, authors conducted a review to identify reports associated with aplasia cutis congenital (ACC) under MTZ/CMZ reported in the literature. In most instances, exposure occurred in the first weeks of gestation. Six familial cases involving siblings were identified. The authors recommend that practitioners should be aware of ACC following MTZ/CMZ exposure in utero [63R]. Another study explored the association of genetics with MMI/CBZ therapy. The case reports 2 siblings with physical features consistent with carbimazole/MMI embryopathy. Also reported is a previously unreported minor dental anomaly in this sibling pair with antenatal exposure of CBZ [64A]. A Danish study looked at the use of MMI/CMZ and PTU in early pregnancy, and its association with an increased prevalence of birth defects. The prevalence of birth defects was higher in children exposed to ATDs in early pregnancy (PTU, 8.0%; MMI/CMZ, 9.1%; MMI/CMZ and PTU, 10.1%; no ATD, 5.4%; nonexposed, 5.7%; $p < 0.001$). Both maternal use of MMI/CMZ (adjusted OR = 1.66 [95% CI 1.35–2.04]) and PTU (1.41 [1.03–1.92]) and maternal shift between MMI/CMZ and PTU in early pregnancy (1.82 [1.08–3.07]) were associated with an increased odds ratio (OR) of birth defects. MMI/CMZ and PTU toxicities were also associated with the urinary system. Choanal atresia, esophageal atresia, omphalocele, omphalomesenteric duct anomalies, and aplasia cutis were common in MMI/CMZ-exposed children (combined, adjusted OR = 21.8 [13.4–35.4]) [37R].

References

[1] France M, Schofield J, Kwok S, et al. Treatment of homozygous familial hypercholesterolemia. Clin Lipidol. 2014;9(1):101–18. http://dx.doi.org/10.2217/clp.13.79 [R].

[2] Angelin B, Kristensen JD, Eriksson M, et al. Reductions in serum levels of LDL cholesterol, apolipoprotein B, triglycerides and lipoprotein(a) in hypercholesterolaemic patients treated with the liver-selective thyroid hormone receptor agonist eprotirome. J Intern Med. 2015;277(3):331–42. http://dx.doi.org/10.1111/joim.12261 [C].

[3] Kelderman-Bolk N, Visser TJ, Tijssen JP, et al. Quality of life in patients with primary hypothyroidism related to BMI. Eur J Endocrinol. 2015;173(4):507–15. http://dx.doi.org/10.1530/eje-15-0395. PubMed PMID: 26169304. Epub 2015/07/15. [R].

[4] Bengtsson C, Padyukov L, Källberg H, et al. Thyroxin substitution and the risk of developing rheumatoid arthritis; results from the Swedish population-based EIRA study. Ann Rheum Dis. 2014;73(6):1096–100. http://dx.doi.org/10.1136/annrheumdis-2013-203354 [R].

[5] Krysiak R, Kowalska B, Okopien B. Serum 25-hydroxyvitamin D and parathyroid hormone levels in non-lactating women with post-partum thyroiditis: the effect of L-thyroxine treatment. Basic Clin Pharmacol Toxicol. 2015;116(6):503–7. http://dx.doi.org/10.1111/bcpt.12349. PubMed PMID: 25395280. Epub 2014/11/15 [C].

[6] Keles MK, Yosma E, Aydogdu IO, et al. Multiple subungual pyogenic granulomas following levothyroxine treatment. J Craniofac Surg. 2015;26(6):e476–7. http://dx.doi.org/10.1097/scs.0000000000001922. PubMed PMID: 26355986. Epub 2015/09/12 [R].

[7] Kim MK, Yun KJ, Kim MH, et al. The effects of thyrotropin-suppressing therapy on bone metabolism in patients with well-differentiated thyroid carcinoma. Bone. 2015;71:101–5. http://dx.doi.org/10.1016/j.bone.2014.10.009. PubMed PMID: 25445448. Epub 2014/12/03 [C].

[8] Nyandege AN, Slattum PW, Harpe SE. Risk of fracture and the concomitant use of bisphosphonates with osteoporosis-inducing medications. Ann Pharmacother. 2015;49(4):437–47. http://dx.doi.org/10.1177/1060028015569594. PubMed PMID: 25667198. Epub 2015/02/11 [R].

[9] Bakiner O, Bozkirli E, Ertugrul D, et al. Plasma fetuin-A levels are reduced in patients with hypothyroidism. Eur J Endocrinol. 2014;170(3):411–8. http://dx.doi.org/10.1530/EJE-13-0831. PubMed PMID: 24366942 [C].

[10] Stuijver DJ, van Zaane B, Squizzato A, et al. The effects of an extremely high dose of levothyroxine on coagulation and fibrinolysis. J Thromb Haemost. 2010;8(6):1427–8. http://dx.doi.org/10.1111/j.1538-7836.2010.03854.x. PubMed PMID: 20345725 [A].

[11] Kreisner E, Lutzky M, Gross JL. Charcoal hemoperfusion in the treatment of levothyroxine intoxication. Thyroid. 2010;20(2):209–12. http://dx.doi.org/10.1089/thy.2009.0054. PubMed PMID: 20151829 [A].

[12] Irving SA, Vadiveloo T, Leese GP. Drugs that interact with levothyroxine: an observational study from the Thyroid Epidemiology, Audit and Research Study (TEARS). Clin Endocrinol (Oxf). 2015;82(1):136–41. http://dx.doi.org/10.1111/cen.12559. PubMed PMID: 25040647. Epub 2014/07/22 [C].

[13] Goldberg AS, Tirona RG, Asher LJ, et al. Ciprofloxacin and rifampin have opposite effects on levothyroxine absorption. Thyroid. 2013;23(11):1374–8. http://dx.doi.org/10.1089/thy.2013.0014. PubMed PMID: 23647409. Epub 2013/05/08 [A].

[14] Fukuhara N, Horiguchi K, Nishioka H, et al. Short-term preoperative octreotide treatment for TSH-secreting pituitary adenoma. Endocr J. 2015;62(1):21–7. http://dx.doi.org/10.1507/endocrj.EJ14-0118. PubMed PMID: 25273395. Epub 2014/10/03 [C].

[15] Nepal AK, Suwal R, Gautam S, et al. Subclinical hypothyroidism and elevated thyroglobulin in infants with chronic excess iodine intake. Thyroid. 2015;25(7):851–9. http://dx.doi.org/10.1089/thy.2015.0153. PubMed PMID: 25950720 [C].

[16] Liua L, Wanga D, Liua P, et al. The relationship between iodine nutrition and thyroid disease in lactating women with different iodine intakes. Br J Nutr. 2015;114(09):1487–95 [C].

[17] Cho YA, Kim J. Dietary factors affecting thyroid cancer risk: a meta-analysis. Nutr Cancer. 2015;67(5):811–7. http://dx.doi.org/10.1080/01635581.2015.1040517. PubMed PMID: 25996474 [M].

[18] Cheetham T, Plumb E, Callaghan J, et al. Dietary restriction causing iodine-deficient goitre. Arch Dis Child. 2015;100(8):784–6. http://dx.doi.org/10.1136/archdischild-2015-308567. PubMed PMID: 26069028 [A].

[19] Simpson ER, Gallie B, Laperrierre N, et al. The American Brachytherapy Society consensus guidelines for plaque brachytherapy of uveal melanoma and retinoblastoma. Brachytherapy. 2014;13(1):1–14. http://dx.doi.org/10.1016/j.brachy.2013.11.008 [S].

[20] Tsui I, Beardsley RM, McCannel TA, et al. Visual acuity, contrast sensitivity and color vision three years after iodine-125 brachytherapy for choroidal and ciliary body melanoma. Open ophthalmol J. 2015;9:131–5. http://dx.doi.org/10.2174/1874364101509010131. Epub 2015/08/28. PubMed PMID:26312123. PMCID: Pmc4541296 [C].

[21] Caminal JM, Padron-Perez N, Arias L, et al. Transscleral resection without hypotensive anaesthesia vs iodine-125 plaque brachytherapy in the treatment of choroidal melanoma. Eye (Lond). 2016;30:833–42. http://dx.doi.org/10.1038/eye.2016.49. PubMed PMID: 27034202. Epub 2016/04/02. [R].

[22] Motiani MV, Almanzor R, McCannel TA. Scleral buckle-associated ciliochoroidal melanoma. Semin Ophthalmol. 2016;1–3. http://dx.doi.org/10.3109/08820538.2015.1115090. PubMed PMID: 27082038. Epub 2016/04/16. [A].

[23] Wilson C, Waterhouse D, Lane SE, et al. Ten-year outcomes using low dose rate brachytherapy for localised prostate cancer: an update to the first Australian experience. J Med Imaging Radiat Oncol. 2016;60:531–8. http://dx.doi.org/10.1111/1754-9485.12453 [R].

[24] Ohashi T, Yorozu A, Saito S, et al. Urinary and rectal toxicity profiles after permanent iodine-125 implant brachytherapy in Japanese men: nationwide J-POPS multi-institutional prospective cohort study. Int J Radiat Oncol Biol Phys. 2015;93(1):141–9. http://dx.doi.org/10.1016/j.ijrobp.2015.05.014 [R].

[25] Keyes M, Pickles T, Crook J, et al. Effect of aging and long-term erectile function after iodine-125 prostate brachytherapy. Brachytherapy. 2015;14(3):334–41. http://dx.doi.org/10.1016/j.brachy.2015.01.001 [R].

[26] Eriguchi T, Yorozu A, Kuroiwa N, et al. Predictive factors for urinary toxicity after iodine-125 prostate brachytherapy with or without supplemental external beam radiotherapy. Brachytherapy. 2016;15:288–95. http://dx.doi.org/10.1016/j.brachy.2015.12.011 [R].

[27] Strom TJ, Cruz AA, Figura NB, et al. Health-related quality-of-life changes due to high-dose-rate brachytherapy, low-dose-rate brachytherapy, or intensity-modulated radiation therapy for prostate cancer. Brachytherapy. 2015;14(6):818–25. http://dx.doi.org/10.1016/j.brachy.2015.08.012 [R].

[28] Luo Y-J, Liu Z-L, Ye P-C, et al. Safety and efficacy of intraoperative iodine-125 seed implantation brachytherapy for rectal cancer patients: a prospective clinical research. J Gastroenterol Hepatol. 2015;31:1076–84. http://dx.doi.org/10.1111/jgh.13261 [C].

[29] Peters M, Hoekstra CJ, van der Voort van Zyp JRN, et al. Rectal dose constraints for salvage iodine-125 prostate brachytherapy. Brachytherapy. 2016;15(1):85–93. http://dx.doi.org/10.1016/j.brachy.2015.10.004 [C].

[30] Rault E, Vandenberghe S, Van Holen R, et al. Comparison of image quality of different iodine isotopes (I-123, I-124, and I-131). Cancer Biother Radiopharm. 2007;22(3):423–30. http://dx.doi.org/10.1089/cbr.2006.323. PubMed PMID: 17651050 [C].

[31] Alexander C, Bader JB, Schaefer A, et al. Intermediate and long-term side effects of high-dose radioiodine therapy for thyroid carcinoma. J Nucl Med. 1998;39(9):1551–4. PubMed PMID: 9744341 [C].

[32] Hadid T, Raufi A, Kafri Z, et al. Safety and efficacy of radioimmunotherapy (RIT) in treatment of non-Hodgkin's lymphoma in the community setting. Nucl Med Biol. 2016;43(4):227–31. http://dx.doi.org/10.1016/j.nucmedbio.2015.12.004 [C].

[33] Husseni MA. The incidence of hypothyroidism following the radioactive iodine treatment of Graves' disease and the predictive factors influencing its development. World J Nucl Med. 2016;15(1):30–7. http://dx.doi.org/10.4103/1450-1147.167582. Epub 2016/02/26. PubMed PMID:26912976. PMCID: Pmc4729012. [C].

[34] Reulen HJ, Poepperl G, Goetz C, et al. Long-term outcome of patients with WHO Grade III and IV gliomas treated by fractionated intracavitary radioimmunotherapy. J Neurosurg. 2015;123(3):760–70. http://dx.doi.org/10.3171/2014.12.jns142168. PubMed PMID: 26140493. Epub 2015/07/04 [R].

[35] Cooper DS. Antithyroid drugs. N Engl J Med. 2005;352(9):905–17. http://dx.doi.org/10.1056/NEJMra042972. PubMed PMID: 15745981 [R].

[36] Werner MC, Romaldini JH, Bromberg N, et al. Adverse effects related to thionamide drugs and their dose regimen. Am J Med Sci. 1989;297(4):216–9. PubMed PMID: 2523194 [C].

[37] Andersen SL, Olsen J, Wu CS, et al. Birth defects after early pregnancy use of antithyroid drugs: a Danish nationwide study. J Clin Endocrinol Metab. 2013;98(11):4373–81. http://dx.doi.org/10.1210/jc.2013-2831. PubMed PMID: 24151287. Epub 2013/10/24 [R].

[38] Watanabe N, Narimatsu H, Noh JY, et al. Antithyroid drug-induced hematopoietic damage: a retrospective cohort study of agranulocytosis and pancytopenia involving 50,385 patients with Graves' disease. J Clin Endocrinol Metab. 2012;97(1): E49–53. http://dx.doi.org/10.1210/jc.2011-2221. PubMed PMID: 22049174 [R].

[39] van Staa TP, Boulton F, Cooper C, et al. Neutropenia and agranulocytosis in England and Wales: incidence and risk factors. Am J Hematol. 2003;72(4):248–54. http://dx.doi.org/10.1002/ajh.10295. PubMed PMID: 12666135 [R].

[40] Kaysin A, Viera AJ. A case of atypical Bartonella henselae infection in a patient with methimazole-induced agranulocytosis. BMJ case rep. 2015;2015: http://dx.doi.org/10.1136/bcr-2015-209314. PubMed PMID: 26315358 [A].

[41] Yang J, Zhang J, Xu Q, et al. Unusual synchronous methimazole-induced agranulocytosis and severe hepatotoxicity in patient with hyperthyroidism: a case report and review of the literature. Int J Endocrinol. 2015;2015:1–6. http://dx.doi.org/10.1155/2015/934726. Article ID 934726, PubMed PMID: 26060496 PMCID: PMC4427828 [A].

[42] Fan XY, Wang WM, Yan XB, et al. Invasive pulmonary aspergillosis accompanied by soft tissue lesions during treatment of a patient with hyperthyroidism: a case report. Cent Eur J Immunol. 2015;40(1):117–21. http://dx.doi.org/10.5114/ceji.2015.50844. PubMed PMID: 26155194 PMCID: PMC4472550. [A].

[43] Cho YY, Joung JY, Jeong H, et al. Postinfectious Guillain-Barre syndrome in a patient with methimazole-induced agranulocytosis. Korean J Intern Med. 2013;28(6):724–7. http://dx.doi.org/10.3904/kjim.2013.28.6.724. Epub 2013/12/07. PubMed PMID:24307850 PMCID: Pmc3847000. [A].

[44] Thomas SK, Sheffield JS, Roberts SW. Thionamide-induced neutropenia and ecthyma in a pregnant patient with hyperthyroidism, Obstet Gynecol. 2013;122(2 Pt 2):490–2. http://dx.doi.org/10.1097/AOG.0b013e3182864370. PubMed PMID: 23884271. Epub 2013/07/26 [A].

[45] Rayner SG, Hosseini F, Adedipe AA. Sepsis mimicking thyroid storm in a patient with methimazole-induced agranulocytosis. BMJ Case Rep. 2013;2013:http://dx.doi.org/10.1136/bcr-2013-200145 PubMed PMID: 23861276. Epub 2013/07/19 [A].

[46] Cheung CL, Sing CW, Tang C, et al. HLA-B*38:02:01 predicts carbimazole/methimazole-induced agranulocytosis. Clin Pharmacol Ther. 2016;99(5):555–61. http://dx.doi.org/10.1002/cpt.309. PubMed PMID: 26599303 [C].

[47] Criado PR, Grizzo Peres Martins AC, Gaviolli CF, et al. Propylthiouracil-induced vasculitis with antineutrophil cytoplasmic antibody. Int J Low Extrem Wounds. 2015;14(2):187–91. http://dx.doi.org/10.1177/1534734614549418. PubMed PMID: 25256279 [R].

[48] Shikha D, Harris J, Resta C, et al. Antineutrophilic cytoplasmic antibody positive vasculitis associated with methimazole use. Case Rep Endocrinol. 2015;2015:3 [A].

[49] Schamp V, Verfaillie C, Bonroy C, et al. Propylthiouracil induced ANCA-associated vasculitis in a 14-year-old girl. Acta Clin Belg. 2015;70(2):127–9. http://dx.doi.org/10.1179/2295333714Y.0000000090. PubMed PMID: 25937486 [A].

[50] Khan TA, Yin Luk FC, Uqdah HT, et al. A fatal case of propylthiouracil-induced ANCA-associated vasculitis resulting in rapidly progressive glomerulonephritis, acute hepatic failure, and cerebral angiitis. Clin Nephrol. 2015;83(5):309–14. http://dx.doi.org/10.5414/CN108322. PubMed PMID: 25208313 [R].

[51] Ortiz-Diaz EO. A 27-year-old woman presenting with refractory hypoxaemic respiratory failure, haemoptysis and thyrotoxicosis: a rare manifestation of propylthiouracil therapy. BMJ Case Rep. 2014;2014:http://dx.doi.org/10.1136/bcr-2014-204915 PubMed PMID: 25150234. Epub 2014/08/26 [A].

[52] Akkurt ZM, Ucmak D, Acar G, et al. Cryoglobulin and antineutrophil cytoplasmic antibody positive cutaneous vasculitis due to propylthiouracil. Indian J Dermatol Venereol Leprol. 2014;80(3):262–4. http://dx.doi.org/10.4103/0378-6323.132261. Epub 2014/05/16. PubMed PMID:24823411 [A].

[53] Bonaci-Nikolic B, Nikolic MM, Andrejevic S, et al. Antineutrophil cytoplasmic antibody (ANCA)-associated autoimmune diseases induced by antithyroid drugs: comparison with idiopathic ANCA vasculitides. Arthritis Res Ther. 2005;7(5):R1072–81. http://dx.doi.org/10.1186/ar1789. PubMed PMID: 16207324 PMCID: 1257438 [R].

[54] Arab DM, Malatjalian DA, Rittmaster RS. Severe cholestatic jaundice in uncomplicated hyperthyroidism treated with methimazole. J Clin Endocrinol Metab. 1995;80(4):1083–5. http://dx.doi.org/10.1210/jcem.80.4.7714072. PubMed PMID: 7714072 [R].

[55] Heidari R, Niknahad H, Jamshidzadeh A, et al. An overview on the proposed mechanisms of antithyroid drugs-induced liver injury. Adv Pharm Bull. 2015;5(1):1–11. http://dx.doi.org/10.5681/apb.2015.001. PubMed PMID: 25789213 PMCID: PMC4352210. [H].

[56] Niculescu DA, Dusceac R, Galoiu SA, et al. Serial changes of liver function tests before and during methimazole treatment in thyrotoxic patients. Endocr Pract. 2016;22:974–9. http://dx.doi.org/10.4158/EP161222. PubMed PMID: 27042749 [R].

[57] Lo JC, Rivkees SA, Chandra M, et al. Gestational thyrotoxicosis, antithyroid drug use and neonatal outcomes within an integrated healthcare delivery system. Thyroid. 2015;25(6):698–705 [R].

[58] Yang M, Qu H, Deng HC. Acute pancreatitis induced by methimazole in a patient with Graves' disease. Thyroid. 2012;22(1):94–6. http://dx.doi.org/10.1089/thy.2011.0210. PubMed PMID: 22136208 [A].

[59] Lai S-W, Lin C-L, Liao K-F. Use of methimazole and risk of acute pancreatitis: a case–control study in Taiwan. Indian J Pharmacol. 2016;48(2):192–5 [C].

[60] Agito K, Manni A. Acute pancreatitis induced by methimazole in a patient with subclinical hyperthyroidism. J Investig Med High Impact Case Rep. 2015;3(2)http://dx.doi.org/10.1177/2324709615592229 2324709615592229. PubMed PMID:26425645 PMCID: PMC4557366. [A].

[61] Mandel SJ, Cooper DS. The use of antithyroid drugs in pregnancy and lactation. J Clin Endocrinol Metab. 2001;86(6):2354–9. http://dx.doi.org/10.1210/jcem.86.6.7573. PubMed PMID: 11397822 [R].

[62] Laurberg P, Andersen SL. Therapy of endocrine disease: antithyroid drug use in early pregnancy and birth defects: time windows of relative safety and high risk?. Eur J Endocrinol. 2014;171(1):R13–20. http://dx.doi.org/10.1530/eje-14-0135. PubMed PMID: 24662319. Epub 2014/03/26. [R].

[63] Sachs C, Tebacher-Alt M, Mark M, et al. Aplasia cutis congenita and antithyroid drugs during pregnancy: case series and literature review. Ann Dermatol Venereol. 2016;143:423–35. http://dx.doi.org/10.1016/j.annder.2016.02.018. Epub 2016/04/02. PubMed PMID:27033749 [R].

[64] Goel H, Dudding T. Carbimazole/methimazole embryopathy in siblings: a possible genetic susceptibility. Birth Defects Res A Clin Mol Teratol. 2013;97(11):755–8. http://dx.doi.org/10.1002/bdra.23200. PubMed PMID: 24265129 Epub 2013/11/23 [A].

40

Insulin Other Hypoglycemic Drugs

Sara N. Trovinger*,1, Sandra L. Hrometz†, Sipan Keshishyan†,
Sidhartha D. Ray†

*Department of Pharmacy Practice, Manchester University College of Pharmacy, Natural and Health Sciences,
Fort Wayne, IN, USA
†Department of Pharmaceutical Sciences, Manchester University College of Pharmacy, Natural and Health Sciences,
Fort Wayne, IN, USA
1Corresponding author: sntrovinger@manchester.edu

INSULINS [SED-15, 1761; SEDA-34, 685; SEDA-36, 645–647; SEDA-37, 521–523]

A 26-week, open-label, controlled, stratified treat to target trial at 45 sites in 5 Asian countries randomized 424 patients to receive either insulin degludec/insulin aspart vs biphasic insulin aspart 30. Both groups showed similar rates of confirmed hypoglycemia (9.6 episodes/patient/year vs 9.5 episodes/patient/year, respectively). Episodes of severe hypoglycemia were also similar across both groups in addition to weight gain (1.3 kg vs 1.67 kg, respectively) [1C].

829 patients participated in a 26-week extension of the BEGIN Basal-Bolus Type 2 trial. This extension showed that degludec insulin was associated with fewer overall episodes of hypoglycemia (estimated rate ratio = 0.76; $p = 0.011$) and a reduction in nocturnal hypoglycemia (estimated rate ratio = 0.69; $p = 0.016$) as compared to insulin glargine [2C].

A meta-analysis of studies conducted from 2005 to August 2014 regarding technosphere insulin revealed less hypoglycemia associated with the drug than with that of rapid-acting insulins (odds ratio = 0.488; $p = 0.0124$ for type 1 diabetics and $p = 0.0943$ for type 2 diabetics). This study also revealed increased respiratory effects associated with technosphere insulin when compared to technosphere powder placebo (45.2% and 35.9%, respectively). Side effects reported most commonly were cough, upper respiratory infection, and nasopharyngitis [3M].

884 patients with type 2 diabetes (T2D) in 15 countries around the world were randomized in a 52-week, open-label, phase 3, non-inferiority trial comparing once-weekly glucagon-like peptide-1 agonist (dulaglutide 1.5 mg, dulaglutide 0.75 mg) to the long-acting insulin, glargine. Glargine was administered once daily at bedtime. Patients in the glargine group showed a statistically significant greater risk of serious adverse events when compared to the dulaglutide 1.5 mg group ($p = 0.0013$), though there was no increased risk of any specific event. The risk of serious adverse events between the dulaglutide 0.75 mg group and the glargine group was not statistically different ($p = 0.29$). Both the dulaglutide 1.5 mg group and the dulaglutide 0.75 mg group showed increased gastrointestinal (GI) events as compared to glargine (respective p values): nausea ($p < 0.001$ for both), diarrhea ($p < 0.0001$, $p = 0.0002$), vomiting ($p < 0.001$ for both), and dyspepsia ($p < 0.001$, $p = 0.006$). Both dulaglutide groups had statistically significant decreases in appetite when compared to glargine ($p < 0.001$) [4C].

A 36-week, randomized, open-label, parallel-arm study conducted in Europe, Asia, the Middle East, and South America randomized 701 patients in a 1:1 ratio to receive either glargine or the intermediate-acting neutral protamine Hagedorn (NPH) insulin. All patients were already being treated with dual therapy of metformin and glimepiride. The insulin was titrated weekly to achieve median prebreakfast and nocturnal plasma glucose levels of ≤5.5 mmol/L, while avoiding values of ≤4.4 mmol/L. Patients in the glargine group had a statistically significant decrease in nocturnal events/person-year as compared to those in the NPH insulin group (0.35 and 0.66, respectively, $p = 0.003$). This study is referred to as the Least One Oral Antidiabetic Drug Treatment (LANCELOT) study [5C].

The Evaluation of insulin glargine versus sitagliptin in insulin-naïve patients (EASIE) trial was a 24-week trial that compared the safety, efficacy, and tolerability of sitagliptin and insulin glargine in type 2 diabetics who were previously uncontrolled on metformin. In a 3-month extension of the EASIE trial, 111 patients who were not controlled on their previous regimen of either metformin and sitagliptin or metformin and glargine were started on all three medications. Patients who were initially on metformin with glargine and had the sitagliptin added later were more likely to experience symptomatic hypoglycemia (6.5 [4.9;8.3]) compared to those who were initially on metformin and sitagliptin, and the glargine was started later (3.2 [2.4;4.1]) [6C].

An open-ended trial in 206 patients, hospitalized with T2D, examined the effect of adding supplemental bedtime insulin to their existing basal-bolus insulin regimens. Patients were randomized to receive supplemental insulin at bedtime for blood glucose greater than 7.8 mmol/L, or no supplemental insulin at bedtime except if blood glucose exceeded 19.4 mmol/L in this open-label trial. Again, all patients were on a basal-bolus insulin regimen. Blood glucose levels were measured via a point-of-care testing device prior to each meal, at bedtime, and at 3 A.M. There were no differences in fasting blood glucoses between the two groups ($p = 0.76$). The incidence of hypoglycemia also did not differ between the two groups ($p = 0.5$) [7C].

An open-label randomized trial compared intravenous (IV) insulin or subcutaneous insulin in 65 patients admitted at a single academic medical center for an exacerbation of congestive heart failure. Hypoglycemia (defined as capillary blood glucose <3.9 mmol/L) was higher in the IV group than in the subcutaneous group (27% vs 2.6% on day 1 and 23% vs 2.6% on day 2, respectively) [8c].

In a prospective, crossover, randomized, multicenter, blinded study, 28 patients received two insulin infusions; one infusion of regular human insulin and one of rapid, short-acting insulin, lispro. All patients were on parenteral nutrition during both infusions. A washout period of at least 6 hours was observed between the two treatments. Insulin treatment was initiated at 0.04 units/kg/hour when the patient's blood glucose reached a level greater than or equal to 180 mg/dL and continued until the blood glucose was less than or equal to 140 mg/dL. Two patients in the regular insulin group developed severe hypoglycemia following discontinuation of the insulin infusion, as compared to none for the lispro group. The lowest average blood glucose reached by participants was statistically significantly lower in the regular insulin group as compared to the lispro group (108.7 vs 117.2, respectively, $p = 0.003$). Blood glucose also increased at a faster rate following discontinuation of

infusion in the lispro group as compared to the regular insulin group ($p < 0.001$) [9c].

97 pregnant women with either preexisting T2D or gestational diabetes mellitus at ≤34 weeks were randomized to receive either long-acting insulin detemir or intermediate-acting NPH for glycemic control in an open-label, noninferiority study. Patients in the NPH group were more likely to have a glucose reading of <60 mg/dL ($p = 0.0128$). They also experienced a greater number of symptomatic events per patient ($p = 0.245$), glucoses <60 mg/dL per patient ($p < 0.001$), symptomatic events per week ($p < 0.001$), and glucoses <60 mg/dL per week ($p < 0.001$) [10c].

A different study comparing therapies in pregnant women compared the use of metformin alone, insulin alone, and metformin in combination with insulin. Women in either insulin group received a combination of both short and intermediate acting human insulins twice daily (before breakfast and dinner). 150 pregnant women completed this parallel open-labeled clinical study in Karachi, Pakistan. Women who received insulin alone experienced a statistically significant weight gain during their pregnancy as compared with women on metformin alone and metformin combined with insulin (12.5, 9.8, and 9.8 kg, respectively; $p = 0.000$). Infants born to mothers who utilized insulin alone were greater in weight as compared to those whose mothers used metformin alone and metformin combined with insulin (3.7, 3.4, 3.3 kg, respectively; $p = 0.002$ and $p = 0.001$, respectively). The infants in the insulin alone group had a statistically significantly greater Apgar score at 5 min as compared to the other two groups (8.6, 8, and 8.2, respectively; $p = 0.000$ and $p = 0.001$, respectively). Despite the above, the infants in the insulin alone group were also more likely to spend greater than 24 hours in the NICU as compared to those in the metformin alone group and the metformin combined with insulin group (13, 2, and 1, respectively; $p = 0.047$ and $p = 0.038$, respectively). The insulin alone infants were also more likely to experience neonatal hypoglycemia as compared to those on metformin alone (16 vs 2, respectively; $p = 0.015$) [11C].

DIPEPTIDYL PEPTIDASE-4 (DPP-4) INHIBITORS [SEDA-36, 648; SEDA-37, 526–528]

Cardiovascular

Two large randomized, placebo-controlled clinical trials (SAVOR TIMI 53 and EXAMINE) reported on the cardiovascular risks of DPP-4 inhibitors. Although published in 2013, much of the 2015 literature seems to be focused on further analysis of these studies.

The 16 492 participants in SAVOR TIMI 53 had a diagnosis of T2D with a history or risk of cardiovascular events. The trial reported that saxagliptin was associated with a 27% increase in hospital admissions for heart failure (HF) compared to placebo when this endpoint was examined separately instead of part of a cohort of composite cardiovascular events ($p = 0.007$). Saxagliptin had no effect on composite cardiovascular events of cardiovascular death, myocardial infarction (MI) or ischemic stroke (primary end point), or the secondary end point which included primary end points, or hospitalization for HF, coronary revascularization, or unstable angina [12MC].

An analysis of the older participants of the SAVOR-TIMI 53 trial divided individuals into four age-dependent subpopulations: <65, ≥65, <75 and ≥75 years of age. The analysis revealed no difference in hospitalization for or due to HF in the <65 compared to the ≥65 groups ($p = 0.76$). Likewise, there was no difference in hospitalization for or due to HF in the <75 compared to the ≥75 age groups ($p = 0.34$). Statistically significant events, although not consistently age-dependent occurred in the saxagliptin groups when compared to age-matched controls receiving a placebo. There was an increase in cardiovascular mortality in the saxagliptin group in the youngest cohort (<65 years versus ≥65 years group, $p = 0.047$). Within the category of "percent with ≥1 treatment-related adverse effect" (including hypoglycemia), an increased incidence occurred in the ≥65 and ≥75 years of age cohorts ($p = 0.015$ and 0.042, respectively). Death due to ≥1 treatment-related serious adverse effects was greater in the <65 years ($p = 0.007$) and ≥75 years ($p = 0.02$) saxagliptin groups compared to placebo. The incidence of hypertension increased only in those <65 years of age ($p = 0.032$). The ≥75 years cohort was the only group with an increase in nausea and urinary tract infection ($p = 0.022$ and 0.021, respectively). Subjects in the saxagliptin <65 years ($p = 0.012$) and <75 years ($p = 0.02$) cohorts reported an increased incidence in cancer (all cancers) compared to placebo. The incidence of pancreatic cancer was higher in the <75-year group only ($p = 0.012$) [13M].

The 5380 subjects in EXAMINE were within 15–90 days of being hospitalized for unstable angina, coronary revascularization, MI or stroke. The authors reported no difference in the primary composite outcomes of cardiovascular death, MI and stroke with alogliptin. Additionally, the all-cause mortality rate was comparable between the groups. EXAMINE did not report on HF, and it was not part of the composite outcomes [14MC].

Risk of cardiovascular death and hospital admission for HF was assessed separately and compositely in a *post hoc* analysis of the EXAMINE trial. The risk of hospital admission for HF was only significantly greater with alogliptin in those who did not have a history of HF at baseline ($p = 0.0260$). There was not a significant difference between alogliptin and placebo in those with a history of HF at baseline ($p = 0.996$). The risk of cardiovascular death was similar between alogliptin and placebo, regardless of baseline HF status. Likewise, when the risk of both cardiovascular death and hospital admission for HF was combined, there was not a significant difference between alogliptin and placebo, regardless of baseline HF status [15M].

Toth performed a meta-analysis on the safety of saxagliptin using 28 clinical trials. According to the authors, after review of existing literature, saxagliptin appears to be safe and is not associated with an increased risk of cardiovascular disease, nor does it reduce the incidence of adverse cardiovascular events in those with T2D and increased cardiovascular risk [16M].

Savarese and colleagues conducted a meta-analysis on 94 trials, enrolling 85 224 patients in order to assess the effects of DPP-4 inhibitors on cardiovascular morbidity and mortality in diabetics. The DPP-4 inhibitors were compared to placebo or other anti-diabetic treatments. The authors concluded that DPP-4 inhibitors do not affect all-cause mortality, cardiovascular mortality and stroke in diabetics. They noted a decrease incidence of MI with short-term treatment (<29 weeks) but an increase in HF risk with long-term treatment (≥29 weeks) [17M].

The Trial to Evaluate Cardiovascular Outcomes after Treatment with Sitagliptin (TECOS) studied 14 671 subjects with T2D and cardiovascular disease. Subjects received sitagliptin ($n = 7332$) or placebo ($n = 7339$) to their existing therapy in this randomized, double-blind study. The primary composite cardiovascular outcomes (the first confirmed event of cardiovascular death, nonfatal MI, nonfatal stroke or hospitalization for unstable angina) were not significantly different between the groups ($p = 0.65$), occurring in 839 receiving sitagliptin and 851 receiving placebo. Additionally, rates of hospitalization for HF did not differ between the two groups ($p = 0.98$), occurring in 228 receiving sitagliptin and 229 receiving placebo. Subjects were followed for a median of 3 years [18MC].

The cardiovascular safety of sitagliptin was evaluated in post-acute MI individuals with comorbidities of chronic kidney disease and T2D. Subjects ($n = 1025$) were identified using the Taiwan National Health Insurance Research Database between 2009 and 2011. Twenty percent ($n = 205$) of identified individuals were placed in the sitagliptin group, and 820 matched controls were in the comparison group. After initiation of the study, follow-up occurred at 3 months, 1 year and after the complete course of the study. The mean age of the entire cohort was 68.7 years, and the mean follow-up period was 1.02 years. The primary composite outcomes were recurrent MI, ischemic stroke or cardiovascular death. Secondary outcomes included death from any cause, hospitalization for HF, coronary revascularization, pancreatitis, hypoglycemia, and diabetic ketoacidosis (DKA) or hyperosmolar hyperglycemic state. When looking at all 3 primary outcome parameters collectively, there was not a significant difference between the sitagliptin and the control group ($p = 0.079$). However, when the composite events were examined individually, the rate of acute MI increased significantly ($p = 0.008$ for the entire course of the study). While an increased rate of MI was seen at the 3 months' follow-up (6.3% for sitagliptin and 3.5% for controls), this was not statistically significant until 1 year after study initiation (13.7% with sitagliptin and 8.4% with control; $p = 0.031$). There was never a significant increase in ischemic stroke or cardiovascular death between the groups. When looking at secondary outcomes, the only parameter affected was the incidence of percutaneous coronary revascularization, which was significantly higher in the sitagliptin group ($p = 0.026$).

A subgroup analysis was also performed in end-stage renal disease (ESRD) individuals on hemodialysis, which complicates the findings a bit. Collectively, the individuals treated with sitagliptin (regardless of concurrent ESRD) had a statistically significant increase in recurrent MI ($p < 0.05$) and percutaneous coronary revascularization ($p < 0.05$). However, a subgroup analysis comparing sitagliptin use in ESRD and non-ESRD patients revealed that, the increased risk of MI only occurred in the ESRD subgroup ($p = 0.002$). Likewise, the significantly increased risk of percutaneous coronary revascularization occurred in the ESRD subgroup ($p = 0.002$), and not the non-ESRD subgroup ($p = 0.927$) [19MC].

Pancreatitis

TECOS reported no significant differences in rates of acute pancreatitis ($p = 0.12$) or pancreatic cancer ($p = 0.85$) with sitagliptin use compared to placebo over a 3 year (median) follow-up period [18MC].

Susceptibility Factors for Pancreatitis

Using the Taiwan National Health Research Insurance Database, a cohort of newly diagnosed type 2 diabetics was identified and followed until onset of acute pancreatitis or the end of the study. The cohort included a total of 114 141 eligible individuals, of which, 10 877 were DPP-4 inhibitor users (44.75% female) and 103 264 were nonusers (43.12% females). Types of DPP-4 inhibitors included sitagliptin, saxagliptin and vildagliptin. Individuals were excluded if they had evidence of acute pancreatitis before diabetes onset and if younger than 18 years of age. During the follow-up period, acute pancreatitis had developed in 25 of the DPP-4 inhibitor users and 486 of the nonusers. After controlling for age, sex, comorbidities and Diabetes Complications Severity Index scores, the risk of acute pancreatitis in the total study population was not significantly different between the DPP-4 inhibitor users and nonusers. However, subgroup analysis revealed that the female DPP-4 inhibitor users >65 years of age had a significantly higher risk of developing acute pancreatitis than female nonusers. Additionally, the risk of acute pancreatitis was significantly higher in DPP-4 inhibitor users (male and female) aged ≥65 years, but not in those <65 years of age. The author's cite caution in interpreting these results since this was a retrospective observational design and some patient information was missing. For instance, although the DPP-4 inhibitor prescriptions were filled, there is no guarantee that patients were compliant [20MC].

Cancer

TECOS did not show a significant difference in the incidence of pancreatic cancer in subjects receiving sitagliptin compared to placebo [18MC].

A 66-year-old male with recurrent metastatic carcinoid tumor involving the duodenum, pancreatic head and mediastinal lymph nodes experienced a rapid progression of his cancer within 3.5 months of starting saxagliptin therapy. Seven years prior, a portion of the tumor was resected, and he had been successfully managed with drug therapy since that time. During a routine checkup, his plasma serotonin levels (which were being used to monitor disease progression) more than doubled after starting saxagliptin therapy. The serotonin level had remained stable for several years. Saxagliptin was immediately discontinued, and serotonin levels returned to baseline within 4 weeks. Other laboratory markers remained unchanged before, during and after saxagliptin was initiated. Although this appears to be the first report of a possible interaction with a DPP-4 inhibitor and carcinoid tumor based upon temporal correlation, the authors commented that there is no literature providing direct evidence of a relationship [21A].

Skin

Vildagliptin-induced bullous pemphigoid was reported in 3 case studies involving elderly individuals. The first case occurred in an 86-year-old woman after 1 month of vildagliptin treatment. She was also taking metformin. Vildagliptin was discontinued and symptoms resolved with clobetasol. The second case was a 79-year-old man taking vildagliptin, metformin and gliclazide for 37 months. Local treatment with clobetasol initially controlled the condition. While clobetasol was being slowly tapered, lesions recurred at 3 months. The authors state that the patient's condition improved after discontinuing vildagliptin, but did not specify when that occurred. In last case, a 77-year-old woman was hospitalized for a 3-month history of extensive lesions. She had been taking gliclazide and vildagliptin for 26 months. Her condition improved with the discontinuation of vildagliptin in addition to the use of topical clobetasol. The authors speculate that a possible mechanism may involve a modified immune response or an alteration of the antigenic properties of the epidermal basement membrane. In two of the cases, the individuals were also taking metformin. In all 3 cases, the lesions regressed with topical clobetasol; however, vildagliptin had to be discontinued in order for sustained remission to occur [22A].

INCRETIN MIMETICS (GLP-1 AGONISTS)
[SEDA-36, 650; SEDA-37, 528–530]

There are currently four glucagon-like peptide-1 (GLP-1) agonists available in both the US and Europe (Europe has a fifth approved GLP-1 agonist). Administration ranges include twice daily (exenatide; Byetta®), once daily (liraglutide; Victoza®) and once-weekly exenatide (Bydureon®), albiglutide (Tanzeum® and Eperzan®) and dulaglutide (Trulicity®) injections. The side effect profiles are similar among the four GLP-1 agonists. The most frequent adverse effect being GI disturbances, namely, nausea, vomiting and diarrhea [23R]. A recent review article on albiglutide added upper respiratory tract infections as one of the most common patient-reported side effects [24R].

Gastrointestinal

A review article of head-to-head studies reported that once-weekly exenatide is associated with less nausea than twice daily exenatide and liraglutide. Dulaglutide and liraglutide have similar rates of nausea, while albiglutide has a lower rate of nausea than liraglutide [23R].

An open-label observational study evaluated the safety and efficacy of adding liraglutide to pre-existing dual therapy (metformin with either a sulfonylurea or pioglitazone) over a 12-month period. The 245 study subjects had inadequate glycemic control on dual therapy. Liraglutide was added to their medication regimen and follow-up occurred at 3-month intervals. Adverse drug reactions occurred in 58 subjects (23.7%). Mild to moderate GI symptoms were the most commonly reported adverse effect ($n = 21$ [11.4%]). Nausea was the most common GI side effect ($n = 17$ [6.9%]). Serious adverse drug reactions were reported in 6 subjects [2.4%]. Hypoglycemia was noted in a few individuals concurrently taking a sulfonylurea. Only one case of major hypoglycemia was recorded. After initiating liraglutide, sulfonylurea treatment was discontinued, or the dose was decreased in 35 subjects (19%). The authors specifically reported that there were no pancreatic events [25C].

A nationwide audit database was used to investigate whether there were specific risk factors that increased the likelihood of GI side effects with liraglutide. A total of 4442 participants were divided into three groups: those who did not report GI side effects ($n = 3905$ [87.9%]), those who reported GI side effects but continued liraglutide use ($n = 297$ [6.7%]) and those who discontinued liraglutide within 26 weeks due to GI side effects ($n = 240$ [5.4%]). GI side effects included nausea, diarrhea, vomiting, crampy abdominal pain, constipation, belching, reflux, flatulence of similar related terms. The authors reported that older age and those who were not taking metformin had more significant GI side effects leading to discontinuation of liraglutide therapy [26MC].

Pancreas

Proliferation of pancreatic ductal cell and pancreatitis has been reported in some animal studies using GLP-1 agonists; however, the mechanism of GLP-1 agonist-induced pancreatitis has not been determined. The only clinical study using humans is a randomized, placebo-controlled, double-blind crossover study in 12 male subjects with type 2 DM. Subjects were infused with exenatide or placebo, and the short-term effects on exocrine pancreatic secretion were examined. Intravenous infusion of exenatide did not appear to have a direct effect on exocrine pancreatic function. Pancreatic secretion volume, secretion rate and changes in pancreatic duct diameter did not differ from that of placebo [27c].

A population-based case control study using medical databases in Denmark reported on the incidence of acute pancreatitis with incretin-based therapy. The study population consisted of 12 868 patients with a first-time hospitalization for acute pancreatitis and 128 680 matched controls. There were 89 pancreatitis patients (0.69%) and 684 controls (0.53%) who were current or had a history of incretin use. Both GLP-1 agonists and DPP-4 inhibitors were considered incretin therapy. The crude OR for acute pancreatitis was 1.36 (95% CI 1.08–1.69) for incretin users, while users of non-incretin antihyperglycemic medications had an OR of 1.44 (95% CI 1.34–1.54). After adjustment for confounding factors (risk factors for acute pancreatitis and morbidity scale ratings), the risk of acute pancreatitis was not found to be increased with DPP-4 inhibitors (OR 1.04 [95% CI 0.80–1.37]), GLP-1 agonists (OR 0.82 [95% CI 0.54–1.23]) or non-incretin antihyperglycemics (OR 1.05 [95% CI 0.98–1.13]), compared to subjects who were non-users of antihyperglycemic medications. The authors concluded that since there was a similar increase in ORs for all antihyperglycemic medications, this possibly demonstrates an association of increased pancreatitis risk in diabetics rather than a specific drug effect [28MC].

Drug Administration

A review article of head-to-head studies summarized the incidence of injection-site reactions to be highest in the once-weekly GLP-1 agonists (albiglutide, dulaglutide and the once-weekly exenatide) compared to the once daily liraglutide and the twice daily exenatide [23R].

Once-weekly exenatide was studied in a 5-year efficacy and safety trial. The initial, controlled phase of the study compared safety and efficacy between twice daily and once-weekly exenatide over a 30-week period. At week 30, all participants continuing into the 230-week extension phase were switched to once-weekly exenatide. Of the 295 subjects in the initial phase, 258 entered the extension phase, and 153 (59.3%) finished the entire 260 weeks (5 year) study. Serious adverse events occurred in 13 (4.4%) participants during the 30-week phase and in 57 (22.1%) of the 258 participants in the extension phase.

The most common serious adverse events by organ system in the open-ended extension between events were cardiac disorders (14 [5.4%]), infections/infestations (14 [5.4%]) and musculoskeletal/connective tissue disorders (9 [3.5%]). Serious adverse effects were defined as those resulting in death, a life-threatening situation, inpatient hospitalization or prolongation of inpatient hospitalization, incapacity or substantial disruption to the ability to conduct normal life functions, congenital anomaly or birth defect, or an important medical event that may jeopardized the patient and required medical or surgical intervention to prevent one of the previously mentioned outcomes. One case of pancreatitis (0.4%), one case of pancreatic carcinoma (0.4%) and 3 cases (1.2%) of acute renal failure were reported in the 5-year extension phase of the trial. The most common adverse events in the extension phase were upper respiratory tract infection (106 [41.1%]), nasopharyngitis (73 [28.3%]), diarrhea (66 [25.6%]), sinusitis (55 [21.3%]), back pain (51 [19.8%]) and arthralgia (47 [18.2%]) [29C].

A 50-year-old female with T2D and dyslipidemia presented with eosinophil-rich granulomatous panniculitis at the sites of her once-weekly exenatide injections. Exenatide had been started 1 month earlier, and she had 3 lesions, with the most recent one appearing 3 days after her last injection. Although two other cases of eosinophil-rich granulomatous panniculitis have been reported at the site of exenatide injection; the histology of her lesion was also found to contain the actual microsphere material that encases exenatide in the once-weekly preparation [30A].

TYPE 2 SODIUM-GLUCOSE COTRANSPORTER (SGLT-2) INHIBITORS [SEDA-36, 652; SEDA-37, 530–531]

In December 2015, the US Food and Drug Administration revised labels for SGLT-2 inhibitors to add warnings concerning the risks of ketoacidosis and serious urinary tract infections, based upon their adverse event reporting system database. Specifically, 73 cases of ketoacidosis occurred in T1D and patients taking SGLT-2 inhibitors. Additionally, 19 cases of SGLT-2 inhibitor-associated urinary tract infections leading to life-threatening urosepsis and pyelonephritis occurred between March 2013 and October 2014 [31S].

Urinary tract and genital mycotic infections are the most common side effects of canagliflozin, occurring frequently in women. Additional potential side effects include nausea, renal impairment, hyperkalemia, and hypoglycemia. The incidence of pancreatitis is 2.7 for 100 mg daily dose and 0.9 for 300 mg daily dose per 1000 patient-years [32S].

Fracture Risk

A nine study (both placebo and active controlled) analysis of fracture risk with canagliflozin involved a total of 10 194 participants with T2D. The incidence and risk of fractures were analyzed three ways: the nine pooled studies collectively (referred to as the "overall population"), the CANVAS study alone and the eight pooled non-CANVAS studies. All of the subjects in the CANVAS study had a prior history of a cardiovascular event (such as MI or stroke) or ≥ 2 risk factors for a future cardiovascular event. In the 8 non-CANVAS studies ($n = 5867$), fracture incidence was similar with canagliflozin (1.7%) and non-canagliflozin subjects (2.6%). In the CANVAS study ($n = 4327$), there was a significantly increased incidence of fracture with canagliflozin (4%) compared to placebo (2.6%). For the overall population (9 pooled studies), the incidence of fracture was higher with canagliflozin (2.7%) versus non-canagliflozin (1.9%). The incidence of reported fall-related adverse events was significantly higher with the canagliflozin group in CANVAS but not in the pooled non-CANVAS studies or the overall population. An explanation for the different results among studies is the differences in participant characteristics. Compared to the pooled non-canagliflozin studies, the participants in CANVAS had a significantly higher mean age (57.6 years vs 62.4 years; $p > 0.001$), BMI (31.7 kg/m2 vs 32.1 kg/m^2; $p = 0.004$), HbA1c (7.9% vs 8.2%; $p < 0.001$) and duration of T2D (8.4 years vs 13.4 years; $p < 0.001$). The amount of participants with a prior history of a cardiovascular event was 10% in the non-CANVAS study and 60% in CANVAS. The number of participants with microvascular complications was 25% in the non-CANVAS group and 44% in CANVAS participants [33M].

Pancreatitis

A case of severe acute pancreatitis was reported in a 33-year-old African American female 2 weeks after initiating canagliflozin. She presented to the emergency room with a 2-day history of progressively worsening nausea, vomiting, and severe abdominal pain. Upon admission, she had a fever, hypotension, tachycardia, leukocytosis, acidosis, and hyperglycemia with elevated anion gap and pancreatic enzymes. Specific labs and vitals were as follows: blood pressure, 79/39; heart rate, 118 bpm; respiratory rate, 27; temperature, 40.3°C; white blood cell count, $23.6 \times 10^3/mm^3$; creatinine, 3.19 mg/dL; calcium, 9.3 mg/dL; amylase, 535 IU/L; lipase, 373 IU/L; blood glucose, 563 mg/dL; HbA1c, 13.5%; anion gap, 19; blood pH, 6.89; PCO2, 48.8; FiO2, 100. Blood alcohol was negative. Urine was positive for ketones, and triglycerides were within normal limits. In addition to the recent canagliflozin, metformin and levothyroxine were her long-term medications. She was given several liters of normal saline in addition to a bicarbonate and insulin drip, since she was initially diagnosed with DKA. She was also started on broad-spectrum antibiotics for her fever and leukocytosis. A computerized tomography (CT) scan of the abdomen showed evidence of acute pancreatitis and chest X-ray revealed bilateral pleural effusions.

She was started on a norepinephrine drip, intubated and admitted to the intensive care unit after she became progressive more hypotensive and unresponsive during aggressive fluid resuscitation. Her renal function deteriorated with decreased urine output and increasing serum creatinine (4.26 mg/dL) with persistent acidosis requiring continuous renal replacement therapy. In the intensive care unit, an APACHE (Acute Physiology and Chronic Health Evaluation) II score was calculated and estimated a mortality rate of 97.2%. Over the next few days, her condition improved and norepinephrine was discontinued. She was successfully extubated after 4 days. After excluding all other causes for her symptoms and given the timing of her presentation, canagliflozin was determined to be the likely cause of her illness. Canagliflozin was discontinued, and she has remained stable since discharge [34A].

METFORMIN [SEDA-15, 506; SEDA-36, 647; SEDA-37, 523–526]

Renal Dosing Adjustments

Per an FDA Drug Safety communication (April 2016), metformin use continues to be contraindicated in men and women with serum creatinine levels of ≥1.5 and ≥1.4 mg/dL, respectively. European guidelines recommend reducing the metformin dose when eGFR is 30–45 mL/min per 1.73 m^2 and discontinued when eGFR drops below this level [35S].

Susceptibility Factors for Gastrointestinal Intolerance

Factors affecting tolerance to metformin-induced GI side effects was studied in a 4-week study. Subjects with T2D were divided into those who were *H. pylori*-positive ($n = 195$) and *H. pylori*-negative ($n = 220$). The investigators reported that the incidence of abdominal pain, nausea, bloating and anorexia was at least twice as high in the *H. pylori*-positive ($p < 0.01$ for each), but there was not a significance difference in the incidence of diarrhea or vomiting. At the beginning of the study, all subjects were started on 500 mg of metformin daily. Gastrointestinal side effects were evaluated weekly, and the dose was progressively increased to 1500 mg/day based upon tolerance and compliance. At the conclusion of the study period, the *H. pylori*-positive individuals were on a significantly lower dose than those who were *H. pylori*-negative ($p < 0.01$). A total of 29.2% of the *H. pylori*-positive and 12.7% of the *H. pylori*-negative subjects did not complete the study related to digestive disturbances ($p < 0.01$). Other independent variables that correlated with a significantly increased incidence of GI disturbances were female gender and increased age. Elevated BMI, triglycerides and low-density-lipoprotein cholesterol were associated with a significant decrease in GI symptoms [36C].

Subjects newly diagnosed with T2D were the targets of a prospective observational cohort study ($n = 92$) investigating the GI side effects of metformin. Subjects were started on metformin as their initial hypoglycemic agent. Gastrointestinal adverse effects (defined as experiencing bloating, abdominal pain, nausea, diarrhea, vomiting and/or diarrhea) were experienced in 43 patients (47%). At the end of the 6-month study period, subjects were genotyped for two common loss-of-function variants in the transporter responsible for intestinal absorption of metformin (organic cation transporter-1 or OCT-1). The number of reduced-function alleles present was associated with metformin-induced GI side effects ($p = 0.034$). The authors also controlled for the concurrent use of OCT-1 inhibiting medications. When looking at additional parameters, both female gender and lower body weight showed a trend (not statistically significant) to increased GI side effects, which is consistent the study above [36C,37c].

Death

A retrospective, observational, cohort study utilized type 2 diabetics was identified in Taiwan's National Health Insurance Database to determine mortality in patients with advanced CKD taking metformin. For inclusion, serum creatinine had to be more than 530 µmol/L (equivalent to 9.54 mg/dL) in order to closely represent stage 5 CKD. A total of 813 metformin users were matched by propensity score to 2439 non-users. Median follow-up in the matched cohorts was 2.1 years (range 0.3–9.8 years). All-cause mortality was reported in 53% of metformin users and 41% of non-users. After multivariate adjustments, metformin use was deemed an independent risk factor for mortality ($p < 0.0001$). The increased risk was dose-dependent, with the highest risk in those taking more than 1000 mg daily. Metformin was not associated with a significantly higher risk of metabolic acidosis compared to non-users (1.6 cases for metformin versus 1.3 cases per 100 patient-years for nonuse; $p = 0.19$). Interestingly, progression to ESRD was significantly slower in the metformin users compared to nonusers ($p < 0.0001$), even after taking into account risk of death before reaching ESRD ($p < 0.0001$) [38MC].

Acid–Base Balance

The risk and incidence of lactic acidosis with metformin continues to be discussed and debated, although it has been licensed in the US for 21 years. Data extracted from the Australian Therapeutic Goals Administration (TGA) were used to estimate the incidence of lactic acidosis occurring with metformin use. The TGA receives reports on adverse events from predominantly pharmaceutical companies, but also on a voluntary basis from hospitals, health care providers and consumers. They identified a total of 152 reported cases between 1997 and 2011. Their analysis revealed an estimated incidence of 2.3 cases per 100 000 patient-years (range was 0.5 and 6.8 cases per 100 000). In this study, 26.5% of cases had at least one pre-existing contraindication for metformin use (the most common being renal insufficiency) and 74.2% reported having at least one clinical condition that could causes acidosis. The author's literature review found the reported incidence of lactic acidosis in those taking metformin ranged from 1.5 to 530 cases per 100 000 patient-years, across multiple countries. The author's recognized that the 2.3 cases per 100 000 patient-years figure may be lower than the actual number due to the likely under-reporting to the TGA [39C].

In a commentary published in the *Journal of Diabetes and Its Complications*, attention was drawn to the term metformin-induced lactic acidosis (MILA) as compared to metformin-associated lactic acidosis (MALA). The authors communicate that in many cases, those taking metformin possess co-morbidities that increase the risk of lactic acidosis, such as hypovolemia and intestinal hypoxia. Additionally, patients are often taking other medications that have been associated with lactic acidosis or metabolic acidosis. Therefore, the clinical literature, which vaguely reports the occurrence of lactic acidosis events with metformin use, is quite confusing and

possibly misleading. Since neither MILA nor MALA is usually specified, it readily lends to the assumption that metformin must be the cause of the lactic acidosis. The authors emphasize that MALA is a preventable complication if it is avoided in those with impaired renal function (eGFR < 45 mL/min per 1.73 m^2), liver failure, severe hypoxia, heart failure, surgery and alcohol use [40r].

Nervous System

A 70-year-old man taking metformin 500 mg twice daily for approximately 1 year experienced multiple episodes of recurrent acute confusion and drowsiness. Except for elevated creatinine levels, other labs, vitals, general and neurological examinations were unremarkable. During these episodes, metformin was routinely discontinued, while serum creatinine levels were actively lowered. Recovery always occurred within 2 days of metformin discontinuation. However, metformin was restarted each time he left the hospital, which resulted in a total of three of these episodes in a 6-month period. After the third episode, he was diagnosed with possible metformin-induced encephalopathy without lactic acidosis. Metformin was permanently discontinued, and he had not experienced further symptoms of encephalopathy. Metformin has been associated with iatrogenic encephalopathy secondary to hypoglycemia, acute liver failure and lactic acidosis, especially in renal impairment. The authors point out that the lack of encephalopathy following metformin discontinuation, despite recurrent episodes of elevated plasma creatinine, dispute the possibility that renal failure was the direct cause of the encephalopathy [41A].

The case presentations of MALA included a 70-year-old male with Stage 3 CKD (defined as GFR 30–60 mL/min per 1.73 m^2 per the Renal Association in the United Kingdom), acute kidney injury and HF who presented with chest pain and progressive shortness of breath. He was being treated with 500 mg metformin twice daily for T2D. His admission labs showed acute kidney injury: serum creatinine, 2.2 mg/dL; lactic acid, 11.1 mmol/L; arterial pH, 7.03; serum bicarbonate, 3.8 mmol/L; anion gap, 26 mEq/L; blood glucose, 206 mg/dL; serum ketones, negative. His metformin level was 25 µg/mL (~10 times elevated). Immediate hemodialysis promptly resolved all metabolic parameters and returned metformin to 1.5 µg/mL (within therapeutic range of 1–2 µg/mL).

Next, a 56-year-old male with T2D, cirrhosis and acute kidney disease presented after a syncopal spell. Further examination revealed jaundice, ascites and pretibial pitting edema. The day before, a liver biopsy was performed in addition to paracentesis and removal of 4 L of ascitic fluid. His admission labs showed acute kidney injury, with a serum creatinine of 2.1 mg/dL (1.1 mg/dL baseline), bicarbonate of 18 mEq/L and anion gap of 12 mEq. Diuretics and lisinopril were held but metformin 500 mg twice daily was continued. On day 3, he developed altered mental status and respiratory failure. Labs were drawn to show worsening renal failure: serum creatinine, 3.2; lactic acid, 10.6 mmol/L; arterial pH, 7.0; PCO_2, 21 mm Hg; serum bicarbonate, 4 mmol/L; anion gap, 47 mEq/L; aspartate aminotransferase, 3598 U/L; alanine aminotransferase, 898 U/L; INR, 7.0. His metformin level was 31 µg/mL. The patient underwent emergency hemodialysis, which resolved the high anion gap, metabolic acidosis and returned his metformin level to 5.4 µg/mL.

The last case of MALA was an intentional metformin overdose. The 60-year-old T2D male was a type 2 diabetic being treated with metformin and insulin (regular and neutral protamine Hagedorn). He reported ingestion of 5000 mg of metformin in addition to alcohol consumption. He was in mild distress with stable vitals upon admission. Treatment consisted of activated charcoal and intravenous hydration. His labs were as follows: serum creatinine, 0.8 mg/dL; lactic acid, 7.4 mmol/L; arterial pH, 7.35; anion gap, 22 mEq/L. He was admitted to the hospital for hemodialysis; however, the metabolic acidosis and his clinical status improved during the next 24 hours [42A].

SULFONYLUREAS [SEDA-36, 652; SEDA-37, 531–532]

Electrolyte Balance

A possible case of syndrome of inappropriate antidiuretic hormone (SIADH) occurred after 1 month of glimepiride therapy in a 62-year-old Japanese man. First-generation sulfonylureas have been associated with SIADH for decades, but this is the first published case for a third-generation agent. His drug regimen included a 3-month history of voglibose (an alpha-glucosidase inhibitor), alogliptin and metformin for T2D. For the previous 3 months, he was also using multiple cardiovascular medications and a proton pump inhibitor. At the initiation of glimepiride, his plasma sodium was normal (138 mmol/L). One month later, he had hyponatremia (125 mmol/L), a plasma osmolality of 276 mOsm/kg (normal <275 mOsm/kg), urine osmolality of 410 mOsm/kg (normal 100 mOsm/kg) and urinary sodium of 134 mmol/L (normal >20 mmol/L). Other parameters measured to help identify the cause of plasma and urine abnormalities included blood urea nitrogen, creatinine, adrenocorticotropic hormone (ACTH), cortisol, thyroid hormone, dehydration, cardiac insufficiency and renal insufficiency. All of these were within normal limits. Glimepiride was immediately discontinued, and the serum sodium returned to normal after 12 days, even without water restriction [43A].

References

[1] Kaneko S, Chow F, Choi DS, et al. Insulin degludec/insulin aspart versus biphasic insulin aspart 30 in Asian patients with type 2 diabetes inadequately controlled on basal or per-/self-mixed insulin: a 26-week, randomized, treat-to-target trial. Diabetes Res Clin Pract. 2015;I07:139–47 [C].

[2] Hollander P, King AB, Del Prato S, et al. Insulin degludec improves long-term glycaemic control similarly to insulin glargine but with fewer hypoglycaemic episodes in patients with advanced type 2 diabetes on basal-bolus insulin therapy. Diabetes Obes Metab. 2015;17:202–6 [C].

[3] Nuffer W, Trujillo JM, Ellis SL. Technosphere insulin (Afrezza): a new, inhaled prandial insulin. Ann Pharmacother. 2015;49(1):99–106 [M].

[4] Blonde L, Jendle J, Gross J, et al. Once-weekly dulaglutide versus bedtime insulin glargine, both in combination with prandial insulin lispro, in patients with type 2 diabetes (AWARD-4): a randomized, open-label, phase 3, non-inferiority study. Lancet. 2015;385:2057–66 [C].

[5] Home PD, Bolli GB, Mathieu C, et al. Modulation of insulin dose titration using a hypoglycaemia-sensitive algorithm: insulin glargine versus neutral protamine Hagedorn insulin in insulin-naïve people with type 2 diabetes. Diabetes Obes Metab. 2015;17:15–22 [C].

[6] Chan JC, Aschner P, Owens DR, et al. Triple combination of insulin glargine, sitagliptin and metformin in type 2 diabetes: the EASIE post-hoc analysis and extension trial. J Diabetes Complications. 2015;29:134–41 [C].

[7] Vellanki P, Bean R, Ovedokun FA, et al. Randomized controlled trial of insulin supplementation for correction of bedtime hyperglycemia in hospitalized patients with type 2 diabetes. Diabetes Care. 2015;38(4):568–74 [C].

[8] Dungan KM, Osei K, Gaillard T, et al. A comparison of continuous intravenous insulin and subcutaneous insulin among patients with type 2 diabetes and congestive heart failure exacerbation. Diabetes Metab Res Rev. 2015;31:93–101 [c].

[9] Bilotta F, Badenes R, Lolli S, et al. Insulin infusion therapy in critical care patients: regular insulin vs short-acting insulin. A prospective, crossover, randomized, multicenter blind study. J Crit Care. 2015;30:437.e1–6 [c].

[10] Herrera KM, Rosenn BM, Foroutan J, et al. Randomized controlled trial of insulin detemir versus NPH for the treatment of pregnant women with diabetes. Am J Obstet Gynecol. 2015;213:426.e1–7 [c].

[11] Sinuddin J, Karim N, Hasan AA, et al. Metformin versus insulin treatment in gestational diabetes in pregnancy in a developing country. A randomized control trial. Diabetes Res Clin Pract. 2015;I07:290–9 [C].

[12] Scirica BM, Bhatt DL, Braunwald E, et al. Saxagliptin and cardiovascular outcome in patients with type 2 diabetes mellitus. N Engl J Med. 2013;369:1317–26 [MC].

[13] Leiter LA, Teoh H, Braunwald E, et al. Efficacy and safety of saxagliptin in older participants in the SAVOR-TIMI 53 trial. Diabetes Care. 2015;38:1145–53 [M].

[14] White WB, Cannon CP, Heller SR, et al. Alogliptin after acute coronary syndrome in patients with type 2 diabetes. N Engl J Med. 2013;369:1327–35 [MC].

[15] Zannad F, Cannon CP, Cushman WC, et al. Heart failure and mortality outcomes in patients with type 2 diabetes taking

alogliptin versus placebo in EXAMINE: a multicenter, randomized, double-blind trial. Lancet. 2015;385:2067–76 [M].

[16] Toth PP. Overview of saxagliptin efficacy and safety in patients with type 2 diabetes and cardiovascular disease or risk factors for cardiovascular disease. Vasc Health Risk Manag. 2015;11:9–23 [M].

[17] Savarese G, Perrone-Filardi P, D'Amore C, et al. Cardiovascular effects of dipeptidyl peptidase-4 inhibitors in diabetic patients: a meta-analysis. Int J Cardiol. 2015;181:239–44 [M].

[18] Green JB, Bethel MA, Armstrong PW, et al. Effect of sitagliptin on cardiovascular outcomes in type 2 diabetes. N Engl J Med. 2015;373:232–42 [MC].

[19] Chen D, Wang S, Mao C, et al. Sitagliptin and cardiovascular outcomes in diabetic patients with chronic kidney disease and acute myocardial infarction: a nationwide cohort study. Int J Cardiol. 2015;181:200–6 [MC].

[20] Lai Y, Hu H, Chen H. Dipeptidyl peptidase-4 inhibitors and the risk of acute pancreatitis in patients with type 2 diabetes in Taiwan. Medicine. 2015;94(43):1–5 [MC].

[21] Pech V, Abusaada K, Alemany C. Dipeptidyl peptidase-4 inhibition may stimulate progression of carcinoid tumor, Case Rep Endocrinol. 2015; http://www.ncbi.nlm.nih.gov/pubmed/?term=Pech+V%2C+Abusaada+K%2C+Alemany+C. Article ID 952019, 3 pages [A].

[22] Béné J, Jacobsoone A, Coupe P, et al. Bullous pemphigoid induced by vildagliptin: a report of three cases. Fundam Clin Pharmacol. 2015;29:112–4 [A].

[23] Madsbad S. Review of head-to-head comparisons of glucagon-like peptide-1 receptor agonists. Diabetes Obes Metab. 2016;18:317–22 [R].

[24] Trujillo JM, Nuffer W. Albiglutide: a new GLP-1 receptor agonist for the treatment of type 2 diabetes. Ann Pharmacother. 2014;48(11):1494–501 [R].

[25] Buysschaert M, D'Hooge D, Preumont V, et al. ROOTS: a multicenter study in Belgium to evaluate the effectiveness and safety of liraglutide (Victoza®) in type 2 diabetic patients. Diabetes Metab Syndr. 2015;9:139–42 [C].

[26] Thong KY, Gupta PS, Blann AD, et al. The influence of age and metformin treatment status on reported gastrointestinal side effects with liraglutide treatment in type 2 diabetes. Diabetes Res Clin Pract. 2015;109(1):124–9 [MC].

[27] Smits MM, Tonneijck L, Musket MHA, et al. Glucagon-like peptide-1 receptor agonist exenatide has no acute effect on MRI-measured exocrine pancreatic function in patients with type 2 diabetes: a randomized trial. Diabetes Obes Metab. 2016;18:281–8 [c].

[28] Thomsen RW, Pedersen L, Møller N, et al. Incretin-based therapy and risk of acute pancreatitis: a nationwide population-based case-control study. Diabetes Care. 2015;38:1089–98 [MC].

[29] Wysham CH, MacConell LA, Maggs DG, et al. Five-year efficacy and safety data of exenatide once weekly: long-term results from the DURATION-1 randomized clinical trial. Mayo Clin Proc. 2015;90(3):356–65 [C].

[30] Andres-Ramos I, Blanco-Barrios S, Fernandez-Lopez E, et al. Exenatide-induced eosinophil-rich granulomatous panniculitis: a novel case showing injected microspheres. Am J Dermatopathol. 2015;37(10):801–2 [A].

[31] Food and Drug Administration. FDA Drug Safety Communication: FDA revises labels of SGLT2 inhibitors for diabetes to include warnings about too much acid in the blood and serious urinary tract infections, http://www.fda.gov/Drugs/DrugSafety/ucm475463.htm. Accessed March 17, 2016 [S].

[32] Invokana® (canagliflozin) [prescribing information, revised December 2015]. Titusville, NJ: Janssen Pharmaceuticals, Inc. [S].

[33] Watts NB, Bilezikian JP, Usiskin K, et al. Effects of canagliflozin on fracture risk in patients with type 2 diabetes mellitus. J Clin Endocrinol Metab. 2016;101:157–66 [M].

[34] Chowdhary M, Kabbani A, Chhabra A. Canagliflozin-induced pancreatitis: a rare side effect of a new drug. Ther Clin Risk Manag. 2015;11:991–4 [A].

[35] ERBP: Guideline development group. Clinical practice guideline on management of patients with diabetes and chronic kidney disease stage 3b or higher (eGFR <45 mL/min). Nephrol Dial Transplant. 2015;30(Suppl 2):ii1–ii142 [S].

[36] Huang Y, Sun J, Wang X, et al. Helicobacter pylori infection decreases metformin tolerance in patients with type 2 diabetes mellitus. Diabetes Technol Ther. 2015;17(2):1–6 [C].

[37] Dujic T, Causevic A, Bego T, et al. Organic cation transporter 1 variants and gastrointestinal side effects of metformin in patients with type 2 diabetes. Diabet Med. 2015;33:511–4 [c].

[38] Hung S, Chang Y, Liu J, et al. Metformin use and mortality in patients with advanced chronic kidney disease: national, retrospective, observational, cohort study. Lancet. 2015;3:605–14 [MC].

[39] Huang W, Castelino RL, Peterson GM. Adverse event notifications implicating metformin with lactic acidosis in Australia. J Diabetes Complications. 2015;29:1261–5 [C].

[40] Mathier C. Metformin associated lactic acidosis: time to let it go? J Diabetes Complications. 2015;29:974–5 [r].

[41] Béjot Y, Bielefield P, Guiboux A, et al. Recurrent encephalopathy induced by metformin in an elderly man. J Am Geriatr Soc. 2015;63(3):620–1 [A].

[42] Pasquel FJ, Klein R, Adigweme A, et al. Metformin-associated lactic acidosis. Am J Med Sci. 2015;39(3):263–7 [A].

[43] Adachi H, Yanai H. Adverse drug reaction: a possible case of glimepiride-induced syndrome of inappropriate antidiuretic hormone secretion. Diabetes Metab. 2015;41:176–7 [A].

41

Miscellaneous Hormones

Renee McCafferty*, *Sidhartha D. Ray*[†,1]

*Department of Pharmacy Practice, Manchester University College of Pharmacy, Natural and Health Sciences, Fort Wayne, IN, USA

[†]Department of Pharmaceutical Sciences, Manchester University College of Pharmacy, Natural and Health Sciences, Fort Wayne, IN, USA

[1]Corresponding author: sdray@manchester.edu

CALCITONIN [SEDA-34, 703; SEDA-35, 789; SEDA-36, 659; SEDA-37, 539]

Osteoarthritis

Two randomized, double-blind, multi-center, placebo-controlled trials evaluate efficacy and safety of oral salmon calcitonin in patients with painful osteoarthritis with structural damage. Adverse events were mainly gastrointestinal (diarrhea, nausea, vomiting) and resolved upon calcitonin discontinuation. FDA recently cautioned against using salmon calcitonin in osteoporosis due to inferior efficacy and possibly more adverse effects when compared to other bone treatments. Authors conclude that the present formulation of salmon calcitonin did not provide reproducible benefits in patients with symptomatic knee osteoarthritis [1C].

GONADOTROPINS (GONADORELIN, GnRH AND ANALOGUES) [SEDA-35, 789; SEDA-36, 660; SEDA-37, 539]

Idiopathic Central Precocious Puberty

Effectiveness and safety of domestic leuprorelin (GnRH analog) and imported leuprorelin were compared in 236 Chinese girls with idiopathic central precocious puberty and found to be comparable [2C].

GONADOTROPHIN-RELEASING HORMONE ANTAGONISTS [SEDA-35, 790; SEDA-36, 661; SEDA-37, 542]

Anti-Inflammatory Effects

Adverse event rates were similar between cetrorelix (GnRH antagonist) and placebo when used for their anti-inflammatory effect against RA [3C].

Advanced Prostate Cancer

GnRH antagonists were compared to standard androgen suppression therapy for advanced prostate cancer in a systematic review. There were more injection-site events with GnRH antagonists but less cardiovascular events [4M].

SOMATROPIN (HUMAN GROWTH HORMONE, hGH) [SEDA-35, 791; SEDA-36, 661; SEDA-37, 542]

Pediatric Clinical Studies

A pilot study was done involving 15 boys with predicted adult short stature who were all given recombinant human growth hormone (rhGH). Authors concluded that rhGH is very likely to be beneficial in late puberty as long as the knee epiphyses are still open. No secondary effects, such as headaches or hyperglycemia, were detected [5c].

A two-phase trial looked at bone mineral density in children with Prader–Willi syndrome treated with growth hormone. No adverse effects were reported. Bone mineral density remained stable during the first phase of the study, 4 years of treatment with GH during pre-pubertal years. During the second study phase, GH continued to be given for a total of 9 years. During longer-term administration (after 4 years), bone mineral density tended to decrease but stayed within the normal range. The authors included recommendations for GH-treated children with Prader–Willi syndrome to increase bone mineral density monitoring, especially during puberty, and stimulate physical activity to increase lean body mass. While stating the need for further study of complex hormonal treatments in this population, recommendations are included regarding optimal timing of concomitant sex hormone replacement [6C].

MELATONIN AND ANALOGUES
[SED-15, 224; SEDA-35, 792; SEDA-36, 664; SEDA-37, 545]

Migraine Prophylaxis

In a study of 60 children suffering from migraine headaches, melatonin 0.3 mg/kg daily for 3 months was given for migraine prophylaxis. Adverse events were reported in a total of 14 children (23.3%) consisting of sleepiness, vomiting, mild hypotension and constipation. Frequency, severity and duration of migraines were all reduced significantly which led the authors to conclude that melatonin may be effective migraine prophylaxis in children without causing life-threatening side effects [7c].

Insomnia Reviews

A review of melatonin used in chronopharmacology of insomnia remarked on its remarkable tolerability and stated that it has been given at very large doses over long periods of time without signs of abuse potential. The authors compare the safety of melatonin to that of other hypnotics and recommend that it be first-line therapy for insomnia in patients 55 years and over. The analog, tasimelteon has emerged for sleep resynchronization in blind patients without light perception. Agomelatine is another new melatonin analog marketed in Europe as an antidepressant [8R].

This review of melatonin's effectiveness to promote healthy sleep reports that most common side effects of melatonin include headache, somnolence, palpitations and abdominal pain. The following adverse events are reported infrequently: nasopharyngitis, arthralgia, tachycardia, dizziness, nausea, vomiting, nightmares, difficulty swallowing and breathing, hypnotic activity, heavy head, heartburn, flatulence, swelling of arms/legs, sweating/hot flash, exanthema, sleeping difficulties, depression, problems with the rectal probe, and sleep walking. Melatonin has been reported to reduce body temperature which could keep the drug from being useful during cold stress. Central nervous system effects (somnolence, headaches, increased frequency of seizures, nightmares) may be caused by melatonin supplementation. In healthy subjects, daytime dosing of melatonin (0.1–1.0 mg) caused drowsiness, fatigue, and performance decrements, peaking at around 3–4 hours. If melatonin is used to promote daytime sleep, circadian phase shifts may occur. If used to promote circadian phase shifts, sleepiness at undesired times may occur. The authors suggest that promotion of daytime sleep may not be appropriate in some military situations. Blood pressure effects (up or down) and dermatologic effects may occur. While this review notes no serious adverse events or health risks with melatonin use, it recommends addressing potential health effects of the drug [9R].

This review focuses more on the pharmacology of melatonin. The point is made melatonin has an immunostimulant effect which may make it problematic, even contraindicated as therapy in patients with autoimmune disorders. Agomelatine is touted as improving sleep as it is used for its antidepressant effects in comparison to some other antidepressants which are known to trigger sleep disorders. Ramelteon has been shown to be highly variable for maintaining sleep in elderly patients. Tasimelteon was approved by the FDA in 2014 for treatment of non-24-hour sleep–wake rhythm disorder in blind adults. Melatonin-controlled release tablets are approved for use in Europe in patients >55 years of age at 2 mg/day. Doses, as high as 300 mg/day for up to 2 years, have been found to be safe in amyotrophic lateral sclerosis patients. One source reported that adverse effects of melatonin include nausea, headache, rebound insomnia and a risk for hepatotoxicity. Withdrawal symptoms may occur if used for 6–12 months [10R].

Melatonin inhibits proliferation of most tumor cells through intracellular signaling. Its potent antioxidant effects are known, but it is hypothesized to have prooxidant effects on some tumor cells, especially Ewing sarcoma cells. The type of tumor cell metabolism seems to determine whether melatonin will cause cell death (Warburg effect) or inhibit cell proliferation. The authors suggest that melatonin could be used as a personalized antitumoral agent if the metabolic profile of a patient's tumor could be characterized [11E].

Agomelatine, a melatonin analogue, has been marketed since 2009 in some countries for its antidepressant effects. It has known potential to cause liver injury associated with elevations in serum transaminase levels >3× upper limit of normal. Serious hepatic reactions such as cytolytic hepatitis, jaundice and liver enzyme levels >10× upper limit of normal are reported to occur at a rate of one in every 1000–10000 persons. Six patients with hepatic risk factors have been reported worldwide to have developed hepatic failure resulting in death or liver transplant. In response, the manufacturer of agomelatine has issued liver monitoring guidance. Authors of this review state that liver injury associated with agomelatine is idiopathic and usually reversible. They suggest warning against factors that may increase risk for liver injury (concomitant alcohol consumption). Patients should be counseled that fatigue, nausea, vomiting and dark urine may indicate liver injury and should be reported immediately [12R].

Case Reports

A 19-year-old experienced severe sedation when melatonin was added to his regimen of citalopram, nortriptyline and oxycodone. His sedation improved upon melatonin discontinuation and worsened when melatonin was reintroduced. Although other meds in his regimen may cause sedation, a melatonin interaction was determined to be "possible" to "likely." A combined additive pharmacodynamics interaction may have occurred. Melatonin is known to inhibit multiple cytochrome p450 isoenzymes and can inhibit the effects of concomitant medications that depend on these isoenzymes for metabolism and clearance. Professionals prescribing, dispensing or recommending melatonin should advise caution in consideration of potentially interacting drugs and if the patient is to be driving or operating heavy machinery [13A].

Ramelteon, a melatonin-receptor agonist, is suspected to have caused nightmares in a 30-year-old male patient with history of attention-deficit hyperactive disorder. He had been treated with dextroamphetamine/amphetamine and zolpidem for years. He had tried over-the-counter melatonin in the past without much relief for his insomnia and was interested in taking an agent for sleep that was not a controlled substance. Zolpidem was tapered from 10 to 5 mg daily at bedtime for a week, and then stopped. The patient reports beginning ramelteon 2–3 days after stopping zolpidem. A few days after starting nightly ramelteon, he developed vivid nightmares which stopped after he discontinued ramelteon. Nightmares have been reported to occur with melatonin therapy. Non-benzodiazepine hypnotics such as zolpidem can decrease REM sleep on EEG. Ramelteon effects on REM sleep are not well characterized. Animal studies have shown that sleep induced by ramelteon and melatonin was indistinguishable from control animals. The authors state that zolpidem discontinuation does not cause withdrawal nightmares as benzodiazepines can. Nightmares have been reported with zolpidem discontinuation so further study could be beneficial [14A].

OXYTOCIN AND ANALOGUES
[SEDA-35, 793; SEDA-36, 665; SEDA-37, 546]

Cardiovascular Effects

Oxytocin is known to cause hypotension and tachycardia. It may also cause nausea and vomiting, myocardial ischaemia and arrhythmias, especially when given in boluses >5 units. Chest pain and pulmonary edema may also occur. It would be highly desirable to prevent these side effects. Phenylephrine 80 mcg co-administered with the oxytocin dose has helped prevent these cardiovascular effects from oxytocin but was found to be excessive. This study co-administered 50 mcg of phenylephrine with oxytocin and found that dose do not reliably prevent hemodynamic effects of the oxytocin bolus [15C].

Autism Risk

Maternal exposure to oxytocin during birth, induction and/or augmentation of labor, has been suspected to increase the rate of autism as the infant develops. A cohort of 557,040 live births was identified according to Denmark's birth registry between January 1, 2000 and December 31, 2009. Of this group, each child living on his first birthday was followed until December 31, 2012. An epidemiological analysis was performed to explore possible association between oxytocin exposures at birth with subsequent development of autism. A modest association between oxytocin-augmented labor and risk for autism was found in males but the therapeutic benefit of oxytocin administration during labor warrants caution in interpretation of these results [16c].

Caloric Intake

A randomized, placebo-controlled crossover study of 25 healthy, fasting men gave a single-dose of intranasal oxytocin (24 IU) or placebo then double portions of a breakfast meal each subject selected from a menu. Content of food consumed was measured along with relevant parameters in the study subjects. Men receiving oxytocin prior to meals consumed less fat and less overall calories while not affecting the caloric content of food ordered from the menu. Increased levels of cholecystokinin were found after oxytocin, unrelated to caloric intake. Indirect calorimetry showed an increased fat utilization and decreased carbohydrate utilization as well as a trend toward a reduction in triglyceride levels following oxytocin administration. Oxytocin also reduced insulin levels without changing glucose levels which implies increased insulin sensitivity. There was a slight decrease in body temperature (-0.3 °F, $p = 0.006$) after oxytocin. A few mild adverse effects were reported with no rate difference between oxytocin and placebo [17C].

SOMATOSTATIN (GROWTH HORMONE RELEASE-INHIBITING HORMONE) AND ANALOGUES [SED-15, 3160; SEDA-35, 794; SEDA-36, 666; SEDA-37, 549]

Pasireotide Clinical Studies

Long-acting release pasireotide, a somatostatin analog, was compared with octreotide long-acting repeatable for managing carcinoid symptoms refractory to first-generation somatostatin analogues. Efficacy was similar but pasireotide was associated with more hyperglycemia, fatigue and nausea. Two patients stopped pasireotide due to grade 4 hyperglycemia [18C].

An open-label extension trial was conducted in 58 patients with Cushing's disease who had been taking pasireotide for 12 months. The initial 12 months of the trial began with 162 Cushing's patients treated with either 600 or 900 mcg pasireotide twice daily. A total of 24 months of pasireotide was completed by 40 patients so its efficacy and safety could be further assessed. Throughout the study period, reductions in urinary free cortisol, serum cortisol and plasma ACTH were maintained. Clinical signs were also consistently improved such as blood pressure, weight and total cholesterol levels. Adverse events were reported by 98.1% of studied patients within the 24-month period. Gastrointestinal disorders were most common at 81.5% of patients (55.6% reported diarrhea, 48.1% nausea). Hyperglycemia was observed in 38.9% of which 11.7% were grade 3 and 8.6% were grade 4. Cholelithiasis occurred in 31.5% and was suspected to be drug related. Over the 24-month period, 42 patients (25.9%) had adverse events that were rated as serious. No patient deaths occurred. Authors conclude that the safety profile of pasireotide was typical for a somatostatin analogue except glucose level changes which they recommended monitoring closely [19C].

VASOPRESSIN RECEPTOR ANTAGONISTS [SEDA-34, 713; SEDA-35, 797; SEDA-36, 668; SEDA-37, 552]

Cirrhosis with Ascites

Three vasopressin receptor antagonists were considered as a group for their use limitations in the treatment of cirrhosis with ascites. When lixivaptan, satavaptan or tolvaptan were compared with placebo, they were found to have good effects at elevating serum sodium levels and improvement of ascites. Monitoring was recommended to avoid treatment-related adverse events such as over-correction of hyponatremia. Authors acknowledge the lack of evidence that vasopressin antagonists extend life in cirrhosis and call for future randomized controlled trials to study survival with each agent [20R].

Tolvaptan

A retrospective study of patients who had received tolvaptan was performed to provide insight into risk factors associated with development of hyponatremia. Keeping the daily dose of tolvaptan <7.5 mg was recommended in short- and long-term treatments. Age >75 years was also found to be predictive of late onset hyponatremia so caution is justified in this age group [21c].

A blinded re-examination of data from multiple tolvaptan trials for autosomal dominant polycystic kidney disease (ADPKD) was performed to better define the clinical pattern of potentially associated liver injury. The risk of liver failure in ADPKD after long-term tolvaptan therapy was estimated at 1:4000 with onset occurring within 3–18 months of receiving tolvaptan. All subjects experiencing hepatic injury recovered with no reports of liver failure. Frequent monitoring of liver function tests is recommended to reduce risk of liver injury during long-term tolvaptan use [22c].

In a meta-analysis of randomized controlled trials using tolvaptan in heart failure was performed to better describe the short- and long-term effects and allow evaluation as to its place in therapy. It was found that while tolvaptan may not bring long-term benefits in heart failure patients, it improves volume overload and hyponatremia without obvious increases in potassium and creatinine [23R].

Interim results of an ongoing study comparing tolvaptan use in heart failure patients >80 years of age with those <80 years. Tolvaptan was found to have similar safety and effectiveness profiles, but higher starting doses were found to be associated with more hypernatremia in those >80. Starting tolvaptan at no more than a 7.5 mg dose contributes to prevention of hypernatremia in heart failure patients >80 years of age [24C].

VASOPRESSIN AND ANALOGUES [SEDA-33, 915; SEDA-34, 714; SEDA-35, 798; SEDA-36, 669; SEDA-37, 552]

Hemodynamic Support

In a retrospective, propensity-matched cohort of septic shock patients, vasopressin was favorably compared to hydrocortisone for hemodynamic support secondary to norepinephrine. Vasopressin was associated with quicker hemodynamic stability and discontinuation of hemodynamic support. Arrhythmias were more frequent with vasopressin, but incidence of superinfection, hyperglycemia and hyponatremia was less frequent when compared to patients receiving hydrocortisone. Authors concluded that vasopressin was a more advantageous endocrine agent for hemodynamic support in septic shock than hydrocortisone [25c].

DESMOPRESSIN (N-DEAMINO-8-D-ARGININE VASOPRESSIN, DDAVP) [SEDA-34, 714; SEDA-35, 798; SEDA-36, 669; SEDA-37, 552]

Dermatologic Reaction

Interstitial Granulomatous Drug Reaction (IGDR) has been reported in a 56-year-old man after he had taken intranasal desmopressin for diabetes insipidus developed after prolactinoma excision. Rechallenge was associated with a recurrence of the IGDR truncal lesions. Both the initial and rechallenge eruptions resolved within 2–3 weeks of desmopressin discontinuation [26A].

References

[1] Karsdal MA, Byrjalsen I, Alexanderson P, et al. Treatment of symptomatic knee osteoarthritis with oral salmon calcitonin: results from two phase 3 trials. Osteoarthr Cartil. 2015;23:532–43 [C].

[2] Li WJ, Gong CX, Guo MJ, et al. Efficacy and safety of domestic leuprorelin in girls with idiopathic central precocious puberty: a multicenter, randomized, parallel, controlled trial. Chin Med J. 2015;128(10):1314–20 [C].

[3] Kass A, Hollan I, Fagerland MW, et al. Rapid anti-inflammatory effects of gonadotropin-releasing hormone antagonism in rheumatoid arthritis patients with high gonadotropin levels in the AGRA trial. PLoS One. 2015;10(10):e0139439 [C].

[4] Kunath F, Borgmann H, Blümle A, et al. Gonadotropin-releasing hormone antagonists versus standard androgen suppression therapy for advanced prostate cancer: a systematic review with meta-analysis. BMJ Open. 2015;5:e008217 [M].

[5] Rothenbuhler A, Ormieres B, Kalifa G, et al. A pilot study of growth hormone administration in boys with predicted adult short stature and near-ending growth. Growth Horm IGF Res. 2015;25:96–102 [c].

[6] Bakker NE, Kuppens RJ, Siemensma EPC, et al. Bone mineral density in children and adolescents with Prader-Willi syndrome: a longitudinal study during puberty and 9 years of growth hormone treatment. J Clin Endocrinol Metab. 2015;100(4):1609–18 [C].

[7] Fallah R, Shoroki FF, Ferdosian F. Safety and efficacy of melatonin in pediatric migraine prophylaxis. Curr Drug Saf. 2015;10(2):132–5 [c].

[8] Golombek DA, Seithikurippu RP, Brown GM, et al. Some implications of melatonin use in chronopharmacology of insomnia. Eur J Pharmacol. 2015;762:42–8 [R].

[9] Costello RB, Lentino CV, Boyd CC, et al. The effectiveness of melatonin for promoting healthy sleep: a rapid evidence assessment of the literature. Nutr J. 2014;13:106 [R].

[10] Emet M, Ozcan H, Ozel L, et al. A review of melatonin, its receptors and drugs. Eurasian J Med. 2016;48:135–41 [R].

[11] Sanchez-Sanchez AM, Antolin I, Puente-Moncada N, et al. Melatonin cytotoxicity is associated to Warburg effect inhibition in Ewing sarcoma cells. PLoS One. 2015;10(8):e0135420. http://dx.doi.org/10.1371/journal.pone.0135420. eCollection 2015. [E].

[12] Freiesleben SD, Furczyk K. A systematic review of agomelatine-induced liver injury. J Mol Psychiatry. 2015;3:4 [R].

[13] Foster BC, Cvijovic K, Boon HS, et al. Melatonin interaction resulting in severe sedation. J Pharm Pharm Sci. 2015;18(2):124–31 [A].

[14] Shah C, Kablinger A. Ramelteon-induced nightmares: a case report. Asian J Psychiatr. 2015;18:111–2 [A].

[15] Rumboll CK, Dyer RA, Lombard CJ. The use of phenylephrine to obtund oxytocin-induced hypotension and tachycardia during caesarean section. Int J Obstet Anesth. 2015;24(4):297–302 [C].

[16] Weisman O, Agerbo E, Carter CS, et al. Oxytocin-augmented labor and risk for autism in males. Behav Brain Res. 2015;284:207–12 [c].

[17] Lawson EA, Marengi DA, DeSanti RL, et al. Oxytocin reduces caloric intake in men. Obesity (Silver Spring). 2015;23(5):950–6 [C].

[18] Wolin EM, Jarzab B, Eriksson B, et al. Phase III study of pasireotide long-acting release in patients with metastatic neuroendocrine tumors and carcinoid symptoms refractory to available somatostatin analogues. Drug Des Devel Ther. 2015;9:5075–86 [C].

[19] Schopohl J, Gu F, Rubens R, et al. Pasireotide can induce sustained decreases in urinary cortisol and provide clinical benefit in patients with Cushing's disease: results from an open-ended, open-label extension trial. Pituitary. 2015;18:604 [C].

[20] Yan L, Xie F, Lu J, et al. The treatment of vasopressin V2-receptor antagonists in cirrhosis patients with ascites: a meta-analysis of randomized controlled trials. BMC Gastroenterol. 2015;15:65 [R].

[21] Hirai K, Shimomura T, Moriwaki H, et al. Risk factors for hypernatremia in patients with short- and long-term tolvaptan treatment. Eur J Clin Pharmacol. 2016;72(10):1177–83. http://dx.doi.org/10.1007/s00228-016-2091-4. [c].

[22] Watkins PB, Lewis JH, Kaplowitz N, et al. Clinical pattern of tolvaptan-associated liver injury in subjects with autosomal dominant polycystic kidney disease: analysis of clinical trials database. Drug Saf. 2015;38(11):1103–13 [c].

[23] Xiong B, Huang Y, Tan J, et al. The short-term and log-term effects of tolvaptan in patients with heart failure: a meta-analysis of randomized controlled trials. Heart Fail Rev. 2015;20(6):633–42. http://dx.doi.org/10.1007/s10741-015-9503-x. [R].

[24] Kinugawa K, Inomata T, Sato N, et al. Effectiveness and adverse events of tolvaptan in octogenarians with heart failure. Int Heart J. 2015;56:137–43 [C].

[25] Bissell BD, Erdman MJ, Smotherman C, et al. The impact of endocrine supplementation on adverse events in septic shock. J Crit Care. 2015;30(6):1169–73 [c].

[26] Vincenzo M, Guiseppe S, Maria O, et al. Interstitial granulomatous drug reaction after intranasal desmopressin administration. Indian J Dermatol. 2016;61(1):125 [A].

42

Drugs That Affect Lipid Metabolism

Robert D. Beckett[1], Andrea L. Wilhite, Nicholas Robinson, Audrey Rosene

Manchester University College of Pharmacy, Natural, and Health Sciences, Fort Wayne, IN, USA
[1]Corresponding author: rdbeckett@manchester.edu

BILE ACID SEQUESTRANTS [SED-15, 1902; SEDA-36, 676; SEDA-37, 559]

Bile acid sequestrants, ion exchange polymers that decrease low-density lipoprotein (LDL), cholesterol and total cholesterol, are not substantially absorbed through the gastrointestinal tract. The most common adverse drug effects are constipation, dyspepsia, nasopharyngitis, and nausea. Serious events such as abdominal distention, dysphagia, fecal impaction, gastrointestinal obstruction, heart disease (colesevelam), pancreatitis, and increased triglycerides (colesevelam) have been reported.

Cholestyramine

No relevant publications from the review period were identified.

Colesevelam

No relevant publications from the review period were identified.

Colestipol

A non-randomized, non-controlled, open-label study treated 26 patients with end-stage kidney disease on hemodialysis with colestipol 1 g tablets (dose varied based on baseline serum phosphate concentration) instead of their stable phosphate binder [1c]. The objective of the study was to determine effects of colestipol on serum phosphate in a pilot study. Adverse event and tolerability data were gathered through weekly assessments of participants. Six participants withdrew from the study; two dropouts were due to adverse effects (gastrointestinal effects [3.8%] and itching [3.8%]).

CHOLESTERYL ESTER TRANSFER PROTEIN INHIBITORS [SEDA-35, 810; SEDA-36, 677; SEDA-37, 560]

Sterol transporter inhibitors, such as ezetimibe, decrease gastrointestinal absorption of cholesterol and other phytosterols, decreasing LDL and total cholesterol, with minor increases in high-density lipoprotein cholesterol (HDL). Ezetimibe is generally well tolerated, but musculoskeletal effects, including myalgia and increased creatine kinase, have been reported in combination with other agents.

Ezetimibe

The Improved Reduction of Outcomes: Vytorin Efficacy International Trial (IMPROVE-IT) was a randomized, double-blind clinical trial of patients with recent hospitalization for acute coronary syndrome with an LDL of at least 50 mg/dL up to 100 mg/dL (previously treated) or 125 mg/dL (previously untreated) [2MC]. Patients were randomized to receive simvastatin 40 mg daily as monotherapy ($n=9077$) or in combination with ezetimibe 10 mg daily ($n=9067$). Cancer, gallbladder-related, and musculoskeletal-related events, as well as creatine kinase concentrations and liver injury tests were analyzed as pre-specified safety endpoints, with cancer and musculoskeletal-related events adjudicated by

Side Effects of Drugs Annual, Volume 38
ISSN: 0378-6080
http://dx.doi.org/10.1016/bs.seda.2016.08.005

blinded independent committees. Results were similar between groups using 7-year estimates as follows: cancer events (10.2% vs. 10.2%, $p=0.57$), cancer deaths (3.6% vs. 3.8%, $p=0.71$), gallbladder-related adverse events (3.5% vs. 3.1%, $p=0.10$), rhabdomyolysis or myopathy (0.3% vs. 0.3%, $p=0.90$), liver injury tests at least three times upper limit of normal (2.3% vs. 2.5%, $p=0.43$). Results for elevated creatine kinase were not provided. Rates of discontinuation due to adverse events were similar (10.1% vs. 10.6%, no p-value provided). Results suggest high tolerability of ezetimibe in combination with simvastatin.

An open-label clinical trial randomized 262 patients with a 12-month history of elective vascular surgery and chronic kidney disease (CKD) to rosuvastatin 10 mg daily ($n=136$) or rosuvastatin 10 mg daily plus ezetimibe 10 mg daily ($n=126$) in order to determine effects of combination therapy on renal function [3C]. Most patients were classified as having Stage 2 (estimated GFR at least 90 mL/min/1.73 m2; 62% vs. 60%) or 3 (estimated GFR 60–89 mL/min; 24% vs. 33%) CKD at baseline. No patients experienced acute renal failure or progressed to end stage CKD during the 12-month treatment period. Mean estimated GFR decreased from 64.6 ± 16.5 and 64.9 ± 16.8 mL/min at baseline to 57.0 ± 15.4 and 58.1 ± 16.9 ($p=0.802$ between groups). Similarly, mean serum creatinine increased from 1.16 ± 0.27 and 1.17 ± 0.28 mg/dL at baseline to 1.30 ± 0.28 and 1.30 ± 0.31 mg/dL ($p=0.642$ between groups). Results suggest that addition of ezetimibe to rosuvastatin did not result in renal-related adverse effects.

Plaque Regression with Cholesterol Absorption Inhibitor or Synthesis Inhibitor Evaluated by Intravascular Ultrasound (PRECISE-IVUS) was a randomized, controlled, single-blind study [4C]. Japanese patients with coronary artery disease, who underwent coronary angiography or percutaneous coronary intervention and had an LDL greater than 100 mg/dL, were randomized to atorvastatin titrated to an LDL goal of less than 70 mg/dL with ($n=122$) or without ($n=124$) ezetimibe 10 mg daily. Two percent of patients in each group ($n=4$) discontinued the study due to adverse drug reactions, including two cases of gastritis and one case each of eczema and numbness. Results from this study provide minimal adverse effects information regarding ezetimibe, but do suggest it was well tolerated.

In a randomized, double-blind clinical trial, patients with heterozygous familial hypercholesterolemia or non-familial hypercholesterolemia and LDL greater than 160 mg/dL who were aged 6–12 years were randomized 2:1 to treatment with ezetimibe 10 mg daily as monotherapy ($n=92$) or placebo ($n=45$) for 12 weeks [5C]. The proportions of patients experiencing at least one adverse event (60.9% vs. 55.6%; absolute risk reduction [ARR] 5.3%, 95% CI −11.9% to 22.8%) and at least one serious event (2.2% vs. 0.0%; ARR 2.2%, 95% CI −5.8% to

7.6%) were similar between groups. There was no difference in terms of pre-specified adverse events of interest (i.e., elevated creatine kinase with and without symptoms, elevated liver injury tests, gallbladder-related events, musculoskeletal events, pancreatitis), with none of the listed events occurring in more than 1 patient per treatment group. Rates of hypersensitivity were similar between groups (7.6% vs. 8.9%; ARR −1.3%, 95% CI −6.9–5.9%). Three discontinuations occurred due to adverse events in the ezetimibe group: one case of elevated alanine aminotransferase (ALT), one case of prurigo, and one congenital epileptic event. No discontinuations due to adverse effects occurred in the placebo group. Results suggest that ezetimibe is well tolerated in this specific pediatric population.

Chinese patients admitted to one hospital for acute coronary syndromes, who also had type 2 diabetes mellitus received treatment with a statin (i.e., atorvastatin 20 mg daily, pravastatin 20 mg daily, rosuvastatin 10 mg daily, or simvastatin 20 mg daily) with ($n=44$) or without ($n=40$) ezetimibe 10 mg daily in a prospective cohort study [6c]. There were no statistically significant differences between groups in baseline characteristics. No treatment-related adverse effects, elevated liver injury tests, other hepatic events, or creatine kinase elevations were reported. No differences in terms of liver injury test or creatine kinase mean values were identified.

NICOTINIC ACID DERIVATIVE [SED-15, 2512; SEDA-35, 815; SEDA-36, 679; SEDA-37, 560]

Niacin (nicotinic acid) is a B3-complex vitamin necessary for lipid metabolism. Niacin is known to reduce total cholesterol and triglycerides, and to increase HDL, through an unknown mechanism. Peripheral vasodilation associated with niacin can manifest as flushing, orthostatic events, pruritus, tingling, and warmth. Sustained-release or controlled release formulations decrease risk, but these formulations have been associated with hepatotoxicity. Laropiprant is a prostaglandin antagonist used in combination with niacin to reduce vasodilation.

Niacin

A subgroup analysis of Atherothrombosis Intervention in Metabolic Syndrome with Low HDL/Triglycerides: Impact on Global Health Outcomes (AIM-HIGH), a double-blind, randomized, placebo-controlled trial of patients age 45 years and older with dyslipidemia and stable cardiovascular disease, evaluated effects of niacin ER on change in kidney function, safety, and tolerability

[7MC]. All patients received simvastatin 40 mg once daily and were randomized to at least 1500 mg total daily dose of niacin extended release (ER) or placebo following a niacin tolerability 4- to 8-week run-in period, where doses were increased in weekly increments. CKD ($n = 505$) was defined as glomerular filtration rate (GFR) less than 60 mL/min/1.73 m2. Mean decrease in estimated GFR was 1.8% ± 22.3% with niacin ER versus 3.3 ± 24.2% with placebo ($p = 0.10$). Study discontinuation was more common with niacin ER (32.7%) versus placebo (22.7%, $p = 0.01$). Of patients who discontinued the study, the most common reasons related to adverse effects were flushing and itching (30.1% vs. 14.0%), increased serum glucose concentration (6.0% vs. 3.5%), and gastrointestinal symptoms (6.0% vs. 1.8%) (p-values not provided). Results from this subgroup are similar to previously reported adverse effects; however, it should be noted that patients had to tolerate niacin ER at least 1500 mg total daily dose to be included in the study. Results may not be generalizable to patients who could not tolerate niacin ER during the run in requirement or at the specified dose.

A 24-week, open-label clinical trial randomized 99 human immunodeficiency virus (HIV)-infected patients with low HDL and high triglycerides to treatment with niacin ER (titrated to 1500 mg daily in 500 mg increments at 4-week intervals) or fenofibrate 200 mg daily in order to evaluate for improved arterial endothelial function and inflammatory biomarkers [8C]. Although no serious adverse events occurred, 72% of patients who received niacin experienced an adverse event of interest compared to 43% of patients who received fenofibrate ($p = 0.007$). The most common of these events were flushing (26% with niacin vs. 0% with fenofibrate) and possible myopathy (10% with niacin vs. 4% with fenofibrate), although no patients experienced persistent myopathy, discontinuation due to myopathy, or myositis. Results from this analysis suggest that the common adverse effects with niacin are similar in HIV-infected patients compared to the general population.

A double-blind clinical trial randomized patients with type 2 diabetes mellitus in a 4:3 ratio to treatment with niacin ER/laropiprant titrated to 2 g/40 mg daily ($n = 432$) or placebo ($n = 336$) for 36 weeks. A subsequent *post-hoc* analysis compared patients who were not under glycemic control at baseline (uncontrolled defined as A1c greater than 6.8%, $n = 376$) and fasting plasma glucose (FPG, uncontrolled defined as greater than 129 mg/dL, $n = 380$) compared to patients who were controlled ($n = 392$ and $n = 388$, respectively) [9C]. Patients who were uncontrolled and in the niacin ER group were more likely to experience worsening of A1c (31.2%) compared to uncontrolled patients on placebo (14.3%), controlled patients on niacin ER (10.1%), and

controlled patients on placebo (7.4%). Results were similar when patient groups were defined in terms of FPG instead of A1c. Rates were similar across subgroups for pre-specified safety events of interest: adjudicated cardiovascular events (all subgroups less than 2%), liver injury tests (all subgroups less than 2%), hepatitis-related events (all groups less than 1%), and creatine kinase elevations (all subgroups 0%). Inferential statistics were not presented. Results suggest that use of niacin ER in combination with laropiprant is associated with worsening blood glucose control in patients with diabetes compared to placebo and that risk increases for patients uncontrolled at baseline.

FIBRIC ACID DERIVATIVES [SED-15, 1358; SEDA-35, 812; SEDA-37, 561]

Fibrates are generally preferred for patients with elevated triglycerides. Literature has not shown that they reduce cardiovascular risk; however, these agents are often used in patients who are at risk for pancreatitis due to high triglyceride levels. Common adverse effects of this class include gastrointestinal disturbances, elevated liver enzymes, and myalgias and myopathy (particularly in combination with statins, in the case of gemfibrozil).

Fenofibrate

Co-Administration with Statins

In one randomized, open-label, crossover pharmacokinetic study, Hispanic patients ($n = 36$) were administered a single dose of atorvastatin 20 mg, followed by the combination of atorvastatin 20 mg and fenofibrate 160 mg to evaluate the effects of co-administration [10c]. Patients' blood samples were drawn at regular time intervals up to 96 hours after administration of the medication(s). This study found that there was an increase in atorvastatin concentration following fenofibrate administration versus atorvastatin alone. This change was similar to those noted in previous studies and was not considered a clinically meaningful change in atorvastatin concentrations (plasma max, area under the curve, or area under the curve extrapolated to infinity). Based on study participants receiving only one dose of each study drug, it is difficult to extrapolate these results to patient responses clinically.

Gemfibrozil

No relevant publications from the review period were identified.

HMG-CoA REDUCTASE INHIBITORS
[SED-15, 1632; SEDA-35, 812; SEDA-37, 562]

HMG-CoA reductase inhibitors (statins) are used to treat dyslipidemia and have demonstrated potential to reduce cardiovascular risk. Statins are considered first-line therapy in patients at risk for cardiovascular disease, as described by national treatment guidelines. It has been widely documented and seen in clinical practice that all statins pose a risk for myopathy, myalgia and very rarely, rhabdomyolysis.

Cataracts

The relationship between statins and cataracts remains controversial in the current literature, with differing results found among randomized, controlled trials and observational studies. Little additional relevant literature has been identified for this review in relationship to the protective or causative effects of statin on cataract development. A sub-study was performed from the Simvastatin and Ezetimibe Aortic Stenosis Study [11c]. In this double-blind placebo controlled trial, patients were randomized to simvastatin 40 mg plus ezetimibe 10 mg versus placebo with a primary end point of incident cataract. The simvastatin plus ezetimibe group was associated with a 44% lower risk of cataract development [HR 0.56; 95% CI 0.33–0.96, $p = 0.034$]. These results should be taken into consideration with the body of literature available which has shown variable results with statins and cataracts.

Diabetes

Previous literature has established an increased risk of new-onset diabetes mellitus for certain statin medications, including atorvastatin, rosuvastatin, and simvastatin [12M]. New evidence suggests the likelihood of this association being variable between individual agents versus a class effect. Although recent literature regarding statins may pose heightened awareness of the risk of new-onset diabetes mellitus, clinicians should consider the risk versus benefit for patients in which a statin is warranted.

In an Asian population, a retrospective study investigated the effect of low-dose atorvastatin (10–20 mg) and the risk of developing new-onset diabetes mellitus (NODM) over 3 years [13C]. A total of 3566 patients who had established cardiovascular disease or cardiovascular risk without a history of DM were divided into two groups: those treated with low-dose atorvastatin ($n = 566$) or no lipid lowering agents (control, $n = 3000$). More patients received 10 mg of atorvastatin vs 20 mg (88% vs 12%, respectively). Propensity score matching

was incorporated to account for potential cofounding variables. Prior to adjustment for baseline cofounding variables, the incidence of NODM was higher in the low-dose atorvastatin group compared with control group (5.8% vs 2.1%, $p < 0.001$). Although the incidence of NODM remained higher in the low-dose atorvastatin group vs the control group after controlling for cofounding variables, there was no statistically significant difference between the two groups (5.9% vs. 3.2%, $p = 0.064$). Although high-dose atorvastatin has been associated with NODM in patients at high risk for developing diabetes, this study suggests that this association may not exist for low-dose atorvastatin.

A meta-analysis of 15 randomized controlled trials evaluated the effects of pitavastatin (dose range, 1–8 mg daily) on glycemic levels and the incidence of NODM in non-diabetic individuals [12M]. 4815 non-diabetic patients (3236 assigned to pitavastatin and 1579 to control) were compared based on HbA1c, fasting blood glucose, and onset of NODM for an average of 12 weeks. Based on BMI, FBG, and age, most patients included in the trials were not considered high risk for the development of diabetes. At the end of follow-up, there were no statistically significant differences found between pitavastatin and control for HbA1c levels (MD −0.03%, 95% CI, −0.11–0.05), the incidence of NODM (RR 0.70, 95% CI, 0.30–1.61), or fasting blood glucose levels (MD −0.01 mg/dL, 95% CI, −0.77–0.74).

Patients with familial hypercholesterolemia (FH) were enrolled in the SAFEHEART study, an open-label, multicenter, prospective study [14C]. Patients with established diabetes were excluded from the study. A total of 3823 patients were included in the analyses. The mean follow-up was 5.9 years, and most patients (59%) were using high-intensity dosed statins with most commonly used statins being atorvastatin and simvastatin. In the group of patients with high intensity statins, new-onset diabetes was 1.7% in the FH group versus 0.2% in the non-FH group ($p = 0.001$). However, when results were adjusted for confounding factors, statin use did not demonstrate an increased risk of new-onset diabetes [OR 1.02; 95% CI 0.95–1.08, $p = 0.31$]. In a multivariate logistic regression, age, HOMA-IR, metabolic syndrome and plasma glucose were statistically significant predictors of new-onset diabetes in the FH group only. These adjusted results demonstrate that there were several factors in the FH group that increased risk of new-onset diabetes; however, statin use was not found to increase this risk in patients with FH.

Pancreatitis

Original observational studies and case reports previously provided evidence that statins may cause pancreatitis. Further studies have not established a causal relationship between statins and pancreatitis; with some evidence pointing towards protective effects and others suggesting causation of pancreatitis. The evidence remains controversial as detailed in the following studies.

In a population-based case–control study, 4376 patients hospitalized for acute pancreatitis were compared to 19 859 hospitalized patient controls from the adult population in Finland with a primary aim of examining the association between statin use and the risk of acute pancreatitis [15c]. A total of 19% and 13% of hospitalized patients were exposed to statins, respectively. It was found that statin use was associated with an increased incidence rate of acute pancreatitis [OR 1.25; 95% CI 1.13–1.39] in this patient population. The increase was most commonly seen during the first 3 months of statin use [OR 1.37; 95% CI 0.94–2.00].

An additional population-based case–control study in Taiwan sought to evaluate the relationship between rosuvastatin use and acute pancreatitis [16C]. A case group of patients were selected based on a first episode of acute pancreatitis ($n = 5728$). A control group of patients was identified as a comparator group ($n = 22 912$). For both the case and control, patients were separated into rosuvastatin users ($n = 21$, $n = 21$, respectively) and non-users ($n = 5616$, $n = 22 656$, respectively). Rosuvastatin use was associated with a higher proportion of acute pancreatitis versus control subjects [Adjusted OR 3.21; 95% CI 0.67–1.19]. This study suggests that rosuvastatin is associated with a slightly increased risk of pancreatitis.

A retrospective cohort study evaluated the relationship between simvastatin and atorvastatin, each independently, and the risk of acute pancreatitis [17C]. The incidence rate of pancreatitis among simvastatin and atorvastatin users was compared with a reference population of adults. The risk of acute pancreatitis was reduced with simvastatin use, crude incidence rate ratio 0.626, 95% CI, 0.588–0.668, $p < 0.0001$. In a subsequent multivariate analysis, simvastatin was independently associated with reduced risk of pancreatitis, adjusted RR 0.29 (95% CI 0.27–0.31). Atorvastatin demonstrated similar results, adjusted RR 0.33 (95% CI 0.29, 0.38). These findings suggest that there is a reduced incidence of pancreatitis, and it may be a class effect.

Exercise

Myopathy and myalgias are well documented in the literature and are clinically common with the use of statins. Some evidence suggests that exercise may exacerbate these statin-related side effects; however, other literature has reported that statins do not reduce exercise level or intensity. A recent subgroup analysis of the National Runners' and Walkers' Health Study found that there was no difference in running distance in statin-treated hypercholesterolemic patients compared to those treated with other medications ($p = 0.64$) or not treated at all ($p = 0.94$) [18c].

A review article evaluating 16 original articles sought to determine the effects of statins in association with acute or chronic exercises on skeletal muscle [19R]. Study results suggested that exacerbations of skeletal muscle injuries were more frequent with intense training or strenuous exercises with the use of a statin in athletes. In contrast, it was found that moderate training did not increase pain reports or elevate CK levels and improved muscle and metabolic functions. These findings suggest that the extent to which statins impact the ability to exercise may depend on the rigor and intensity of the workout the patient is engaged.

Cancer

Although past research in this area has been controversial, recent literature supports a trend of reduced risk of cancer among patients prescribed statin medications. A case–control study evaluated whether the long-term use of statins (>5 years) is associated with a reduced risk of renal cell carcinoma in Denmark between 2002 and 2012 [20C]. A total of 4606 patients were matched in 1:10 fashion to cancer-free controls. Statins were not found to be linked to any chemopreventative effects against the incidence of renal cell carcinoma (OR 1.06, 95% CI, 0.91–1.23).

A second case–control study compared 311 cases of esophageal cancer to 856 controls and prescriptions for statins and non-statin lipid lowering medications in patients diagnosed with Barrett's esophagus [21C]. Patients who developed esophageal cancer were less likely to use a statin than control patients (40.2% vs 54%, $p < 0.01$). The average daily dose of simvastatin (the primary statin analyzed, representing 86.9% of prescriptions) was lower in cases than in the control group (21–40 mg/day, 9.3% vs. 14.5%, respectively, and >40 mg/day, 8.4% vs. 12.6%, respectively, $p < 0.01$). Statin use was found to be inversely associated with the development of esophageal adenocarcinoma (OR 0.65; 95% CI, 0.47–0.91), specifically late-stage esophageal adenocarcinoma (OR 0.44, 95% CI, 0.25–0.79).

Another population-based case–control study evaluated 3174 cholangiocarcinoma patients against 3174 controls and the association between the risk of cholangiocarcinoma and statin use by type of statin and dose [22C]. Fewer patients with cholangiocarcinoma reported use of statins (22.7% vs 26.5%, $p < 0.001$). The adjusted OR of statin use associated with cholangiocarcinoma was 0.80 (95% CI, 0.71–0.90). A dose–response relationship between statin use and the risk of developing cancer was also identified, with stronger doses associated with a lower risk of cholangiocarcinoma.

Two cohort studies evaluating statin use and effects in prostate cancer found similar positive results [23C,24C]. Statins were found to not only possess a modest protective effect against the development of prostate cancer, but statin use among prostate cancer patients was associated with significantly decreased all-cause mortality (adjusted HR = 0.65, 95% CI, 0.60–0.71). The results also supported a dose–response relationship as both low- and high-dose groups were found to have significantly decreased death rates compared with the control group of prostate cancer patients who did not use statins.

Fewer studies report an increased risk of cancer in patients who use statins [25C]. A recent case–control study including 500 individuals with thyroid cancer as cases and 2500 controls found a significantly increased risk of thyroid cancer associated with previous regular statin use (OR 1.40, 9% CI, 1.05–1.86). This association, however, was only significant for females versus males (OR 1.43, 95% CI, 1.07–1.90 vs OR 1.28, 95% CI, 0.75–2.17, respectively). Of note, in patients who reported previous irregular statin use, the risk of developing thyroid cancer was insignificant (OR 1.35, 95% CI, 0.88–2.07). This finding suggests potential for statins increasing risk of thyroid cancers.

PROPROTEIN CONVERTASE SUBTILISIN/ KEXIN TYPE 9 (PCSK9) INHIBITORS

Two proprotein convertase subtilisin/kexin type 9 (PCSK9) inhibitors were approved by the US Food and Drug Administration in 2015: alirocumab and evolocumab [26R]. Both of these drugs are injectable monoclonal antibodies used to reduce LDL. These medications act to inactivate the PCSK9 enzyme. PCSK9 binds to LDL receptors on the hepatic surface and promotes LDL receptor degradation. Inactivation of PCSK9 decreases LDL receptor degradation, increasing recirculation of the receptor to the surface of the hepatocytes, and causing lowering of LDL cholesterol levels in the bloodstream. This class of medication generates a 40–70% relative reduction in LDL when given in combination with a statin.

Clinical trial experience to date suggests that alirocumab and evolocumab are generally safe, well tolerated, and similar in safety profile to ezetimibe [26R]. However, long-term clinical trials have yet to reach completion. The most common reported adverse effects were back pain, influenza symptoms, nasopharyngitis, and upper respiratory tract infections; however, these generally occurred at the same rate as control. Despite the subcutaneous route of administration, injection site reactions were not common. Several types of hypersensitivity-related adverse events have been reported, including cutaneous leucocytoclastic vasculitis, delayed-type rash, pruritis.

For this reason, clinical trials have focused on gathering hypersensitivity data.

Considering that PCSK9 inhibitors have been associated with substantial LDL reduction in clinical trials (one study reached a mean LDL of 34 ± 16 mg/dL), in many cases even following treatment with statins, concerns have been raised regarding risks that could be associated with excessive LDL reduction [26C]. Postulated risks associated with very low LDL concentrations (e.g., hemorrhagic stroke, neurocognitive impairment) have not manifested in clinical trials to date. One potential reason that these concerns have not manifested may be that intracellular LDL, rather than plasma, plays a more essential role in hormone and vitamin synthesis.

The following sections describe specific results from clinical studies evaluating alirocumab and evolocumab, focusing on results for common and severe adverse events.

Alirocumab

In a randomized, double-blind, phase 3 parallel group clinical trial, adults with heterozygous familial hypercholesterolemia, coronary heart disease, or coronary heart disease risk equivalent with LDL cholesterol levels greater than or equal to 70 mg/dL were randomized in a 2:1 ratio to receive alirocumab ($n = 1553$) or placebo (saline injection, $n = 788$) for 78 weeks [27MC]. Adverse events were reported in 81% of alirocumab patients and 82.5% of placebo patients, with 7.2% in alirocumab and 5.8% of placebo leading to study discontinuation. The most common adverse events were general allergic reaction (10.1% vs. 9.5%), local injection site reactions (5.9% vs. 4.2%), myalgia (5.4% vs. 2.9%) and worsening of diabetes (12.9% vs. 13.6%). The following occurred more commonly in alirocumab: neurocognitive disorder (1.2% vs. 0.5%) and ophthalmologic events (2.9% vs. 1.9%) along with the more common occurrences of general allergic reaction, local injection site reaction and myalgia. None of the adverse event reports were statistically significant with the exception of myalgia ($p = 0.006$).

In a 24-week, double-blind, randomized clinical trial patients were randomized to add-on alirocumab 75 or 150 mg every 2 weeks with atorvastatin 20 mg ($n = 57$) or atorvastatin 40 mg ($n = 47$) compared with add-on ezetimibe 10 mg plus atorvastatin 20, 40, 80 mg, or rosuvastatin 40 mg ($n = 149$) [28C]. Adverse effects were assessed by reporting, laboratory parameters, vital signs, physical exam, and electrocardiogram (ECG). Treatment Emergent Adverse Effects (TEAEs) were reported in 65.4% of patients taking alirocumab and 63.8% of patients in the control groups. Patients experiencing TEAEs leading to discontinuation was 6.7% with alirocumab versus 5.4% with placebo. The most common events reported were back pain (6.7% vs. 4.0%), nasopharyngitis

(4.8% vs. 5.4%), hypertension (4.8% vs. 0.7%), urinary tract infection (2.9% vs. 5.4%), diarrhea (1.9% vs. 5.4%), nausea (1% vs. 7.4%) and creatine kinase greater than three times upper limit of normal (3% vs. 5.4%). The following appeared to be more common with alirocumab: injection site reactions (2.9% vs. 2.0%), neurological events (2.9% vs. 2.0%), hypertension and back pain. Inferential statistics were not conducted.

In a 52-week, double-blind, randomized clinical trial, 316 patients were randomized 2:1 to receive alirocumab 75 mg Q2 weeks ($n = 209$) or placebo (saline injection, $n = 107$) [29C]. All patients were receiving a maximally tolerated statin dose of either atorvastatin 40 mg, atorvastatin 80 mg or rosuvastatin 20 mg or rosuvastatin 40 mg or simvastatin 80 mg. TEAEs were reported in 157 (75.8%) of alirocumab patients and 81 (75.7%) of placebo patients. The most common events reported were upper respiratory tract infection (7.7% vs. 10.3%), arthralgia (3.9% vs 7.5%), nasopharyngitis (7.2% vs. 4.7%), urinary tract infection (6.3% vs. 3.7%), dizziness (5.3% vs. 5.6%), non-cardiac chest pain (1% vs. 6.5%), sinusitis (5.3% vs. 3.7%), local injection site reactions (5.3% vs. 2.8%) and potential general allergic reaction events (8.7% vs. 6.5%). The following occurred more commonly in alirocumab: nasopharyngitis, urinary tract infection, sinusitis, injection site reaction, potential general allergic reaction events and neurologic events (2.4% vs. 1.9%). Inferential statistics were not conducted.

In a 52-week, double-blind, double-dummy randomized control trial 720 patients were randomized 2:1 receiving alirocumab 75 mg plus oral placebo ($n = 479$) or 10 mg oral ezetimibe plus subcutaneous placebo ($n = 241$) [30C]. TEAEs were reported in 71.2% of alirocumab patients and 67.2% of ezetimibe patients. The most commonly reported events were accidental overdose (6.3% vs. 6.6%), upper respiratory tract infection (6.5% vs. 5.8%), dizziness (4.8% vs. 5.4%) and myalgia (4.4% vs. 5.0%). The following occurred more frequently in alirocumab: upper respiratory tract infection, injection site pain, and creatine kinase greater than three times upper limit of normal (2.8% vs. 2.5%). There is a planned evaluation for this study at 104 weeks.

The adverse events that appeared to be most common among trials with alirocumab were injection site reactions, nasopharyngitis, urinary tract infection, and upper respiratory tract infection. Neurological adverse events were consistently, but less commonly, present. One study suggested statistically significant increased risk for myalgia compared to control (5.4% vs. 2.9%, $p = 0.006$).

Evolocumab

In a pooled study of two open-label, randomized trials, 4465 patients were randomized in a 2:1 ratio to receive either evolocumab 140 mg every 2 weeks or 420 mg once a month based on patient preference (evolocumab group, $n = 2976$) or to the standard of care therapy group ($n = 1489$) [31MC]. The most common events reported were musculoskeletal related (6.4% vs. 6.0%). The events that occurred more commonly in evolocumab groups were injection site reaction (4.3% vs. not applicable [no control injection was administered to the standard of care group]), neurocognitive events (0.9% vs. 0.3%), arthralgia (4.6% vs. 3.2%), headache (3.6% vs. 2.1%), limb pain (3.3% vs. 2.1%) and fatigue (2.8% vs. 1.0%). Inferential statistics were not conducted.

In a double-blind, placebo-controlled multicenter trial, 331 patients were randomized in a 2:2:1:1 ratio to receive either evolocumab 140 mg every 2 weeks ($n = 111$), evolocumab 420 mg monthly ($n = 110$), placebo every 2 weeks ($n = 55$), or monthly placebo ($n = 55$) [32C]. Adverse events were reported in 55% of evolocumab 140 mg every 2 weeks group, 57% of evolocumab 420 mg monthly group, 43% of placebo every 2 weeks group and 55% of monthly placebo group. The most commonly reported events were nasopharyngitis (7% and 10% vs. 4% and 5%), headache (4% and 5% vs. 2% and 5%), contusion (5% and 4% vs. 0% and 2%), back pain (2% and 5% vs. 0% and 2%), nausea (5% and 3% vs. 0% and 2%), potential injection site adverse events (5% and 7% vs. 4% and 4%) and musculoskeletal-related adverse events (7% and 2% vs. 0% and 1%) for the evolocumab and placebo groups, respectively. The following events appeared to occur more frequently in evolocumab groups: nasopharyngitis, contusion, back pain, nausea, muscle-related adverse events, and potential injection site adverse events. Inferential statistics were not conducted.

A double-blind, phase 3, placebo and ezetimibe controlled study examined 307 patients randomized 2:2:1:1 to evolocumab 140 mg every 2 weeks ($n = 103$) or 420 mg once a month ($n = 102$) or ezetimibe daily with placebo every 2 weeks ($n = 51$) or ezetimibe and monthly placebo ($n = 51$) [33C]. Groups were combined to evolocumab ($n = 205$) and placebo ($n = 102$) for analysis. The most commonly reported adverse events were headache (8% vs. 9%), myalgia (8% vs. 18%), pain in extremities (7% vs. 1%), muscle spasms (6% vs. 4%), fatigue (4% vs. 10%), nausea (4% vs. 7%), and diarrhea (2% vs. 7%). The following appeared to occur more frequently in evolocumab: pain in extremities and muscle spasms. Inferential statistics were not conducted.

In a 52-week randomized, double-blind, phase 3 clinical trial patients were randomized 2:1 receiving evolocumab 420 mg once a month ($n = 599$) or placebo ($n = 302$) [34C]. Adverse events were reported in 74.8% of patients with evolocumab and 74.2% with placebo. The most common adverse effects were nasopharyngitis (10.5% vs. 9.6%), upper respiratory tract infection (9.3% vs. 6.5%), influenza (7.5% vs. 6.3%), and back pain (6.2% vs.

5.6%). The following occurred more frequently in evolocumab: nasopharyngitis, upper respiratory tract infection, influenza, back pain, sinusitis (4.2% vs. 3.0%), myalgia (4.0% vs. 3.0%), dizziness (3.7% vs. 2.6%), gastroenteritis (3.0% vs. 2.0%), oropharyngeal pain (2.5% vs. 1.3%), upper abdominal pain (2.2% vs. 0.7%), dyspepsia (1.8% vs. 0.7%), rash (1.8% vs. 0.3%), anxiety (1.7% vs. 0.7%). Inferential statistics were not conducted.

In a 12-week, phase II, double-blind, randomized, placebo controlled study, 310 Japanese patients were randomized to 6 groups: placebo every 2 weeks ($n=52$), evolocumab 70 mg every 2 weeks ($n=49$), evolocumab 140 mg every 2 weeks ($n=52$), placebo once monthly ($n=50$), evolocumab 280 mg once monthly ($n=51$) and evolocumab 420 mg once monthly ($n=53$) [35C]. TEAEs occurred as follows: placebo every 2 weeks (34.6%) of patients, evolocumab 70 mg every 2 weeks (49%), evolocumab 140 mg every 2 weeks (53.8%), placebo once monthly (42%), evolocumab 280 mg once monthly (41.2%) and evolocumab 420 mg once monthly (58.5%). The most common TEAE for all groups was nasopharyngitis (no values provided). TEAEs led to discontinuation for 2% of evolocumab 70 mg, 1.9% of evolocumab 140 mg and 3.8% of evolocumab 420 mg versus 0% with placebo. Potential injection site reactions were reported in placebo (1.9%), evolocumab 70 mg (2%), evolocumab 140 mg (3.8%) and evolocumab 420 mg (1.9%). ALT or aspartate aminotransferase (AST) greater than three times upper limit of normal was reported in evolocumab 70 mg (2%). Creatine kinase greater than five times upper limit of normal was reported in the monthly placebo group (2%) and evolocumab 280 mg (2%). Inferential statistics were not conducted.

A 12-week randomized, double-blind, placebo controlled phase 3 clinical trial enrolled 50 patients in a 2:1 ratio to evolocumab 420 mg Q4 weeks ($n=33$) or placebo ($n=17$) [36c]. TEAEs were reported in 36% of the evolocumab group and 63% of the placebo group. The most common events were upper respiratory tract infection (9% vs. 6%), influenza (9% vs. 0%), gastroenteritis (6% vs. 0%), nasopharyngitis (6% vs. 0%), nausea (0% vs. 13%), potential injection site reactions (0% vs. 6%), creatine kinase greater than five times upper limit of normal (3% vs. 6%), and ALT or AST greater than three times upper limit of normal (6% vs. 6%). The events that appeared more frequently in evolocumab were upper respiratory tract infection, influenza, gastroenteritis, nasopharyngitis and musculoskeletal pain (3% vs. 0%). Inferential statistics were not conducted.

The adverse events that appeared to be most common based on the above evolocumab studies were injection site reaction, nasopharyngitis, muscle related or myalgia, upper respiratory tract infection and influenza. No inferential statistics were performed for the safety data for these trials.

Overall, it appears that adverse effects were more frequently reported in the evolocumab trials compared to alirocumab; however, there was general inconsistency among evolocumab trials as to which were most often reported. The most frequent adverse effects common to alirocumab and evolocumab were injection site reactions, myalgia or muscle related, upper respiratory tract infection, and nasopharyngitis. Neurocognitive effects were reported in small rates with each drug but were more than placebo (when reported). However, inferential statistics were not conducted. Evolocumab appears to have influenza reported more frequently than alirocumab.

References

[1] Hood CJ, Wolley MJ, Kam AL, et al. Feasibility study of colestipol as an oral phosphate binder in hemodialysis patients. Nephrology. 2015;20(4):250–6 [c].

[2] Cannon CP, Blazing MA, Giugliano RP, et al. Ezetimibe added to statin therapy after acute coronary syndromes. New Engl J Med. 2015;372(25):2387–97 [MC].

[3] Kouvelos GN, Arnaoutoglou EM, Milionis JH, et al. The effect of adding ezetimibe to rosuvastatin on renal function in patients undergoing elective vascular surgery. Angiology. 2015;66(2):128–35 [C].

[4] Tsujita K, Sugiyama S, Sumida H, et al. Impact of dual lipid-lowering strategy with ezetimibe and atorvastatin on coronary plaque regression in patients with percutaneous coronary intervention. J Am Coll Cardiol. 2015;66(5):495–507 [C].

[5] Kusters DM, Caceres M, Coll M, et al. Efficacy and safety of ezetimibe monotherapy in children with heterozygous familial or nonfamilial hypercholesterolemia. J Pediatr. 2015;166(6):1377–84 [C].

[6] Li L, Zhang M, Su F, et al. Combination therapy analysis of ezetimibe and statins in Chinese patients with acute coronary syndrome and type 2 diabetes. Lipids Health Dis. 2015;14(1). http://dx.doi.org/10.1186/s12944-015-0004-7 [c].

[7] Kalil RS, Wang JH, de Boer IH, et al. Effect of extended release niacin on cardiovascular events and kidney function in chronic kidney disease: a post-hoc analysis of the AIM-HIGH trial. Kidney Int. 2015;87(6):1250–7 [MC].

[8] Dube MP, Komarow L, Fichtenbaum CJ, et al. Extended-release niacin versus fenofibrate in HIV-infected participants with low high-density lipoprotein cholesterol: effects on endothelial function, lipoproteins, and inflammation. Clin Infect Dis. 2015;61(5):840–9 [C].

[9] Bays HE, Brinton EA, Triscari J, et al. Extended-release niacin/laropiprant significantly improves lipid levels in type 2 diabetes mellitus irrespective of baseline glycemic control. Vasc Health Risk Manag. 2015;11:165–72 [C].

[10] Patino-Rodriguez O, Martinex-Medina RM, Torres-Roque I, et al. Absence of a significant pharmacokinetic interaction between atorvastatin and fenofibrate: a randomized, crossover, study of a fixed-dose formulation in healthy Mexican subjects. Front Pharmacol. 2015;6(4):1–6 [c].

[11] Bang CN, Greve AM, La Cour M, et al. Effect of randomized lipid lowering with simvastatin and ezetimibe on cataract development (from the simvastatin and ezetimibe in aortic stenosis study). Am J Cardiol. 2015;116(12):1840–4 [c].

[12] Vallejo-Vaz AJ, Kondapally SR, Kurogi K, et al. Effect of pitavastatin on glucose, HbA1c and incident diabetes: a meta-analysis of randomized controlled clinical trials in individuals without diabetes. Atherosclerosis. 2015;24(2):409–18 [M].

[13] Park JY, Rha SW, Choi B, et al. Impact of low dose atorvastatin on development of new-onset diabetes mellitus in Asian population: three-year clinical outcomes. Int J Cardiol. 2015;184:502–6 [C].

[14] Fuentes F, Alcala-Diaz JF, Watts GF, et al. Statins do not increase the risk of developing type 2 diabetes in familial hypercholesterolemia: the SAFEHEART study. Int J Cardiol. 2015;201:79–84 [C].

[15] Kuoppala J, Pulkkinen J, Kastarinen H, et al. Use of statins and the risk of acute pancreatitis: a population-based case–control study. Pharmacoepidemiol Drug Saf. 2015;24(10):1085–92 [C].

[16] Lai SW, Lin CL, Liao KF. Rosuvastatin and risk of acute pancreatitis in a population-based case–control study. Int J Cardiol. 2015;187:417–20 [C].

[17] Wu BU, Pandol SJ, Lio IL. Simvastatin is associated with reduced risk of acute pancreatitis: findings from a regional integrated healthcare system. Gut. 2015;64(1):133–8 [C].

[18] Williams PT, Thompson PD. Effects of statin therapy on exercise levels in participants in the national runners' and walkers' health study. Mayo Clin Proc. 2015;90(10):1338–47 [c].

[19] Bonfim MR, Oliverira AS, Amaral S, et al. Treatment of dyslipidemia with statins and physical exercises; recent findings of skeletal muscle responses. Arq Bras Cardiol. 2015;104(4):324–32 [R].

[20] Pottegard A, Clark P, Friis S, et al. Long-term use of statins and risk of renal cell carcinoma: a population-based case–control study. Eur Urol. 2015;15:1001–5 [C].

[21] Nguyen T, Duan Z, Naik AD, et al. Statin use reduces risk of esophageal adenocarcinoma in US veterans with barrett's esophagus: a nested case–control study. Gastroenterology. 2015;149(6):1392–8 [C].

[22] Peng YC, Lin CL, Hsu WY, et al. Statins are associated with a reduced risk of cholangiocarcinoma: a population-based case–control study. Br J Clin Pharmacol. 2015;80(4):755–61 [C].

[23] Kantor ED, Lipworth L, Fowke JH, et al. Statin use and risk of prostate cancer: results from the southern community cohort study. Prostate. 2015;75(13):1384–93 [C].

[24] Sun LM, Lin MC, Lin CL, et al. Statin use reduces prostate cancer all-cause mortality: a nationwide population-based cohort study. Medicine (Baltimore). 2015;94(39):e1644. http://dx.doi.org/10.1097/MD.0000000000001644.

[25] Hung SH, Lin HC, Chung SD. Statin use and thyroid cancer: a population-based case–control study. Clin Endocrinol. 2015;83(1):111–6 [C].

[26] Latimer J, Batty JA, Neely DD, et al. PCSK9 inhibitors in the prevention of cardiovascular disease. J Thromb Thrombolysis. 2016. http://dx.doi.org/10.1007/s11239-016-1363-1. Epub ahead of print.

[27] Robinson JG, Farnier M, Krempf M, et al. Efficacy and safety of alirocumab in reducing lipids and cardiovascular events. N Engl J Med. 2015;372(16):1489–99 [MC].

[28] Bays H, Gaudet D, Weiss R, et al. Alirocumab as add-on to atorvastatin versus other lipid treatment strategies. J Clin Endocrinol Metab. 2015;100(8):3140–8 [C].

[29] Kereiakes DJ, Robinson JG, Cannon CP, et al. Efficacy and safety of the proprotein convertase subtilisin/kexin type 9 inhibitor alirocumab among high cardiovascular risk patients on maximally tolerated statin therapy. Am Heart J. 2015;169(6):906–15 [C].

[30] Cannon CP, Cariou B, Blom D, et al. Efficacy and safety of alirocumab in high cardiovascular risk patients with inadequately controlled hypercholesterolaemia on maximally tolerated doses of statins. Eur Heart J. 2015;36(19):1186–94 [C].

[31] Sabatine MS, Giugliano RP, Wiviott SD. Efficacy and safety of evolocumab in reducing lipids and cardiovascular events. N Engl J Med. 2015;372(16):1500–9 [MC].

[32] Raal FJ, Stein EA, Dufour R, et al. PCSK9 inhibition with evolocumab (AMG 145) in heterozygous familial hypercholesterolaemia (RUTHERFORD-2): a randomised, double-blind, placebo-controlled trial. Lancet. 2015;385(9965):331–40 [C].

[33] Stroes E, Colghoun D, Sullivan D, et al. Anti-PCSK9 antibody effectively lowers cholesterol in patients with statin intolerance: the GAUSS-2 randomized, placebo-controlled phase 3 clinical trial of evolocumab. J Am Coll Cardiol. 2014;63(23):2541–8 [C].

[34] Blom DJ, Hala T, Bolognese M, et al. A 52-week placebo-controlled trial of evolocumab in hyperlipidemia. N Engl J Med. 2014;370(19):1809–19 [C].

[35] Hirayama A, Honarpour N, Yoshida M, et al. Effects of evolocumab (AMG 145), a monoclonal antibody to PCSK9, in hypercholesterolemic, statin-treated Japanese patients at high cardiovascular risk—primary results from the phase 2 YUKAWA study. Circ J. 2014;78(5):1073–82 [C].

[36] Raal FJ, Honarpour N, Blom DJ, et al. Inhibition of PCSK9 with evolocumab in homozygous familial hypercholesterolaemia (TESLA Part B): a randomised, double-blind, placebo-controlled trial. Lancet. 2015;385(9965):341–50 [c].

43

Cytostatic Agents—Tyrosine Kinase Inhibitors Utilized in the Treatment of Solid Malignancies

David Reeves[1]

Department of Pharmacy Practice, College of Pharmacy and Health Sciences, Butler University, Indianapolis, IN, USA

Department of Pharmacy, St. Vincent Indianapolis Hospital, Indianapolis, IN, USA

[1]Corresponding author: dreeves@butler.edu

INTRODUCTION

Malignant cells have many genomic alterations which have become increasingly important in the treatment and control of various cancers. Therapies targeted at these alterations have much appeal and have garnered much momentum over the past decade. One of the earlier targeted therapies, imatinib, transformed the treatment of chronic myeloid leukemia (CML) and has led to the long-term control of this difficult to treat malignancy [1C]. Though the results with targeted therapies in other malignancies have largely not been as dramatic or consistent as imatinib's effect on the natural history of CML, they have become a mainstay of treatment in multiple malignancies and continue to be investigated in many settings. Unlike traditional chemotherapeutic medications, these drugs are targeted to alterations in cancer cells, many blocking upregulated signaling pathways specifically within the malignant cells. With this specificity, adverse effects of targeted therapies differ greatly from those observed with chemotherapy.

Targeted therapies utilized for the treatment of malignancies encompass a heterogeneous group of medications including tyrosine kinase inhibitors, monoclonal antibodies, and other small molecule inhibitors specifically targeted to alterations in cancer cells. This chapter will focus on tyrosine kinase inhibitors (TKI) utilized for the treatment of solid tumors, specifically inhibitors of vascular endothelial growth factor (VEGF), epidermal growth factor receptor (EGFR), anaplastic lymphoma kinase (ALK), and mitogen-activated protein (MAP) kinase pathways. TKI exert their effects on cancer cells by inhibiting signaling pathways within the cell which are usually upregulated, leading to decreased cell growth and proliferation. Each class of medications has a unique side effect profile which patients may be at risk for experiencing for prolonged periods, considering these medications are generally administered orally on a routine basis until disease progression or intolerance. This chapter will focus on developments related to the tolerability of these medications which have been published in the literature between December 1, 2014 and January 31, 2016.

VASCULAR ENDOTHELIAL GROWTH FACTOR (VEGF) INHIBITORS

Currently, multiple TKI target the VEGF pathway and are utilized for many malignancies. A hallmark of these medications is their ability to block the VEGF receptor signaling, inhibiting angiogenesis. Those included in this review consist of: axitinib, cabozantinib, pazopanib, regorafenib, sorafenib, sunitinib, and vandetanib. In recent large trials, the most common adverse effects reported included fatigue, diarrhea, hand foot syndrome, nausea, and hypertension [2MC,3MC,4C,5C].

In a worldwide treatment use trial of sunitinib in patients with imatinib resistant advanced gastrointestinal stromal tumor, the most common adverse effects of any grade were fatigue (42%), diarrhea (40%), hand foot syndrome (32%) and nausea (29%) [2MC]. Common grade 3 and 4 adverse effects included hand foot syndrome (11%), fatigue (9%), hypertension (7%), and diarrhea (5%). Hypothyroidism was reported in 13%, and cardiac adverse effects occurred in ≤1%. Overall 2% experienced grade 5 adverse effects (death), while 53% required dose interruption or dose decrease. Similar adverse effects were also noted in patients randomized to the sorafenib arm of a phase III trial comparing it to linifanib for hepatocellular carcinoma [3MC]. Grade 3 or higher adverse effects occurred in 75%, with hypertension (10.6%), hand foot syndrome (14.8%), elevated aspartate aminotransferase (AST) concentrations (12.5%), and diarrhea (9.2%) being most common. Again, 50% required dose interruption.

A more recently approved VEGF pathway inhibitor, cabozantinib was compared to everolimus for the treatment of renal cell carcinoma in a phase III trial in which 60% required dose reductions and 9% discontinued the medication [4C]. All patients experienced adverse effects during treatment with 68% experiencing grade 3 or 4 adverse effects (hypertension—15%, diarrhea—11%, fatigue—9%). Grade 5 reactions occurred in 7%. Another study in which all patients experienced an adverse effect was a phase III study of regorafenib in metastatic colorectal cancer [5C]. Grade 3 or higher adverse effects occurred in 54% with hand foot syndrome (16%), hypertension (11%), hyperbilirubinemia (7%), hypophosphatemia (7%) and elevated alanine aminotransferase (ALT) concentrations (7%) being most common. Discontinuation occurred in 14% of the population, while 63% required dose interruption and 40% required dose reduction.

Despite benefits in clinical endpoints observed with these medications, adverse effects remain burdensome. In a health-related quality of life (HRQoL) study of pazopanib in soft tissue sarcoma, HRQoL did not improve or decline with treatment despite significantly worse symptom scores for diarrhea, loss of appetite, nausea, and fatigue in those receiving pazopanib [6C].

Cardiovascular

Cardiac adverse effects are a concern shared by many who utilize drugs targeting the VEGF pathway. Three meta-analyses have been published describing cardiovascular outcomes among the VEGF TKI [7M,8M,9c]. In one analysis, the effects of sorafenib, sunitinib, vandetanib, axitinib, and pazopanib on the incidence of congestive heart failure (CHF) were analyzed from 16 studies including 10647 patients [7M]. All grade CHF was increased among those receiving the VEGF TKI compared to those not (2.39% vs 0.75%, respectively; RR 2.69, 95% CI: 1.86–3.87, $p < 0.001$). High grade CHF was also increased, however, not significantly (1.19% vs. 0.65%, respectively; RR 1.65, 95% CI: 0.76–3.70, $p = 0.227$). Another meta-analysis of 11612 patients enrolled in studies investigating sunitinib, axitinib, cediranib, and regorafenib demonstrated in increased risk of all grade hypertension (RR 1.93, 95% CI: 2.03–3.81, $p < 0.00001$) and bleeding (RR 1.93, 95% CI: 1.41–2.64, $p < 0.00001$) [8M]. High grade hypertension and bleeding were also significantly

increased in those receiving the VEGF TKI. When individual agents were analyzed, the greatest bleeding risk appeared to be with sunitinib (RR 2.80, 95% CI: 2.01–3.91, $p < 0.00001$). Interestingly, this meta-analysis did not demonstrate a significant increase in left ventricular (LV) dysfunction or thrombosis with the VEGF TKI. The last meta-analysis included sunitinib, sorafenib, pazopanib, axitinib, vandetanib, cabozantinib, and regorafenib and investigated the effect of these medications on QTc interval [10M]. The incidence of all grade QTc prolongation with these VEGF TKI was 4.4%, significantly greater than the control group (RR 8.66, 95% CI: 4.92–15.2, $p < 0.001$). High grade QTc prolongation was also increased at an incidence of 0.83%. The risk of QTc prolongation was not related to length of therapy and appeared to be highest in those receiving vandetanib or sunitinib and lowest in those receiving pazopanib or axitinib. Contrary to the findings of this meta-analysis, two small studies of patients receiving regorafenib and axitinib did not demonstrate clinically significant effects on QTc interval [9c,11c].

In an analysis of patients enrolled in a large trial comparing axitinib to sorafenib in those with renal cell carcinoma ($n = 723$), hypertension was fairly common (40.4% axitinib vs. 29.0% sorafenib) [12C]. Grade 3 hypertension occurred in 15.3% of those receiving axitinib and 10.7% of those receiving sorafenib, while grade 4 hypertension occurred in 0.3% of both groups. Despite this common adverse effect which was also observed in the aforementioned meta-analysis, hypertension rarely led to treatment discontinuation or adverse cardiovascular outcomes.

Two case reports of patients experiencing aortic dissection while receiving VEGF TKI were also published [13A,14A]. Both patients were being treated for renal cell carcinoma, one with axitinib and one with sunitinib. The patient receiving axitinib had recently been switched from sunitinib after experiencing palmar/plantar erythrodysesthesia. Ten days after starting axitinib in one patient and 20 days after starting sunitinib in the other, they experienced chest pain and were determined to have an aortic dissection. The patient receiving axitinib had a Stanford type A dissection from the ascending aorta to the left external iliac artery, and the patient receiving sunitinib had a Stanford type B dissection from the aortic arch to the abdominal aorta. Both patients received necessary emergent care and survived. Additional case reports describing cardiovascular adverse effects included a report of acute myocardial infarction in 3 patients receiving sorafenib and Takotsubo cardiomyopathy occurring in a patient within 24 hours of starting axitinib therapy [15A,16A].

Gastrointestinal

Gastrointestinal adverse effects have been described with VEGF TKI, most commonly diarrhea; however, two recent case reports describe patients experiencing unique gastrointestinal distress. The first report described a 71-year-old male with hepatitis B and hepatocellular carcinoma who experienced pneumoperitoneum, pneumoretroperitoneum, and pneumatosis intestinalis of the jejunum [17A]. The patient was receiving sorafenib for 4 weeks when he began to experience progressive abdominal distension. Symptoms resolved upon discontinuation of the sorafenib and did not reoccur when resumed at a lower dosage. The second report was of a 50-year-old female with small intestinal stromal tumor, receiving regorafenib after failing imatinib and sunitinib [18A]. Ten days after starting regorafenib, the patient experienced liver failure and an elevated LDH, which was determined to be consistent with impaired blood flow. The patient improved with plasma exchange and steroids.

A recent meta-analysis also investigated the incidence of pancreatitis with VEGF pathway inhibitors (sunitinib, sorafenib, pazopanib, axitinib, vandetanib, cabozantinib, ponatinib, regorafenib) [19M]. All grade pancreatitis was elevated in those receiving these medications (HR 1.95, 95% CI 1.02–3.70, $p = 0.042$); however, high grade pancreatitis was not significantly elevated (HR 1.89, 95% CI 0.95–373, $p = 0.069$). Malignancy type and agent did not appear to impact the rate of pancreatitis.

Endocrine

Thyroid toxicity associated with the VEGF TKI has been reported in prior studies and was found to occur in 13% of those in the worldwide treatment use trial described above [2MC]. Furthermore, a retrospective evaluation of 62 patients receiving sunitinib demonstrated hypothyroidism in 19% which was preceded by thyrotoxicosis in 2 patients (3.2%) [20c]. On top of the thyroid toxicity associated with sunitinib, hypoglycemia was reported in a 60-year-old male receiving sunitinib for renal cell carcinoma [21A]. The patient had a history of type 2 diabetes mellitus and was receiving glimepiride. Fourteen days after starting sunitinib, the patient had grade 3 thrombocytopenia and hypoglycemia. At that time, glimepiride was discontinued. Five days later, the patient was admitted to the ED with loss of consciousness and blood glucose of 42 mg/dL. Hypoglycemia continued despite oral intake and dextrose infusion. Over the next 2 weeks, the glucose gradually rose, and the patient was discharged. Sunitinib was restarted at a lower dosage, and the patient did not have any further issues; nor did he require any further anti-diabetic medications.

Dermatologic

Hand foot syndrome has been described with many of the VEGF TKI and continues to be reported as a significant adverse effect, along with other dermatologic reactions. In a phase II trial of cabozantinib in urothelial carcinoma, 73% of the 41 patients enrolled developed skin toxic effects [22c]. Most common dermatologic effects reported included hand foot syndrome (44%), hair depigmentation (44%), xerosis (20%), scrotal erythema/ulceration (15%), and nail splinter hemorrhages (12%). Thirty percent required dose reductions which led to decreased symptoms; however, the dermatologic reactions did not resolve fully until the drug was discontinued.

Due to the problematic nature of these dermatologic reactions, management strategies are necessary. Two studies were published describing management options for hand foot syndrome. The first study investigated the prophylactic use of urea-based cream in patients receiving sorafenib [23C]. Patients were randomized to receive either 10% urea-based cream three times daily or supportive care without creams. Any grade hand foot skin reaction was reduced in those receiving the urea-based cream (56% vs 73.6%, $p < 0.001$), as were grade 2 or higher reactions (20.7% vs 29.2%, $p = 0.004$). Time to hand foot skin reactions was also increased to 84 days compared to 34 days ($p < 0.001$). Despite these benefits, there was no effect on the rate of dose reduction or interruption (9.1% vs. 11.8%, $p = 0.1937$). From this study, it remains a question whether urea-based creams would be better than the current standard of care, use of prophylactic basic emollients. The second study utilized a 1% sildenafil cream to treat patients with grade 1–3 hand foot syndrome due to capecitabine or sunitinib [24c]. It is believed that sildenafil may provide relief via its effects on the nitric oxide pathway. Patients served as their own control, using the sildenafil cream on one extremity and placebo on the other. Of the 9 evaluable patients, 5 described some improvement in symptoms, but there was no difference in pain scores or grading of the hand foot syndrome. One patient described improvement in tactile function.

In addition to the typical dermatologic reactions described above, case reports have described other reactions including a photoallergic reaction and Stevens–Johnson syndrome [25A,26A]. The patient experiencing the photoallergic reaction was a 51-year-old Caucasian female with follicular thyroid carcinoma, receiving vandetanib in combination with everolimus [25A]. The reaction developed over 3–4 days, approximately 1 month after starting the vandetanib. Erythematous eczematous plaques with vesication spread over sun exposed area. The patient had experienced heavy sun exposure 2 weeks prior during which time she wore long sleeves and pants and applied SPF 50 sunscreen. Subsequently, the patient had daily sun exposure without sunscreen. The vandetanib and everolimus were discontinued, and the patient was given methylprednisolone, hydroxyzine, clobetasol shampoo, triamcinolone cream and antibiotics. Erythema decreased over the next week, and the patient was restarted on therapy once the steroid course was complete. The patient experiencing Stevens–Johnson syndrome experienced the reaction 9 days after starting regorafenib for recurrent rectal carcinoma [26A]. Resolution of the reaction occurred after stopping the medication and administering oral and topical steroids.

Lupus erythematosus and subcorneal pustular dermatosis have also been reported to occur with VEGF TKI. A 67-year-old male receiving pazopanib for renal cell carcinoma developed wide spread photo distributed erythematous annular and polycyclic scaly lesions 30 days after starting the drug [27A]. Biopsy, antinuclear antibody (ANA) of 1:160 and positive anti-Ro/SSA antibodies led to a diagnosis of lupus erythematous. Pazopanib was discontinued, and the patient was given topical betamethasone and sun protection. Lesions improved after 3 weeks but did not resolve completely. After 3 months, lesions were still mild, and the anti-Ro/SSA remained positive. The patient with subcorneal pustular dermatosis occurring within 70 days of starting sorafenib was a 76-year-old male who experienced multiple erythematous skin eruptions in a circular or linear pattern with itching and pain on extremities [28A]. The reaction persisted for 7 months despite treatment with topical steroid and a sorafenib dose reduction. The reaction did not resolve until sorafenib was discontinued.

Muscloskeletal

Pediatric data regarding TKI use are often limited; however, a report of growth abnormalities in pediatric patients during VEGF TKI administration was recently published [29c]. In an analysis of 53 pediatric patients receiving anti-VEGF therapy (35 receiving TKI, 13 receiving monoclonal antibodies, and 5 receiving angiopoietin), 9.4% developed growth plate abnormalities. One patient was receiving sunitinib, and 4 patients were receiving pazopanib. Four patients experienced growth plate widening, and an additional patient experienced both widening and physeal cartilage hypertrophy. Reversal of abnormalities was observed after discontinuation.

Pharmacogenomics

A case report provided some insight into those who may be at increased risk for adverse effects due to sunitinib [30A]. The patient was a Japanese woman with metastatic renal cell carcinoma, receiving sunitinib 50 mg daily. On day 11, the patient developed fever and was found to have severe thrombocytopenia and elevated transaminases which persisted for 1 week. Sunitinib was discontinued on day 12. The patient further developed a pleural effusion and edema. On day 14, the sunitinib level along with the level of its major active metabolite were found to be elevated. On day 25, toxicities resolved. Genomic testing was completed to check for SNPs in CYP 3A5, ABCB1, and ABCG2. The patient was found to be homozygous for the variant allele of ABCG2 421 C > A. This variant is threefold more common in Asians than in Caucasians and may be related to the altered metabolism and subsequent toxicity observed in this patient.

EPIDERMAL GROWTH FACTOR RECEPTOR (EGFR) INHIBITORS

Similar to the group of medications targeting the VEGF pathway, there are also multiple inhibitors of the EGFR pathway with multiple indications. Inhibitors of EGFR prevent downstream signaling from the EGFR receptors. Included in this review are afatinib, erlotinib, osimertinib, and gefitinib. This group also includes the inhibitor of the HER2 tyrosine kinase, lapatinib, as the HER2 receptor is part of the EGFR family. Recent large trials showed that acneiform rash, nail effects, diarrhea, and stomatitis were the most common adverse effects [31C,32C,33C,34C,35C,36MC]. The incidence of grade 3 adverse effects and serious adverse effects varied depending on the trial with 12.3–40% experiencing grade 3 or higher adverse effects and 6–36.9% experienced serious adverse effects [31C,32C,35C,36MC]. The most common grade 3 or higher adverse effects included diarrhea, rash, and acne. Adverse effects resulting in dose reductions were common, occurring in 32–75% of the population. Drug discontinuation due to adverse effects was necessary in 7–18.5% [31C,33C]. In a trial comparing afatinib and erlotinib, grade 3 diarrhea and stomatitis were more common with afatinib, while grade 3 rash and acne were more common with erlotinib [34C]. Serious adverse events occurred in 12% of those receiving afatinib and 6% of those receiving erlotinib. Likewise, dose reduction was necessary more often in those receiving afatinib (27% vs. 14%).

EGFR mutations occur more frequently in the Asian population with non-small cell lung cancer (NSCLC), and TKI are considered first-line therapy in those with mutations. Two studies included an Asian population receiving erlotinib for NSCLC, one with 519 Chinese patients and the other with 10708 Japanese patients [37C,38MC]. In the study of Chinese patients, 23% experienced adverse effects with 7.7% developing grade 3 or 4 adverse effects [37C]. There was one death due to interstitial lung disease and few serious adverse events (perianal abscess, grade 3 liver dysfunction, interstitial lung disease). In the Japanese population, 79% developed adverse effects with the majority being skin disorders (67%), rash

(61%), diarrhea (22%), and hepatic dysfunction (10%) [38MC]. The median times to onset for common adverse effects include 9 days for rash, 8 days for diarrhea, and 13 days for hepatic dysfunction. Another subgroup analysis of a Japanese population in a larger lung cancer population showed similar trends with the most common adverse effects being diarrhea, rash, acne, nail effects, and stomatitis [33C].

In a study of 62 patients receiving erlotinib for NSCLC with a focus on patient experience and adherence, mean adherence was 96.8% [39c]. The most common symptoms reported include fatigue (91%), rash (86%), and cough (77%). Severe symptoms reported after 1 month of treatment included rash (39%), fatigue (32%), sleeping problems (29%), and anorexia (21%). Stomatitis was a risk factor for taking erlotinib incorrectly; however, other symptoms described did not appear to impact adherence.

In a HRQoL study of lapatinib, quality of life (QOL) score decreased in both those receiving lapatinib and those receiving placebo without reaching significance [40MC]. Despite similar decreases in quality of life, patients receiving lapatinib experienced an increased incidence of diarrhea and rash. Lapatinib also significantly decreased scores for social functioning.

Dermatologic

Skin adverse effects, mainly acneiform rash, are common occurrences with EGFR inhibitors and have been associated with response. Despite this, they can be serious requiring dose reduction or interruption. Multiple meta-analyses describing the incidence of rash have been performed. In one meta-analysis of 17 trials of TKI vs. chemotherapy for NSCLC, rash was more common in those receiving the EGFR TKI in the first- or second-line setting (OR 24.54, 95% CI 6.81–88.47, $p < 0.0001$ for first-line therapy and OR 7.72, 95% CI 3.7–16.11, $p < 0.0001$ for second line therapy) [41M]. In another meta-analysis of 8 studies, including 2962 patients receiving EGFR TKI or chemotherapy for first-line treatment of NSCLC, grade 3 rash occurred more commonly in those receiving an EGFR TKI (HR 11.79, 95% CI 4.68–29.66, $p < 0.001$) [42M]. Furthermore, in a pooled safety analysis of 21 phase II/III trials including 1468 patients receiving EGFR TKI for the treatment of NSCLC, rash was one of the most commonly observed adverse effects [43M]. Interestingly, grade 3 rash occurred more frequently with afatinib compared to erlotinib (15% vs. 8.8%, respectively, $p = 0.003$) and more frequently with erlotinib compared to gefitinib (8.8% vs 3.5%, respectively, $p = 0.0008$). There were no differences in incidence related to whether the TKI were being administered for first-line therapy or for second-line treatment and beyond. There were also no differences in the incidence of rash between Asians and

non-Asians. In yet another meta-analysis of 9 trials including 1774 patients receiving EGFR TKI or chemotherapy, rash occurred more frequently in those receiving the TKI [44M]. Both gefitinib and erlotinib had a lower risk of rash compared to afatinib, similar to the other meta-analysis (RR 0.41, 95% CI 0.25–0.65 for gefitinib vs afatinib; RR 0.41, 95% CI 0.26–0.66 for erlotinib vs afatinib). The previously described meta-analyses did not include lapatinib. In a meta-analysis specific to lapatinib trials, all grade skin rash, hand foot syndrome, and pruritus were increased (RR 3.04, 95% CI 2.33–3.96, $p < 0.001$ for skin rash; RR 4.45, 95% CI 1.15–17.19, $p = 0.03$ for hand foot syndrome; RR 2.02, 95% CI 1.46–2.8, $p < 0.001$ for pruritus) [45M].

In addition to the large meta-analyses describing dermatologic adverse effects associated with EGFR TKI, two case reports were published, one with erlotinib and one with gefitinib. The case report involving erlotinib for the treatment of NSCLC in a 56-year-old male described the occurrence of papulovesicular skin lesions, present on FDG PET/CT as multiple areas of uptake [46A]. The areas corresponded to subcutaneous nodules on CT and pustular nodules on exam. It was noted that without correct characterization of the lesions, they could be mistakenly interpreted as cutaneous metastases. The second case report involved a 42-year-old female receiving gefitinib, pemetrexed, and cisplatin for the treatment of metastatic NSCLC [47A]. On the eighth day of gefitinib, the patient developed an acne-like rash, oral ulcers, conjunctivitis, and fever. The rash evolved into blisters and ulcerated. The gefitinib was discontinued, and the patient was started on steroids and immunoglobulin. Re-epithelization of denuded skin occurred within 40 days. The patient was retreated with another EGFR TKI (icotinib, available in China) without recurrence.

Gastrointestinal

Similar to rash, gastrointestinal adverse effects, particularly diarrhea, have been reported in prior trials of EGFR TKI. In a recent meta-analysis of EGFR TKI for first-line treatment of NSCLC including 8 studies and 2962 patients, grade 3 diarrhea was more common in those receiving TKI compared to chemotherapy (HR 5.69, 95% 1.69–19.60, $p < 0.001$) [42M]. Interestingly, in the pooled safety analysis described previously, grade 3 diarrhea was more common with afatinib and equivalent with erlotinib and gefitinib (9.6% vs 2.7%, $p < 0.001$, afatinib vs. erlotinib, respectively; 2.7% vs. 1.1%, $p = 0.10$, erlotinib vs. gefitinib, respectively) [43M]. There was no difference in the incidence of diarrhea between Asians and non-Asians. This study also investigated the incidence of hepatotoxicity. Grade 3 hepatotoxicity was more common in gefitinib compared to erlotinib (18% vs 5.4%,

$p < 0.001$) and more common in erlotinib compared to afatinib (5.4% vs. 1.7%, $p = 0.037$). There was an increased incidence of hepatotoxicity in Asians compared to non-Asians (18.5% vs. 3.2%, $p = 0.027$). Another meta-analysis demonstrated that diarrhea was more common in those receiving TKI compared to those receiving chemotherapy [44M]. In this same meta-analysis, afatinib again showed a higher risk for diarrhea (RR 0.29, 95% CI 0.2–0.41 for gefitinib vs. afatinib; 0.36, 95% CI 0.25–0.54 for erlotinib vs. afatinib) and gefitinib showed a higher risk for elevated transaminases compared to both erlotinib and afatinib (RR 2.02, 95% CI 1.17–3.46 for gefitinib vs. afatinib; RR 2.29, 95% CI 1.63–3.23 for gefitinib vs. erlotinib). A meta-analysis including only erlotinib for NSCLC echoed the above results [48M]. This analysis included 19 trials and 7524 patients. All grade diarrhea (RR 2.96, 95% CI 2.37–3.8, $p < 0.001$) and stomatitis (RR 3.62, 95% CI 2.43–5.39, $p = 0.00001$) and high grade diarrhea (RR 4.65, 95% CI 3.3–6.55, $p < 0.001$) occurred more frequently in those receiving erlotinib. A meta-analysis of lapatinib studies also demonstrated an elevated risk of all grade stomatitis (RR 1.67, 95% CI 1.02–2.3, $p < 0.04$) with this medication [45M].

Two case reports were also published describing unique gastrointestinal adverse effects. A 55-year-old female receiving erlotinib for metastatic NSCLC cancer developed coffee-ground emesis, sepsis, and multi-organ failure after experiencing dysphasia and epigastric pain for 3 days [49A]. An esophagogastroduodenoscopy (EGD) demonstrated a black esophagus also known as acute esophageal necrosis. The patient passed away due to sepsis and multi-organ failure. A 57-year-old male with pancreatic cancer who was receiving erlotinib and capecitabine for 2 months experienced maroon stools shortly after discontinuation of the regimen [50A]. An EGD was completed, and the patient was found to have radiation gastritis (the patient previously received radiation with capecitabine). The patient was treated with argon plasma coagulation and required multiple admissions over the next 2 months due to gastrointestinal bleeds requiring repeat EGDs and transfusions. Radiation recall gastritis was attributed to the erlotinib therapy in this case.

Pulmonary

Interstitial lung disease (ILD) has been reported at a low frequency in trials of EGFR TKI and can be fatal as demonstrated in a recent case report of a 67-year-old with pancreatic cancer receiving erlotinib and gemcitabine [51A]. In a meta-analysis of gefitinib, erlotinib, and afatinib use, all grade ILD occurred in 1.6% with grade 3 or higher occurring in 0.9% [52M]. The ILD resulted in death in 13% of the cases. Compared to control, TKI increased the risk of all grade (OR 1.74, 95% CI 1.25–2.43, $p = 0.001$) and high grade (OR 4.38, 95% CI 2.18–8.79, $p < 0.001$) ILD. No differences were noted in the risk of ILD between agents. These results were echoed in the previously described pooled safety analysis which found there was no difference between the agents in the risk of ILD [43M]. In the same analysis, Asian patients were compared to non-Asians and found to have a similar incidence of interstitial lung disease (2.5% vs. 0.9%, $p = 0.11$). However, when comparing Japanese to non-Japanese Asians, those of Japanese descent had an increased risk for ILD (3.8% vs. 0.3%, $p = 0.0009$).

Management of ILD usually involves discontinuation of the offending agent and administration of high dose steroids. It is largely unclear whether or not patients can be safely restarted on the offending agent after resolution. In a case report of a 63-year-old male, with EGFR mutated NSCLC, the patient was started on erlotinib as second-line therapy [53A]. Two weeks after therapy initiation, the patient developed rapidly progressive dyspnea, cough and fever. One week later, he was admitted to the hospital due to acute respiratory distress. CT demonstrated bilateral interstitial lung density, and the patient required intubation and high dose steroids. The patient recovered and was discharged 2 months later. Due to good disease response to erlotinib, the decision was made to restart the drug at a reduced dose (50 mg daily) in combination with prednisone. The patient tolerated this, and the dose was increased to 100 mg daily without any further lung toxicity. Due to disease progression, the drug was discontinued and restarted 2 months later at a dose of 150 mg daily in combination with bevacizumab and prednisone 5 mg daily. The patient tolerated treatment for 10 months at this dose. This case demonstrates that restarting the offending medication may be considered in select cases in combination with continued steroid use.

Ophthalmic

Ophthalmic adverse effects have been described in clinical trials of EGFR inhibitors. In two of the more recent trials of afatinib, grade 1 and 2 conjunctivitis was described to occur in one trial in 5% (grade 3 occurred in <1% or 2 of the 322 patients receiving afatinib) and ocular effects occurred in 42.6% of Japanese patients in a subgroup analysis of a large phase III trial (most adverse effects were grade 1 or 2; grade 3 ocular effects occurred in 1.9% or 1 of the 54 patients receiving afatinib) [31C,33C]. In addition to being observed in these clinical trials, a case report was published describing ocular effects in a 74-year-old female receiving erlotinib for NSCLC [54A]. The patient developed irritation, excessive elongation of eyelashes, blepharitis, and tear film dysfunction. She was able to tolerate therapy for 6 months with supportive care including monthly eyelash trimming and intensive topical lubrication.

Renal

Renal adverse effects are rarely reported with EGFR TKI. Nevertheless, a case report of a renal adverse effect in a 57-year-old female with metastatic NSCLC receiving gefitinib was published [55A]. Six months after starting gefitinib, the patient experienced edema of the lower limbs, weight gain, hypoalbuminemia, hyperlipidemia, and proteinuria. She was diagnosed with nephrotic syndrome. Gefitinib was discontinued and within 2 months, urine protein decreased while albumin increased. The patient did not receive any additional treatment besides gefitinib discontinuation for the nephrotic syndrome. A few months after resolution, erlotinib was started without further renal effects.

ANAPLASTIC LYMPHOMA KINASE (ALK) INHIBITOR

ALK inhibitors represent a newer group of medications utilized mostly for the treatment of NSCLC expressing the ELM4–ALK fusion gene. Inhibition of these mutated tyrosine kinases prevents intracellular signaling from the ALK mutation, leading to decreased cellular proliferation. Medications reviewed here include: crizotinib, ceritinib, and alectinib. In a phase III trial of first-line crizotinib for treatment of ALK mutated NSCLC, the most common adverse effects observed in the crizotinib arm included: visual disorder (71%), diarrhea (61%), nausea (56%), and edema (49%) [56C]. Grade 3 and 4 aminotransferase elevations occurred in 15% and 11% experienced neutropenia. One case of fatal pneumonitis was observed. Overall, despite the adverse effects, there was a reduction in lung cancer symptoms and improved QOL compared to chemotherapy. In an analysis of 3 patients receiving ceritinib for anaplastic large-cell lymphoma, adverse effects observed included diarrhea, fatigue, aminotransferase elevations, vomiting, diarrhea, and acute pericarditis [57c].

Pulmonary

One patient in the phase III trial described above experienced fatal ILD [56C]. A case report of a 75-year-old female with metastatic NSCLC receiving third-line therapy with alectinib was also published describing this pulmonary toxicity [58A]. After 102 days of alectinib therapy, a chest CT demonstrated patchy/diffuse ground glass opacities. The patient was asymptomatic and

diagnosed with grade 1 ILD. Alectinib was discontinued and azithromycin was started. The report did not mention any further issues or complications after alectinib discontinuation.

Hypersensitivity

Two reports of hypersensitivity were published recently describing reactions with crizotinib. The first occurred in a 78-year-old female with ALK mutated NSCLC [59A]. Forty days after starting crizotinib, the patient experienced hives on the head, chest and back 4 hours after ingesting her morning dose. One hour after the evening dose, the reaction intensified with facial edema. The patient received dexchlorpheniramine intramuscularly and cetirizine orally and the symptoms resolved within 10 hours. The decision was made to continue crizotinib via a rapid oral desensitization protocol. The patient received dexchlorpheniramine and methylprednisolone intramuscularly followed by increasing doses of a crizotinib suspension. Doses were administered at 30 minute intervals until a cumulative dose of 200 mg was administered. After receiving this desensitization protocol, the patient tolerated crizotinib for 7 months. In a second case report, a 63-year-old female with ALK mutated NSCLC experienced erythema multiforme 1 week after initiation of crizotinib [60A]. The offending agent was discontinued, and topical clobetasol ointment was initiated. The patient improved within 1 week without developing severe complications such as Steven's–Johnson syndrome.

Gastrointestinal

Gastrointestinal adverse effects are frequently observed with ALK TKI, including diarrhea observed in 61% and nausea in 56% of those in the most recent phase III trial of crizotinib [565C]. Besides these, case reports have been published describing an esophageal injury and dysgeusia [61A, 62A]. A 69-year male with NSCLC receiving crizotinib developed pneumonia and crizotinib was held [61A]. Crizotinib was restarted upon resolution and 19 days after resuming therapy, the patient developed retrosternal pain. An EGD revealed an esophageal lesion with ulceration likely due to retention of a medication tablet within the esophagus. It was determined that crizotinib was the most likely cause of the ulceration; therefore, administration with the patient in the upright position with plenty of fluids may be necessary to prevent such injuries. In a 54-year-old female with NSCLC receiving crizotinib, the patient noticed dysgeusia 5 days after therapy initiation [62A]. This deteriorated to a grade 3 toxicity and progressive appetite loss. The patient was unable to discern between salty, sweet, sour, and bitter.

She experienced a 2 kg weight loss in 2 weeks. Crizotinib was discontinued and symptoms improved after 2 weeks. Upon re-initiation of crizotinib, dysgeusia returned, and the patient was changed to alectinib without any further taste alterations.

Neurologic

Vision disorders were the most common adverse effect in the most recent phase III trial occurring in 71% [56C]. In this trial, vision disorders included visual impairment, photopsia, blurred vision, vitreous floaters, reduced visual acuity, diplopia, and photophobia. The majority of visual disorders were mild (grade 1 and 2) with grade 3 and 4 vision disorders occurring in 10%. In a case report of a 69-year-old female receiving crizotinib for NSCLC, the patient developed progressive vision loss [63]. The patient had a history of brain metastases which were stable. Mild visual shadows were experienced 3 weeks after crizotinib initiation followed by progressive vision loss 3 months later. MRI demonstrated optic neuropathy. Crizotinib was discontinued and the visual field defects persisted. After stabilization of the visual field defects (approximately 3 months later), crizotinib was restarted. Upon re-initiation, the patient once again developed visual field deficits of the right optic pathway.

INHIBITORS OF THE MITOGEN-ACTIVATED PROTEIN (MAP) KINASE PATHWAY (B-Raf AND MEK INHIBITORS)

B-Raf TKI and MEK TKI inhibit the MAP kinase pathway which is activated in those with certain malignancies, especially those with B-Raf mutations. Inhibition of the B-Raf kinase with TKI may be instituted alone or in combination with MEK inhibition. Dabrafenib has been successfully combined with trametinib, while vemurafenib has been combined with cobimetinib. Trametinib has also been utilized as a single agent. Combination therapy is often administered because resistance to B-Raf inhibition can occur due to reactivation of the MAP kinase pathway which is further blocked by the MEK TKI. Additionally, the adverse effect profile is altered with combination therapy. Two large phase III trials of patients with melanoma and B-Raf V600E or B-Raf V600K mutations were published comparing combination therapy (dabrafenib + trametinib) and monotherapy with either dabrafenib or vemurafenib [64C,65C]. The vemurafenib monotherapy trial included 352 patients in each group, and the dabrafenib monotherapy trial included 211 in the combination

group and 212 in the monotherapy group. The adverse effect profiles were similar in both trials. Adverse effects occurring in more than 20% of the population receiving combination therapy were: pyrexia, nausea, diarrhea, chills, vomiting, arthralgia, rash, and fatigue. Patients receiving B-Raf inhibitor monotherapy experienced the following in more than 20% of the population: pyrexia, fatigue, rash, nausea, diarrhea, arthralgia, hyperkeratosis, hand foot syndrome, alopecia, skin papilloma, photosensitivity, and cutaneous squamous cell carcinoma (cSCC). Though there were overlapping toxicities observed in the combination and monotherapy groups, patients in the monotherapy group experienced more dermatologic adverse effects, especially in the occurrence of cSCC which was observed in 20% of the population receiving dabrafenib and 18% receiving vemurafenib compared to 1–3% receiving combination therapy. This difference is likely due to the fact that with monotherapy, cells lacking B-Raf mutations have a contrary reaction, in which the MAP kinase pathway becomes activated resulting in secondary skin tumors. Overall adverse effect rates were similar between groups (87–98% with combination therapy and 90–99% with monotherapy). In the vemurafenib trial, grade 3 or higher adverse effects occurred in 52% receiving the combination compared to 63% receiving monotherapy [64C]. Likewise, grade 3 adverse effects in the dabrafenib trial occurred in 32% receiving combination therapy compared to 30% receiving monotherapy [65C]. In an additional small trial ($n = 13$) of dabrafenib for 14 days followed by combination therapy for 14 days prior to surgery for melanoma, adverse effects were similar with fatigue, rash, nausea, myalgia, pyrexia and hand foot syndrome being reported [66c].

In addition to the description of adverse effects in the combination vs. monotherapy trials described above, HRQoL results were published for these trials [67C,68C]. In the dabrafenib vs. dabrafenib + trametinib trial, the combination therapy resulted in significantly increased global health dimension scores [67C]. The functional domains represented in the European Organization for Research and Treatment of Cancer Quality of Life Questionaire-C30 (physical, role, emotional, cognitive, and social functioning) all trended in favor of the combination arm. Moreover, pain scores were significantly improved with the combination. Symptom scores related to nausea/vomiting, dyspnea, constipation, and diarrhea trended in favor of dabrafenib monotherapy. Similarly, the trial of vemurafenib vs. dabrafenib + trametinib demonstrated a significant increase in global health status scores and higher scores for physical, role, emotional, cognitive, and social functioning [68C]. Symptoms scores were also significantly lower in favor of the combination for pain, fatigue, nausea/vomiting, insomnia, appetite loss, and diarrhea.

SPECIAL REVIEW

Dermatologic

Dermatologic reactions are common, particularly in those receiving monotherapy with the B-Raf inhibitors. In the phase III trials, the incidence of rash with monotherapy was 43% with vemurafenib and 20% with dabrafenib [64C,65C]. In a case series of 5 patients with melanoma receiving vemurafenib, dermatologic adverse effects included: photosensitivity, keratoacanthoma, actinic keratosis, and alopecia in a 66-year-old female; cSCC in a 76-year-old male; keratosis pilaris-like rash, thinning of the hair, plantar hyperkeratosis, verrucous papilloma, and cSCC in a 71-year-old male; melanoma in situ in a 49-year-old male; erythema nodosum and photosensitivity in a 35-year-old male [69A].

Photosensitivity was also commonly observed in vemurafenib clinical trials, occurring in 22%. Not only has photosensitivity been reported with sun exposure, but also with indoor lighting. A 45-year-old female, a 32-year-old male, and a 53-year-old male experienced photosensitivity while receiving vemurafenib for metastatic melanoma [70A]. The patients were all exposed to indoor fluorescent lamps. One patient's symptoms resolved by changing to LED lighting, while the others resolved with avoidance and wearing a baseball cap. Fluorescent lighting emits UVA radiation, and these cases demonstrate that minimal amounts of UV radiation may cause photosensitivity with vemurafenib. Another case of photosensitivity 1 week after starting vemurafenib for the treatment of melanoma in a 41-year-old male was reported [71A]. The patient developed a photosensitivity reaction with blistering and skin erosion on sun exposed areas. Despite sun avoidance and topical steroids, minimal improvement was observed; therefore, the patient was started on oral steroids for 3 weeks followed by a tapering of the dosing. Nine months later, the patient was still receiving dexamethasone 4 mg daily and still experiencing persistent blistering, erosions, and erythema on both hands. New lesions developed 1 month later on the forearm and chest. Further investigation demonstrated Trichophyton rubrum. Topical clotrimazole and ultimately a course of oral itraconazole decreased the severity of the lesions.

Secondary skin malignancies, likely due to paradoxically increased MAP kinase pathway signaling in the absence of concomitant MEK inhibition in cells without B-Raf mutations, were observed in phase III trials and have been described in case reports. In a 67-year-old female receiving vemurafenib for the treatment of melanoma, skin lesions developed within 2 weeks of starting the medication [72A]. The patient experienced a grade 2 folliculocentric eruption on the body and face which was treated successfully with topical clobetasol. The patient went on to develop 3 hyperkeratotic lesions on the neck and trunk within the first 6 weeks of therapy which when excised, one was squamous cell carcinoma. The patient also developed 3 hyperkeratotic lesions on her lower extremity which were again excised and determined to be keratoacanthoma-like squamous

cell carcinoma, well-differentiated squamous cell carcinoma and hyperkeratotic squamoproliferative lesion with squamous cell carcinoma. The patient further developed three additional lesions consistent with squamous cell carcinoma on the opposite lower extremity which were unable to be excised. Treatment with topical fluorouracil 5% cream daily was instituted, and the patient experienced a complete resolution of the skin lesions within 7 weeks. In another patient, a 45-year-old female receiving vemurafenib for the treatment of melanoma, secondary malignancies were observed [73A]. In the first year of treatment with vemurafenib, the patient developed 6 primary melanomas (two tested negative for B-Raf mutations), 2 atypical melanocytic proliferations, and 9 dysplastic nevi. These cutaneous changes, though not squamous cell carcinoma, were believed to be secondary to the vemurafenib treatment.

Multiple case reports have been published describing additional cutaneous adverse effects of B-Raf TKI monotherapy. A 70-year-old male receiving vemurafenib for metastatic melanoma developed pruritic eruptions on the upper trunk and extremities 2 weeks after starting therapy [74A]. Biopsy results demonstrated eccrine squamous syringometaplasia with marked follicular hyperplasia. Two weeks later, the patient had new lesions on his chest, back, and lower extremities, several of which were determined to be well-differentiated squamous cell carcinomas and keratoacanthomas. The patient was started on acitretin 10 mg daily which led to decreased pruritus and improvement of his initial follicular eruption within 4 weeks. Moreover, his keratoacanthomas decreased in size over this time. Another 50-year-old male receiving vemurafenib for melanoma developed an asymptomatic skin eruption characterized by white, globular, follicular bound, superficial keratinous cysts on his face, chest, and upper back within 7 weeks of starting therapy [75A]. The patient refused treatment for the lesions. Within 10 weeks, the patient developed several keratoacanthoma and squamous cancer in sun exposed areas. The patient continued treatment with vemurafenib for 8 months in total without treatment for his asymptomatic skin lesions. In a 15-year-old female with brainstem glioma, vemurafenib for 10 months led to tender axillary and lower extremity lesions [76A]. Biopsy demonstrated neutrophilic panniculitis. The patient did not receive any treatment and the symptoms slowly improved despite continuing vemurafenib therapy. Radiation recall was also observed in a patient with melanoma when vemurafenib was initiated 5 weeks after completing radiation [77A]. The dermatitis appeared 1 week after initiation of the vemurafenib and resolved over the next 2 months with topical therapies and continuation of vemurafenib. A more common adverse effect, hand foot syndrome, occurred in a 50-year-old male receiving dabrafenib for melanoma [78A]. The patient developed a grade 2 reaction within 1 week of treatment initiation and progressed to grade 3 within 1 month. The patient received multiple topical therapies without improvement including tazarolen, lidocaine, urea, and clobetasol. The patient eventually required opiates to control pain. Dabrafenib was held and the patient experienced symptom relief within 2 *weeks. Dabrafenib therapy was resumed at half the dose, and the patient still required oral opiates to control pain. Pregabalin was started and within 1 week pain improved despite continuing dabrafenib. Lastly, a case series described multiple dermatologic adverse effects in patients receiving MEK inhibitors with or without B-Raf TKI [79A]. Three patients were included in the series, a male in his 60s and two females, one in her 40s and one in her 50s. The male had pancreatic cancer and was receiving treatment with selumetinib, a MEK inhibitor, in combination with an AKT inhibitor. Twelve days after starting, the patient experienced a generalized eruption characterized by diffuse targetoid patches with central duskiness and mild pruritus. The patient was started on topical steroids, and the medications were discontinued with resolution of symptoms observed after 4 weeks. In one of the females, the patient received vemurafenib and cobimetinib for metastatic melanoma. On day 28, she experienced a diffuse eruption with coalescing urticarial patches with surrounding duskiness. The medications were discontinued and oral prednisone was administered. Once symptoms resolved, the patient was restarted on cobimetinib at a decreased dose in combination with prednisone without any reoccurrence after 1 year. In the other female patient, dabrafenib and trametinib were initiated for melanoma. On week 7 of therapy, the patient experienced a pruritic eruption characterized by urticarial patches and plaques with surrounding diffuse duskiness. Trametinib was discontinued and oral prednisone administered. Trametinib was restarted 1 week later without recurrence.*

Many of the case reports above describe adverse cutaneous effects occurring relatively quickly upon therapy initiation. In a report of patients receiving long-term therapy (>52 weeks) with B-Raf TKI or the combination of B-Raf TKI and MEK inhibitors, 48 patients received therapy for greater than 52 weeks [80c]. Cutaneous adverse effects occurring in the B-Raf monotherapy group (n=38) included acantholytic dermatosis (45%), plantar hyperkeratosis (45%), actinic keratosis (26%), verrucal keratosis (18%), and cutaneous squamous cell carcinoma (16%). In the combination therapy group (n=10), cutaneous adverse effects included an acneiform eruption (40%), cyst formation (20%), and plantar hyperkeratosis (30%). This study demonstrates that despite the extent of cutaneous adverse effects and the rapidity with which they developed in the case reports above, some are able to tolerate these medications for prolonged periods of time.

Hypersensitivity

A 47-year-old female receiving vemurafenib for melanoma developed a severe reaction (urticaria, throat swelling, and dyspnea) to the medication within 5 days of initiation [81A]. She was switched to dabrafenib, and within 2 doses, she experienced another rash along with facial and throat selling. Due to these reactions, the patient received a desensitization protocol utilizing escalating doses of dabrafenib from 15 to 300 mg over 15 days.

Premedication included oral prednisone 40 mg daily and promethazine 25 mg twice daily. The prednisone was decreased to 5 mg every 4 days once the patient was tolerating the dabrafenib and she ended up tolerating it for 3 months. A similar case of vemurafenib-induced rash was also successfully mitigated via a slow desensitization which led to tolerability of the medication [82A].

Ocular

Ocular adverse effects have been reported in large phase III trials, including in the large trial described above of vemurafenib vs. dabrafenib + trametinib [73A]. In this study, 2 patients experienced grade 1 chorioretinopathy in the combination arm and 1 experienced this with vemurafenib monotherapy. In addition, a grade 2 retinal vein occlusion occurred in one patient receiving vemurafenib monotherapy. A small case series was also published describing the occurrence and severity of uveitis with vemurafenib treatment [83c]. Uveitis was observed in 7 patients with an average time to ocular signs of 5.6 months. The severity of the uveitis ranged from mild or low grade anterior uveitis to severe panuveitis with retinal detachment. All patients experienced uveitis bilaterally, and a majority were managed with local corticosteroids.

Myelosuppression

Myelosuppression was not reported in the large phase III trials; however, a case report of a 64-year-old female receiving vemurafenib for metastatic melanoma has been published [84A]. She developed severe leukopenia and neutropenia 5 weeks after starting therapy with normal red blood cell and platelet counts. The patient was changed to dabrafenib and the counts recovered within 4 days.

Renal

Fanconi syndrome was reported to be related to vemurafenib therapy in a case report of a 70-year-old male with metastatic melanoma [85A]. On day 9 of therapy, the patient developed fever and an erythematous maculopapular eruption with keratosis pilaris on his extremities and trunk along with photosensitivity on his face. His dose was reduced from 960 to 720 mg twice daily. On day 12, a decline in his potassium, phosphorus, and uric acid were noted and the patient was determined to have Fanconi Syndrome. Vemurafenib was discontinued on day 19 and the electrolytes normalized. On day 29, vemurafenib was restarted at half the dose, and on day 50, the patient again developed hypokalemia and hypouricemia. Vemurafenib was discontinued once again and electrolytes normalized. The patient was switched to dabrafenib and did not have any issues for 5 months.

Pyrexia

Pyrexia was observed in both phase III trials described previously [64C,65C]. It occurred in the combination arms more frequently and led to dose reductions, dose interruptions, and drug discontinuations. In a description of pyrexia occurring in a phase I/II trial with 201 patients receiving dabrafenib and trametinib, pyrexia occurred in 59% of the population [86c]. Pyrexia was grade 2 or higher in 60% of those experiencing this adverse effect, and the median time to onset was 19 days with a median duration of 9 days.

Cardiovascular

Cardiotoxicity was also reported in the large phase III trials, with a decrease in ejection fraction being observed in 8% of patients receiving combination therapy in one trial [64C] and led to permanent discontinuation in 1% of the population of both groups in the other trial [65C]. Furthermore, in a case report of an 11-year-old male receiving trametinib for relapsed neuroblastoma, the patient experienced grade 3 LV systolic dysfunction 13 days after starting therapy despite a normal baseline cardiac workup [87A]. Trametinib was discontinued on day 15, and the patient received lisinopril. The LV function improved to baseline after 35 days but echocardiogram demonstrated a persistent septal hypokinesis of the inferior ventral septum.

CONCLUSION

Tyrosine kinase inhibitors are quickly moving to the forefront of therapy for multiple malignancies. Although they lack the traditional adverse effects observed with cytotoxic chemotherapeutic agents, toxicity can be severe with these medications. Many of the adverse effects are unique to the TKI utilized; however, there is much overlap of toxicities within each subclass. As more are utilized, it is important to remember that patients may tolerate one better than another as demonstrated in many of the case reports described above. Due to the frequency of adverse effects with these medications, patients need to be followed closely and educated regarding potential side effects prior to starting therapy.

References

[1] Hochhaus A, O'Brien SG, Guilhot F, et al. Six-year follow-up of patients receiving imatinib for the first-line treatment of chronic myeloid leukemia. Leukemia. 2009;23(6):1054–61 [C].

[2] Reichardt P, Kang YK, Rukdowski P, et al. Clinical outcomes of patients with advanced gastrointestinal stromal tumors: safety and efficacy in a worldwide treatment-use trial of sunitinib. Cancer. 2015;121(9):1405–13 [MC].

[3] Cainap C, Qin S, Huang WT, et al. Linifanib versus sorafenib in patients with advanced hepatocellular carcinoma: results of a randomized phase III trial. J Clin Oncol. 2015;33(2):172–9 [MC].

[4] Choueiri TK, Escudier B, Powles T, et al. Cabozantinib versus everolimus in advanced renal-cell carcinoma. New Engl J Med. 2015;373:1814–23 [C].

[5] Li J, Qin S, Xu R, et al. Regorafenib plus best supportive care versus placebo plus best supportive care in Asian patients with previously treated metastatic colorectal cancer (CONCUR): a randomized, double-blind, placebo-controlled, phase 3 trial. Lancet Oncol. 2015;16:619–29 [C].

[6] Coens C, van der Graff WTA, Blay JY, et al. Health-related quality-of-life results from PALETTE: a randomized, double-blind, phase three trial of pazopanib versus placebo in patients with soft tissue sarcoma whose disease has progressed during or after prior chemotherapy-a European Organization for Research and Treatment of cancer soft tissue and bone sarcoma group global network study (EORTC 62072). Cancer. 2015;121:2933–41 [C].

[7] Ghatalia P, Morgan CJ, Je Y, et al. Congestive heart failure with vascular endothelial growth factor tyrosine kinase inhibitors. Crit Rev Oncol Hematol. 2015;94:228–37 [M].

[8] Abdel-Rahman O, Fouad M. Risk of cardiovascular toxicities in patients with solid tumors treated with sunitinib, axitinib, cediranib or regorafenib: an updated systematic review and comparative meta-analysis. Crit Rev Oncol Hematol. 2014;92:194–207 [M].

[9] Jones RL, Bendell JC, Smith DC, et al. A phase I open-label trial evaluating the cardiovascular safety of regorafenib in patients with advanced cancer. Cancer Chemother Pharmacol. 2015;76:777–84 [c].

[10] Ghatalia P, Je Y, Kaymakcalan MD, et al. QTc interval prolongation with vascular endothelial growth factor receptor tyrosine kinase inhibitors. Br J Cancer. 2015;112:296–305 [M].

[11] Ruiz-Garcia A, Houk BE, Pithavala YK, et al. Effect of axitinib on the QT interval in healthy volunteers. Cancer Chemother Pharmacol. 2015;75:619–28 [c].

[12] Rini BI, Quinn DI, Baum M, et al. Hypertension among patients with renal cell carcinoma receiving axitinib or sorafenib: analysis from the randomized phase III AXIS trial. Target Oncol. 2015;10:45–53 [C].

[13] Niwa N, Nishiyama T, Ozu C, et al. Acute aortic dissection in a patient with metastatic renal cell carcinoma treated with axitinib. Acta Oncol. 2015;34(4):561–2 [A].

[14] Formiga MN, Fanelli MF. Aortic dissection during antiangiogenic therapy with sunitinib. A case report. Sao Paulo Med J. 2015;133(3):275–7 [A].

[15] Takagi K, Takai M, Kawata K, et al. Three patients with acute myocardial infarction association with targeted therapy of sorafenib for metastatic renal cell carcinoma: case report. Hinyokika Kiyo. 2015;61(9):347–51 [A].

[16] Ovadia D, Esquenazi Y, Bucay M, et al. Association between takotsubo cardiomyopathy and axitinib: case report and review of the literature. J Clin Oncol. 2015;33(1):e1–3 [A].

[17] Huang YH, Siao FY, Yen HH. Abdominal distension in a patient with hepatocellular carcinoma. Gastroenterology. 2015;149:e12–3 [A].

[18] Akamine T, Ando K, Oki E, et al. Acute liver failure due to regorafenib may be caused by impaired liver blood flow: A case report. Anticancer Res. 2015;35(7):4037–41 [A].

[19] Ghatalia P, Morgan CJ, Choueiri TK, et al. Pancreatitis with vascular endothelial growth factor receptor tyrosine kinase inhibitors. Crit Rev Oncol Hematol. 2015;94:136–45 [M].

[20] Jazvic M, Prpic M, Jukic T, et al. Sunitinib-induced thyrotoxicosis—a not so rare entity. Anticancer Res. 2015;35(1):481–5 [c].

[21] Demirci A, Bal O, Durnali A, et al. Sunitinib-induced severe hypoglycemia in a diabetic patient. J Oncol Pharm Pract. 2014;20(6):469–72 [A].

[22] Zou RC, Apolo AB, DiGiovana JJ, et al. Cutaneous adverse effects associated with the tyrosine-kinase inhibitor cabozantinib. JAMA Dermatol. 2015;151(2):170–7 [c].

[23] Ren ZG, Zhu KS, Kang HY, et al. Randomized controlled trial of the prophylactic effect of urea-based cream on sorafenib-associated hand-foot skin reactions in patients with advanced hepatocellular carcinoma. J Clin Oncol. 2015;33(8):894–900 [C].

[24] Meadows KL, Rushing C, Honeycutt W, et al. Treatment of palmar-plantar erythrodysesthesia (PPE) with topical sildenafil: a pilot study. Support Care Cancer. 2015;23:1311–9 [c].

[25] Goldstein J, Patel AB, Curry JL, et al. Photoallergic reaction in a patient receiving vandetanib for metastatic follicular thyroid carcinoma: a case report. BMC Dermatol. 2015;15:2–5 [A].

[26] Mihara Y, Yamaguchi K, Nakama T, et al. Steven–Johnson syndrome induced by regorafenib in a patient with progressive recurrent rectal carcinoma. Gan To Kaguku Ryoho. 2015;42(2):233–6 [A].

[27] Casado-Verrier B, Perez-Santos S, Delgado Mucientes C, et al. Subacute cutaneous lupus erythematosus induced by the new multikinase inhibitor pazopanib. Br J Dermatol. 2014;171:1555–608 [A].

[28] Tajiri K, Nakajima T, Kawai K, et al. Sneddon-Wilkinson disease induced by sorafenib in a patient with advanced hepatocellular carcinoma. Intern Med. 2015;54:597–600 [A].

[29] Voss SD, Glade-Bender J, Spunt SL. Growth plate abnormalities in pediatric cancer patients undergoing phase 1 anti-angiogenic therapy: a report from the Children's Oncology Group phase 1 consortium. Pediatr Blood Cancer. 2015;62(1):45–51 [c].

[30] Miura Y, Imamura CK, Fukunaga K, et al. Sunitinib-induced severe toxicities in a Japanese patient with the ABCG2 421 AA genotype. BMC Cancer. 2014;14:964 [A].

[31] Michiels JH, Haddad RI, Fayette J, et al. Afatinib versus methotrexate as second-line treatment in patients with recurrent or metastatic squamous-cell carcinoma of the head and neck progressing on or after platinum-based therapy (LUX-Head & Neck 1): an open-label, randomized phase 3 trial. Lancet Oncol. 2015;16:583–94 [C].

[32] Yang JC, Wu YL, Schuler M, et al. Afatinib versus cisplatin-based chemotherapy for EGFR mutation-positive lung adenocarcinoma (LUX-Lung 3 and LUX-Lung 6): analysis of overall survival data from two randomized, phase 3 trials. Lancet Oncol. 2015;16:141–51 [C].

[33] Kato T, Yoshioka H, Okamoto I, et al. Afatinib versus cisplatin plus pemetrexed in Japanese patients with advanced non-small cell lung cancer harboring activating EGFR mutations: subgroup analysis of LUX-Lung 3. Cancer Sci. 2015;106:1202–22 [C].

[34] Soria JC, Felip E, Cobo M, et al. Afatinib versus erlotinib as second-line treatment of patients with advanced squamous cell carcinoma of the lung (LUX-Lung8): an open-label randomized controlled phase 3 trial. Lancet Oncol. 2015;16:897–907 [C].

[35] Zhou Q, Cheng Y, Yang JJ, et al. Pemetrexed versus gefitinib as a second-line treatment in advanced nonsquamous nonsmall-cell lung cancer patients harboring wild-type EGFR (CTONG0806): a multicenter randomized trial. Ann Oncol. 2014;25:2385–91 [C].

[36] Scagliotti G, von Pawel J, Novello S, et al. Phase III multinational, randomized, double-blind, placebo-controlled study of tivantinib (ARQ 197) plus erlotinib versus erlotinib alone in previously treated patients with locally advanced or metastatic nonsquamous non-small-cell lung cancer. J Clin Oncol. 2015;33:2667–74 [MC].

[37] Huang Y, Zhang L, Shi Y, et al. Efficacy of erlotinib in previously treated patients with advanced non-small cell lung cancer: analysis of the Chinese subpopulation in the TRUST study. Jpn J Clin Oncol. 2015;45(6):569–75 [C].

[38] Gemma A, Kudoh S, Ando M, et al. Final safety and efficacy of erlotinib in the phase 4 POLARSTAR surveillance study of 10,708 Japanese patients with non-small-cell lung cancer. Cancer Sci. 2014;105(12):1584–90 [MC].

[39] Timmers L, Boons CCLM, Moes-ten Hove J, et al. Adherence, exposure and patients' experiences with the use of erlotinib in non-small cell lung cancer. J Cancer Res Clin Oncol. 2015;141: 1481–91 [c].

[40] Boyle FM, Smith IE, O'Shaughnessy J, et al. Health related quality of life of women in TEACH, a randomized placebo controlled adjuvant trial of lapatinib in early stage Human Epidermal Growth Factor Receptor (HER2) overexpressing breast cancer. Eur J Cancer. 2015;51:685–96 [MC].

[41] Zhang WQ, Li T, Li H. Efficacy of EGFR tyrosine kinase inhibitors in non-small-cell lung cancer patients with/without EGFR-mutation: evidence based on recent phase III randomized trials. Med Sci Monit. 2014;20:2666–76 [M].

[42] Normando SR, Cruz FM, del Giglio A. Cumulative meta-analysis of epidermal growth factor receptor-tyrosine kinase inhibitors as first-line therapy in metastatic non-small-cell lung cancer. Anticancer Drugs. 2015;26:559–1003 [M].

[43] Takeda M, Okamoto I, Nakagawa K. Pooled safety analysis of EGFR-TKI treatment for EGFR mutation-positive non-small cell lung cancer. Lung Cancer. 2015;88:74–9 [M].

[44] Haspinger ER, Agustoni F, Torri V, et al. Is there evidence for different effects among EGFR-TKIs? Systemic review and meta-analysis of EGFR tyrosine kinase inhibitors (TKIs) versus chemotherapy as first-line treatment for patients harboring EGFR mutations. Crit Rev Oncol Hematol. 2015;94:213–27 [M].

[45] Abdel-Rahman O, Fouad M. Risk of mucocutaneous toxicities in patients with solid tumors treated with lapatinib: a systemic review and meta-analysis. Curr Med Res Opin. 2015;31(5):975–86 [M].

[46] Kumar K, Singh H, Gupta RK, et al. Erlotinib-induced cutaneous toxicity: findings on ^{18}F-FDG PET/CT imaging. Clin Nucl Med. 2015;40:e251–2 [A].

[47] Huang JJ, Ma SX, Hou X, et al. Toxic epidermal necrolysis related to AP (pemetrexed plus cisplatin) and gefitinib combination therapy in a patient with metastatic non-small cell lung cancer. Chin J Cancer. 2015;34(2):94–8 [A].

[48] Abdel-Rahman O, Fouad M. Risk of gastrointestinal toxicities in patients with advanced non-small cell lung cancer receiving erlotinib: a systemic review and meta-analysis. Expert Rev Anticancer Ther. 2015;15(4):465–75 [M].

[49] Klair JS, Abraham RR, Jones J, et al. A 'shock-ing' endoscopic finding on esophagogastroduodenoscopy, BMJ Case Rep. 2015; http://casereports.bmj.com/content/2015/bcr-2014-205599. long [A].

[50] Graziani C, Hedge S, Saif MW. Radiation recall gastritis secondary to erlotinib in a patient with pancreatic cancer. Anticancer Res. 2014;34(12):7339–43 [A].

[51] Macerelli M, Mazzer M, Foltran L, et al. Erlotinib-associated interstitial lung disease in advanced pancreatic carcinoma: a case report and literature review. Tumori. 2015;101(4):e122–7 [A].

[52] Qi WX, Sun YJ, Shen Z, et al. Risk of interstitial lung disease associated with EGFR-TKIs in advanced non-small-cell lung cancer: a meta-analysis of 24 patients III clinical trials. J Chemother. 2015;27(1):40–51 [M].

[53] Buges C, Carcereny E, Moran T, et al. Interstitial lung disease arising from erlotinib treatment in a Caucasian patient. Clin Lung Cancer. 2015;16(2):e1–3 [A].

[54] Celik T, Kosker M. Ocular side effects and trichomegaly of eyelashes induced by erlotinib: a case report and review of the literature. Cont Lens Anterior Eye. 2015;38:59–60 [A].

[55] Maruyama K, Chinda J, Kuroshima T, et al. Minimal change nephrotic syndrome associated with gefitinib and a successful switch to erlotinib. Intern Med. 2015;54:823–6 [A].

[56] Solomon BJ, Mok T, Kim DW, et al. First-line crizotinib versus chemotherapy in ALK-positive lung cancer. N Engl J Med. 2014;371:2167–77 [C].

[57] Richly H, Kim TM, Schuler M, et al. Ceritinib in patients with advanced anaplastic lymphoma kinase-rearranged anaplastic large-cell lymphoma. Blood. 2015;126(10):1257–8 [c].

[58] Ikeda S, Yoshioka H, Arita M, et al. Interstitial lung disease induced by alectinib (CH5424802/RO5424802). Jpn J Clin Oncol. 2015;45(2):221–4 [A].

[59] Sanchez-Lopez J, Vinolas N, Munoz-Cano R, et al. Successful oral desensitization in a patient with hypersensitivity reaction to crizotinib. J Investig Allergol Clin Immunol. 2015;25(4):295–315 [A].

[60] Sawamura S, Kajihara I, Ichihara A, et al. Crizotinib-associated erythema multiforme in a lung cancer patient. Drug Discov Ther. 2015;9(2):142–5 [A].

[61] Sawada T, Maeno K, Joh T. Esophageal ulcer in a lung cancer patient. Gastroenterology. 2015;149(2):e6–7 [A].

[62] Koizumi T, Fukushima T, Tatai T, et al. Successful treatment of crizotinib-induced dysgeusia by switching to alectinib in ALK-positive non-small cell lung cancer. Lung Cancer. 2015;88:112–3 [A].

[63] Chun SG, Iyengar P, Gerber DE, et al. Optic neuropathy and blindness associated with crizotinib for non-small-cell lung cancer with ELM4-ALK translocation. J Clin Oncol. 2015;33(5):e25–6.

[64] Robert C, Karasczewska B, Schachter J, et al. Improved overall in melanoma with combined dabrafenib an trametinib. N Engl J Med. 2015;372:30–9 [C].

[65] Long GV, Stroyakovskiy D, Gogas H, et al. Dabrafenib and trametinib versus dabrafenib and placebo for Val600 BRAF-mutant melanoma: a multicenter, double-blind, phase 3 randomized controlled trial. Lancet. 2015;386(9992):444–51 [C].

[66] Johnson AS, Crandall H, Dahlman K, et al. Preliminary results from a prospective trial of preoperative combined BRAF and MEK-targeted therapy in advanced BRAF mutation-positive melanoma. J Am Coll Surg. 2015;220:581–95 [c].

[67] Schadendorf D, Amonkar MM, Stroyakovskiy D, et al. Health-related quality of life impact in a randomized phase III study of the combination of dabrafenib and trametinib versus drabrafenib monotherapy in patients with BRAF V600 metastatic melanoma. Eur J Cancer. 2015;51:833–40 [C].

[68] Grob JJ, Amonkar MM, Karaskewska B, et al. Comparison of dabrafenib and trametinib combination therapy with vemurafenib monotherapy on health-related quality of life in patients with unresectable or metastatic cutaneous BRAF Val600-mutation-positive melanoma (COMBI-v): results of a phase 3, open-label, randomized trial. Lancet Oncol. 2015;16:1389–98 [C].

[69] Silva G, deMacedo M, Gibbons IL, et al. Vemurafenib and cutaneous adverse events—report of five cases. An Bras Dermatol. 2015;90(3 Suppl 1):S242–6 [A].

[70] Boudewijns S, Gerritsen WR, Koornstra RHT. Case series: indoor-photosensitivity caused by fluorescent lamps in patients treated with vemurafenib for metastatic melanoma. BMC Cancer. 2014;14:967–70 [A].

[71] Anforth R, Carlos G, Eiris N, et al. Tinea hidden by a vemurafenib-induced phototoxic reaction in a patient with metastatic melanoma taking dexamethasone. Med J Aust. 2015;203(1):41–2 [A].

[72] Sinha R, Larkin J, Fearfield L. Clinical resolution of vemurafenib-induced squamous cell carcinoma with topical 5-fluorouracil. Br J Dermatol. 2015;172:1132–64 [A].

[73] Brackeen J, Jamerson J, Bracekkn A. Metastatic melanoma patient on vemurafenib develops multiple primary cutaneous melanomas. J Drugs Dermatol. 2015;14(3):316–8 [A].

[74] Yu J, Ravikumar S, Plaza JA, et al. Targeting the adnexal epithelium: an unusual case of syringometaplasia in a patient on vemurafenib. Am J Dermatopathol. 2015;37(5):e57–60 [A].

[75] Gebhardt C, Staub J, Schmieder A, et al. Multiple white cysts on face and trunk of a melanoma patient treated with vemurafenib. Acta Derm Venereol. 2015;95:96–7 [A].

[76] West ES, Williams VL, Morelli JG. Vemurafenib-induced neutrophilic panniculitis in a child with a brainstem glioma. Pediatr Dermatol. 2015;32(1):153–4 [A].

[77] Conen K, Mosna-Firlejczyk K, Rochiltz C, et al. Vemurafenib-induced radiation recall dermatitis: case report and review of the literature. Dermatology. 2015;230(1):1–4 [A].

[78] Lilly E, Burke M, Kluger H, et al. Pregabalin for the treatment of painful hand-foot skin reaction associated with dabrafenib. JAMA Dermatol. 2015;151(1):102–3 [A].

[79] Patel U, Cornelius L, Anadkat MJ. MEK inhibitor-induced dusky erythema: characteristic drug hypersensitivity manifestation in 3 patients. JAMA Dermatol. 2015;151(1):78–81 [A].

[80] Anforth R, Carlos G, Clements A, et al. Cutaneous adverse events in patients treated with BRAF inhibitor-based therapies for metastatic melanoma for longer than 52 weeks. Br J Dermatol. 2015;172:239–43 [c].

[81] Bar-Sela G, Abu-Amna M, Hadad S, et al. Successful desensitization protocol for hypersensitivity reaction probably caused by dabrafenib in a patient with metastatic melanoma. Jpn J Clin Oncol. 2015;45(9):881–3 A.

[82] Klossowski N, Kislat A, Homey B, et al. Successful drug desensitization after vemurafenib-induced rash. Hautartz. 2015;66(4):221–3 [A].

[83] Guedj M, Queant A, Funck-Brentano E, et al. Uveitis in patients with late-stage cutaneous melanoma treated with vemurafenib. JAMA Ophthalmol. 2014;123(12):1421–5 [c].

[84] Orouji E, Ziegler B, Umansky V, et al. Leukocyte count restoration under dabrafenib treatment in a melanoma patient with vemurafenib-induced leukopenia. Medicine. 2014;93(28) e161 [A].

[85] Denis D, Franck N, Fichel F, et al. Fanconi syndrome induced by vemurafenib: a new renal adverse event. JAMA Dermatol. 2015;151(4):453–4 [A].

[86] Menzies AM, Ashworth MT, Swann S, et al. Characteristics of pyrexia in BRAFV600E/K metastatic melanoma patients treated with combined dabrafenib and trametinib in a phase I/II clinical trial. Ann Oncol. 2015;26(2):415–21 [c].

[87] Modak S, Asante-Korang A, Steinherz LJ, et al. Trametinib-induced left ventricular dysfunction in a child with relapsed neuroblastoma. J Pediatr Hematol Oncol. 2015;37(6):e381–3 [A].

44

Radiological Contrast Agents and Radiopharmaceuticals

Makoto Hasegawa, Tatsuya Gomi[1]

Department of Radiology, Ohashi Medical Center, Toho University, Tokyo, Japan
[1]Corresponding author: gomi@oha.toho-u.ac.jp

INTRODUCTION

Contrast agents are widely used in clinical practice to improve diagnostic performance of medical imaging. Various types of contrast agents exist; iodinated contrast agents which absorb more X-rays than human tissue are used for radiographic examinations such as computed tomography (CT), gadolinium-based agents which have T1 relaxation time shortening effects are used for magnetic resonance imaging (MRI), and microbubbles which have a higher echogenecity compared to human tissue are used for ultrasound (US). Although these agents are indispensable in medical imaging, they are not risk free.

Adverse reactions to contrast agents can be classified as acute, late and very late by the timing of the reaction after administration of the agent. Acute reactions can be categorized as allergic-like or physiological by the type of reaction, and mild, moderate, or severe by the severity. Adverse reactions may affect various organ systems. Recent publications which cover various aspects of adverse reactions to contrast agents will be discussed in this chapter, including the recently reported gadolinium accumulation.

WATER-SOLUBLE INTRAVASCULAR IODINATED CONTRAST AGENTS [SED-15, 1848; SEDA-33, 963; SEDA-34, 749; SEDA-35, 863]

There are four types of iodinated water-soluble contrast media, classified according to their physicochemical properties (Table 1). They are mainly used intravascularly, but can also be injected into body cavities, particularly the low-osmolar contrast agents. Some are also used for oral or rectal administration, and the high-osmolar water-soluble contrast agent diatrizoate is suitable only for these purposes. Low osmolar and iso-osmolar iodinated contrast media have almost completely replaced high osmolar agents for intravascular use and administration into body cavities.

Drug Interactions

Metformin, a biguanide oral antihyperglycaemic agent, is used to treat patients with noninsulin-dependent diabetes mellitus. Metformin is thought to act by decreasing hepatic glucose production and enhancing peripheral glucose uptake as a result of increased sensitivity of peripheral tissues to insulin.

The most significant adverse effect of metformin therapy is the potential for the development of metformin-associated lactic acidosis in the susceptible patient. In the presence of certain comorbidities, which lead to decreased metabolism of lactate or increased anaerobic metabolism, *metformin should be discontinued at the time of an examination or procedure using IV iodinated contrast media.* Ideally, it should be withheld for 48 h and administration can resume after reassessment of renal function [1M].

Types of Reactions

Adverse reactions that occur after contrast media injection typically occur within 20 min of the injection. An acute adverse reaction is an adverse reaction that occurs within 1 h of injection. Acute reactions are classified as being of mild, moderate, and severe intensity. Types of

TABLE 1   List of Few Iodinated Water-Soluble Contrast Media

Properties	Examples (INNs)	Brand names
High-osmolar ionic monomers	Diatrizoate	Angiografin, Hypaque, Gastrografin, Renografin, Urografin
	Iotalamic acid	Conray
	Ioxitalamic acid	Telebrix
	Metrizoate	Isopaque, Triosil
Low-osmolar ionic dimers	Ioxaglic acid	Hexabrix
Low-osmolar non-ionic monomers	Iobitridol	Xenetrix
	Iohexol	Omnipaque
	Iomeprol	Iomeron
	Iopamidol	Isovue, Niopam, Solutrast
	Iopentol	Imagopaque
	Iopromide	Ultravist
	Ioversol	Optiray
	Metrizamide	Amipaque
Iso-osmolar non-ionic dimers	Iodixanol	Visipaque
	Iosimenol	Iosmin
	Iotrolan	Isovist

reactions include mild symptoms such as nausea and itching and severe reactions such as hypotensive shock and convulsions. A late adverse reaction to contrast medium is defined as a reaction that occurs at 1 h to 1 week after injection. Maculopapular rashes, erythema, and pruritus are the most common types of late reactions. A very late adverse reaction is a reaction that occurs at more than 1 week after contrast injection; this includes reactions such as thyrotoxicosis [2R].

The incidence of severe reactions has been reported to be low. A recent study analyzed the incidence of adverse reactions in 109 255 cases who underwent enhanced CT examination. A total of 375 (0.34%) patients had acute reactions (281 mild (0.26%); 80 moderate (0.07%); and 14 severe (0.01%)). No death was found. 302 (80.53%) adverse reactions occurred within 15 min after contrast media administration. Female patients (180 cases, 0.40%; $P < 0.01$) or outpatients had significantly higher incidence rates of adverse reactions. The symptoms and signs of most of the adverse reactions were resolved spontaneously within 24 h after appropriate treatment without sequelae. The incidences from the report were consistent with previous reports [3C].

Endocrine

Thyrotoxicosis is a type of very late adverse reaction seen after iodine-based contrast media. Untreated Graves' disease and multinodular goiter and thyroid autonomy are risks for this adverse reaction. Patients with hyperthyroidism are usually advised not to have iodinated contrast media injection. Patients with normal thyroid function are thought to be at low risk for this condition [4M].

Data on the incidence of contrast-induced hyperthyroidism and hypothyroidism are limited. Also, the incidence may vary between iodine-deficient and -sufficient regions. A prospective study in an adult population undergoing an outpatient CT with iodinated contrast media investigated this incidence in an iodine-deficient region. The study included 102 patients whose thyroid function tests and urine iodine measurements were obtained before, 4 and 8 weeks after contrast media administration. TSH levels dropped ($P = 0.0002$), and free T3 (FT3) levels increased ($P = 0.04$) between baseline and week 4 with normalization by week 8; however, these changes were not considered clinically significant. Only 2% of patients developed subclinical hyperthyroidism following a standard dose of iodinated contrast media [5c]. A retrospective cohort study of an Asian population which included a total of 19 642 cases and 78 568 matched controls found that adjusted hazard ratios of hyperthyroidism and hypothyroidism compared with controls were 1.22 (95% CI, 1.04–1.44) and 2.00 (95% CI, 1.65–2.44), respectively [6C].

Neonatal exposure to intravenously administered iodinated contrast media to the mother has previously been reported to have no significant adverse clinical risk of thyroid function abnormalities to the fetus [7c]. Yet, cases of neonatal dysfunction have been previously reported in patients born from mothers who underwent maternal hysterosalpingography (HSG) using oil-soluble iodinated contrast medium. A study investigated the incidence of neonatal thyroid dysfunction following HSG. The report included 212 infants born to mothers who underwent HSG. The study found 5 of the 212 infants tested positive during congenital hypothyroidism screening. The frequency (2.4%) was higher than the recall rate among first congenital hypothyroidism screening results (0.7%) in Tokyo, Japan. Two of the 5 screening-positive infants showed hypothyroidism, and 3 showed hyperthyrotropinemia. The dose of ethiodized oil was significantly higher in the thyroid dysfunction group compared to the normal thyroid function group (20 vs. 8 ml, $P = 0.033$), which suggests a dose dependency. The authors suggest that contrast medium dose should be as low as possible to minimize the risk of neonatal thyroid dysfunction [8c].

Hematologic

Contrast media-induced thrombosis has previously been described in literature [9C,10r]. A case of a 50-year-old patient whose myocardial infarction was possibly induced by thrombosis due to contrast media injection has been reported [11c,12r,13r].

Nervous System

Transient neurological symptoms including cortical blindness have been previously reported in literature [14r,15c]. A case of a 76-year-old man with spinal arteriovenous fistula experienced repeated reversible paraplegia after administration of iomeprol for spinal digital subtraction angiography, and contrast-enhanced CT angiography. Symptoms resolved after administration of dexamethasone [16c].

Radiation

Radiation dose increase in iodine-charged tissue has previously been reported in *in vitro* and *in vivo* experiments [17E,18E,19E,20r]. This may result in induction of DNA double-strand break induction [21E]. This effect has been demonstrated in a study of 179 patients who underwent contrast enhanced, and 66 patients who underwent unenhanced CT. From the blood samples obtained from these patients, gammaH2AX foci levels were increased in both groups after CT. Furthermore, patients who underwent contrast-enhanced CT had an increased amount of DNA radiation damage, compared to the non-enhanced CT group [22c].

Radiation recall is a rare clinical syndrome characterized by an acute inflammatory reaction at the site of prior radiation exposure. It is precipitated by the use of triggering agents, most commonly chemotherapeutic agents [23r,24c,25c,26c]. A case suspected of radiation recall precipitated by iodinated nonionic contrast media has been reported. The case was a 63-year-old woman with previous a history of previous adverse reaction to iodinated contrast media, penicillins and sulfa drugs was diagnosed with breast cancer. The patient received neoadjuvant chemotherapy and mastectomy, and completed postmastectomy radiation. The patient underwent contrast-enhanced CT 7 weeks, 18 weeks and 2 years after radiation therapy for various reasons. The patient developed well-demarcated erythema in the distribution of radiated areas after these scans which were suspected to be radiation recall dermatitis precipitated by the contrast media injections [27c].

Iodinated Radiocontrast-Induced Nephropathy

Contrast-induced nephropathy (CIN) is defined as renal hypofunction with an increase in the serum creatinine (SCr) concentration of 25% or more, or by 44 μmol/l (0.5 mg/dl) or more, developing within 3 days after injection of an intravascular contrast medium in the absence of other causes.

Prevalence

Kidney transplant recipients (KTRs) may be at higher risk of CIN due to high prevalence of chronic kidney disease, DM, and cardiovascular disease and the concurrent use of a nephrotoxic calcineurin inhibitor (CNI) for immunosuppression. To investigate the prevalence in these patients, 124 consecutive KTRs who received intravascular contrast and had stable kidney function before contrast administration were enrolled. CIN developed in 7/124 patients (5.64%). There was no significant association between CIN and age, race, gender, DM, hypertension, baseline serum creatinine level or eGFR, use of angiotensin-converting enzyme inhibitor (ACEi) or angiotensin receptor blocker (ARB), diuretic, and prophylaxis or volume of contrast used. In KTR with eGFR >70 ml/min/1.73 m2, administration of hypo-osmolar contrast does not appear to be associated with a high incidence of CIN [28c].

The prevalence of renal insufficiency among cancer patients is high, and many of them are on nephrotoxic chemotherapeutic agents. To investigate the prevalence of CIN among these patients, a study which included 820 adult patients with active cancer presented and who received CECT were enrolled. The incidence of CIN was 8.0%. Serial CT examination [OR 4.09; 95% CI 1.34–12.56], hypotension before the CT scan (OR 3.95; 95% CI 1.77–8.83), liver cirrhosis (OR 2.82; 95% CI 1.06–7.55), BUN/creatinine >20 (OR 2.54; 95% CI 1.44–4.46), and peritoneal carcinomatosis (OR 1.75; 95% CI 1.01–3.00) were independently associated with CIN [29C].

139 patients underwent endovascular aortic aneurysm repair were enrolled. CIN was detected in 39 of 139 patients (28%). Low preoperative eGFR (eGFR <60 ml/min/1.73 m2) and high preoperative and postoperative urea and creatinine levels were found to be significant for CIN, indicating that precautions should be taken in patients with abnormal preoperative renal functions. In multivariate analysis, postoperative serum urea levels were found to be significant. Other variables, including increased contrast medium doses and the complex endovascular operations, were not found to be significant risk factors for CIN [30c].

The risk of CIN among patients with normal renal function and those with mild to moderate chronic renal impairment is extraordinarily low, if not zero. The evaluation of CIN requires to various attention [31R].

Serum β2-microglobulin has previously been investigated for evaluation of renal injury. A study investigated the application of β2-microglobulin for the prediction of CIN. A total of 424 consecutive inpatients undergoing contrasted coronary computed tomography angiography (CCTA) were enrolled. Fifty-two (12.26%) of them developed CIN. Before CCTA, CIN was predicted by both baseline β2-microglobulin (area under the receiver operating characteristic curve [AUC], 0.791; $P < 0.001$) and cystatin C (AUC, 0.781; $P < 0.001$), whereas creatinine and eGFR were not predictive. Multivariate regression analysis confirmed that baseline β2-microglobulin (OR, 2.137; 95% CI, 1.805–3.109; $P < 0.001$) and cystatin C (OR, 1.873; 95% CI, 1.667–2.341; $P = 0.003$) were independent predictors for CIN [32c].

A number of clinical studies have investigated of neutrophil gelatinase-associated lipocalin (NGAL) for CIN. 10 articles were used for analysis. These 10 articles involved 1310 participants. Overall, the diagnostic odds ratio (DOR)/area under the curve for the receiver operating characteristic (AUROC) for NGAL level to predict CIN was 20.56 [95% CI, 9.67–43.74]/0.87 (95% CI, 0.84–0.90), with sensitivity and specificity of 0.80 (95% CI, 0.74–0.85) and 0.83 (95% CI, 0.73–0.90), respectively. Subgroup analysis showed that the diagnostic performance of the DOR/AUROC of urinary NGAL [29.48 (95% CI, 12.19–71.27)/0.87 (95% CI, 0.84–0.90)] was better than that of plasma/serum NGAL [14.63 (95% CI, 4.51–47.38)/0.85 (95% CI, 0.82–0.88)] (DOR, $P = 0.005$, and AUROC, $P = 0.04$, respectively). Plasma/serum and urinary NGAL levels seem to be useful biomarkers in the early prediction of CIN. Moreover, urinary NGAL levels perform better than plasma/serum NGAL [33M].

Prevention

Various methods of prevention including hydration and administration of sodium bicarbonate have been previously investigated. A study investigated the use of oral sodium citrate to prevent CIN. 130 patients were enrolled in this study. Patients were randomized to receive IV sodium bicarbonate (group I), oral sodium citrate (group II) or nonspecific hydration (group III) before contrast administration. Incidence of CI-AKI was 9.2% with no differences found between hydration groups: 7.0% in sodium bicarbonate group, 11.6% in oral sodium citrate group and 9.1% in the nonspecific hydration group. Hydration with oral sodium citrate may provide a safe, inexpensive and practical method for preventing CI-AKI in low-risk patients [34c].

Fenoldopam mesylate (FP) demonstrated some renoprotective benefit in a pilot trial. Pooled analyses of clinical trials comparing intravenous FP with Saline/Placebo/N-acetyl cysteine (NAC) for the prevention of CIN were reviewed. Five articles involved 719 patients (353 in treatment arm; 366 in control arm). There were

a total of 85 cases of CIN among 353 patients in IV Fenoldopam group, while 73 events occurred among 366 patients in the control arm. The risk ratio for the development of CIN in the Fenoldopam group was 1.19 compared to the control group. This was not statistically significant. Fenoldopamis was found no better than Placebo/Saline or NAC in preventing CIN, but much larger randomized controlled studies may be required [35M].

Susceptibility Factors, Diagnosis and Prevention of Adverse Reaction

In patients who are at risk for an adverse reaction (patients who previously had moderate or severe acute reaction to an iodine-based contrast agent, patients with asthma or any allergy requiring medical treatment), premedication should be considered. In patients who have previously reacted to iodinated contrast media, European Society of Urogenital Radiology guidelines on contrast media suggest the use of a different agent. Although clinical evidence of premedication is limited, the use of prednisolone 30 mg or methylprednisolone 32 mg orally 12 and 2 h before the contrast agent should be considered for patients at risk [4M].

A retrospective study investigated the protective effect of pre-medications and changing contrast media. The study included 771 cases of patients with previous adverse reactions to contrast media. 491 (220 without premedication "control group", and 271 with premedication "premedication only group") of these patients were administered with the same contrast media that caused the adverse reaction previously. 280 patients (58 without premedication "changing only group", and 222 with premedication "changing with premedication group") received a different contrast media. The study found that the control group had 61 repeat adverse reactions, the premedication only group had 47, the changing only group 3, and changing with premedication group had 6 adverse reactions, respectively. The authors suggest that premedication prior to contrast for patients with previous adverse reactions may be protective; however, changing CM was more effective in preventing adverse reactions [36C].

Currently, there is no good clinical mechanism to predict the occurrence of adverse reaction to iodinated contrast agents. Skin tests are known to have a limited sensitivity and high specificity for patients with hypersensitivity. Preliminary intradermal skin testing with contrast agents is not predictive of adverse reactions, may itself be dangerous, and is not recommended [37C]. They may have a modest utility in retrospectively evaluating severe adverse reactions. In vitro tests, such as basophil activation test, lymphocyte transformation test, and lymphocyte activation test, have been reported to be useful in previous reactors. However, the sensitivity and specificity of these tests have not been firmly established.

A meta-analysis of 21 studies to investigate the role of skin tests in patients with hypersensitivity reactions to contrast media reported that the pooled per-patient positive rates of skin tests were 17% (95% CI, 10–26%) in patients with immediate hypersensitivity reactions, and up to 52% (95% CI, 31–72%) when confined to severe reactions. Among patients with nonimmediate reactions, the positive rate was 26% (95% CI, 15–41%). Cross-reactivity rate was higher in nonimmediate reactions (68%; 95% CI, 48–83%) than that in immediate reactions (39%; 95% CI, 29–50%). Recurrence rates of hypersensitivity reactions to skin test-negative ICM were 7% (95% CI, 4–14%) in immediate HSR and 35% (95% CI, 19–55%) in nonimmediate reactions. The authors of this study suggest that skin tests may be helpful in diagnosing and managing patients with hypersensitivity reactions to contrast media, especially in patients with severe immediate hypersensitivity reactions [38M]. Another study evaluated the utility of skin prick tests and intradermal tests in patients with hypersensitivity. The study included 23 patients (17 immediate and 6 delayed reactions). Six commonly used contrast media including iopromide, iohexol, ioversol, iomeprol, iopamidol and iodixanol were tested. Of 10 patients with anaphylaxis, 3 (30.0%) and 6 (60.0%) were positive, respectively, on skin prick and intradermal tests with the culprit agent. In total, 11 (64.7%) had positive on either skin prick or intradermal tests. Three of 6 patients with delayed rashes were positive on patch test and/or delayed intradermaltests. Five patients (3 anaphylaxis, 1 urticaria and 1 delayed rash) underwent subsequent radiological examinations, 3 patients administered alternative contrast media from the results of skin testing with no adverse reaction. However, two patients developed anaphylaxis after being administered with the culprit contrast media. The sensitivity of skin tests was 64.7% (11/17) for immediate and 50% (3/6) for delayed hypersensitivity reactions in this study, which was consistent with previously reported sensitivities [39c]. These tests may be useful for selecting an alternative contrast media in patients with prior hypersensitivity reactions.

MRI CONTRAST MEDIA

Gadolinium Salts [SED-15, 1469; SEDA-33, 968; SEDA-34, 754; SEDA-35, 866; SEDA-36, 701]

Contrast enhancement is obtained by the T1 relaxation time shortening characteristics of gadolinium (Gd). From the type of use, these agents can be categorized into extracellular fluid agents, blood pool agents, and organ-specific agents. Extracellular gadolinium-based contrast agents can be categorized as non-ionic and ionic from their charge, and linear or macrocyclic structure. Blood pool agents can be categorized into albumin binding gadolinium complexes such as gadofosveset and gadocoletic acid, and polymeric gadolinium complexes such as gadomelitol. The gadolinium salts that are used as contrast media in magnetic resonance imaging (MRI) and that have been assigned International Nonproprietary Names (INNs) by the WHO are listed in Table 2.

Gadolinium agents are considered to have no nephrotoxicity at approved dosages for MRI. Therefore, MR with gadolinium has been used instead of contrast-enhanced CT in those at risk for developing worse renal failure if exposed to iodinated contrast media.

Observational Studies

A phase 3 efficacy and safety trial of gadobutrol confirmed the safety of profile of the agent. The study included 343 patients, out of which 14 patients (4.1%) experienced at least one adverse event that was considered to be drug-related and was consistent previously published literature. All treatment-related adverse events were not serious. The most common drug-related adverse event was nausea ($n=6$) [40C].

Multiorgan Damage

Nephrogenic systemic fibrosis (NSF) is a multisystemic disease in patients with renal insufficiency.

TABLE 2 Gadolinium Salts That Have Been Used as Contrast Media in Magnetic Resonance Imaging

Name (INN)	Brand name	Charge	Structure
Gadobenic acid	Multihance	Ionic	Linear
Gadobutrol	Gadovist	Non-ionic	Macrocyclic
Gadocoletic acid			
Gadodenterate			
Gadodiamide	Omniscan	Non-ionic	Linear
Gadofosveset	Ablavar	Ionic	Linear
Gadomelitol	Vistarem		
Gadopenamide			
Gadopentetic acid	Magnevist	Ionic	Linear
Gadoteric acid	Dotarem	Ionic	Macrocyclic
Gadoteridol	Prohance	Non-ionic	Macrocyclic
Gadoversetamide	OptiMARK	Ionic	Linear
Gadoxetic acid	Eovist, Primovist	Ionic	Ionic

TABLE 3   Risks of Systemic Fibrosis from Gadolinium-Containing Salts

Name (INN)	Chelate	Charge	Structure	Risk
Gadodiamide	DTPA–BMA	Non-ionic	Linear	High (3–7%)
Gadopentetic acid	DTPA	Ionic	Linear	High (0.1–1%)
Gadoversetamide	DTPA–BMEA	Non-ionic	Linear	High
Gadobenic acid	BOPTA	Ionic	Linear	Intermediate
Gadofosveset	DTPA–DPCP	Ionic	Linear	Intermediate
Gadoxetic acid	EOB–DTPA	Ionic	Linear	Intermediate
Gadobutrol	BT-DO3A	Non-ionic	Cyclic	Low
Gadoteric acid	DOTA	Ionic	Cyclic	Low
Gadoteridol	HP-DO3A	Non-ionic	Cyclic	Low

DPTA, diethylene triamine penta-acetic acid; BMA, 5,8-bis(carboxymethyl)-11-[2-(methylamino)-2-oxoethyl]-3-oxo-2,5,8,11-tetra-azatridecan-13-oic acid; BMEA, N,N′-bis(methoxyethylamide); BOPTA, benzyloxypropionic tetra-acetic-acid; DPCP, N,N′-bis(pyridoxal-5-phosphate)-*trans*-1,2-cyclohexyldiamine-N,N′-diacetic acid; EOB-DTPA, ethoxybenzyldiethylene triamine penta-acetic acid; BT-DO3A, 10-(2,3-dihydroxy-1-hydroxymethylpropyl)-1,4,7,10-tetra-azacyclododecane-1,4,7-triacetic acid; HP-DO3A, 10-(2-hydroxypropyl)-1,4,7-tetra-azacyclododecane-1,4,7-triacetic acid; DOTA, 1,4,7,10-tetra-azacyclododecane-N,N′,N″,N‴-tetra-acetic acid.

Administration of gadolinium-based contrast agents, especially linear-structured agents, has been associated with the development of NSF (Table 3). After the restriction of gadolinium-based agents in high-risk patients in guidelines, the number of new cases has decreased sharply. *Yet, clinicians should continue to be cautious when administering gadolinium-based contrast agents; renal insufficiency should be screened for patients prior to administration* [41r,42,43C,44R].

There is no specific treatment for NSF. Improvement of skin lesions after recovery of renal function [45c] and response to therapeutic plasma exchange have previously been reported [46c].

℞

Special Review

Gadolinium Accumulation

In vitro investigations have found that the chemical stability of gadolinium contrast agents are different according to their structure, with macrocyclic chelates being the most stable, and non-ionic linear chelates the least stable. Ionic agents are more stable than non-ionic agents. Evidence of stability has been demonstrated in in vivo experiments which found evidence that more gadolinium retention are found in animals administered with non-ionic linear agent gadodiamide than ionic linear agent gadopentetate dimeglumine. Very small amounts of gadolinium were retained after macrocyclic agent administration [47R].

Free gadolinium is toxic in tissues, and acts as an inorganic blocker of voltage-gated calcium channels [48R,49R,50E]. *Cell membrane modification has also been reported in an in vitro study* [51E]. *The retention of gadolinium has been previously reported in a rat model* [52E] *and in human bone tissue* [53c]. *A study comparing 19 patients who underwent contrast-enhanced MRI and 16 patients who underwent unenhanced MRI has found a higher signal intensity in the dentate nucleus and globus pallidus on unenhanced T1-weighted MRI, with relation to cumulative dose of gadolinium contrast agents, which suggested gadolinium accumulation in these areas* [54C]. *This was also demonstrated in a pediatric patients* [55,56c]. *This was confirmed in two studies which investigated postmortem tissue samples to determine the deposition. These studies used inductively coupled mass spectrometry to quantify gadolinium deposition. Gadolinium was detected in all patients from the gadolinium-based contrast agent group. All patients in the contrast group had relatively normal renal function at the time of MR examination* [57c,58]. *The accumulation of gadolinium in the dentate nucleus and globus pallidus may vary between structures of the agent used. Studies comparing the hyperintensity of the dentate nucleus and/or globus pallidus on unenhanced T1-weighted images between linear and macrocyclic agents found that high intensity of the dentate nucleus had a strong association with previous administration of linear agents, while no association was found with macrocyclic agents* [59C,60c,61c]. *However, a study evaluating the high signal intensity of the dentate nucleus and globus pallidus in patients who received multiple administrations of gadobutrol, a macrocyclic agent, found that the signal intensity increased after multiple gadobutrol administrations which also correlated with the number of administrations. This study suggests that deposition of gadolinium occurs in macrocyclic agents* [62c]. *Another study of 69 patients compared the high signal in of the globus pallidus and dentate nucleus in two different linear gadolinium-based contrast agents. The study found that there was a significant increase in signal intensity for gadodiamide-enhanced studies, but not with gadobenate dimeglumine-enhanced studies, which may be due to the difference of stability of these agents [63c]. Dose dependency has been demonstrated previously [64c]. Analysis of skin samples in a patient with NSF revealed that gadolinium may be deposited as GdPO4 as well as intact gadolinium-based contrast media (Gd-HP-DO3A) 8 years after the administration [65E]. There is lack in knowledge of the long-term effects of gadolinium retention in these areas. Yet, clinician should be aware of the accumulation, and caution may be necessary when using linear agents as well as macrocylic agents.*

Observational Studies

A phase 3 efficacy and safety trial of gadobutrol confirmed the safety of profile of the agent. The study included 343 patients, out of which 14 patients (4.1%) experienced at least one adverse event that was considered to be drug-related and was consistent previously published literature. All treatment-related adverse events were not serious. The most common drug-related adverse event was nausea (1.7%) [40C].

The renal safety of gadobenate dimeglumine was assessed in a study of 352 patients with decompensated cirrhosis awaiting liver transplant. The study found that the pre- and post-MRI serum creatinine values did not demonstrate a clinically significant difference (mean change $= 0.017$ mg/dl; $P = 0.38$), including those patients with a pre-MRI serum creatinine ≥ 1.5 mg/dl. Thus, gadobenate dimeglumine can be considered non-nephrotoxic and may be used in patients waiting for liver transplant, even in patients with concomitant renal insufficiency [66C].

SUPERPARAMAGNETIC IRON OXIDE (SPIO) MRI CONTRAST AGENTS [SEDA-33, 970; SEDA-34, 757]

Iron oxide-containing contrast agents consist of suspended colloids of iron oxide nanoparticles, which reduce T2 MRI signals. They are taken up by the reticuloendothelial system. Superparamagnetic iron oxide (SPIO) contrast agents are taken up by the liver and spleen. The ultrasmall superparamagnetic iron oxide (USPIO) contrast agents have a longer plasma circulation time and have greater uptake into marrow and lymph nodes. They also have a greater T1 shortening effect than SPIO contrast agents. For these characteristics, they have been investigated for liver imaging, macrophage imaging or blood pool agents.

Ferumoxytol is an intravenously injected superparamagnetic iron oxide coated with polyglucose sorbitol carboxymethylether, which is used for the treatment of anemia caused by low levels of iron in patients with chronic kidney disease. It has previously been used in the magnetic resonance imaging (MRI) of the central nervous system and lower extremities [67c,68c,69M,70c,71]. A report investigated the efficacy of ferumoxytol for vascular assessment of lower extremity arterial disease in patients. The study included 10 patients suspected with arterial occlusive disease. Five patients with renal insufficiency were scanned with ferumoxytol, and 5 with gadolinium. No adverse reactions were found in both groups [72c].

Ultrasound Contrast Agents [SED-15, 3543; SEDA-32, 855; SEDA-33, 971; SEDA-34, 758; SEDA-35, 869; SEDA-36, 703]

A study investigated the safety profile of intravenous second-generation ultrasound contrast agents (UCAs) containing sulfur hexafluoride in 137 pediatric patients. The study found one severe anaphylactic reaction was observed in 0.6% ($n = 1$). No other adverse events during or after intravenous administration of contrast were observed. Although ultrasound contrast agents are considered safe, further studies are necessary to investigate the safety profile of these agents [73c].

References

[1] ACR Manual on Contrast Media, Version 9. American College of Radiology; 2013 [M].

[2] Morcos SK, Thomsen HS. Adverse reactions to iodinated contrast media. Eur Radiol. 2001;11(7):1267–75 [R].

[3] Li X, Chen J, Zhang L, et al. Clinical observation of the adverse drug reactions caused by non-ionic iodinated contrast media: results from 109,255 cases who underwent enhanced CT examination in Chongqing, China. Br J Radiol. 2015;88(1047):20140491 [C].

[4] ESUR guidelines on contrasts media 8.1 European Society of Urogenital Radiology, Available from: http://www.esur.org/guidelines/; 2013 [M].

[5] Jarvis C, Simcox K, Tamatea JA, et al. A low incidence of iodine-induced hyperthyroidism following administration of iodinated contrast in an iodine-deficient region. Clin Endocrinol (Oxf). 2016;84(4):558–63 [c].

[6] Kornelius E, Chiou JY, Yang YS, et al. Iodinated contrast media increased the risk of thyroid dysfunction: a 6-year retrospective cohort study. J Clin Endocrinol Metab. 2015;100(9):3372–9 [C].

[7] Kochi MH, Kaloudis EV, Ahmed W, et al. Effect of in utero exposure of iodinated intravenous contrast on neonatal thyroid function. J Comput Assist Tomogr. 2012;36(2):165–9 [c].

[8] Satoh M, Aso K, Katagiri Y. Thyroid dysfunction in neonates born to mothers who have undergone hysterosalpingography involving an oil-soluble iodinated contrast medium. Horm Res Paediatr. 2015;84(6):370–5 [c].

[9] Davidson CJ, Mark DB, Pieper KS, et al. Thrombotic and cardiovascular complications related to nonionic contrast media during cardiac catheterization: analysis of 8,517 patients. Am J Cardiol. 1990;65(22):1481–4 [C].

[10] Efe SC, Ozturk S, Gurbuz AS, et al. Contrast-induced thrombosis: are we aware? J Vasc Interv Radiol. 2015;26(3):446–8 [r].

[11] Aksu U, Topcu S. Contrast media induced myocardial infarction in patient with subtotal LAD occlusion. Int J Cardiol. 2015;191:231–2 [c].

[12] Aksu U, Topcu S. Contrast media and thrombosis. Int J Cardiol. 2015;197:279 [r].

[13] Kirat T, Kose N, Altun I, et al. The thrombogenic potential of contrast media and thrombotic complications after coronary angiography. Int J Cardiol. 2015;194:1 [r].

[14] Junck L, Marshall WH. Neurotoxicity of radiological contrast agents. Ann Neurol. 1983;13(5):469–84 [r].

[15] Mentzel HJ, Blume J, Malich A, et al. Cortical blindness after contrast-enhanced CT: complication in a patient with diabetes insipidus. AJNR Am J Neuroradiol. 2003;24(6):1114–1116 [c].

[16] Mielke D, Kallenberg K, Hartmann M, et al. Paraplegia after contrast media application: a transient or devastating rare complication? Case report. J Neurosurg Spine. 2016;24:806–9 [c].

[17] Santos Mello R, Callisen H, Winter J, et al. Radiation dose enhancement in tumors with iodine. Med Phys. 1983;10(1):75–8 [E].

[18] Iwamoto KS, Cochran ST, Winter J, et al. Radiation dose enhancement therapy with iodine in rabbit VX-2 brain tumors. Radiother Oncol. 1987;8(2):161–70 [E].

[19] Mesa AV, Norman A, Solberg TD, et al. Dose distributions using kilovoltage x-rays and dose enhancement from iodine contrast agents. Phys Med Biol. 1999;44(8):1955–68 [E].

[20] Riley P. Does iodinated contrast medium amplify DNA damage during exposure to radiation. Br J Radiol. 2015;88(1055):20150474 [r].

[21] Deinzer CK, Danova D, Kleb B, et al. Influence of different iodinated contrast media on the induction of DNA double-strand breaks after in vitro X-ray irradiation. Contrast Media Mol Imaging. 2014;9(4):259–67 [E].

[22] Piechowiak EI, Peter JF, Kleb B, et al. Intravenous iodinated contrast agents amplify DNA radiation damage at CT. Radiology. 2015;275(3):692–7 [c].

[23] Burris 3rd HA, Hurtig J. Radiation recall with anticancer agents. Oncologist. 2010;15(11):1227–37 [r].

[24] Guarneri C, Guarneri B. Radiation recall dermatitis. Can Med Assoc J. 2010;182(3):E150 [c].

[25] Heirwegh G, Bruyeer E, Renard M, et al. Radiation-recall myositis presenting as low-back pain (2010: 4b). Eur Radiol. 2010;20(7):1799–801 [c].

[26] Wernicke AG, Swistel AJ, Parashar B, et al. Levofloxacin-induced radiation recall dermatitis: a case report and a review of the literature. Clin Breast Cancer. 2010;10(5):404–6 [c].

[27] Lau SK, Rahimi A. Radiation recall precipitated by iodinated nonionic contrast. Pract Radiat Oncol. 2015;5:263–6 [c].

[28] Haider M, Yessayan L, Venkat KK, et al. Incidence of contrast-induced nephropathy in kidney transplant recipients. Transplant Proc. 2015;47(2):379–83 [c].

[29] Hong SI, Ahn S, Lee YS, et al. Contrast-induced nephropathy in patients with active cancer undergoing contrast-enhanced computed tomography. Support Care Cancer. 2016;24:1011–7 [C].

[30] Guneyli S, Bozkaya H, Cinar C, et al. The incidence of contrast medium-induced nephropathy following endovascular aortic aneurysm repair: assessment of risk factors. Jpn J Radiol. 2015;33(5):253–9 [c].

[31] McDonald RJ, McDonald JS, Newhouse JH, et al. Controversies in contrast material-induced acute kidney injury: closing in on the truth? Radiology. 2015;277(3):627–32 [R].

[32] Li S, Zheng Z, Tang X, et al. Preprocedure and postprocedure predictive values of serum beta2-microglobulin for contrast-induced nephropathy in patients undergoing coronary computed tomography angiography: a comparison with creatinine-based parameters and cystatin C. J Comput Assist Tomogr. 2015;39(6):969–74 [c].

[33] Tong J, Li H, Zhang H, et al. Neutrophil gelatinase-associated lipocalin in the prediction of contrast-induced nephropathy: a systemic review and meta-analysis. J Cardiovasc Pharmacol. 2015;66(3):239–45 [M].

[34] Martin-Moreno PL, Varo N, Martinez-Anso E, et al. Comparison of intravenous and oral hydration in the prevention of contrast-induced acute kidney injury in low-risk patients: a randomized trial. Nephron. 2015;131(1):51–8 [c].

[35] Naeem M, McEnteggart GE, Murphy TP, et al. Fenoldopam for the prevention of contrast-induced nephropathy (CIN)-do we need more trials? A meta-analysis. Clin Imaging. 2015;39(5):759–64 [M].

[36] Abe S, Fukuda H, Tobe K, et al. Protective effect against repeat adverse reactions to iodinated contrast medium: premedication vs. changing the contrast medium. Eur Radiol. 2016;26:2148–54 [C].

[37] Yamaguchi K, Katayama H, Takashima T, et al. Prediction of severe adverse reactions to ionic and nonionic contrast media in Japan: evaluation of pretesting. A report from the Japanese Committee on the Safety of Contrast Media. Radiology. 1991;178(2):363–7 [C].

[38] Yoon SH, Lee SY, Kang HR, et al. Skin tests in patients with hypersensitivity reaction to iodinated contrast media: a meta-analysis. Allergy. 2015;70(6):625–37 [M].

[39] Ahn YH, Koh YI, Kim JH, et al. The potential utility of iodinated contrast media (ICM) skin testing in patients with ICM hypersensitivity. J Korean Med Sci. 2015;30(3):245–51 [c].

[40] Gutierrez JE, Rosenberg M, Duhaney M, et al. Phase 3 efficacy and safety trial of gadobutrol, a 1.0 molar macrocyclic MR imaging contrast agent, in patients referred for contrast-enhanced MR imaging of the central nervous system. J Magn Reson Imaging. 2015;41:788–96 [C].

[41] Weller A, Barber JL, Olsen OE. Gadolinium and nephrogenic systemic fibrosis: an update. Pediatr Nephrol. 2014;29:1927–37 [r].

[42] Thomsen HS, Morcos SK, Almen T, et al. Nephrogenic systemic fibrosis and gadolinium-based contrast media: updated ESUR Contrast Medium Safety Committee guidelines. Eur Radiol. 2013;23(2):307–18.

[43] Edwards BJ, Laumann AE, Nardone B, et al. Advancing pharmacovigilance through academic-legal collaboration: the case of gadolinium-based contrast agents and nephrogenic systemic fibrosis—a Research on Adverse Drug Events and Reports (RADAR) report. Br J Radiol. 2014;87(1042):20140307 [C].

[44] Canga A, Kislikova M, Martinez-Galvez M, et al. Renal function, nephrogenic systemic fibrosis and other adverse reactions associated with gadolinium-based contrast media. Nefrologia. 2014;34(4):428–38 [R].

[45] Schad SG, Heitland P, Kuhn-Velten WN, et al. Time-dependent decrement of dermal gadolinium deposits and significant improvement of skin symptoms in a patient with nephrogenic systemic fibrosis after temporary renal failure. J Cutan Pathol. 2013;40(11):935–44 [c].

[46] Poisson JL, Low A, Park YA. The treatment of nephrogenic systemic fibrosis with therapeutic plasma exchange. J Clin Apher. 2013;28(4):317–20 [c].

[47] Thomsen HS, Morcos SK, Almen T, et al. Nephrogenic systemic fibrosis and gadolinium-based contrast media: updated ESUR Contrast Medium Safety Committee guidelines. Eur Radiol. 2013;23(2):307–18 [R].

[48] Idee JM, Fretellier N, Robic C, et al. The role of gadolinium chelates in the mechanism of nephrogenic systemic fibrosis: a critical update. Crit Rev Toxicol. 2014;44(10):895–913 [R].

[49] Idee JM, Port M, Dencausse A, et al. Involvement of gadolinium chelates in the mechanism of nephrogenic systemic fibrosis: an update. Radiol Clin N Am. 2009;47(5):855–69. vii. [R].

[50] Okada E, Yamanaka M, Ishikawa O. New insights into the mechanism of abnormal calcification in nephrogenic systemic fibrosis—gadolinium promotes calcium deposition of mesenchymal stem cells and dermal fibroblasts. J Dermatol Sci. 2011;62(1):58–63 [E].

[51] Gianulis EC, Pakhomov AG. Gadolinium modifies the cell membrane to inhibit permeabilization by nanosecond electric pulses. Arch Biochem Biophys. 2015;570:1–7 [E].

[52] Hope TA, Doherty A, Fu Y, et al. Gadolinium accumulation and fibrosis in the liver after administration of gadoxetate disodium in a rat model of active hepatic fibrosis. Radiology. 2012;264(2):423–7 [E].

[53] White GW, Gibby WA, Tweedle MF. Comparison of Gd(DTPA-BMA) (Omniscan) versus Gd(HP-DO3A) (ProHance) relative to gadolinium retention in human bone tissue by inductively coupled plasma mass spectroscopy. Investig Radiol. 2006;41(3):272–8 [c].

[54] Kanda T, Ishii K, Kawaguchi H, et al. High signal intensity in the dentate nucleus and globus pallidus on unenhanced T1-weighted MR images: relationship with increasing cumulative dose of a gadolinium-based contrast material. Radiology. 2014;270(3):834–41 [C].

[55] Roberts DR, Holden KR. Progressive increase of T1 signal intensity in the dentate nucleus and globus pallidus on unenhanced T1-weighted MR images in the pediatric brain exposed to multiple doses of gadolinium contrast. Brain Dev. 2016;38:331–6.

[56] Miller JH, Hu HH, Pokorney A, et al. MRI brain signal intensity changes of a child during the course of 35 gadolinium contrast examinations. Pediatrics. 2015;136(6):e1637–40 [c].

[57] McDonald RJ, McDonald JS, Kallmes DF, et al. Intracranial gadolinium deposition after contrast-enhanced MR imaging. Radiology. 2015;275(3):772–82 [c].

[58] Kanda T, Fukusato T, Matsuda M, et al. Gadolinium-based contrast agent accumulates in the brain even in subjects without severe renal dysfunction: evaluation of autopsy brain specimens with inductively coupled plasma mass spectroscopy. Radiology. 2015;276(1):228–32.

[59] Kanda T, Osawa M, Oba H, et al. High signal intensity in dentate nucleus on unenhanced T1-weighted MR images: association with linear versus macrocyclic gadolinium chelate administration. Radiology. 2015;275:803–9. 140364. [C].

[60] Radbruch A, Weberling LD, Kieslich PJ, et al. Gadolinium retention in the dentate nucleus and globus pallidus is dependent on the class of contrast agent. Radiology. 2015;275(3):783–91 [c].

[61] Radbruch A, Weberling LD, Kieslich PJ, et al. High-signal intensity in the dentate nucleus and globus pallidus on unenhanced T1-weighted images: evaluation of the macrocyclic gadolinium-based contrast agent gadobutrol. Investig Radiol. 2015;50(12):805–10 [c].

[62] Stojanov DA, Aracki-Trenkic A, Vojinovic S, et al. Increasing signal intensity within the dentate nucleus and globus pallidus on unenhanced T1W magnetic resonance images in patients with relapsing-remitting multiple sclerosis: correlation with cumulative dose of a macrocyclic gadolinium-based contrast agent, gadobutrol. Eur Radiol. 2016;26:818–9 [c].

[63] Ramalho J, Castillo M, AlObaidy M, et al. High signal intensity in globus pallidus and dentate nucleus on unenhanced T1-weighted MR images: evaluation of two linear gadolinium-based contrast agents. Radiology. 2015;276(3):836–44 [c].

[64] Errante Y, Cirimele V, Mallio CA, et al. Progressive increase of T1 signal intensity of the dentate nucleus on unenhanced magnetic resonance images is associated with cumulative doses of intravenously administered gadodiamide in patients with normal renal function, suggesting dechelation. Investig Radiol. 2014;49(10):685–90 [c].

[65] Birka M, Wentker KS, Lusmoller E, et al. Diagnosis of nephrogenic systemic fibrosis by means of elemental bioimaging and speciation analysis. Anal Chem. 2015;87(6):3321–8 [E].

[66] Shaffer KM, Parikh MR, Runge TM, et al. Renal safety of intrasmall gadolinium-enhanced magnetic resonance imaging in patients awaiting liver transplantation. Liver Transpl. 2015;21(11):1340–6 [C].

[67] Li W, Tutton S, Vu AT, et al. First-pass contrast-enhanced magnetic resonance angiography in humans using ferumoxytol, a novel ultrasmall superparamagnetic iron oxide (USPIO)-based blood pool agent. J Magn Reson Imaging. 2005;21(1):46–52 [c].

[68] Neuwelt EA, Varallyay CG, Manninger S, et al. The potential of ferumoxytol nanoparticle magnetic resonance imaging, perfusion, and angiography in central nervous system malignancy: a pilot study. Neurosurgery. 2007;60(4):601–11. discussion 611–612. [c].

[69] Stabi KL, Bendz LM. Ferumoxytol use as an intravenous contrast agent for magnetic resonance angiography. Ann Pharmacother. 2011;45(12):1571–5 [M].

[70] Ruangwattanapaisarn N, Hsiao A, Vasanawala SS. Ferumoxytol as an off-label contrast agent in body 3T MR angiography: a pilot study in children. Pediatr Radiol. 2015;45:831–9 [c].

[71] Bashir MR, Bhatti L, Marin D, et al. Emerging applications for ferumoxytol as a contrast agent in MRI. J Magn Reson Imaging. 2015;41(4):884–98.

[72] Walker JP, Nosova E, Sigovan M, et al. Ferumoxytol-enhanced magnetic resonance angiography is a feasible method for the clinical evaluation of lower extremity arterial disease. Ann Vasc Surg. 2015;29(1):63–8 [c].

[73] Piskunowicz M, Kosiak W, Batko T, et al. Safety of intravenous application of second-generation ultrasound contrast agent in children: prospective analysis. Ultrasound Med Biol. 2015;41(4):1095–9 [c].

45

Drugs Used in Ocular Treatment

Lisa V. Stottlemyer*,†,1, and Alan Polnariev‡,1

*Wilmington VA Medical Center, Wilmington, DE, USA
†Pennsylvania College of Optometry, Elkins Park, PA, USA
‡College of Pharmacy, University of Florida, Gainesville, FL, USA
1Corresponding authors: lisa.stottlemyer@va.gov; apolnariev@gmail.com

Many different classes of drugs are utilized for the treatment of ocular disease and all pose risk of side effects, some severe. Ocular medications can be administered topically, orally or injected into the eye, and each route allows for potential of local and systemic side effects. For example, the most common side effects of any topically applied eye drops are burning upon instillation and conjunctival hyperemia, which may be related to either the therapeutic agent or preservatives [1M], while medication injected into the vitreous cavity often leaves the patient reporting floaters or a spot in their vision as they can appreciate the shadow of the depot of drug [2A].

Drug delivery to the intended site of action can be a challenge because pharmacologic agents must overcome anatomic and physiologic barriers that serve to protect the eye [3,4]. The viscosity, concentration, chemical structure of a compound and frequency of application all impact the bioavailability of a topically applied ophthalmic medication. For example, more viscous formulations of eye drops are less affected by tear dilution which allows for longer ocular contact time to maximize absorption. Similarly, the multiple layers of the cornea form a natural barrier that is more easily breached by the lipid solubility of prednisolone acetate than prednisolone phosphate, which is more hydrophilic [5]. The presence of the blood ocular barrier, comprised of the blood–aqueous and blood–retinal barriers, poses another challenge to drug delivery, accounting for the reason that systemic and IV medications are infrequently employed for the treatment of eye disease. However, improvements on the use of biomaterials and nanotechnology as non-invasive drug distribution techniques offer major advancements in ocular delivery systems [4]. For example,

investigators have demonstrated how 20-nm gold nanoparticles, when administered intravenously, can safely permeate the blood–retinal barrier and distribute throughout the retinal layers sparing the eye of structural damage or increased cell death [4].

By far, topical application is the most common route of administration of medications used for the treatment of ocular disease and some conditions, such as glaucoma, require frequent, chronic dosing. Often the preservatives therein contribute to ocular surface disease [1M]. Symptoms such as redness, stinging, burning and foreign body sensation are reported to be present in up to 60% of patients using topical anti-glaucoma medications [6A].

There are several classic side effects for each class of medications that are so prevalent, we almost expect them. For example, beta blockers classically cause bradycardia even when topically applied, and steroids are well known to cause increased IOP and posterior sub-capsular cataracts. Systemic side effects of topically applied ocular medications have been attributed to the "first pass" effect in that up to 80% of topically applied medication drains through the nasolacrimal system and is absorbed into the bloodstream through the nasal mucosa. By this route, organ systems are exposed to concentration of drug prior to the drugs first pass through the liver where many are metabolized [7A,8A]. Infants and children may be more at risk for serious systemic side effects due to the fact that there is often no weight adjusted dose available and struggling with an uncooperative child may lead to a greater number of drops instilled [8A]. This chapter is meant to serve as a review of both the common and lesser occurring side effects of ocular medications reported in the literature.

Anti-Vascular Endothelial Growth Factor (VEGF) Medications

Pegaptanib, Bevacizumab, Aflibercept, Ranibizumab
GENERAL

Anti-VEGF medications are injected into the vitreous cavity through the pars plana and are used for the treatment of many conditions including age-related macular degeneration (AMD), central retinal vein occlusion, diabetic macular edema and proliferative diabetic retinopathy, and retinopathy of prematurity (ROP). Reported adverse events following anti-VEGF injections include endophthalmitis, intraocular inflammation, retinal detachment, increased intraocular pressure, ocular hemorrhage [9R] as well as systemic events such as blood pressure elevation, myocardial infarction, stroke and death.

Corneal complications of ant-VEGF injections include corneal edema, delayed healing and limbal insufficiency [10A].

A comparison of age-related treatment trials (CATT) reported the incidence of endophthalmitis after intravitreal injection of anti-VEGF to be 0.085% [11M]. Sterile intraocular inflammation has been reported with all intravitreal anti-VEGF medications injected intravitreally. A review of the literature of large-scale clinical trials showed that enrolled patients that were treated with ranibizumab experienced inflammation rates of 1.4–2.9%. Lower rates of inflammation, 0.09–0.4%, were reported for those treated with bevacizumab [9R].

The overall risk of rhegmatogenous retinal detachment is low. Meyer et al. reviewed 35 942 injections of either 0.05 ml of ranibizumab, 0.05–0.1 ml of bevacizumab or 0.05 bevacizumab rtPA combined with 0.2 ml SF-6 gas. Five retinal detachments occurred between day 2 and day 6 post injection (4 of the 5 occurring in myopic eyes) yielding an overall incidence of 0.013% per injection [12c].

Tractional retinal detachments have also been reported with anti-VEGF medications (ranibizumab and bevacizumab) [12c,13M,14R] and are thought to result from contraction of fibrovascular tissue following a brisk halt to proliferating neovascular vessels.

Elevated intraocular pressure is an important risk factor for the development of glaucoma. Increased post-injection intraocular pressure (IOP) is common and has been reported with all anti-VEGF drugs; however, it is generally a transient rise in IOP that resolves within several hours without treatment [9R,15M]. Possible risk factors for sustained increase in IOP, and therefore increased risk of developing glaucoma, are the following: increased number of injections, pre-existing glaucoma, male gender and frequency of repeat injection within 8 weeks or less [9R,16C]. It has been theorized that the recurrent stress to the endothelium of Schlemm's canal from repeated injections causes the IOP to rise [17R].

Ocular hemorrhages have also been reported with the use of anti-VEGF medications (ranibizumab and bevacizumab). Of note, Ladas et al. report nearly a 10% incidence of subconjunctival hemorrhage after injection with greatest frequency among patients concurrently taking aspirin [18C]. Sub-retinal and vitreous hemorrhages have also been reported with the use of ranibizumab and bevacizumab.

BEVACIZUMAB

Significantly higher serum levels have been detected following intravitreal injection with bevacizumab as compared to similar injections with pegaptanib and ranibizumab [14R,19M]. Frequently reported systemic adverse events with bevacizumab include blood pressure increases, deep vein thrombosis, transient ischemic attack, congestive heart failures and myocardial infarction [14R,17R]. Lesser reported complications include repeated fever of several days duration after injection, tonic–clonic seizures, transient global amnesia, erectile dysfunction and acute decrease in kidney function [9R,14R].

In recent years, bevacizumab has been investigated for the treatment of ROP, and while treatment response is promising, there is some concern for the effects of systemically absorbed drug on developing pre-term infants as VEGF plays an important role in blood vessel and organ development [20c]. A retrospective case series of 37 premature infants that were treated with 0.625 mg bevacizumab in 0.025 ml injected intravitreally, reported no local (e.g. cataract, endophthalmitis, vitreous hemorrhage, or retinal detachment). Additionally, patients were followed for systemic effects such as compromised development of brain, lungs, kidneys and skeleton and reported no such adverse effects. Still, they recommend lowest effective dose and further large scale studies to evaluate systemic toxicity given this developmentally fragile patient base [20c].

A case of choroidal ischemia resulting in hypotony and exudative retinal detachment occurred in a 6-week-old preterm infant hours after injection of bevacizumab for the treatment of severe retinopathy of prematurity [21A]. A case has been reported where a 63-year-old man developed dendritic keratitis 3 days after injection of bevacizumab for the treatment of diabetic retinopathy and macular edema. VEGF is found in the corneal epithelium and is thought to play a role in corneal immunity. It is speculated that blocking VEGF may have allowed for reactivation of herpes simplex virus in this patient, resulting in corneal infection [22A].

A retrospective cohort study of 174 patients (201 eyes) reported a sustained rise in intraocular pressure occurred in 11% of patients treated with bevacizumab. It is postulated that the rise in intraocular pressure is related to mechanical obstruction of aqueous outflow due to the repackaging of bevacizumab in plastic syringes and that these syringes may cause contamination with materials such as silicone oil [16C].

A data analysis of Medicare claims performed by Gower et al. identified an 11% higher risk of overall mortality and a 57% higher risk of hemorrhagic cerebrovascular accidents in patients treated with bevacizumab when compared to those treated with ranibizumab [23M].

Onoda et al. reported two cases of severe gastrointestinal effects post intravitreal injection of bevacizumab (1.25 mg/0.05 ml). The first, a 78-year-old woman with a distant history of colon cancer and post-operative ischemic colitis suffered a recurrence of ischemic colitis 1 day after injection. The second, a 64-year-old man experienced abdominal pain 2 days after injection. Nine days later he was given a second injection after vitrectomy surgery and the following day developed paralytic ileus with symptoms of vomiting and severe abdominal pain and distention. The authors hypothesize that systemically absorbed drug reduced nitric oxide production which resulted in vasoconstriction and ultimately decreased gastrointestinal blood flow. Both patients were admitted to the hospital for treatment and symptoms improved without surgery [24A].

RANIBIZUMAB

Although the most common side effect of ranibizumab is uveitis [14R], other drug-induced effects may occur.

Bosanquet et al. reported a case of acute generalized exanthematous pustulosis, a cutaneous drug reaction, in a 90-year-old female. Four days after receiving an intravitreal injection of ranibizumab, she developed malaise and a progressive erythematous rash involving the torso and limbs. Early in the course, the rash spread despite treatment with topical and oral corticosteroid before finally resolving spontaneously 6 weeks after the initial appearance [25A].

A case of marginal keratitis developed in a 56-year-old man being treated with ranibizumab for diabetic macular edema. One day after injection, he presented with pain, redness and pain in the injected eye. Multiple peripheral subepithelial infiltrates and a mild anterior chamber reaction were present. This case of marginal keratitis is thought to be related to a hypersensitivity reaction to reflux of ranibizumab onto the ocular surface. The patient was treated with topical moxifloxacin and dexamethasone eye drops and condition resolved over the course of a week [10A].

Reports of lower serum anti-VEGF levels in adults after intravitreal ranibizumab injections when compared to bevacizumab prompted a small case study to evaluate the safety and efficacy of ranibizumab for the treatment of zone 2, stage 3 retinopathy of prematurity with plus disease. Six eyes (of 4 premature infants) were given injections of ranibizumab (0.3 mg in 0.03 ml) and monitored closely for regression of disease as well as ocular and systemic complications. While all patients had rapid regression of the ROP, three of the six eyes developed significantly elevated IOP that required paracentesis to reduce the pressure and one patient developed nasopharyngitis noted as a possible side effect of the drug [26A]. Larger prospective trials are needed to adequately assess the safety of this emerging ROP treatment.

THE FUTURE OF AMD TREATMENT

Novel treatments are being developed to target known features of AMD including: blocking the complement and other inflammatory pathways, lessening oxidative stress, protecting and regenerating retinal pigment epithelial cells and restoring choroidal blood flow [27]. Some of these therapeutic options, especially regenerative therapy, are derived from stem cell research and offer enormous potential to develop a cure for this debilitating disease [28]. Recently, breakthroughs in research have helped clinicians better understand the role of individual and genetic factors in the development of AMD and how to design more effective treatment modalities [29].

MEDICATIONS USED TO TREAT GLAUCOMA

Topical therapy is the mainstay of glaucoma management. Life threatening adverse events including central nervous system depression and cardiogenic shock are described in two infants treated with topical antiglaucoma medications (brimonidine and timolol) [8A]. These cases highlight the fact that systemic absorption and lack of weight adjusted dosages likely subject infants to greater risk of systemic side effects.

Prostaglandin Analogues

Latanoprost, Bimatoprost, Travoprost, Latanoprostene Bunod

GENERAL

Prostaglandin analogue side effects are local and involve hyperemia, increased lash growth, periocular skin pigmentation and increased iris pigmentation [30c]. One small ($n = 69$) prospective observational case study reported statistically significant increase of periocular skin hyperpigmentation in patients treated with bimatoprost and latanoprost after 3 months of treatment, occurring more frequently and to a greater degree with the bimatoprost-treated group [31c]. Deepening of the superior lid sulcus [30c] and sunken eye appearance [32A] has also been described. No systemic adverse events have been attributed to prostaglandin therapy [33C].

The VOYAGER trial, a randomized, investigator masked, parallel group, dose-ranging study ($n=413$) compared the safety and efficacy of four different concentrations of latanoprostene bunod (LBN 0.006%, 0.012%, 0.024%, and 0.040%) to latanoprost 0.005%. Subjects were treated with one drop in the study eye once daily for 28 days. The most commonly reported side effect of all four LBN-treated groups was installation site pain occurring in 14.6% (LBN 0.006%), 16.7% (LBN 0.012%), 12.0% (LBN 0.024%) and 17.3% (LBN 0.040%) of subjects, compared to 6.1% of subjects in the latanoprost-treated group. Ocular hyperemia, however, was more commonly reported in the latanoprost group, occurring in 8.5% of subjects versus 1.2% (LBN 0.006%), 6.0% (LBN 0.012%), 2.4% (LBN 0.024%) and 4.9% (LBN 0.040%) of subjects treated with LBN. Additionally, there was one patient with a headache in the latanoprost group that was considered to be related to the drug [34c].

Two different randomized trials comparing travoprost 0.004% to bimatoprost 0.01% reported an increased occurrence of mild to moderate ocular hyperemia in the bimatoprost-treated group [35c,36c]. In a prospective, randomized, investigator-masked, multicenter clinical trial, patients were randomized to treatment once daily with either 0.03% bimatoprost ($n=131$) or 0.004% travoprost ($n=135$). Ocular hyperemia was the most commonly reported treatment-related adverse event occurring in 3.1% of bimatoprost-treated subjects and 1.5% of travoprost-treated subjects [35c]. Similar findings were reported by investigators who conducted a 12-week, phase 4, randomized, investigator-masked, crossover study ($n=84$) comparing the tolerability of travoprost 0.004% to bimatoprost 0.01%. Subjects were randomized to once daily use of either travoprost or bimatoprost for 6 weeks and then crossed over to the alternate treatment for 6 weeks. Mild ocular hyperemia was reported in 31% of subjects in the travoprost-treated group versus 39% of subjects treated with bimatoprost. Moderate hyperemia was reported in 2% of subjects treated with bimatoprost. No moderate hyperemia was noted in the travoprost-treated group [36c].

Prostaglandin analogues have also been reported to cause nongranulomatous, and to a far lesser extent granulomatous, anterior uveitis presumably because the prostaglandin activity causes a pro-inflammatory state [37A].

Latanoprost is considered etiologic in a case of bilateral serous macular retinal detachments that promptly resolved upon discontinuation of treatment [38A].

Benzalkonium chloride (BAK) is a commonly used preservative for ocular medications and is associated with conjunctival inflammation and corneal compromise [33C]. A recent multi-center, double-masked, randomized, two treatment equivalence clinical trial compared polyquarternium-1 preserved travoprost 0.003% to BAK preserved travoprost 0.004% to determine whether a lower concentration of travoprost preserved with an alternate preservative would lead to better tolerability of the drug while offering equivalent IOP control. The study demonstrated equivalent IOP lowering and safety profiles in both groups with hyperemia occurring in 12% of travoprost 0.003% vs. 15% of travoprost 0.004% treated group [33C].

Beta Blockers

While common localized side effects of beta blockers are in keeping with the other classes of glaucoma medications (predominantly burning upon instillation of drops and conjunctival hyperemia), the prevalence of systemic effects is a frequent limitation of these agents [1M]. Beta blockers' effect on heart rate and respiration is widely reported and includes bradycardia, blood pressure decreases, worsening of asthma attacks and chronic obstructive pulmonary disease (COPD). Rana et al. highlight serious systemic effects in a case report of an 84-year-old male with hypertension, diabetes and hypercholesterolemia who developed a bradycardia arrhythmia, confusion and hypoglycemia that required ICU admission while being treated with a topical beta blocker (Timolol) for the treatment of open angle glaucoma [39A].

TIMOLOL

A recent comparative, phase III study ($n=175$) comparing preservative-free 0.1% Timolol gel with a preserved 0.1% Timolol gel reported the most common ocular side effect was blur and systemic side effects included upper abdominal pain, dry mouth, osteoarthritis, nightmares, dyspnea and erectile dysfunction [40c].

A self-controlled case series study reported an increased risk of hospitalization due to bradycardia in the second to sixth month after initiation of medication [41A].

LEVOBUNOLOL

A case recently reported an 88-year-old man developed symptomatic bradycardia after instillation of drops, which resolved with discontinuation of drug, highlights the potential cardiac side effects of topical beta blockers [42A].

Carbonic Anhydrase Inhibitors (CAI)

Patient on topical CAIs often report a bitter or metallic taste after instillation, stinging of the eyes and conjunctival hyperemia [43A].

Sympathetic α2-Receptor Antagonists

Local ocular side effects of sympathomimetic agents include conjunctival hyperemia, irritation, pupil dilation and allergic conjunctivitis [1M].

In a case recently reported by Shah et al., a patient developed diffuse conjunctival hyperemia with a combined papillary and follicular response on the palpebral conjunctiva, non-staining superior corneal limbal infiltrates and scattered punctate epithelial erosions of the cornea. These monocular findings, reminiscent of vernal keratoconjunctivitis, were attributed to brimonidine allergy as brimonidine was initiated in the right eye only, 2 weeks prior to this presentation [6A].

More serious systemic side effects can result from systemic absorption of the topically applied formulations and can be severe in pediatric patients. A small case series reports four children who experienced somnolence minutes after topical administration of brimonidine. The central nervous system depression is speculated to be the result of poor ability to metabolize the systemically absorbed drug and/or an immature blood–brain barrier [44A].

Combinations

A patient developed a hemorrhagic choroidal detachment and severely reduced visual acuity 1 day after initiation of treated with fixed combination 0.5% timolol maleate/0.004% travoprost. This effect was attributed to the sudden decrease in intraocular pressure [45A]. Treatment was immediately discontinued; full resolution and visual recovery occurred within the following 4 months.

A 12-week prospective, interventional, single-arm study ($n = 47$) evaluating the efficacy and safety of adding fixed combination brinzolamide/timolol to existing prostaglandin therapy reported the most common side effect was headache. Other noteworthy side effects reported were allergic conjunctivitis, burning, eyelid swelling blur, conjunctival discomfort, metallic taste, ocular foreign body sensation and one serious side effect of pseudostenocardia which required patient to be removed from the study [46c].

In a prospective, open, randomized, comparative controlled study ($n = 90$) evaluating safety and efficacy of brimonidine/timolol fixed combination versus monotherapy, no statistically significant effect on blood pressure was noted in any of the groups. Furthermore there was equal statistically significant reduction in heart rate in all patients treated with timolol (both timolol only and timolol in combination). There was no heart rate reduction in the brimonidine only group [47c]. Ocular side effects were not reported in this paper.

In an observer masked, crossover comparative study evaluating 24-h efficacy of dorzolamide/timolol fixed combination compared to brimonidine/timolol fixed combination, the most notable side effect was at bitter taste occurring in 18.3% of patients on the dorzolamide containing regimen versus 0% in the brimonidine-treated group [48c]. Ocular stinging, conjunctival hyperemia and itching were also reported in both treatment groups.

Antimicrobials

Sulfonamides

Sulfacetamide: A 15-year-old boy was hospitalized with Toxic Epidermal Necrolysis (TEN) 3 days after using sulfacetamide eye drops for conjunctivitis. He presented with a fever, widespread blistering rash and severe ocular inflammation with cicatricial lid changes, symblepharon and reduced vision. Over the next few days, the rash spread to involve greater than 30% of his body with erosions on all mucosal membranes. The exact pathogenesis is unknown, although most patients with TEN are noted to have abnormal metabolism of the drug. It is unusual for topical medications to incite TEN. This case highlights the importance of a strong history given that this medication was acquired over-the-counter [49A].

Aminoglycosides

Gentamicin is the most toxic antibiotic used in ophthalmology and toxicity can mimic a retinal vaso-occlusive event involving macular infarction and optic atrophy [50A,51A]. One such case was presented by Lartey et al. wherein total loss of vision occurred after a routine cataract surgery utilizing the use of a sub-conjunctival gentamicin injection (20 mg in 0.5 ml) for endophthalmitis prophylaxis. The vision loss was the result of macular infarction noted on post-operative day 1, followed by notable optic atrophy 2 months later [50A]. This effect may occur if gentamicin, when injected sub-conjunctivally, enters the interior of the eye through the corneal scleral wound [52A]. A similar case of suspected aminoglycoside toxicity occurred in a 52-year-old male who developed severe vision loss after sutureless vitrectomy with sub-conjunctival injection of 0.5 ml of 0.4 mg/ml gentamicin [53A]. Fundus examination revealed extensive retinal hemorrhages, retinal edema and micro-infarcts and fluorescein angiography demonstrated capillary non-perfusion, mostly in the posterior pole consistent with this patient's dense central scotoma and poor visual acuity. The authors believe that this clinical presentation resulted from toxicity to the gentamicin which gained access to eye through the sutureless sclerotomies [53A].

Additionally, two patients developed toxic anterior segment syndrome (TASS) within 2 weeks after a single subconjunctival injection of gentamicin (20 mg in 0.5 ml) used during routine cataract surgery. The associated effects were corneal edema, dilated pupil, cystoid macular edema and uveitis [54A]. The corneal edema, macular edema (present in only one of the two reported cases) and uveitis resolved slowly in the following months; in both cases, however, the pupil dilation was permanent.

Topical gentamicin has been implicated in the development of acute renal failure in a 67-year-old woman being treated for endophthalmitis. Once topical gentamicin and fortified vancomycin were discontinued, the patient experienced a dramatic improvement in renal status prompting her physicians to suspect toxicity. Serum gentamicin levels were 0.34 mg/l 2 days after discontinuation of the drug, the first ever report of measurable serum gentamicin resulting from topical administration. Acute renal failure completely resolved after her eye drops were stopped [55A].

Fluoroquinolones

GENERAL

Corneal precipitates with topical fluoroquinolone use are widely reported, occurring in approximately 15% of patients treated with ciprofloxacin but also with ofloxacin, norfloxacin and gatifloxacin [56A]. Precipitates appear to occur with greater frequency in older patients and while they do not slow the rate of infection resolution, they may result in a delay of re-epithelialization [56A,57r].

CIPROFLOXACIN

While oral and IV administrations of ciprofloxacin have been noted to decrease serum levels of phenytoin and decrease seizure threshold, Malladi et al. report a case of topical flanoquinolone administration where use of 0.3% ciprofloxacin eye drops four times a day for 2 weeks led to reduced serum phenytoin levels and increased seizure activity [58A]; serum levels rose steadily upon discontinuation of the eye drops and were back to therapeutic levels within a week.

LEVOFLOXACIN

Contact urticaria syndrome characterized by conjunctival hyperemia, nasal discharge, sneezing, facial edema, pruritic rash, and mild dyspnea was reported in a patient prescribed topical administration of 0.5% levofloxacin hydrate eye drops for bacterial conjunctivitis [59A]. Symptoms of conjunctival hyperemia, nasal discharge and sneezing developed immediately, followed by the other symptoms.

Vancomycin

A retrospective case series reviewed cases of postoperative hemorrhagic occlusive retinal vasculitis (HORV) after cataract surgery and reported that all (11/11 eyes) were treated with intercameral vancomycin (1 mg/0.1 ml) for endophthalmitis prophylaxis. All patients experienced painless vision loss, uveitis, vasculitis and extensive retinal hemorrhages between post-operative

day 1 and 14. Authors speculate that HORV represents a type III hypersensitivity reaction to vancomycin [60c].

Mydriatics/Cycloplegics

Mydriatics and cycloplegics cause pupillary dilation and congestion of the anterior chamber angle yielding increased risk for acute angle closure in at-risk patients. Additional side effects include potential central nervous system toxicity which can induce seizures, coma and death [61A].

ATROPINE/HOMATROPINE

A small case series report reminds clinicians that children are particularly at risk for systemic side effects. A 6-month-old boy was admitted to the ER with acute urinary retention for greater than 36 hours. Symptoms began 3 hours after instillation of 2 drops homatropine 1% and a 2-year-old boy was admitted for drowsiness, thirst and dry mouth which occurred after being given 3 drops of atropine 1% [62A]. Maximum concentration of 0.3% atropine is recommended for infants to reduce risk of systemic side effects.

Delirium, a feature of anti-cholinergic syndrome, was reported in a 55-year-old male. Onset of delirium occurred 30 minutes after 0.6-mg injection of atropine given as a pre-anesthetic medication prior to bronchoscopy. Patient was treated immediately with psychiatric medications and symptoms resolved. One day later, the patient was given a single drop of atropine 1% in each eye for fundus evaluation and again developed delirium [63A]. The delirium resolved promptly after 8 mg of midazolam was given intravenously [63A].

A lethal dose of atropine is between 100 and 200 mg. Atropine eye drops are up to 10 times more concentrated than oral and injectable formulations and a massive oral dose of eye drops has been cited in an intentional case of homicide by poisoning. Based on toxicological analysis of the decedent's peripheral blood, urine and tissue samples, the administered dose was estimated to be the equivalent of 200–500 mg of atropine. A 172-mg dose is the equivalent of ingesting two 10-ml bottles of atropine eye drops; evidence in the case revealed those charged with the crime purchased three 10-ml bottle of atropine 1% 1 month before the crime [64A].

CYCLOPENTOLATE

In a recent survey of pediatric ophthalmologists, Wygnanski-Jaffe et al. report 5 cases of epileptic seizures resulting from administration of 1.0% cyclopentolate eye drops. Seizures occurred within the first hour of dosing in all 5 cases. The median age of patients was 5 years, and patients had no prior history of seizure activity. Lower body weight and immaturity of the central nervous system in children is thought to predispose patients to the toxic effects of cycloplegic agents [61A]. The susceptibility of children to central nervous system effects of cyclopentolate was further evidenced in a case where a 4-year-old boy experienced the inability to walk, disequilibrium, dysarthria and disorientation 3 hours after the instillation of 6 drops of 1% cyclopentolate in both eye [65A].

Anti-cholinergic addiction has been reported with cyclopentolate eye drops [66A]. The eye drops were initially prescribed for the treatment of uveitis; however, the patient enjoyed the "tingling" feeling and "felt high" when he used them. He gradually increased the dose over a period of 10 years, ultimately using 300–400 drops per day to achieve the desired high. He was unable to go more than a few hours without the drops because he would experience withdrawal symptoms of anxiety, sweating and nausea. He was admitted to an alcohol and drug treatment center to address the addiction [66A].

Recently, a case of fatal necrotizing enterocolitis was reported in a preterm infant dilated with 0.5% cyclopentolate and 1.25% phenylephrine. While necrotizing enteral colitis is commonly feared in preterm infants, it is thought that the cyclopentolate-induced parasympatholytic effect on the gut and the phenylephrine-induced vasoconstriction are important risk factors for this condition [67A].

CYCLOMIDRIL (0.2% CYCLOPENTOLATE AND 1% PHENYLEPHRINE COMBINATION)

Cardiopulmonary arrest was reported in a pre-term infant after topical administration of cyclomidril to effect dilation for a retinopathy of prematurity (ROP) screening [7A]. Three sets of eye drops were administered at 15-minute intervals. Fifteen minutes after the third set, the baby became unresponsive. The baby was resuscitated but experienced a second event 3 hours later. Follow-up ROP screenings with 1.0% tropicamide and 2.5% phenylephrine (instead of cyclomidril) were uneventful [7A].

PHENYLEPHRINE

Topical phenylephrine is widely reported to cause a transient rise in blood pressure and bradycardia; however, a systematic review and meta-analysis including eight randomized clinical trials with a total of 918 patients concluded that phenylephrine 2.5% leads to no clinically relevant rise in blood pressure, and the elevation associated with 10% phenylephrine is short-lived [68M].

Corticosteroids

It is widely known that topical corticosteroids frequently cause elevated intraocular pressure, decreased

corneal healing and posterior sub-capsular cataracts. Elevated intraocular pressure usually occurs within the first 4 weeks of treatment; however, delayed onset has been reported with difluprednate 0.05% emulsion dosed two to four times daily for 1 year prior to the significant IOP rise [69A].

Fluorometholone (FML) has recently been noted to have caused a manic episode in a 76-year-old man, marking the first report of psychiatric side effects of topical administration [70A], and growth suppression was observed in a small case series of children, aged 6–10, treated with one drop FML in each eye three times a daily for allergic conjunctivitis [71A].

A 35-year-old man developed central serous chorioretinopathy days after using dexamethasone 0.1% eye drops intranasally for the treatment of rhinitis. The conditions spontaneously resolved but recurred several times over the course of the year, each time occurring 5–7 days after intranasal use of dexamethasone eye drops [72A].

Intravitreal injections and implants offer high potency and sustained dose of corticosteroid, and major concerns with use are elevated intraocular pressure and cataract formation, although more severe side effects are reported. Of note, one case of scleral melt over the site of the fluocinolone implant is reported. This effect occurred in a 42-year-old female 18 months after the placement of the implant and required treatment with a scleral graft [73A]. Furthermore, local intraocular immune suppression is suggested as causative for reactivation of viral eye disease. A case of cytomegalovirus endotheliitis developed 4 months after a fluocinolone acetonide implant was inserted into the eye of a 40-year-old immunocompetent patient [74A] and acute retinal necrosis developed in a 52-year-old woman 1 month after intravitreal dexamethasone implantation [75A]. A retrospective case series reviewed 30 cases of viral retinitis occurring after local corticosteroid administration and reported that 70% of retinitis occurred after intravitreal injection of triamcinolone, 13.3% after sub-tenon's injection of triamcinolone, 10% after fluocinolone acetonide implant and 3.3% after anterior subconjunctival injection of triamcinolone [76M].

SPECIAL REVIEW ON PHARMACOGENETICS

The phenotypic manifestation of ocular diseases is characteristically maintained by the arrangement of genetic variations via: polymorphic changes, mutations, copy number variations or epigenetic changes [77]. Recent research in genome-wide association studies (GWAS) and next-generation sequencing has dramatically improved our understanding of how genetic variants are linked to several retinal disorders including AMD and retinitis pigmentosa [77]. During the late 1980s and 1990s, genetic linkage studies were conducted to determine the prevalence of common single-gene disorders such as sickle cell disease and Marfan syndrome [78]. Beginning in the early 2000s, researchers began to shift their attention towards GWAS's in order to identify more specific genetic associations found in patient populations thought to be afflicted with the same condition [78]. Results from the first successfully conducted GWAS were published in *Science* in 2005. In this landmark study, 96 patients with polymorphisms associated with AMD and 50 control subjects were evaluated [79]. Researchers determined that, among the 116 204 SNPs genotyped, a common intronic variant in the *complement factor H* (*CFH*) gene, located on chromosome 1, was found to be correlated with AMD and has since been confirmed in multiple family-based studies. In fact, individuals that are homozygous for the particular risk allele possess a 7.4 times greater likelihood of developing the disease [79]. Another genomic study identified at least 25 genes that may be influential in the risk of AMD, including *CFH, ARMS2* and *HTRA1* [80]. Currently, more than 185 genetic loci are linked to human retinal dystrophies yet these known loci represent only one half of all genetic defects in patients, leaving a large proportion of loci left to be identified. The practice of genotyping can confirm the diagnosis of a disease at the molecular level, to allow for a more precise prognosis of an individual's potential for the development of a disease [81].

Several new micro-array technologies have greatly expanded over the last 20 years affording scientists the ability to analyze entire genomes quicker than ever before, and this has implications in providing more cost-effective and accessible genotyping [82]. These micro-chips can be used to effectively detail genetic code for conditions such as: Stargardt dystrophy, Leber's congenital amaurosis (LCA), Usher syndrome and retinitis pigmentosa. A patient's DNA can be screened and all known mutations can be loaded onto a chip within a matter of hours. Koenekoop et al. reported that identification rates (identifying at least one disease-associated mutation) are approximately: 70% in Stargardt dystrophy, 60–70% in LCA and 45% in Usher syndrome subtype 1 [81]. This practice can then be combined with genotype–phenotype correlations to help identify the causal gene associated with the clinical condition (e.g. preserved para-arteriolar retinal pigment epithelium infers involvement of the CRB1 gene in Leber's congenital amaurosis) [81]. These genetic associations have the potential to facilitate gene-replacement strategies and treatments necessary for several genetically acquired retinal diseases [82]. As medicine evolves to become more personalized, testing an individual's genetic makeup and biomarker profile will become customary and complementary to traditional ophthalmic examinations in clinical practice. This approach will have the potential to include all facets of patient care; from genetic counseling to treating diseases with DNA-based therapies [83]. Understanding the genetic profile of a disease not only helps in diagnostics but also in gene therapy in genetically linked conditions, as recently shown for LCA [77,84].

References

[1] Inoue K. Managing adverse effects of glaucoma medications. Clin Ophthalmol. 2014;8:903–13 [M].

[2] Charalampidou S, Nolan J, Ormonde GO, et al. Visual perceptions induced by intravitreous injections of therapeutic agents. Eye. 2011;25(4):494–501 [A].

[3] Fraunfelder FT, Fraunfelder FW, Chambers WA. Drug-induced ocular side effects: clinical ocular toxicology. 7th ed. Philadelphia: Elsevier; 2015.

[4] Gaudana R, Ananthula HK, Parenky A, et al. Ocular drug delivery. AAPS J. 2010;12(3):348–60. http://dx.doi.org/10.1208/s12248-010-9183-3.

[5] Stringer W, Bryant R. Dose uniformity of topical corticosteroid preparations: difluprednate ophthalmic emulsion 0.05% versus branded and generic prednisolone acetate ophthalmic suspension 1%. Clin Ophthalmol. 2010;4:1119–24. http://dx.doi.org/10.2147/OPTH.S12441.

[6] Shah A, Modi Y, Wellik S, et al. Brimonidine allergy presenting as vernal-like keratoconjunctivitis. J Glaucoma. 2015;24(1):89–91 [A].

[7] Lee J, Kodsi S, Gaffar M, et al. Cardiopulmonary arrest following administration of cyclomydril eyedrops for outpatient retinopathy of prematurity screening. J AAPOS. 2014;18(2):183–4 [A].

[8] Kiryazov K, Stefova M, Iotova V. Can ophthalmic drops cause central nervous system depression and cardiogenic shock in infants? Pediatr Emerg Care. 2013;29(11):1207–9 [A].

[9] Falavarjani K, Nguyen Q. Adverse events and complications associated with intravitreal injection of anti-VegF agents: a review of literature. Eye. 2013;27:787–94 [R].

[10] Bayhan S, Bayhan H, Adam M, et al. Marginal keratitis after intravitreal injection of ranibizumab. Cornea. 2014;33(11):1238–9 [A].

[11] Haddock L, Ramsey D, Young L. Complications of subspecialty ophthalmic care: endophthalmitis after intra-vitreal injections of anti-vascular endothelial growth factor medications. Semin Ophthalmol. 2014;29(5–6):257–62 [M].

[12] Meyer CH, Michels S, Rodrigues EB, et al. Incidence of rhegmatogenous retinal detachments after intravitreal avascular endothelial factor injections. Acta Ophthalmol. 2011;89:70–5 [c].

[13] Arevalo F, Maia M, Flynn HW, et al. Tractional retinal detachment following intravitreal bevacizumab in patients with severe proliferative diabetic retinopathy. Br J Ophthalmol. 2008;92:213–6 [M].

[14] Tolentino M. Systemic and ocular safety of intravitreal anti-vegF therapies for ocular neovascular disease. Surv Ophthalmol. 2011;56(2):95–113 [R].

[15] Gismondi M, Salati C, Salvetat ML, et al. Short-term effect of intravitreal ranibizumab on intraocular pressure. J Glaucoma. 2009;18(9):658–61 [M].

[16] Mathalone N, Arodi-Golan A, Sar A, et al. Sustained elevation of intraocular pressure after intravitreal injections of bevacizumab in eyes with neovascular age-related macular degeneration. Graefes Arch Clin Exp Ophthalmol. 2012;250:1435–40 [C].

[17] Ziemssen F, Sobolewska B, Deissler H, et al. Safety of monoclonal antibodies and related therapeutic proteins for the treatment of neovascular macular degeneration: addressing outstanding issues. Expert Opin Drug Saf. 2015;15(1):1–13 [R].

[18] Ladas ID, Karagiannas DA, Rouvas AA, et al. Safety of repeat intravitreal injections of bevacizumab versus ranibizumab: our experience after 2000 injections. Retina. 2009;29(3):313–8 [C].

[19] Hard A, Hellstrom A. On safety, pharmacokinetics and dosage of bevacizumab in ROP treatment—a review. Acta Paediatr. 2011;100:1523–7 [M].

[20] Nicoara SD, Nascutzy C, Cristian C, et al. Outcomes and prognostic factors of intravitreal bevacizumab monotherapy in zone I stage 3+ and aggressive posterior retinopathy of prematurity. J Ophthalmol. 2015;2015. Article ID 102582, 8 p. [c].

[21] Chhablani J, Rani PK, Balakrishnan D, et al. Unusual adverse choroidal reaction to intravitreal bevacizumab in aggressive posterior retinopathy of prematurity: the Indian Twin Cities ROP screening (ITCROPS) Data Base Report #7. Semin Ophthalmol. 2014;29(4):222–5 [A].

[22] Khalili M, Mehdizadeh M, Mehryar M. Herpetic epithelial keratitis after intravitreal injection of bevacizumab. Cornea. 2009;28(3):360–1 [A].

[23] Gower EW, Cassard S, Chu L, et al. Adverse event rates following intravitreal injection of Avastin or Lucentis for treating age-related macular degeneration. Invest Ophthalmol Vis Sci. 2011;52:6644 [M].

[24] Onoda Y, Shiba T, Hori Y, et al. Two cases of acute abdomen after intravitreal injection of bevacizumab. Case Rep Ophthalmol. 2015;6:110–4 [A].

[25] Bosanquet DC, Davies WL, May K, et al. Acute generalized exanthematous pustulosis following intravitreal ranibizumab. Int Wound J. 2011;8:317–9 [A].

[26] Menke M, Framme C, Nelle M, et al. Intravitreal ranibizumab monotherapy to treat retinopathy of prematurity zone II, stage 3 with plus disease. BMC Ophthalmol. 2015;15:20 [A].

[27] Hanus J, Zhao F, Wang S. Current therapeutic developments in atrophic age-related macular degeneration. Br J Ophthalmol. 2016;100(1):122–7.

[28] Blenkinsop TA, Corneo B, Temple S, et al. Ophthalmologic stem cell transplantation therapies. Regen Med. 2012;7(6 Suppl):32–9. http://dx.doi.org/10.2217/rme.12.77.

[29] Grassmann F, Fauser S, Weber BH. The genetics of age-related macular degeneration (AMD)—novel targets for designing treatment options? Eur J Pharm Biopharm. 2015;95(Pt B):194–202. http://dx.doi.org/10.1016/j.ejpb.2015.04.039.

[30] Nakakura A, Tabuchi H, Kiuchi Y. Latanoprost therapy after sunken eyes caused by travoprost or bimatoprost. Optom Vis Sci. 2011;88(9):1140–4 [c].

[31] Karslioglu MZ, Hosal MB, Tekeli O. Periocular changes in topical bimatoprost and latanoprost use. Turk J Med Sci. 2015;45(4):925–30 [c].

[32] Ung T, Currie Z. Periocular changes following long-term administration of latanoprost 0.005%. Ophthal Plast Reconstr Surg. 2012;28(2):e42–4 [A].

[33] Peace J, Ahlberg P, Wagner M, et al. Polyquaternium-1-preserved travoprost 0.003% or benzalkonium chloride-preserved travoprost 0.004% for glaucoma and ocular hypertension. Am J Ophthalmol. 2015;60(2):266–74 [C].

[34] Weinreb RN, Ong T, Sforzolini BS, et al. A randomised, controlled comparison of latanoprostene bunod and latanoprost 0.005% in the treatment of ocular hypertension and open angle glaucoma: the VOYAGER study. Br J Ophthalmol. 2015;99(6):738–45 [c].

[35] Kammer JA, Katzman B, Ackerman SL, et al. Efficacy and tolerability of bimatoprost versus travoprost in patients previously on latanoprost: a 3-month, randomised, masked-evaluator, multicenter study. Br J Ophthalmol. 2010;94(1):74–9 [c].

[36] DuBiner HB, Hubatch DA. Late-day intraocular pressure-lowering efficacy and tolerability of travoprost 0.004% versus bimatoprost 0.01% in patients with open-angle glaucoma or ocular hypertension: a randomized trial. BMC Ophthalmol. 2014;14:151 [c].

[37] Chiam P. Travoprost induced granulomatous anterior uveitis. Case Rep Ophthalmol Med. 2011;2011. Article ID 507073; 2 p. [A].

[38] Tuzcu EA, Keskin U, Coskun M, et al. Bilateral serous detachment associated with latanoprost/timolol fixed combination use: a report of one phakic case. Case Rep Ophthalmol Med. 2012;2012. Article ID 305379, 3 p. [A].

[39] Rana MA, Mady AF, Rehman BA, et al. From eyedrops to ICU, a case report of 3 side effects of ophthalmic timolol maleate in the same patient. Case Rep Crit Care. 2015;2015. Article ID 714919, 4 p. [A].

[40] Easty DL, Nemet-Wasmer G, Vounatsos J-P, et al. Comparison of a non-preserved 0.1% T-Gel eye gel (single dose unit) with a preserved 0.1% T-Gel eye gel (multidose) in ocular hypertension and glaucomatous patients. Br J Ophthalmol. 2006;90(5):574–8 [c].

[41] Pratt N, Ramsay E, Ellett L, et al. Association between ophthalmic timolol and hospitalization for bradycardia. J Ophthalmol. 2015;2015. Article ID 567387, 6 p. [A].

[42] Lin L, Wang Y, Chen Y, et al. Bradyarrhythmias secondary to topical levobunolol hydrochloride solution. Clin Interv Aging. 2014;9:1741–5 [A].

[43] Sharpe ED, Day DG, Beischel CJ, et al. Brimonidine. 0.15% versus dorzolamide 2% each given twice daily to reduce intraocular pressure in subjects with open-angle glaucoma or ocular hypertension. Br J Ophthalmol. 2004;88:953–6 [A].

[44] Levy Y, Zadok D. Systemic side effects of ophthalmic drops. Clin Pediatr. 2004;43(1):99–101 [A].

[45] Coban DT, Erol MK, Yucel O. Hemorrhagic choroidal detachment after use of anti-glaucomatous eyedrops: case report. Arq Bras Oftalmol. 2013;76(5):309–10 [A].

[46] Hommer A, Hubatsch DA, Cano-Parra J. Safety and efficacy of adding fixed-combination brinzolamide/timolol maleate to prostaglandin therapy for treatment of ocular hypertension or glaucoma. J Ophthalmol. 2015;2015. Article ID 131970, 7 p. [c].

[47] Joshi SR, Akat PB, Ramanand JB, et al. Evaluation of brimonidine–timolol fixed combination in patients of primary open-angle glaucoma. Indian J Ophthalmol. 2013;61(12):765–7 [c].

[48] Konstas AGP, Quaranta L, Yan DB, et al. Twenty-four hour efficacy with the dorzolamide/timolol-fixed combination compared with the brimonidine/timolol-fixed combination in primary open angle glaucoma. Eye. 2012;26(1):80–7 [c].

[49] Byrom L, Zappala T, Muir J. Toxic epidermal necrolysis caused by over the counter eye drops. Aust J Dermatol. 2013;54:144–6 [A].

[50] Lartey S, Armah P, Ampong A. A sudden total loss of vision after routine cataract surgery. Ghana Med J. 2013;47(2):96–9 [A].

[51] Kuo H, Lee J. Macular infarction after 23-gauge trans-conjunctival sutureless vitrectomy and sub-conjunctival gentamicin for macular pucker: a case report. Can J Ophthalmol. 2009;44(6):720–1 [A].

[52] Salati C, Migliorati G, Brusin P. Sclero-retinal necrosis after a sub-conjunctival injection of gentamicin in a patient with surgically repaired episcleral retinal detachment. Eur J Ophthalmol. 2004;14(6):575–7 [A].

[53] Brouzas D, Moschos M, Koutsandrea C, et al. Gentamicin-induced macular toxicity in 25-gauge sutureless vitrectomy. Cutan Ocul Toxicol. 2013;32(3):258–9 [A].

[54] Litwin A. Toxic anterior segment syndrome after cataract surgery secondary to sub-conjunctival gentamicin. J Cataract Refract Surg. 2012;38:2196–7 [A].

[55] Tang R, Tse R. Acute renal failure after topical fortified gentamicin and vancomycin eyedrops. J Ocul Pharmacol Ther. 2011;27(4):411–3 [A].

[56] Wilhelmus K, Abshire R. Corneal ciprofloxacin precipitation during bacterial keratitis. Am J Ophthalmol. 2003;136(6):1032–7 [A].

[57] Patwardhan A, Khan M. Topical ciprofloxacin can delay recovery from viral ocular surface infection. J R Soc Med. 2005;98:274–5 [r].

[58] Malladi A, Liew E, Ng X, et al. Ciprofloxacin eyedrops-induced subtherapeutic serum phenytoin levels resulting in breakthrough seizures. Singapore Med J. 2014;55(7):e114–5 [A].

[59] Saito M, Nakada T. Contact urticaria syndrome from eyedrops: levofloxacin hydrate ophthalmic solution. J Dermatol. 2013;40(2):130–1 [A].

[60] Witkin AJ, Shah AR, Engstrom RE, et al. Postoperative hemorrhagic occlusive retinal vasculitis. Expanding the clinical spectrum and possible association with vancomycin. Ophthalmology. 2015;122:1438–51 [c].

[61] Wygnanski-Jaffe T, Nucci P, Goldchmit M, et al. Epileptic seizures induced by cycloplegic eyedrops. Cutan Ocul Toxicol. 2014;33(2):103–8 [A].

[62] Princelle A, Hue V, Pruvost I, et al. Systemic adverse effects of topical ocular instillation of atropine in 2 children. Arch Pediatr. 2013;20:391–4 [A].

[63] Panchasara A, Mandavia D, Anovadiya A, et al. Central anti-cholinergic syndrome induced by single therapeutic dose of atropine. Curr Drug Saf. 2012;7:35–6 [A].

[64] Carlier J, Escard E, Peoch M, et al. Atropine eyedrops: an unusual homicidal poisoning. J Forensic Sci. 2014;59(3):859–64 [A].

[65] Derinoz O, Anil E. Inability to walk, disequilibrium, incoherent speech, disorientation following the instillation of 1% cyclopentolate eyedrops: case report. Pediatr Emerg Care. 2012;28(1):59–60 [A].

[66] Darcin A, Dilbaz N, Yilmaz S, et al. Cyclopentolate hydrochloride eyedrops addiction: a case report. J Addict Med. 2011;5(1):84–5 [A].

[67] Ozgun U, Demet T, Ozge A, et al. Fatal necrotizing enterocolitis due to mydriatic eyedrops. J Coll Physicians Surg Pak. 2014;24(Special Suppl 2):S147–9 [A].

[68] Stavert B, McGuinness M, Harper A, et al. Cardiovascular adverse effects of phenylephrine eyedrops. A systematic review and meta-analysis. JAMA Ophthalmol. 2015;133(6):647–52 [M].

[69] Kurz P, Chheda L, Kurz D. Effects of twice daily topical difluprednate 0.05% emulsion in a child with pars planitis. Ocul Immunol Inflamm. 2011;19(1):84–5 [A].

[70] Kumagi R, Ichimiya Y. Manic episode induced by steroid (fluorometholone) eye drops in an elderly patient. Psychiatry Clin Neurosci. 2014;68:652–3 [A].

[71] Wolthers O. Growth suppression caused by corticosteroid eyedrops. J Pediatr Endocrinol Metab. 2011;24(5–6):393–4 [A].

[72] Prakash G, Shephali J, Tirupati N, et al. Recurrent central serous chorioretinopathy with dexamethasone eyedrops used nasally for rhinitis. Middle East Afr J Ophthalmol. 2013;20(4):363–5 [A].

[73] Georgalas I, Koutsandrea C, Papaconstantinou D, et al. Scleral melt following Retisert intravitreal fluocinolone implant. Drug Des Devel Ther. 2014;8:2373–5 [A].

[74] Park U, Kim S, Yu H. Cytomegalovirus endotheliitis after fluocinolone acetonide (Retisert) implant in a patient with Behçet uveitis. Ocul Immunol Inflamm. 2011;19(4):282–3 [A].

[75] Kucukevcilioglu M, Eren M, Sobaci G. Acute retinal necrosis following intravitreal dexamethasone implant. Arq Bras Oftalmol. 2015;78(2):118–9 [A].

[76] Takakura A, Tessler HH, Goldstein DA, et al. Viral retinitis following intraocular or periocular corticosteroid administration: a case series and comprehensive review of the literature. Ocul Immunol Inflamm. 2014;22(3):175–82 [M].

[77] Riaz M, Baird PN. Genetics in retinal diseases. Dev Ophthalmol. 2016;55.57–62. 2015 Oct 26.

[78] Priya RR, Chew E, Swaroop A. Genetic studies of age-related macular degeneration. Lessons, challenges and opportunities for disease management. Ophthalmology. 2012;119(12):2526–36.

[79] Klein RJ, Zeiss C, Chew EY, et al. Complement factor H polymorphism in age-related macular degeneration. Science. 2005;308(5720):385–9. http://dx.doi.org/10.1126/science.1109557.

[80] DeAngelis NM, Silveira AC, Carr EA, et al. Genetics of age-related macular degeneration current concepts, future directions. Semin Ophthalmol. 2011;26(3):77–93.

[81] Koenekoop RK, Lopez I, den Hollander AI, et al. Genetic testing for retinal dystrophies and dysfunctions: benefits, dilemmas and solutions. Clin Experiment Ophthalmol. 2007;35(5):473–85.

[82] Lamy P, Grove J, Wiuf C. A review of software for microarray genotyping. Hum Genomics. 2011;5(4):304–9. http://dx.doi.org/10.1186/1479-7364-5-4-304.

[83] Porter L, Black G. Personalized ophthalmology. Clin Genet. 2014;86(1):1–11. http://dx.doi.org/10.1111/cge.12389.

[84] Boye SE, Boye SL, Lewin AS, et al. A comprehensive review of retinal gene therapy. Mol Ther. 2013;21(3):509–19.

46

Safety of Complementary and Alternative Medicine (CAM) Treatments and Practices

R.A. Bellanger*,1, S. Ramsinghani†, C. Franklin†, C. Seeger‡

*Department of Pharmacy Practice, University of the Incarnate Word, Feik School of Pharmacy, San Antonio, TX, USA
†Department of Pharmaceutical Sciences, University of the Incarnate Word, Feik School of Pharmacy, San Antonio, TX, USA
‡University of the Incarnate Word, Feik School of Pharmacy, San Antonio, TX, USA
1Corresponding author: bellange@uiwtx.edu

INTRODUCTION

The World Health Organization (WHO) defines traditional medicine as a culmination of knowledge, skills and practices used to maintain health or prevent, diagnose, improve or treat human illness that is indigenous to differing cultures. WHO considers integrative, complementary and alternative medicine (CAM) as interchangeable terms to refer to health care practices that are not integral to a country's own traditions or dominant health care system [1S].

The United States Department of Health and Human Services, National Institutes of Health, National Center for Complementary and Integrative Health (NCCIH) considers complementary practices those that use health care approaches developed outside of mainstream Western conventional medicine along with conventional practices. Integrative health practice coordinates conventional and complementary approaches within care settings. Alternative medicine would be the sole use of traditional systems from outside of the Western conventional medicine practice [2S,3S].

CAM treatments and practices are divided by NCCIH into sectors of mind/body practices, biologic-based therapies and alternative systems. Mind and body practices include yoga, meditation, relaxation techniques (e.g., deep breathing exercises, guided imagery), massage, and chiropractic or osteopathic manipulation. Biologic-based therapies include vitamins, minerals, natural dietary supplements and probiotics. Alternative medical systems would include homeopathy, naturopathy, Ayurvedic medicine, and traditional Chinese medicine [4S].

This approach informs the United States National Health Interview Survey (NHIS) which is answered by tens of thousands of US citizens every year. The survey requests information on the use of complementary health approaches every 5 years. In 2012, the most recent data were collected and reported, and the use of complementary health practices was reported by 33.2% of adults and 11.6% of children, aged 4–17 years [2S,3S]. In the United States, 34 billion dollars a year was spent on CAM self-care therapies, classes, and practitioners, estimated at over 11% of total out of pocket healthcare expenses [5S].

CAM health practices often have been around for centuries but not accepted by many practitioners of Western conventional health practice, even in countries where some of these practices originated, e.g. Germany. WHO published guidelines for research and evaluation of traditional medicine practices in 2000 with the purpose of standardizing and improving the quality of research methodologies and thus, acceptance of the data generated by healthcare practitioners and the public [1S]. According to WHO estimates, 80% of the world's population relies primarily on traditional medicine. WHO estimates that the demand for medicinal plants is $14 billion annually (2012 data). The increase in global demand has raised concerns for the safety of using medicinal herbs [6R].

Safety of complementary therapies, both biologically based and mind–body based, is found in mainstream medical literature. Mind–body therapy safety concerns including serious side effects are not reported with the frequency of those for natural dietary supplements. This may be due to the lack of standardization of adverse effect nomenclature [7R], the rise of self-care for many of these techniques, including yoga [8M], and the lack of regulations or structure for reporting for both the public and providers of touch and manipulative therapies [9M]. The reports of safety concerns of dietary supplement use and interactions with prescription medications and/or existing disease states are more frequent but less than would be projected by the number of substances available and the population size and diversity [10C]. The mechanisms and structure for reporting adverse reactions or other concerns regarding dietary supplements in the US and other countries do not give a complete collection of data from all potential adverse effects. It is estimated that less than 10% of all adverse events due to taking dietary supplements are ever reported to companies or governments. Reasons for the reduced number of complaints may be due to the perception by the consumer of the natural origins and low risks of dietary supplement intake, leading to discounting of association of any adverse effects with the product [11R].

METHODS

A literature search of PubMed, Google Scholar, NIH and WHO databases for meta-analyses, case studies, and case reports published in English from October 2014 through January 2016 included the terms: CAM therapies, herbal therapies, mind–body therapy, yoga, tai chi, chiropractic, manipulative therapy, acupuncture, traditional Chinese medicine, and adverse effects (neurologic, psychiatric, cardiac, renal, gastrointestinal, nephrotoxicity, hepatotoxicity), side effects, adverse reactions, contaminants. Specific products searched include: soybean, *Camellia sinensis*, *Gingko biloba*, *Citrus aurantium* (bitter orange), *Cinnamomum verum* (cinnamon), *Cimcifuga racemosa* (black cohosh), *Echinacea purpurea*, *Vitex agnus castus* (chaste tree), *Hypericum perforatum* (St. John's wort), *Panax ginseng*, *Panax* species, *Valerian officinalis*, *Serenoa repens* (Saw palmetto), *Silybum marianum* (Milk thistle), *Amorphophallus konjac*, *Paullinia cupana* (Guarana), *Primrose*, *Acai*, *Garcinia cambogia*, *Cascara sagrada* are included in this document by body system.

NATURAL DIETARY AND HERBAL SUPPLEMENTS

In the United States, under FDA regulations, the manufacturers of dietary supplements are responsible for safeguarding their products' quality by following current good manufacturing practices and providing truthful, not misleading, labeling information. However, the dietary supplement manufacturer does not have to provide the FDA with demonstrations of safety or efficacy of the product prior to marketing [12R].

In the U.S., claims about dietary supplements can be made by the manufacturer about effects on health, describing the link between structure of the dietary supplement and function, or nutrient content. If a dietary supplement manufacturer makes a claim about a product's effects, the manufacturer must have data to support the claim. Claims about how a supplement affects the structure or function of the body must be followed by the words "This statement has not been evaluated by the U.S. Food and Drug Administration (FDA). This product is not intended to diagnose, treat, cure, or prevent any disease." Post marketing surveillance of dietary supplements is conducted by the FDA. The agency evaluates safety by conducting or assessing published research on the product and monitoring reports of side effects from consumers, health care providers, and supplement companies. Unsafe products can be removed from the market or a warning can be given to the manufacturer regarding safety, health claim or labeling violations [13S].

Govindaraghavan and Sucher [12R] describe current best practices to provide consistent quality, safety and efficacy of herbal dietary supplements (HDS). Quality of the raw ingredients, including the accurate identification and authentication of all components, identification of any contaminants and assurance of good manufacturing practices, lack consistent definitions, legal requirements, and quality assurance practices in the international dietary supplement industry. The industry currently relies on identification of the plant not the parts, powders or extracts mostly found in the manufacturing process. Documentation of each batch of raw product for site of collection, botanical authentication, and management of cultivation practices (irrigation, fertilization, harvesting, processing and storage and a quality control check at each level of processing) would increase the quality of the end product. These practices are not routinely used within the industry. New techniques of DNA barcoding and phytochemical profiling of plant parts may increase the ability to identify raw ingredients before manufacture. Extracts should be obtained using a standardized extracting method on authenticated raw material and be standardized to an active ingredient marker. Transparency of the process from identification and gathering of the plant to the end product that is marketed to consumers should be the goal of all manufacturers to ensure quality and safety to the people who purchase their products [11R,12R].

Safety of HDS is determined by the quality of the process from cultivation or wild gathering through manufacture of the end product marketed to consumers. It is also determined by the marketing strategies used to convince the public that they need these supplements [10C]. These processes are not subject to international guidelines or uniform standards throughout the industry [12R].

Geller and colleagues [10C] gathered abstracted data from 63 emergency departments in the US of incidences of allergic or adverse events attributed to dietary supplements. The study excluded products considered to be food or drinks (including energy drinks and herbal teas). The authors identified greater than 3600 cases over a 9-year period. In more than 88% of cases, the adverse event that led to the emergency department visit was due to ingestion of a single dietary supplement. The majority of visits were by female patients. The mean age of patients was 32 years of age. Patients over the age of 65 years were twice more likely to be hospitalized than younger patients, and over 30% of supplement-associated adverse events were due to micronutrients (iron, potassium and calcium). Swallowing problems and choking due to calcium supplements were common in this age group. Children most often ingested vitamin and mineral products without supervision. Energy drinks and weight-loss products were the most common product listed to cause cardiovascular, central nervous system and gastrointestinal adverse reactions due to supplements in patients visiting emergency departments in the 5–34 years of age groups. From the data gathered, the authors estimate that 23000 emergency department visits annually in the US are due to adverse events from ingestion of dietary supplements [10C].

Adverse Effects: Central Nervous System and Cardiac Systems

Risks and adverse effects associated with energy drink use are thought to be due to the sympathomimetic effects from excess caffeine consumption. Other ingredients, taken in excess, may play a role in some of the adverse outcomes—guarana, taurine, glucuronolactone and B vitamins. Caffeine in overdose can cause seizures, psychosis, cardiac arrhythmias and, rarely, death. Alcohol mixed with energy drinks is popular with young adults. The subject misperceives their level of intoxication because of the stimulant effects of the energy drink, and this can lead to increases in the total amount of alcohol consumed [14M].

The cardiovascular and cerebrovascular effects of a popular energy drink, containing sugars, caffeine, taurine and B vitamins, were evaluated on healthy female subjects aged 19–29 years in a crossover study. Noninvasive monitors were used to detect changes in blood pressure, heart rate, cerebral blood flow velocity and stroke volume at baseline and after imbibing the energy drink or water. Mental stress was evaluated with a math exercise and Likert scale of perceived stress. The energy drink increased heart rate, blood pressure, cardiac output, cerebrovascular resistance, and decreased cerebral blood flow velocity from pre-drink baseline over that induced after water ingestion. Adding a mental task at 80 minutes after ingestion of either drink caused increases in all cardiovascular parameters but more in the energy drink subjects. The decrease in cerebral blood flow velocity was most pronounced in the energy drink subjects throughout the study period. Subjects on the energy drink or water answered the mental task questions similarly, but stress was more pronounced in the energy drink group. The authors question the ability of energy drinks to improve mental task outcomes or coping skills [15C].

Energy shots containing caffeine, amino acids, B vitamins, and glucuronolactone were given in a randomized double-blinded crossover study to 26 healthy active-duty young military personnel. Study subjects were given the active energy shot product or placebo liquid twice daily for a week, had a washout period of 7 days, then were switched to the alternative product twice daily for a week. Blood pressure, heart rate and electrocardiograms were conducted on days 1 and 7 of each arm of the study. Increases in blood pressure, but not heart rate or EKG findings, were found on day 1 of the active moiety but not on day 7 [16C].

The hemocoagulability of 32 healthy subjects (aged 24–29 years) was evaluated after energy drink consumption. Contents of the energy drink included 140 mg of caffeine with a "proprietary blend" containing taurine, *Panax ginseng*, L-carnitine, glucuronolactone, inositol and guarana. No participants had any history of coagulopathy or platelet disorder or any adverse effects from consuming energy drinks. Water in the same volume was used as a control liquid. Energy drink consumption was associated only with arachidonic acid-induced platelet activation ($p < 0.018$) compared with the water group. Arachidonic acid induced activation at 1 hour after energy drink consumption increased the peak ($p < 0.026$) and the velocity of ($p < 0.008$) platelet aggregation [17c].

Asian red ginseng was associated with manic psychosis including hallucinations in two patients [18A]. Both patients had an estimated ingestion of over 15 g of ginseng per day for over a week before symptoms were exhibited. They both recovered after discontinuation of the product.

Weight loss products causing adverse psychiatric effects were reviewed by Bersani and colleagues [19R]. Many HDS products proposed to promote weight loss *Panax ginseng*, *Ma huang*, *Guarana*, and *Yohimbe* are associated with euphoria, nervousness, anxiety, sleeplessness and other mood disturbances. Interactions of herbal weight loss preparations with prescription psychiatric medications are also reported due to similarities in chemical structure or alteration of absorption or metabolism [19R,20M].

Adverse Effects: Pulmonary

Panax quinquefolium (American ginseng) was noted to be the cause of pulmonary embolism in a 41-year-old woman. The patient had used an intentional overdose of a *Panax* supplement prior to symptoms. She had taken the same supplement in recommended doses without incident prior to admission to the emergency department [21A].

Adverse Effects: Renal

Multiple HDS and other dietary supplement use was assessed for safety in an outpatient population with chronic kidney disease (CKD) and an estimated glomerular filtration rate of less than 60 ml/minute per 1.73 m^2 at baseline. Interviews of the 357 renal patients with documentation of associated laboratory assessments were conducted over a one-year timeframe. The authors found no differences in the progression of chronic kidney disease in study patients taking herbal and dietary supplements at least three times a week and the comparator group who reported no dietary supplement use. There were two patients that had an acute kidney injury during the study period associated with an herbal product, a traditional Chinese medicine combination product or *Tradescantia fluminensis* (river spiderwort), used for a month. The use of herbal and dietary supplements was also associated with uncontrolled hyperphosphatemia in the study population. Since the study did not control for the number or type of herbal or dietary supplement consumed, the cause is uncertain [22C].

Rhabdomyolysis and severe acute kidney injury by tubular injury and a thickened basement membrane are associated with creatine supplements. Protein supplements containing creatine ethyl ester may also be associated with elevated plasma creatinine levels and potentially result in an inaccurate measure of renal function in individuals. Oxalate stones can form in the renal tubules of some persons after high doses of vitamin C, ascorbic acid, causing flank pain and hematuria [23M].

Adverse Effects: Endocrine

Hypericum perforatum (St John's wort, SJW) is a popular HDS used by patients with mild to moderate depression, among other health concerns. The effect of SJW on glucose tolerance was assessed in 10 healthy male subjects (aged 18–40 years) with normal glucose metabolism. Laboratory samples of the subjects' blood were drawn at baseline without exposure to SJW, after 21 days of treatment with SJW (240–294 mg dry extract of SJW and 900 mcg hypericin) twice daily and then at 6 weeks after the treatment period ended. A 75 g glucose bolus was administered to each subject after a 12-hour fast, then laboratory values were obtained including HbA1c, fasting plasma glucose, serum insulin, C-peptide levels and glucose levels at multiple points within 2 hours of ingestion.

Fasting levels of glucose, serum insulin and C-peptide did not differ from pre-SJW to post-SJW. The total and incremental AUC of serum glucose at 2 hours after the 75 g bolus increased over baseline in the treatment period and the increase continued into the post treatment phase of the study. The authors state that SJW causes reduced glucose-stimulated insulin secretion and glucose intolerance during treatment and after a 6-week break in treatment [24c].

Adverse Effects: Hepatic

Hepatotoxicity is one of the most frequent toxicities of HDS. In Western countries, HDS are the second highest cause of drug-induced liver injury (DILI). Between 2008 and 2013, 15.5% of the 839 DILI cases in the United States were due to HDS. In contrast, that number is much higher in the Eastern world where HDS are more popular. For example, a Korean study on DILI revealed 62.5% of the 371 cases were of HDS-induced liver injury (HILI) in nature [25r].

There are three types of DILI (or HILI)—hepatocellular, cholestatic, and mixed type. The hepatocellular injury is the most common type and is characterized by elevated serum concentration of liver enzymes alanine aminotransferase (ALT) and aspartate aminotransferase (AST) as the first diagnostic biomarker. This is followed by elevation of total bilirubin and alkaline phosphatase (ALP). In the cholestatic injury, the movement of bile through the bile canalicular system is impeded. The impedance causes accumulation of toxic bile and excretion products. Serum elevation of alkaline phosphatase precedes that of aminotransferase. The mixed type injury can start as hepatocellular or cholestatic and spread very rapidly to all parts of the liver [26R]. The *R*-value helps in determining the type of liver injury and is the ratio of ALT to ALP, both expressed as multiples of upper limit of normal (ULP) of each. A value of $R \geq 5$ indicates hepatocellular, $R < 2$ indicates cholestatic, and R between 2 and 5, indicates mixed type injury [25r]. Some presentations of liver injury are nausea, vomiting, abdominal pain, fatigue, jaundice, dark urine, pale-colored stool, and pruritus depending on the type of liver damage [26R].

Establishing causality for HILI is challenging. Clinicians often fail to question patients about HDS use that could link to liver injury. Conversely, patients are not often forthcoming about HDS use because they perceive them as safe alternatives and may also feel they could be reprimanded for self-use. With lack of confirmatory tests, diagnosis is generally made by excluding non-DILI causes [27r]. Retrospective analysis of case reports is the predominant method of causality assessment [28R]. In a recent study, reassessment of 100 DILI cases into different categories by three independent observers gave moderate inter-observer reliability, but high agreement within one category [29c]. In the drug-induced liver injury network (DILIN), about 15% of the cases can be attributed to HDS [30S].

HDS use for weight loss is one of the most reported causes of hepatotoxicity. Zheng reviewed liver injury reported for weight loss/fat-burning products sold under the labels of Hydroxycut and Oxyelite Pro (OEP) brands [31R]. *Camellia sinensis* (green tea) is a frequent component of weight loss supplements. (−)-Epigallocatechin-3-gallate (EGCG), a major constituent of green tea, is linked to many health benefits. The consumption of green tea in various forms has grown significantly due to description of its health promoting effects in cardiovascular disease, diabetes, obesity, cancer, etc. However, 19 cases of hepatotoxicity were reported between 2009 and 2015 [32M]. Studies in mice have implicated high-dose EGCG to hepatotoxicity [33E,34E].

Polygonum multiflorum (He Shou Wu; HSW) root in raw or processed form has been used for treating hair loss or grey hair. A systematic review of case studies and case reports for liver damage revealed that when the daily dose was less than 12 g, the median time for liver damage was 60 days, while at doses higher than 12 g/day, the median time for liver damage was 30 days. Thus, the herb demonstrated a "dose-time-toxicity" relationship [35M].

Cascara sagrada is commonly used for relieving constipation. The active constituent is an anthranoid glycoside called senna. It is metabolized by the intestinal flora to produce an aglycone that stimulates intestinal motility and secretary activity. Although relatively safe, extended use or large quantities have been linked to hepatotoxicity [36A].

A 77-year-old Japanese woman with a history of hypertension, hyperlipidemia, and diabetes used an over-the-counter herbal supplement of *Cascara sagrada* to relieve her constipation. The patient had never taken the supplement before. She took 3 capsules of 250 mg each on the first day, increasing to 4 capsules for the next 2 days. Constipation was relieved on the third day at which time the patient discontinued the use of the supplement. The patient noted pale, clay-colored stool and clear, dark orange-colored urine. The stool color returned to normal within a week but the urine color did not. On day 10, the patient presented to the primary care physician with 2 days of fatigue and yellow-tinged skin. Physical exam indicated jaundice without hepatomegaly. Metabolic panel and CBC were within normal limits. Urinalysis showed abnormal orange-yellow color, and elevated (2+) bilirubin. Liver enzymes were elevated as was bilirubin. Hepatitis serologies were negative. The herbal supplement was discontinued, and the patient was held for follow-up observation. Abdominal ultrasound revealed diffuse hepatocellular injury, consistent with DILI. However, the ultrasound suggested a distal obstruction which was diagnosed as extrahepatic cholangiocarcinoma, not causally liked to *Cascara sagrada* and was subsequently removed surgically [36A].

Kratom obtained from South Asian *Mitragyna* trees is consumed to relieve pain, fatigue, and muscle aches, or manage diarrhea or opioid withdrawal. At low doses, *kratom* promotes alertness, while at high doses, it causes sedation. The leaves can be directly chewed or extracted to make a powder or tablets. The active constituents are alkaloids mitragynine and 7-hydroxymitragynine, the latter having a 13-fold higher potency than morphine. The active alkaloids bind to mu, delta, and kappa opioid receptors. Interestingly, *kratom* has been used safely in South East Asia, while it has caused liver injuries in Western countries [37A].

A 58-year-old Caucasian male undergoing treatment for schizoaffective disorder with psychotropic medications consumed 1 tablespoonful of *kratom* powder daily for 3 months. The psychiatrist noticed jaundice and confirmed it by laboratory analysis. The patient was advised to discontinue *kratom*. Liver abnormalities resolved over time. About a year later, the patient noticed dark urine and sought medical help. Jaundice developed in a few days. The patient had resumed taking *kratom* for about a month. Patient's vital signs were normal. He had mild confusion but no edema or ascites. Laboratory tests were elevated in liver enzymes. Ammonia levels were more than four times the normal value. Ultrasound revealed irregular hepatic texture but no biliary obstruction. *Kratom* was discontinued and patient stabilized in the following 2 days [37A].

Ranunculus ficaria (Lesser celandine), a perennial herbaceous plant with yellow flowers, has knotty tubers that resemble piles. Because of this appearance, it has been used to treat piles and is called pilewort. While Greater celandine is well associated with hepatotoxicity, the first worldwide case of hepatotoxicity was only recently reported for lesser celandine [38A].

A 36-year-old woman with no significant disease and no history of alcohol or drug abuse was admitted to the hospital for acute hepatitis. Physical examination revealed jaundice of the sclera. Liver enzymes and bilirubin were highly elevated. Anti-HB IgG was positive, while antibodies to HCV, HAV and HEV were negative. There was no evidence of other viral infections. The patient had consumed 1 cup per day of lesser celandine tea for 3 days. Lesser celandine was immediately discontinued, and the patient recovered within a period of 3 weeks and liver enzymes normalized [38A].

Conjugated linoleic acid (CLA) is a polyunsaturated fatty acid that is an essential fatty acid in the absence of arachidonic acid. CLA has been shown to have many beneficial effects such as stimulating immune response, improving insulin sensitivity and modifying lipid metabolism. CLA has been used as a dietary supplement to assist in weight loss. The first case of CLA-induced hepatitis in the United States and third worldwide was reported recently [39A].

A 26-year-old female on a strict diet and exercise program to lose weight presented to the hospital with pain in the right upper quadrant and vomiting for 1 day. The patient had been using CLA for a week prior to the hospital visit. The liver enzymes and bilirubin were elevated but other findings were unremarkable. Liver biopsy revealed sinusoidal infiltration with macrophages and lymphocytes. A diagnosis of acute hepatitis was made, and CLA was discontinued. Liver enzymes stabilized to normal within 2 weeks [39A].

Cinnamon has been used by patients to help with the treatment of diabetes as an herbal alternative in conjunction with other medications. Cinnamon contains coumarin, and it has been proposed that its metabolite, o-hydroxyphenylacetic acid could be hepatotoxic. Cinnamon should be avoided with other drugs that may be hepatotoxic. A case of acute hepatitis was reported in a patient who consumed cinnamon for about a week to treat her diabetes. The patient was on a number of medications (rosuvastatin, paroxetine, amlodipine, aspirin, clopidogrel, insulin, losartan, metoprolol, and pantoprazole). Cinnamon and high-dose rosuvastatin were withheld and symptoms resolved. Rosuvastatin was reintroduced without renewal of pain or elevation in liver enzymes. The clinical opinion was that cinnamon combined with high-dose rosuvastatin could potentially be hepatotoxic [40A].

Mistletoe (Viscum album) has been used as a homeopathic remedy in the treatment of hypertension, epilepsy, thromboembolism, rheumatoid arthritis, and immunosuppressant. Kudzu (Pueraria lobata) root has been used in Southeastern Asia to treat diabetes, hyperlipidemia, cardiovascular disease, and liver disease. Only one case of mistletoe and two cases of kudzu-related hepatotoxicity had been reported thus far [41A].

Mistletoe and kudzu root extract were found to cause acute hepatitis in a 55-year-old Korean man who was admitted to hospital with epigastric and right-quadrant pain, mild fever, and brownish urine. The patient's past medical history was not significant and he was using the mistletoe and kudzu root extract for general well-being. His understanding was that the herbal extract was "safe as water". Laboratory analysis revealed highly elevated liver enzymes (AST, ALT, alkaline phosphatase) and total bilirubin and negative serology. The herbal extract was discontinued, and the patient improved over the next 8 days [41A].

CONCERNS WITH HERBAL PRODUCT CONTAMINATION

During growth, harvest, processing, and storage, natural products can be polluted by molds, pesticides, heavy metals, and other chemicals, resulting in contamination. Mycotoxins are secondary metabolites produced by certain fungi during growth in the field, processing, transport, or storage. These may cause cancer, abnormalities, neurological problems, stillbirths, neural tube defects, cardiovascular problems, and in some cases, death. Pesticides are among the most widely used chemicals in the world and the most dangerous contaminates for humans. Pesticide residues on HDS can result in many health problems, such as skin rashes, asthma attacks, emphysema and cancer. Heavy metals found in some water and soil sources used in growing botanicals or processing HDS can lead to contamination with lead, cadmium, mercury, and arsenic. Exposure to heavy metals may result in a variety of diseases, such as neurological damage, renal damage, and cancer. Other foreign matter, including sulfide residues and herbicides can also lead to the external contamination of herbal medicines. Some unscrupulous manufacturers of HDS can illegally add pharmaceutical grade ingredients to enhance a specific activity that would be less pronounced with the HDS alone [42R,6R,43R].

Analysis was conducted on 150 dietary supplements marketed to increase sexual performance, 61% included unlabeled phosphodiesterase-5 inhibitors (sildenafil, tadalafil, veradenafil, and 34% modified analogues) with a concern that 25% of them had higher than the maximum recommended dose. Another 5.5% found other drug treatments used for sexual dysfunction (yohimbine, flibanserin, phentolamine, dehydroepiandrosterone or testosterone). A further 2.5% contained products from plants known to improve sexual performance. Only 31% of the samples could be considered as true herbal/natural product. The authors state that contamination is possible due to inadequate cleaning of the manufacturing chain, presence of impurities or degradation products, various compositions of a given dietary supplement with the same batch number, and inadequate labelling [44E].

Di Lorenzo and colleagues [45M] reviewed the literature for causality of adverse effects from common ingredients of HDS. Adverse effects were reported for 39 of the 66 botanical substances selected to be included in their search. Most of the noted adverse effects (86.6%) were associated with 14 plants, including Glycine max/soybean (19.3%), Glycyrrhiza glabra/liquorice (12.2%), Camellia sinensis/green tea (8.7%) and Ginkgo biloba/gingko (8.5%). Reports of adulterated HDS included in the study:

(1) Camellia sinensis (L.) Kuntze (green tea) had reports of associated acute hepatotoxicity caused by catechins and their gallic esters. However, two reports indicated that the acute hepatotoxicity was due to Chinese herbal supplements containing green tea and an adulterant, N-nitroso-fenfluramine, the probable hepatotoxic agent. (2) Citrum aurantium (bitter orange) causes specific adverse effect and interactions when combined with

conventional pharmaceuticals. Alone, the natural presence of sympathomimetic stimulant amines, such as synephrine, may be causative of the numerous adverse cardiovascular effects. When bitter orange was used in combination with caffeine, ephedrine, yohimbine, phenyl ethylamine, and thyroxine, enhancement of the cardiovascular adverse effects was reported, such as tachycardia, hypertension, ventricular fibrillation, angina, acute myocardial infraction, ischemic stroke, and exercise-induced syncope. (3) *Glycine max* (soybean) in the form of soy milk containing high levels of iodine is reported to cause thyroid dysfunction [45M].

Adulteration of HDS was recently reviewed [46R] highlighting concerns of augmentation with pharmaceutical drugs and active analogs to improve HDS product activity. The marketed products are often in weight loss, sexual enhancement, and performance enhancement categories. The products are often not labelled with all ingredients and do not undergo the rigorous testing required by the FDA or other regulatory agencies for these pharmaceutic drugs. The FDA and the European Union (E.U.) recalled hundreds of weight loss products during 2010–2015 due to safety concerns of illegal addition of sibutramine, a substance banned in the U.S. and the E.U. due to association of use with serious cardiovascular events, stroke or heart attack. Other recalled HDS weight loss products contained unlabeled phenolphthalein, a laxative, and fluoxetine, an antidepressant. Hundreds of notifications have been issued by the FDA for sexual enhancement dietary supplements due to positive detections of approved PDE-5 inhibitors or its analogs. The EU also sent out notifications for similar products and those containing stimulants such as alkaloids, ephedrine and synephrine. Patients hospitalized in Hong Kong were reported to have traces of sibutramine, fenfluramine analogs in blood samples after taking adulterated weight loss products. Evaluation of HDS products after recall continued to show the presence of banned or unlabeled drugs. Many remained available for purchase containing the same adulterant previously identified by the FDA and several products contained a different analog, or the same compound added with a new adulterant [46R].

A synthetic stimulant—1,3-dimethylbutylamine (DMBA)—is an intentional contaminant in herbal products labeled as AMP citrate, 4-amino-2-methylpentane citrate, Pentergy and others. Cohen et al. determined that at least 12 dietary supplements labeled to contain one or more of these ingredients also contained DMBA. The suggested serving size on the product could deliver between 13 and 120 mg of DMBA per serving which could cause potential health risks [47E].

A hospital in Connecticut notified the CDC and the Connecticut Department of Public Health of a fatal case of gastrointestinal mucormycosis in a preterm infant. Unopened bottles of ABC Dophilus Powder were tested and yielded *Rhizopus* species, a saprophytic fungus capable of causing this gastrointestinal toxicity. The product was voluntarily recalled by the manufacturer due to the safety hazard to the high risk pediatric populations that would receive this treatment [48A].

An investigation of store brand herbal supplements from four major retailers in New York found that only 21% of the products, when tested through DNA analysis, contained the herbs indicated on the label. For the retailer with the poorest outcome, only 4% of the products contained the herb(s) listed on the label. Contaminants included items like rice, bean, asparagus, primrose, wheat, etc. The herbal manufacturing industry contested this finding by observing that DNA can be damaged during processing of herbal supplements, leading to incorrect DNA analysis [49r].

Melamine, used to fraudulently enhance test results for protein content of foods and supplements, can potentially cause urate stones and nephropathy in persons ingesting this adulterant. These supplements were tested in 2008 in China. Almost 300 000 infants were screened and diagnosed with urinary tract stones and sand-like calculi associated with melamine in milk products. Of these, 50 000 infants were hospitalized, with six associated deaths. The study also reported that another source of contamination in these products could be pesticide residues such as cyromazine [50E].

A study reported liquid herbal supplement products contaminated with fecal coliforms, *Klebsiella* species and *Enterobacter* species, in Mwanza city. The contamination was associated with low socioeconomic conditions, lack of formal training in preparation of HDS, lack of registration with the ministry of health, lack of appropriate packaging of products, and use of solvents that were not sanitized before or during preparation. This was observed by doing a cross-sectional study involving 59 workers and 109 liquid HDS products[51E].

MIND–BODY THERAPIES

Adverse Effects: Manipulative Therapy, Chiropractic Therapy

Spinal manipulative therapy of the lower back is recommended in guidelines for treatment of lower back pain. Most common concerns after treatment are considered benign and self-limiting within 24 hours. Reporting of serious harm in the primary literature from chiropractic intervention is poor; however, the overall incidence of serious adverse events is presumed low. The authors defined a serious adverse event as "an untoward occurrence that results in death or is life threatening, requires hospitalization or results in permanent disability." In the 41 studies from the Europe, North America, Australia and Asia that were included, 77 serious adverse events were reported including cauda equine syndrome (38%), lumbar disc herniation (30%) or fracture (9%) and hematoma or hemorrhagic cyst (8%). Other serious adverse events (16%) were reported as neurologic or vascular compromise, soft tissue trauma, muscle abscess formation, disrupted fracture healing and esophageal rupture. A majority of patients with serious adverse events were women with an average age of 50 years. Of the cases where subsequent treatment was listed, 53 cases were treated with surgery [9M]. Chiropractic manipulation in the pediatric population was reviewed to determine the consistency of safety terminology. The rate of adverse reactions from manipulations of spine, cranium, and myofascial ranged from 0.23% to 9% of patients per year. The author suggests classification and terminology of terms used to describe adverse effects and side effects of manipulative therapies be structured in a common database would increase the number and quality of reports [7R].

Although reports of adverse effects with manipulative therapy are scant, a case report of brachial plexus injury causing paralysis of the left shoulder following massage therapy was published. The middle-aged woman had received deep tissue massage targeting the left shoulder twice weekly for 2 weeks before she experienced worsening symptoms of shoulder numbness and weakness. The symptoms progressed to paralysis of the upper arm and shoulder. The patient recovered after a year of rehabilitation and guided exercise [52A].

Adverse Effects: Acupuncture

Acupuncture is practiced in many countries to relieve pain and nausea. A recent review of the literature on the use of acupuncture in pregnancy concluded that adverse event reporting is poor and lack the use of validated scales to assess harm to the woman or fetus/infant, although reports of minor and serious adverse events occur and are reported. Minor effects attributed to the use of acupuncture during pregnancy include altered taste, hematoma, treatment discomfort, uterine contractions and being placed on bed rest. Premature labor was reported in one study as being due to the procedure, other serious adverse events are listed as not attributable to the study in acupuncture patients, including premature delivery, pregnancy loss, pre-eclampsia and stillbirth. The authors state that serious adverse events occur in 1 in 1193 women or per >7300 sessions. Acupuncture vs. sham non-penetrating acupuncture did not show differences in adverse events, mild or serious [20M].

The efficacy and safety of acupuncture for symptoms of dizziness and vertigo were assessed in an emergency department in Taiwan. The patients were randomized to receive acupuncture or sham acupuncture with seed patches at non-acupoints. Outcomes were measured by the dizziness handicap inventory (DHI), a visual analog scale (VAS) of dizziness and vertigo and heart rate variability. Baseline characteristics were similar between groups. Efficacy of acupuncture was only shown on the VAS at 30 minutes and at 7 days. No adverse effects were reported by patients or caregivers after treatment [53C].

Pneumothorax due to acupuncture for chronic back pain in a 66-year-old man was reported to alert practitioners to a rare but potentially serious complications of this practice. The patient presented to an emergency room for shortness of breath after returning home from an acupuncture session. The patient had suffered a pneumothorax but was not hospitalized. It was stated that the patient had not been informed of any potential risk of complications prior to acupuncture procedure [54A].

Adverse Effects: Tai Chi

Wayne and colleagues discovered limited adverse effect reporting in studies of Tai Chi. Out of 153 studies identified as randomized controlled trials, only 50 included reporting of adverse effects and only 18 of those had a monitoring protocol developed for adverse effects in which adverse effects were reported, an additional 3 studies had a protocol but did not report any adverse effects. No serious adverse events were attributable to Tai Chi. Minor complaints included increased muscle aches, pain, headache and dizziness [55M].

Adverse Effects: Yoga

Yoga techniques are considered to aid in the prevention of fall injury by giving the practitioner increased ability to balance. Participants of a more encompassing women's health study, women aged 59–64 years were asked about falls and fall-related injury, as well as, participation in yoga or meditative practices. Over 10 000 Australian women replied, of those, 4413 had slipped, tripped or stumbled in the past year, and 2770 had fallen to the ground. Of these, 1398 had been injured due to the fall and 901 had sought medical attention for this injury. Women who self-reported as regularly practicing yoga or other meditation in the past year were less likely to have had any occurrences than those who did not. No significant differences between groups were found for any of the falls-related events [8M].

CONCLUSIONS

Use of CAM practices is increasing around the world due to perceived health benefits, low cost and relatively low risk. Safety of CAM practices and treatments is being researched in many countries. Standardization of HDS product efficacy and safety markers or reporting does not exist globally or even regionally. Limited information on the adverse effects of mind–body practices is available due to no official public or governmental reporting mechanisms as compared to HDS. In many cases, there is a lack of information until complaints against a particular product or practice are brought to governmental authorities. Healthcare providers should familiarize themselves with CAM practices and their benefits and risks to best care for their patient population.

References

[1] World Health Organization. General guidelines for methodologies on research and evaluation of traditional medicine; 2000, http://apps.who.int/medicinedocs/en/d/Jwhozip42e/. Accessed April 5, 2016. [S].

[2] Black LI, Clarke TC, Barnes PM. Use of complementary health approaches among children aged 4–17 years in the United States: National health interview survey, 2007–2012. Natl Health Stat Report. 2015;78:1–17 [S].

[3] Clarke TC, Black LI, Stussman BJ, et al. Trends in the use of complementary health approaches among adults: United states, 2002–2012. Natl Health Stat Report. 2015;79:1–16 [S].

[4] National Center for Complementary and Alternative Medicine. Complementary, alternative, or integrative health: what's in a name? 2013, https://nccih.nih.gov/health/integrative-health. Accessed April 5, 2016. [S].

[5] National Institutes of Health. National Center for Complementary and Alternative Medicine. The use of complementary and alternative medicine in the United States: cost data; 2016, https://nccih.nih.gov/sites/nccam.nih.gov/files/NHIS_costdata.pdf. Accessed April 5, 2016. [S].

[6] Tripathy V, Basak B, Varghese TS, et al. Residues and contaminants in medicinal herbs—a review. Phytochem Lett. 2015;14:67–78 [R].

[7] Marchand AM. A literature review of pediatric spinal manipulation and chiropractic manipulative therapy: evaluation of consistent use of safety terminology. J Manipulative Physiol Ther. 2015;38(9):692–8 [R].

[8] Cramer H, Ward L, Saper R, et al. The safety of yoga: a systematic review and meta-analysis of randomized controlled trials. Am J Epidemiol. 2015;182(4):281–93 [M].

[9] Hebert J, Stomski NJ, French SD, et al. Serious adverse events and spinal manipulative therapy of the low back region: a systematic review of cases. J Manipulative Physiol Ther. 2015;38(9):677–91 [M].

[10] Geller AI, Shehab N, Weidle NJ, et al. Emergency department visits for adverse events related to dietary supplements. N Engl J Med. 2015;373(16):1531–40 [C].

[11] Wegener T, Deitelhoff B, Silber-Mankowsky A. Drug safety aspects of herbal medicinal products. Wien Med Wochenschr. 2015;165(11–12):243–50 [R].

[12] Govindaraghavan S, Sucher NJ. Quality assessment of medicinal herbs and their extracts: criteria and prerequisites for consistent safety and efficacy of herbal medicines. Epilepsy Behav. 2015;52:363–71 [R].

[13] National Center for Complementary and Integrative Health. Using dietary supplements wisely; 2009, https://nccih.nih.gov/sites/nccam.nih.gov/files/Using_Dietary_Supplements_Wisely_10-06-2015%20(2).pdf. Updated June 2014. Accessed April 5, 2016, 2016. [S].

[14] Breda JJ, Whiting SH, Encarnacao R, et al. Energy drink consumption in Europe: a review of the risks, adverse health effects, and policy options to respond. Front Public Health. 2014;2:134 [M].

[15] Grasser EK, Dulloo AG, Montani J. Cardiovascular and cerebrovascular effects in response to red bull consumption combined with mental stress. Am J Cardiol. 2015;115(2):183–9 [C].

[16] Shah SA, Dargush AE, Potts V, et al. Effects of single and multiple energy shots on blood pressure and electrocardiographic parameters. Am J Cardiol. 2016;117(3):465–8 [C].

[17] Pommerening MJ, Cardenas JC, Radwan ZA, et al. Hypercoagulability after energy drink consumption. J Surg Res. 2015;199(2):635–40 [c].

[18] Norelli LJ, Xu C. Manic psychosis associated with ginseng: a report of two cases and discussion of the literature. J Diet Suppl. 2015;12(2):119–25 [A].

[19] Bersani FS, Coviello M, Imperatori C, et al. Adverse psychiatric effects associated with herbal weight-loss products. Biomed Res Int. 2015;2015:120679 [R].

[20] Clarkson CE, O'Mahony D, Jones DE. Adverse event reporting in studies of penetrating acupuncture during pregnancy: a systematic review. Acta Obstet Gynecol Scand. 2015;94(5):453–64 [M].

[21] Yigit M, Cevik E. A rare cause of pulmonary embolism: Panax. Am J Emerg Med. 2015;33(2):311.e1–2 [A].

[22] Tangkiatkumjai M, Boardman H, Praditpornsilpa K, et al. Prevalence of herbal and dietary supplement usage in Thai outpatients with chronic kidney disease: a cross-sectional survey. BMC Complement Altern Med. 2013;13:153 [C].

[23] Nauffal M, Gabardi S. Nephrotoxicity of natural products. Blood Purif. 2016;41(1–3):123–9 [M].

[24] Stage TB, Damkier P, Christensen MM, et al. Impaired glucose tolerance in healthy men treated with St. John's Wort. Basic Clin Pharmacol Toxicol. 2016;118(3):219–24 [c].

[25] Stournaras E, Tziomalos K. Herbal medicine-related hepatotoxicity. World J Hepatol. 2015;7(19):2189 [r].

[26] Sreya Kosanam RB. Drug-induced liver injury: a review. Int J Pharmacol Res. 2015;5(2):24–30 [R].

[27] Stickel F, Shouval D. Hepatotoxicity of herbal and dietary supplements: an update. Arch Toxicol. 2015;89(6):851–65 [r].

[28] Calitz C, du Plessis L, Gouws C, et al. Herbal hepatotoxicity: current status, examples, and challenges. Expert Opin Drug Metab Toxicol. 2015;11(10):1551–65 [R].

[29] Hayashi PH, Barnhart HX, Fontana RJ, et al. Reliability of causality assessment for drug, herbal and dietary supplement hepatotoxicity in the drug-induced liver injury network (DILIN). Liver Int. 2015;35(5):1623–32 [c].

[30] Vuppalanchi R, Navarro V, Vega M, et al. Herbal dietary supplement associated hepatotoxicity: an upcoming workshop and need for research. Gastroenterology. 2015;148(3):480–2 [S].

[31] Zheng EX, Navarro VJ. Liver injury from herbal, dietary, and weight loss supplements: a review. J Clin Transl Hepatol. 2015;3(2):93–8 [R].

[32] Mazzanti G, Di Sotto A, Vitalone A. Hepatotoxicity of green tea: an update. Arch Toxicol. 2015;89(8):1175–91 [M].

[33] Wang D, Wang Y, Wan X, et al. Green tea polyphenol (-)-epigallocatechin-3-gallate triggered hepatotoxicity in mice: responses of major antioxidant enzymes and the Nrf2 rescue pathway. Toxicol Appl Pharmacol. 2015;283(1):65 [E].

[34] Church RJ, Gatti DM, Urban TJ, et al. Sensitivity to hepatotoxicity due to epigallocatechin gallate is affected by genetic background in diversity outbred mice. Food Chem Toxicol. 2015;76:19–26 [E].

[35] Lei X, Chen J, Ren J, et al. Liver damage associated with polygonum multiflorum thunb: a systematic review of case reports and case series. Evid Based Complement Alternat Med. 2015;2015, article 4597949 [M].

[36] Nakasone ES, Tokeshi J. A serendipitous find: a case of cholangiocarcinoma identified incidentally after acute liver injury due to cascara sagrada ingestion. Hawaii J Med Public Health. 2015;74(6):200 [A].

[37] Dorman C, Wong M, Khan A. Cholestatic hepatitis from prolonged kratom use: a case report. Hepatology. 2015;61(3):1086–7 [A].

[38] Yilmaz B, Yilmaz B, Aktaş B, et al. Lesser celandine (pilewort) induced acute toxic liver injury: the first case report worldwide. World J Hepatol. 2015;7(2):285 [A].

[39] Bilal M, Patel Y, Burkitt M, et al. Linoleic acid induced acute hepatitis: a case report and review of the literature. Case Reports Hepatol. 2015;2015, article 807354 [A].

[40] Brancheau D, Patel B, Zughaib M. Do cinnamon supplements cause acute hepatitis? Am J Case Rep. 2015;16:250 [A].

[41] Kim HJ, Kim H, Ahn JH, et al. Liver injury induced by herbal extracts containing mistletoe and kudzu. J Altern Complement Med. 2015;21(3):180 [A].

[42] Wang Z, Huang L. Panax quinquefolius: An overview of the contaminants. Phytochem Lett. 2015;11:89–94 [R].

[43] Liu SH, Chuang WC, Lam W, et al. Safety surveillance of traditional Chinese medicine: current and future. Drug Saf. 2015;38(2):117–28 [R].

[44] Gilard V, Balayssac S, Tinaugus A, et al. Detection, identification and quantification by 1 H NMR of adulterants in 150 herbal dietary supplements marketed for improving sexual performance. J Pharm Biomed Anal. 2015;102:476–93 [E].

[45] Di Lorenzo C, Ceschi A, Kupferschmidt H, et al. Adverse effects of plant food supplements and botanical preparations: a systematic review with critical evaluation of causality. Br J Clin Pharmacol. 2015;79(4):578–92 [M].

[46] Rocha T, Amaral JS, Oliveira MBP. Adulteration of dietary supplements by the illegal addition of synthetic drugs: a review. Compr Rev Food Sci Food Saf. 2016;15(1):43–62 [R].

[47] Cohen PA, Travis JC, Venhuis BJ. A synthetic stimulant never tested in humans, 1,3-dimethylbutylamine (DMBA), is identified in multiple dietary supplements. Drug Test Anal. 2015;7(1):83–7 [E].

[48] Vallabhaneni S, Walker TA, Lockhart SR, et al. Notes from the field: fatal gastrointestinal mucormycosis in a premature infant associated with a contaminated dietary supplement— Connecticut, 2014. MMWR Morb Mortal Wkly Rep. 2015;64(6):155–6 [A].

[49] Herbal supplements filled with fake ingredients, New York attorney general Eric Schneiderman finds—CBS news. http://www.cbsnews.com/news/herbal-supplements-targeted-by-new-york-attorney-general/. February 3, 2015. Accessed April 12, 2016. [r].

[50] Gabriels G, Lambert M, Smith P, et al. Melamine contamination in nutritional supplements—is it an alarm bell for the general consumer, athletes, and 'Weekend warriors'? Nutr J. 2015;14(1):1 [E].

[51] Walther C, Marwa KJ, Seni J, et al. Microbial contamination of traditional liquid herbal medicinal products marketed in Mwanza city: magnitude and risk factors. Pan Afr Med J. 2016;23:65 [E].

[52] Chang CY, Wu YT, Chen LC, et al. Massage-induced brachial plexus injury. Phys Ther. 2015;95(1):109–16 [A].

[53] Chiu CW, Lee TC, Hsu PC, et al. Efficacy and safety of acupuncture for dizziness and vertigo in emergency department: a pilot cohort study. BMC Complement Altern Med. 2015;15, article 173 [C].

[54] Brogan RJ, Mushtaq F. Acupuncture-induced pneumothorax: the hidden complication. Scott Med J. 2015;60(2):e11–3 [A].

[55] Wayne PM, Berkowitz DL, Litrownik DE, et al. What do we really know about the safety of tai chi? A systematic review of adverse event reports in randomized trials. Arch Phys Med Rehabil. 2014;95(12):2470–83 [M].

47

Miscellaneous Drugs, Materials, Medical Devices and Techniques

Anjan Nan[1]

Department of Pharmaceutical Sciences, University of Maryland Eastern Shore School of Pharmacy, Princess Anne, MD, USA

[1]Corresponding author: anan@umes.edu

ALUMINUM

Aluminum (Al) and Al-containing compounds have long been extensively used in industry, water purification, medications, food additives and vaccines. The human body is easily exposed to a significant amount of Al and recent reports suggest that chronic Al exposure may lead to a risk of Alzheimer's disease (AD). However, these reports are not always consistent due to differences in study populations, Al exposure levels and study designs. Wang et al. reported a systematic review and meta-analysis of several epidemiological studies to examine the extent of association of chronic Al exposure with AD. This analysis included a systematic literature search of PubMed, Web of Knowledge, Elsevier Science Direct and Springer databases for human epidemiological studies up to June, 2015. The quality of included studies was determined to be high based on the Newcastle–Ottawa Scale (NOS) (score of 7 or higher). The meta-analysis included 8 cohort and case–control studies, with a total of 10567 individuals. Follow-up duration of the cohort studies varied from 8 to 48 years. Q test and I2 statistic were used to demonstrate no significant heterogeneity between selected studies. The overall odds ratio (OR) was calculated. Two types of Al exposure were reported: drinking water and occupational exposure. Al exposure was defined by a concentration equal to or greater than 100 µg Al/L in the drinking water [1M].

The results of this study showed that individuals chronically exposed to Al were 71% more likely to develop AD (OR: 1.71, 95% CI, 1.35–2.18). Sensitivity analysis demonstrated that the overall OR is not influenced by any individual study. Publication bias was also excluded by the analysis. The pooled OR among individuals who drank water containing an Al level at or higher than 100 µg/L was 1.95 (95% CI, 1.47–2.59) compared to those who drank water containing less than 100 µg/L.

Studies have demonstrated that the brain is sensitive to Al, due to the non-dividing nature of most neurons susceptibility to oxidative stress ability to cross the blood–brain barrier and slow clearance from the brain. The positively charged Al can easily bind with the metal-binding amino acids of various proteins. Al can form a complex with amyloid beta (Aβ) and inhibit their degradation, thus enhancing the production and aggregation of Aβ. The extracellular accumulation of Aβ in the brain is regarded as an early event in the development of AD. Several studies have suggested that the AD brain can elicit a neuroinflammatory response and lead to formation of reactive oxygen species (ROS) in the brain.

Chronic exposure to Al at a level routinely ingested by humans has exhibited profound memory loss in elderly patients as evidenced by analysis of brain autopsy samples from AD patients. To this effect Al chelation therapy in AD patients has been reported as beneficial. While many available studies look at acute effects, the present study demonstrates a positive link between chronic Al exposure and AD. However, the limitations of the meta-analysis must be considered as it was not possible to consider every report of Al exposure including drinking water, occupational exposure, drugs, processed foods, vaccinations, sun protection lotions, deodorants and other sources. The practical challenges of obtaining accurate record of human data for chronic (decades) exposure, lack of dose-dependent response studies and the limited number of studies (8) included in the meta-analysis further limit the scope of this work.

A recent study is reported by Elserougy and coworkers that indicate harmful effects of Al on respiratory health and pulmonary functions of occupationally exposed workers. It investigated the possible relationship between inhalation exposure to Al fumes and levels of C-reactive protein (CRP) and alpha-1-antitrypsin (A1AT). In this study 56 male Al workers with a mean duration of occupational exposure of 10.1 ± 9.5 years were compared with 52 male participants who were not exposed to Al fumes (control). All participants underwent full clinical examination. Blood samples were collected for the determination of serum CRP and A1AT and urine samples for measuring Al. Results showed that urinary Al (UAl) was significantly higher in Al workers compared with controls ($p < 0.05$). A1AT was significantly lowered in Al workers compared with the controls ($p < 0.000$). Serum CRP was positive in only two (3.6%) of the exposed workers. In addition smoking resulted in higher UAl and lower A1AT in both groups. Smokers of both groups (exposed and controls) showed significantly higher UAl and lower A1AT compared with non-smokers. There was a significant negative correlation between the duration of exposure and A1AT ($p < 0.05$) and a positive significant correlation between smoking index (SI) and UAl. There was also a significant negative correlation between SI and some of the pulmonary function tests, namely, the percentage of predicted forced vital capacity, forced expiratory volume in the first second and peak expiratory flow in the exposed group. Those correlations point to the importance of the combined effect of smoking and Al exposure on the impairment of lung functions. The authors of the study recommend the determination of CRP and A1AT in Al-exposed workers as these parameters may undergo changes before reduction in pulmonary functions takes place [2c].

Risk of Al Toxicity in Pediatric Patients

Unlike the United States, there are no regulations regarding Al content of large- and small-volume parenterals in Canada. A recent study measured plasma Al concentrations in pediatric patients who receive long-term parenteral nutrition. These children are believed to be at higher risk of Al toxicity and possibly impaired neurological development because the infusion bypasses the gastrointestinal tract. In this study plasma Al concentration was retrospectively gathered from the charts of 27 patients with intestinal failure (IF) receiving long-term PN at The Hospital for Sick Children, Toronto, Canada, and compared with age- and sex-matched controls for comparison. In addition, Al concentration was measured in PN samples collected from 10 randomly selected

patients with IF and used to determine their Al intake. The plasma Al concentration of children with IF receiving long-term PN was found to be significantly higher than that of control patients (1195 ± 710 vs 142 ± 63 nmol/L; $p < 0.0001$). In 10 patients for whom Al intake from their PN solution was determined, mean Al intake from PN was $15.4 \pm 15\,\mu g/kg$, which was threefold higher than the US Food and Drug Administration upper recommended intake level. Al intake was also significantly related to plasma Al concentration ($p = 0.02$, $r(2) = 0.52$). The study therefore concluded that pediatric patients receiving long-term PN for IF in Canada are at risk for Al toxicity [3c].

CALCIUM

Recent evidence suggests that calcium (Ca) supplements increase the risk of cardiovascular events, but the mechanism(s) by which this occurs is not clear. Bristow and coworkers evaluated the effects of various Ca supplements on blood Ca levels, and blood pressure and their acute effects on blood coagulation. 100 postmenopausal women were randomized to 1 g/day of Ca or placebo. Blood pressure was measured at baseline and every 2 h up to 8 h after their first dose and after 3 months of supplementation. Blood pressure was found to decline over 8 h in both the groups. The reduction in systolic blood pressure was smaller in the Ca group compared with the control group by >5 mm Hg between 2 and 6 h ($p \leq 0.02$), and the reduction in diastolic blood pressure was smaller at 2 h (difference 4.5 mm Hg, $p = 0.004$). Blood coagulability was assessed by thromboelastography (TEG) and found to increase from baseline over 8 h in the calcium and control groups. At 4 h, the increase in the coagulation index was greater in the Ca group compared with the control group ($p = 0.03$), which could be due to a reduction in the time to clot initiation. These data collectively suggest that Ca supplements may acutely influence blood pressure and blood coagulation [4c].

CATHETER

Catheter-related bloodstream infections are often a cause of significant morbidity and mortality in hemodialysis patients. While these are commonly associated with Gram-positive Staphylococcus aureus and other skin bacteria, Gram-negative organisms e.g. Pseudomonas are also identified in patients with frequent exposures with health care environment. Kataria et al. reported catheter-related bacteremia by the Gram bacillus, *Stenotrophomonas maltophilia* in three hemodialysis patients that were successfully treated with dialysis catheter removal and antibiotic therapy. The patients presented with acute onset of fever without any localizing symptom. All patients had tunneled internal jugular catheters for dialysis access but showed no evidence of tunnel infection. Blood cultures from all the tunneled catheters grew *S. maltophilia* within 1–3 days of incubation. The strains were sensitive to ampicillin–sulbactam, levofloxacin and trimethoprim–sulfamethoxazole (TMP-SMX). The bacteremia persisted despite treatment with dual antibiotic therapy for 4–5 days, necessitating catheter removal. Subsequently, the patients recovered and repeat blood cultures were sterile [5r].

The study is of high importance as *S. maltophilia* can form biofilm on the catheters and other *in situ*-devices. Risk factors for infection with *S. maltophilia* include hospitalization, HIV infection, malignancy, neutropenia, mechanical ventilation and presence of central venous catheters. These strains are frequently resistant to a number of antibiotics including aminoglycosides and carbapenems.

Catheter-Associated Mycobacteremia

Case Report

Mycobacterium fortuitum is a rapidly growing *Mycobacterium* ubiquitous in nature that is known to form biofilms and colonize the *in situ* central line catheters. Catheter-associated mycobacteremia is a rare condition caused by rapidly growing Mycobacteria in central venous devices (TID). Rathor and coworkers report the case of a 48-year-old female cancer patient who reported clinical illness and neutropenia while on chemotherapy via totally implanted central venous device, 6 months post laparoscopic-assisted right hemicolectomy. She had persistent fever which was not embolization related as evidenced by chest X-ray and echocardiography. Urine R/E and immunological tests all came back negative against malaria, dengue, herpes or CMV. On the fourth day blood sample which was taken from the chemo port revealed irregularly staining Gram-positive bacilli. An Ehrlich–Ziehl–Neelsen stain was done, and acid-fast bacilli were seen. Upon the suspicion of a rapidly growing nontuberculous Mycobacterium (RGM) spp. the isolate was analyzed and identified as *M. fortuitum*. The patient was subsequently administered chemotherapy via a peripheral line, as a matter of caution to prevent the possible impending bacteremia. Repeat blood cultures from the chemo port and peripheral line were collected. On the fourth day the chemo port cultures were positive again for acid-fast bacilli. The diagnosis of chemo port colonization was made and removal of chemo port was planned [6A].

RGM is not virulent or life threatening but has a high predisposition to create biofilms and thus to colonize and infect intravascular catheters. Fever with or without chills and rigors in a patient who has received chemotherapy via a TID/CVC in the past 3 months is a subtle indicator of the underlying infection.

CONTINUOUS RENAL REPLACEMENT THERAPY

Intensive care unit patients who require continuous renal replacement therapy (CRRT) experience a high incidence of adverse events (AEs), according to a new study. A team at Mayo Clinic in Rochester, Minn., led by Kianoush Kashani, MD, carried out a retrospective study consisting of 595 Caucasian adult patients (≥18 years) who underwent CRRT from January 1, 2007 to December 31, 2009. Regional citrate anticoagulation was used in these patients. The clinicians found that the most common clinically significant electrolyte derangements were ionized hypocalcemia (22%), ionized hypercalcemia (23%), and hyperphosphatemia (44%). 97% of the patients had at least one additional AE including new onset hypotension (within the first hour after CRRT initiation) (43%), hypothermia (44%), new onset arrhythmias (29%), new onset anemia (31%) and thrombocytopenia (40%). The study concluded that although the extent to which these complications are attributable to CRRT is not known, clinicians need to be cautious and aware of their high prevalence in this patient population [7R].

CHLORHEXIDINE

Chlorhexidine is a broad-spectrum topical antimicrobial agent that is used to bathe hospitalized patients to reduce bacterial infections and multidrug resistant organisms (MDROs). While chlorhexidine bathing is routinely practiced to reduce MDRO acquisition and hospital-acquired bloodstream infections, the effect on other infections is unclear. There is a concern that overexposure may result in the development of resistance. Noto and coworkers conducted a cluster-randomized trial to evaluate the effect of chlorhexidine bathing on the rates of multiple healthcare-associated infections among critically ill adults. The trial population included 9340 patients admitted to 5 adult intensive care units of a tertiary medical center in Nashville, Tennessee, from July 2012 through July 2013. Once-daily bathing of all patients with disposable cloths impregnated with 2% chlorhexidine or non-antimicrobial cloths as a control was studied for a 10-week period followed by a 2-week washout period during which patients were bathed with non-antimicrobial disposable cloths, before crossover to the alternate bathing treatment for 10 weeks. Each unit crossed over between bathing assignments 3 times during the study.

The primary outcomes monitored were: central line-associated bloodstream infections (CLABSIs), catheter-associated urinary tract infections (CAUTIs), ventilator-associated pneumonia (VAP), and Clostridium difficile infections. Secondary outcomes included rates of clinical cultures that tested positive for MDROs, blood culture contamination, health care-associated bloodstream infections, and rates of the primary outcome by ICU [8c].

It was observed that Chlorhexidine bathing did not change rates of either the primary or secondary outcomes in any individual intensive care unit. The findings of this trial therefore did not support daily bathing of critically ill patients with chlorhexidine. A word of caution is to be noted here as the study may have overestimated the chlorhexidine intervention effects. As pointed out in a related commentary by Pittet et al., Chlorhexidine bathing could result in lower blood culture contamination rather than actual infection rates [9r].

VITAMIN D SUPPLEMENT

Due to public concerns about vitamin D deficiency there is a widespread use of over the counter (OTC) vitamin D (-D3 or -D2) supplements, containing up to 10 000 IU/unit dose (400 IU = 10 µg). Such doses can be toxic and cause hypercalcemia particularly in the vulnerable infant population. There is a wide variability in Vitamin D content in OTC supplements which are not strictly regulated by the FDA. Vitamin D-induced hypercalcemia is also related to genetic factors such as mutations in the CYP24A1 gene. Therefore, differential diagnosis of hypercalcemia should include both dose-dependent and genetic etiologies.

Case Report
A 4-month-old female who was exclusively breast-fed and received an oral liquid vitamin D3 supplement was reported as a case of vitamin D3-associated toxicity. The vitamin D3 content of the supplement was threefold higher (6000 IU of D/drop) than the label recommendation (2000 IU). Therefore, the infant received 50 000 IU/day for 2 months which resulted in severe hypercalcemia (serum Ca = 18. 7 mg/dL), suppressed PTH (<6 pg/mL), hypercalciuria and nephrocalcinosis (result of chronic exposure to high 25(OH)D3). The hypercalcemia in the infant was eventually managed during her hospital stay by fluids and calcitonin and bisphosphonates administration. Her serum calcium and 25(OH)D3 levels (marker of vitamin D3 status) decreased progressively to reach normal range over the next 3–3.5 months. Genetic

cause of hypercalcemia, hypercalciuria and nephrocalcinosis was ruled out on the basis of normal 24,25 (OH)2D3 to 25(OH)D3 ratio which is indicative of normal CYP24A1 function. The study points out that safety parameters have to be established for long-term high dose vitamin D3 supplementation. There is a need for stricter regulation of vitamin D3 content in OTC supplements and prominent warning labels regarding maximum allowable daily doses [10A].

DAPSONE GEL

Case Report 1
Dapsone (diaminodiphenyl sulphone or DDS) is an anti-inflammatory compound used in the treatment of leprosy-associated dermatoses. Generally reported adverse reactions of this drug include acneiform eruptions and toxic epidermal necrolysis. A recent rare side effect was reported by Karjigi et al. in a 30-year-old woman who was treated with paucibacillary multi drug therapy that included dapsone as the main constituent. She developed itchy skin lesions over the both forearms, 'V' area of the neck and upper back after 1 week of the drug administration. The condition appeared to be photosensitive as it worsened upon exposure to sunlight. A clinical diagnosis of dapsone-induced photosensitive dermatitis was confirmed by histopathology and recurrence of symptoms and signs after re-exposure to the drug. The patient also had an unusually early onset compared to the previously reported cases [11A].

Case Report 2
This is the only reported case of acute dapsone poisoning out of 21 000 consecutive intoxications treated in the Clinical Toxicology Clinic at St George University hospital, Plovdiv, Bulgaria, between 1999 and 2013. A 37-year-old Caucasian woman ingested 45 tablets (100 mg) of dapsone and 30 tablets (10 mg) of olanzapine in suicidal self-poisoning. Fifteen minutes later her general condition worsened and she lost consciousness for 40 minutes 9 h after the ingestion, her methemoglobin level was 51.7%. Dapsone is well known to produce methemoglobinemia (>30%) [13A,14A,15A,16r], depending on the ingested quantity or individual susceptibility [12A].

Other factors that led to confirmatory diagnosis of dapsone poisoning were: cyanosis, tachycardia, and brown color of blood. In this patient the estimated dapsonemia was 24.4096 µg/mL (based on methemoglobinemia), which was consistent with severe dapsone intoxication due to effective absorption of ~17–19 tablets of the drug. The patient recovered 8 days later after receiving several treatments including intubation, ventilation, repeated gastric lavage, hemodialysis, blood exchange transfusion and antidote treatment with methylene blue.

There are several recent reports of dapsone-induced hypersensitivity side effects [17A,18A,19r].

DISULFIRAM

Disulfiram (tetraethylthiuram disulfide) is a drug used for treating alcohol dependency for over 60 years. Known side effects of this drug include neurological toxicity, postural hypotension, circulatory collapse and mental confusion.

Case Report 1

Vrishabhendraiah et al. report a rare case of disulfiram-induced seizures in a 35-year-old male patient who was dependent on alcohol for 10 years. He was detoxified in the hospital and administered disulfiram 250 mg twice daily for initial 5 days then once daily for 10 days. The patient was completely abstinent from alcohol as confirmed by his serum gamma-glutamyl transferase levels (15 IU/L) suggestive of no recent intake of alcohol. The patient's mother reported that the he had one episode of loss of consciousness with the movement of limbs suggestive of generalized tonic–clonic seizures. There was no past or family history of seizures. No neurological abnormalities were found as well. Once disulfiram was discontinued, there was no further history of seizures for 1 month. Investigations such as complete blood count, urea, creatinine, serum electrolytes—sodium, potassium, chloride, hepatic transaminases, blood sugar, urine analysis, thyroid function, and uric acid levels were all within normal limits ruling out other causes of seizures. Only few studies reported the case of seizures in patients on disulfiram therapy particularly in context of clinical delirium over 5–6 weeks. Such reports could open up areas for further research on mechanisms by which disulfiram causes seizures with convulsions and about prevention [20A].

Case Report 2

Neuropathy is one of the most severe side effects of disulfiram therapy. A 35-year-old male with complaint of daily alcohol intake of 250–750 mL (40% alcohol by volume) for the last 10 years was administered disulfiram 250 mg twice daily for 2 months, while the patient abstained from alcohol. The patient complained of numbness and tingling sensation of soles of the feet since last 1 month. Nerve conduction studies revealed small fiber axonal degeneration predominantly sensory type. After withdrawing disulfiram, the patient improved within the next 2 weeks, and by 6 weeks, numbness and tingling sensation of soles of the feet disappeared completely. Nerve conduction studies did not reveal any abnormality at 8 weeks of discontinuation of disulfiram [21A].

Axonal degeneration is a pathological hallmark of disulfiram toxicity. It is very important to differentiate disulfiram neuropathy from alcoholic neuropathy as it develops in the absence of ongoing alcohol use and predominantly affects large-diameter sensory fibers. Distal paresthesia and numbness are often initial manifestations of disulfiram neuropathy. The reported patient also had tobacco dependence for the last 6 years which is of significance as both drugs are CYP 450 substrates possibly leading to more chances of side effects. The patient also developed sensory neuropathy upon receiving 500 mg daily dose of disulfiram. Based on literature reports the lowest effective dose to avoid peripheral neuropathy should be less than 250 mg daily.

Overall considering the wide use of disulfiram for alcoholism, regular neurological monitoring may be useful to detect such adverse effects at early stages.

FIBRIN

Fibrin glue is a biodegradable and absorbable biological agent, which is widely used in abdominal operations to close the wound, reduce leakage and bleeding, promote wound healing, and prevent adhesion. Yang reported a case of a 65-year-old man, whose common bile duct was injured by fibrin glue. The patient was initially admitted for icteric skin and sclera caused by common bile duct stones. Preoperative ultrasound, computed tomography and magnetic resonance cholangiopancreatography indicated multiple stones in the extrahepatic bile duct and common bile duct, dilated intrahepatic bile duct, and cholecystectomy change. Pathological analysis confirmed calcified biliary mucosa. Open surgery was performed to clear the stones by a choledochoscopic procedure and the injury of the common bile duct was repaired by liver round ligament. The study highlights that use of fibrin glue should strictly be controlled in surgery, and large doses of fibrin glue for bleeding and bile duct bile leakage should be carefully monitored [22A].

GELFOAM

Gelfoam is primarily composed of purified porcine gelatin. In dentistry, Gelfoam is used to help hemostasis after extraction by helping to keep the formed blood clot in place. A rare case of anaphylaxis under anesthesia was reported implicating Gelfoam sponges. A 2-year-old, 11-kg female patient with William's syndrome was admitted for dental rehabilitation under general anesthesia. She had undergone 3 prior general anesthetics because of her syndrome but no anesthetic difficulties were experienced. The patient was induced general anesthesia with sevoflurane and 60% nitrous oxide. The dental treatment consisted of composite and glass ionomer restorations, stainless-steel crown placement, and extractions. After 45 minutes from induction, close to the end of treatment, the pediatric dentist placed Gelfoam sponges in the extraction sockets along with placement of sutures. In 2 minutes, her blood pressure dropped to 50/30 mm Hg and the heart rate began to decline to the low 80s. Atropine 50 μg was given, which resulted in a rise in heart rate. Upon placing her on IV fluid a blood pressure reading of 30/10 mm Hg was obtained. Periorbital and lip edema and puffy hands were observed indicative of anaphylaxis. 4 g of epinephrine was given intravenously which raised the systolic pressure to 60 mm Hg. Subsequently, 5 mg of diphenhydramine and 15 mg of hydrocortisone were given. Vitals continued to improve over the next 5 minutes, with a systolic blood pressure reading of 85 mm Hg. She did not require further hemodynamic support with epinephrine. Post-anesthesia the patient received hydralazine overnight for high blood pressure and she was discharged the next day. Seven weeks later, the patient received skin prick and intradermal testing for all of the drugs administered and suspected agents. Testing was negative for all agents except Gelfoam, which caused a 5-mm by 5-mm reaction. The patient's mother was skin prick tested for Gelfoam to act as a control, as there is no standardized testing for Gelfoam. She developed a 3-mm by 3-mm reaction. It was recommended by the immunologist that the patient avoid Gelfoam in the future.

Gelfoam is primarily composed of purified porcine gelatin. The patient's family followed a vegetarian diet, so it was unlikely that the child would have been sensitized by a food source. Reactions by children following vaccination containing porcine or bovine gelatin are known and may be sensitizing events [23A].

A related case of a life-threatening intraoperative anaphylaxis to gelatin in Floseal (used to reduce bleeding) was recently reported during spinal surgery in a pediatric subject. Upon Floseal injection a 9-year-old boy went into tachycardia. It was determined that, during a spinal operation 8 years prior, the patient had an episode of less-severe anaphylaxis. Although the cause of the reaction was unclear at that time, Floseal had been administered. Post anaphylaxis analysis revealed an elevated tryptase level and increased IgE level to bovine gelatin. As was the case with this patient who was also atopic, asthmatic, and allergic, these subjects are more likely to develop hypersensitivity than individuals who are not allergic [24Ar].

GLYCOLS

A 29-year-old African man, nonsmoker, with no significant medical history was admitted experiencing nausea, abdominal pain, weakness, hyporexia, hypertension (blood pressure, 170/100 mm Hg), and anuria. Laboratory values indicated severe kidney failure (KF). Analysis of laboratory findings indicated elevated levels of all the KF parameters (serum creatinine: 15.5 mg/dL; estimated GFR, 4.3 mL/min/1.73 m^2). This patient also presented metabolic acidosis (bicarbonate, 16.4 mEq/L) with mildly elevated anion gap (23 mmol/L), and high levels of serum lipase (3027; reference, <216 IU/L), transaminases (ALT: 98 IU/L; AST: 100 IU/L), and C-reactive protein (131; reference, <5 mg/L). Possibilities of chronic kidney disease, urinary tract obstruction, renal artery stenosis, and renal vein thrombosis were eliminated via Renal and Doppler sonography. It was reported that the patient had been smearing his skin with brake fluid for the past few months to treat a "dermatitis." The brake fluid was class DOT3 (Department of Transportation), with a mean diethylene glycol concentration of 10%. Over the next 3 h, the patient developed progressive drowsiness, hypotension (systolic blood pressure, 100 mm Hg), and respiratory failure requiring intubation and ventilator support in the intensive care unit. Kidney biopsy specimen exhibited acute toxic proximal tubular necrosis indicative of diethylene glycol intoxication. Over the next several days, the patient's neurologic situation progressively worsened: paralysis, loss of corneal, vestibulo-ocular, and gag reflexes, and absence of auditory evoked potentials; electroencephalography showed depression of activity in the cerebral cortex. Later, progressive improvements in kidney and neurologic function occurred [25A].

Diethylene glycol intoxication usually is associated with ingestion of counterfeit drugs, so it could be a public health threat, particularly considering the spread of the illegal internet drug market. Diethylene glycol poisoning leads to death in more than two-thirds of patients. Many of the survivors do not recover kidney function. The reported patient survived with almost full recovery of kidney and neurologic function possibly due to lower absorption through the skin.

LATEX

Case Report

Natural latex rubber products have been known to cause severe anaphylactic reactions during surgery but are still used in pediatric surgery. A healthy 4.5-year-old boy developed severe hypotension, tachycardia and bronchospasm during surgery. An allergy test showed natural latex rubber as the trigger for this severe intraoperative anaphylactic reaction. There was no previous clinical evidence of natural latex rubber allergy. The child had been previously exposed to natural latex rubber as his mother worked as a cosmetician at home using latex gloves. Such contact could have had a slight sensitizing effect that manifested after the initial contact with the conjunctiva through the surgeon's natural latex rubber gloves. Avoiding natural latex rubber products is very important to reduce allergic reactions in children [26A].

MELATONIN

Melatonin is a natural health product (NHP) that is generally regarded as safe by the FDA. However, there is increasing body of evidence that NHPs can have clinically significant adverse effects and interactions with each other as well as with biologics, drugs, over-the-counter products and traditional medicines. The Pharmacy Study of Natural health product Adverse Reactions (SONAR), a multi-center study to identify adverse reactions related to NHPs reported a patient who presented with severe sedation after intake of melatonin concurrently with two antidepressants (citalopram and nortriptyline) and one opioid analgesic (oxycodone).

The sedation improved when melatonin was discontinued. *In vitro* testing of the patient's melatonin demonstrated that it had the potential to interact with other drugs. Mechanistic studies confirmed that melatonin strongly inhibits CYP isozymes and can therefore enhance the effects of medications metabolized by this isozyme, including their adverse effects. Furthermore, melatonin seems to also inhibit CYP3A7 activity, which might be relevant in pregnancy, for neonates and infants. In summary health care professionals prescribing melatonin should advise caution in patients who are also taking other health products that may either reduce efficacy or enhance risk. Future research and extensive pharmacovigilance is required to examine potential melatonin interactions with health products having similar metabolic pathways [27A].

METHYLENE BLUE

Vasoplegia, occurs during cardiopulmonary bypass, leads to vasodilatation via an increase in cGMP that blocks calcium from entering the smooth muscle cells. Methylene blue is a cGMP blocker that leads to higher intracellular calcium concentrations and increases vascular responsiveness. Methylene blue is commonly used to treat vasoplegia. Despite its favorable safety profile, there have been reports of methylene blue-induced encephalopathy and serotonin syndrome in patients undergoing parathyroidectomy. Methylene blue and its metabolite azure B are reversible inhibitors of monoamine oxidase A, which, in combination with selective serotonin reuptake inhibitors (SSRIs), have been linked to increased serotonin levels in the brain and serotonin toxicity. Smith et al. reported a case of serotonin syndrome (SS) following methylene blue administration in a cardiothoracic surgery patient. A 59-year-old woman taking preoperative venlafaxine and trazodone was given a single dose of 2 mg/kg methylene blue (167 mg) during a coronary artery bypass and mitral valve repair. Postoperatively, she had fever and developed full-body tremors, rhythmic twitching of the perioral muscles, slow conjugate roving eye movements, and spontaneous movements of the upper extremities. Electroencephalography revealed generalized diffuse slowing consistent with toxic encephalopathy. The patient's symptoms were consistent with a methylene blue-induced serotonin syndrome. Such cases are very rarely reported and could be precipitated by concomitant administration of methylene blue with serotonin-modulating agents [28A].

PHENOL/PHTHALATE

Phthalates, a group of endocrine disruptors, have attracted public attention due to their possible adverse environmental and human health effects. Epidemiological studies reveal increased phthalate metabolites in urine correlated with abdominal obesity and insulin resistance in adolescents and adult males. Infants and toddlers are the most vulnerable because they exhibit more hand-to-mouth activity and consume the most food as a percent of their body weight.

The plasticizer benzyl butyl phthalate (BBP) for example is a known endocrine disruptor that in HepG2 cells, significantly down-regulated Sirt1 and Sirt3 gene expression at low concentrations thus impairing two vital epigenetic regulators and mitochondrial biogenesis regulators in liver cells.

Werner et al. examined the association of urinary phthalate metabolite concentrations during pregnancy with maternal blood pressure and risk of pregnancy-induced hypertensive diseases. They analyzed maternal urine samples collected at 16 and 26 weeks gestation for 9 phthalate monoester metabolites reflecting exposure to 6 phthalate diesters. Of the phthalate metabolites evaluated, only mono-benzyl phthalate (MBzP) concentrations in urine were significantly associated with maternal diastolic blood pressure at <20 weeks gestation and risk of pregnancy-induced hypertensive diseases [29M].

A longitudinal cohort study of pregnant women in Mexico City and their offspring was carried out to explore associations between *in utero* and peripubertal urinary phthalate metabolite and bisphenol A (BPA) concentrations and markers of peripubertal metabolic homeostasis. Phthalate metabolites and BPA were associated with metabolism biomarkers at age 8–14 years in patterns that varied by sex, pubertal status, and exposure timing. These include lower insulin secretion, higher or lower IGF-1 insulin resistance, and higher or lower leptin. It is believed that exposure to endocrine-disrupting chemicals (EDC) during development may play a role in the increasing prevalence of metabolic syndrome and type 2 diabetes among children and adolescents by interfering with metabolic homeostasis [30R].

Recent *in vitro* and *in vivo* studies strongly suggest the role of phthalates in the pathogenesis of endometriosis. For example the effect of di-(2-ethylhexyl)-phthalate (DEHP) on endometrial cells showed significant increases of MMP-2 and 9 activities, cellular invasiveness, Erk phosphorylation, and p21-activated kinase 4 expression. In mice studies DEHP treatment led to larger size of the endometrial implant. A prospective case–control study for human sample analyses showed that urinary concentration of the metabolites of DEHP was significantly higher in women with endometriosis [31E].

For additional case studies of exposure to phthalate and related chemicals in personal care and consumer products, the readers are encouraged to see the recent comprehensive review by Calafat et al. [32R]. Another systematic review of the effects of phthalate exposure on the neurodevelopment in children is recently published [33R].

SCLEROTHERAPY

Sclerotherapy is a medical procedure used to eliminate varicose veins and spider veins. The procedure involves an injection of a solution (generally a salt solution of 1% polidocanol or sodium tetradecyl sulfate) directly into the vein. The solution irritates the lining of the blood vessel, causing it to swell and stick together, and the blood to clot. Over time, the vessel turns into scar tissue that fades from view.

A 71-year-old woman with primary myelofibrosis and esophageal varices was admitted for her first rubber band ligation procedure (platelet count, 58000/mm^3; partial thromboplastin time, 33.4 seconds; international normalized ratio, 1.28). At endoscopy, the esophageal mucosa was extremely fragile and difficult to aspirate into the ligation device. Three of the six rubber bands placed at the gastroesophageal junction slipped off, leaving oozing blood. This was treated by injecting 3.5 mL of polidocanol. During withdrawal of the endoscope, several areas with bluish bullous lesions (each <1 cm in diameter) were observed in the upper two-thirds of the esophagus. One of these lesions, which showed slight oozing of blood, was injected with 1 mL of polidocanol. Hematemesis developed 4 h later, with a drop in the hemoglobin concentration of 0.8–10.2 g/dL. At second look endoscopy, the submucosal bullae involved up to half of the circumference of the esophagus and more than two-thirds of its length. One of these bullae had ruptured and was covered by a clot. The rubber bands were still in place. There was no ongoing bleeding. Within the next 18 h, the hemoglobin concentration decreased to 7.6 g/dL, and the patient received two thrombocyte concentrates. At follow-up endoscopy after 6 weeks, the mucosa of the upper two-thirds of the esophagus was normal. Varices were still present in the lowest third. Intramural hematoma of the esophagus is a rare entity. It may occur spontaneously; be secondary to a coagulopathy, as in myelofibrosis; or develop after variceal sclerotherapy. In our patient, low platelet counts, abnormal platelet function, sclerosis of the esophageal mucosa, and sclerotherapy may have been contributing factors. In summary, intramural hematoma of the esophagus is a rare complication that can result in severe blood loss [34A].

SEVELAMER

Sevelamer is a commonly used phosphate binder that is composed of a carbon backbone bound to ammonia (NH$_3$). It works by becoming protonated in the stomach to NH$_4$$^+$, which binds to phosphates (PO$_4$$^-$). There have been several reports of gastrointestinal side effects of Sevelamer such as bleeding. Okwara et al. reports a case of a 79-year-old Korean man with a history of end-stage renal disease on dialysis as well as diabetes mellitus and ischemic heart disease who complained of non-bloody diarrhea, intermittent abdominal pain and fever. Abdominal examination found significant tenderness on palpation in the right lower quadrant. Laboratory test results on admission showed an increased white blood cell count of 13400/μL [35A].

Computed tomographic imaging of the abdomen showed irregular circumferential thickening of the cecum. Colonoscopy showed a large circumferential polypoid mass in the cecum occluding 40% of the lumen. A biopsy was performed on this lesion, which found extensive necrosis and ischemic changes. In addition, there was crystalline material consistent with sevelamer crystals.

Mass formation in the setting of colitis has been attributed to submucosal hemorrhage.

SILICONE OIL

Case Report

Silicone oil (polydimethylsiloxane, PDMS) is used as a tamponade agent in retinal detachment surgery to displace the retina towards the eye wall by surface tension and close retinal breaks due to lower specific gravity (than the vitreous humor). Numerous mechanisms of vision loss in silicone oil-filled eyes have been described in the literature. Silicone oil can cause keratopathy, glaucoma, optic neuropathy, and cataract. There have been reports of severe vision loss with long-term use of silicone oil tamponade. Imaging and histological studies show that oil droplets infiltrate various ocular tissues, including the retina. Other reports have documented the migration of silicone oil into the brain. Some have suggested that infiltration of oil droplets into the neuroretina causes macular degeneration [36Ar,37A].

A 60-year-old man experienced a marked unilateral myopic shift of 20 diopters during attempted removal of intravitreal heavy silicone oil used in the treatment of inferior proliferative vitreoretinopathy following retinal detachment. Examination revealed heavy silicone oil adherent to the corneal endothelium and forming a convex interface with the aqueous, obscuring the entire pupil. Surgical intervention was required to restore visual acuity. The case highlights the potential ocular complications associated with silicone oil migration into the anterior chamber, including corneal endothelial decompensation and a significant increase in myopia.

SODIUM BENZOATE

Sodium benzoate is a widely used preservative found in many foods and soft drinks. It is metabolized within mitochondria to produce hippurate, which is then cleared by the kidneys. Ingestion of sodium benzoate at the generally regarded as safe (GRAS) dose leads to a robust excursion in the plasma hippurate level. Few previous reports have demonstrated adverse effects of benzoate and hippurate on glucose homeostasis in cells and animal models.

In one recent study the effect of acute exposure to GRAS levels of sodium benzoate on insulin and glucose homeostasis was evaluated in a randomized, controlled, cross-over study of 14 overweight subjects. Serial blood samples were collected following an oral glucose challenge, in the presence or absence of sodium benzoate.

No statistically significant effect was found however of the 146 metabolites targeted, four changed significantly in response to benzoate, including the expected rise in benzoate and hippurate. In addition, anthranilic acid, a tryptophan metabolite, exhibited a robust rise, while acetyl glycine dropped. Although this study shows that GRAS doses of benzoate do not have an acute, adverse effect on glucose homeostasis, future studies will be necessary to explore the metabolic impact of chronic benzoate exposure [38c].

References

[1] Wang Z, Wei X, Yang J, et al. Chronic exposure to aluminum and risk of Alzheimer's disease: a meta-analysis. Neurosci Lett. 2016;610:200–6. Epub 2015/11/26. [M].

[2] Elserougy S, Mahdy-Abdallah H, Hafez SF, et al. Impact of aluminum exposure on lung. Toxicol Ind Health. 2015;31(1):73–8. Epub 2012/12/22. [c].

[3] Courtney-Martin G, Kosar C, Campbell A, et al. Plasma aluminum concentrations in pediatric patients receiving long-term parenteral nutrition. JPEN J Parenter Enteral Nutr. 2015;39(5):578–85. Epub 2014/04/20. [c].

[4] Bristow SM, Gamble GD, Stewart A, et al. Acute effects of calcium supplements on blood pressure and blood coagulation: secondary analysis of a randomised controlled trial in post-menopausal women. Br J Nutr. 2015;114(11):1868–74. Epub 2015/10/01. [c].

[5] Kataria A, Lata S, Khillan V. Hemodialysis catheter-related bacteremia caused by Stenotrophomonas maltophilia. Indian J Nephrol. 2015;25(5):318–9. Epub 2015/12/03. [r].

[6] Rathor N, Khillan V, Panda D. Catheter associated mycobacteremia: opening new fronts in infection control. Indian J Crit Care Med. 2015;19(6):350–2. Epub 2015/07/22. [A].

[7] Akhoundi A, Singh B, Vela M, et al. Incidence of adverse events during continuous renal replacement therapy. Blood Purif. 2015;39(4):333–9. Epub 2015/05/30. [R].

[8] Noto MJ, Domenico HJ, Byrne DW, et al. Chlorhexidine bathing and health care-associated infections: a randomized clinical trial. JAMA. 2015;313(4):369–78. Epub 2015/01/21. [c].

[9] Pittet D, Angus DC. Daily chlorhexidine bathing for critically ill patients: a note of caution. JAMA. 2015;313(4):365–6. Epub 2015/01/21. [r].

[10] Ketha H, Wadams H, Lteif A, et al. Iatrogenic vitamin D toxicity in an infant—a case report and review of literature. J Steroid Biochem Mol Biol. 2015;148:14–8. Epub 2015/02/01. [A].

[11] Karjigi S, Murthy SC, Kallappa H, et al. Early onset dapsone-induced photosensitive dermatitis: a rare side effect of a common drug. Indian J Lepr. 2015;87(3):161–4. Epub 2016/03/24. [A].

[12] Iliev YT, Zagorov MY, Grudeva-Popova JG. Acute poisoning with dapsone and olanzapine: severe methemoglobinemia and coma with a favourable outcome. Folia Med. 2015;57(2):122–6. Epub 2016/03/05. [A].

[13] Furuta K, Ikeo S, Takaiwa T, et al. Identifying the cause of the "saturation gap": two cases of dapsone-induced methemoglobinemia. Intern Med. 2015;54(13):1639–41. Epub 2015/07/03. [A].

[14] Hanuschk D, Kozyreff A, Tafzi N, et al. Acute visual loss following dapsone-induced methemoglobinemia and hemolysis. Clin Toxicol. 2015;53(5):489–92. Epub 2015/04/11. [A].

[15] Swartzentruber GS, Yanta JH, Pizon AF. Methemoglobinemia as a complication of topical dapsone. N Engl J Med. 2015;372(5):491–2. Epub 2015/01/30. [A].

[16] Watton C, Smith K, Carter E. Methemoglobinemia as a complication of topical dapsone. N Engl J Med. 2015;372(5):492. Epub 2015/01/30. [r].

[17] Gavilanes MC, Palacio AL, Chellini PR, et al. Dapsone hypersensitivity syndrome in a lepromatous leprosy patient—a case report. Lepr Rev. 2015;86(2):186–90. Epub 2015/10/28. [A].

[18] Kinehara Y, Kijima T, Inoue K, et al. Dapsone hypersensitivity syndrome-related lung injury without eosinophilia in the bronchoalveolar lavage fluid. Intern Med. 2015;54(7):827–31. Epub 2015/04/04. [A].

[19] Sauvetre G, MahEvas M, Limal N, et al. Cutaneous rash and dapsone-induced hypersensitivity syndrome a common manifestation in adult immune thrombocytopenia. Presentation and outcome in 16 cases. Am J Hematol. 2015;90(10):E201–2. Epub 2015/06/30. [r].

[20] Vrishabhendraiah SS, Gopal Das CM, Jagadeesh MK, et al. Disulfiram-induced seizures with convulsions in a young male patient: a case study. Indian J Psychiatry. 2015;57(3):309–10. Epub 2015/11/26. [A].

[21] Mohapatra S, Sahoo MR, Rath N. Disulfiram-induced neuropathy: a case report. Gen Hosp Psychiatry. 2015;37(1):97.e5–6. Epub 2014/12/03. [A].

[22] Yang YL, Zhang C, Zhang HW, et al. Common bile duct injury by fibrin glue: report of a rare complication. World J Gastroenterol. 2015;21(9):2854–7. Epub 2015/03/12. [A].

[23] Ji J, Barrett EJ. Suspected intraoperative anaphylaxis to gelatin absorbable hemostatic sponge. Anesth Prog. 2015;62(1):22–4. Epub 2015/04/08. [A].

[24] Agarwal NS, Spalding C, Nassef M. Life-threatening intraoperative anaphylaxis to gelatin in Floseal during pediatric spinal surgery. J Allergy Clin Immunol Pract. 2015;3(1):110–1. Epub 2015/01/13. [Ar].

[25] Devoti E, Marta E, Belotti E, et al. Diethylene glycol poisoning from transcutaneous absorption. Am J Kidney Dis. 2015;65(4):603–6. Epub 2014/12/03. [A].

[26] Malsy M, Leberle R, Ehehalt K, et al. Anaphylactic reaction 5 minutes after the start of surgery: a case report. BMC Res Notes. 2015;8:117. Epub 2015/04/19. [A].

[27] Foster BC, Cvijovic K, Boon HS, et al. Melatonin interaction resulting in severe sedation. J Pharm Pharm Sci. 2015;18(2):124–31. Epub 2015/07/15. [A].

[28] Smith CJ, Wang D, Sgambelluri A, et al. Serotonin syndrome following methylene blue administration during cardiothoracic surgery. J Pharm Pract. 2015;28(2):207–11. Epub 2015/01/24. [A].

[29] Werner EF, Braun JM, Yolton K, et al. The association between maternal urinary phthalate concentrations and blood pressure in pregnancy: the HOME study. Environ Health. 2015;14:75. Epub 2015/09/19. [M].

[30] Watkins DJ, Peterson KE, Ferguson KK, et al. Relating phthalate and BPA exposure to metabolism in peripubescence: the role of exposure timing, sex, and puberty. J Clin Endocrinol Metab. 2016;101(1):79–88. Epub 2015/11/04. [R].

[31] Kim SH, Cho S, Ihm HJ, et al. Possible role of phthalate in the pathogenesis of endometriosis: in vitro, animal, and human data. J Clin Endocrinol Metab. 2015;100(12):E1502–11. Epub 2015/10/07. [E].

[32] Calafat AM, Valentin-Blasini L, Ye X. Trends in exposure to chemicals in personal care and consumer products. Curr Environ Health Rep. 2015;2(4):348–55. Epub 2015/09/08.[R].

[33] Ejaredar M, Nyanza EC, Ten Eycke K, et al. Phthalate exposure and childrens neurodevelopment: a systematic review. Environ Res. 2015;142:51–60. Epub 2015/06/24. [R].

[34] Durchschein F, Krones E, Eherer AJ, et al. Sclerotherapy-associated esophageal hematoma in a patient with myelofibrosis and portal hypertension. Endoscopy. 2015;47(Suppl 1 UCTN):E20–1. Epub 2015/01/21. [A].

[35] Okwara C, Choi C, Park JY. Sevelamer-induced colitis presenting as a pseudotumor. Clin Gastroenterol Hepatol. 2015;13(7):A39–40. Epub 2015/02/24. [A].

[36] Nicholson BP, Bakri SJ. Silicone oil emulsification at the fovea as a reversible cause of vision loss. JAMA Ophthalmol. 2015;133(4):484–6. Epub 2015/01/16. [Ar].

[37] Vincent SJ, Vincent RA, Manning LM, et al. Persistent anterior chamber silicone oil and myopia. J Cataract Refract Surg. 2015;41(7):1527–9. Epub 2015/08/20. [A].

[38] Lennerz BS, Vafai SB, Delaney NF, et al. Effects of sodium benzoate, a widely used food preservative, on glucose homeostasis and metabolic profiles in humans. Mol Genet Metab. 2015;114(1):73–9. Epub 2014/12/17. [c].

Reviewers List

Name	Surname	Affiliation
Asima	Ali, PharmD, BCPS	Clinical Assistant Professor, Pharmacy Practice, Campbell University College of Pharmacy and Health Sciences, Wake Forest University Baptist Medical Center, North Carolina, USA
Renee	Belanger	Associate Professor, Pharmacy Practice, University of the Incarnate Word, Feik School of Pharmacy, San Antonio, TX
Adrian	Black	Senior Regulatory Authoring Analyst- 3E Company and Adjunct Faculty at the Institute of Public Health of New York Medical College, Valhalla, NY 7173, North Crest Court Warrenton, VA 20187
Alison	Brophy, PharmD, BCPS	Critical Care Pharmacist, Saint Barnabas Medical Center, Clinical Assistant Professor, Ernest Mario School of Pharmacy, Rutgers, The State University of New Jersey, USA
Saira B.	Chaudhry, PharmD, MPH	Infectious Diseases Pharmacotherapy Specialist Clinical, Assistant Professor, Ernest Mario School of Pharmacy, Rutgers, The State University of New Jersey, Shore University Medical Center, Robert Wood Johnson Medical School, USA
Monica	Donnelley, PharmD, BCPS-AQ ID	Assistant Professor, College of Pharmacy OP, Department of Clinical Sciences, Touro University California College of Pharmacy
Josh G.	Gray, PhD	Department of Chemistry & Biochemistry, United States Coast Guard Academy, New London, CT, USA
Joshua P.	Gray, PhD	Associate Professor of Chemistry, United States Coast Guard Academy, Department of Science, Chemistry, 27 Mohegan Ave, New London, CT 06320, USA
Herb J.	Halley, PharmD	Director of Experiential Education, Manchester University College of Pharmacy, 10627 Diebold Road, Fort Wayne, IN 46845

Name	Surname	Affiliation
Jennifer	Henrickson, PharmD	Assistant Dean/Associate Professor of Pharmacy Practice, Manchester University College of Pharmacy, Natural & Health Sciences, 10627 Diebold Road, Fort Wayne, Indiana 46845
Jason	Isch, PharmD	Ambulatory Care Pharmacy Resident, Saint Joseph Regional Medical Center, 611 E Douglas Rd. #412, Mishawaka, IN 46545
Timothy	Maher, PhD	Professor of Pharmacology, Associate Dean of Graduate Studies- School of Pharmacy, School of Pharmacy, MCPHS University, Boston, USA
Cassandra	Maynard, PharmD, BCPS	Clinical Pharmacy Specialist - IM/Cardiology, St. Mary's Health Center, Clinical Associate Professor, SIUE - School of Pharmacy, Edwardsville, IL
Oleg	Opsha, MD	Maimonides Medical Center, Department of Radiology, Chief of Musculoskeletal Section, 10 Schindler terrace, West Orange, NJ 07052, USA
Yekaterina	Opsha, PharmD, BCPS	Clinical Assistant Professor, Ernest Mario School of Pharmacy, Rutgers, The State University of NJ, Clinical Specialist-Cardiovascular Medicine, Saint Barnabas Medical Center, Livingston, NJ, USA
Sreekumar	Othumpangat, PhD	Sr. Scientist, Allergy and Clinical Immunology Branch, HELD/NIOSH/CDC, 1095 Willowdale Road, Morgantown, WV 26505, USA
Hanna	Raber, PharmD, BCPS	Assistant Professor/Dept of Clinical Sciences, University of Utah School of Medicine, Pharmacotherapy Specialist, Salt Lake City, UT 84112, USA
Sidhartha D.	Ray, PhD	Professor, Department of Pharmaceutical Sciences, College of Pharmacy, Manchester University, USA

Name	Surname	Affiliation
Mona	Shah, PharmD, BCPS	Emergency Medicine Clinical Pharmacy Specialist, PGY2 Pharmacy Residency Director, Inova Fairfax Hospital, 3300 Gallows Road, Falls Church, VA, 22042, USA
Thomas	Smith, PharmD	Assistant Professor of Pharmacy Practice, Manchester University College of Pharmacy, 10627 Diebold Road, Fort Wayne, IN 46845, USA
Brian	Spoelhoff, PharmD, BCPS	Neurocritical Care and Neurosciences, Johns Hopkins Bayview Medical Center, Department of Pharmacy, 4940 Eastern Ave, Baltimore, MD 21224

Name	Surname	Affiliation
Kelan	Thomas, PharmD, BCPS	Assistant Professor of Clinical Sciences, Touro University California College of Pharmacy, Psychiatric Pharmacist, St. Helena Hospital Center for Behavioral Health, LifeLong Medical Care - Downtown Oakland, CA, USA
Jennifer	Kim, PharmD, BCPS, BCACP, CPP	Assistant Director of Pharmacy Education, AHEC Assistant Professor of Clinical Education, UNC Eshelman School of Pharmacy, Chapel Hill, NC, USA
Deborah	Zeitlin, PharmD	Butler University College of Pharmacy and Health Sciences, 4600 Sunset Avenue, Indianapolis, IN 46208

Index of Drugs

For drug–drug interactions see the separate index. In pages 545–546.

Index of Drug-Drug Interactions

Index of Adverse Effects and Adverse Reactions